£85.50

REFERENCE ONLY

Wolff's ANATOMY
—OF THE—
EYE AND ORBIT

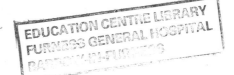

Wolff's ANATOMY

—OF THE—

EYE AND ORBIT

Eighth edition

ANTHONY J. BRON BSc, FRCS, FCOphth

Professor of Ophthalmology, University of Oxford, Oxford, UK

RAMESH C. TRIPATHI MD, PhD, FACS, MS Ophth, DORCP&S,

FRCPath, FICS, FNAS(I)

Professor and Chairman, Department of Ophthalmology, University of South Carolina
School of Medicine, South Carolina Eye Institute, Columbia, SC, USA

BRENDA J. TRIPATHI PhD

Professor of Pathology and Adjunct Professor of Ophthalmology, University of South

Carolina School of Medicine, Columbia, SC, USA

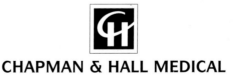

CHAPMAN & HALL MEDICAL

London · Weinheim · New York · Tokyo · Melbourne · Madras

Published by Chapman & Hall, 2–6 Boundary Row, London SE1 8HN, UK

Chapman & Hall, 2–6 Boundary Row, London SE1 8HN, UK

Chapman & Hall GmbH, Pappelallee 3, 69469 Weinheim, Germany

Chapman & Hall USA, 115 Fifth Avenue, New York, NY 10003, USA

Chapman & Hall Japan, ITP-Japan, Kyowa Building, 3F, 2-2-1 Hirakawacho, Chiyoda-ku, Tokyo 102, Japan

Chapman & Hall Australia, 102 Dodds Street, South Melbourne, Victoria 3205, Australia

Chapman & Hall India, R. Seshadri, 32 Second Main Road, CIT East, Madras 600 035, India

First edition 1933

Eighth edition 1997

© 1997 Anthony J. Bron, Ramesh C. Tripathi and Brenda J. Tripathi

Typeset in 10/12 Palatino by Keyset Composition, Colchester, Essex

Printed in Spain

ISBN 0 412 41010 9 (HB)

611 84 BRO

A catalogue record for this book is available from the British Library

Library of Congress Catalog Card Number: 96 84205

Contents

4 The extraocular muscles and ocular movements

5 Innervation and nerves of the orbit

12   The lens and zonules

13   The vitreous

14   The retina

15   The visual pathway

16 Autonomic, aminergic, peptidergic and nitrergic innervation of the eye

17 Development of the human eye

References and further reading

Index

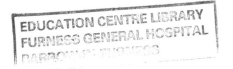

Preface to the seventh edition

Eugene Wolff's book has now passed through six editions and ten reprints in less than forty years, growing in pages from 309 to 553 and in illustrations from 173 (initially none in colour) to 467 (56 in colour). Both text and illustrations contain much that is of historical interest, and – like my predecessor – I have wished to avoid tampering unnecessarily with the author's creation. However, very considerable changes have been necessary which have entailed a rewriting of about a quarter of the text. Only the chapters on the osseous orbit and comparative anatomy have required less extensive deletions and replacement by new writing. In all sections many old citations (limited in interest and often undocumented) have been omitted; and yet the Bibliography has almost doubled in length, a measure of the injection of new contributions. The accumulations of knowledge, particularly in such fields as the ultrastructural detail of ocular tissues, analysis of ocular movements, and organization in the visual pathways, have demanded particular attention; and it is to these that revision has been deliberately directed. These and other fields of study have evoked many highly specialized monographs and a countless legion of original papers, many of which can only be quoted briefly. But it is my belief that readers of such a generalized textbook as this will thus find useful signposts by which to look elsewhere for further detail.

There are 75 new illustrations in this edition, the majority being replacements. In this regard I am much indebted to my friend, Mr Richard E. M. Moore, DFA(London), MMAA, FRSA, who works in my own department; he has contributed 28 new illustrations and diagrams. I am also most grateful to Dr John Marshall and his assistant, Mr P. L. Ansell (both of the Institute of Ophthalmology, University of London), who have provided much improved substitutes for 40 electron- and photo-micrographs. I must also thank Dr N. A. Locket (of the same Institute) for the loan of preparations for photomicrography. My colleagues, Mr Kevin Fitzpatrick and Mr Joe Curtis, have also helped in the replacement of several illustrations. Dr Gordon Ruskell (The City University, London) has helped with much useful criticism. From the publishing staff, and particularly Mr John Goodhall, I have received most efficient and patient support. Despite all this help I am solely responsible for any inaccuracies and omissions in this text. While hoping that readers will find it improved in its usefulness, I hope equally that they will volunteer their criticisms and suggestions.

Roger Warwick
Guy's Hospital Medical School,
University of London
February 1976

Extracts from
Preface to the first edition

This *Anatomy of the Eye and Orbit* is based mainly on lectures and demonstrations which I have had the honour to give during ten years as Demonstrator of Anatomy at University College, and for the last three years as Pathologist and Lecturer in Anatomy to the Royal Westminster Ophthalmic Hospital.

It is an attempt to present to the Student and Ophthalmic Surgeon the essentials of the structure, development, and comparative anatomy of the visual apparatus in conjunction with some of their clinical applications. The motor nerves to the eye muscles have received special attention, as have also the illustrations, many of which are from my own preparations.

Eugene Wolff
Harley Street, London
1933

Preface

Revision of Eugene Wolff's *Anatomy of the Eye and Orbit* has been a very considerable task and one which we have enjoyed. This new edition builds on the strengths of its predecessors while reflecting the increase in our knowledge since the seventh edition was published over twenty years ago.

The larger format of this edition permits the use of double columns, and gives far greater flexibility to the display of illustrations. The text is now over 600 pages long, despite the omission of the chapter on comparative anatomy. The number of illustrations, many of them with multiple parts, has been increased to 667, of which 570 are new or have been redrawn. Many of the old figures have been reannotated where possible, to give a consistency of style.

In order to do justice to the expansion of knowledge of the anatomy of the eye and its related structures, seven new chapters have been added: the cornea and sclera, the iris, the ciliary body and choroid, the drainage angle and the lens and the retina have each been given independent status. Although we have retained parts of the old text, most has been extensively revised. In many respects the book is entirely new; new topics include: the innervation and classification of the extraocular muscles, the ocular mucins, the collagens and proteoglycans of the ocular coats, the properties of the trabecular cells, stereology of the lens, the detailed anatomy of the ocular circulations, the morphology and connectivity of the retinal cells, the functions of the retinal pigment epithelium and current views on the topography of the visual pathway and the role of the visual and prestriate cortices.

We are indebted to the many scientists who have provided illustrations for this book and would like to thank the following individuals, in particular, who were most generous with material and with their time and advice. They include: M. P. Bergen; M. van Buskirk; M. B. Carpenter; O. Earley; G. Eisner; A. W. Fryckowski; T. F. Freddo; I. K. Gipson; I. Grierson; J. Jonas; H. Kolb; L. Koornneef; J. R. Kuszak; D. Landon; E. Lütjen-Drecoll; N. R. Miller; J. M. Olver; Y. Pouliquen; A. C. Rhoton; G. L. Ruskell; J. Sebag; K. Sellheyer; B. W. Streeten; E. R. Tamm; G. Vrensen; S. Zeki and E. van der Zypen.

From the inception of this new edition of Wolff's Anatomy, until his death, Roger Warwick, who revised several previous editions, was a constant source of encouragement and inspiration. We hope that we did not stray too far from his wishes. We would like to thank our publishers, Chapman and Hall, in particular Nick Dunton, for their support and forebearance, and also Jane Bryant and Sue Deeley for the copy editing and project management, respectively.

We are aware that, despite our best efforts, this book has many deficiencies and we welcome the comments and criticisms of our readers.

Anthony J. Bron
Ramesh C. Tripathi
Brenda J. Tripathi
Oxford, UK and Columbia, SC
March 1997

CHAPTER ONE

The bony orbit and paranasal sinuses

1.1 THE BONY ORBIT

The human orbital cavities, following the bilateral symmetry of other vertebrates, flank the sagittal plane of the skull between its cranial and facial parts (Fig. 1.1), encroaching about equally on both (Whitnall, 1932; Dutton, 1994).

Above them is the anterior cranial fossa, between them the nasal cavity and ethmoidal air sinuses, below each a maxillary sinus (antrum), and laterally from behind forwards are the middle cranial and temporal fossae.

The orbit is essentially a socket for the eyeball, containing the muscles, nerves and vessels proper to it. Moreover, it transmits certain vessels and nerves to supply areas around the orbital aperture. Seven bones form the orbit: the maxillary, palatine, frontal, sphenoid, zygomatic, ethmoid and lacrimal bones.

The orbit resembles a quadrilateral pyramid whose base, directed forwards, laterally and slightly downwards, corresponds to the orbital margin, and whose apex is between the optic foramen and medial end of the superior orbital fissure (Whitnall, 1911). Comparison with a quadrilateral pyramid fails with the floor (which is the shortest orbital wall), which does not reach the apex, the cavity being triangular in section in this region.

Also, because the orbit is developed around the eye, and is bulged out by the lacrimal gland, it tends towards spheroidal form, and its widest part is not at the orbital margin but about 1.5 cm behind it. Its four walls are for the most part separated by ill-defined rounded borders, and Whitnall compares the orbit to a pear whose stalk is the optic canal. Note that the medial walls of the orbits are almost parallel, whereas the lateral walls make an angle of about 90° with each other. The orbital axes thus run from behind forwards, laterally and slightly downwards.

THE ROOF OR VAULT OF THE ORBIT

The roof of the orbit is triangular and formed largely by the triangular orbital plate of the frontal bone, and behind this by the lesser wing of the sphenoid. It faces downwards and slightly forwards. It is markedly concave anteriorly and flatter posteriorly, the concavity being greatest about 1.5 cm from the orbital margin, corresponding to the equator of the globe.

The lacrimal fossa

The fossa for the lacrimal gland lies behind the zygomatic process of the frontal bone, as a slight increase in the general concavity of the anterior and lateral part of the roof, and is better appreciated by touch than by sight. The fossa contains not only the lacrimal gland but also some orbital fat, principally at its posterior part (accessory fossa of Rochon-Duvigneaud). It is bounded below by the zygomaticofrontal suture, at the junction of roof and lateral wall of the orbit. The fossa is usually

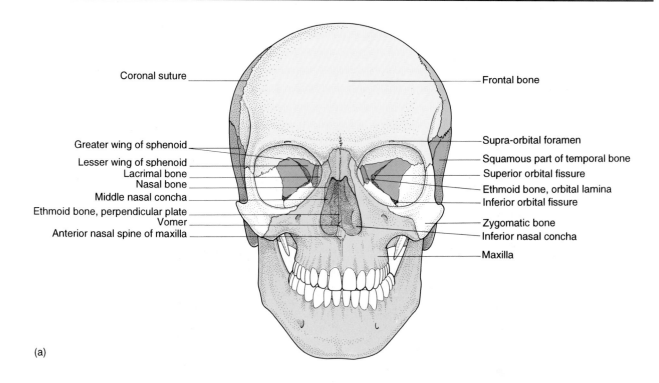

(a)

Fig. 1.1 The skull. (a) Anterior aspect. (Redrawn from Williams, P.L. *et al.* (eds) (1995) *Gray's Anatomy*, 38th edition, published by Churchill Livingstone.)

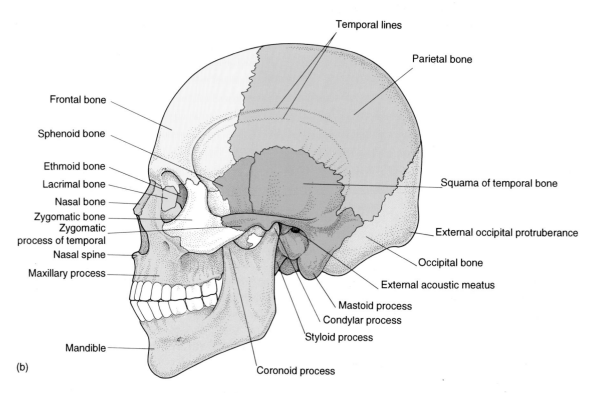

(b)

Fig. 1.1 (b) Left lateral aspect. (Redrawn from Williams, P.L. *et al.* (eds) (1995) *Gray's Anatomy*, 38th edition, published by Churchill Livingstone.)

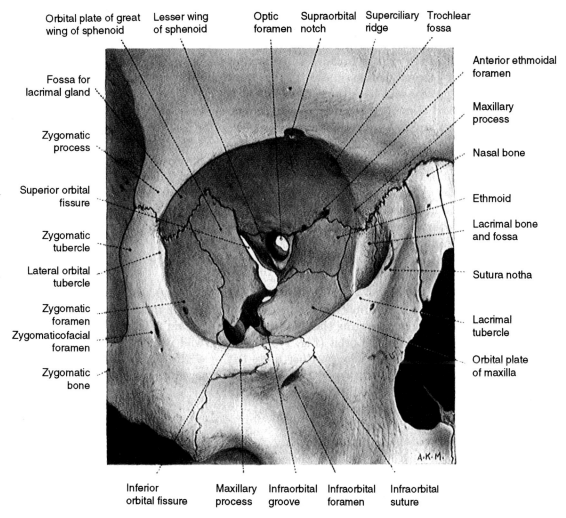

Orbital plate of great wing of sphenoid   Lesser wing of sphenoid   Optic foramen   Supraorbital notch   Superciliary ridge   Trochlear fossa

Fossa for lacrimal gland

Zygomatic process

Superior orbital fissure

Zygomatic tubercle

Lateral orbital tubercle

Zygomatic foramen

Zygomaticofacial foramen

Zygomatic bone

Anterior ethmoidal foramen

Maxillary process

Nasal bone

Ethmoid

Lacrimal bone and fossa

Sutura notha

Lacrimal tubercle

Orbital plate of maxilla

Inferior orbital fissure   Maxillary process   Infraorbital groove   Infraorbital foramen   Infraorbital suture

Fig. 1.2   The right orbit, viewed along its axis.

smooth, but is pitted by attachment of the suspensory ligament of the lacrimal gland when this is well developed.

The fovea

The fovea for the **trochlea** of the superior oblique muscle is a small depression close to the fronto-lacrimal suture about 4 mm from the orbital margin (Figs 1.2 and 1.3). Sometimes (in about 10% of cases) the ligaments which attach the U-shaped cartilage of the pulley to it are ossified; then the fovea shows, more often posteriorly, a spicule of bone (the spina trochlearis). Rarely, a ring of bone, representing the completely ossified trochlea, may be seen (Winckler). Above the fovea the frontal sinus separates the two plates of the frontal bone, extending posterolaterally from the fovea to a variable extent.

The frontosphenoidal suture

Usually obliterated in the adult, this suture lies between the orbital plate of the frontal bone and the lesser wing of the sphenoid.

The roof of the orbit is demarcated from the medial wall by fine sutures between the frontal bone above and ethmoid and lacrimal bones and frontal process of the maxilla below. In, or just above, the frontoethmoidal suture, the anterior and posterior ethmoidal canals open (Figs 1.2 and 1.3). Posteriorly the superior orbital fissure separates roof from lateral wall, anteriorly the slight ridge of the fron-tozygomatic suture intervenes. The orbital aspect of the roof is usually smooth but may be marked by small apertures and depressions. The apertures, the cribra orbitalia, are most commonly medial to the anterior part of the lacrimal fossa. They are not always present and are most marked in the fetus and

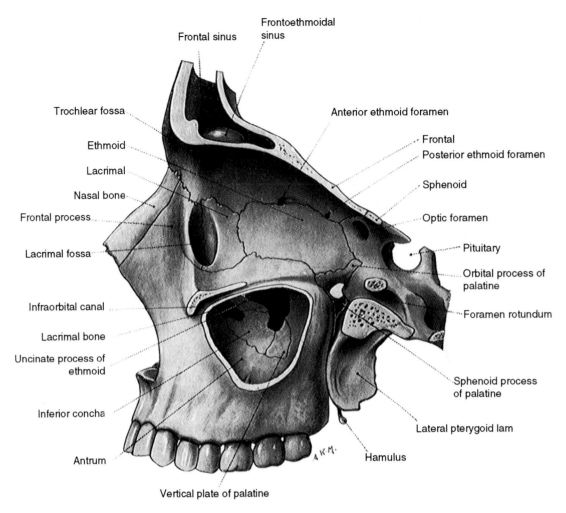

Frontal sinus
Frontoethmoidal sinus
Trochlear fossa
Ethmoid
Lacrimal
Nasal bone
Frontal process
Lacrimal fossa
Infraorbital canal
Lacrimal bone
Uncinate process of ethmoid
Inferior concha
Antrum
Vertical plate of palatine
Anterior ethmoid foramen
Frontal
Posterior ethmoid foramen
Sphenoid
Optic foramen
Pituitary
Orbital process of palatine
Foramen rotundum
Sphenoid process of palatine
Lateral pterygoid lam
Hamulus

Fig. 1.3 The medial wall of the orbit.

infant (Winckler). The apertures impart a porous appearance to the bone, and allow veins to pass from the diploë to the orbit.

In the posterior part of the orbit, in or near the lateral part of the lesser sphenoidal wing, small orifices may serve as vascular communications between the orbit and cranial dura mater. Numerous small grooves made by vessels or nerves lead to these orifices.

Very rarely, an anteroposterior fissure may be up to 14 mm long, filled with periorbita and dura mater.

Structure

The roof of the orbit is thin, translucent and fragile except where formed by the lesser wing of the sphenoid, which is 3 mm thick. By transmitted light the ridges and depressions on the cranial aspect can be seen to correspond to the sulci and gyri of the frontal lobe, especially in the posterior two-thirds. The translucency of the anterior third shows up the orbital extension of the frontal sinus.

Occasionally in old age parts of the roof may be absorbed, bringing the periorbita into direct contact with the dura mater of the anterior cranial fossa. In the dried skull the roof of the orbit can be easily broken.

Penetrating wounds through the lids, inflicted by pointed objects, are sometimes complicated by orbital fracture and injury to the frontal lobe of the cerebrum.

The roof of the orbit is variably invaded by the frontal sinus and sometimes the ethmoidal sinuses. The frontal sinus may extend laterally to the zygomatic process and posteriorly close to the optic foramen. The sphenoidal or posterior ethmoidal sinuses sometimes invade the lesser wing of the sphenoid and the frontal sinus may surround, more or less completely, the optic canal.

Relations

The frontal nerve is in contact with the periorbita along the whole roof (Figs 5.17 and 5.18). The supraorbital artery accompanies it only in the anterior half. Inferior to both are levator palpebrae and the superior rectus.

The trochlear nerve lies medially, in contact with the periorbita, on its way to the superior oblique muscle.

The lacrimal gland adjoins the lacrimal fossa and the superior oblique the junction of roof and medial wall.

Invading the roof to a variable extent are the frontal and ethmoidal sinuses; the former usually reaches the roof's mid point. Above the roof are the frontal lobe of the cerebrum and its meninges (Fig. 5.22).

THE MEDIAL WALL OF THE ORBIT

This wall, shown in Fig. 1.3, is the only wall which is not obviously triangular: approximately oblong, it is flat or slightly convex. It lies parallel to the sagittal plane, and consists, from the front backwards, of four bones united by vertical sutures:

- the frontal process of the maxilla;
- the lacrimal bone;
- the orbital plate of the ethmoid;
- a small part of the body of the sphenoid.

Of these, the orbital plate of the ethmoid is the largest. It usually shows a mosaic of light and dark areas. The dark areas correspond to the ethmoidal sinuses, the light lines to the partitions between them (Fig. 1.19).

Anteriorly is the **lacrimal fossa**, formed by the frontal process of the maxilla and the lacrimal bone. It is bounded by the **anterior** and **posterior lacrimal crests**. There is no definite boundary above, while below the fossa is continuous with the osseous nasolacrimal canal. At their junction the hamulus of the lacrimal bone curves round from the posterior to the anterior lacrimal crest and bounds the fossa to the lateral side (Fig. 1.3). Here the fossa is some 5 mm deep, gradually becoming shallower as it ascends. It is about 14 mm high. The lacrimal bone and maxillary frontal process vary on formation of the fossa; and

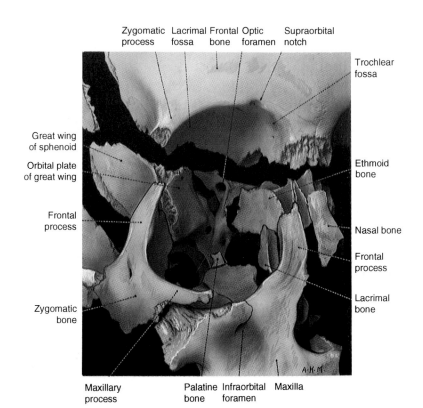

Zygomatic process Lacrimal fossa Frontal bone Optic foramen Supraorbital notch

Trochlear fossa

Great wing of sphenoid

Orbital plate of great wing

Frontal process

Zygomatic bone

Ethmoid bone

Nasal bone

Frontal process

Lacrimal bone

Maxillary process Palatine bone Infraorbital foramen Maxilla

Fig. 1.4 The bones of the right orbit in situ, but separated.

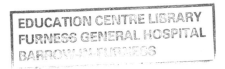

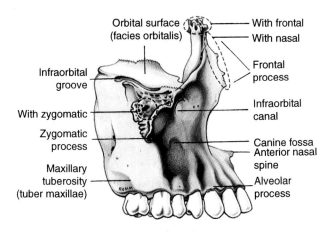

Fig. 1.5 Right maxilla (lateral aspect).

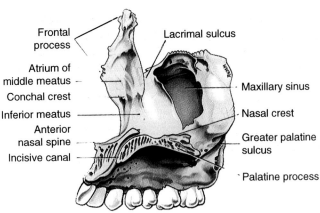

Fig. 1.8 Right maxilla (medial aspect).

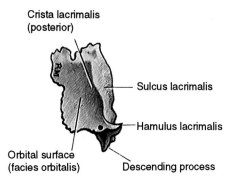

Fig. 1.6 Right lacrimal bone (lateral aspect).

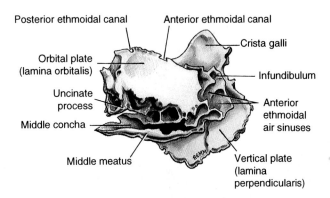

Fig. 1.7 The ethmoid bone (right lateral aspect).

hence the vertical suture between them also varies in position.

The anterior lacrimal crest on the frontal process of the maxilla is ill defined above but well marked below, where it continues as the lower orbital margin, where there is often a **lacrimal tubercle** (Fig. 1.2).

The lacrimal bone separates the upper half of the fossa from the anterior ethmoidal sinuses, and the lower part from the middle meatus of the nose (see also p.49).

Structure

The medial wall is the thinnest orbital wall (0.2–0.4 mm thick). It is translucent, so that the ethmoidal sinuses are visible as a mosaic pattern upon the wall.

The orbital plate of the ethmoid (lamina papyracea) is as thin as paper. Infection of the ethmoidal sinuses can easily extend into the orbit and is said to be the most common cause of orbital cellulitis. However, the orbital plate rarely shows senile absorption, whereas the thicker lacrimal bone, especially in the lacrimal fossa, is often absorbed.

Variations

The lacrimal bone may be divided by accessory sutures into several parts. A sutural bone may be developed in its upper part. An accessory lacrimal bone, constant in many lower animals, may appear anteriorly. The hamulus may be separate, double or absent.

Relations

Medially, running from the front backwards (Fig. 1.4), are the lateral nasal wall, infundibulum, ethmoidal sinuses, and sphenoidal air sinus. The optic foramen is located at the posterior end of the medial wall (Fig. 1.3).

The superior oblique muscle is in the angle between roof and medial wall; the medial rectus adjoins the wall, while between the two muscles are the anterior and posterior ethmoidal and infratrochlear nerves and the termination of the ophthalmic artery (Fig. 5.18).

Anteriorly, the lacrimal sac, in its fossa, is surrounded by lacrimal fascia, behind which are attached the lacrimal fibres of orbicularis oculi (Horner's muscle), septum orbitale, and the check ligament of the medial rectus (Fig. 2.67).

THE FLOOR OF THE ORBIT

Like the roof, the floor of the orbit is triangular. It slopes slightly downwards and laterally. Its lowest part is an anterolateral concavity about 3 mm deep.

The floor, 47.6 mm, is the shortest orbital boundary and is formed by three bones:

- the orbital plate of the **maxilla**;
- the orbital surface of the **zygomatic bone**;
- the orbital process of the **palatine bone**.

The maxillary area is the largest, the zygomatic is anterolateral, and the palatine, most posterior, is smallest.

The floor is traversed by the **infraorbital sulcus**, which runs forwards from the inferior orbital (sphenomaxillary) fissure. Usually near the floor's mid point the sulcus becomes a canal completed by a plate of bone passing from its lateral side to the medial at the infraorbital suture which (Fig. 1.4) can be traced over the orbital margin into the medial side of the infraorbital foramen (Fig. 1.2). It may intersect the zygomaticomaxillary suture.

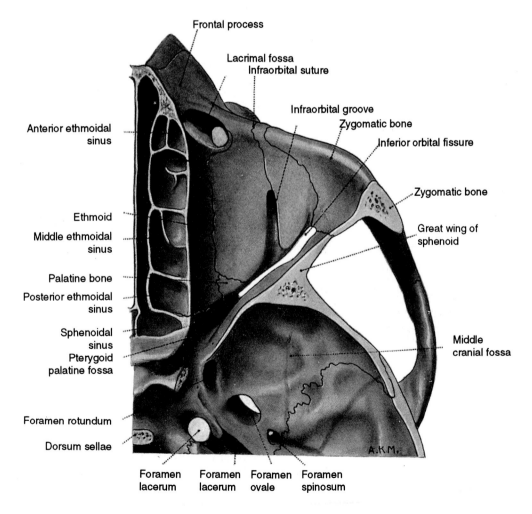

Fig. 1.9 The floor of the orbit.

The infraorbital canal descends in the orbital floor to open at the infraorbital foramen about 4 mm below the orbital margin. It transmits the infraorbital vessels and nerve, which here have middle and anterior superior alveolar (dental) branches occupying correspondingly named canals.

Lateral to the opening of the nasolacrimal canal a small pit or rough area occasionally marks attachment of the inferior oblique muscle.

Between the orbital floor and medial wall is a fine suture; posteriorly the lateral wall is separated from it by the inferior orbital (sphenomaxillary) fissure, but is continuous with it anteriorly (Fig. 1.4).

Variations

The roof of the infraorbital canal and its floor may be incomplete, but the floor of the orbit rarely shows senile absorption. Langer noted three cases where the infraorbital canal was in the suture between the maxilla and the zygomatic bone. The infraorbital foramen is multiple in 2–18% of different populations (Harris, 1933; Berry, 1975).

Relations and structure

Below most of the floor of the orbit is the maxillary sinus. Because the bone is only 0.5–1 mm thick here, tumours of the sinus can easily invade the orbit, causing proptosis. It is thinnest at the infraorbital groove and canal (Fig. 1.15).

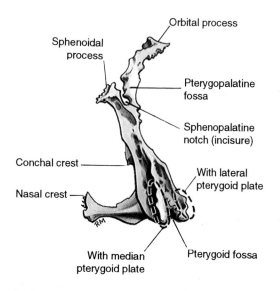

Fig. 1.10 Right palatine bone (posterior aspect).

Posteriorly, a small sinus in the orbital process of the palatine bone (and sometimes extensions from the ethmoidal sinuses) invade the floor.

The inferior rectus adjoins the floor near the apex of the orbit, but is separated from it anteriorly by the inferior oblique muscle and fat. At the lateral edge of the inferior rectus, or between it and the lateral rectus, is the nerve to the inferior oblique (Fig. 5.24).

The inferior oblique arises at the lateral edge of the opening of the nasolacrimal canal and passes posterolaterally and up near the floor (Fig. 5.20).

The infraorbital vessels and nerve occupy their sulcus and canal.

THE LATERAL WALL OF THE ORBIT

This wall is triangular; its base is anterior. It makes an angle of 45° with the median plane and faces anteromedially and slightly up in its lower part. It is slightly convex posteriorly, flat at its centre, while anteriorly (orbital surface of the zygomatic), behind the orbital margin, it is deeply concave.

The lateral wall is formed by two bones:

- posteriorly by the orbital surface of the greater wing of the sphenoid;
- anteriorly by the orbital surface of the zygomatic bone.

The **sphenoidal** area is separated from roof and floor by the superior and inferior orbital fissures.

The **zygomatic** area merges with the floor, and joins the roof at the frontozygomatic suture, approximately horizontal and often marked by a slight ridge. The sphenozygomatic suture is vertical (Fig. 1.2).

The spina musculi recti lateralis

This small bony projection, on the inferior margin of the superior orbital fissure at the junction of its wide and narrow portions, may be pointed, round or grooved. It is produced mainly by a groove for the superior ophthalmic vein, which is prolonged upwards anterior to the spine. A part of the lateral rectus muscle is attached to it. The spine may be double.

The zygomatic groove and foramen

The groove for the zygomatic nerve and vessels runs from the anterior end of the inferior orbital fissure to a foramen in the zygomatic bone. This leads into a canal which divides one branch opening on the face, the other in the temporal fossa. If the nerve divides before entering its canal, there may be two or even three grooves and foramina in the orbit.

The lateral orbital tubercle (Whitnall, 1932)

This is a small elevation on the orbital surface of the zygomatic bone behind the lateral orbital margin and about 11 mm below the frontozygomatic suture. It gives attachment to:

- the check ligament of the lateral rectus muscle;
- the suspensory ligament of the eyeball;
- the aponeurosis of the levator palpebrae superioris (Fig. 5.20).

Frequently a foramen in or near the suture between the greater wing of the sphenoid and the frontal bone, near the lateral end of the superior orbital fissure, leads from the orbit to the middle cranial fossa, and transmits a branch of the meningeal artery and a small vein.

Structure

Being much exposed to stress, the lateral wall is the thickest orbital wall, especially at the orbital margin. Behind the margin the wall thins a little, thickens again, and finally thins once again where it adjoins the middle cranial fossa (Fig. 1.4). At this site, around the sphenozygomatic suture, it is only 1 mm thick and is translucent. In 30% of skulls, according to Nippert (1931), supplementary fissures in this area represent primitive communications between the orbit and temporal fossa.

Relations

The lateral wall separates the orbit anteriorly from the temporal fossa and muscle, posteriorly from the middle cranial fossa and temporal lobe of the cerebrum (Fig. 1.4).

The lateral rectus muscle is in contact with the whole of this wall, with the lacrimal nerve and artery above it.

The inferior pole of the **lacrimal gland** reaches the lateral wall, where the **lacrimal nerve** receives a parasympathetic branch from the zygomatic, which, with its vessels, also adjoins the wall (Fig. 5.24).

THE SUPERIOR ORBITAL (SPHENOIDAL) FISSURE

The sphenoid fissure lies between the roof and the lateral wall, separating the lesser and greater wings of the sphenoid, and is closed laterally by the frontal bone.

Wider at the medial end below the optic foramen, the superior orbital fissure is often described as comma-shaped. Sometimes it tapers regularly towards its lateral extremity, but usually it shows a narrow lateral and a wider medial part, at the junction of which is the spine for the **lateral rectus** (Fig. 1.2).

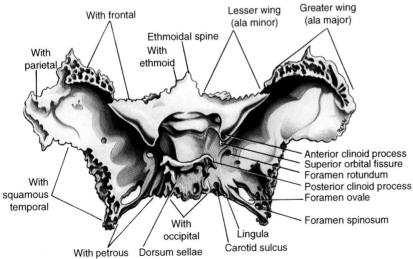

Fig. 1.11 The sphenoid bone (superior, endocranial aspect).

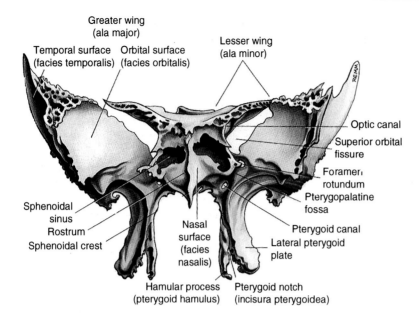

Greater wing
(ala major)

Temporal surface   Orbital surface
(facies temporalis) (facies orbitalis)

Lesser wing
(ala minor)

Optic canal

Superior orbital
fissure

Foramen
rotundum

Pterygopalatine
fossa

Sphenoidal
sinus
Rostrum
Sphenoidal crest

Nasal
surface
(facies
nasalis)

Pterygoid canal

Lateral pterygoid
plate

Hamular process   Pterygoid notch
(pterygoid hamulus) (incisura pterygoidea)

Fig. 1.12 The sphenoid bone (anterior aspect).

The fissure is about 22 mm long, and is the largest communication between the orbit and middle cranial fossa. Its tip is 30–40 mm from the frontozygomatic suture. The medial end is separated from the optic foramen by the posterior root of the lesser wing of the sphenoid, on which is the infraoptic tubercle below and lateral to the optic foramen (Fig. 1.2). Beyond the lateral edge of the fissure one or more frontosphenoidal foramina may appear in the suture between the frontal bone and the greater wing, forming a communication between the lacrimal and middle meningeal arteries. A sulcus, possibly for an anastomotic vessel between the middle meningeal

and infraorbital arteries, extends from the summit of the fissure towards the orbital floor in about one-third of skulls (Royle, 1973).

The common tendinous ring (annulus tendineus communis) of the rectus muscles spans the superior orbital fissure between its medial and lateral parts. The lateral rectus is attached here to both margins of the fissure.

According to Hovelacque (1927) and Wolff (1954) the lateral limb is closed by dura mater and nothing passes through it (Figs 5.4 and 5.5). Above the annulus are the trochlear, frontal, and lacrimal nerves, superior ophthalmic vein, and the recurrent lacrimal artery.

Within the annulus or between the two heads of the lateral rectus are the superior division of the oculomotor nerve, nasociliary and sympathetic roots of the ciliary ganglion, inferior division of the oculomotor, abducent nerve and sometimes the ophthalmic vein or veins – these run from above downwards. The abducent nerve ascends above the inferior division of the oculomotor to lie lateral to and between the two divisions (Fig. 5.6). Only the inferior ophthalmic vein is, occasionally, below the annulus.

THE INFERIOR ORBITAL (SPHENOMAXILLARY) FISSURE

This fissure lies between the lateral wall and the floor of the orbit and joins the orbit to the pterygopalatine and infratemporal fossae. It commences inferolateral

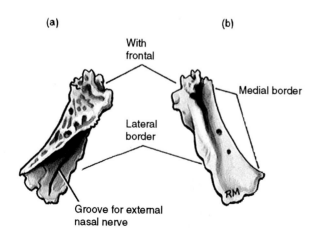

(a)   **(b)**

With
frontal

Medial border

Lateral
border

Groove for external
nasal nerve

Fig. 1.13 The right nasal bone. (a) Medial aspect; (b) lateral aspect.

to the optic foramen, at the medial end of the superior orbital fissure, and runs anterolaterally for 20 mm to end about 2 cm from the inferior orbital margin (Figs 1.2 and 1.4).

The fissure is bounded anteriorly by the maxilla and orbital process of the palatine bone, posteriorly by the whole lower margin of the orbital surface of the greater wing of the sphenoid. It is usually closed anteriorly by the zygomatic bone and is narrower centrally than at its ends, the anterior end being sometimes markedly widened.

The width of the fissure depends on the developmental stage of the maxillary sinus and thus is relatively wide in the fetus and infant. The lateral border is sharp and may have grooves above and below it; it is higher than the medial border anteriorly, lower posteriorly and closed by periorbita and the muscle of Müller.

The inferior orbital fissure is close to the foramen rotundum and the sphenopalatine foramen (Figs 1.2 and 1.3). It transmits the infraorbital and zygomatic nerves, orbital periosteal branches from the pterygopalatine ganglion, and a branch from the inferior ophthalmic vein to the pterygoid plexus (Fig. 5.23).

THE ETHMOIDAL FORAMINA

The ethmoidal foramina, between the roof and medial wall of the orbit, are in the frontoethmoidal suture or in the frontal bone. They open into canals formed largely by the frontal, but completed by the ethmoidal bones (Figs 1.2, 1.3, 1.10 and 1.19).

THE ANTERIOR ETHMOIDAL CANAL

The anterior ethmoidal canal is inclined posterolaterally. Its posterior border forms a groove on the orbital plate of the ethmoid. It opens in the anterior cranial fossa at the side of the cribriform plate, and transmits the anterior ethmoidal nerve and artery.

THE POSTERIOR ETHMOIDAL CANAL

This canal transmits the posterior ethmoidal nerve and artery. Supplementary foramina are common, and their positions are variable (see Berry, 1975, for extensive review).

THE OPTIC FORAMEN

The optic foramen, or rather **optic canal**, connects the middle cranial fossa to the apex of the orbit, and is

formed by the two roots of the lesser wing of the sphenoid. The canal is directed anterolaterally, and slightly downwards, at an angle of about 36° with the median plane. If projected forwards, its axis passes approximately through the middle of the inferolateral quadrant of the orbital opening. Hence it differs from the axes of the orbit and lateral wall. Projected backwards the two optic axes meet on the dorsum sellae at about 90°. The canal is infundibular, the mouth of the funnel being anterior, oval in shape, its longer diameter vertical. The cranial opening is flattened transversely, the middle part of the canal being circular. The upper and lower borders of the intracranial end are sharp, the medial and lateral borders rounded. The interoptic groove is thus smoothly continuous with the medial walls of both canals (Fig. 1.11). Rarely, the optic foramen may be double (Warwick).

The lateral border of the orbital opening is variably defined as the anterior border of the posterior root of the lesser wing of the sphenoid. The medial border (formed by the anterior root) is less defined.

The distance between the intracranial openings is 25 mm; between the orbital openings 30 mm.

Anteriorly the roof of each canal extends more than its floor, while posteriorly the floor projects beyond the roof, this gap being filled in by dura mater with a posterior edge (the falciform fold) (Fig. 5.16).

The optic canal is close to the sphenoidal air sinus and sometimes to a posterior ethmoidal sinus. According to Fazakas (1933), the longer the optic canal, the thinner its medial wall and the more likely it is to encroach on a posterior ethmoidal sinus. The bone between canal and sinuses is often very thin, and the canal may ridge the interior of a sinus. The sphenoidal or a posterior ethmoidal sinus may variably invade the lesser wing and may surround the canal completely. The posterior part of the gyrus rectus and olfactory tract are superior to the canal.

The optic canal is separated from the medial end of the superior orbital fissure by a bar of bone, on which the annulus tendineus is attached (Fig. 1.2).

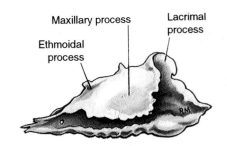

Maxillary process Lacrimal process Ethmoidal process

Fig. 1.14 The right inferior concha (lateral aspect).

The canal transmits the optic nerve and its meningeal coverings (Figs 15.27 and 15.31), the ophthalmic artery, located at first below, then lateral to the nerve and embedded in its dural sheath (Figs 15.27 and 15.28), and branches from the periarterial sympathetic plexus. Separating the artery and nerve is a layer of fibrous tissue, which may be ossified.

Average measurements of the optic canal

The orbital opening is 6–6.5 mm vertically and 4.5–5 mm horizontally. In the middle portion it is 5 × 5 mm. The canal is further narrowed by the periosteum.

The lateral wall is 5–7 mm long (width of the posterior root of the lesser wing of the sphenoid). The roof, 10–12 mm in length, varies with the development of the lesser wing between the anterior clinoid process and body of the sphenoid. The upper and medial walls are longer. The longer the optic canal, the narrower it is, and vice versa (Fazakas, 1933). See also Kier (1966) for further details.

THE ORBITAL MARGIN

The orbital margin is most commonly quadrilateral with rounded corners, and is usually spiral, the inferior orbital margin being continuous with the anterior lacrimal crest, the superior with the posterior lacrimal crest. The lacrimal fossa thus lies within the orbital margin.

Each side measures about 40 mm, but usually the width is greater than the height; the relation between the two is the **orbital index,*** which varies in different races. The opening is directed slightly laterally, and its upper and lower margins descend gently to the lateral side.

The orbital margin is formed by frontal, zygomatic, and maxillary elements.

The superior orbital margin

This margin is formed solely by the orbital arch of the frontal bone. It is concave downwards, convex

---

*The orbital index (of Broca)

$$= \frac{\text{Height of orbit} \times 100}{\text{Width of orbit}}$$

Three classes of orbit are recognized. (1) Megaseme (large): the index is 89 or more, as is characteristic of Mongolian races, except the Esquimaux. The opening is round. (2) Mesoseme (intermediate): index between 89 and 83, as in Caucasians (European 87, English 88.4), according to Flower, 1907. (3) Microseme (small): index 83 or less; a negroid characteristic. The orbital opening is rectangular.

forwards, sharp in its lateral two-thirds and rounded in the medial third. About 25 mm from the mid line and at the summit of the arch is the **supraorbital notch**, whose lateral border is usually the sharper. This is occasionally converted into a foramen by ossification of ligament which spans it, opening 3–6 mm behind the orbital margin. It transmits the supraorbital nerve and vessels. The notch or foramen is palpable in the living.

Sometimes medial to the supraorbital notch a second notch or foramen occurs and transmits the medial branches of the supraorbital nerves and vessels where these have divided inside the orbit.

Supraorbital grooves leading from these notches or foramina are sometimes seen. Berry (1975) has reviewed variations in supraorbital notches and foramina; a foramen occurs in 15–87% in different ethnic groups (e.g. 51% of Mexican skulls).

A groove may also occur about 10 mm medial to the supraorbital notch for the supratrochlear nerve and artery.

A **supraciliary canal** (Ward, 1858) appears in about 50% of skulls (Fig. 1.2). It has a small opening near the supraorbital notch, and transmits a nutrient artery and a branch of the supraorbital nerve to the frontal air sinus.

The lateral orbital margin

This margin is the strongest part of the orbital outlet. It is formed by the zygomatic process of the frontal and by the zygomatic bone. It is concave when viewed laterally and is posterior to the medial margin.

The inferior orbital margin

This margin is raised slightly above the floor of the orbit. It is formed by the zygomatic bone and maxilla, usually in equal amounts.

The zygomatic part is a long thin spur (the maxillary or marginal process) which overlaps the maxilla (Figs 1.2 and 1.5). The suture between the two, sometimes marked by a tubercle, can be felt about half-way along the margin just above the infraorbital foramen (Fig. 1.2).

Sometimes the zygomatic (spur) may reach the anterior lacrimal crest, excluding the maxilla, or it may be reduced to a small part of the margin.

The medial margin

The medial margin is the anterior lacrimal crest on the frontal process of the maxilla and posterior lacrimal crest on the lacrimal. These crests overlap; the medial margin is thus not continuous, but is considered to ascend from the anterior crest over the maxillary frontal process to the superior margin (Fig. 1.2).

Variations

In the sphenozygomatic suture accessory (sutural or Wormian) ossicles may occur. Another suture occurs in 21.1% of Japanese skulls, in which the zygomatic bone may be in two parts (Os Japonicum).

1.2 AGE AND SEX CHANGES

Changes in the orbit during growth depend partly on general cranial and facial development, and partly on that of the neighbouring air sinuses.

The orbital margin is sharp and well ossified at birth. 'The eyeball is therefore well protected from stress and injury during parturition. When we recollect the relatively large size and the advanced stage of development of the eye at birth, it is clearly specially desirable that such protection should be afforded; that it is efficacious, the rarity of birth injuries of the globe in cases of unassisted labour can testify' (Fisher, 1904).

At 7 years of age, except in its upper part, the margin is less sharp, the superomedial and inferolateral angles are more defined and hence the orbital opening tends to be somewhat trapezoidal.

In coronal section behind the orbital margin the orbit is quadrilateral with rounded corners. In the newborn it is ellipsoid and higher on the lateral.

The infantile orbits diverge more than the adult, i.e. their axes, from the middle of the orbital opening to the optic foramen, make an angle of 115°, and, if projected backwards, meet at the nasal septum. In the adult these axes make an angle of 40–45°, and meet at the upper part of the clivus of the sphenoid. These axes are horizontal in the infant, but slope down and backwards at 15–20°.

The superior orbital fissures are relatively large in children, the greater wing of the sphenoid being relatively narrower, and the wide and narrow parts are less distinct.

The orbital index is high in children, the vertical diameter being almost the same as the horizontal, but in adults the latter increases (see table 1.1). The orbits grow little after the age of 7 years.

In children the interorbital distance is small. Children are not infrequently considered to squint when this is really due to the narrow interorbital distance, which makes the eyes look too close

together. With the growth of frontal and ethmoidal sinuses the distance increases, and the 'squint' disappears.

The infraorbital foramen is usually present at birth; but it may be a terminal notch of an infraorbital groove whose roof has not yet grown over it to form a canal.

The orbital process of the zygomatic bone may almost reach the lacrimal fossa, and this condition may persist through childhood or even into adult years.

The roof of the orbit is relatively much larger than its floor at birth, because the fetal skull has a large cranium (orbital roof) and a small face (orbital floor). The fossa for the lacrimal gland is shallow, but the accessory fossa is well marked.

The optic canal is at birth actually a foramen; at 1 year its length is 4 mm. The axis also changes with age: while directed anterolaterally, as in the adult, it is inclined more downwards.

Table 1.1 gives a résumé of the changes in the orbital opening with age (Winckler).

The periosteum or periorbita is much thicker and stronger at birth than in the adult.

Table 1.1 Changes in the orbital opening with age

	Form	Height (mm)	Width (mm)	Index
Fetus (8 months)	Oval	14	18	77.7
Newborn (6 months)	= Rounded	27	27	100
Child (7 years)	Quadrilateral	28	33	84.8
Adult	Quadrilateral	35	39	89.7

SENILE CHANGES

Senile changes are largely due to absorption of bone. Thus, in elderly skulls holes sometimes occur in the roof of the orbit, the periorbita being in direct contact with dura mater.

The **medial wall**, although normally thin, rarely shows absorption in its ethmoidal area, but its lacrimal part usually does.

The **lateral wall** often displays absorption or marked thinning.

In the **floor**, senile changes rarely produce holes, except those in the roof or floor of the infraorbital canal.

The **orbital fissures**, especially the inferior, are widened by absorption of their margins.

In long-headed (dolichocephalic) skulls the orbits tend to look more laterally than in the short-headed (brachycephalic) (Mannhardt, 1871).

MENSURATION

There is a great difference between the measurements given by different authorities. The following are average:

Depth of orbit	40 mm
Height of orbital opening	35 mm
Width of orbital opening	40 mm
Interorbital distance	25 mm
Volume	30 ml
Ratio of volume of orbit: volume of globe	4.5:1
	(Ovio)

SEX DIFFERENCES

Up to puberty sexual differences between the orbits, as in the whole skull, are slight. Thereafter the male skull begins to develop secondary sexual characters, especially in the mandible and frontal region.

The female skull remains more infantile in form. The orbits remain rounder and the upper margin sharper than in the male. The glabella and superciliary ridges are less marked or almost absent. The forehead is more vertical and the frontal eminences more obvious. The contours of the region are rounder and the bones smoother. The zygomatic process of the frontal bone is more slender and pointed. The female orbit is more elongated and relatively larger than the male (Merkel, 1885). In contrast, greater development of the frontal sinuses in the male produces distinct superciliary ridges, and hence a less vertical forehead and less pronounced frontal eminences.

1.3 THE PERIORBITA (Figs 1.15 and 5.17)

The periorbita or orbital periosteum invests every surface of the bones of the orbit, to which it is in general loosely adherent, so that it may be lifted from them by blood or pus or during operations.

At various points, however, it is firmly fixed:

- at the orbital margin, where it is thickened to form the arcus marginale and continuous with the periosteum of the face;
- at the sutures, where it is continuous with sutural 'ligaments';
- at fissures and foramina;
- at the lacrimal fossa.

Through the superior orbital fissure, the optic foramen, and anterior ethmoidal canal (Fig. 5.17) the periorbita is continuous with the dura mater.

In the superior orbital fissure the periorbita is dense but allows various structures to pass through.

In the optic foramen the dural sheath of the optic nerve is adherent to periosteum. Here the periorbita splits, becoming in part continuous with the dural sheath, and also providing attachment for muscles and sending processes along their sheaths. Fine processes also pass from the periorbita, to divide fat into lobules and to form coverings for vessels and nerves.

Through the inferior orbital fissure the periorbita blends with periosteum in the infratemporal and pterygopalatine fossae, through the temporal canal with that of the temporal fossa, and via the zygomatic canal with that on the zygomatic bone.

It is adherent to the posterior lacrimal crest, and here divides to enclose the lacrimal fossa, separated from the sac by loose areolar tissue. It thence descends the duct to merge with periosteum in the inferior meatus.

These facts are important in exenteration of the orbit. After division of periosteum at the orbital margin, the periosteal cone is easily detached except at the sites, as noted above, where attachments must be divided.

The periorbita consists of two layers. Next to bone oblique fibres predominate. They are not obvious in the inner zone, which is much weaker and gives covering to the frontal and lacrimal nerves and forms the space for the lacrimal gland.

The periorbita is liable to ossification where it roofs over the infraorbital canal and where it is attached to the posterior lacrimal crest.

Orbital periosteum, like that elsewhere, is sensitive. It is supplied by those trigeminal nerve branches which lie in contact with it – frontal, lacrimal zygomatic, infraorbital and ethmoidal.

THE ORBITAL MUSCLE OF MÜLLER (MUSCULUS ORBITALIS)

Associated with the periorbita, near the inferior orbital fissure, is an aggregation of non-striated muscle fibres, the orbital muscle (of Müller), which not only spans the fissure but also extends back, deep to the annular tendon as far as the cavernous sinus. Anteriorly it fades away in the periorbita. Its action in the human is doubtful. In certain mammals having no lateral wall between the orbit and the temporal fossa the muscle is large and replaces the body wall (Fig. 1.17). Scattered smooth muscle is also found within the connective tissue 'pulleys' of the recti.

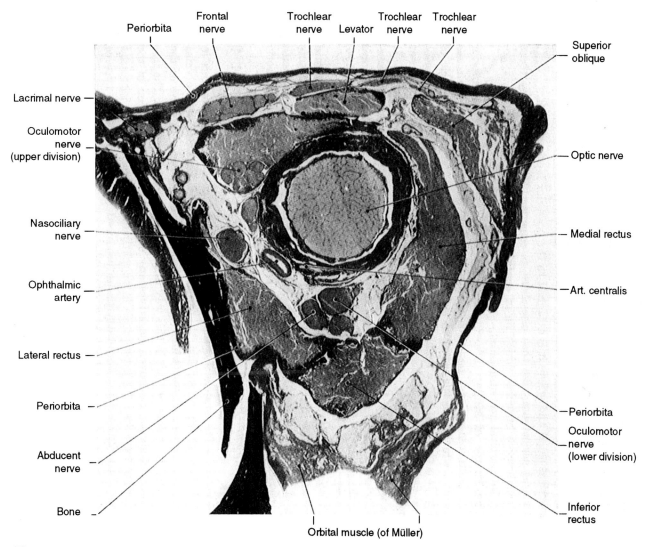

Fig. 1.15 Coronal section of the right orbit, near apex.

Relations

Above is orbital fat containing the inferior ophthalmic vein and its tributaries, and below is fatty tissue of the pterygopalatine fossa in which are the infraorbital nerve, pterygopalatine ganglion with arteries and veins surrounding it. Through the muscle pass veins connecting the ophthalmic vein and pterygoid plexus.

Nerve supply

The orbital muscle of Müller is supplied by a branch from the pterygopalatine ganglion (sympathetic).

Function

The muscle was once considered to cause proptosis in exophthalmic goitre, either directly or by pressure on veins passing through it. But while the muscle may protrude the eye in some animals, it does not do so in humans, in whom it is vestigial. Moreover, venous compression would be bypassed. Hyperthyroid proptosis is probably due to oedema of orbital fat. Apparent exophthalmos is a widening of the palpebral fissure caused by overaction of striated muscle in levator palpebrae superioris.

1.4 SURFACE ANATOMY OF THE ORBITAL REGION

THE SUPERCILIARY RIDGES

These ridges, elevations above the orbital margins, meet in the **glabella**, the prominence above the nose. Their development is not a direct indication of the size of the frontal sinuses. The supraciliary ridges are

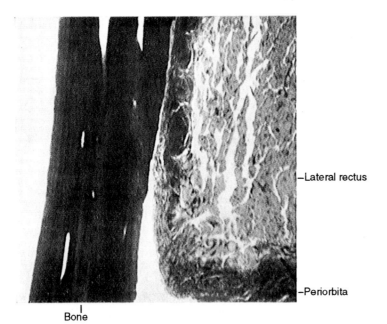

−Lateral rectus

−Periorbita

Bone

Fig. 1.16 Detail of Fig. 1.15. Note how loosely attached the periorbita is to the bone.

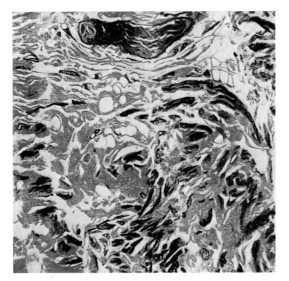

Fig. 1.17 Detail of Fig. 1.15, to show fibres of the orbital muscle of Müller.

larger in the male than in the female and absent in childhood.

THE FRONTAL EMINENCES

The frontal eminences are paired protrusions of the frontal bone about 5 cm above each orbit; they are more prominent in the female than the male, and are even more so in the infant.

THE INFRAORBITAL FORAMEN

This foramen lies 4–5 mm below the tubercle on the orbital margin marking the junction of zygomatic bone and maxilla. It is usually oval, and is directed anteroinferiorly. The foramen may be double: indeed, up to five have been described.

The supraorbital notch, infraorbital foramen and mental foramen are all near a vertical line between the premolar teeth.

THE TEMPORAL CREST

The temporal crest runs posterosuperiorly from the frontal zygomatic process into the temporal lines on the parietal bone.

THE SUTURA NOTHA

As can be seen in Fig. 1.2, this is a groove on the frontal process of the maxilla, parallel with the anterior lacrimal crest, for a branch of the infraorbital artery.

THE SUPERIOR ORBITAL MARGIN

This is an easily palpable prominence, sharp laterally and more rounded medially.

The **eyebrow** corresponds in position only in part to the margin. The head of the eyebrow is largely inferior to the medial part of the margin, and is palpated by upward pressure. The body lies along the margin, while the tail is above its lateral part, palpable and usually visible below it.

The **frontal zygomatic process** forms a marked subcutaneous prominence.

THE SUPRAORBITAL NOTCH

This notch can be felt at the junction of lateral two-thirds with medial one-third of the orbit, and the supraorbital nerve can often be rolled under the finger here.

THE LATERAL ORBITAL MARGIN

This margin is visible only above the orbit, but is palpable in its whole extent.

THE INFERIOR ORBITAL MARGIN

The inferior margin is not visible, because the skin of the lower lid passes smoothly into that of the cheek showing, especially in the old, the nasojugal and malar furrows. Its sharp ridge is easily palpated, and laterally a fingertip can push into the orbit for about a centimetre or so.

THE LACRIMAL TUBERCLE

The tubercle can be felt on the sharp anterior lacrimal crest, as can the tubercle of the inferior margin marking the suture between zygomatic bone and maxilla.

The **trochlea** of the superior oblique is easily felt posterior to the superomedial angle of the orbital margin.

THE LATERAL ORBITAL TUBERCLE

The lateral orbital tubercle (of Whitnall) can be felt just within the lateral orbital margin at its mid point.

THE INFRAORBITAL FORAMEN

The foramen can be identified by its sharp superior margin 4–5 mm below the tubercle of the lower orbital margin.

THE ZYGOMATIC TUBERCLE

This tubercle is felt posteroinferior to the frontal zygomatic process; a V-shaped interval marks the frontozygomatic suture.

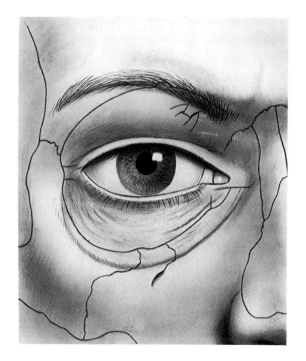

Fig. 1.18 Surface projection of the orbital opening.

THE ANTERIOR LACRIMAL CREST

The crest is easily felt, and posterior to it lie the lacrimal fossa and posterior crest. Note that the examining finger is below the medial angle of the eye and not the ridge made by the medial palpebral ligament.

THE TEMPORAL CREST

This crest can be traced posteriorly from the frontal zygomatic process.

THE NASAL BONE

Medial to the frontal process of the maxilla, the nasal bone can be palpated to its lower end, where it joins the lateral nasal cartilage.

1.5   THE PARANASAL SINUSES (Figs 1.19–1.21)

THE MAXILLARY SINUS

The maxillary sinus is a pyramidal cavity in the maxilla (Figs 1.3, 1.19).

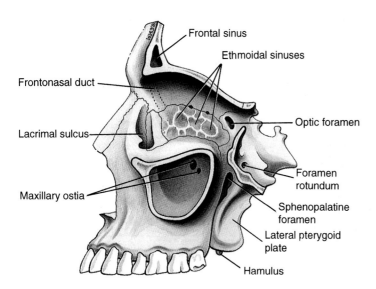

Fig. 1.19 The left paranasal sinuses.

Base

The base of the maxillary sinus forms part of the lateral wall of the nose; its apex adjoins or enters the zygomatic bone. The base presents a large opening, partly closed in the articulated skull by the uncinate process of the ethmoid above, inferior concha below, palatine behind, and lacrimal in front (Fig. 1.3). The mucous membrane further closes this, leaving a small aperture or **ostium** (sometimes two) near the roof of the sinus, drainage of which is poor. The ostium opens into the middle nasal meatus in the hiatus semilunaris (Fig. 1.20). The nasolacrimal duct forms a ridge in the anterior part of the base (Fig. 1.20).

Walls

The anterolateral wall, reached by everting the upper lip, contains the anterior and middle superior alveolar (dental) nerves and their canals (Fig. 5.29).

The posterior wall adjoins the infratemporal fossa, forming its anterior wall. In it are canals for the posterior superior alveolar (dental) nerves.

Roof

The roof of the maxillary sinus is formed by the orbital plate of the maxilla, the floor of the orbit. The roof contains the infraorbital canal which provides passage for the infraorbital nerve and vessels ridging the front part of the roof.

Floor

The floor, formed by the maxillary alveolar process, is about 1.25 cm below the floor of the nose. The sinus lies above the premolars and molars, the roots of which may produce elevations on its floor. With advancing age the floor undergoes absorption, which may expose the roots, especially of the first molar.

THE FRONTAL SINUSES

These are cavities of variable extent between the two plates of the frontal bone (Figs 1.3, 5.17 and 5.21), and are separated by a septum, which is usually deviated to one side. In the peripheral parts of the sinus small partitions form loculi. Some frontal sinuses extend laterally to the zygomatic process; others, especially if the septum is much to one side, may be mere slits.

On average (Logan-Turner, 1901, 1908a,b), the height of the frontal sinus is 3 cm, the breadth 2.5 cm and depth 2 cm.

Posteroinferiorly the ethmoidal and frontal sinuses are separated by a thin plate of bone, and a **frontoethmoidal** sinus may project into the frontal sinus (Fig. 1.3).

The sinus drains into the nose by the **infundibulum**, a narrow canal between the anterior ethmoidal sinuses and hiatus semilunaris in the middle meatus, anterior to the anterior ethmoidal and maxillary sinuses (Fig. 1.20). This favours spread of infection between sinuses.

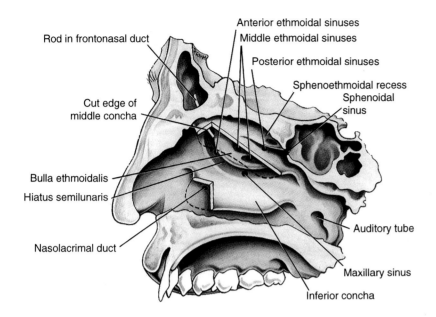

Fig. 1.20 The right lateral wall of the nasal cavity to show the openings of the paranasal sinuses and nasolacrimal duct.

Walls

The posterior wall is thin, but contains each diploë, and separates the sinus from the meninges and frontal lobes of the cerebrum.

The anterior wall is thicker and also contains diploë. Osteomyelitis spreads more readily in this than the posterior wall.

Floor

The floor of the frontal sinus separates it from the orbit and nasal cavity.

THE ETHMOIDAL SINUSES

The ethmoidal sinuses are mostly situated in the lateral mass of the ethmoid, but are completed by the frontal, palatine, sphenoid, maxillary and lacrimal bones. Collectively they form an **ethmoid labyrinth**.

Above them are the meninges and cerebrum in the anterior cranial fossa. In front is the infundibulum of the frontal sinus, behind the sphenoidal sinus. Below is the nasal cavity, laterally the orbit and lacrimal fossa (Figs 1.4 and 5.17).

The sinuses are separated from these regions by very thin plates of bone, favouring spread of infection (ethmoiditis is the most common cause of orbital cellulitis).

The sinuses are divided by irregular septa into anterior, middle, and posterior groups (Fig. 1.19).

The anterior and middle sinuses open into the middle meatus, the anterior in the hiatus semilunaris, the middle on the bulla ethmoidalis (Fig. 1.20). The posterior sinuses lie anteromedial to the optic canal and open into the superior meatus.

THE SPHENOIDAL AIR SINUSES

The two sphenoidal sinuses are in the body of the sphenoid bone (Figs 1.20, 3.16 and 15.57), separated by a vertical septum often deviated from the mid line. A variable transverse septum also occurs in each sinus, usually inclined anteroinferiorly as the 'carotid buttress' (Cushing) a useful landmark for the internal carotid artery in the nasal approach to the hypophysis. It can often be seen in radiographs of the region. The sphenoidal sinus lies in front of the hypophyseal (pituitary) fossa. The sinus enlarges by resorption of bone as age advances, extending below the fossa and into the root of the lesser wing. It may excavate the basisphenoid and basiocciput till close to the anterior margin of the foramen magnum.

Above the sphenoidal sinuses are the hypophysis and optic nerves, which often ridge each sinus. This close relation explains involvement of the nerve in sinusitis, causing sudden loss of vision (retrobulbar neuritis) (Fig. 15.27).

Below is the nasal cavity, and in its floor the pterygoid canal, which may ridge it.

In front are the ethmoidal sinuses, the posterior often bulging into the sphenoidal.

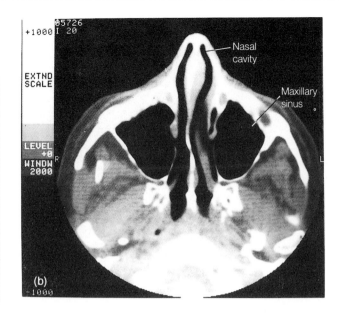

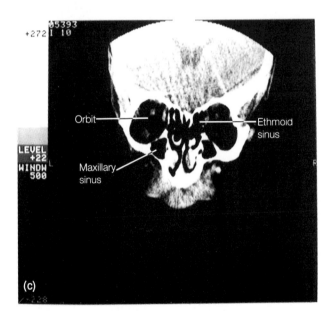

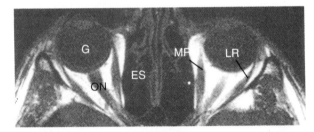

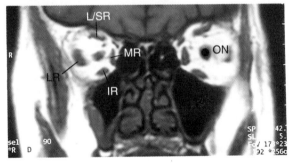

Fig. 1.21 Computed axial tomography of the skull. (a) Horizontal view of the orbits; (b) horizontal view of the maxillary sinuses; (c) coronal view. (Courtesy of Dr M. Golding.) Magnetic resonance imaging of the orbits. (i) Horizontal section; (ii) coronal section. ES, ethmoid sinus; G, globe; IR, inferior rectus; L, levator; LR, lateral rectus; MR, medial rectus; ON, optic nerve. (Courtesy of J. Byrne.)

Laterally are the cavernous sinuses, each containing an internal carotid artery and abducent nerve. In front of this the body of the sphenoid bone forms the medial wall of the orbit.

Each sphenoidal sinus opens into its sphenoethmoidal recess. When large this may extend between the foramina rotundum and ovale, which may explain involvement of the contained nerves in disease of the sinus.

1.6 NERVE SUPPLY TO THE SINUSES

THE MAXILLARY SINUS

The maxillary sinus receives many branches from the maxillary nerve: from the infraorbital nerve to the roof by perforating branches; from the superior alveolar nerves, on their way to the teeth, to the posterior, lateral and anterior walls. The anterior

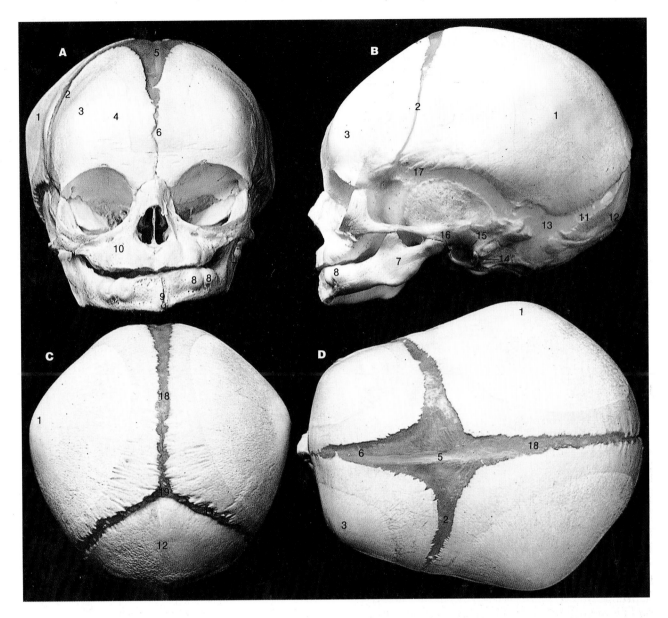

Fig. 1.22 The skull of a full-term fetus (A) from the front; (B) from the left and slightly below; (C) from behind; (D) from above.

1 = Parietal tuberosity;
2 = coronal suture;
3 = frontal tuberosity;
4 = half of frontal bone;
5 = anterior fontanelle;

6 = frontal suture;
7 = ramus of mandible;
8 = elevations of deciduous teeth
   in body of mandible;
9 = symphysis menti;

10 = maxilla;
11 = lambdoid suture;
12 = occipital bone;
13 = mastoid fontanelle;
14 = stylomastoid foramen;

15 = external acoustic meatus;
16 = tympanic ring;
17 = sphenoidal fontanelle;
18 = sagittal suture;
19 = posterior fontanelle.

The face at birth forms a smaller proportion of the cranium than in the adult (about one-eighth compared to one-half), because of the small size of the nasal cavity and maxillary sinuses and the lack of erupted teeth. The posterior fontanelle (C, 19) closes about 2 months after birth, the anterior fontanelle (A, 5; D, 5) in the second year. Because of the lack of the mastoid process (which does not develop until the second year) the stylomastoid foramen (B, 14) and the emerging facial nerve are relatively near the surface and are unprotected. (From McMinn, R.M.H. and Hutchings, R.T. (1988), published by Wolfe Medical Publications Ltd., with permission)

superior alveolar nerve supplies the nasal wall near the nasolacrimal duct, and behind this the anterior (greater) palatine nerve supplies nasal wall and maxillary ostium.

THE FRONTAL SINUS

The frontal sinus is supplied by the supraorbital nerve.

THE ETHMOIDAL SINUSES

The anterior and middle ethmoidal sinuses are supplied by the anterior ethmoidal nerve, the posterior ethmoidal and sphenoidal sinus by the posterior ethmoidal nerve.

1.7   LYMPH DRAINAGE OF THE SINUSES

The sphenoidal and posterior ethmoidal air sinuses drain back to retropharyngeal lymph nodes; the middle and anterior ethmoidal, frontal and maxillary sinuses drain to submandibular nodes.

1.8   DEVELOPMENT OF THE SINUSES

The accessory sinuses of the nose are all evaginations from the nasal cavity. They are rudimentary at birth (Fig. 1.22).

FRONTAL SINUSES

The rudiment of each frontal sinus grows upwards from the ethmoid bone, reaching the frontal at 1 year. Its stalk forms the infundibulum. At 7 years the frontal sinus is about the size of a pea, growing rapidly thereafter, to reach its full size at about 25 years.

ETHMOIDAL SINUSES

At birth the ethmoidal sinuses are small depressions, and grow rapidly after 7 years.

SPHENOIDAL SINUSES

The sphenoidal sinus is extending into the sphenoidal concha at the time of birth; but at 2 years the sphenoid body is still trabecular, each sinus being a mere depression at its future opening. Active growth is delayed until late childhood and is largely complete at adolescence, though senile absorption may further enlarge the sinus.

MAXILLARY SINUSES

The maxillary sinus appears as a shallow groove in each lateral nasal wall during the fourth or fifth month of intrauterine life. At 1 year it reaches the infraorbital canal. The sinus grows rapidly with the second dentition, so that at 12 years it is nearly adult size, but slow growth continues until 18 years.

1.9   THE CRANIAL CAVITY

CALVARIA

The calva or skull cap is composed of parts of the frontal and parietal bones and the upper squama of the occipital. Anteriorly the **frontal crest** projects between the cerebral hemispheres in the median plane and gives attachment to the falx cerebri. The **sagittal sulcus**, accommodating the superior sagittal sinus, widens as it passes posteriorly in the mid line.

The frontal branch of the meningeal vein (and less so, the accompanying artery) grooves the cranial vault deeply behind the cranial suture.

BASE OF THE SKULL (Figs 1.22–1.26)

The floor of the base of the skull is divided into anterior, middle and posterior fossae, which support the cerebral and cerebellar hemispheres and transmit nerves and vessels between the cranial cavity and the exterior.

The anterior cranial fossa

The bones which contribute to the anterior fossa are the frontal, the cribriform plate of the ethmoid, and the lesser wing and anterior body of the sphenoid.

Centrally is the **cribriform plate**, which presents a median eminence (the crista galli), and exhibits on either side of this numerous fine foramina for the olfactory nerves passing from nasal mucosa to olfactory bulb. The **foramen caecum**, a depression between the crista galli and frontal crest, rarely transmits a vein. The **anterior ethmoidal canal** opens on the line of suture between the frontal bone and the cribriform plate, whose medial edge overlaps it above. Directed medially, this canal transmits the anterior ethmoidal nerves and vessels, which run deep to dura, to gain the nasal cavity via a slit at the side of the crista galli.

At the posterolateral corner of the cribriform plate is the **posterior ethmoidal canal**, overhung by the anterior border of the sphenoid. It transmits the posterior ethmoidal vessels.

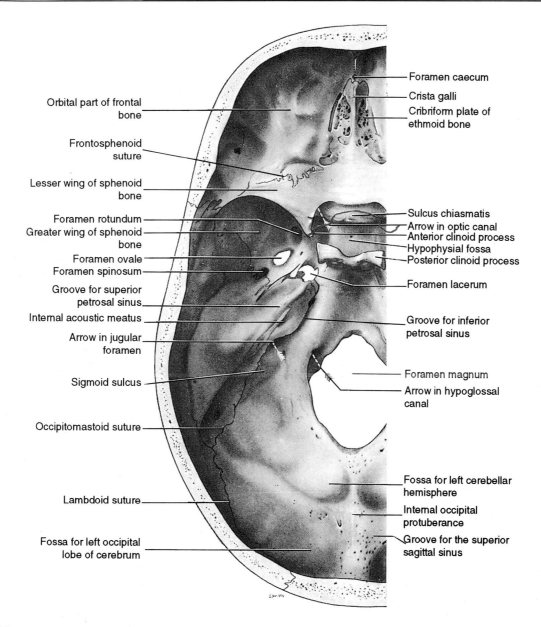

Orbital part of frontal bone

Frontosphenoid suture

Lesser wing of sphenoid bone

Foramen rotundum

Greater wing of sphenoid bone

Foramen ovale

Foramen spinosum

Groove for superior petrosal sinus

Internal acoustic meatus

Arrow in jugular foramen

Sigmoid sulcus

Occipitomastoid suture

Lambdoid suture

Fossa for left occipital lobe of cerebrum

Foramen caecum

Crista galli

Cribriform plate of ethmoid bone

Sulcus chiasmatis

Arrow in optic canal

Anterior clinoid process

Hypophysial fossa

Posterior clinoid process

Foramen lacerum

Groove for inferior petrosal sinus

Foramen magnum

Arrow in hypoglossal canal

Fossa for left cerebellar hemisphere

Internal occipital protuberance

Groove for the superior sagittal sinus

Fig. 1.23 The internal (endocranial) surface of the left half of the base of the skull. (From Williams, P.L. *et al.* (eds) (1995) *Gray's Anatomy*, 38th edition, published by Churchill Livingstone.)

On each side of the median plane the orbital part of the frontal bone forms the greater part of the floor and separates the orbit from the inferior surface of the frontal lobe. Its convex cranial surface is marked with impressions for the cerebral gyri and one or two meningeal vascular grooves. Its anteromedial laminae are separated by the frontal sinus while its medial part separates the ethmoidal labyrinth from the fossa.

Behind the cribriform plate the **jugum sphenoidale**, the upper surface of the anterior sphenoid body, separates the sphenoidal air sinuses from the fossa. Its sharp posterior edge forms the anterior margin of the sulcus chiasmaticus. The jugum sphenoidale underlies the gyri recti and olfactory tracts. Lateral to the jugum is the **lesser wing of the sphenoid**, whose posterior free margin curves laterally and forwards and overhangs the middle cranial fossa. Laterally it tapers, to end at or near the end of the superior orbital fissure. Its posteromedial extremity forms the **anterior clinoid process**. The lesser wing is related to the inferior

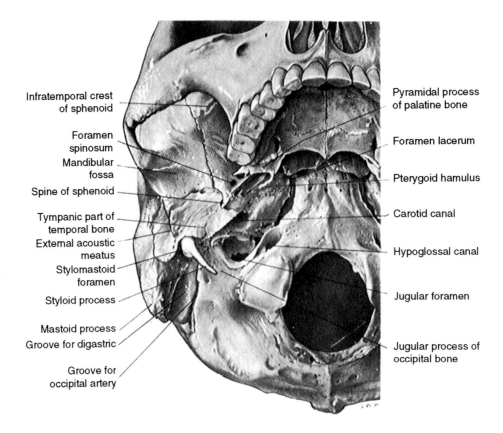

Infratemporal crest of sphenoid

Foramen spinosum

Mandibular fossa

Spine of sphenoid

Tympanic part of temporal bone

External acoustic meatus

Stylomastoid foramen

Styloid process

Mastoid process

Groove for digastric

Groove for occipital artery

Pyramidal process of palatine bone

Foramen lacerum

Pterygoid hamulus

Carotid canal

Hypoglossal canal

Jugular foramen

Jugular process of occipital bone

Fig. 1.24 The right and part of the left side of the basal aspect of the skull. To show some features to better advantage, the anterior end of the skull has been elevated so that the Frankfurt plane is tilted to an angle of about 45° to the horizontal. (From Williams, P.L. *et al.* (eds) (1995) *Gray's Anatomy*, 38th edition, published by Churchill Livingstone.)

surface of the frontal lobe above, and more medially to the anterior perforated substance. Below, it forms the upper border of the superior orbital fissure. The anterior clinoid process is grooved medially by the internal carotid artery as it pierces the roof of the cavernous sinus, and receives the attachment of the free border of the tentorium cerebelli. The **middle clinoid processes**, which complete the anterior boundary of the sella turcica, may each be connected to an anterior clinoid process by a thin bar of bone, to form a **caroticoclinoid foramen**.

Two roots connect the lesser wing medially to the body of the sphenoid. The broad, flat anterior root is continuous with the jugum sphenoidale; the smaller, thicker, posterior root is connected to the sphenoid body opposite the posterior border of the **chiasmal sulcus**. Between the two lies the optic canal.

The middle cranial fossa

The bones contributing to the middle fossa are the sphenoid, temporal and parietal bones.

Centrally, the floor is formed by the body of the sphenoid. Anteriorly, the chiasmal sulcus leads from one optic canal to the other. It rarely makes contact with the optic chiasm, which is usually above and behind it. The optic canal between the roots of the lesser wing and body of the sphenoid extends forwards, laterally and somewhat downwards with its contained optic nerve, ophthalmic artery and meninges.

Behind the chiasmal sulcus is the saddle-shaped upper surface of the sphenoid body (**sella turcica**) whose anterior slope bears a median eminence, the **tuberculum sellae**. Behind this is the **hypophyseal fossa** which houses the **hypophysis cerebri** (pituitary gland) and forms part of the roof of the sphenoidal sinuses. Its posterior margin is formed by the **dorsum sellae**, a plate of bone projecting upwards and forwards from the body of the sphenoid, and whose superolateral angles are expanded into the **posterior clinoid processes**. These receive the anterior attachment of the tentorium cerebelli and that of the petroclinoid ligaments. The lower end of the latter attaches to a spicule of bone, with the abducent nerve

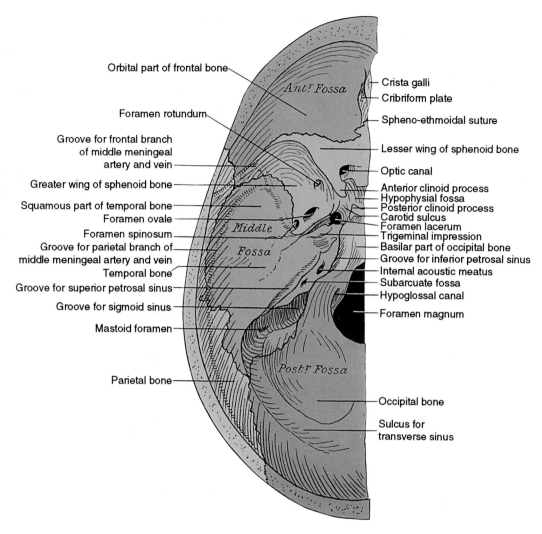

Orbital part of frontal bone
Ant.^r Fossa
Crista galli
Cribriform plate
Foramen rotundum
Spheno-ethmoidal suture
Groove for frontal branch
of middle meningeal
artery and vein
Lesser wing of sphenoid bone
Greater wing of sphenoid bone
Optic canal
Anterior clinoid process
Squamous part of temporal bone
Hypophysial fossa
Posterior clinoid process
Foramen ovale
Carotid sulcus
Foramen spinosum
Foramen lacerum
Groove for parietal branch of
Trigeminal impression
middle meningeal artery and vein
Basilar part of occipital bone
Temporal bone
Groove for inferior petrosal sinus
Middle
Internal acoustic meatus
Fossa
Groove for superior petrosal sinus
Subarcuate fossa
Hypoglossal canal
Groove for sigmoid sinus
Foramen magnum
Mastoid foramen
Post.^r Fossa
Parietal bone
Occipital bone
Sulcus for
transverse sinus

Fig. 1.25 The internal surface of the left half of the base of the skull.

immediately in front, between ligament and dorsum sellae; behind, a notch accommodates the roots of the trigeminal nerve.

The body of the sphenoid, lateral to the sella turcica is grooved by the internal carotid artery, running forward to the foramen lacerum. The lateral margin of the groove may be deepened by a projection, the **lingula**, while the **middle clinoid process** forms an elevation at its anteromedial margin.

Laterally, the middle fossa is deep and houses the temporal lobe of the cerebrum. The anterior boundary of the fossa is the greater wing of the sphenoid; laterally is the temporal squama and posteriorly the petrous temporal bone. It is related to the orbital apex in front, the temporal fossa laterally and to the infratemporal fossa below.

Various foramina communicate with the exterior of the skull.

The middle fossa communicates with the orbit anteriorly through the superior orbital fissure bounded by the lesser wing of the sphenoid above, the greater below and the body medially. The wedge-shaped slit has its base medial and its apex directed upwards, laterally and forwards. It transmits the ophthalmic veins and smaller vessels, the oculomotor, trochlear and abducent nerves and branches of the ophthalmic division of the trigeminal nerve.

The optic canal is described on p.11.

The foramina

The **foramen rotundum** pierces the greater wing of the sphenoid immediately below and behind the medial end of the superior orbital fissure; it conducts the maxillary nerve forwards to the **pterygopalatine fossa**. Developmentally it is formed from the fissure itself.

The **foramen ovale**, directly behind the foramen rotundum, is lateral to the lingula and posterior end of the carotid groove. It transmits the mandibular nerve to the infratemporal region, the accessory meningeal artery, and sometimes the lesser petrosal nerve. An occasional medial emissary foramen is found medial to the foramen ovale, which transmits an emissary vein from the cavernous sinus.

The **foramen spinosum**, just posterolateral to the foramen ovale, transmits the middle meningeal artery and a small meningeal nerve. The artery passes laterally, grooving the temporal squama with its vein; its frontal branch passes upwards across the pterion to reach the anterior parietal bone. The parietal branch runs posterosuperiorly across the temporal squama to the posterior temporal bone.

The **foramen lacerum** lies behind the posterior end of the carotid groove, posteromedial to the foramen ovale. It is bounded by the apex of the petrous temporal bone behind and the body of the sphenoid and posterior border of its greater wing in front. The posterior wall of the foramen is pierced by the carotid artery, which ascends with its sympathetic and venous plexuses through its upper opening. The greater petrosal nerve leaves its groove on the anterior surface of the petrous temporal bone, turns downward into the foramen lacerum, lateral to the carotid artery, and is joined by the deep petrosal nerve (sympathetic) to form the nerve of the pterygoid canal. The nerve passes from this region into the pterygopalatine fossa via the pterygoid canal in the anterior wall of the foramen lacerum.

Behind the foramen lacerum is the shallow depression for the trigeminal ganglion on the anterior surface of the petrous temporal bone. A further depression posterolateral to this is bounded by the **arcuate eminence**, overlying the anterior semicircular canal. The **tegmen tympani**, a thin bony plate forming the roof of the tympanic cavity and part of the mastoid antrum, lies anterolateral.

Lateral to the trigeminal impression is the groove for the greater petrosal nerve, which descends forwards from its hiatus. The hiatus for the lesser petrosal nerve is lateral to this.

The superior border of the petrous temporal is grooved by the superior petrosal sinus, which connects the cavernous to the sigmoid sinuses. The cavernous sinus extends on each side of the body of the sphenoid sinus, from the medial end of the superior orbital fissure to the apex of the petrous bone. The sinuses are connected anteriorly and posteriorly across the tuberculum and dorsum sellae. The **diaphragma sellae** is a connective tissue sheet enclosing the infundibulum and roofing over the hypophysis cerebri, attached to the tuberculum sellae in front and the dorsum sellae behind.

The posterior cranial fossa

The posterior fossa is the largest and deepest cranial fossa. Contributing bones are the occipital and temporal, and a small portion of the parietal bone. It houses the pons and medulla in front and the cerebellar hemispheres behind and on each side.

The **foramen magnum**, which pierces the floor of the fossa in the sagittal plane, is completely encompassed by the occipital bone. It is oval, and narrows anteriorly where it is encroached by the occipital condyles. Behind, it is wider and communicates with the vertebral canal. It transmits the medulla oblongata at its transition into spinal cord. The anterior margin of the foramen magnum receives attachment of the apical ligament of the dens inferiorly; the membrana tectoria stretches across this and is attached more anteriorly to the basilar part of the occipital bone. The alar ligaments of the dens attach to the roughened medial parts of the condyles.

The **clivus**, embodying the basilar part of the occipital bone, the posterior part of the sphenoid body and the dorsum sellae, slopes forwards and upwards from the foramen magnum and supports the pons and medulla. Across its surface, the inferior petrosal sinuses are connected by a basilar plexus of veins which communicate below with the vertebral plexus (Fig. 1.26).

The **jugular foramen** lies at the posterior end of the petro-occipital suture which is grooved to receive the inferior petrosal sinus. The foramen is directed forwards, downwards and laterally. Its posterior part contains the sigmoid sinus, which is in continuity below with the internal jugular vein. Its sharp upper border is notched by the glossopharyngeal nerve and may be further divided into two or three compartments. The accessory, vagus and glossopharyngeal nerves from behind forwards, traverse the foramen in front of the vein.

The **hypoglossal canal** pierces the occipital bone at the junction of its basal and lateral parts, just lateral to the foramen magnum and anterior to its transverse diameter. It transmits the hypoglossal nerve and sometimes a meningeal branch of the ascending pharyngeal artery. Behind, a condylar canal may transmit an emissary vein from the sigmoid sinus.

The petrous temporal bone forms a large part of the anterolateral wall of the fossa.

The **internal acoustic meatus**, just above the jugular foramen, traverses directly laterally for 1 cm to a perforated plate of bone which separates it from

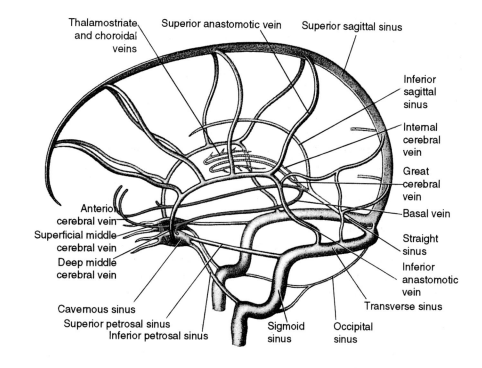

(a)

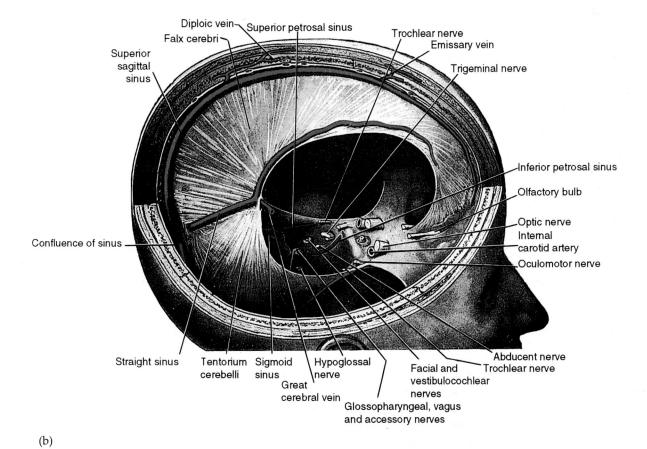

(b)

Fig. 1.26 (a) Schema of the venous sinuses of the dura mater and their connections with the cerebral veins. The more deeply placed cerebral veins are shown in blue, and those inside the brain are shown in interrupted blue; (b) the dura mater, its processes and venous sinuses, right aspect;

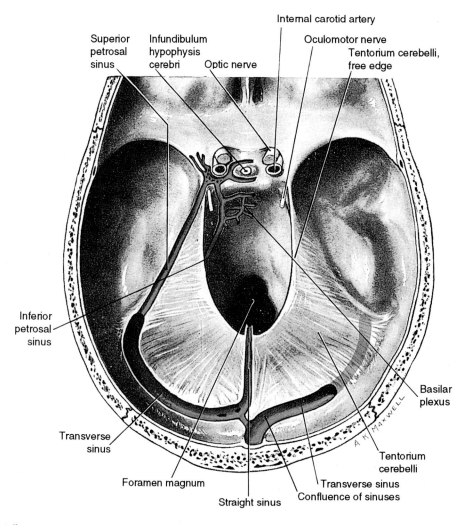

Fig. 1.26 (contd) (c) the tentorium cerebelli and venous sinuses, superior aspect. (From Williams, P.L. *et al.* (eds) (1995) *Gray's Anatomy*, 38th edition, published by Churchill Livingstone.)

the middle ear. It transmits the facial and vestibulocochlear nerves, the nervus intermedius and the labyrinthine vessels. The plate is divided unequally by a transverse crest, above which the bone is pierced by the **facial canal**, conducting the facial nerve (Fig. 1.27). A depression behind this (the superior vestibular area) transmits nerves to the utricle and anterior and lateral semicircular ducts. Below the crest, the spiral openings in the cochlear area anteriorly constitute the **tractus spiralis foraminosus**. Behind this, the inferior vestibular area transmits nerves for the saccule; below and behind the nerve to the posterior semicircular duct passes through the **foramen singulare**.

The **sigmoid sinus** grooves the mastoid part of the temporal bone, descending behind the mastoid antrum to the jugular foramen. A mastoid foramen

within the grove transmits an emissary vein and a meningeal branch of the occipital artery.

Near the mid line behind the foramen magnum is the **internal occipital crest**, to which the falx cerebelli is attached. It leads upwards to the irregular **internal occipital protuberance** underlying the confluence of the sinuses. To either side of this the occipital bone is grooved by the **transverse sinus**, continuous laterally with the sigmoid sinus.

Below the transverse sinus the internal occipital crest divides the occipital bone into two gentle hollows, adapted to the cerebellar hemispheres.

1.10   INJURY TO THE FACE AND ORBIT

Blunt injury to the skull may cause fractures at points of weakness. 'Blow-out' fracture of the ethmoidal or

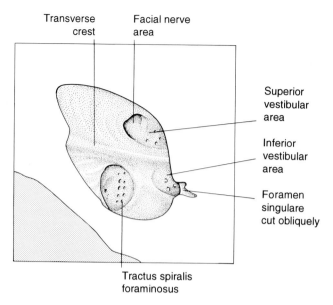

Transverse crest

Facial nerve area

Superior vestibular area

Inferior vestibular area

Foramen singulare cut obliquely

Tractus spiralis foraminosus

Fig. 1.27 The fundus of the right internal acoustic meatus, exposed by a section through the petrous part of the right temporal bone nearly parallel to the line of its superior border.

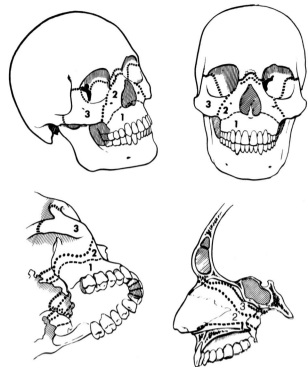

Fig. 1.28 Fractures of the face. 1 = Le Fort I (transverse fracture); 2 = Le Fort II (paramedial fracture); 3 = Le Fort III (craniofacial disjunction). (From Dingman, R.O. and Natvig, P. (1964) *The Surgery of Facial Fractures*, published by W.B. Saunders.)

maxillary sinus results from closed injury to the orbit and fracture of the medial orbital wall (lamina papyracea of the ethmoid), or floor of the orbit (medial to the infraorbital canal) respectively.

Le Fort (1901) described anatomical lines of weakness in the facial skeleton which render it susceptible to fracture, on frontal impact. This has given title to two forms of fracture which follows these lines (Fig. 1.28).

The Le Fort type II fracture runs across the nasal bones, extending on both sides across the frontal process of the maxilla and the nasolacrimal canal. The line of fracture traverses the floor of the orbit and crosses the lower orbital margin in the region of the maxillary zygomatic suture to involve the lateral wall of the maxillary antrum and pterygoid laminae.

In a Le Fort type III fracture the line of fracture starts at the upper part of the nasal bones, close to the front and nasal suture (sometimes associated with dislocation of the nasal lines here and disruption of the cribriform plate of the ethmoid). The fracture runs backwards through the medial wall of the orbit near the front and maxillary suture, and extends back to the inferior orbital fissure. Here the fracture line bifurcates; one line runs forward in the lateral wall of the orbit to a point below the frontomalar suture; the other runs down and back from the pterygomaxillary fissure to the roots of the pterygoid laminae.

CHAPTER TWO

The ocular appendages: eyelids, conjunctiva and lacrimal apparatus

2.1 THE EYELIDS OR PALPEBRAE

The eyelids help to keep the corneas moist, and protect against injury and excessive light, regulating the amount of light reaching the retina. When they are closed, stimulation of visual cortex ceases. The lids are essential for distribution and drainage of the tears: the upper lid restores the preocular tear film at each blink and blinking has a pumping effect on the lacrimal sac.

The upper eyelid extends over the orbital margin to the eyebrow above, the lower more smoothly into the cheek, where nasojugal and malar sulci may limit it (Fig. 2.1); these folds increase with age, and here the skin is tied to periosteum. At the nasojugal sulcus a band of connective tissue passes between or-

bicularis oculi and levator labii superioris. The sulci mark the junctions between the loose palpebral and denser tissues in the cheek, hence limiting oedema and demarcating adipose herniation.

Lines of 'minimal tension' occur in facial skin as elsewhere (Fig. 2.2), formed by two kinds of force: the first group are due to habitual expression, e.g. frontal furrows near the glabella, circumpalpebral sulci, nasolabial folds, circumoral and preauricular lines; the second group are lines due to relaxation of the palpebral skin itself. Elective skin incisions are often made in lines of minimal tension, but in order to forestall palpebral eversion (ectropion) during healing, palpebral incisions, especially inferior, are usually orthogonal to lines of minimal tension and the palpebral margin.

The upper lid is the most mobile, and is raised in the vertical plane by an elevator muscle (levator palpebral superioris). In forward gaze the upper lid just overlaps the cornea, in closure it covers it. In contrast, the lower lid lies just below the cornea when the eye is open, on closure merely reaching it (see Table 2.1). The opened lids enclose an elliptical **palpebral fissure** between their margins, which meet at medial and lateral angles or canthi.

The canthi

The **lateral canthus** is acute, about 30–40°, or 60° with the lids wide open. It often continues into an inferolateral groove in the line of the upper palpebral margin; around this small furrows or 'crow's feet' occur with age. The lateral canthus is 5–7 mm medial

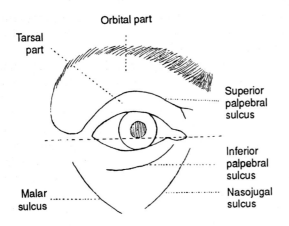

Fig. 2.1 The surface anatomy of the eyelids.

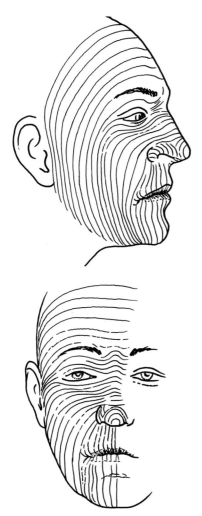

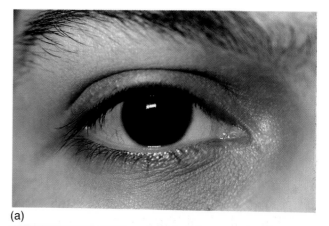

(a)

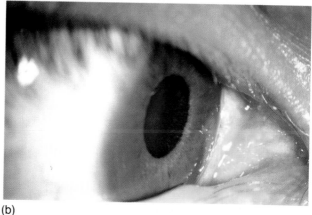

(b)

Fig. 2.3 (a) The interpalpebral fissure, showing the right eye in the primary position; (b) the inner canthus during adduction of the eye, showing recession of the caruncle.

Fig. 2.2 The lines of minimal tension of the face (Langer's lines). These are generated by two mechanisms: 1, lines of habitual expression (e.g. in the forehead, at the glabella region, around the eyelids and nasolabial fold and other lines of expression around the mouth and preauricular region); 2, lines of skin relaxation in flexion and extension (e.g. circular lines formed in the neck in flexion and at the back of the neck in extension). (From Converse, J.M. (1964) *Reconstructive Plastic Surgery Vol. 1*, published by W.B. Saunders.)

to the orbital margin and 1 cm from the frontozygomatic suture (Fig. 1.18).

The **medial canthus**, more obtuse, has a horizontal inferior lower rim and a superior rim sloping inferomedially; their contained canaliculi accord with this configuration. The canthus continues medially into a visible ridge produced by the **medial palpebral ligament** (Fig. 1.18).

The **lateral canthus** is in contact with the globe, the medial separated from it by a small 'tear lake', the lacus lacrimalis. A yellowish conjunctival fold, the **lacrimal caruncle** projects into the lacus, and lateral to it is the pink **plica semilunaris**. The lacrimal caruncle is a small area of tissue derived from skin and contains large modified sweat glands, and sebaceous glands opening into the follicles of fine hairs. The plica semilunaris represents the membrana nictitans ('third eyelid') of many other vertebrates. It often contains non-striated muscle. Along each palpebral margin, opposite the plica, a small **lacrimal papilla** bears the punctum lacrimale, which conducts tear fluid into the lacrimal canaliculi. The puncta divide the margins into ciliary and lacrimal parts (Fig. 2.3).

Although eyeballs vary little in size, palpebral fissures do, forming the feature which popularly defines the size of the 'eye'. In Caucasians with the lids open, the lateral canthus is about 2 mm above the medial, thus imparting an inferomedial slope to the fissure, an obliquity increased in Mongolian races, who also show a dermal fold across the medial canthus (the **epicanthus**), which can overlap the caruncle (Fig. 2.4).

Epicanthi are normal in all races in fetal life, disappearing as the nasal bridge develops. The presence of canthi have been associated with flat

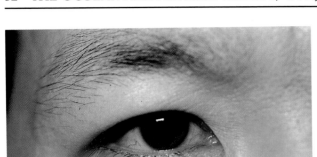

Fig. 2.4 Epicanthal folds in a Chinese man.

nasal bones, but Duckworth (1904) noted that they are absent in Negroes, who have nasal bones flatter than in Mongols. The presence of canthi may be associated with congenital ptosis.

With the lids open the palpebral fissures are about 30 mm long by 15 mm high (see Table 2.1) and are asymmetrical. The greatest height above an intercanthal line is medial; below it is lateral (Fig. 2.1). The cornea, iris and pupil, a lateral triangle and medial crescent of sclera, the caruncle and plica, are all visible in the fissure.

When the lids close, the lateral canthus drops below the medial and the fissure becomes sinuous, and concave upwards centrally. The lash line follows the fissure except medially, where it is horizontal. Laterally the lateral canthus slopes downwards.

Interpalpebral areas of conjunctiva and cornea, particularly lower central cornea, form the most exposed ocular regions. These are hence the common sites of congestion, degeneration or injury due to exposure to chemical and physical agents, including drying and radiation. Lid closure in response to threat or injury is accompanied by reflex elevation of the eyeball (Bell's phenomenon); hence lower areas are most affected by thermal and caustic injuries. Imperfect closure in coma or facial palsy also exposes this lower area to damage (*coma vigilence*).

Table 2.1 summarizes the dimensions and relations of palpebral fissures at different ages. Note that the ocular area visible between the lids decreases with age.

The palpebral margin

The palpebral margin is about 2 mm wide measured from its posterior margin to the posterior lash line. In the adult, there is no change in width with age, or between the sexes, but the margin is narrower in children (Table 2.1). Lid margin vascularity increases with age in adults, particularly in women, and telangiectatic vessels are seen with increasing frequency on the lower lid margin with increasing age (Hykin and Bron, 1992). From its rounded anterior border project the eyelashes (**cilia**) in two or three rows. The superior cilia, longer and more numerous, curl up, while the lower curl down; hence the cilia do not interlace in lid closure. Cilia are usually darker than other hairs and remain so except in certain diseases (e.g. alopecia areata). Each lash survives for about 5 months; its replacement is fully grown in 10 weeks. Young cilia are clubbed, and may remain so in chronic inflammatory conditions. They are longer and more curled in childhood.

Table 2.1 Some characteristics of the palpebral opening and its relation to certain parts of the globe

	Length (mm)	Height (mm)	Pupil	Cornea	Lacus and plica lacrimales	Position of transverse axis
Newborn	18.5–19	10	Touches free border of lower eyelid	Upper border at level of free margin of upper eyelid	Not visible	Middle of pupil
Infant	24–25	13	Equidistant from free borders of eyelids	Upper and lower borders covered to same extent	Slightly visible	Below middle of pupil
Adult	28–30	14–15	Near free border of upper eyelid	Lower border at level of free margin of lower eyelid	Visible	Lower border of pupil
Old age	28	11–12	Touches free margin of upper eyelid	Lower border a little distance from free margin of lower eyelid	Very visible	Near lower border of cornea

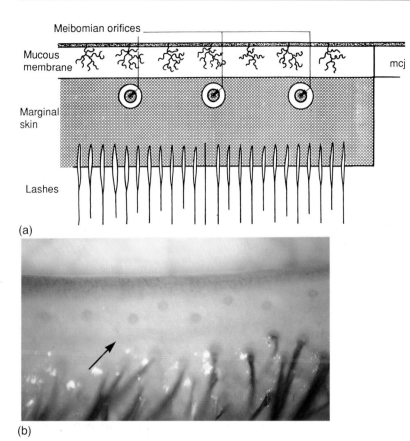

(a)

(b)

Fig. 2.5 (a) Disposition of the meibomian orifices behind the mucocutaneous junction (mcj) of the lid margin (the 'grey line'); (b) micrograph of meibomian orifices of the lower lid of a normal Caucasian subject. The 'grey line' is arrowed.

Ciliary follicles

Unlike other hairs, cilia have no erector muscles; they are set obliquely, anterior to the palpebral muscle, reach the tarsal plate, and have a sensory innervation.

The sharp posterior border is apposed to the globe. Anterior to it are the orifices of tarsal glands. Between this and the cilia is a narrow **grey line**, marking an avascular palpebral plane (Fig. 2.5).

The ciliary part of the palpebral rim bears lashes. Medial to the puncta is the lacrimal part of the palpebral rim, containing the **lacrimal canaliculus**; this part is rounded, has no tarsal glands and rarely has cilia.

STRUCTURE

Palpebral tissues, from the front to back, are:

1. skin;
2. subcutaneous areolar tissue;
3. striated muscle (orbicularis oculi);
4. submuscular areolar tissue;
5. tarsal plates and fibrous tissue;
6. septum orbitale;
7. non-striated muscle;
8. conjunctiva.

Skin

The palpebral skin is thin (less than 1 mm thick) and almost transparent, folding and wrinkling easily. A fold often exists laterally in the upper lid in old age, and may overhang the lid margin. The skin is very elastic and recovers rapidly after oedema. As the upper lid is raised a superior tarsal sulcus develops at the superior tarsal border, caused by attachments of levator palpebrae superioris. The upper palpebral skin is thus partly buried when the upper lid is raised, wholly in view only when it is lowered. A similar, inferior tarsal sulcus is poorly developed. Palpebral skin is attached to the orbital margin and palpebral ligaments, particularly the medial.

The skin of the medial part of the eyelid (Fig. 2.6) differs markedly from that of the temporal (Fig. 2.7). It is smoother and more oily and while it has only a few rudimentary hairs and associated sebaceous glands, the unicellular sebaceous glands in the basal epidermis are plentiful (Wolff, 1951) (Fig. 2.8).

Structure

Although the epithelium is thin, it has a stratum corneum, stratum granulosum, and stratum mucosum of three or four layers. The basal layer (stratum germinativum) rests on a basement

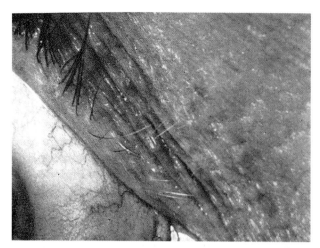

Fig. 2.6 Skin of nasal portion of the right upper eyelid. Note that it is almost devoid of hairs, apart from lashes.

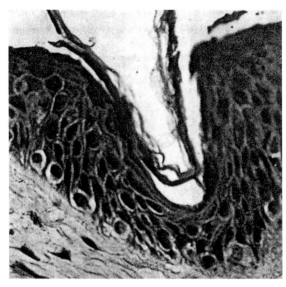

Fig. 2.8 Section of skin from the nasal side of the eyelid to show numerous unicellular sebaceous glands in the basal layer of the epidermis.

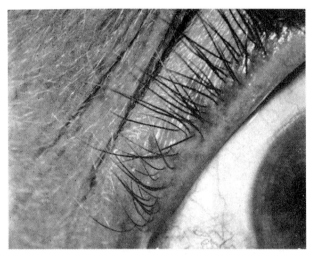

Fig. 2.7 Skin of lateral portion of upper eyelid. Note numerous hairs, in addition to the lashes.

membrane. Epithelium at the palpebral margin thickens, when traced backwards, to contain between seven and ten layers, and the dermis becomes denser, more elastic and folded into high, narrow papillae.

The **mucocutaneous junction** is just behind the openings of the tarsal glands, i.e. at the junction of 'wettable' and 'non-wettable' surfaces, representing the anterior limit of the marginal strip of tear fluid (Fig. 2.9).

Palpebral hairs

Palpebral hairs, large in the fetus, are very fine in adults: they have small sebaceous and sweat glands.

There are always large pigment cells in perivascular connective tissue and hair follicles, more abundant here than elsewhere. More numerous in brunettes than blondes, the pigment cells contain a golden yellow or brown pigment. Such melanocytes are mobile and may, by accumulation, produce colour changes in the lids.

Subcutaneous areolar tissue

The subcutaneous areolar tissue is loose and contains no fat; the skin is mobile on the subjacent muscle and is easily distended by oedema or haemorrhage. It is absent near the ciliary margin and palpebral sulci, and at the canthi where skin adheres to the palpebral ligaments.

Striated muscle

The striated muscle is the palpebral part of the orbicularis palpebrarum. The muscle fibres encircle the palpebral opening, are obliquely interrelated, and overlap each other. Filling almost the whole thickness of the lid margin is its ciliary part (muscle of Riolan) (Fig. 2.10), traversed by ciliary follicles, glands of Moll and excretory ducts of tarsal glands (Fig. 2.11).

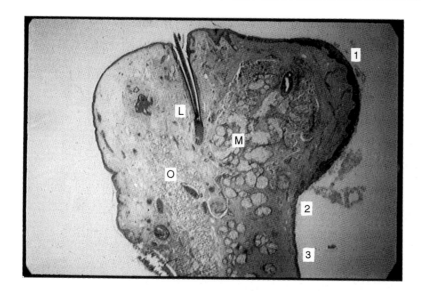

Fig. 2.9 Vertical section through the eyelid (Masson trichome stain). Original magnification ×2. (Courtesy of Dr D. Lucas.)

Submuscular areolar tissue

The submuscular areolar tissue lies between the orbicularis and tarsal plate, and communicates with the subaponeurotic stratum of the scalp. Hence pus or blood can enter the upper lid from the scalp. Through this plane, entered by incision at the grey line, the lid may be split into anterior and posterior layers. It is traversed by fibres of the levator, some passing to the skin through orbicularis, others to the lower third of the tarsus (but see p.37). The stems of the palpebral nerves are in this plane; therefore any local anaesthetic must be injected deep to the orbicularis.

In the lower lid the submuscular areolar tissue is in a single stratum (the preseptal space) in front of the septum orbitale. In the upper lid it is divided by the levator into pretarsal and preseptal spaces.

The small **pretarsal space** encloses the peripheral arterial arcade (Figs 2.10 and 2.52), bounded anteriorly by the levator tendon and orbicularis, posteriorly by the tarsal plate and palpebral muscle. It is limited above by the origin of this muscle from the levator and below by the attachment of levator to the tarsal plate (but see p.39).

The **preseptal space** is triangular in section, bounded in front by orbicularis, behind by the orbital septum and tendinous fibres of levator piercing orbicularis. Above is the **preseptal mass of fat**, which is distinct from the general subcutaneous fat. It lies largely in front of the septum and behind the orbicularis as a crescent along the orbital margin, which it may overlap. Its lower border adjoins the upper palpebral furrow. It is adherent to orbicularis and epicranial aponeurosis, which thus separates the preseptal 'space' from the so-called 'dangerous area' of the scalp. The premuscular and retromuscular levels communicate through the orbicularis, but the septum and tarsal plates isolate them from the orbit.

Tarsal plates and fibrous tissue

The fibrous layer is the framework of the lids. It is thick centrally as the **tarsal plates**, thin peripherally as the **septum orbitale**. The two regions are continuous and, when the lids are closed, form a shutter for the orbital opening, incomplete only at the palpebral fissure.

The tarsal plates maintain the shape and firmness of the lids. They contain no cartilage, but consist of dense fibrous tissue and some elastic tissue, particularly around the tarsal glands. They extend from a point 7 mm from the lateral orbital tubercle to the lacrimal puncta, 9 mm from the anterior lacrimal crest.

Both tarsi are well delimited, but laterally at the palpebral margin they are united with the connective tissue of ciliary follicles to form the ciliary mass of Whitnall.

The superior tarsus, transversely crescentic, is larger, being 11 mm in height at its middle; the inferior tarsus, somewhat oblong, is 5 mm high. Both are about 29 mm long and 1 mm thick.

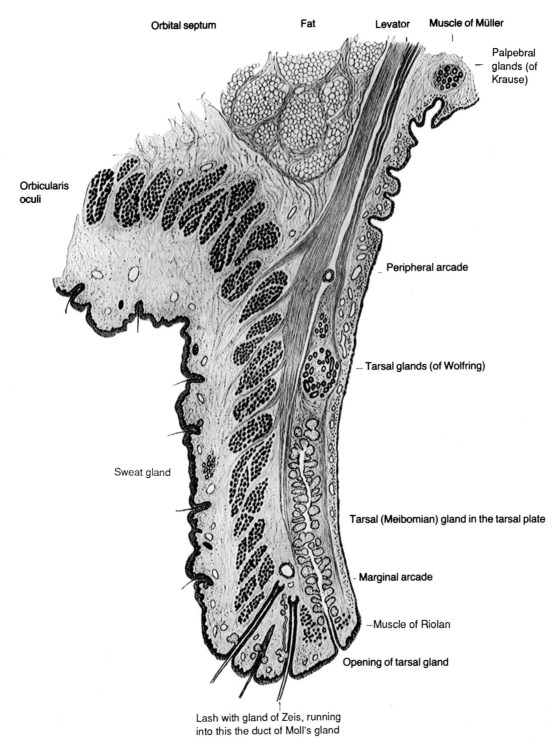

Fig. 2.10   Vertical section through the upper lid (Wolff's preparations).

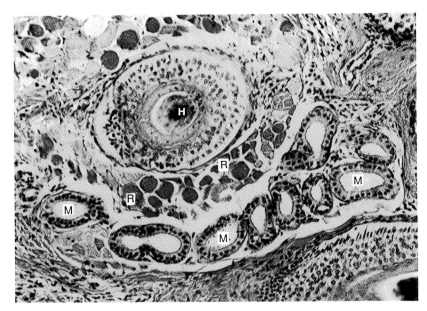

Fig. 2.11 Section of lid margin showing muscle bundles of Riolan (R) traversed by hair follicle (H). Note the associated coiled gland of Moll (M). Original magnification ×205. (From Tripathi, R. C. and Tripathi, B. J. in Davson, H. (ed.) (1984) *The Eye, Vol. 1A*, 2nd edition, published by Academic Press.)

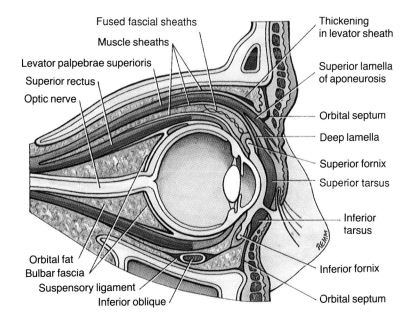

Fused fascial sheaths
Muscle sheaths
Levator palpebrae superioris
Superior rectus
Optic nerve

Thickening in levator sheath
Superior lamella of aponeurosis
Orbital septum
Deep lamella
Superior fornix
Superior tarsus
Inferior tarsus

Orbital fat
Bulbar fascia
Suspensory ligament
Inferior oblique
Inferior fornix
Orbital septum

Fig. 2.12 Vertical anteroposterior section of the orbit.

Surfaces of the tarsi

The **anterior** surface is convex and separated from orbicularis by areolar tissue, facilitating independent movement. The **posterior** surface is concave, adherent to the conjunctiva and shaped to the eyeball. The **'free' border** at the margin of the lid is thick, horizontal and coextensive with the ciliary part of the margin; the **'attached' border** is thin, and continuous with the septum orbitale, except where pierced by the levator in the upper lid and the inferior rectus in the lower (see below). Palpebral muscles are attached to the superior and inferior borders of the corresponding tarsi (Figs 2.10 and 2.12).

The **ends** of both plates are attached to the orbital margin by ligaments.

The medial palpebral ligament

Somewhat triangular in shape, this is attached to the maxilla from the anterior lacrimal crest nearly to its suture with the nasal bone (Figs 1.18, 2.68, 5.19 and 5.36). It has a lower border, below which pass some fibres of orbicularis; above it is continuous with the periosteum. Its base is at the anterior lacrimal crest, where the ligament divides. The posterior part is continuous with the lacrimal fascia, covering the upper part of the lacrimal sac.

The anterior part divides at the medial canthus into two bands, crossing the lacrimal fossa (but not in contact with the sac), to blend with the medial ends of the tarsal plates. These bands form a 'Y' on its side with the main ligament. The two branches correspond to the lacrimal parts of the lid margins and contain the lacrimal canaliculi, enclosing the caruncle and bounding the medial canthus.

The anterior surface of the ligament is adherent to skin and faces anterolaterally while its branches face anteromedially, together making an obtuse angle.

A deep or reflected part of the ligament is said to arise as it crosses the lacrimal sac to attach behind it: some, however, regard this as a fascial expansion (Whitnall, 1932).

Superolateral traction of the lateral canthus makes the medial palpebral ligament prominent. This prominence is almost entirely on the frontal process of the maxilla.

A fingertip placed in the lacrimal fossa will lie below the position of medial canthus, which some consider to correspond to the anterior lacrimal crest. If a vertical incision is made 2 mm medial to the medial canthus, the lacrimal sac is exposed under its lateral lip.

Therefore the lower, prominent part of the medial palpebral ligament is not much in front of the sac; a probe pressed backwards below it will hit bone, not the sac.

The lateral palpebral ligament

Attached to the orbital tubercle 11 mm below the frontozygomatic suture, this ligament is 7 mm long and 2.5 mm broad. Its fibrous tissue is not very dense. It is quite unlike the well-developed medial palpebral ligament, being little more than the areolar tissue of the septum orbitale behind the lateral palpebral raphe.

The lateral palpebral ligament is deeper and less prominent than the medial ligament. Its anterior surface is fused with preciliary fibres of the orbicularis. Superficial to the lateral palpebral ligament lie a few lobules of the lacrimal gland and the lateral palpebral raphe, formed by orbicularis fused with the orbital septum. Posterior to it is the lateral check ligament, separated from it by a lobule of lacrimal gland (Fig. 4.41). The upper border is united with the levator (Fig. 5.20), its lower with an expansion from the inferior oblique and inferior rectus.

The septum orbitale (Figs 2.12, 2.13 and 5.36)

The septum orbitale (palpebral fascia) is attached to the orbital margin at the **arcus marginale**, where the periorbita is continuous with extraorbital periosteum; centrally it is continuous with the tarsal plates, except where pierced by fibres of the levator in the upper lid and an expansion from the inferior rectus in the lower. However, its continuity with the superior tarsus between fibres of levator is difficult to demonstrate and is denied by many. Part of the septum is carried forwards with the levator, part reflected along its upper surface (Fig. 2.10).

The septum is a flexible fascia which follows all movements of the lids; some consider it the deep fascia of the palpebral part of orbicularis. Its fibres run in arcades, which cross at right-angles.

The septum is thicker laterally and stronger in the upper lid, where two tendinous slips from its lateral side gradually diminish medially.

Weak areas in the septum orbitale determine the sites of herniation of orbital fat. Such herniae are frequent, especially in old people.

The attachment of the septum does not exactly follow the orbital margin (Fig. 2.13). Laterally the attachment is separated from the lateral palpebral ligament and its orbital tubercle by loose connective tissue and fat. Ascending, it crosses the frontozygomatic suture and then follows the orbital margin to the supraorbital notch which it spans, creating a foramen. Thence it descends along the margin, in front of the trochlea, crossing the supratrochlear vessels and nerve to reach bone again behind the posterior lacrimal crest. It descends on the lacrimal bone behind the pars lacrimalis of orbicularis, lacrimal sac and medial palpebral ligament and in front of the medial check ligament (Fig. 2.68). The attachment crosses the lacrimal fascia to the anterior lacrimal crest, level with the lacrimal tubercle, following the orbital margin to the zygomatic bone. Here it leaves the margin on its facial aspect by a few millimetres, forming an osteofibrous pocket, the premarginal recess of Eisler, which contains fat. The attachment then returns to the orbital margin below the lateral orbital tubercle.

Laterally the septum is superficial, anterior to the lateral palpebral ligament, while medially it is behind the lacrimal part of orbicularis oculi (Fig. 2.12). Where this lacrimal muscle diverges into the eyelids the corresponding parts of the septum meet behind the caruncle and plica, between which lies the medial inferior palpebral artery (Fig. 2.13).

Relations

In the upper eyelid the septum is mainly in contact with orbital fat which separates it from the lacrimal gland, levator and tendon of superior oblique.

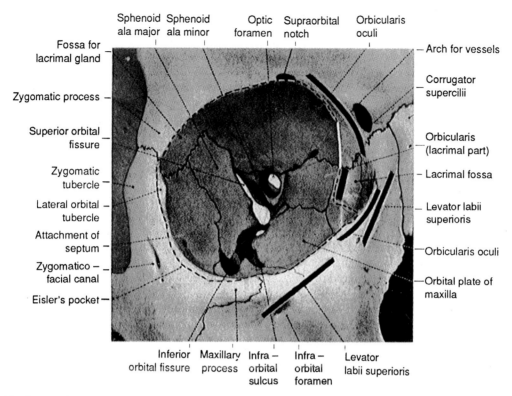

Fig. 2.13 Attachment of septum orbitale and the muscles around the orbit.

Medially it is in contact with orbital fat between the trochlea and medial palpebral ligament (Fig. 4.47).

In the lower eyelid the septum lies in contact with orbital fat and the expansions of inferior rectus and inferior oblique (Figs 2.12 and 4.39).

In the lower lid there is only one 'space', between the septum and tarsal plate behind and orbicularis in front (Fig. 2.14).

The septum orbitale is pierced by:

- lacrimal vessels and nerves;
- supraorbital vessels and nerves;
- supratrochlear nerve and artery;
- infratrochlear nerve;
- anastomosis between the angular and ophthalmic veins;
- superior and inferior palpebral arteries above and below the medial palpebral ligament;
- levator palpebrae superioris in the upper and a prolongation of inferior rectus in the lower lid.

Non-striated muscle

The layer of non-striated muscle fibres, the palpebral muscle of Müller, is just behind the septum orbitale in both lids; its fibres are mostly vertical and are derived from the levator muscle (in the upper lid) and the inferior rectus (in the lower), and are attached to

the orbital margins of the tarsal plates (Figs 2.10, 2.12 and 4.39). The inferior muscle may be visible through the conjunctiva. The whole muscle is supplied by sympathetic nerve fibres. It widens the palpebral fissure. Non-striated muscle also crosses the inferior orbital fissure and occurs in the fascia bulbi. The whole system represents the retractor bulbi of some mammals. For further detail of orbital smooth muscle see Chapter 4.

Conjunctiva

The conjunctiva of the lids, the palpebral conjunctiva, is firmly adherent to the tarsus.

2.2 THE PALPEBRAL GLANDS

Apart from cutaneous glands and those of the conjunctiva, there are various tarsal glands, named eponymously after Meibomius, Moll and Zeis.

MEIBOMIAN GLANDS

The tarsal glands (meibomian glands) are long sebaceous glands unconnected with hairs, though they may represent an extinct row of lashes. They lie within the tarsal plates, which they almost completely traverse (Figs 2.10 and 2.14); the upper ones are therefore longer. Arranged vertically, about 25 in the upper lid and 20 in the lower, they consist of a central canal, into which open numerous rounded acini secreting sebum. The small orifices of the canals open on the margin of the lid just in front of the mucocutaneous junction (Fig. 2.15).

The meibomian secretion prevents overflow of tears by reason of its hydrophobic properties, prevents tears from macerating the skin, and after blinking leaves an oily film over the tears to retard evaporation. Each canal is lined by four layers of cells and a basement membrane. At its mouth there are six layers, the deepest being cylindrical. Keratinization increases towards the lid margin. The acini are usually globular, 10–15 in number and are placed irregularly along the central canal almost to its orifice, like a chain of onions (Figs 2.16–2.19). The glands show through the conjunctiva as yellow streaks; the globular arrangement is quite visible in the young. (See Obata (1994) for further morphological details).

In the monkey, the blands are richly innervated. Many nerve fibres encircle the acini and ducts and appear to be apposed to the acinar basement membranes (Chung *et al.*, 1996). This differs from sebaceous gland elsewhere, which are not innervated. There is a rich innervation with smooth and varicose nerve endings immunoreactive to neuropeptide Y (NPY) and vasointestinal peptide (VIP) suggesting a predominantly parasympathetic innervation, although it should be noted that NPY-reactive fibres may also have sympathetic and other origins. Fibres staining for tyrosine hydroxylase (TH), calcitonin gene-related peptide (CGRP) and substance (SP) are present, but relatively sparse. TH innervation is more associated with vessels, whereas CGRP and SP-reactivity is associated with sensory nerves running in the trigeminal ganglion. The implication is that the glands are neuromodulated. Like the lacrimal acini, they also possess androgen receptors and appear to be under endocrine control (Sullivan *et al.*, 1996). Delivery of meibomian oil onto the lid margin is the result of secretion, supplemented by the muscular action of each blink (Bron, 1996).

CILIARY GLANDS

The ciliary glands (of Moll) are simple tubules which begin in a spiral (not in a glomerulus like the sweat glands); they resemble sweat glands arrested in development. They are 1.5–2 mm long and set obliquely in contact with the bulbs of cilia. They are more numerous in the lower lid, but not as numerous as cilia. Each has a fundus, body, ampullary part and neck. The lumen is large (Figs 2.20–2.22) but narrows at the neck. The duct traverses dermis and epidermis and opens between cilia into a ciliary follicle or a sebaceous gland of Zeis (Fig. 2.10).

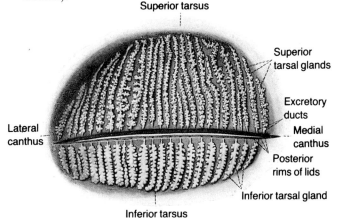

Superior tarsus

Superior tarsal glands

Excretory ducts

Lateral canthus

Medial canthus

Posterior rims of lids

Inferior tarsal gland

Inferior tarsus

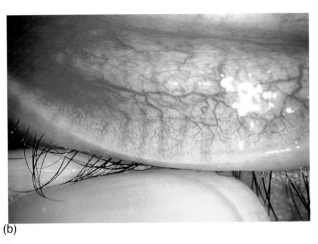

(b)

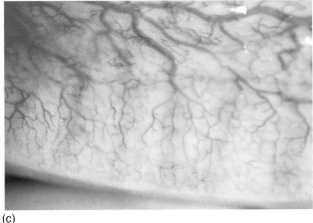

(c)

Fig. 2.14 (a) The posterior surface of the two eyelids which have been made transparent by soda-glycerine to show the tarsal glands (of Meibomius); (b) lower tarsal plate of young adult to show the arrangement of conjunctival vessels and the meibomian glands (arrows); (c) higher magnification of (b).

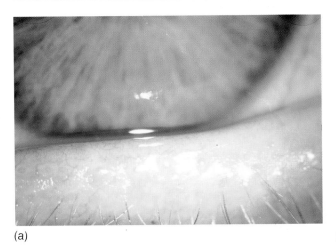

(a)

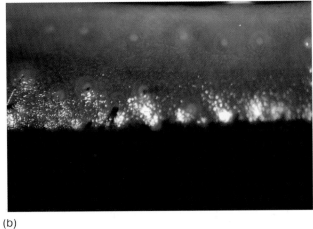

(b)

Fig. 2.15 The lower lid margin in a pigmented subject. Note the clear demonstration of the oil gland orifices (in b) (compare with Fig. 2.5).

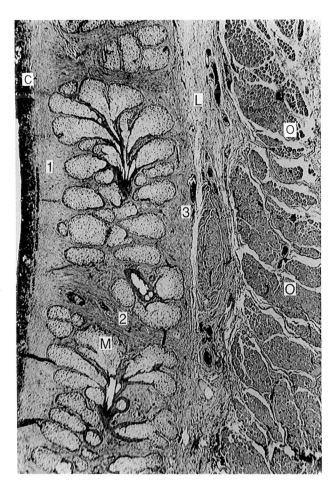

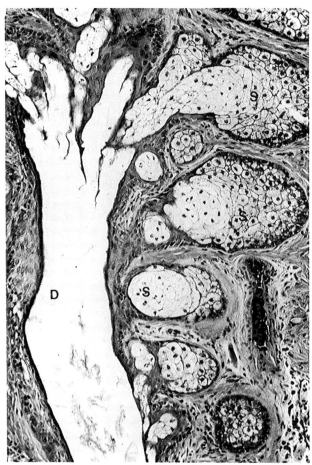

Fig. 2.16 Vertical section of lid, showing the tarsal plate containing meibomian glands (M). Note the vertical orientation of compact connective tissue on the inner (1) and outer (3) surfaces of the plate and sagittal orientation of the central zone (2). C = conjunctiva; L = levator aponeurosis; O = orbicularis oculi muscle bundles. Original magnification ×51. (From Tripathi, R. C. and Tripathi, B. J. in Davson, H. (ed.) (1984) *The Eye, Vol. 1A*, 2nd edition, published by Academic Press.)

Fig. 2.17 Section of meibomian gland showing a number of saccules (S) with disintegrating secretory cells. The resulting meibomian secretion is poured into the duct (D), which is lined by stratified squamous epithelium. Original magnification ×205. (From Tripathi, R. C. in Davson, H. (ed.) (1984) *The Eye, Vol. 1A*, 2nd edition, published by Academic Press.)

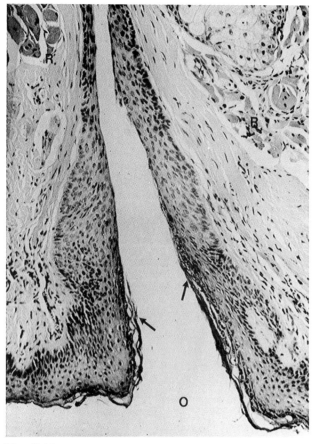

Fig. 2.18 Section of lid passing through opening of the tarsal gland. Towards the external orifice (O), the duct epithelium thickens and the surface cells show keratinization (arrows). R = Muscle of Riolan. Original magnification ×205. (From Tripathi, R. C. in Davson, H. (ed.) (1984) *The Eye, Vol. 1A*, 2nd edition, published by Academic Press.)

Tarsal plate

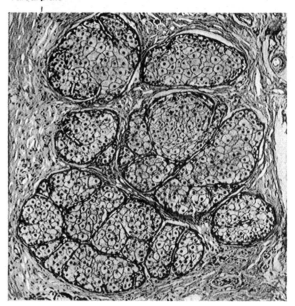

Fig. 2.19 Lobules of a tarsal (meibomian) gland. (Wolff's preparation.)

Structure

The secretory part is lined by cylindrical cells containing secretory granules and fatty granulations; between these and their basement membrane is an ill-defined stratum of longitudinal or obliquely placed myoepithelial cells. The lining of the duct is similar, but lacks myoepithelial cells.

Tarsal (Meibomian) gland   Orbicularis oculi   Ciliary gland of Moll

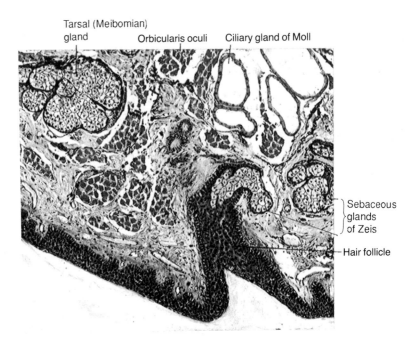

Sebaceous glands of Zeis

Hair follicle

Fig. 2.20 Section of the lid margin to show the three types of gland. (Wolff's preparation.)

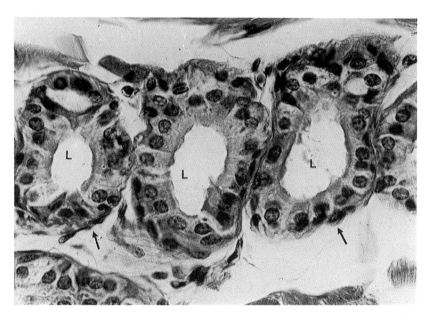

Fig. 2.21 Section of ciliary gland of Moll showing lumen (L) lined by cylindrical epithelial cells supported by a layer of flattened myoepithelial cells and basement membrane (arrows). Original magnification × 820. (From Tripathi, R. C. in Davson, H. (ed.) (1984) *The Eye, Vol. 1A*, 2nd edition, published by Academic Press.)

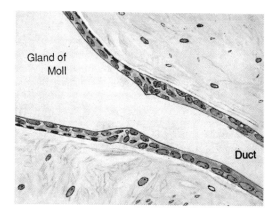

Fig. 2.22 Junction of ciliary gland (of Moll) and duct. Note the funnel-shaped termination of the gland.

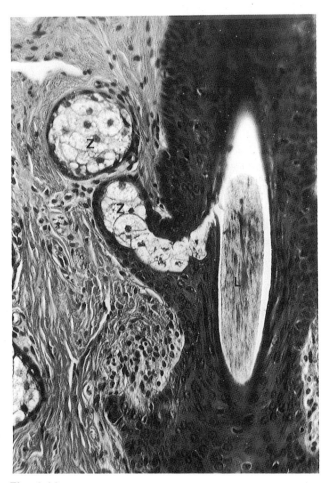

Fig. 2.23 Section to show a gland of Zeiss (Z) emptying into a lash follicle (L). Note how there is nuclear fragmentation and loss of cellular definition as the follicle is approached.

SEBACEOUS GLANDS

The sebaceous glands (of Zeis) discharge directly into and adjoin ciliary follicles, usually two to each follicle (Figs 2.20, 2.23 and 2.24). Each consists of one to three acini (there are usually 10–20 in ordinary sebaceous glands). The epithelium, resting on a basement membrane, consists of actively dividing cubical cells whose polygonal progeny develop granules of a sebaceous nature. The nuclei become rounded, paler, diminish in size, stain more densely, and finally disappear. The degenerating cells lose their walls and are pushed centrally and then towards the duct. The sebum so formed exudes into the ciliary

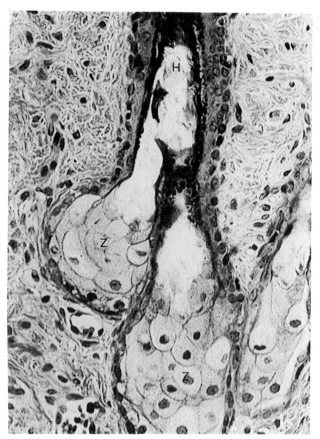

Fig. 2.24 Section of ciliary gland of Zeiss (Z). The glands are associated with the hair follicles (H) by short ducts. Original magnification ×512. (From Tripathi, R. C. in Davson, H. (ed.) (1984) *The Eye, Vol. 1A*, 2nd edition, published by Academic Press.)

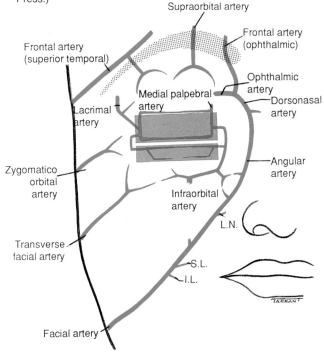

Fig. 2.25 The anastomoses of arteries of internal and external carotid origin around the orbital opening.

follicle. As elsewhere, it prevents the hairs from becoming dry and brittle.

2.3 THE PALPEBRAL BLOOD VESSELS

ARTERIES

The medial and lateral **palpebral arteries** are branches of the ophthalmic and lacrimal arteries, respectively (Fig. 2.20).

The medial palpebral arteries – superior and inferior – pierce the septum orbitale above and below the medial palpebral ligament (Fig. 2.48). Each anastomoses with the corresponding lateral palpebral artery to form the **tarsal arcades** in the submuscular areolar tissue (i.e. between the orbicularis and tarsal plate), close to the lid margin (Figs 2.25 and 2.26). The *tarsal arcades* anastomose with branches of the superficial temporal, transverse facial, and infraorbital arteries.

In the upper lid a **second arterial arcade** (arcus tarseus superior) is formed from the superior branch of the medial palpebral in front of the upper margin of the tarsal plate (Figs 2.10 and 2.25).

Branches of the arcades supply the orbicularis and skin, conjunctiva and tarsal glands.

VEINS

The palpebral veins are larger and more numerous than the arteries and are arranged in pretarsal and posttarsal strata. They form a dense plexus (visible in the living) near the upper and lower conjunctival fornices. Some drain into frontal and temporal veins, others traverse orbicularis to become tributaries of the ophthalmic veins.

LYMPHATICS

The lymphatic channels also form pre- and posttarsal plexuses, connected by cross-channels. According to Fuchs the former have many valves, the latter none. The posttarsal plexus drains the conjunctiva and tarsal glands, the pretarsal the skin and its appendages. Both groups drain as follows: those for the lateral side run to the preauricular and deep parotid nodes and thence to the deep cervical chain; the medial parts of the lids, especially the lower, drain to the submandibular lymph nodes and thence to the deep cervical (Fig. 2.27). Small lymphoid nodules have been described in the palpebral connective tissue (Fig. 2.27).

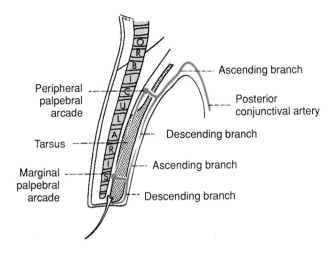

Fig. 2.26 Schematic vertical section of the upper lid to show the disposition of the peripheral and marginal palpebral arcades and their ascending and descending branches.

NERVES

Motor

The orbicularis is served by the facial nerve, the levator by the upper division of the oculomotor nerve, and non-striated muscle by sympathetic nerves.

Sensory

The upper lid is served mainly by the supraorbital nerve, assisted medially by the supra- and infra-trochlear, and laterally by lacrimal branches of the ophthalmic nerve. The lower lid is innervated by the infraorbital nerve, with slight overlap near the canthi by lacrimal and infratrochlear nerves. The plane of the main branches of the nerves is between the orbicularis and the tarsal plate (Fig. 2.28).

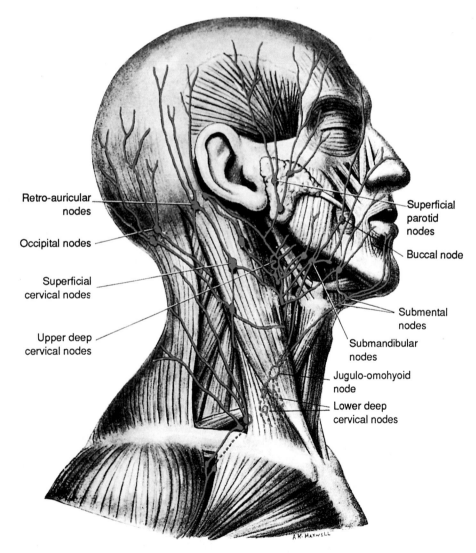

(a)

Fig. 2.27 (a) The superficial lymph nodes and lymph vessels of the head and neck;

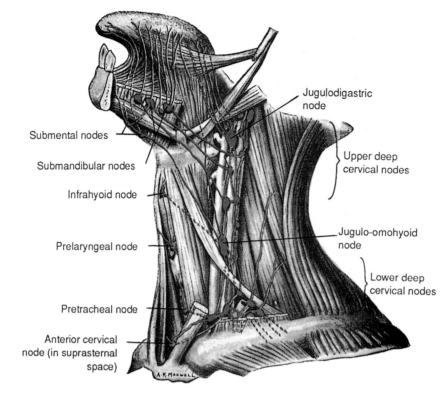

(b)

Fig. 2.27 (contd) (b) Deep dissection to show the whole chain of the cervical nodes and the lymphatic drainage of the tongue. (From Williams, P.R. *et al.* (eds) (1995) *Gray's Anatomy*, 38th edition, published by Churchill Livingstone.)

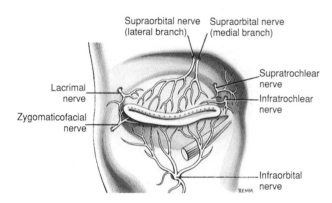

Fig. 2.28 Nerves of the eyelids of the right eye.

2.4 MUSCLES OF THE PALPEBRAL REGION

ORBICULARIS OCULI

Orbicularis oculi is the palpebral sphincter. It is an elliptical sheet extending from the lids, where it surrounds the palpebral fissure, to the brow, temple and cheek. It consists of two main parts: palpebral; orbital (Fig. 2.29).

Palpebral part

The palpebral part of orbicularis oculi is central and confined to the lids. It consists of pale fibres and may divide into **pretarsal** and **preseptal strata**, which are joined, by the thinnest parts of the muscle, at the superior and inferior palpebral sulci.

It diverges from the medial palpebral ligament and neighbouring bone, and curves across the lids in a series of half ellipses, which interlace beyond the lateral canthus as the **lateral palpebral raphe** which is strengthened by the septum orbitale.

Orbital part

The orbital part has a curved origin from the upper orbital margin medial to the supraorbital notch, the

Fig. 2.29 (facing page) (a) Diagram to show the arrangement of orbicularis. The palpebral portion comprises (**a**) the pretarsal muscle; (**b**) the preseptal muscle. The orbital part (**c**) surrounds the orbital rim; (From Collin (1983) *A Manual of Systematic Eyelid Surgery*, published by Churchill Livingstone) (b) the lids and palpebral aperture in the primary position of gaze of a 20-year-old man. Note the well-marked superior lid fold; (c) light lid closure. Note the gentle curve of the lid margin and the persistence of the superior lid fold as a fine crease; (d) the outer canthus; (e) the inner canthus; (f) the palpebral apertures in the primary position of gaze of a 70-year-old woman; (g) inner canthus of the subject shown in (f). Note the accentuated concavity of the canthus and resulting prominence of the punctum, due to atrophy of pericanalicular tissue;

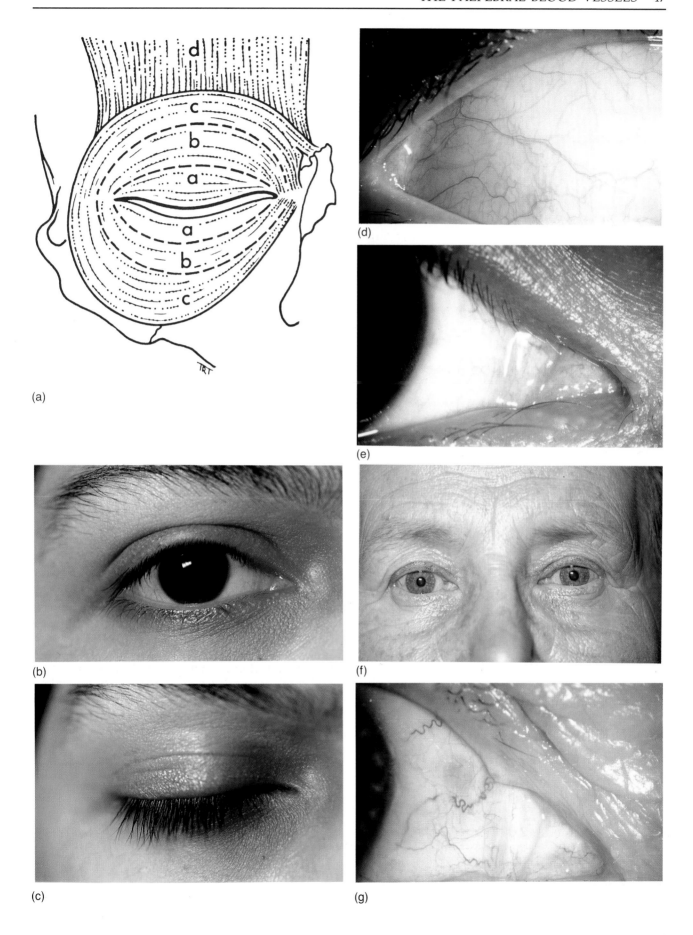

(a)

(b)

(c)

(d)

(e)

(f)

(g)

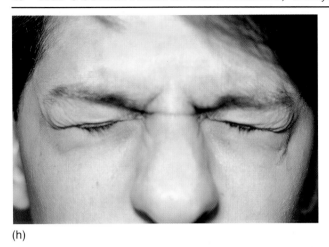

(h)

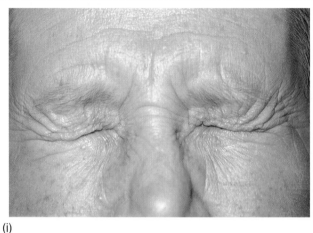

(i)

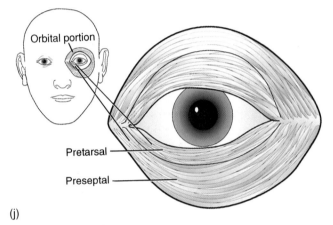

(j)

Fig. 2.29 (contd) (h) forced lid closure in a 20-year-old; (i) forced lid closure in a 70-year-old. Note the exaggerated periorbital skin creases; (j) schematic diagram comparing the relative lengths of individual muscle fibres in the pretarsal and preseptal regions of the palpebral portion of the human orbicularis oculi muscle. The pretarsal portion is comprised of short fibres of heterogeneous length in its medial, middle and lateral portions. The preseptal portion is comprised of shorter fibres in its medial and lateral portions than its middle portion. Individual muscle fibres do not appear to extend the entire length of the muscle. The fibre distribution of the orbital portion has not been determined. (From Wirtschafter *et al.* (1995).)

maxillary process of the frontal bone and the frontal process of the maxilla, from the medial palpebral ligament, and from the lower orbital margin medial to the infraorbital foramen. This attachment is musculotendinous and discontinuous. Peripheral fibres sweep across the orbital margin in concentric loops, the more central ones forming almost complete rings.

Recent studies of volume reconstructions of the orbicularis muscle and the distribution of the motor end plates suggest that both its palpebral and orbital parts are made up of short muscle fibres averaging 1.1 mm long (0.4–2.1 mm) connected by myomyous junctions which interrupt the course of the muscle bundles (Fig. 2.29j) (Wirtschafter *et al.*, 1995). Neuromuscular junctions are arranged in staggered clusters along the entire length of the muscle. This arrangement has implications for the use of

botulinum A toxin in the treatment of blepharospasm, since it implies that the toxin must be diffused through the lids to achieve a maximum result.

Information is available as to orbicularis muscle fibre size and type (Wirtschafter *et al.*, 1995). It contains myofibres with the smallest diameters of any facial muscle (Polgar *et al.*, 1973). At increasing distance from the eyelid margin, there is a gradual increase in fibre diameter and in the proportion of type 1 fibres. These are slow twitch, fatigable oxidative fibres and make up 10–15% of the muscle. Fast twitch, glycolytic type 2 fibres represent almost 100% of the pretarsal fibres, and have a cross-sectional area of 400 μm^2; only 3–4% are type 1. In the preseptal region, 8–15% are type 1 and the average cross-sectional area is about 550 μm^2 (McLoon and Wirtschafter, 1991; Porter, Burns and May, 1989). These topographic differences may influence the orbicularis contraction during the blink and forced eye closure.

Relations

The palpebral part has areolar tissue but no fat on both aspects. Anteriorly, this separates it from skin; posteriorly, the submuscular areolar layer separates it from tarsal plates and palpebral fascia, containing main vessels and nerves and fibres of levator. This part is adherent to dermis at the medial and lateral canthi. Fibres of the levator pass through it to the skin (Fig. 2.10).

The orbital part spreads above on the forehead (contributing to the structure of the eyebrow and covering corrugator supercilii), laterally on the temple (covering the anterior part of the temporal fascia), and below on the cheek (overlapping the zygomatic bone and elevator muscles of the upper lip and nostril). Anteriorly it is separated from the skin by a layer of fat, to which it is adherent, and thus to skin.

Peripheral fibres of orbicularis attached to skin are **musculus superciliaris** (Merkel, 1887), a depressor of the medial end of the eyebrow (Arlt, 1863), to the skin of which some superomedial peripheral fibres are attached; **musculus malaris** (Henle, 1853) formed by some medial and lateral peripheral fibres attached to the skin of the cheek. Some fibres are attached to skin round the medial canthus, wrinkling the medial part of the lids (Merkel, 1887).

A third part of the orbicularis oculi is a recognizable entity, the **pars lacrimalis** (tensor tarsi), often named Horner's muscle, although it was earlier recorded by Duverney (1749) and Gerlach (1880). It is a thin layer attached behind the lacrimal sac to the upper posterior lacrimal crest (Figs 2.66 and 2.67) and the lacrimal fascia. Passing anterolaterally, it divides into two, slips around the canaliculi and blends with the pretarsal and ciliary parts of orbicularis oculi in both lids.

The **pars ciliaris** (muscle of Riolan), formed of fine striated muscle fibres, is in the dense tissue of the palpebral margins. The ciliary glands (of Moll) are between these fibres and palpebral parts of orbicularis (Fig. 2.10). They also surround the tarsal (meibomian) glands (Figs 2.10 and 2.69). Medially the ciliary and lacrimal parts are continuous (Fig. 2.66).

Actions

The palpebral part closes the lids gently, as in blinking, which is often involuntary and frequently without obvious stimulus. Reflex blinking is stimulated by visible threats and loud noises. Voluntary blinking, to clarify vision or to break eye contact, also occurs. Reflex blinking is stimulated by drying of the cornea; it spreads tear fluid, and the pars lacrimalis helps to empty the sac (p.84).

The orbital part closes the lids firmly, and draws the skin of the forehead, temple and cheek medially, which forms radial furrows around the lateral canthus. These are temporary in youth, but become permanent later ('crow's feet'). The muscle also contracts during short but powerful expiration, as in crying, coughing, blowing the nose, sneezing, and excessive laughter. Contraction of the orbital part depresses the eyebrow to reduce excessive light from above, the relaxed palpebral part allowing the lids to remain open. When both parts contract the eyelids are 'screwed up'.

The two parts of the muscle affect the volume of the conjunctival sac differently: the palpebral part does not diminish its volume, so that no tears spill, but the orbital fibres compress the sac, and tears spill over the cheek. Contraction of the orbital part, pressing the puckered lids against the globe, is more effective against external violence than mere blinking.

The palpebral part is opposed by levator palpebrae superioris, the orbital by occipitofrontalis.

Nerve supply

Orbicularis oculi is innervated by the **facial nerve**, through its temporal and zygomatic branches which enter the muscle from its lateral side and deep aspect. Several temporal branches ascend across the zygoma and pass above the lateral canthus to supply the upper half of orbicularis, assisted by upper zygomatic branches, the lower of which cross the zygomatic bone to reach its lower part. As these nerves penetrate the muscle they divide further (Fig. 5.35). Because any nerve may be affected by disease or injury, paralysis may be local: for example, paralysis of the lower palpebral part allows the lower lid to evert (ectropion), leading to epiphora.

CORRUGATOR SUPERCILII (Fig. 5.36)

This muscle is situated at the medial end of the eyebrow deep to frontalis and orbicularis. Attached at the medial end of the superciliary ridge, it passes superolaterally through the overlying muscles, to the skin of the eyebrow near its mid point.

Action

The two corrugators pull the eyebrows towards the nose, making them project over the medial canthus, producing vertical furrows above the bridge of the nose, and sometimes a depression at their dermal attachments.

The corrugator supercilius muscle is used primarily to reduce glare. It is well developed in outdoor workers and even in children who wear no hats who, acquire vertical furrows at an early age. In facial expression it is the basis of frowning, evident in crying, sorrow, pain, and when attempting mental recall.

Nerve supply

The corrugators are supplied by the facial nerve, through its superior zygomatic branch.

OCCIPITOFRONTALIS

Occipitofrontalis consists of paired occipital and frontal muscles, united by the large, thin, epicranial aponeurosis, covering most of the cranial vault.

Each **occipitalis**, small and quadrilateral, is attached to the lateral two-thirds of the highest nuchal line and to the mastoid process, immediately superior to the sternocleidomastoid. Its parallel fascicles pass into the epicranial aponeurosis.

Frontalis, also quadrilateral, is attached to the epicranial aponeurosis mid-way between the coronal suture and the orbital margin and to the skin of the eyebrows, mingling with orbicularis and corrugator. Above, a distinct triangular interval separates the frontal muscles; below, the medial fibres converge to blend with the procerus, which is ascending and is hence the antagonist of frontalis.

Action

Frontalis elevates the eyebrows and draws the scalp forwards, wrinkling the forehead transversely in variable furrows, often convex upwards laterally and centrally concave or absent. Occipitalis retracts the scalp in opposition to frontalis.

Occipitofrontalis opposes the orbital part of orbicularis oculi to elevate the eyebrows in upward gaze; levator palpebrae superioris opposes the palpebral part.

Occipitofrontalis increases access of light to the eye – and also reflection, thus animating expression. Frontalis is contracted when vision is difficult due to distance or insufficient light. It expresses surprise, admiration, fear and horror, in all of which the element of 'attention' is present, as Duchenne (1883) noted. Raised eyebrows, with lids half-closed, suggest forced attention, or craftiness!

Nerve supply

The occipato-frontalis is supplied by the facial nerve, through its posterior auricular and temporal branches.

MUSCULUS PROCERUS

The paired proceri, close together near the mid line, occupy the bridge of the nose and an interval between the lower fibres of frontalis. They are attached inferiorly to the nasal bones and lateral nasal cartilages and pass to blend with the dermis near the bridge of the nose (Fig. 5.36). Pulling on this skin they create transverse furrows in the lower central part of the forehead and root of the nose. Hence also the frequent concave mid point to the transverse furrows of the forehead.

The procerus acts with corrugator supercilii to increase prominence of the eyebrows to reduce bright light. Duchenne named it 'the muscle of aggression' (Duchenne, 1883), but it may also express anguish.

Frontalis, orbicularis oculi, corrugator supercilii and procerus were regarded by Howe (1907) as accessory muscles of accommodation, contracting when vision is difficult (presumably to achieve stenopoeic viewing). The continuity of frontalis and occipitalis may sometimes explain occipital headache associated with eye strain.

2.5 THE EYEBROWS (SUPERCILII)

Each eyebrow (supercilium) is a transverse elevation studded with hairs between the forehead and upper lid. It resembles the scalp, consisting of skin, subcutaneous connective tissue, a muscular stratum, submuscular areolar tissue, and pericranium. The latter is adherent to the variably prominent part of the frontal bone which shapes the region. Its size is obviously influenced by that of the frontal sinus.

SKIN

The skin of the forehead and eyebrows is thick and mobile, with many sebaceous glands, and adherent to the superficial fascia.

The hairs of the eyebrow are stiff and form a comma-like area, the head of which (with vertical hairs) is medial and typically below the orbital margin, the body lying along the margin (with oblique or horizontal hairs). The tail is usually above the orbital margin. However, there is much variation; the eyebrow may be high or low, much curved or almost horizontal. Many muscles are attached to the mobile superciliary skin, so that they may be elevated, depressed, displaced medially, and so on, contributing much to expression.

Usually the space between the eyebrows is hairless – hence the term **glabella**. The eyebrows are sometimes continuous across the mid line.

SUBCUTANEOUS TISSUES

The subcutaneous tissue contains little fat and much fibrous tissue which connects the dermis to the underlying muscles. Thus the skin, subcutaneous and muscle layers move together.

MUSCLE LAYER

This contains vertical fibres of frontalis, arched horizontal fibres of orbicularis, and the oblique fibres of corrugator supercilii.

SUBMUSCULAR AREOLAR LAYER

This is a continuation of the so-called 'dangerous' area of the scalp, and also continues into the upper lid between the septum orbitale and orbicularis. However, a deep part of the epicranial aponeurosis may, by attachment to the orbital margin, cut off this area from the lids.

The arterial supply of the superciliary region is from the supraorbital and superficial temporal arteries, the venous drainage is to the same veins and also the angular vein. The lymphatic capillaries drain into the submandibular and parotid nodes.

Functionally this layer is important in allowing the skin, subcutaneous tissue and muscle layer to move freely upon it.

2.6 THE CONJUNCTIVA

The conjunctiva is a thin, translucent mucous membrane which joins the eyeball to the lids: hence its name. It covers the lids posteriorly, is reflected anteriorly to the sclera, becoming continuous with the corneal epithelium. The **conjunctival sac** thus formed is open at the palpebral fissure. It normally contains about 7 µl of tear fluid but can accommodate up to 30 µl. Instilled eyedrops in excess of this volume are either drained by the lacrimal sac or overflow the lids.

Although the conjunctiva is continuous, it is con-

veniently described in three regions: palpebral, bulbar, and fornical.

THE PALPEBRAL CONJUNCTIVA

This may be subdivided into the marginal, tarsal and orbital zones.

Marginal conjunctiva

The marginal conjunctiva is a transition zone between skin and the conjunctiva proper. Its structure is continued on the back of the lid for about 2 mm (Parsons) to a shallow **subtarsal fold**, near which the perforating vessels traverse the tarsus to conjunctiva.

The puncta open in the marginal zone, and thus the conjunctival sac is continuous with the nasal inferior meatus via the lacrimal passages. Thus conjunctival infection may spread to the nose and *vice versa*.

Tarsal conjunctiva

The tarsal conjunctiva is thin, adherent and very vascular; its consequent reddish colour is a convenient clinical indicator. The tarsal glands appear as yellow streaks through the translucent tarsal conjunctiva, which is intimately adherent to the superior tarsus and almost impossible to separate by dissection, which makes surgical repairs here very difficult. Unlike the upper tarsal conjunctiva the lower is adherent for only half the tarsal width.

Orbital conjunctiva

The orbital conjunctiva of the upper lid is between the tarsal upper border and fornix. It is loosely attached to the subjacent non-striated muscle (Fig. 2.10). It is folded horizontally by movement, most when the eyes are open and least when they are shut. The folds are a postnatal development.

Low magnification shows, just above the superior tarsal plate, a series of shallow grooves, which create a mosaic of low elevations (Stieda's plateaux and grooves), which are not true papillae. This area may encroach up to halfway across the tarsal conjunctiva.

THE CONJUNCTIVAL FORNIX

This is a continuous annular cul-de-sac. It is artificially but conveniently divided into superior, inferior, lateral and medial regions (Fig. 2.30).

The **superior fornix** reaches the orbital margin,

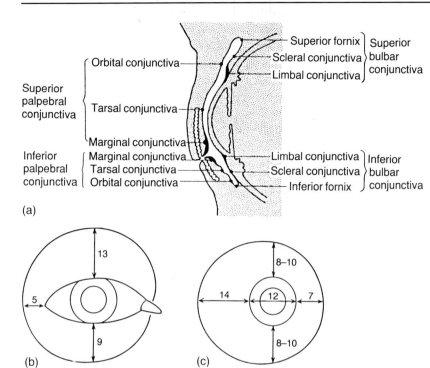

(a)

(b)   (c)

Fig. 2.30 (a) Diagrammatic representation of the conjunctival sac in vertical section of the closed eye; (b) dimensions (in millimetres) of human conjunctival sac measured from lid margins with the palpebral aperture open (after Whitnall, 1921); (c) dimensions (in millimetres) of human conjunctival sac measured from the limbus with an assumed corneal diameter of 12 mm (after Whitnall, 1921). (From Tripathi, R. C. in Davson, H. (ed.) (1984) *The Eye*, *Vol. 1A*, 2nd edition, published by Academic Press.)

8–10 mm from the limbus; the **inferior fornix** to within a few millimetres of the inferior orbital margin, 8 mm from the limbus; the **lateral fornix**, 5 mm from the surface and 14 mm from the limbus, extends just posterior to the equator. The **medial fornix** is the most shallow, comprising medial ends of the superior and inferior fornices.

Fornical conjunctiva is adherent to areolar tissue, which is continuous with expansions from the sheaths of the levator and rectus muscles, whose contractions can therefore deepen the fornices; it also continues into the tarsi. It contains conjunctival glands (of Krause) and palpebral muscles (of Müller).

In intertendinous intervals behind the fornices the conjunctiva adjoins orbital fat, and haemorrhage (e.g. from a basal cranial fracture) can advance under the conjunctiva to the limbus.

The whole fornix is well vascularized; its venous plexus and aponeurotic expansions from inferior rectus and oblique are visible in its inferior part.

Incisions at the superior fornix enter areolar tissue between levator and superior rectus; at the inferior fornix they enter between the inferior palpebral and inferior rectus muscles and expansions from inferior ocular muscles (Figs 2.12 and 4.28).

THE BULBAR CONJUNCTIVA

Thin, and so translucent that underlying sclera appears white, the bulbar conjunctiva is tied to subjacent structures by areolar tissue, and is thus mobile enough to allow ocular movements. Bulbar conjunctiva is in contact with tendons of the recti, covered by **fascia bulbi** (Tenon's capsule); both are divided to expose the tendons, anterior to which the conjunctiva covers the anterior part of the bulbar fascia. They are separated, to about 3 mm from the cornea, by areolar tissue containing subconjunctival vessels. Between conjunctiva and sclera is loose episcleral tissue. In this episcleral region lie the anterior ciliary arteries, forming a pericorneal plexus, and tendons of the recti.

At about 3 mm from the cornea, conjunctiva fascia bulbi and sclera are adherent. Because the conjunctiva here is less mobile, a firmer hold of the globe can be obtained at surgery. At this union conjunctiva sometimes forms a slight ridge, obvious in some infections – the **limbal conjunctiva**. At the limbus, between conjunctiva and sclera, the conjunctival dermis, fascia bulbi, and episcleral connective tissue are densely fused.

STRUCTURE

Conjunctival structure varies from region to region, and this may affect pathological processes. Only neonatal conjunctiva is pristine; it is exposed to pathological vagaries from an early age. As a mucous membrane, conjunctiva has an epithelium and submucosal lamina propria.

Epithelium

Most of the **palpebral margin** is covered by keratinized stratified epithelium. The mucocutaneous junction (Figs 2.9, 2.31 and 2.32) is posterior to openings of the tarsal glands, i.e. at the junction of 'dry' and 'moist' regions where the marginal strips of tear fluid end. Here the skin changes abruptly to non-keratinized squamous cells in about five strata, all nucleated. The basal epithelium retains papillae.

The deepest layer is of cylindrical cells, as in epidermis, with intermediate layers of polyhedral cells, the most superficial being flat but indented. Squamous cells are gradually replaced by columnar and cubical cells in the direction of the conjunctival sac. The number of layers is also reduced, but deepest cells remain cylindrical. Goblet cells, absent at the mucocutaneous junction, begin to appear and are very numerous beyond the subtarsal fold (Kessing, 1968).

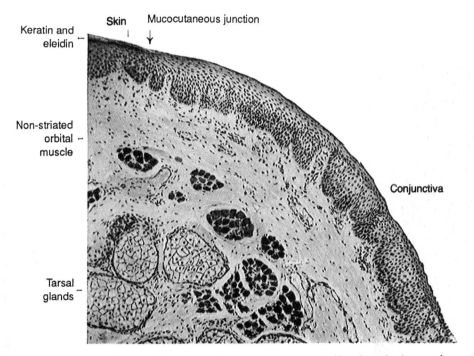

Fig. 2.31 Vertical section of the posterior edge of the lower lid margin (low power). Note how the layers of squamous cells diminish in number when traced to the right.

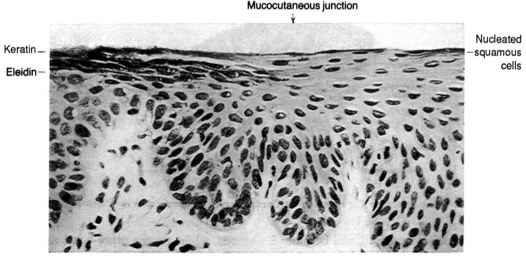

Fig. 2.32 Vertical section of the mucocutaneous junction of the lower eyelid. Note the sudden termination of keratin and eleidin layers at arrow. To the right are nucleated squamous cells.

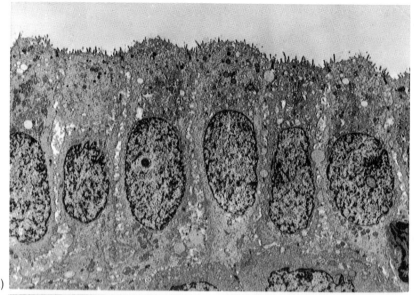

(a)

Fig. 2.33 (a) TEM of fornical conjunctiva of a 45-year-old, showing tall columnar cells, with long straight apical microvilli, numerous liposomes (black arrow) in the apical cytoplasm, and wide intercellular spaces containing amorphous material (white arrow). Original magnification ×2500;

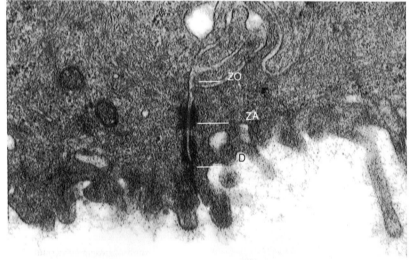

(b)

(b) TEM of the junctional zone of two superficial epithelial cells. The apicolateral cell junction consists of a zonula occludens (ZO) (tight junction), a zonula adherens (ZA) and a desmosome (D). The apical microvilli are covered by an elaborate glycocalyx. Original magnification ×30 000;

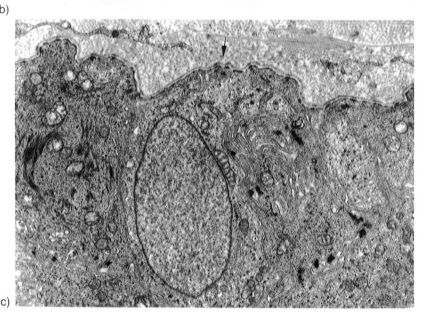

(c)

(c) TEM of the basal region of bulbar conjunctival epithelium, showing dense intermediate filaments (IF) and numerous hemidesmosomes forming attachment to the basement membrane (arrow). Profiles of collagen bundles are seen in the lamina propria. The cell nucleus is unusually euchromatic. Original magnification ×6000. (Courtesy of Dr O. Earley.)

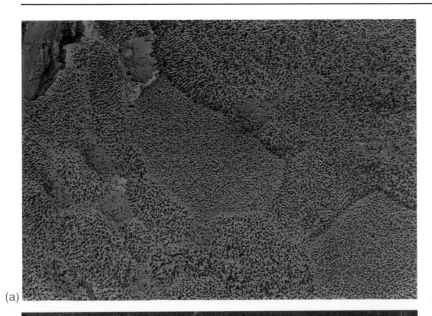

Fig. 2.34 (a) SEM of the surface of the conjunctiva from a normal eye showing a hole from which a cell has recently been sloughed off. Note the differing microvillous population and the shallow nature of the hole. Field width 36 μm;

(a)

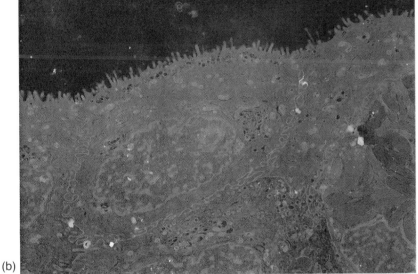

(b) Thiery's method showing branching chains of silver granules extending outwards from the microvilli and cell surface;

(b)

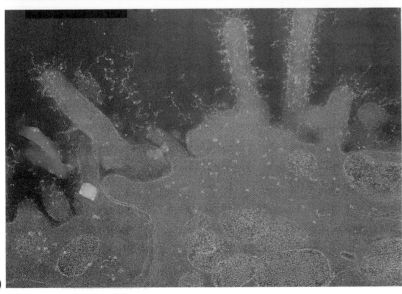

(c) Micrograph showing the spacing of anchoring sites both on the cell surface and upon the microvilli. The identical nature of most of the staining is well shown. The circle includes an area of surface anchor sites;

(c)

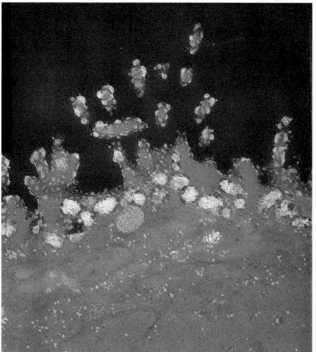

(d)

Fig. 2.34 (contd)   (d) Normal conjunctival surface cell showing subsurface vesicles and microvilli. (From Dilley, P.N. (1985) *Trans. Ophthal. Soc. UK*, **104**, 381.)

The epithelium of the superior **tarsal conjunctiva** is bilaminar, with a deeper layer of cubical cells (whose oval nuclei have their long axes parallel to the surface) and a superficial layer of cylindrical cells, whose oval nuclei are basal and perpendicular to the surface. Towards the fornix a third, intermediate, layer of polyhedral cells begins to appear; at the **fornix**, although epithelium is otherwise unchanged, there are often three layers. Epithelium of inferior tarsal conjunctiva has three or four layers in most of its extent, but sometimes two and, rarely, five. Basal cells are cubical; as in all save juxtamarginal conjunctiva they are followed by layers of polygonal cuneiform and conical cells. The surface cells possess a glycocalyx (Figs 2.33 and 2.34) that stains positively for glycoprotein and is difficult to distinguish from mucin, which is thought by some to be adsorbed onto the epithelial surface (Figs 2.35 and 2.36).

From fornix to limbus, epithelium becomes less glandular, losing its goblet cells, and more epidermal in type; but it is never keratinized. More polyhedral layers appear, superficial cells become flatter, deeper ones taller. At the **limbus**, the epithelium is stratified, and papillae form, giving the deep aspect a characteristic sinuous profile. Basal cells here are small, cylindrical or cubical, with little protoplasm and dense nuclei which produce the dark line characteristic of limbal conjunctiva (Figs 2.33, 6.18 and 7.48(a).

They often contain pigment granules. There are several layers of polygonal cells and one or two layers of squamous cells with oval nuclei parallel to the surface. The polygonal cells, unlike those in the cornea, lack intercellular bridges.

Fine structure of the conjunctival epithelium

Epithelial cells are attached to one another by desmosomes across highly interdigitating borders. The intercellular spaces are wider than those of the corneal epithelium.

The **basal cells** contain large electron-dense nuclei surrounded by a perinuclear halo which is free of organelles (Abdel-Khalek, Williamson and Lee, 1978). The basal aspect of the cells attaches to an undulating basal lamina by hemidesmosomes. A prominent network of intermediate filaments inserts into the attachment structures. The percentage of basal membrane occupied by hemidesmosomes is greater in central cornea (27.9 ± 9.2%) than at the limbus (14.9 ± 3.5%) (Caroll and Kuwabara, 1968; Gipson, 1989). Mitochondria, rough endoplasmic reticulum and Golgi membranes are sparse, and usually perinuclear. Mitoses are uncommon (Lee *et al.*, 1981). Conjunctival cell density falls with age. Earley (1991) has shown an almost twofold increase in mean cell area at the surface comparing subjects under 21 years of age with those over 80 years. Intermediate cells are polygonal and have less condensed cytoplasm. Mitochondria are larger and denser than in the basal layer while intermediate filaments are sparser and less aggregated (Breitbach and Spitznas, 1988). The majority of cells ('dark cells') are of high electron density, with fewer 'light' cells. Some cells contain electron-dense, rod-shaped bodies (Abdel-Khalek, Williamson and Lee, 1978). The superficial cells are joined at their anterior contiguous borders by junctional complexes (comprising zonulae occludentae, zonulae adherentae, and maculae adherentae) which seal the intercellular space anteriorly (Fig. 2.33). This confers the property of a semipermeable membrane on the conjunctival epithelium (as with the corneal epithelium) facilitating the passage of lipid-soluble molecules from the tears to the conjunctiva and obstructing the movement of water-soluble molecules and ions. This favours the entry of lipid-soluble drugs (such as chloramphenicol) into the conjunctiva, and is also a barrier to the movement of protein across the conjunctiva from the extracellular space into the tears.

Scanning electron microscopy (SEM) shows the **surface epithelial cells** to be polygonal, mostly hexagonal, often with a petalloid arrangement

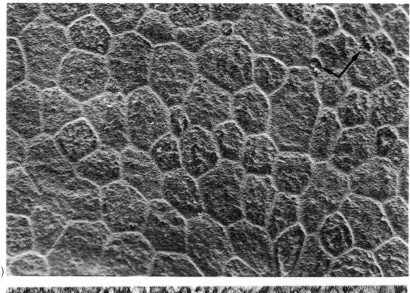

(a)

Fig. 2.35 (a) SEM of conjunctival epithelium of a 30-year-old shows regular small polygonal cells (mean area 46.98 μm^2) and interspersed goblet cells (arrows). Original magnification ×1500.

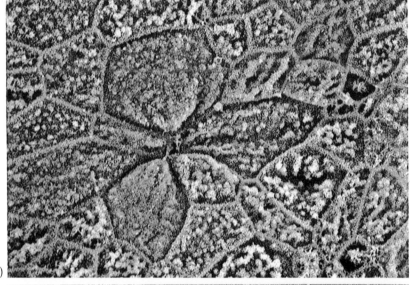

(b)

(b) SEM of conjunctival epithelium of a 54-year-old showing cellular pleomorphism, variegate microvillar pattern and well-defined cell borders. Goblet cell stomas appear as small dark craters interposed between the epithelial cells. The mean cell area measured 118.43 μm^2. A 'dark' cell shows short regular tightly compacted microvilli. Original magnification ×1500.

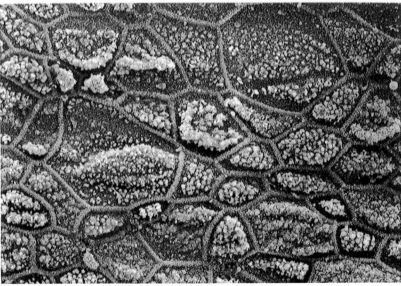

(c)

(c) SEM of conjunctival epithelium of a 77-year-old. The epithelial cells are pleomorphic (mean cell area 84.2 μm^2) and the microvilli show gross clumping and centralization. The cell borders are particularly prominent and there is a notable absence of goblet cells. Original magnification ×1500.

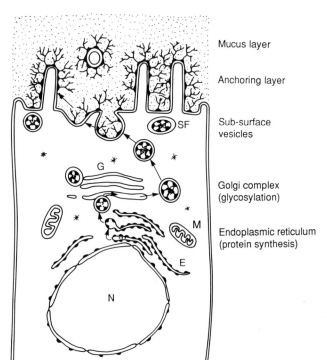

(d)

Fig. 2.35 (contd) (d) SEM of conjunctival epithelium of a 30-year-old showing a presecretory goblet cell stoma (diameter 4 μm) containing a central tuft of microvilli. Radial microvilli traverse the stomal opening and the border is delineated by a row of tall microvilli. Original magnification ×6000. (Courtesy of Dr O. Earley.)

Mucus layer

Anchoring layer

Sub-surface vesicles

Golgi complex (glycosylation)

Endoplasmic reticulum (protein synthesis)

Fig. 2.36 Diagrammatic representation of a surface conjunctival cell of the conjunctival epithelium. A proposed pathway of exocytosis, and fate of a subsurface vesicle is indicated by arrows. AF = Anchored fibrils; AS = sites of anchorage to cell membrane; C = clumped microvilli; D = dense microvilli; E = endoplasmic reticulum; EX = exterior surface of eye; F = fibrils associated with the cell surface and microvilli; G = Golgi complex; GC = long microvilli; M = mitochondrion; MV = microvillus; N = nucleus; RF = released fibrils; S = subsurface vesicle; SP = sparse microvilli; ST = short microvilli. (From Dilley, P.N. (1985) *Trans. Ophthal. Soc. UK*, **104**, 381.)

around a central core of cells (Blumcke and Morgenroth, 1967; Pfister, 1975). They are 3–20 μm wide at the limbus, and 6–10 μm on the tarsus (Greiner, Covington and Allansmith, 1979). The cells are studded with a carpet of shaggy microvilli or, to a lesser extent, microplicae, whose density, size and location determine an appearance of 'light' and 'dark' cells. Greiner, Covington and Allansmith (1979) and Earley (1991) attribute the light appearance to a high density of microvilli, while Pfister (1975) found fewer microvilli on light cells, but a greater mucus coating; the mucus coat on SEM is greater in young subjects (Earley, 1991). The dark cells of the tarsal conjunctiva are slightly depressed below the surface, larger and with shorter, broader microvilli (Greiner, Covington and Allansmith, 1977).

Microvilli are about 0.5–1 μm high and about 0.5 μm thick, with an intervillous gap of 0.5–1 μm (Schwarz, 1971; Dilly, 1985). **Microplicae**, which may be fused microvilli (Steuhl, 1989), are only 0.5 μm in height and width and up to 3 μm in length. On the upper tarsus (Greiner *et al.*, 1980a, 1982) they may be branched, or tufted (5% greater than 1 μm). They are longer in the lower fornix (Nichols, Dawson and Togni, 1983), and elongated microvilli may bridge over goblet orifices (Greiner, Covington and Allansmith, 1977, 1979) or lymphoid collections.

Actin filaments pass from within the microvilli into a horizontal condensation – the terminal web, which anchors the cell membrane to the cytoskeleton (Gipson and Anderson, 1977). Nichols, Dawson and Togni (1983) postulated a contractile function in relation to the microvilli.

The **apical cytoplasm** of the surface cells contains numerous vesicles (sometimes referred to as

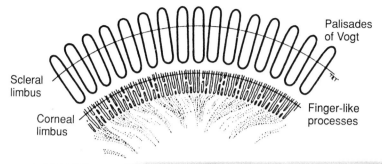

(a)

Fig. 2.37 (a) Schematic drawing of the upper limbus in a pigmented subject to show the relationship between the limbus, the palisades of Vogt, the finger-like radial processes which may sometimes be seen and pigment epithelial slide onto the cornea itself. (From Bron, A.J. (1973) *Trans. Ophthalmol. Soc. UK*, **93**, 455.)

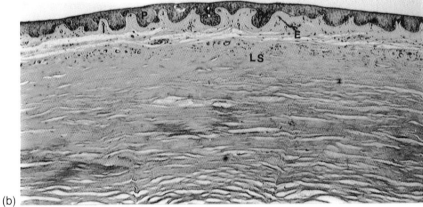

(b)

(b) Low-power view of transverse section of the limbal palisades. The palisades (PP) are composed of epithelial rete pegs. The interpalisades (IP) contain vessels, nerves and lymphocytes. E = Episclera and episcleral vessels; LS = limbal sclera. Original magnification ×110.

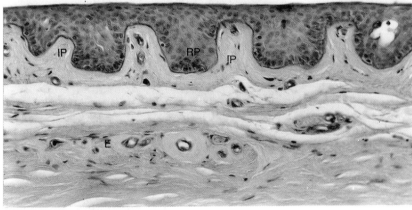

(c)

(c) Transverse section of upper limbus in higher power. RP = rete peg of the palisade; IP = interpalisade.

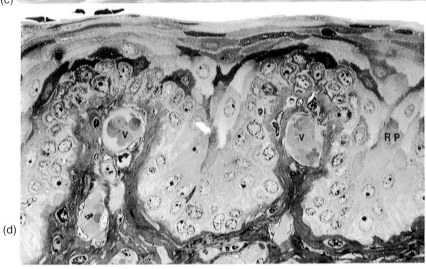

(d)

(d) High-power view of the palisade region showing a blood vessel (V) derived from the episcleral vessel system in the interpalisade region. The organization of the rete pegs (RP) is well shown. P = Palisade cells. Original magnification ×700. (From Tripathi, R. C. in Ruben, M. (ed.) (1972) *A Textbook of Contact Lens Practice*, published by Baillière Tindall.)

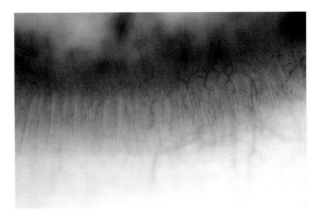

Fig. 2.39 Upper limbus in a pigmented subject. The pigment within the epithelial cells of the rete peg demarcate each palisade. The margins of the palisade are most clearly defined because of the higher amount of the pigment within the basal cells.

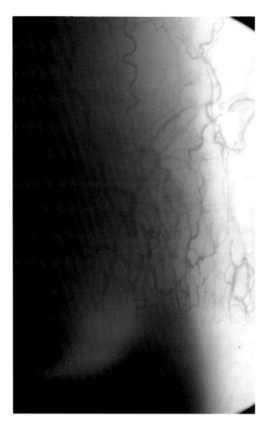

Fig. 2.38 Lower limbus in a Caucasian subject, showing vascular loops within the limbal palisades.

'subsurface vesicles'), 0.4–0.8 μm wide and surrounded by a unit membrane (Srinivasan *et al.*, 1977; Greiner *et al.*, 1980a). Dilly (1985) has studied these using Ruthenium red and silver stains and has demonstrated the presence of a 'mucoprotein' anchored to the inner membrane of the vesicle and histochemically identical to the material attached to the outer surface of the epithelial cells (Fig. 2.36).

This mucoprotein is distinct from the contents of the goblet cells and from surface mucin. Dilly (1985) has proposed that a 'mucoprotein' synthesized in the cells is packaged by the Golgi apparatus, transferred to vesicles, and then transported to the cell surface after fusion with the cell membrane. He has suggested that intermediate filaments in the cell (keratin/tonofilaments) may play a dynamic role in selecting or conducting vesicles to the surface.

There is an increase in conjunctival vesicles in vernal catarrh (Takakusaki, 1969), contact lens allergy (Greiner *et al.*, 1980b) and the denervated eye (Dilly and Mackie, 1981). This has led to a view that the vesicles provide an additional mucin secretory source, but their product is histochemically different from goblet cell mucin and ocular surface 'mucin'.

Although goblet cells and conjunctival vesicles stain positively with PAS and Alcian blue, only the vesicles and the conjunctival membrane-associated material stain by Thiery's (silver) method. Also, the intervillous and supravillous mucus stain differently to each other with colloidal iron (Wright and Mackie, 1977; Dilly and Mackie, 1981).

Histochemical staining suggests that the vesicular material is a glycoprotein, but does not provide evidence that it is a mucin. It is reasonably regarded as the basis of a surface **glycocalyx** which is responsible for the wettability of the ocular surface and binds physically to the overlying goblet cell mucin (Liotet *et al.*, 1987; Tiffany, 1990a, b).

Evidence for the nature of the ocular surface mucins has been suggested recently by Gipson, on the basis of studies using immunohistochemical technqiues and *in-situ* hybridisation, which have shown that three of the nine cloned mucin genes are expressed at the ocular surface (Watanabe *et al.*, 1995; Inatomi *et al.*, 1995; 1996), MUC 1, a membrane-spanning mucin is expressed by the stratified corneal and conjunctival epithelia, excluding the goblet cells. The conjunctiva also expresses two secretory mucins; MUC 4 in the stratified epithelium but not goblet cells and MUC5 in the goblet cell alone.

The **limbal epithelium** is about ten cells deep, about twice as thick as in the cornea, forming the papillae of the **limbal palisades** (of Vogt), whose distinctive feature, in the upper and lower limbus, is their radial arrangement (Figs 2.37 and 2.38). This is particularly obvious in pigmented subjects (Fig. 2.39). A separate vascular supply, with elongated vascular loops, extends in submucous capillary connective tissue from episcleral arteries. It is obvious by slit-lamp (Graves, 1934; Bron and Goldberg, 1980),

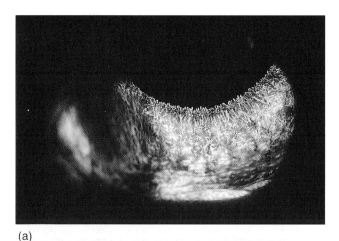

(a)

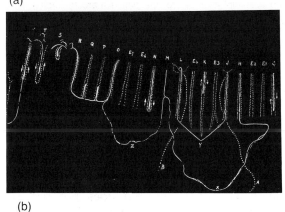

(b)

Fig. 2.40 (a) Fluorescein angiogram of the limbal region, showing the marginal arcades and the short segments of vessels within the palisades; (b) Drawings of the limbal arcades. Linear magnification ×36. (From Graves, B. (1934) *Br. J. Ophthalmol.*, **18**, 305.)

and appears during fluorescein angiography (Fig. 2.40). The epithelium of the palisade zone provides the generative zone for the corneal epithelium.

Goblet cells

These occur throughout conjunctiva, especially the plica semilunaris, singly or in association with epithelial crypts (Figs 2.41 and 2.54). They are most dense nasally, least dense in upper temporal fornix, and absent at the palpebral mucocutaneous junction and the limbus (Kessing, 1966, 1968). The goblet cells are the chief source of tear mucin, and are essential for moistening the ocular surface (the lacrimal gland and conjunctival epithelium have been proposed as other sources). Goblet cells probably arise from the basal layer of epithelium and tend to retain attachment to its basement membrane. Round or oval in shape, 10–20 μm wide, with flat basal nuclei (Figs 2.42–2.44), the cells become larger and more oval as they approach the surface, where they develop a

stoma and discharge their mucin content. They are finally shed, unlike intestinal goblet cells which they otherwise resemble. Electron microscopy demonstrates an electron-dense basal nucleus with relatively dense cytoplasm in which rough endoplasmic reticulum, mitochondria and a well-developed Golgi apparatus are embedded. They are attached by desmosomes to neighbouring epithelial cells. Goblet cells have abundant secretory granules 0.4–10 nm in diameter, with the largest granules closest to the apical membrane. The content of these large granules is more homogeneous and less electron dense than that of the deeper granules. When the apical aspect of the goblet cell reaches the epithelial surface, it presents a number of surface microvilli which are gradually lost as the cell distends prior to disgorging (Pfister, 1975; Greiner *et al.*, 1981) (Figs 2.35 and 2.44). This may be related to loss of microfilamentary anchors passing between the microvilli and the terminal web, a latticework of fine filamentous material lying subjacent to the microvilli. Ultimately the apical plasma membrane ruptures and the mucous secretory granules are released to the surface. Goblet cell openings are 1–3 μm on the tarsus, and 2–5 μm elsewhere. They may be bridged by microvillous processes (Greiner, Covington and Allansmith, 1979; Greiner *et al.*, 1981).

Hyaline bodies found in 25% of elderly, normal bulbar conjunctivae are thought by some to represent degenerate goblet cells (Abdel-Khalek, Williamson and Lee, 1978). On transmission electron microscopy (TEM) they are electron dense centrally, with an electron lucent periphery rimmed by trilamellar membrane (Earley, 1991). They make up about 15% of the superficial epithelial cell population (Steuhl, 1989), and 8% of the basal epithelial cell population in children (Rao *et al.*, 1987). Their mean linear density is 10 cells/mm (Kessing, 1968).

Although goblet cells have been regarded as terminally differentiated cells which discharge their contents, including nuclei and organelles with their (holocrine) secretions, there is a view that they may be apocrine glands capable of replenishing their secretion after discharge (Wanko, Lloyd and Matthews, 1964). Recently Wei, Sun and Lavker (1990) have identified 'label-retaining' goblet cells in radiolabelling experiments, which suggests that they have a proliferative capacity. Goblet cells are thought to form basally and lose their connection with basal lamina early, before migration to the surface (Kessing, 1968) which is supported by the observation of paired, basal, 'presecretory' goblet cells during conjunctival resurfacing of cornea in rabbit experiments (Aitken *et al.*, 1988).

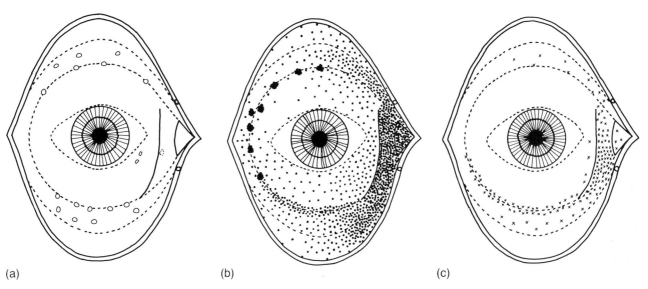

(a)   (b)   (c)

Fig. 2.41 (a) Diagram of the relative topographic distribution of the goblet cells. Right eye with semilunar fold and Krause's accessory lacrimal glands in the upper and lower fornical areas, which are indicated by dotted lines. Tarsal margins are also indicated by dotted lines;

(b) schematic drawing of the distribution of saccular and branched crypts in the right eye;

(c) schematic representation of the distribution of the intra-epithelial mucus crypts in the right eye;

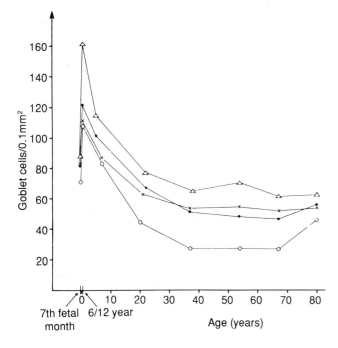

(d)

(d) age variation in goblet cell density in the bulbar area. Note that the highest density at all ages is in the lower nasal quadrant. △ = Lower nasal quadrant; ● = upper nasal quadrant; × = lower temporal quadrant; ○ = upper temporal quadrant. (From Kessing (1986) *Acta Ophthalmol. Suppl.* **95**, 1 with permission.)

Various mucous crypts have been described in the conjunctiva (Kessing, 1968). The net-shaped crypts (of Henle) are best developed in the upper tarsal area. These are tubular structures with lumina of 15–30 μm which contain a few goblet cells. Saccular and branched crypts have been considered as rudimentary accessory lacrimal glands. They occur in the upper and lower fornices and orbital zone with a density of 1–5 crypts/20 mm². Similar structures are seen on the free margin of the plica and inferonasal to the limbus in youth. They contain small numbers of goblet cells. The intraepithelial mucous crypts consist of clusters of goblet cells arranged around a central lumen and with an overall diameter of 50 μm. They predominate in the lower fornix and on the plica with a density of 10–100 crypts/20 mm². Their numbers increase in chronic inflammation, and decrease in dry eye, pemphigoid and vitamin A deficiency. Loss of goblet cells affects the wetting of the ocular surface, even when tear fluid is adequate.

Melanocytes

Melanocytes occur at the limbus, fornix, plica and caruncle, and at sites of perforation of the anterior ciliary vessels (Montagna, 1967). In highly pigmented

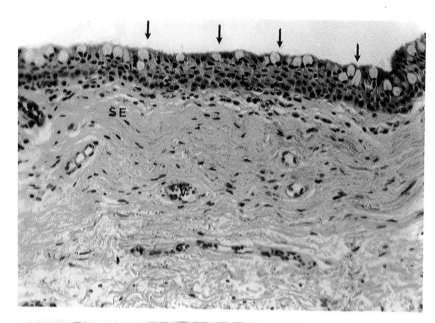

Fig. 2.42 Light micrograph of human bulbar epithelium showing mature goblet cells (arrowed) at the epithelial surface. SE = Subepithelial connective tissue; V = episcleral vessel.

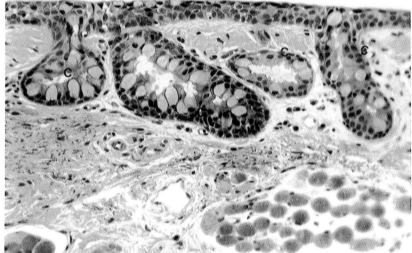

Fig. 2.43 Goblet cell crypts (C) of the bulbar conjunctiva.

races they give the conjunctival surface a brown tinge; in Caucasians they are usually amelanotic, although melanin can be demonstrated by the dopa reaction (Fig. 2.45).

Langerhans cells

The cells of Langerhans are cells of the so-called 'dendritic system' (Stingl, Tamaki and Katz, 1980) which includes epidermal and mucosal cells of Langerhans and dendritic cells in thymus and lymph nodes. They appear to represent a highly differentiated cell line from bone marrow related to the monocyte–macrophage–histiocyte series: like these, they have surface receptors for the Fc component of

IgG, the third component of complement and surface HLA-DR (Ia) antigen; unlike them they are not phagocytic, but function in antigenic presentation, lymphokine and prostaglandin production, and stimulation of T lymphocytes. They are involved in allograft rejection of the cornea, and in contact hypersensitivity of the skin.

Cells of Langerhans were originally described in humans as dendritic cells in the basal corneal epithelium (Engelman, 1867) and further described by Sugiura, Waku and Kondo (1962) as part of a 'polygonal cell' system present in all vertebrates. They are also present in the human limbus (Sugiura, Waku and Kondo, 1962) and in the conjunctival epithelium (Gillette, Chandler and Greiner, 1982). In

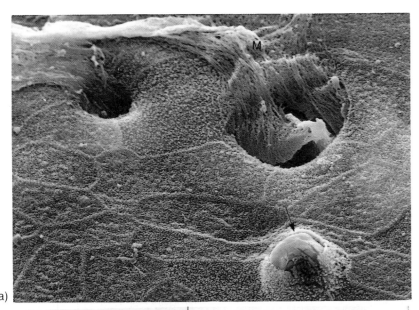

(a)

Fig. 2.44 (a) SEM of conjunctival epithelium of a 5-year-old, showing goblet cells at different stages of mucus secretion. The presecretory goblet cell stoma (arrow) is smaller than those actively engaged in mucus secretion (M). Original magnification ×1500.

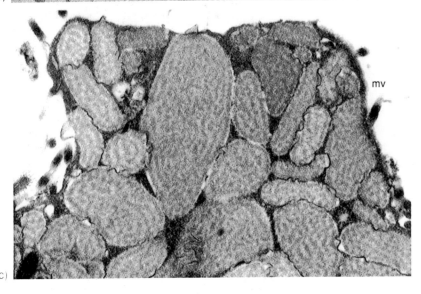

(b)

(b) TEM of bulbar conjunctiva of a 77-year-old, showing a secretory goblet cell discharging packets of intact mucus granules on to the cell surface. Original magnification ×5000.

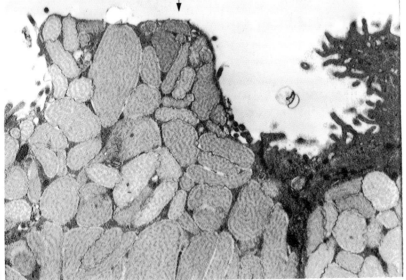

(c)

(c) SEM profile of the apical part of a secretory goblet cell, showing tightly packed mucus secretory granules about to erupt through the attenuated apical cytoplasm (arrow). Adjacent epithelial cells have a well-formed filamentous glycocalyx. mv = microvilli. Original magnification ×10 000.

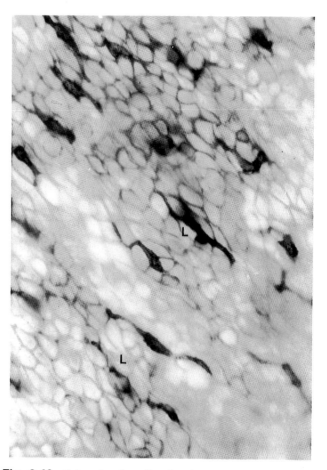

the absence of corneal injury or inflammation cells of Langerhans are present in the peripheral but rarely central corneal epithelium (Vantrappen *et al.*, 1985). Their density in skin is 500/mm^2 and in peripheral cornea 15–20/mm^2 (Rodrigues *et al.*, 1981).

The highest density of Langerhans cells was found in the tarsal conjunctiva by Steuhl *et al.* (1995) (lower central: 4.7 cells/mm^2), followed by the fornix (upper central: 3.1 cells/mm^2) and the bulbar conjunctiva (upper lateral: 1.0 cells/mm^2). The numbers decreased with age from an average of 4.4 cells/mm^2 in those under 20 years of age, to 1.2 cells/mm^2 in those over 60 years of age.

They exhibit a unique ultrastructural feature, the Birbeck granule, which stains positively for ATPase, and express T-6, S-100 and HLA-DR antigens at their surface (which may be detected by immunohistochemical techniques). They can thus be readily differentiated from surrounding epithelial cells (Fig. 2.46) (Braude and Chandler, 1983). Cells of Langerhans no desmosomes.

(d)

Fig. 2.44 (contd)   (d) Higher magnification of the region shown in (c), to show individual secretory granules bound by a membrane. The thin apical plasma membrane bears a few microvilli (mv). Original magnification ×19 000. (Courtesy of Dr O. Earley.)

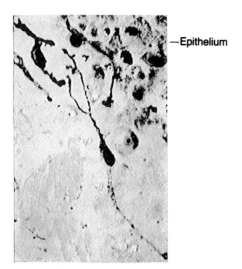

—Epithelium

Fig. 2.45   Flat section at the limbus, to show subconjunctival melanocytes (Bielchowsky stain).

Fig. 2.46   Rat conjunctiva. Abundant Langerhan's cells (L) (ATPase stain).

The accessory lacrimal glands

Two groups of accessory lacrimal glands are associated with the conjunctiva.

Glands of Krause

The glands of Krause lie mainly in the deep subjunctival tissue of the upper fornix (about 42), between the palpebral part of the lacrimal gland and the tarsal plate, and also in the lower fornix (6–8) (Krause, 1867). Their ductules unite into a single duct which empties into the fornix. Similar glands occur on the caruncle. Gobbels and Spitznas showed that the glands of Krause are innervated.

Glands of Wolfring

The glands of Wolfring are larger than those of Krause. There are two to five above the superior tarsus or within its upper border near the mid point and two within the lower edge of the inferior tarsus. Their short, wide, excretory ducts are lined by a layer of cubical basal cells and superficial cylindrical cells like those of conjunctiva (Fig. 2.47).

Henle's 'glands' are merely folds of mucous membrane between the fornices and tarsal plates. The **glands of Manz**, present at the limbus in some ungulates, are not found in humans.

The conjunctival submucosa

The submucosa has superficial lymphoid and deep fibrous layers which extend to the limbus. The lymphoid layer appears first in the fornices at 3–4 months of age, and its development and that of the conjunctiva produce folds in the tarsal conjunctiva at the fifth month.

Lymphoid layer

The lymphoid layer is a fine connective tissue reticulum, containing many lymphocytes, which is thickest in the fornices (50–70 μm, Villard, 1896) and ends at the subtarsal fold, so that lymphocytes are absent from the marginal conjunctiva.

Lymphocytic nodules occur near the canthi but diminish in the conjunctival periphery; the true follicles found in the inferior fornix of the dog, cat and rabbit do not occur in humans. Expansions of these foci may cause visible surface swellings in follicular conjunctivitis of viral or allergic origin.

Lymphocytes, predominantly T cells, are found in substantia propria and epithelium, in a ratio of about 2:3. Neutrophils are also found in the epithelium and submucosa, while plasma cells and mast cells (which preponderate in the perilimbal and tarsal regions) are found only in the submucosa (Allansmith, Greiner and Baird, 1978).

Lymphoid aggregations corresponding to the mucosal associated lymphoid tissue (MALT) of the gut and bronchi are also found in the conjunctiva. The conjunctival associated lymphoid tissue (CALT) consists of T and B lymphocytes, without plasma cells. The stratified architecture of the epithelium overlying these lymphoid nodules is partly obscured by infiltrating lymphocytes. The epithelium lacks goblet cells and exhibits exaggerated microvillous

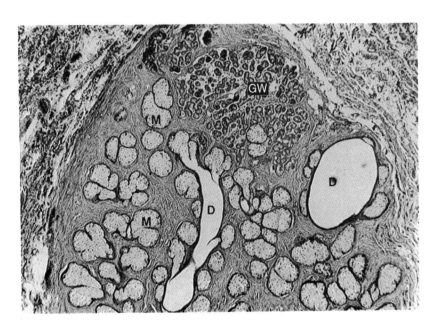

Fig. 2.47 Vertical section of the upper lid showing the location of the glands of Wolfring (GW) in the upper portion of the tarsal plate in close vicinity to the meibomian gland (M). Original magnification ×72. (From Tripathi, R. C. and Tripathi, B. J. in Davson, H. (ed.) (1984) *The Eye, Vol. 1A*, 2nd edition, published by Academic Press.)

processes (Chandler and Gillette, 1983; Franklin and Remus, 1984).

Fibrous layer

The fibrous layer is generally thicker than the lymphoid layer, except over the tarsal plate, with which it blends. It contains the conjunctival vessels and nerves and glands of Krause.

CONJUNCTIVAL PAPILLAE

True papillae occur only at the limbus and in the marginal conjunctiva. The limbal papillae form the upper and lower palisades of Vogt (Fig. 2.37) where fingerlike columns of epithelium interdigitate with long extensions of the submucosa while the surface of the epithelium remains flat. Focal vascular papillary elevations occur, particularly over the upper tarsus, in chronic conjunctivitis or allergic eye disease.

ARTERIES

The arterial supply of the conjunctiva is from:

1. the peripheral tarsal arcades;
2. the marginal tarsal arcades;
3. the anterior ciliary arteries;
4. the deep ciliary system.

Peripheral tarsal arcade

The peripheral tarsal arcade in the tarsal plate, fornix and proximal bulbar conjunctiva runs at the upper border of the tarsus between the two parts of the levator (Figs 2.10, 2.25, 2.26 and 2.48). Its peripheral perforating branches pass above the tarsal plate, pierce the palpebral muscle and divide into ascending and descending conjunctival branches.

The descending branches supply the proximal two-thirds of the tarsal conjunctiva, anastomosing with the shorter branches of the marginal artery which have pierced the tarsal plate at the subtarsal fold. The ascending branches pass up over the fornix to the globe, where they become the **posterior conjunctival arteries** (Fig. 2.49). These anastomose with the **anterior conjunctival arteries** about 4 mm from the limbus and together they supply the bulbar conjunctiva.

The peripheral arcade of the lower lid, when present, lies in front of the inferior palpebral muscle of Müller and is distributed like that of the upper lid. It may arise from the lacrimal, the transverse facial or superficial temporal arteries. It is often absent, and the inferior tarsal plate, fornix or bulbar conjunctiva are then supplied by the marginal arcade or muscular arteries to the inferior rectus.

Marginal tarsal arcade

The marginal arcades send perforating branches through the tarsus to the conjunctiva at the subtarsal

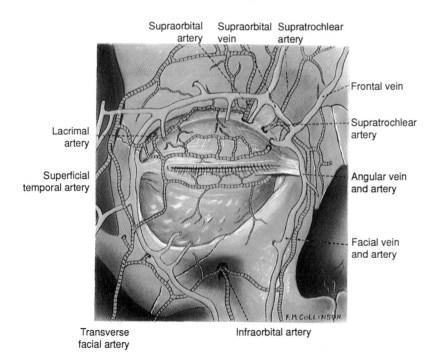

Fig. 2.48 The blood supply of the eyelids.

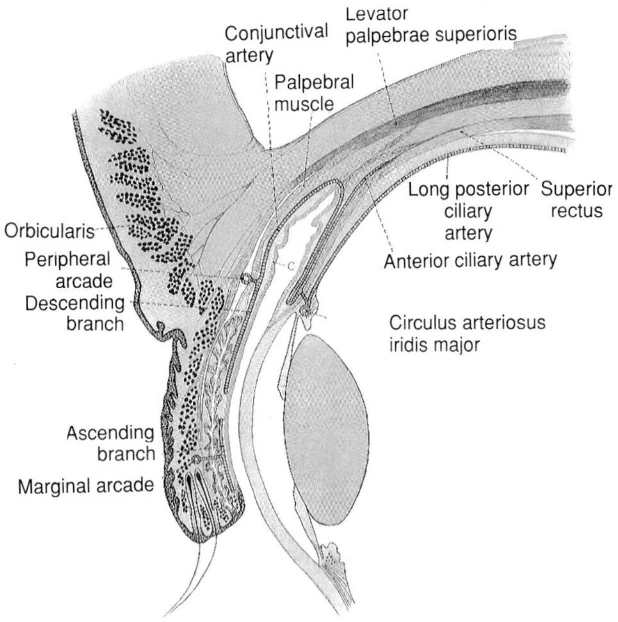

Fig. 2.49 Section of the upper lid and anterior portion of the eye to show the blood supply to the conjunctiva (C).

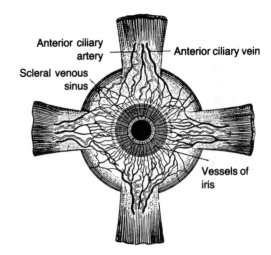

Fig. 2.50 Anterior ciliary arteries and veins.

fold. These divide into marginal and tarsal twigs, which run perpendicularly either to feed the very vascular zone at the lid margin or to meet with corresponding branches of the peripheral arcade.

The tarsal conjunctiva is thus well supplied with blood, hence its red colour. The fornix is red and the bulbar conjunctiva is colourless unless congested.

The vascular supply of the anterior segment

According to Leber, the anterior segment of the human eye has deep and superficial circulations which arise from the ophthalmic artery and are in communication anteriorly. This has been borne out in recent years by vascular casting studies (Ashton and Smith, 1953; Morrison and van Buskirk, 1983), and by low-dose fluorescein angiography and studies in red-free light (Meyer and Watson, 1987; Meyer, 1989).

The ophthalmic artery provides two sagittal systems (Fig. 10.25). The **deep sagittal system**, of medial and lateral long posterior ciliary arteries, supplies a **deep coronal arterial circle** made up of the major arterial circle of the iris and the ciliary intramuscular circle. This system communicates, through perforating scleral arteries, with the superficial episcleral arterial circle derived from the anterior ciliary arteries. Usually (in about 60% of vessels) flow is from the deep to the superficial system in both the vertical and horizontal meridia (Meyer, 1989). This is of interest,

because fluorescein angiography demonstrates unexplained iris perfusion defects after vertical (but not horizontal) muscle surgery (Hayreh and Scott, 1978).

The **superficial sagittal system** is composed of the muscular arteries of the recti and their anterior ciliary branches (Figs 2.49, 2.50, 10.25 and 10.26). Each muscular artery gives off two anterior ciliary arteries except that to the lateral rectus which supplies only one. The anterior ciliary arteries appear darker than the conjunctival. They run forwards in the episclera and pierce the sclera to join the circulus iridis major which they help to form (Fig. 10.25). The scleral foramina are often marked by pigment. At this point the anterior ciliaries give off episcleral arteries which pass forward to form the **episcleral arterial** circle, 1–5 mm behind the limbus. In humans this may have superficial and deep components, giving an appearance of discontinuity.

Episcleral branches anastomose to form the deep episcleral capillary net of the pericorneal plexus. These do not move with the conjunctiva. At the limbus the episcleral arteries make a hairpin bend, and enter the bulbar conjunctiva as the anterior conjunctival arteries, which run to anastomose with branches of the posterior conjunctival artery about 4 mm from the limbus. Its perilimbal branches in the conjunctiva form the superficial or conjunctival part of the pericorneal plexus. At the limbus, the episcleral arteries give rise to **marginal corneal arcades**, which extend subepithelially to the peripheral edge of Bowman's layer of the cornea. They also give off fine loops to the palisades of Vogt at the upper and lower limbus (Bron and Goldberg,

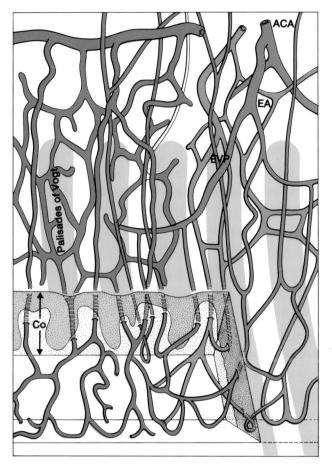

Fig. 2.51 Drawing of the peripheral corneal vascular arcades and palisades of Vogt. Bowman's layer terminates at the periphery of the cornea (Co). Cross-section of the conjunctiva shows the palisades of Vogt. Palisades are formed by stromal papillae and epithelial rete pegs. An anterior ciliary artery (ACA) is seen in the upper right corner: it forms the episcleral arteries (EA). Two sets of vessels originate from the superficial marginal arterial plexus of the limbus: terminal, forming the peripheral corneal arcades near the termination of Bowman's layer; and recurrent, which also form part of the peripheral arcades. These run posteriorly through the palisades to supply the perilimbal conjunctiva. The recurrent vessels anastomose with the conjunctival vessels from the fornices. The episcleral venous plexus (EVP) is deep to the palisades of Vogt. The lymphatics are coloured green: two groups of lymphatics (superficial and deep) extend through the palisades of Vogt. (From Alvarado, J.A. and Weddell, J.E. (1971) *Histology of the Human Eye*, published by W.B. Saunders.)

1980) (Fig. 2.51). Each limbal arteriole supplies between one and three superficial limbal capillaries which form a network of vessels one to four tiers deep. These vessels are less leaky on fluorescein angiography than those of the bulbar and tarsal conjunctiva, because the limbal capillaries have a thicker endothelium and fewer fenestrations (Iwamoto and Smelser, 1965).

These vascular anatomical arrangements explain different patterns of redness which occur in inflammatory disease of the external eye. The tarsal conjunctiva, fornix and posterior bulbar conjunctiva are supplied by the palpebral arcades. The perilimbal bulbar conjunctiva, limbus and episclera are supplied by the deep ciliary arterial circle via the scleral perforating arteries, in addition to the anterior ciliary arteries. In conjunctivitis the bulbar conjunctiva becomes brick-red and the redness increases towards the fornix and tarsal plate; the episcleral system is spared. The congested bulbar vessels are seen to move with the conjunctiva and blanch poorly on pressure.

In affections of the anterior uvea or cornea (anterior uveitis, keratitis) the ciliary system is congested. Dilatation of the episcleral and limbal vessels gives rise to a characteristic 'circumcorneal' or 'ciliary injection'; clinically the vessels do not move when the conjunctiva is moved, but blanch on pressure. In interstitial keratitis, the vessels which invade the deep cornea arise within the sclera from the deep portion of the anterior ciliary arteries.

THE CONJUNCTIVAL VEINS

The conjunctival veins accompany and outnumber the corresponding arteries. The palpebral veins drain the tarsal conjunctiva, fornix and posterior bulbar conjunctiva. In the upper lid, a venous plexus between the tendons of the levator drains into the veins of the levator and superior rectus and thence into the ophthalmic.

Immediately behind the limbal arcades and anterior to the episcleral arterial circle lies a **perilimbal venous circle**, composed of up to three communicating parallel vessels. These collect blood from the limbus, marginal corneal arcades and the anterior conjunctival veins, which are more conspicuous than their corresponding arteries. They drain into **radial episcleral collecting veins**, and then into the veins of the rectus muscles. They receive blood from the episcleral veins and from veins which emerge from the sclera, presumably draining deeper structures, and also drain the larger ciliary emissary veins which emerge from the scleral foramina. The veins leave the anterior surface of the globe, over the rectus muscles. They dilate in hyperaemia.

LYMPHATICS

A superficial plexus of small vessels extends beneath the vascular capillaries. A deep plexus of large vessels, in the fibrous layer of the conjunctiva, receives lymph from this. It drains towards the canthi, joining the lympathics of the lids: the lateral channels drain to the parotid nodes, the medial to the submandibular (Fig. 2.27).

NERVES

The nerves supplying the conjunctiva are from the same sources as for the lids, but the long ciliary nerves supply the circumcorneal conjunctiva (and cornea) and the lacrimal and infratrochlear nerves supply a larger proportion of conjunctiva than skin. Nerve endings are either simple (naked or 'free') or specialized (e.g. end bulbs), such as the 'end bulbs' of Krause.

Free nerve endings

Nerve fibres lose their myelin sheaths and form a subepithelial plexus in the superficial substantia propria. They then form an intraepithelial plexus around the bases of the epithelial cells, sending free fibrils between them.

End bulbs

The end bulbs of Krause (Fig. 2.52) are round and 20–100 µm long. Each is surrounded by a capsule continuous with the nerve sheath and lined by

endothelial cells containing a twisted mass of fibrils. One or two nerves enter each capsule, losing their myelin sheath. The classic papers (Weddell, 1941; Weddell, Palmer and Pallie, 1955; Sinclair, 1967) on the sensibility of skin and cornea have considerably modified views on nerve endings and their functioning in the conjunctiva. According to these observers the so-called 'end bulb of Krause' is but a stage in the cycle of growth and decay of such specialized organs. Moreover, these special endings are comparatively rare and variable in distribution in the human conjunctiva, 'free' endings being much more numerous and widespread.

2.7 THE CARUNCLE (Figs 1.18, 2.53 and 2.54)

The caruncle (from Latin *caro* = flesh) is a soft, pink, ovoid body, about 5 mm high and 3 mm broad, situated in the lacus lacrimalis medial to the plica semilunaris. It is attached to the plica, and fibres of the medial rectus sheath enter its deep surface. Thus, it is most prominent on lateral gaze and is retracted on medial gaze. Deeply, abundant connective tissue is in contact with the septum orbitale and medial check ligament.

The caruncle is modified skin, bearing goblet cells and lacrimal tissue in addition to hairs, sebaceous and sweat glands. The epithelium is non-keratinized, stratified squamous, the sebaceous glands are like those of the lids and the hairs (about 15) are fine, colourless and directed medially. Modified lacrimal glands (of Krause), surrounded by a thin layer of fat, are often conspicuous in the centre of the caruncle, with a tubuloacinous structure and a duct opening near the plica. Near the conjunctiva, single goblet cells are found, or groups which form a kind of acinus.

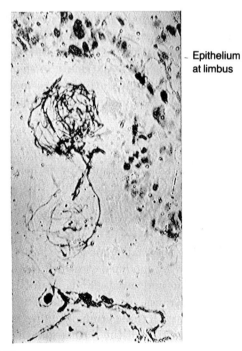

Epithelium at limbus

Fig. 2.52 Flat section at the limbus to show the end bulb of Krause (Bielchowsky stain).

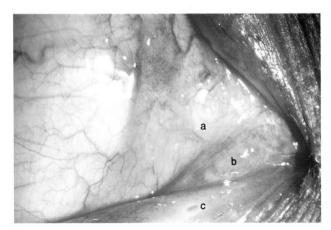

Fig. 2.53 The nasal canthus region, showing (a) the plica, (b) the caruncle and (c) the lower puncta.

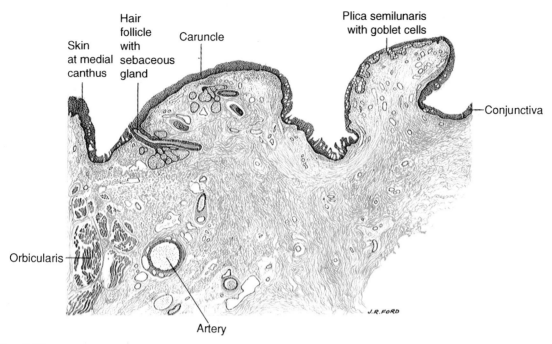

Skin at medial canthus | Hair follicle with sebaceous gland | Caruncle | Plica semilunaris with goblet cells

Conjunctiva

Orbicularis

Artery

Fig. 2.54 Horizontal section through the caruncle and plica semilunaris (Wolff's preparation).

BLOOD SUPPLY

The caruncle is supplied by the superior medial palpebral arteries. The branches pass through deep connective tissue, which may maintain their patency when cut and encourage bleeding.

LYMPHATICS

These drain into the submandibular lymph nodes.

NERVE SUPPLY

The infratrochlear nerve supplies the caruncle.

2.8   THE PLICA SEMILUNARIS

The plica is a narrow crescentic fold of conjunctiva, concave laterally, lying lateral to and partly behind the caruncle. It reaches the middle of the inferior fornix below and extends less far above. The free lateral border is separated from the bulbar conjunctiva by a 2 mm recess, which almost disappears when the eye looks laterally. Its pink, vascular colour contrasts with the white of the sclera. In structure it resembles bulbar conjunctiva but it has eight to ten (not six) epithelial layers and a cylindrical (not cuboidal) basal layer. Goblet cells are numerous (Fig.

2.54) and may be superficial or grouped, with a narrow duct (intraepithelial gland of Tourneux) (Fig. 2.55). Melanophores are always present, but may be non-pigmented in blonde individuals.

The connective tissue stroma is loose and vascular and may contain a nodule of fibrocartilage. The plica may represent the nictitating membrane of many vertebrates, but see Stibbe (1928).

A simpler view is that the plica is an inevitable formation. The conjunctival area at the medial can-

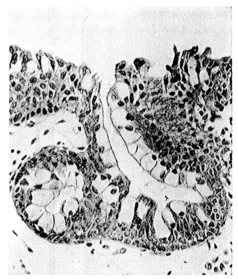

Fig. 2.55 Section of a portion of plica semilunaris to show the gland of Tourneux.

thus must be lax enough to allow full lateral ocular rotation, producing a fold in medial rotation. No such arrangement exists laterally; here the fornix is deep. The shallow medial fornix enables the puncta to dip into tear fluid.

2.9 THE LACRIMAL APPARATUS AND TEARS

The lacrimal gland, above and anterolateral to the eyeball, secretes tears through a series of ducts into the superior fornix. The gland appears in all vertebrates except fish, where ambient water replaces the tears.

The tears moisten the surface epithelia of the cornea and conjunctiva, lubricate the apposed surfaces of lid and globe and supply the first and major refractive interface of the eye, between the air and precorneal tear film, which contributes 43 dioptres of the total 50 dioptres refractive power of the eye. The tears contain substances such as immunoglobulins, complement, lysozyme, lactoferrin and ceruloplasmin, which have a role in combating infection and in the inflammatory response at the ocular surface (Bron and Seal, 1986).

The lacrimal gland (Figs 5.20, 5.23 and 5.24) consists of:

- a large orbital or superior part;
- a small palpebral or inferior part in continuity with the superior part.

The orbital (superior) part

The orbital part is in a fossa on the anterolateral area of the orbital roof. Shaped like an almond, it displays superior and inferior surfaces, anterior and posterior borders, medial and lateral extremities.

The **superior surface** is convex and lies in the fossa on the frontal bone, connected to it by weak trabeculae. The **inferior surface**, slightly concave, lies successively on the levator, its expansion and the lateral rectus (Figs 5.15 and 5.22). The **anterior border** is well-defined and in contact with the septum orbitale. Hence skin, orbicularis and septum orbitale must be divided to reach the gland. The **posterior border**, more rounded, is in contact with the orbital fat and level with the posterior pole of the eye. The **medial extremity** rests on levator and the **lateral extremity** on the lateral rectus. Connective tissue attachments are found: to the bony fossa of the lacrimal gland above; to the zygomatic bone below; to the periorbita behind; and to the accompanying ducts within.

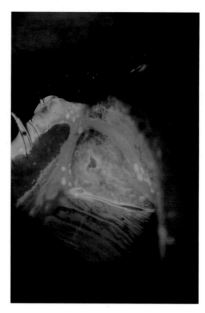

Fig. 2.56 A demonstration of the streaming of lacrimal fluid from the aperture of the palpebral portion of the lacrimal gland. The streams are viewed in light blue with 2% fluorescein in the conjunctival sac. The margin of each stream is highly fluorescent as the fresh lacrimal fluid dilutes the fluorescein.

The palpebral (inferior) part

The palpebral part is also flattened horizontally, and is one-third the size of the orbital part, with its anterior border just above the lateral border of the upper fornix. Thus, it is visible through the conjunctiva when the upper lid is everted and up to 12 ductular openings may be seen with biomicroscopy, or made visible with 2% fluorescein (Bron, 1986) (Fig. 2.56). It lies mainly on the fornix, palpebral conjunctiva and the superior palpebral muscle. The lateral expansion of the levator separates the two parts, which are otherwise continuous behind it (Fig. 5.22).

The **conjunctival glands of Krause** (Fig. 2.10) are accessory lacrimal glands lying between the fornix and convex border of the tarsus as a downward continuation of the palpebral part.

STRUCTURE OF THE LACRIMAL GLAND

The lacrimal gland is tubuloacinar with short, branched tubules, resembling the parotid gland in structure (Fig. 2.57). Its lobules, each the size of a pin-head, are not sharply differentiated from surrounding fat, which extends between them. The **acini** are made up of pyramidal secretory cells with their apices directed towards a central lumen (Fig. 2.58). The basal portion of the acinus is separated from a basement membrane by myoepithelial cells. The

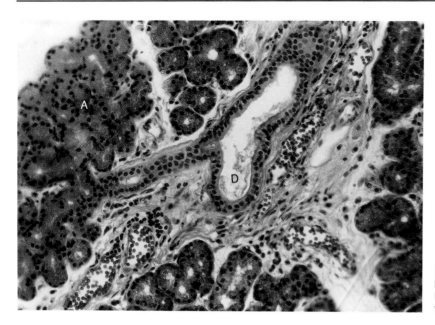

Fig. 2.57 Light micrograph of the human lacrimal gland. A = lacrimal gland acini; D = lacrimal ductule. Note the highly vascular stroma of the gland.

interlobular and interacinar connective tissue contains many small vessels, unmyelinated nerves (Orzalesi, Riva and Testa, 1971) and plasma cells (Allansmith *et al.*, 1976) and is poorly developed in the young.

In each acinus, adjacent secretory cells are joined near their lumen by junctional complexes; more basally, where there is extensive interdigitation of plasma membranes, there are rare desmosomes (Fig. 2.59). Apical microvilli, about 0.5 μm in length, extend into the lumen (Egeberg and Jensen, 1969). The nucleus and rough endoplasmic reticulum are basal in the cells. Scattered Golgi complexes lie laterally here and also in the apical part of the cell (Kuhnel, 1968a; Essner, 1971). The most prominent features are the abundant **secretory granules**, which extend from the apex up to and surrounding the nucleus. Granules range in size from 0.5 to 1.4 μm (Ruskell, 1975) and contain a finely granular material with indistinct limiting membranes (Fig. 2.60). It is not agreed whether different serous and mucous types of cell exist in the lacrimal gland (Essner, 1971), but the studies of Ito and Shibasaki (1964), Kuhnel (1968) and Allen, Wright and Reid (1972) support the presence of a mucus-secreting cell. Ultrastructural differences in granule density and type have been discussed by various authors, but their significance is uncertain (Kobayashi, 1958; Egeberg and Jensen, 1969; Ruskell, 1975). Myoepithelial cells are elongated, with flattened nuclei and numerous fibrils resembling those of smooth muscle cells. They are regarded as contractile and may aid the expulsion of secretion (Scott and Pease, 1959).

The **ducts** show two or three cell layers and

numerous microvilli at the luminal surface. Organelles are less well developed than in secretory cells and the nucleus is central. Adjacent cell membranes show complex interdigitation. Egeberg and Jensen (1969) demonstrated intact secretory granules within the duct lumen suggesting an apocrine mode of secretion (Fig. 2.60).

Plasma cells of the interstitial space are an important source of immunoglobulins secreted into the tears. Allansmith *et al.* (1976) have estimated that human lacrimal glands contain over three million plasma cells. Franklin (1973) and Gillette *et al.* (1980) have shown IgA-secreting (and fewer IgG-, IgM-, IgE-, and IgD-secreting) cells by immunofluorescent staining (Fig. 2.61).

In tears, as in other exocrine secretions, IgA is the chief immunoglobulin. Secretory IgA is dimeric in form, two molecules of IgA being linked by a polypeptide J chain, also of plasma cell origin (Tomasi, 1976). Lacrimal acinar cells synthesize a secretory component (SC) which becomes membrane associated and may provide a binding site for the J chain of dimeric IgA (Koshland, 1975). It is suggested that the IgA-SC complex enters the acinar cell by adsorptive pinocytosis (Brandtzaeg and Baklien, 1977) and is transported to the acinar lumen.

VESSELS

The **lacrimal artery** enters at the posterior border from the neurovascular hilus; sometimes the **transverse facial artery** supplies a branch. The **lacrimal vein** joins the superior ophthalmic.

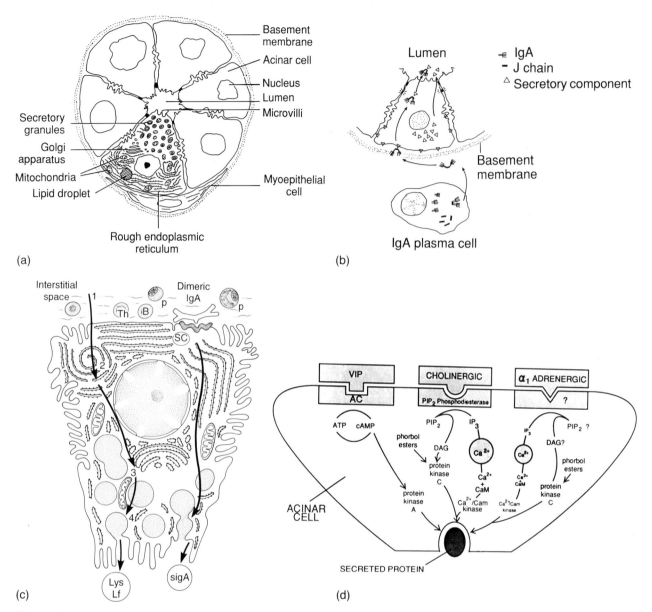

Fig. 2.58 (a) Schematic drawing of the lacrimal acinus. (b) Secretion of secretory IgA. (c) Illustration of the secretory process. The left-hand side of the drawing shows the process of secretion of lacrimal proteins such as lysozyme (lys) and lactoferrin (lf). 1. Amino acids are taken up into the cell from the interstitium, 2. proteins are synthesized in the rough endoplasmic reticulum, 3. modified in the Golgi apparatus and 4. released from the secretory granules. The right-hand side of the drawing illustrates the translocation of secretory IgA (sIgA) from the basolateral membrane; to the lacrimal acinar lumen. T-helper lymphocytes (Th) are thought to stimulate IgA-specific B lymphocytes (B) to differentiate into the IgA-specific plasma cells. Dimeric IgA binds to secretory component (SC), which acts as membrane-bound receptors for IgA. This is internalized and involved in the transport of sIgA to the lumen for secretion. (Modified from J. Murube del Castillo.) (d) The following model for protein secretion has been proposed by Dartt (1989). Three separate pathways can be utilized to stimulate lacrimal gland protein secretion: cAMP-dependent (activated by VIP, β-adrenergic agonists, α-MSH, (ACTH), IP_3/Ca^{2+}/Protein kinase C-dependent (cholinergic agonists), and other (α_1-adrenergic agonists). The cAMP-dependent agonists stimulate secretion by interacting with specific receptors on the basolateral membranes of acinar cells. This activates adenylate cyclase, most likely via a stimulatory G protein, to produce cAMP. cAMP, perhaps via cAMP-dependent protein kinases (protein kinase A), causes exocytosis. Cholinergic agonists stimulate protein secretion by interacting with the muscarinic receptor (glandular M_4) on the basolateral membranes of the acinar cell. This interaction via a G protein activates phospholipase C to generate IP_3 and DAG diacyl glycerol from PIP_2. IP_3 causes Ca^{2+} release from an intracellular store which is probably endoplasmic reticulum related. The Ca^{2+} activates Ca^{2+} calmodulin-dependent protein kinases which presumably cause exocytosis. The DAG generated by cholinergic agonists causes a translocation of protein kinase C from cytosol to membranes where it is activated and probably causes exocytosis. The VIP and cholinergic pathways, the ACTH and cholinergic pathways, and the α_1- and β-adrenergic pathways can interact to potentiate secretion. This interaction occurs after the rise in second messengers. α_1-adrenergic agonists stimulate protein secretion by interacting with specific receptors on the basolateral membranes of lacrimal glands acinar cells. These receptors are α_1-adrenergic receptors, although they are somewhat uncharacteristic. (Courtesy of D. Dartt.)

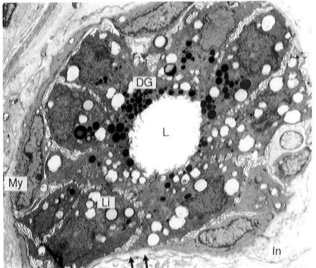

(a)

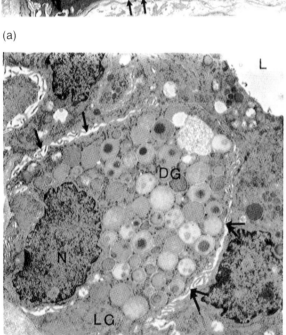

(b)

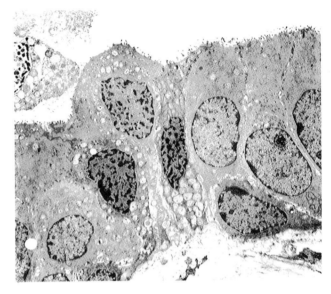

Fig. 2.60 TEM of lacrimal duct structure. Original magnification ×5400. (Courtesy of Mr B. Damato.)

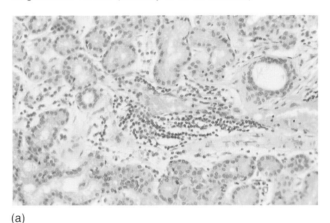

(a)

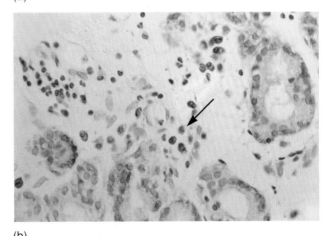

(b)

Fig. 2.59 (a) TEM of lacrimal acinus and surrounding interstitial space (In). Each acinar cell contains a well-defined basal nucleus and a number of electron-dense secretory granules (DG) as well as lipid inclusions (Li). The intercellular spaces (arrows) are wide, but narrow towards the apical ends of the cells where junctional complexes are present (not shown). There are profuse microvillus interdigitations of the plasmalemmas of adjacent cells, and microvilli project from the apical ends into the intra-acinar lumen (L). Myoepithelial cells containing myofilaments and electron-dense fusiform densities lie at the basal aspect of the acinus (My). Original magnification ×4200. (Courtesy of Mr B. Damato.) (b) TEM of a lacrimal acinar cell showing an accumulation of electron-lucent (LG) and electron-dense (DG) secretory granules. N = Nucleus; L = acinar lumen; arrows indicate intercellular space. Original magnification ×8850.

Fig. 2.61 (a) Light micrograph of a human lacrimal gland, stained with haematoxylin and eosin, to show the interstitial space lying between the acini and the ductules; (b) high-power light micrograph of human lacrimal gland, stained with methyl green/pyronine, showing lymphocytes and plasma cells (arrowed).

LYMPHATICS

These pass from the gland to the conjunctival channels and thence to preauricular nodes.

NERVES

The lacrimal gland is innervated by the lacrimal, greater (superficial) petrosal, and cervical sympathetic trunk. The fibres of the greater (superficial) petrosal, the 'nerve of tear secretion', are axons of neurons in the so-called 'superior salivatory nucleus'. They travel in the nervus intermedius to the geniculate ganglion and, without synapse, form the greater (superficial) petrosal nerve. This occupies a groove on the front of the petrous temporal (Fig. 5.16), passes under the trigeminal ganglion to join (in the foramen lacerum) the deep petrosal (from the sympathetic plexus round the internal carotid artery) and forms the nerve of the pterygoid canal (Figs 5.5 and 5.30).

The nerve of the pterygoid canal (vidian nerve), containing parasympathetic (secretomotor) and sympathetic (vasomotor) fibres, joins the pterygo-palatine (sphenopalatine) ganglion, in which only the parasympathetic fibres relay. The postganglionic secretomotor fibres have in the past been said to enter the zygomatic nerve and reach the lacrimal gland via a connection with the lacrimal nerve. This orthodox description may require modification. Ruskell (1971a) has reviewed the evidence of his own researches in primates. He describes a parasympathetic pathway through orbital branches of the pterygopalatine ganglion, which join a 'retro-orbital plexus', whose rami lacrimales carry non-myelinated postganglionic fibres, both sympathetic and parasympathetic. Postganglionic sympathetic fibres may reach the gland by several routes: along the lacrimal artery (from the internal carotid plexus); through the deep petrosal nerve (and hence also from the same plexus); and through the lacrimal nerve. Ruskell has identified sympathetic fibres in the adventitia of the lacrimal artery and (to a very limited extent) in the lacrimal nerve (Fig. 2.62).

The **sensory fibres** are carried by the lacrimal nerve from nerve cells in the trigeminal ganglion, but most of these reach the skin.

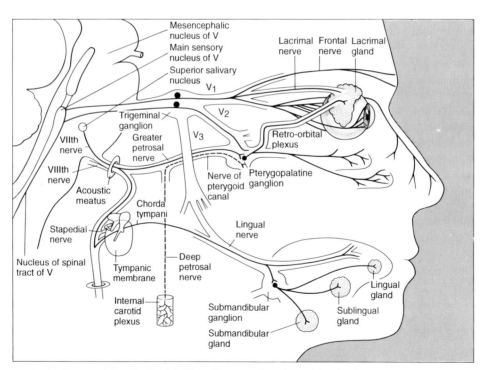

Fig. 2.62 The lacrimal reflex arc (after Kurihashi). The afferent path is formed by the first and second branches of the trigeminal nerve. The efferent path proceeds from the lacrimal nucleus, near the superior salivary nucleus via the facial nerve (nervus intermedius) through the geniculate ganglion, the greater superficial petrosal nerve and the nerve of the kerogloid canal (where it is joined by sympathetic fibres of the deep petrosal nerve). The nerve passes to the pterygopalatine ganglion where it synapses with third order neurones which rejoin the maxillary nerve to supply the lacrimal gland via fibres which form the retro-orbital plexus of nerves. These carry parasympathetic and VIPergic nerve fibres to the gland.

THE PUNCTA

Each punctum lacrimale is a small, round or oval orifice on the summit of an elevation, the **papilla lacrimalis**, near the medial end of the lid margin at the junction of its ciliated and non-ciliated parts. It is in a line with the openings of the ducts of the tarsal glands, the nearest of which is within 0.5–1 mm. The puncta are relatively avascular and thus paler than surrounding areas, a pallor accentuated by lateral tension on the lower lid – an aid in finding a stenosed punctum (Fig. 2.63).

The upper punctum is slightly medial to the lower, respective distances from the medial canthus being 6 and 6.5 mm. However, in lid closure the puncta often make contact (Doane, 1980, 1981). The upper punctum opens inferoposteriorly, the lower superoposteriorly. Hence normal puncta are visible only when lids are everted.

Each punctum, with lids open or shut, faces into the groove between the plica semilunaris and globe,

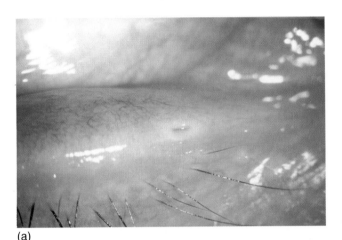

(a)

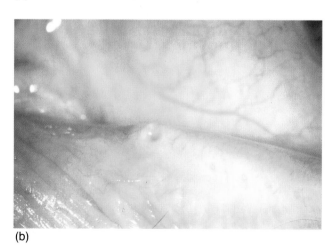

(b)

Fig. 2.63 Lacrimal puncta. (a) Lower, everted, in a 20-year-old man; (b) upper, everted, in a 70-year-old woman.

its patency maintained by surrounding dense fibrous tissue continuous with the adjacent tarsal plate. Fibres of the orbicularis also press the punctum towards the lacus lacrimalis; muscle atrophy makes the papilla more prominent, commonly so in the aged.

THE LACRIMAL CANALICULI

Each canaliculus is first vertical and then horizontal, facts of importance in passing a probe. The vertical part is about 2 mm long and turns medially at roughly a right-angle to become the horizontal part, almost 8 mm in length. At the angle is a dilatation or **ampulla**. Both horizontal parts converge towards medial canthus, the upper slightly downwards, the lower slightly upwards, both being in a lid margin; the upper is the shorter.

The canaliculi pierce the fascia (i.e. the periorbita covering the lacrimal sac) separately, uniting to enter a small diverticulum of the sac, the lacrimal sinus of Maier (Fig. 2.45) at a point on the posterolateral surface of the sac about 2.5 mm from its apex.

Structure

The canalicular lining is stratified squamous epithelium (Figs 2.64 and 2.65) supported by elastic tissue. The wall is so thin and elastic that canaliculi can be dilated to three times normal diameter, which is 0.5 mm, and lateral traction on the lids easily straightens them to facilitate probing. Coloured fluid injected into a canaliculus can be seen through the translucent tissue of the lid's margin.

Like its punctum a canaliculus is surrounded by fibres of orbicularis, which invert the punctum inwards in the lower lid.

The medial third of the canaliculi are covered in front by the two bands which connect the medial palpebral ligaments to the tarsi, while behind is the lacrimal part of orbicularis oculi (Horner's muscle) (Figs 2.66 and 2.67).

THE LACRIMAL SAC

The membranous lacrimal sac occupies a hollow (the lacrimal fossa) formed by the lacrimal bone and frontal process of the maxilla near the anterior border of the medial orbital wall. The sac, closed above and open below, is continuous with the nasolacrimal duct, a mere constriction marking their junction. Their common axis (indicated by a line from the

Hair follicle with
ciliary gland of Zeis

Skin —

Orbicularis
oculi —

Tarsal —
glands

(Medial)

(a)   Conjunctival aspect   (b)

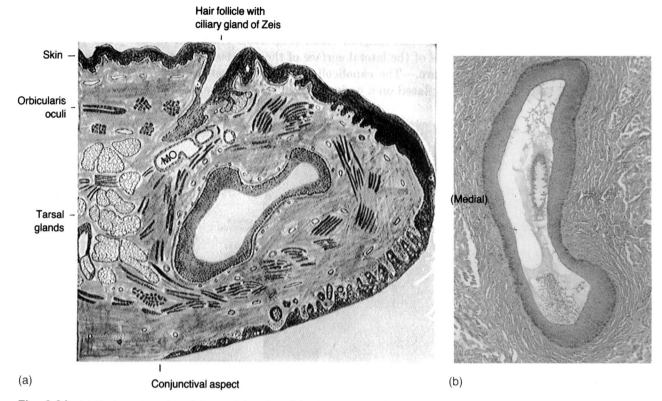

Fig. 2.64 (a) Horizontal section of the medial region of the lower eyelid, showing the lacrimal canaliculus at the junction of the vertical and horizontal portions, surrounded by fibres of orbicularis. MO = Ciliary gland of Möll. Note goblet cells in the conjunctiva. (Wolff's preparation.) (b) High-power view of horizontal section of lacrimal canaliculus (haematoxylin and eosin stain, original magnification × 85). (Courtesy of D. Lucas.)

medial canthus to the first upper molar tooth) slopes down and backwards at 15–25°; but from the front there is a slight angle between their axes, the sac sloping slightly more laterally than the duct, although both are nearly vertical (Fig. 2.68).

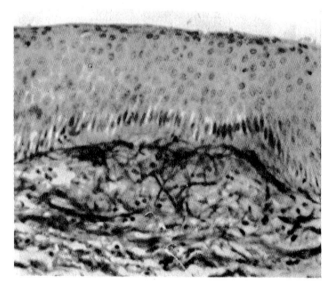

Fig. 2.65 Portion of the wall of the canaliculus. Note the elastic fibres deep to the epithelium.

The sac is enclosed by a periorbita, which splits at the posterior lacrimal crest, encloses the sac, reuniting at the anterior crest, and thus forms the **lacrimal fascia** (Figs 2.66–2.68). This fascia is separated from the sac by areolar tissue containing a fine plexus of veins continued around the duct, except at the fundus where it is closely adherent, and sometimes on its medial aspect.

Relations

Medial to the sac, separated by periorbita and bone, are the anterior ethmoid sinuses (Fig. 1.4), which may extend behind or in front of the sac, and below this the nasal middle meatus. Lateral to it are skin, part of orbicularis oculi, and lacrimal fascia, attached to which are a few fibres of the inferior oblique. Anterior are the medial palpebral ligament and angular vein.

The angular vein complicates the surgical approach to the lacrimal sac. It crosses the ligament subcutaneously 8 mm from the medial canthus. Sometimes a tributary crosses the ligament between the medial canthus and parent vein. Incision for removal

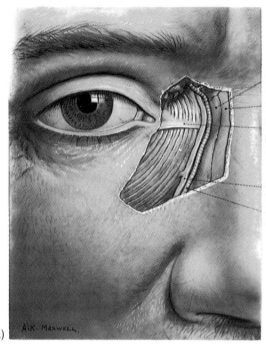

Frontal
process

Nasal bone

Medial
palpebral
ligament

Angular
vein

Angular
artery

(a)

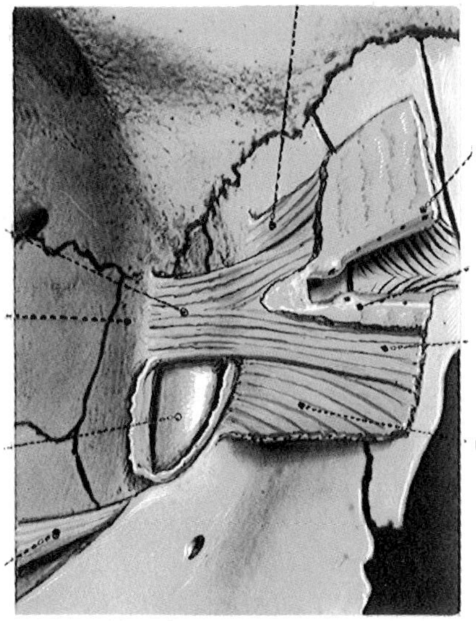

A.K. MAXWELL,

Orbicularis

Horner's
muscle

Lacrimal
bone

Lacrimal
sac

Inferior
oblique

Upper lid

Lower
punctum

Ciliary
bundle
(of Riolan)

Orbicularis

(b)

Fig. 2.66(a)   Dissection to show lacrimal apparatus. Relation of angular vein and artery to medial palpebral ligament (Wolff's dissection). (b) The relations of the lacrimal sac and the pars lacrimalis (Horner's muscle). (Wolff's dissection.)

of the sac should not be more than 2–3 mm medial to the medial canthus.

The inferior edge of the medial palpebral ligament is free, but a sheet of areolar tissue ascends laterally from it to blend with the lacrimal fascia covering the fundus of the sac (Fig. 2.67). This attachment may

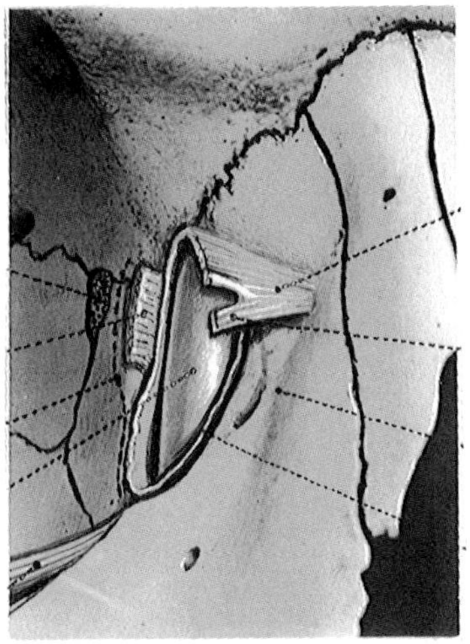

Lateral
prolongation
of sheath of
medial rectus

Lacrimal
muscle

Septum
orbitale

Lacrimal sac

Inferior
oblique

Medial
palpebral
ligament

Prolongation
to the tarsus

Groove in
frontal process
and
sutura notha

Lacrimal fascia

Fig. 2.67   The relations of the lacrimal sac. (Wolff's dissection.)

explain how relatively slight blows to the eye may lead to swelling of the lids on blowing the nose. A sudden strain on the ligament may tear the sac. Below the level of the ligament only fibres of orbicularis are anterior and can securely resist distension of the lacrimal sac. Hence abscesses and fistulas will open below the ligament.

Posterior to the sac are the lacrimal fascia and muscle; the latter, attached to the upper half of the posterior lacrimal crest, passes laterally behind the sac and covers posteriorly the medial third of the canaliculi. Further posterior are the septum orbitale and check ligament of the medial rectus (Fig. 4.42).

The **lacrimal sinus** (of Maier) is a diverticulum of the upper part of the sac behind the middle of the lateral surface into which the canaliculi open either together or separately (Fig. 2.69).

THE NASOLACRIMAL DUCT

The nasolacrimal duct, the continuation of the lacrimal sac from its so-called 'neck' to the inferior meatus in the nose, is only 15 mm in length. It lies in a canal formed mainly by the maxilla (Figs 1.4 and 1.7) and completed by the lacrimal bone and lacrimal process of the inferior concha. It descends posterolaterally, a surface indication being a line from the medial canthus to the first upper molar. Its inferior orifice varies greatly. When it corresponds to the opening of the bony canal at the highest part of the inferior meatus it is rounded; but it may be prolonged as a membranous submucous tube opening at varying levels on the lateral meatal wall and

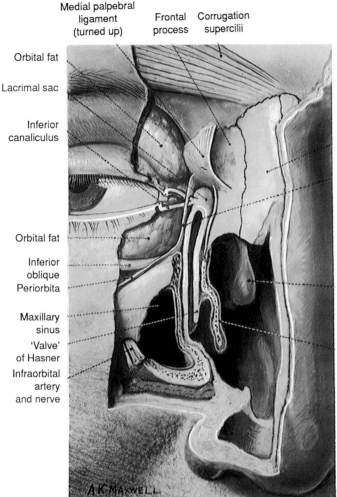

Medial palpebral ligament (turned up)

Frontal process

Corrugation supercilii

Orbital fat

Lacrimal sac

Inferior canaliculus

Orbital fat

Inferior oblique

Periorbita

Maxillary sinus

'Valve' of Hasner

Infraorbital artery and nerve

Nasal bone

Lacrimal fascia

Middle concha

Inferior concha

Fig. 2.68 Dissection to show the relations of the lacrimal sac and the nasolacrimal duct from the front. (Wolff's preparation.)

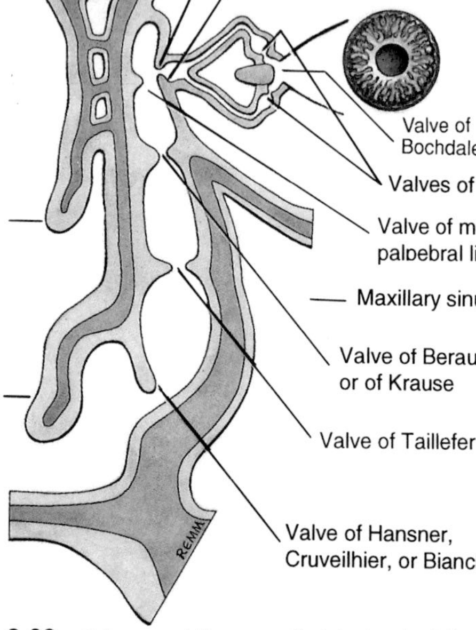

Valve of Rosenmüller

Valve of Huschke

Middle concha

Inferior concha

Valve of Bochdalek

Valves of Foltz

Valve of medial palpebral ligament

Maxillary sinus

Valve of Beraud or of Krause

Valve of Taillefer

Valve of Hansner, Cruveilhier, or Bianchi

Fig. 2.69 Scheme of the so-called 'valves' of the nasolacrimal canal.

becoming more slit-like as it descends. It may be very difficult to find.

The duct is lateral to the middle meatus (Fig. 2.68). It may make a ridge in the maxillary sinus (Fig. 1.19).

The valves

Numerous valves have been described in the nasolacrimal duct. They are folds of mucous membrane with no valvular function, because fluids can be blown up the duct to emerge at the puncta. The most constant is the 'valve' of Hasner (plica lacrimalis) at the lower end, a relic of the fetal septum (Figs 2.68 and 2.69). Usually well developed, the plica may prevent a sudden blast of air (when blowing the nose) from entering the lacrimal sac.

Structure

The lacrimal sac and duct have a double-layered epithelium, the superficial layer composed of

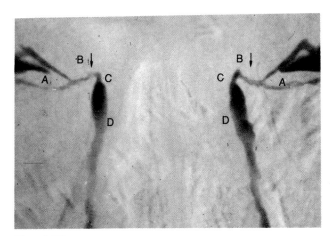

Fig. 2.70 Dacryocystogram demonstrating the nasolacrimal system using a subtraction technique. A = common canaliculi; B (arrow) = common canaliculus; C = upper pole of the lacrimal sac; D = nasolacrimal duct. (Courtesy of Dr Glyn Lloyd.)

columnar cells, the deeper cells being flatter. The bases of the columnar cells reach the basement membrane; they are never ciliated, but goblet cells, in variable numbers, and sometimes mucous glands, occur. Subepithelial lymphocytes occur and may be aggregated pathologically into follicles. The membranous wall of the sac is of fibroelastic tissue, the elastic element being continued around the canaliculi. Around the nasolacrimal duct is a curious plexus of vessels, forming erectile tissue like that on the inferior concha. Engorgement of these vessels is said to be sufficient to obstruct the duct.

In its upper part the nasolacrimal duct is easily separable from bone; below it is closely adherent, forming a mucoperiosteum, which may facilitate spread of infection. The course of the lacrimal sac and duct can be demonstrated by dacryocystography (Fig. 2.70).

Vessels

The **arteries** are supplied from palpebral branches of the ophthalmic (Fig. 5.20), angular and infraorbital arteries and nasal branch of the sphenopalatine. The **veins** drain into the angular and infraorbital vessels above, below into the nasal veins. The **lymphatics** pass to the submandibular and deep cervical nodes.

Nerves

The nasolacrimal duct is innervated by the infratrochlear and anterior superior alveolar nerves.

THE PREOCULAR TEAR FILM

The preocular tear film is the sheet of tears which covers the exposed interpalpebral portion of the globe and cornea. That portion overlying the cornea is the precorneal tear film. The tear film has for many years been regarded as about 7 μm thick (Mishima et al., 1966) and (as Wolff proposed) composed of three layers: a deep mucin layer, an aqueous layer and a surface oily layer.

Recent measurements of the precorneal tear film in humans indicate a thickness of up to 40 μm, and the mucin layer (which had been thought to be about 0.03 μm) was found to be in the region of 30 μm (Prydal, 1990; Prydal and Campbell, 1992). For many years our concept of the structure and function of the tear film was based on the model of Holly and Lemp (1971, 1977). The corneal surface was thought to be hydrophobic, and intrinsically non-wettable. The role of goblet cell mucin was to achieve wettability. Recent studies have suggested that the ocular surface does remain wettable even in the absence of goblet cell mucin (Cope et al., 1986; Liotet et al., 1987; Tiffany, 1990a,b) and that the ocular surface is intrinsically wettable by reason of the highly glycosylated glycocalyx of its surface cells (Dilly, 1985; Nichols, Chiappino and Dawson, 1985).

The deep mucin layer

This is said to be bonded to the glycocalyx of the surface epithelial cells and is demonstrable in the living eye by Alcian blue drops instilled in the tear sac and in ultrastructural studies by staining with ruthenium red and other dyes (Dilly, 1985).

The aqueous layer

This layer is the major component, carrying dissolved salts, proteins, enzymes and antimicrobial substances (Bron and Seal, 1986). It also contains dissolved mucin. The lacrimal and accessory lacrimal glands make the chief contribution to the aqueous content, but constituents are added by all the glands which abut the conjunctival sac.

The surface oily layer

The surface layer is an oily film, 0.1 μm thick, derived chiefly from the meibomian oil glands but also from the glands of Zeiss. With dim illumination and using the tear film as a mirror surface, the oily layer may be seen as a multicoloured interference pattern. The lipid constituents vary but consist chiefly of wax and cholesterol esters with some phospholipid and hydrocarbons (Andrews, 1973). The oil film can be stretched or compressed by widening or narrowing the palpebral aperture.

The preocular tear film is re-established with each blink, about once every 5 s. Between blinks the film thins, partly because of evaporation, and partly due to the flow of aqueous tears into the neighbouring marginal tear strips. If blinking is deliberately prevented, the tear film will break up in a random fashion as the lipid layer approaches and then contaminates the surface epithelium. In normal subjects the break-up time is 15–34 s, but is very variable.

The preocular film is compressible and elastic. It has clinging properties that preserve its stability, and spreading properties that ensure clear vision immediately after blinking. The tear lipids are fluid at lid temperature and spread readily from their origin just anterior to the mucocutaneous junction, across the watery surface of the tear film. They retard evaporation (Mishima and Maurice, 1961). If the lid margins are everted (as by the operating speculum) the preocular film spreads, thins and evaporates more quickly than normal.

In the act of blinking the upper lid descends and the marginal strip of tears sweeps over the cornea. The goblet cells of the tarsal conjunctiva release packets of mucus which coat its smooth surface and spread a mucin layer on to the surface of the corneal epithelium to form its deepest layer (Wolff, 1951). This mechanism is thought also to be important in the removal of unwanted mucin, cells and foreign debris, which are collected together as a mucous thread in the lower fornix (Norn, 1966, 1974; Adams, 1979). The blink is probably important in delivering tear oil to the lid margins.

The glands responsible for the secretion and maintenance of the precorneal tear film do not lie in the cornea itself. In this way the cornea is protected while its optical homogeneity is preserved.

DISTRIBUTION OF THE TEARS

Tears are found in the conjunctival fornices (4.5 μl), preocular tear film (1.1 μl), and along the marginal tear strips (2–9 μl) (Mishima and Maurice, 1961; Mishima, 1965). The marginal tear strips are wedge-shaped tear menisci which run along the posterior borders of upper and lower lids at their points of apposition to the globe (Fig. 2.71). They become continuous temporally at the lateral canthus (Fig. 2.72) and nasally at the medial canthus, running around the groove between the lacrimal parts of the

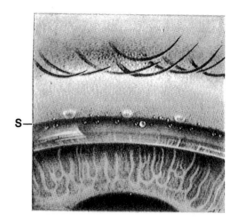

Fig. 2.71 The superior marginal strip (S). Note the oil droplets in it and also some air bubbles.

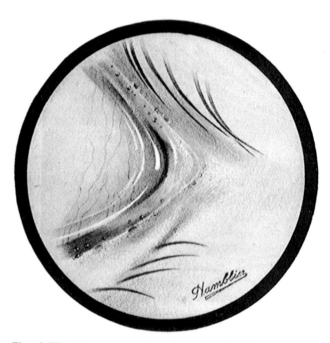

Fig. 2.72 Schematic drawing of the tear film. Recent studies have suggested that the mucin layer may be up to about 30 μm in thickness so that the total thickness of the tear film may be as great as 40 μm.

lid margin, and the plica and caruncle (Figs 2.73 and 2.74). The marginal tear strips can be seen to have a concave anterior border in the optical section of the slit-lamp, and this curved mirror face is responsible for the bright linear reflex which they present when viewed with diffuse illumination (Fig. 2.75). The normally apposed lacrimal puncta dip at all times into the marginal strip of tears. In lateral or straight-ahead gaze they are related to the strips bordering the lacus lacrimalis; in medial gaze, when the lacus is recessed backwards, the puncta are in contact with the precorneal portion of the marginal strips.

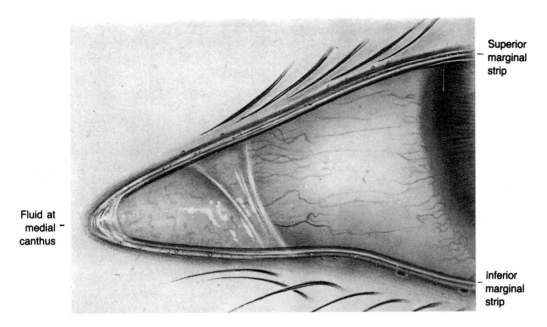

Fig. 2.73 With the eye looking laterally the marginal strips are continued medially between the lid margin on one hand and the plica and caruncle on the other. They join at the medial canthus.

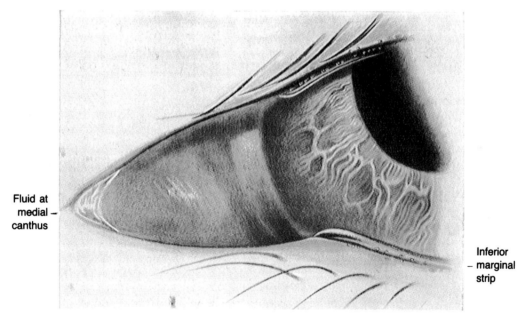

Fig. 2.74 With the eye looking medially a cavity appears deep to each lacrimal portion of the lid margin and the marginal strips stop short. (From Wolff (1946) *Trans. Ophthalmol. Soc. UK*, **66**, 291.)

At the lid margin it can be seen that the anterior limit of the marginal strip is the mucocutaneous junction of the lid, which, running just posterior to the origin of the tarsal gland orifices, is spread with meibomian lipid on its cutaneous aspect and thus affords a non-wettable surface which repulses the tears and prevents them 'brimming over'. In this way

too, the tear lipid, which proves the anterior layer of the tear film, is readily replenished with each blink.

By staining the tears with fluorescein the marginal tear strips may be demonstrated using a blue light source. This shows that there is a zone of thinning, or black line, at the junction of the preocular tear film

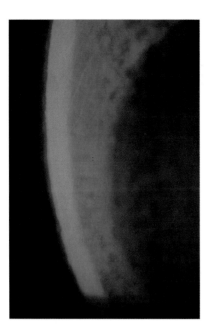

Fig. 2.75 The marginal strip of tears or tear meniscus, stained with fluorescein.

with the marginal strips as they pass into continuity on the surface of the globe. This is due to the lower hydrostatic pressure in the meniscus than within the preocular film. The superior strip extends for a millimetre or so on to the upper cornea and ends as a sharp demarcation line. A similar line is seen below and in contact lens wearers may be reinforced by the ring of meniscus-induced thinning at the lens edge. This may lead to dry spots over the interpalpebral conjunctiva (McDonald and Brubacker, 1971). The marginal strip of tears is noticeably swollen by lacrimation, or reduced in volume when lacrimal gland function is impaired (i.e. 'dry eye').

CONDUCTION OF THE TEARS

Tears are lost from the conjunctival sac partly by the absorption of water through the conjunctiva, partly by evaporation at the surface, and partly by flow into the nasolacrimal system (Frieberg, 1918) as an active process. Tears drain without the aid of gravity and can do so when the head is inverted. Between each blink, fluid flows from the preocular film into the nearest marginal strip of tears. Tears, secreted largely by the lacrimal gland, flow into the lateral part of the upper fornix and enter the upper and lower marginal strip of tears. In this way, tears may be conducted

to the lacrimal puncta; forward spillage is prevented by sebaceous secretion at the mucocutaneous junctions of the lids which render the skin non-wettable.

Tears enter the canaliculi partly by capillarity and partly by a reduction of pressure in the system. The precise mechanism is not agreed upon, but various proposals have been made. Jones (1961) postulated a 'lacrimal pump' in which the canaliculi, filled with tear fluid, become shortened during each blink, and force fluid into the sac. It has also been suggested that contraction of orbicularis dilates the sac, partly by pulling on the medial palpebral ligament which is attached to the sac and partly by contraction of the lacrimal portion of orbicularis which is attached posteriorly to the fascia of the sac. This is thought to create a negative pressure which aspirates fluid into the sac from the canaliculi. Movement of fluid into the puncta can be observed after each blink, or after an adduction of the globe. The pumping action of orbicularis is exaggerated during the blinking and forcible lid closure which accompanies excess lacrimation. It has also been suggested that the 'elastic recoil' of the sac after dilatation drives the tear fluid down the nasolacrimal duct, but there is little evidence for this. It is more likely that the tears entering the duct are in fact absorbed through the mucosa, so that little reaches the nasal cavity except when there is excess tearing (Maurice, 1973).

Recordings of the duct (Frieberg, 1918; Rosengren, 1928) and canaliculi (Wilson, 1976) have confirmed a pressure rise during lid closure which may drive fluid into the nasolacrimal duct. Chavis, Welham and Maisey (1978), using scintillography, suggested that transfer of fluid from the canaliculi to the sac is an active process while flow in the nasolacrimal duct is passive. Studies of particle flow in the marginal strip and high-speed cinematography have shown that the punctal orifices elevate towards each other during blinking and usually meet and occlude when the lid is half-way down. However, meeting is not essential to punctal closure. It is thought that canalicular and sac pressure rise during the remainder of the blink and force the contained fluid through the drainage system. The elastic expansion of the canaliculi in the first few seconds after the blink creates a vacuum within the system which draws in tears when the puncta separate and open (Doane, 1980, 1981; Lemp and Weiler, 1983). Tear fluid enters both lacrimal canaliculi after each blink. Krebiel flow also acts to draw fluid up across the inferior punctum, over the caruncle, into the superior punctum.

CHAPTER THREE

The orbital and cerebral vessels

3.1 THE ORBITAL VESSELS

The orbital contents are supplied chiefly by the **internal carotid artery** via its ophthalmic branch and, to a minor extent, by the **external carotid artery** via the infraorbital artery. Venous drainage is via the ophthalmic veins and tributaries, mainly into the cavernous sinus, but also into the facial veins. There are other minor but distinct extraorbital connections, for example with the pterygoid plexus of veins.

Earliest arterial descriptions were by Cassebohm (1734), Mayer (1877), Zinn (1780), von Haller (1781) and Meyer (1887, a classic account) with substantial contributions in recent times by Hayreh (Hayreh, 1962, 1963, 1972; Hayreh and Dass, 1962 a,b). Although known to Vesalius, the veins received no systematic study until those of Zinn (1755), Walter (1778), Soemmering (1801) and later Sesemann (1869), Festal (1887) and Gurwitsch (1883). Bergen (1981, 1982) has summarized the orbital vascular system and its spatial arrangements.

SPATIAL ARRANGEMENTS

Although even contemporary accounts state that the course and tributaries of the ophthalmic veins mirror those of the ophthalmic artery and its branches (Henle, 1876; Cruveilhier, 1877; Sappey, 1888; Duke-Elder, 1961) it is now accepted that the veins take their own course (Soemmering, 1801; Gurwitsch, 1883; Festal, 1887; Bergen, 1982). This is supported by angiographic studies (Dilenge, Fischgold and David, 1961; Lombardi and Passerini, 1968; Haye, Clay and Bignaud, 1970; Vignaud, Clay and Aubin, 1972; Vignaud, Clay and Bilaniuk, 1974; Vignaud *et al.*, 1974, 1975). Bergen (1982) applied reconstructive photographic techniques (Los, 1970, 1973) to the organization of the orbital vessels and showed distinct differences in the relations of arteries and veins to connective tissue septa (Koorneef, 1976) (Fig. 3.1). Both show limited dichotomous branching.

The **arteries** run within the adipose compartments of the orbit, piercing the septa on passing from one to another; their course is predominantly radial from a centre at the orbital apex (Fig. 3.2). The **veins** are embedded in the septa and other connective tissues for most of their course. The superior ophthalmic vein runs in a sort of hammock in a septum inferior to the superior rectus muscle, while in the posterior orbit all veins are encased in the dense connective tissue of the bony fissures (Figs 3.3 and 3.15(a)). The inferior tributary of the superior ophthalmic vein is partly incorporated into orbicularis oculi, while the inferior ophthalmic vein lies posteriorly, within Müller's orbital muscle. These veins form a series of interconnected rings inside and outside the muscle cone, with the superior ophthalmic vein, most of the medial vein, and the posterior part of the inferior ophthalmic vein running near the surface of the orbital walls. Drainage is from centre to periphery, finally leaving by the cavernous sinus posteriorly and the angular and facial veins anteriorly.

The **microvessels** of the orbit form a complex network whose density increases from orbital apex towards the globe. They are confined chiefly to the adipose compartments with limited connections between compartments but with long anastomotic capillary loops, often parallel to septa when near to them (Bergen, 1982).

3.2 THE ARTERIES

The cervical portion of the internal carotid artery has no branches. Branches from other parts of the internal carotid are:

1. petrous part
    (a) caroticotympanic;
    (b) pterygoid;
2. cavernous part
    (c) cavernous;

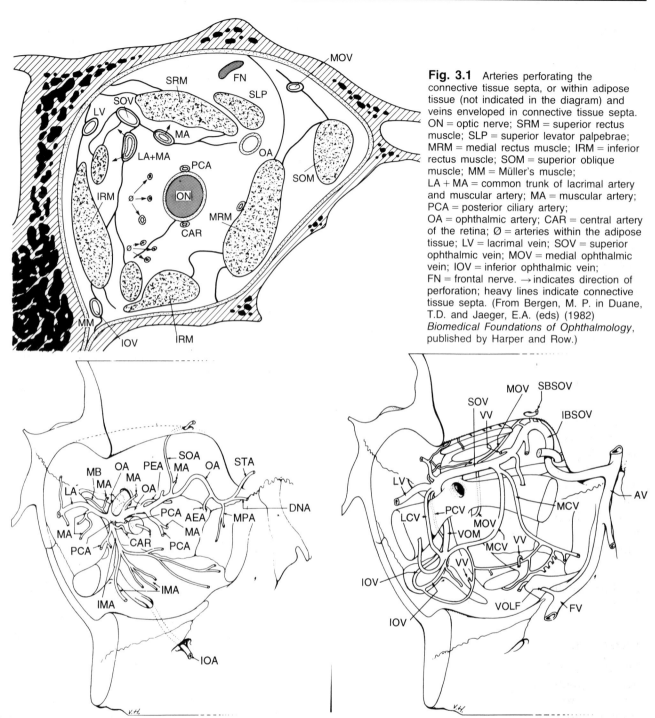

Fig. 3.1 Arteries perforating the connective tissue septa, or within adipose tissue (not indicated in the diagram) and veins enveloped in connective tissue septa. ON = optic nerve; SRM = superior rectus muscle; SLP = superior levator palpebrae; MRM = medial rectus muscle; IRM = inferior rectus muscle; SOM = superior oblique muscle; MM = Müller's muscle; LA + MA = common trunk of lacrimal artery and muscular artery; MA = muscular artery; PCA = posterior ciliary artery; OA = ophthalmic artery; CAR = central artery of the retina; Ø = arteries within the adipose tissue; LV = lacrimal vein; SOV = superior ophthalmic vein; MOV = medial ophthalmic vein; IOV = inferior ophthalmic vein; FN = frontal nerve. → indicates direction of perforation; heavy lines indicate connective tissue septa. (From Bergen, M. P. in Duane, T.D. and Jaeger, E.A. (eds) (1982) *Biomedical Foundations of Ophthalmology*, published by Harper and Row.)

Fig. 3.2 The orbital arteries after a spatial reconstruction made from a series of 60 μm frontal sections. In this series the inferior muscular artery originates laterally to the optic nerve. LA = lacrimal artery; OA = ophthalmic artery; MB = meningeal branch; PEA = posterior ethmoidal artery; SOA = supraorbital artery; PCA = posterior ciliary artery; AEA = anterior ethmoidal artery; MPA = medial palpebral arteries; STA = supratrochlear artery; DNA = dorsal nasal artery; IMA = inferior muscular artery; CAR = central artery of the retina; IOA = infraorbital artery. (From Bergen, M. P. in Duane, T.D. and Jaeger, E.A. (eds) (1982) *Biomedical Foundations of Ophthalmology*, published by Harper and Row.)

Fig. 3.3 The orbital veins after a spatial reconstruction made from a series of 60 50 m frontal sections. No anterior collateral vein could be identified in this series; a double medial collateral vein is present (notice the muscular branches). LV = lacrimal vein; SOV = superior ophthalmic vein; SBSOV = superior root of the superior ophthalmic vein; IBSOV = inferior root of the superior ophthalmic vein; MOV = medial ophthalmic vein; MCV = medial collateral vein; IOV = inferior ophthalmic vein; VOM = 'veine ophthalmique moyenne'; LCV = lateral collateral vein; PCV = posterior collateral vein; VV = vorticose veins; AV = angular vein; FV = facial vein. (From Bergen, M. P. in Duane, T.D. and Jaeger, E.A. (eds) (1982) *Biomedical Foundations of Ophthalmology*, published by Harper and Row.)

(d) hypophyseal;
(e) meningeal;

3. cerebral part
   (f) ophthalmic;
   (g) anterior cerebral;
   (h) middle cerebral;
   (i) posterior communicating;
   (j) anterior choroidal.

The **vertebral** arteries give rise to:

1. anterior and posterior spinal;
2. posterior inferior cerebellar;
3. medullary;

and combine to form the basilar whose branches include:

1. pontine;
2. labyrinthine (internal auditory);
3. anterior inferior and superior cerebellar;
4. posterior cerebral.

THE OPHTHALMIC ARTERY

The ophthalmic artery supplies the orbit and scalp. One branch transcends all others in importance – the central artery of the retina. This is an end artery and its loss (e.g. from embolism) results in complete and irrevocable blindness. Beyond the orbit the ophthalmic artery supplies the forehead to the vertex and the lateral wall of the nose. Here, especially in the scalp, exists a field of anastomosis between the external and internal carotid arteries. The artery is described in three parts:

1. intracranial;
2. intracanalicular;
3. intraorbital.

Intracranial

The intracranial part of the ophthalmic artery arises from the medial, convex side of the fifth bend of the internal carotid as it emerges from the cavernous sinus through its dural roof, medial to the anterior clinoid process and inferior to the mid point of the optic nerve (Figs 5.17, 5.18 and 15.31). The internal carotid narrows after its origin, which may perhaps maintain a high ophthalmic arterial pressure (Whitnall, 1932; Schurr, 1951).

The initial short limb (1–2 mm) of the ophthalmic artery passes forwards horizontally below the optic nerve (Fawcett, 1895; Hayreh, 1963, 1972), ascends briefly, and then bends forward at a right-angle under the medial side of the nerve for a few millimetres; its long limb passes anterolaterally to the inferolateral surface of the nerve (Fig. 3.4). (Because of the anterior direction of the short arterial limb and anterolateral course of the nerve, the nearer at its origin the artery is to the optic foramen the more likely it is to reach the nerve's medial side before crossing laterally.)

There are spiral, intimal cushions of smooth muscle cells and elastic tissue near the artery's origin, for which a regulatory vascular role has been mooted (Bock and Schwarz-Karsten, 1953).

Intracanalicular

At the optic foramen the artery leaves its subdural location to enter the optic nerve sheath, passing forwards between dura and periosteum, which here are fused within the optic canal (Meyer, 1887). The artery does not adhere strongly to the sheath and leaves it near the canal's orbital end (Hayreh and Dass, 1962b). The internal carotid artery is anchored to the dural sheath by its ophthalmic branch, and also indirectly to the optic nerve by the sheaths and by branches to the nerve from the ophthalmic artery (Figs 15.27 and 15.28). The diameter of the ophthalmic artery is diminished in the canal (Dilenge, Fischgold and David, 1961; Vignaud, Clay and Aubin, 1972).

Intraorbital

The first part of this part runs forwards, closely related to the optic nerve's inferolateral surface and attached to it by connective tissue. It forms an 'angle' at the nerve's lateral margin (obtuse 120–135° in 56% of people, right-angled in 40% and acute in 4%; Hayreh, 1972); from which the second part ascends lateral to the nerve, to course medially over it (in 82.6% of subjects) deep to superior rectus. In 17.4% of cases the artery spirals medially under the nerve to reach its superomedial aspect (Fig. 3.4; Hayreh and Dass, 1962b). Sudakevitch (1947) and Bergen and Los (1978) find the vessel firmly attached at the angle, but this is denied by Hayreh and Dass (1962b). The third part of the artery begins at a well-defined bend as it crosses the tendon of the superior oblique to reach the medial orbital wall close to the anterior ethmoidal foramen. It is anchored here by its anterior ethmoidal branch. It passes forwards and upwards, between the medial rectus and superior oblique, narrowing rapidly (Dilenge, Fischgold and David, 1961), runs below the trochlea, and ends at the superomedial orbital angle, behind the maxillary

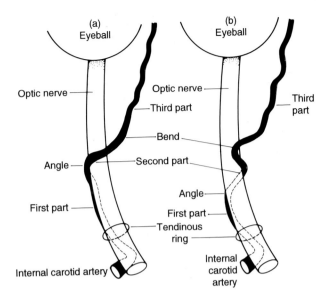

Fig. 3.4 Course of the left ophthalmic artery seen from above. (a) The ophthalmic artery crosses over the optic nerve, the most common situation; (b) the ophthalmic artery crosses under the optic nerve. (From Hayreh, S.S. and Dass, R. (1962) *Br. J. Ophthalmol.*, **46**, 165.)

frontal process, half-way between the medial palpebral ligament and the upper orbital margin.

Posteriorly the artery is in the cone of muscles, with the ciliary ganglion and lateral rectus lateral and optic nerve medial (Figs 5.21 and 5.23). Its third part accompanies the nasociliary nerve between the optic nerve and superior rectus (Fig. 5.21).

This marked tortuosity of the ophthalmic artery permits unrestricted ocular movements without impairing blood supply.

Distribution and branches

The ophthalmic artery supplies most orbital structures, the scalp to its vertex and the nasal wall. It provides considerable anastomosis between external and internal carotid arteries, especially in the scalp.

The marked variation in origin and order of its branches depends on their composite fetal derivation (p.000). The initial section of the ophthalmic artery, including its first ophthalmic part, the lateral posterior ciliary and central retinal arteries, is all derived from the primitive dorsal ophthalmic artery (4 mm fetus); the medial posterior ciliary is from the ventral ophthalmic (5.5 mm fetus), and all other orbital branches are derived from the stapedial artery (16–18 mm fetus) (Hayreh, 1963).

If the ophthalmic artery passes over the optic nerve the central retinal artery is its first branch, alone or

with the medial posterior ciliary or some other branch. If it passes under the nerve the lateral posterior ciliary is the first branch, rarely with some other. The lacrimal (Denonvilliers, 1837), or medial posterior ciliary arteries (Wood Jones, 1949) have also been reported as first branches (Fig. 3.5).

The muscular and ciliary arteries are the most variable (Thane, 1892; Henry, 1959); the central retinal and posterior ciliary arteries are the most tortuous (Rouviere, 1967; Henry, 1959). The central retinal artery is an end artery and its occlusion (for example, by embolism) causes permanent and complete blindness.

The usual order of appearance of branches of this artery is:

1. central retinal;
2. medial and lateral posterior ciliary;
3. lacrimal (and lateral palpebral);
4. recurrent meningeal;
5. muscular (and anterior ciliary);
6. posterior ethmoidal;
7. supraorbital;
8. adipose;
9. anterior ethmoidal;
10. medial palpebral;
11. collaterals to optic nerve sheath;
12. periosteal;
13. dorsal nasal (terminal);
14. supratrochlear (terminal).

The central retinal artery

The terminal branches of this artery anastomose to a limited extent with the arterial circle of Zinn at the optic disc.

The posterior ciliary arteries

These arise below the optic nerve as two to four trunks, usually medial and lateral, which divide into 10–20 branches (Meyer, 1887; Hayreh, 1962). These branches run forwards, surround the optic nerve and pierce the eyeball close to it. Most branches, the **short ciliary arteries**, enter the choroid. Two **long posterior ciliary arteries** pierce the sclera medial and lateral to the nerve (Fig. 5.21) and pass between the sclera and choroid to supply the ciliary body, anastomosing with **anterior ciliary arteries** to form the circulus arteriosus iridis major, supplying the iris.

The lacrimal artery

The lacrimal artery leaves the ophthalmic artery lateral to the optic nerve, and proceeds with the

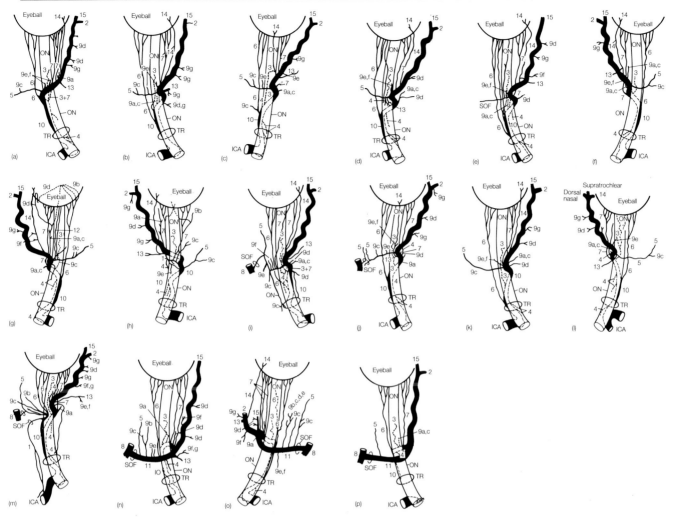

Fig. 3.5 Variations in origin, course, and branches of the ophthalmic artery. (a) Usual pattern; (b)–(p) ophthalmic artery crosses under the optic nerve; (n, o) the ophthalmic artery arises from the internal carotid as usual, but the major contribution comes from the middle meningeal artery; (p) the only source of blood is the middle meningeal artery, as the connection of this with the internal carotid is absent. Because of the incomplete injection of this specimen, small branches could not be traced. 1 = Anastomotic channel; 2 = anterior ethmoid; 3 = central retinal; 4 = collateral branch; 5 = lacrimal; 6 = lateral posterior ciliary; 7 = medial posterior ciliary; 8 = middle meningeal; 9 = muscular arteries to: (a) medial and inferior recti and inferior oblique; (b) inferior rectus; (c) lateral rectus; (d) medial rectus; (e) superior rectus; (f) levator palpebrae superioris; (g) superior oblique; 10 = ophthalmic artery trunk from internal carotid; 11 = ophthalmic artery trunk from middle meningeal (8); 12 = posterior ciliary; 13 = posterior ethmoid; 14 = supraorbital; 15 = main continuation of ophthalmic artery. ICA = Internal carotid artery; ON = optic nerve; SOF = superior orbital fissure; TR = tendinous ring. (From Hayreh, S.S. and Dass, R. (1962) *Br. J. Ophthalmol.*, **46**, 165.)

lacrimal nerve at the upper border of lateral rectus to supply the lacrimal gland. It traverses the gland and supplies the eyelids and the conjunctiva through its lateral palpebral branches and forms superior and inferior anastomotic arcades with the medial palpebral arteries (Figs 5.18 and 5.21).

Other branchlets include two or three muscular branches (to lateral and superior rectus and, less often, inferior and medial recti and inferior oblique), a zygomaticotemporal branch, and anastomoses to the infraorbital artery.

The recurrent meningeal artery

This branch passes posteriorly through the superior orbital fissure of a small foramen in the sphenoidal bone's greater wing to anastomose with the middle meningeal branch of the maxillary (external carotid) artery, thus linking the internal and external carotids. It may be large, replacing the ophthalmic or middle meningeal in part (Fig. 3.5), or may be double, its deeper part representing a vestige of the dorsal ophthalmic artery of the embryo (Lasjaunias *et al.*,

1978). Hayreh (1962) found the artery in 10% of cases, usually in the absence of a lacrimal artery, and always when the ophthalmic artery passed over the optic nerve.

The muscular arteries

The muscular arteries are subdivided into three groups: the **superior** artery, rarely independent, and present in less than one-fifth of orbits, supplies the superior and lateral recti, levator and superior oblique (Hayreh, 1962). The **inferior** artery, present in 98% of specimens, is the largest branch on the orbital floor, arising independently near the 'bend' of the ophthalmic artery and pursuing a fairly constant course. It supplies the inferior and medial recti, inferior oblique and sometimes the lateral rectus (Hayreh, 1962). A variable number of **independent vessels** arise from the main artery and also from the lacrimal and supraorbital.

The muscular arteries of the recti run forward within their tendons and pierce the sclera to anastomose with posterior ciliary arteries. Their anterior ciliary rami pass forward in the episclera to supply the subconjunctival, marginal corneal and perilimbal conjunctival networks (Fig. 9.15a).

The posterior ethmoidal artery

This is the smaller of the ethmoidal arteries, although their widths are usually reciprocal (Fig. 5.21). It supplies the superior oblique as it passes between this muscle and the levator, then enters the posterior ethmoidal canal with the posterior ethmoidal nerve (when present). It supplies the mucous membrane of the posterior ethmoid sinuses, the meninges of the anterior cranial fossa, and the upper nasal mucosa (Hyrtl, 1875). Occasional branches supply the periosteum and orbital tissue.

The supraorbital artery (Figs 5.17 and 5.21)

The supraorbital artery leaves the ophthalmic artery above the optic nerve, passes medial to superior rectus and levator and then between levator and the orbital roof (Vignaud *et al.*, 1974). It joins the supraorbital nerve, accompanies it in the anterior two-thirds of the orbit, and traverses the supraorbital notch or foramen to reach areolar tissue of the scalp deep to frontalis. Here the artery anastomoses with the superficial temporal and supratrochlear arteries. It supplies levator, upper eyelid, scalp, periorbita and diplöe of the frontal bone. Occasional twigs supply

adipose tissue and, rarely, the trochlea and dura of the anterior cranial fossa (Hayreh, 1962).

Adipose branches

Adipose branches arise close to the origin of the anterior ethmoidal artery and supply adipose areolar tissue and the fascias of some muscles (Henry, 1959).

The anterior ethmoidal artery (Figs 5.18 and 5.21)

This branch is larger than the posterior branch although their sizes are reciprocal (Sappey, 1888). It arises from the ophthalmic artery between the superior oblique and medial rectus. With the anterior ethmoidal nerve it traverses the anterior ethmoidal canal to enter the anterior cranial fossa on the cribriform plate. It leaves this by a slit to reach a groove on the deep surface of the nasal bone, appearing on the face between the lateral nasal cartilage and the nasal bone to supply the dorsum of the nasal root. A small branch enters the frontal sinus. Its anterior meningeal branch supplies dura mater in the anterior fossa, including the anterior falx cerebri (Kuhn, 1961; Müller, 1977), mucous membrane anteriorly in the nasal cavity, the anterior ethmoidal air sinuses and nasal skin. Orbital branches supply superior oblique, occasionally medial rectus and inferior oblique, and rarely periosteum and adipose tissue at the medial side of the orbit (Meyer, 1887; Hayreh, 1962).

The medial palpebral arteries

One for each eyelid, these arise separately or together from the main ophthalmic trunk or its dorsal nasal branch. They enter the lids, above and below the medial palpebral ligament; the inferior artery is always the larger. They anastomose with the lateral palpebral arteries (see above) to form superior and inferior arcades in each lid and supply all lid tissues, including skin, muscle, glands, and conjunctiva. These branches also supply the lacrimal caruncle and sac, rarely the nasolacrimal duct, and occasionally levator, the orbital floor and the medial wall (Hayreh, 1962).

Collaterals to the optic nerve sheath

These arise anywhere from the first to proximal third part of the ophthalmic artery.

Periosteal branches

There may be one to four of these branches, which supply the anterior medial orbital wall (Hayreh, 1962) but otherwise arise as a plexus of tiny branches from the ethmoidal, supraorbital and infraorbital arteries, and lacrimal and levator networks (Henry, 1959).

The terminal part of the ophthalmic artery continues to the anterior orbital margin and divides into its **terminal branches**.

The dorsal nasal artery

This branch pierces the orbital septum between the medial palpebral ligament and trochlea, and anastomoses with angular and nasal branches of the facial artery. It supplies skin of the nasal root, the lacrimal sac (perhaps infrequently; Hayreh, 1962), and may give rise to the medial palpebral arteries.

The supratrochlear artery (Figs 2.48 and 5.19)

This is usually the larger terminal branch and pierces the orbital septum with the supratrochlear nerve. It may arise anterior to the septum. It ascends round the supraorbital margin about 1.25 cm from the mid line and supplies skin, muscles and periosteum of the medial frontal scalp. It anastomoses with the supraorbital and opposite supratrochlear arteries, occasionally giving off the superior medial palpebral artery (Hayreh, 1962).

Episcleral and **conjunctival arteries**, and other small branches, are derived from the larger rami mentioned above. For example, small temporal and zygomatic arteries, branches of the lacrimal artery, pass into the canals of the corresponding branches of the zygomatic ramus of the trigeminal nerve.

Variations in the ophthalmic artery (Fig. 3.5)

1. The ophthalmic artery in 15% of cases crosses inferior to the optic nerve.
2. It may enter the orbit through the superior orbital fissure.
3. The lacrimal branch often, and the ophthalmic rarely, may arise from the middle meningeal artery by an enlargement of a recurrent lacrimal anastomosis with the middle meningeal.
4. The lacrimal may be reinforced by the anterior deep temporal.
5. The supraorbital and posterior ethmoidal are both inconstant, and often have accessory ciliary trunks. The dorsal nasal branch may partly replace the facial artery.

For further information consult Meyer (1887); Quain (1908); Whitnall (1932); Hayreh and Dass (1962b).

THE INFRAORBITAL ARTERY

This arises from the maxillary artery (external carotid) in the pterygopalatine fossa and enters the orbit through the posterior end of the inferior orbital fissure (Whitnall, 1932). It runs forward in the inferior orbital sulcus and canal to emerge on the face via the infraorbital foramen. It supplies the inferior orbit to a minor extent with branches to inferior rectus and oblique muscles, lacrimal gland and sac, orbicularis muscle and nasolacrimal duct and soft tissues of the orbital floor (Salamon, Raybund and Grisoli, 1971).

THE GREAT VESSELS OF THE NECK

The aortic arch gives off three branches from its upper aspect: the brachiocephalic trunk (innominate artery), the left common carotid artery, and the left subclavian artery. The right common carotid artery arises as the brachiocephalic trunk divides, behind the right sternoclavicular joint; the left arises from the aortic arch in the thorax, behind and to the left of the brachiocephalic trunk and ascends to the level of the left sternoclavicular joint, after which the course of the two common carotid arteries are similar (Williams and Warwick, 1980).

Each artery passes upwards and slightly laterally to the level of the upper border of the thyroid cartilage, where it divides into its internal and external divisions. The carotid sinus is present at its point of division, while the carotid body lies behind. In the lower neck the arteries are separated by the trachea and above by the thyroid gland, larynx and pharynx. The carotid artery is enclosed within the carotid sheath, which contains the internal jugular vein laterally and the vagus nerve posteriorly and between the two. Anteriorly, sometimes embedded in its sheath, is the superior root of the ansa cervicalis, joined by its inferior root. Posteriorly it is separated from the transverse processes of the fourth, fifth and sixth cervical vertebrae by the longus colli, longus capitis, the origin of the scalenus anterior and the sympathetic trunk. On the right side, the recurrent laryngeal nerve passes behind the lower part of the artery.

External carotid

The external carotid artery passes upwards and forwards, and then inclines backwards to a point behind the neck of the mandible, where it divides in the substance of the parotid gland into its terminal branches: the superficial temporal and maxillary arteries. Its other branches are the superior thyroid, ascending pharyngeal, lingual, facial, occipital and the posterior auricular arteries.

Internal carotid

The internal carotid artery ascends to the base of the skull from its origin at the carotid bifurcation and enters the skull through the carotid canal of the petrous part of the temporal bone. In the neck it lies anterior to the transverse processes of the upper three cervical vertebrae, lying at first superficial and then passing deeply, medial to the posterior belly of the digastric. Below the digastric is the hypoglossal nerve; above the digastric it is separated from the external carotid artery by the styloid process and its attached muscles. Posteriorly it is separated from the longus capitis by the superior cervical ganglion. Medially are the pharynx and the superior laryngeal nerve. Below the base of the skull the jugular vein and vagus lie laterally to the artery; at the base of the skull the vein lies posteriorly, separated from the artery by the glossopharyngeal, vagus, accessory and hypoglossal nerves. Within the petrous bone the internal carotid ascends and then passes forwards, to enter the cranial cavity above the fibrocartilage of the foramen lacerum. It lies at first anterior to the cochlea and tympanic cavity, separated from the latter and from the auditory tube by a thin lamella which may be absorbed in old age. It is separated from the trigeminal ganglion by a thin plate of bone, which may be deficient, the roof of the carotid canal, and the floor of the trigeminal impression. The artery is surrounded by a plexus of small veins, and by the carotid plexus of nerves, derived in part from the internal carotid branch of the superior cervical ganglion.

In the cavernous sinus the carotid artery is covered by the lining endothelium of the venous channels. It at first ascends to the side of the posterior clinoid process and then passes forwards on the side of the sphenoid. It then passes upwards medial to the anterior clinoid process, and exits the cavernous sinus through its dural roof. The artery is surrounded by the carotid plexus of nerves; the oculomotor, trochlear, ophthalmic, and abducent nerves lie lateral to it.

After perforating the dura the artery turns backwards below the optic nerve and runs between the optic and oculomotor nerves to the anterior per-

forated substance. Here it divides into **anterior** and **middle cerebral** arteries.

The internal carotid artery gives off caroticotympanic and pterygoid branches in its petrous part and cavernous, hypophyseal and meningeal branches in its cavernous part. The branches from its cerebral part are the ophthalmic, posterior communicating, anterior choroidal, anterior cerebral and middle cerebral arteries.

Vertebral arteries

The vertebral arteries arise from the first part of the subclavian arteries. Each artery ascends through the foramina of the transverse process of all but the seventh cervical vertebrae, winds behind the lateral mass of the atlas, and enters the skull through the foramen magnum. At the lower border of the pons the two vertebrals join to form the basilar artery. The vertebral arteries give off muscular, spinal, meningeal and medullary branches. The largest branch is the posterior inferior cerebellar artery. Thrombosis of the anterior spinal artery causes the medial medullary syndrome; that of the posterior inferior cerebellar artery causes a lateral medullary syndrome.

THE CEREBRAL ARTERIES (Figs 3.6, 15.68 and 15.30)

The anterior cerebral artery

The anterior cerebral artery leaves the internal carotid near the anterior perforated substance, crosses above the optic nerve, approaches and joins its fellow through the **anterior communicating artery**, about 4 mm long. It then curls round the front (or genu) of the corpus callosum, over which it runs to the splenium, where it anastomoses with the posterior cerebral artery (Figs 3.7 and 3.8).

This artery supplies the front of the caudate nucleus via the anterior perforated substance, the corpus callosum, medial aspect of the hemisphere as far as the parieto-occipital sulcus, a strip of its superolateral surface, and medial part of the inferior surface of the frontal lobe (Figs 3.9 and 3.10).

Note that the anterior cerebral artery supplies the upper aspect of the chiasma and intracranial part of the optic nerve.

The middle cerebral artery

This is the largest branch of the internal carotid, being its direct continuation, and runs laterally into the lateral sulcus and divides on the insula to supply

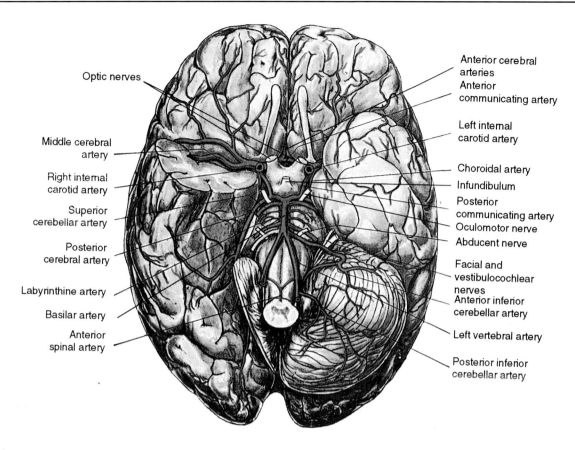

Optic nerves

Middle cerebral artery

Right internal carotid artery

Superior cerebellar artery

Posterior cerebral artery

Labyrinthine artery

Basilar artery

Anterior spinal artery

Anterior cerebral arteries

Anterior communicating artery

Left internal carotid artery

Choroidal artery

Infundibulum

Posterior communicating artery

Oculomotor nerve

Abducent nerve

Facial and vestibulocochlear nerves

Anterior inferior cerebellar artery

Left vertebral artery

Posterior inferior cerebellar artery

Fig. 3.6 The arteries at the base of the brain. The right temporal pole and right hemisphere of the cerebellum have been removed. (From Williams, P.L. *et al.* (eds) (1995) *Gray's Anatomy*, 38th edition, published by Churchill Livingstone.)

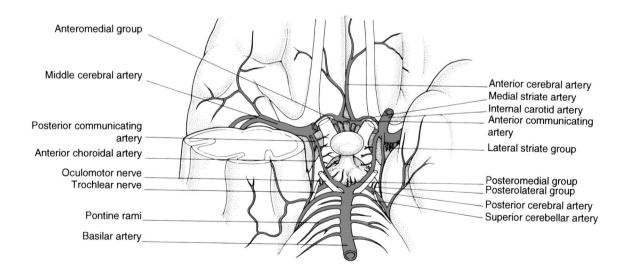

Anteromedial group

Middle cerebral artery

Posterior communicating artery

Anterior choroidal artery

Oculomotor nerve

Trochlear nerve

Pontine rami

Basilar artery

Anterior cerebral artery

Medial striate artery

Internal carotid artery

Anterior communicating artery

Lateral striate group

Posteromedial group

Posterolateral group

Posterior cerebral artery

Superior cerebellar artery

Fig. 3.7 The cerebral arterial circle (Willis) at the base of the brain showing the distribution of the ganglionic branches. These vessels form anteromedial, posteromedial, posterolatreal and lateral striated groups. The medial striate and anterior choroidal arteries are also shown. (Redrawn from Carpenter, M.B. (1976) *Human Neuroanatomy*, 7th edition, published by Williams & Wilkins.)

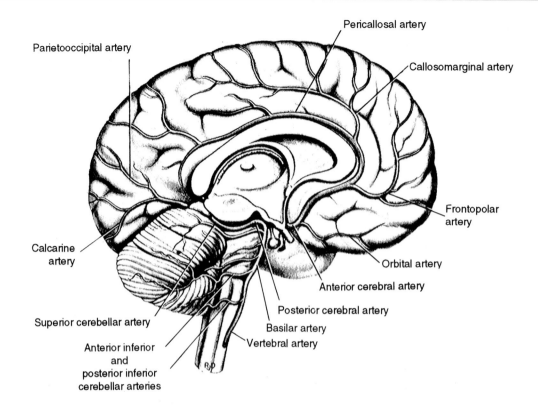

Fig. 3.8 Principal arteries on the medial surface of the cerebrum shown together with the arteries of the brain stem and cerebellum. (From Carpenter, M.B. (1976) *Human Neuroanatomy*, 7th edition, published by Williams & Wilkins.)

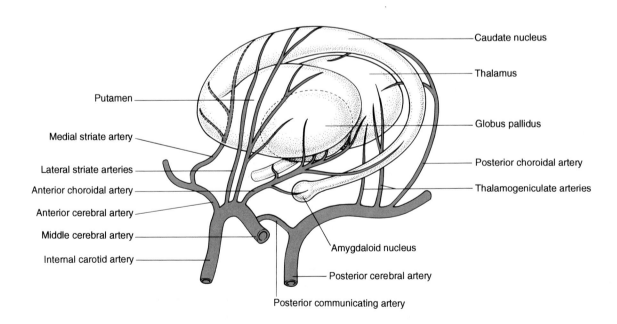

Fig. 3.9 Diagrammatic representation of the arterial supply of the corpus striatum and thalamus. (Redrawn from Carpenter, M.B. (1976) *Human Neuroanatomy*, 7th edition, published by Williams & Wilkins.)

the lateral aspect of the hemisphere, except along its superior (anterior cerebral) and lower (posterior cerebral) borders (Figs 3.11 and 3.12).

Its medial and lateral striate branches enter the brain via the anterior perforated substance. The **medial striate arteries** traverse and supply the medial part of the lentiform nucleus, and also send branches to the caudate nucleus and internal capsule. The **lateral striate arteries** pass between the lentiform nucleus and the external capsule. The largest was called by Charcot the 'artery of cerebral haemorrhage': Abbie (1933–34), however, emphasizes the

crowding of all branches of the middle cerebral artery at the base of the external capsule in the human brain, which may explain the common occurrence of haemorrhage at this site.

The middle cerebral artery supplies the inferolateral aspect of the chiasma and the anterior part of the optic tract. Its deep optic branch supplies the optic radiation. Its cortical branches anastomose with the calcarine branch of the posterior cerebral to supply a small area of striate cortex, concerned with macular vision.

The **deep optic artery** (Abbie, 1933) is a member

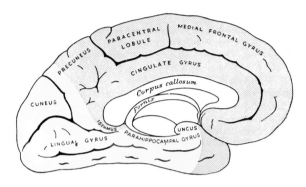

Fig. 3.10 Lateral surface of the left cerebral hemisphere showing areas supplied by the cerebral arteries. Blue = anterior cerebral artery territory; pink = middle cerebral artery territory; yellow = posterior cerebral artery territory. (From Williams, P.L. *et al.* (eds) (1995) *Gray's Anatomy*, 38th edition, published by Churchill Livingstone.)

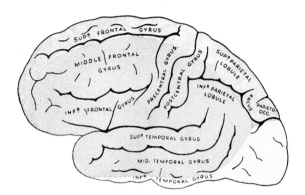

Fig. 3.12 Lateral surface of the left cerebral hemisphere showing areas supplied by the cerebral arteries. Key as in Fig. 3.10. (From Williams, P.L. *et al.* (eds) (1995) *Gray's Anatomy*, 38th edition, published by Churchill Livingstone.)

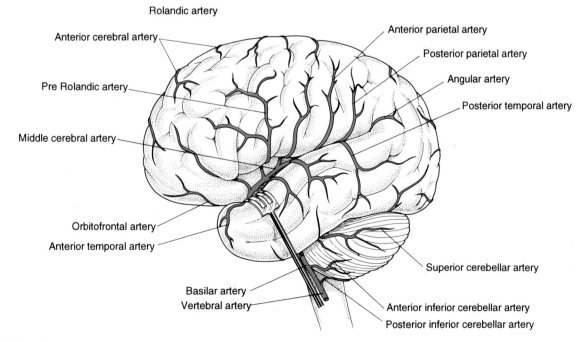

Fig. 3.11 Principal arteries on the lateral surface of the cerebrum and cerebellum. (Redrawn from Carpenter, M.B. (1976) *Human Neuroanatomy*, 7th edition, published by Williams & Wilkins.)

of the lateral striate group and turns posteriorly, partly passing through the putamen, to reach fibres from the infralenticular and retrolenticular parts of the internal capsule, thus supplying the auditory and optic radiations as they leave the capsule (Figs 15.69 and 15.70).

The posterior communicating artery

The posterior communicating artery arises from the internal carotid close to the origin of the middle cerebral. It is usually small, but may be so large that its continuation appears to be the posterior cerebral artery. It may be absent, and the right and left arteries are frequently unequal.

This artery passes horizontally and postero-medially to join the posterior cerebral artery, a branch of the basilar artery, at the superior border of the cerebral peduncle, thus forming an anastomosis between the internal carotid and vertebral arteries. It crosses medially under the posterolateral angle of the chiasma or beginning of the optic tract (Figs 15.30, 15.68 and 15.79). Near the cerebral peduncle it crosses medially above the oculomotor nerve (Fig. 5.2), which may thus be compressed by an aneurysm at this site. It supplies the genu and anterior third of the posterior limb of the internal capsule, and sends branches to the globus pallidus and thalamus.

Note that the posterior communicating artery supplies the inferior part of the chiasma and anterior third of the optic tract.

The anterior choroidal and posterior communicating arteries, like most of the vessels of the interpeduncular space, vary reciprocally: thus one or other may predominate to the almost complete exclusion of the other, and either may usurp the stem of the posterior cerebral artery which then arises from the internal carotid and takes over the whole of the supply to the posterior cerebral field (Abbie, 1934) (see also Gillilan, 1959; Alper, Berry and Paddison, 1959). There is also often asymmetry between these paired vessels.

The anterior choroidal artery

This arises from the internal carotid just beyond the posterior communicating, lateral to the start of the optic tract (Figs 15.30, 15.68, 15.69 and 15.89) (see Abbie, 1934; Carpenter, Noback and Ross, 1954; Herman, 1966).

It runs posteromedially, crossing under the optic tract and its medial side. At the anterior part of the lateral geniculate body it turns laterally, across the optic tract, and divides into branches which enter the inferior horn of the lateral ventricle to reach the anteroinferior part of the choroid plexus. As it passes posteriorly the artery's branches pierce or curl medial and lateral to the optic tract (Fig. 15.30).

Next to the internal carotid, the anterior choroidal artery is the main supply of the internal capsule, vascularizing more than the posterior two-thirds of the posterior limb, and also all its infralenticular and retrolenticular parts, containing the auditory and optic radiations. It also gives branches to the middle third of the cerebral peduncle, the tail of the caudate nucleus, the thalamus and globus pallidus and other structures in the interpeduncular region.

Note that, apart from twigs to the pial network supplying the chiasma, the anterior choroidal artery is the main supply to the optic tract (posterior two-thirds), and supplies the anterolateral part of the lateral geniculate body, and the commencement of the optic radiation (Fig. 15.70). The supply to the tract is mainly via the pial plexus.

The arterial circle

The arterial circle (of Willis) (Figs 3.13, 5.2, 15.30 and 15.79) is the anastomosis of the two internal carotid and basilar arteries. It is the most important bypass when internal carotid or vertebral arteries are blocked.

Set in the subarachnoid space, around the periphery of the interpeduncular cistern, it is formed posteriorly by the two posterior cerebral arteries at the termination of the basilar, and anteriorly by the anterior cerebral arteries, linked by the anterior communicating artery. On each side a **posterior communicating artery** connects the end of the internal carotid or middle cerebral to the posterior cerebral artery. The 'circle', which is somewhat hexagonal, is very variable in the size of its sources. (For further details and variations, see Fawcett and Blachford, 1906; Watts, 1934; Paget, 1945; Kuhn, 1961; Gillilan, 1962, 1972).

The basilar artery

This branch is formed by union of the two vertebral arteries ventral to the pons. It runs upwards between the median groove of the pons and cranial base to bifurcate into the two posterior cerebral arteries at the superior pontine border of the pons.

Bilateral branches of the basilar artery

Pontine   Several on each side penetrate the pons.

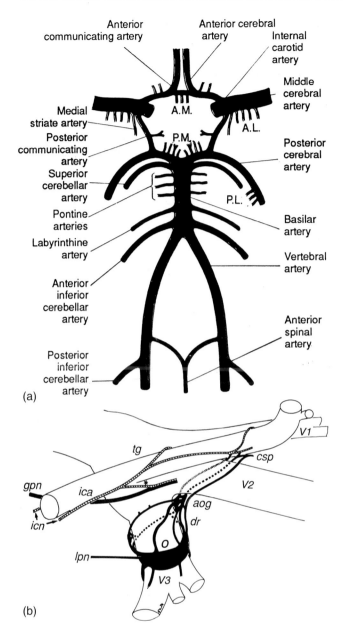

(a)

(b)

Fig. 3.13 (a) The arteries at the base of the brain, showing the constitution of the arterial circle. AL = Anterolateral central branches; AM = anteromedial central branches; PL = posterolateral central branches; PM = posteromedial central branches. (From Williams, P.L. *et al.* (eds) (1995) *Gray's Anatomy*, 38th edition, published by Churchill Livingstone.) (b) Drawing of the trigeminal nerve, the otic ganglion and a representative sample of its dorsal rami viewed from the medial aspect. The solid, broken and shaded lines crossing the maxillary nerve (*V2*) are dorsal otic rami passing medial to, through and lateral to the nerve. *aog*, Accessory otic ganglion; *csp*, cavernous sinus plexus; *dr*, dorsal rami; *gpn*, greater petrosal nerve; *ica*, internal carotid artery; *icn*, internal carotid nerve branches; *lpn*, lesser petrosal nerve; *o*, otic ganglion; *tg*, trigeminal ganglion; *V1, V2, V3*, ophthalmic, maxillary and mandibular nerves. The asterisk indicates the junction of the deep petrosal and greater petrosal nerves to form the nerve of the pterygoid canal – the nerve is cut at its point of entry into the canal. (From Ruskell, G. L. and Simons, T. (1992) *Brain Res.*, **595**, 116 with permission.)

Labyrinthine (internal auditory) This is more often derived from the anterior inferior cerebellar artery, passes laterally with the facial and vestibulocochlear nerves into the internal auditory meatus to supply the labyrinth.

The posterior cerebral artery

Each is formed at the bifurcation of the basilar (Figs 3.7 and 3.13a) and winds round the inferior border of its cerebral peduncle (Figs 15.30, 15.68, 15.69, 15.79 and 15.89). It runs below and parallel to the optic tract, which is at the upper border of the brain stem, and also below the uncus and hippocampal gyrus. Inferior to it is the superior cerebellar artery, and between the two are the oculomotor and trochlear nerves. The artery lies anterior to or among the radicles of the oculomotor and next to the trochlear at the side of the mid brain.

Continuing back above the margin of the tentorium cerebelli, the posterior cerebral artery passes under the splenium and enters the anterior end of the calcarine sulcus, whence its branches run to the parieto-occipital and posterior part of the calcarine sulci. Note that the central branches of these superficial 'feeders' do not anastomose (Gillilan, 1959, 1962).

The **calcarine artery** runs posteriorly, deep in its sulcus (Fig. 15.68), to the occipital pole, curving round this into the lateral calcarine sulcus (if present) to reach the lateral surface of the occipital lobe. Arterial twigs emerge from the sulcus and extend above and below to the limits of the striate area. On the lateral surface the artery supplies all the striate cortex except the peripheral fringe, where the supply is by anastomosing twigs from the middle cerebral (Shellshear, 1927; Abbie, 1933).

The calcarine artery also sends perforating **posterolateral central arteries** to the posterior part of the optic radiation as it diverges towards the cortex.

Near the lateral geniculate body the posterior cerebral artery gives off the **posterior choroidal arteries** (Abbie, 1933), one of which commonly ramifies in the geniculate body.

The posterior cerebral artery thus supplies: the medial surface and posterior lateral surface of the occipital lobe; the posterior part of the optic radiation; the tentorial surface of the cerebrum, except its temporal pole; and the thalamus, internal capsule, red nucleus, geniculate bodies, tela choroidea and choroid plexus of the lateral ventricle.

Note that it supplies the posteromedial part of the lateral geniculate body, most of the visual cortex, and the posterior region of the optic radiation. Hence, blockage of, say, a right posterior cerebral artery may cause destruction of nerve fibres from the right side of each retina, leading to left homonymous hemianopia, sensory aphasia and sometimes hemianaesthesia, by involvement of the posterior part of the internal capsule.

INNERVATION OF THE CEREBRAL ARTERIES

Most of the nerve terminals serving the cerebral arteries are autonomic motor, from the superior cervical, pterygopalatine and possibly the otic ganglia. The sympathetic neurotransmitters induce vasoconstriction and the parasympathetic neuro-transmitters induce vasodilatation. The vascular innervation density is greater in the anterior part of the circle of Willis for adrenergic, cholinergic and peptidergic nerves in a variety of mammals. In the monkey, the adventitia of the internal carotid artery within the carotid canal is continuous with that of the surrounding venous sleeve. The sleeve is bridged by trabeculae, in one of which the internal carotid nerve runs. The nerve divides into two, and gives off fine twigs, which cross the trabeculae to enter the artery; there are few arterial terminals within the canal or in the region of the foramen lacerum. Within the cavernous sinus there is a sharp increase in the number of terminals which, with some variation between animals, constitutes a nerve terminal sleeve (Ruskell and Simon, 1992). This reaches a maximum at the base of the carotid siphon and there is then a sharp fall in density of innervation as the artery leaves the sinus. Innervation densities in the basilar artery and at the circle of Willis are low. Ruskell has speculated that some of these nerve terminals are vasomotor in function, and could explain the vasoconstriction of the internal carotid artery which has been reported in patients suffering from cluster headaches (Ekbom and Greits, 1970) or ophthalmic migraine (Walsh and O'Doherty, 1960). Distension of the internal carotid artery occurs in classical migraine (Friberg et al., 1991), and the pain of distension may be reproduced experimentally by balloon inflation of the middle cerebral artery (Nichols et al., 1990). Trigeminal terminals are relatively infrequent on the cerebral vessels, but are known to be nociceptive (Moskowitz, 1984) and responsible for the pain induced by stimulation of large arteries at the base of the brain (Nichols et al., 1990). Trigeminal terminals innervate the internal carotid artery in the cavernous sinus in monkeys, and could mediate pain at this site in humans.

The otic ganglion is part of the classically accepted cerebral parasympathetic outflow, populated by cholinergic and VIPergic neurones (Edvisson et al., 1989; Suzuki et al., 1990). Postganglionic fibres enter the auriculotemporal branch of the mandibular nerve and terminate in the parotid gland (Williams et al., 1989). In addition to these branches of the ganglion, there are also two dorsal rami, one of which penetrates the pterygoid canal to join the vidian nerve, the other joining the trigeminal ganglion (Fig. 3.13b) (Hovelaque, 1927). In 1922, Rousset described only one dorsal branch, passing to the middle meningeal artery. Andes and Kautzky (1955, 1956) identified dorsal branches in human embryonic tissue, one passing to a small ganglion in the cavernous sinus, another joining the vidian nerve.

There is now little doubt that otic ganglion fibres pass to the cerebral vasculature (Fig. 3.13b). The ganglion straddles the mandibular nerve and receives chiefly myelinated fibres. In addition to those fibres (which it gives off to the mandibular nerve) it gives rise, for instance in the monkey, to a number of nerves, which enter the cranium through the foramen lacerum closely associated with the mandibular nerve. Most rami are myelinated but a few are unmyelinated. Cell bodies are disposed in groups along the rami, and close to the trigeminal ganglion form an accessory otic ganglion. Synapses are only found in the otic and accessory otic ganglion. A small plexus is formed by the accessory otic ganglion, which receives recurrent branches from the mandibular nerve. The dorsal rami continue beyond the plexus and carry postganglionic parasympathetic, and mandibular sensory fibres to the cavernous sinus plexus which receives its sympathetic supply from the internal carotid nerve. This distribution provides parasympathetic, sympathetic and sensory fibres to the cerebral arteries, and to orbital structures via the retroorbital plexus (Ruskell, 1985).

3.3 THE VEINS OF THE ORBIT

THE ANGULAR VEIN

This is formed at a junction of the frontal, orbital, and facial veins by the union of the supraorbital and supratrochlear veins. It descends lateral to the nose with the angular artery, across the nasal edge of the medial palpebral ligament, 8 mm from the medial canthus (Fig. 2.63). It is subcutaneous, and is often visible as a blue ridge until it pierces the orbicularis. The vein (or one of its palpebral branches) complicates surgical approaches to the lacrimal sac. It

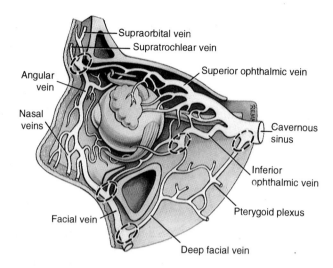

Fig. 3.14 Scheme of the veins of the orbit.

communicates freely with the superior ophthalmic vein and hence the cavernous sinus, and is continuous with the facial vein (Fig. 3.14).

Tributaries of the angular vein

The supraorbital vein

This vein runs along the superior orbital margin deep to orbicularis, which it pierces medially to join the supratrochlear and form the angular vein. It communicates with the superior ophthalmic vein through the supraorbital notch, receiving here a vein from the frontal sinus and diplöe.

The supratrochlear vein

The supratrochlear vein descends the forehead with the supratrochlear artery.

The superior and inferior superficial palpebral veins

These drain into the supraorbital vein. One of the superior group often crosses the medial palpebral ligament between the angular vein and the medial canthus, and is visible through the skin.

Superficial nasal branches

These drain nasal skin.

THE FACIAL VEIN

The facial vein descends obliquely backwards in the face, lateral and superficial to its accompanying artery. It crosses the mandible, and joins the **posterior facial** (retromandibular) **vein** to form the **common facial vein**, which ends in the **internal jugular vein**.

The facial vein communicates with the pterygoid venous plexus (Fig. 3.14), and thus with the cavernous sinus.

The flow from the frontal region is into the angular and facial veins, but it is easy to occlude the facial vein (e.g. by lying face down on a soft pillow), and then blood may flow via the angular vein into the ophthalmic veins: hence the danger of sepsis spreading from forehead and face to the cavernous sinus.

The orbit is drained by the superior and associated ophthalmic veins. They and their tributaries, like most head veins, have no valves, are tortuous, and form plexiform anastomoses. They communicate with the facial and nasal veins and pterygoid plexus and end in the cavernous sinus. The superior ophthalmic vein is the largest and most constant and drains the inferior and middle ophthalmic veins, among others. Two **venous networks**, of which the inferior is the larger, are connected to these veins by collaterals (Figs 3.3 and 3.15).

The veins of the orbit are:

1. superior ophthalmic;
2. inferior ophthalmic;
3. middle ophthalmic;
4. medial ophthalmic;
5. central retinal;
6. tributaries and connections of the ophthalmic veins
   (a) vorticose;
   (b) lacrimal;
   (c) transverse supraoptic;
   (d) muscular;
   (e) ethmoidal;
   (f) palpebral;
7. inferior and superior venous networks;
8. collateral system.

THE SUPERIOR OPHTHALMIC VEIN

This has two roots. The superior root connects with the **supraorbital vein** via or medial to the supraorbital notch. It passes posteromedially under the orbital roof and joins the inferior root, a few millimetres behind the reflected superior oblique tendon. The inferior root connects with the **angular vein**. It arises in the orbit above the medial palpebral ligament and

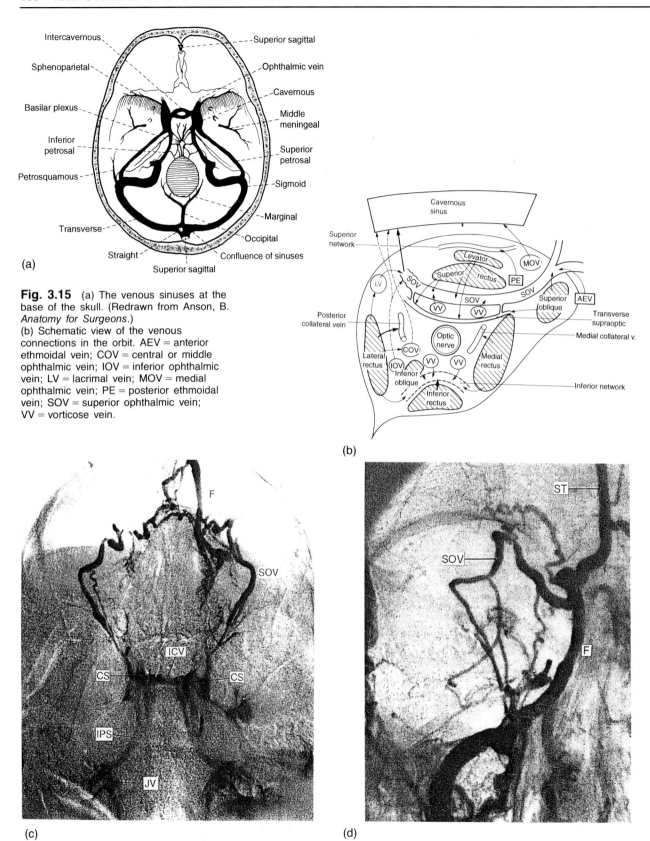

Fig. 3.15 (a) The venous sinuses at the base of the skull. (Redrawn from Anson, B. *Anatomy for Surgeons.*)
(b) Schematic view of the venous connections in the orbit. AEV = anterior ethmoidal vein; COV = central or middle ophthalmic vein; IOV = inferior ophthalmic vein; LV = lacrimal vein; MOV = medial ophthalmic vein; PE = posterior ethmoidal vein; SOV = superior ophthalmic vein; VV = vorticose vein.

(c) Orbital venogram, basal view. F = facial vein; SOV = superior orbital vein; C = cavernous sinus; ICV = intercavernous vein; JV = jugular vein; IPS = inferior petrosal sinus. (Courtesy of Dr G. Lloyd.) (d) Orbital venogram, anteroposterior view. S = supratrochlear; SOV = superior orbital vein; F = facial vein. (Courtesy of Dr G. Lloyd.)

accompanies the ophthalmic artery between the optic nerve and superior rectus to the superior orbital fissure, by which it leaves the orbit to enter the cavernous sinus. Commonly it is joined by the inferior ophthalmic vein.

In the superior fissure the superior ophthalmic vein is usually above the annular tendon, but may pass between the two heads of the lateral rectus or below the tendon (Fig. 3.3). In conditions of raised cavernous sinus pressure (such as caroticocavernous fistula) its engorged state is apparent on orbital venography.

Three parts of the vein are described:

First part

The first part runs posteriorly in adipose tissue to the medial border of the superior rectus within a condensation of connective tissue connecting it to neighbouring structures (Henry 1959; Renard, Lemasson and Saraux, 1965).

Second part

The second part passes posterolaterally in a connective tissue 'hammock' (Koorneef, 1987) to the lateral border of the superior rectus.

Third part

The third part passes dorsomedially to the superior orbital fissure, entering the cavernous sinus through the dense dural tissue which fills it. In its course an aponeurosis from the superior and lateral recti connects the vein to the dura (Henry, 1959).

THE INFERIOR OPHTHALMIC VEIN

This vein is a short trunk which arises anteriorly on the floor of the orbit from the inferior venous network within the muscle cone (Seseman, 1869; Festal, 1887). It runs backwards on inferior rectus and drains into the cavernous sinus directly, or via the ophthalmic vein. It lies in close contact with Müller's orbital muscle (Frund, 1911). While Rouviere (1967) describes the vein as arising anteromedially, Huber (1975) found it only as a venous network.

THE MIDDLE OPHTHALMIC VEIN

The middle ophthalmic vein arises near the lateral side of the medial rectus, the inferior margin of the lateral rectus, or the lateral collateral vein. It drains the inferior venous network and, leaving the muscle cone, joins the confluence of the superior ophthalmic

vein with the cavernous sinus (Henry, 1959). Brismar (1974) regards it as a second inferior ophthalmic vein, with a higher course and connected to it by collaterals. It is present in 1–20% of orbits (Jo and Trauzettel, 1974; Brismar, 1974).

MEDIAL OPHTHALMIC VEIN

A medial ophthalmic vein was described by Brismar (1974) in 40% of phlebograms. It arises from the inferior root or first segment of the superior ophthalmic vein, follows the orbital roof backwards close to the medial orbital wall, and descends to the cavernous sinus (Gurwitsch, 1883).

CENTRAL RETINAL VEIN

The central vein of the retina leaves the optic sheath anterior to the central retinal artery, and joins a network of venules from the sheath, the ophthalmic artery and adipose tissue. It drains, usually, into the superior ophthalmic or posterior collateral vein, occasionally the inferior ophthalmic and rarely (Whitnall, 1932) if ever (Henry, 1959) into the cavernous sinus.

TRIBUTARIES AND CONNECTIONS OF THE OPHTHALMIC VEINS

Vortex veins

There are usually four or more veins. The **superomedial** drains into the first part of the superior ophthalmic (Renard, Lemasson and Saraux, 1965), while the **superolateral** enters its third part between its bend at the lateral margin of the optic nerve and the lateral orbital wall (Henry, 1959). The **inferior** veins join to form the inferior venous plexus.

The lacrimal vein

The lacrimal vein is formed by confluence of a principal lacrimal vein and muscular veins from the superior and lateral rectus. It connects with the lateral palpebral, conjunctival and extraorbital veins, draining into the superior ophthalmic vein's third part (Henry, 1959) or occasionally into the cavernous sinus (Duke-Elder, 1961). Its posterior part is seen in about 75% of phlebograms (Brismar, 1974).

The transverse supraoptic vein

Lying lateral to the superior ophthalmic vein, the transverse supraoptic vein is parallel with it above the optic nerve and joins it posteriorly (Henry, 1959; Renard, Lemasson and Saraux, 1965).

The muscular veins

Numbering three or four, the muscular veins form a rich network from the levator entering the superior ophthalmic vein along its course. Tributaries from the superior oblique and rectus join the supraoptic vein, or the roots or second part respectively of the superior ophthalmic vein. Branches from the lateral rectus drain chiefly into the posterior collateral vein, and also into the lacrimal and middle vein as well as the inferior network, which also drains the inferior and medial rectus. The **medial collateral vein** also receives tributaries from the medial rectus (Henry, 1959).

The presence of **anterior ciliary veins** has been queried (Seseman, 1869), but Bedrossian (1958) and Henry (1959) describe them as collateral to the anterior ciliary arteries and as joining the muscular veins.

Ethmoidal veins

These correspond to the arteries. The **anterior ethmoidal vein** enters the inferior root of the superior ophthalmic or its first part the **posterior ethmoidal vein** joins the superior network above the superior rectus and levator.

Palpebral veins

The **medial palpebral veins** drain into the inferior root of the superior ophthalmic or supraorbital vein. One of the upper group often crosses the medial palpebral ligament between the angular vein and the medial canthus and is visible under the skin. **Lateral palpebral veins** connect with the lacrimal group (Henry, 1959). The veins of the lacrimal sac and nasolacrimal duct enter the inferior venous network, the sac veins also draining into the inferior root of the superior ophthalmic (Renard, Lemasson and Saraux, 1965).

INFERIOR AND SUPERIOR VENOUS NETWORK

The **inferior venous network** lies in an anteromedial to posterolateral axis near the orbital floor. Anteriorly it lies between the inferior and medial recti; its inferior part is between inferior rectus and the globe in the muscle cone, and extends posterolaterally (Henry, 1959). The **superior network** is smaller and is above the levator.

COLLATERAL SYSTEM

The collateral veins form an anastomotic loop between the superior and inferior ophthalmic veins, participating in the inferior venous network. The **anterior collateral vein** joins the inferior root of the superior ophthalmic vein at the anterior medial orbital wall while the **medial collateral vein** links the inferior network to its first part. Laterally, an **anteroexternal vein** runs between globe and lateral rectus from the inferior network to the lacrimal vein. A **posteroexternal** vein joins this network to the superior ophthalmic near the lateral orbital wall (Henry, 1959).

3.4 THE CAVERNOUS SINUSES

The cavernous sinuses are paired structures on each side of the pituitary fossa (Fig. 3.16). They were once thought to lie, like other intracranial venous sinuses, within a dural compartment. The apparent division of the main compartment by fine fibrous trabeculae gave rise to the name of 'cavernous' sinus. However, though it retains this title it is now considered that the 'sinus' is a venous plexus interspersed by delicate connective tissue and some fat cells. It is bounded anteriorly by the medial part of the superior orbital fissure, superiorly by anterior and posterior clinoid processes, posteriorly by the dorsum sellae and inferiorly by the foramina lacerum, ovale and rotundum. Inferomedially lie the sphenoid sinus and part of the frontal bone, while superomedially is the pituitary fossa. Corrosion casts reveal a structure about 3 cm long, 1.05 cm high, 0.5 cm wide and tapering inferiorly and anteriorly to less than 1 mm. The cavernous sinus is contained in a dural compartment which is thickest in its outermost leaf (the inferior and lateral walls) and thinnest medially, where it invests the sphenoid bone. The outer leaf, where it is traversed by the third, fourth and fifth nerves is thinnest on its innermost aspect.

In each sinus lies the internal carotid artery and, laterally, an abducent nerve. The internal carotid artery enters the sinus by ascending from the end of the carotid canal medial in the foramen lacerum, between the lingula and petrosal process of the sphenoid (Figs 1.11 and 5.5). It then turns forwards in a groove on the body of the sphenoid medial to the anterior clinoid process, where it turns to pierce the roof of the sinus between the optic and oculomotor nerves (Fig. 5.2). In the sinus it is surrounded by sympathetic plexus filaments. Its presence in the sinus explains how arteriovenous aneurysms may arise after fracture of the cranial base.

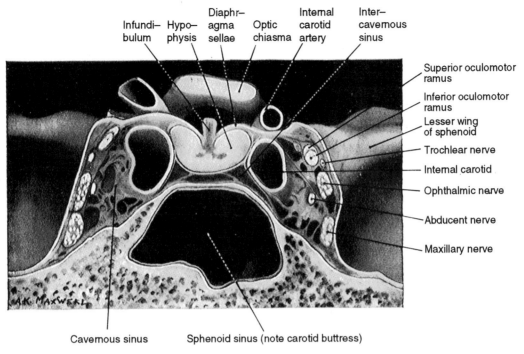

Infundi-bulum, Hypo-physis, Diaphr-agma sellae, Optic chiasma, Internal carotid artery, Inter-cavernous sinus

Superior oculomotor ramus
Inferior oculomotor ramus
Lesser wing of sphenoid
Trochlear nerve
Internal carotid
Ophthalmic nerve
Abducent nerve
Maxillary nerve

Cavernous sinus   Sphenoid sinus (note carotid buttress)

Fig. 3.16 The cavernous sinuses. (After Elliot Smith. Dissection in the Moorfields Hospital Pathological Museum.)

In its lateral wall, from above down, are the oculomotor, trochlear, ophthalmic and maxillary nerves, which pass forwards to the superior orbital fissure and foramen rotundum. Anterior in the sinus the trochlear nerve is above the oculomotor.

Further lateral to and in contact with the lateral wall of the sinus are the trigeminal ganglion (Fig. 5.16) and the temporal lobe of the cerebral hemisphere.

The carotid artery within the cavernous sinus has several branches (Fig. 3.17) (Parkinson, 1972).

THE MENINGOHYPOPHYSEAL ARTERY

This branch arises from the dorsum of the cavernous part of the artery just at, or proximal to, the apogee of its first forward curve. It splits at once into three vessels of nearly equal calibre (the tentorial, dorsal meningeal and inferior hypophyseal arteries). Here it is closely adherent to the wall of the carotid by delicate connective tissue.

Tentorial artery

The tentorial artery passes posterolaterally, and in the sinus supplies the third and fourth cranial nerves for a variable distance. It sends rami forward to the roof of the sinus to anastomose with ophthalmic meningeal branches. It leaves the sinus between two dural layers below the entry of the trochlear, to enter the tentorium to the lateral sinus for 5–8 cm up the falx, and anastomoses across the mid line.

Dorsal meningeal artery

The dorsal meningeal artery runs posteroinferiorly around the dorsum and down the clivus. It anastomoses with its fellow at the root of the dorsum sellae and with meningeal branches of the vertebral and cervical arteries down to the foramen magnum. A branch of varying size runs with the abducent nerve in Dorello's canal.

The inferior hypophyseal artery

This passes medially and slightly anteriorly to bifurcate or trifurcate near the floor of the sella turcica. The main branch lies along the floor of the sella between dural layers. The artery anastomoses directly with its fellow and sends small branches to the posterior hypophyseal lobe and to dura around the upper part of the posterior clinoid process. A variable anterior branch supplies cavernous structures.

The inferior hypophyseal and dorsal meningeal arteries form short, direct anastomoses with their opposite numbers, completing an **anterior circle** around the base of the dorsum sellae.

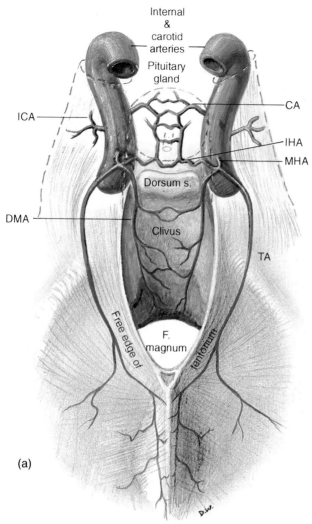

(a)

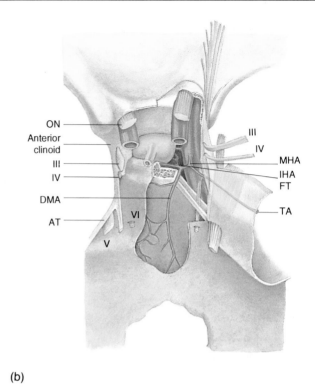

(b)

Fig. 3.17 Arteries arising from the carotid artery in the cavernous sinus.

INFERIOR CAVERNOUS SINUS

In about 80% of dissections an artery of the inferior cavernous sinus arises inferolaterally from the carotid 5 mm anterior to the meningohypophyseal (Fig. 3.17). It supplies the cavernous contents and dura inferiorly. It descends over the abducent nerve and beneath the trigeminal ganglion, supplying it. It also supplies the oculomotor, trochlear, and abducent nerves through most of its length and anastomoses with middle and accessory meningeal arteries near the foramen spinosum. The branches are mainly to dura deep to the ganglion.

CAPSULAR ARTERY

The capsular artery arises inferomedially from the carotid artery, 2–3 mm anterior to the inferior cavernous artery, and has one or two branches which run medially in the floor of the sella and anastomoses beneath the dura with their opposite numbers. They supply fine branches to the dura and anterior

pituitary. They may be absent, or arise from the inferior hypophyseal (McConnell, 1953).

Persistent trigeminal artery

An anomalous persistent trigeminal artery is occasionally found which departs below all the ocular motor nerves, unlike the foregoing arteries which depart above. It arises 5 mm proximal to the meningohypophyseal nerve and runs posterolaterally through the clival dura to anastomose directly with the basilar. It may be the site of saccular aneurysms.

STRUCTURE OF THE CAVERNOUS SINUS

Parkinson (1972) emphasized certain features. The plexus of veins making up the 'sinus' has no constant pattern and the confluence of smaller channels into the larger is inferior. As elsewhere in the head region, the veins have no valves, and they do not completely surround the carotid artery. Finally, the intracranial carotid artery is next to a variety of venous channels well before it enters the cavernous sinus.

Tributaries

Anteriorly, the ophthalmic veins and the sphenoparietal sinus lie along the lesser wing of the sphenoid. Superiorly, there is the superficial middle cerebral vein.

Drainage

The cavernous sinus is drained by superior and inferior petrosal sinuses and emissary veins through the foramen ovale and the foramen of Vesalius.

Communications

Communications of the cavernous sinus include: the intercavernous plexuses; the ophthalmic veins communicate with the angular vein on the face (thus a focus of infection in the upper face may produce thrombosis in the cavernous sinus, though this is now rare); the sphenoparietal sinus drains structures in the side and vault of the skull. The superficial middle cerebral vein drains the cerebral cortex adjoining the lateral sulcus. Thrombosis in the cavernous sinus may involve this vein.

NERVES OF THE CAVERNOUS SINUS (Figs 5.4, 5.5, 5.16 and 5.22)

The oculomotor and trochlear nerves enter the sinus posterosuperiorly through separate openings in a small concavity between the free tentorial edge and posterior clinoid process. They quickly come to lie in the same dural tunnel, with a thin inner dural sheet separating them from the cavernous compartment.

The trigeminal nerve is also lateral in the dural wall within the arachnoid and dural outpouching, the trigeminal cave (of Meckel). The arachnoid space sometimes extends externally anterior to each division of the nerve for a millimetre or so with a short sleeve. The dura propria of the cave can be dissected away from the lateral wall of the sinus; these layers are more firmly blended anteriorly but the trigeminal divisions can easily be separated from the lateral wall as far as the superior orbital fissure. The dura is thickest external to the nerve.

The abducent nerve as it leaves Dorello's canal curves sharply around the lateral aspect of the first part of the carotid artery and then ascends anteriorly,

deep to the ophthalmic division towards the superior orbital fissure. The oculomotor and trochlear nerves pass forwards and gradually downward, and with the trigeminal and abducent nerves form a triangle in the lateral wall of the sinus which is constant and affords a safe surgical approach to structures in the sinus.

LYMPHATICS

Posterior to the orbital septum the orbit contains no lymphatics or lymphoid tissue. The mode of return of orbital tissue fluids to the veins remains uncertain.

THE SUPERIOR PETROSAL SINUS

This skirts the upper border of the petrous temporal bone in the attached margin of the tentorum cerebelli. It crosses above the trigeminal and abducent nerves and drains the cavernous into the transverse sinus. It is usually small.

THE INFERIOR PETROSAL SINUS

This lies in a groove between the petrous temporal and basioccipital bones (Figs 3.18 and 5.15). It is often traversed by the abducent nerve and receives veins from the internal ear, and drains the cavernous sinus into the beginning of the internal jugular vein below the cranial base. This explains how cavernous thrombosis may spread to the transverse sinus, and may finally also produce postauricular swelling via the mastoid emissary vein. This vein traverses a foramen in the mastoid part of the temporal bone, and unites the sigmoid sinus to the posterior auricular vein. The communication between internal auditory veins and the inferior petrosal sinus is a route for spread of infection from the labyrinth to cavernous sinus.

EMISSARY VEIN

The emissary vein, which passes through the foramen of Vesalius, drains to the pterygoid plexus; so also do veins passing via the foramina ovale et lacerum. Moreover, there are indirect connections with the pterygoid plexus via the deep facial vein which unite it to the anterior facial vein, the continuation of the angular, and also via the branch which the inferior ophthalmic vein sends to the plexus, through the inferior orbital fissure (Fig. 3.14).

The pterygoid plexus corresponds to the second

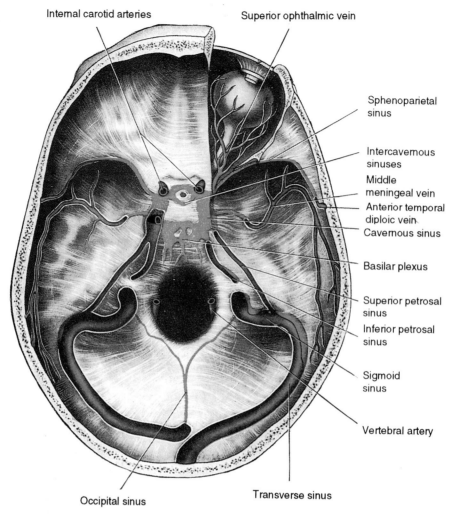

Internal carotid arteries

Superior ophthalmic vein

Sphenoparietal sinus

Intercavernous sinuses

Middle meningeal vein

Anterior temporal diploic vein

Cavernous sinus

Basilar plexus

Superior petrosal sinus

Inferior petrosal sinus

Sigmoid sinus

Vertebral artery

Occipital sinus

Transverse sinus

Fig. 3.18 The sinuses at the base of the skull. The sinuses coloured dark blue have been opened up. (From WIlliams, P.L. *et al.* (eds) (1995) *Gray's Anatomy*, 38th edition, published by Churchill Livingstone.)

and third parts of the maxillary artery and covers both surfaces of the lateral pterygoid muscle and deep surface of the medial pterygoid. This explains how a cavernous thrombosis may spread to the plexus and sometimes produce an abscess in the tonsillar region, which is found at *post mortem* in this condition.

CHAPTER FOUR

The extraocular muscles and ocular movements

The six **extrinsic** or extraocular muscles of the eyeball are striated and thereby distinguished from the **intrinsic** muscles (dilator and sphincter pupillae and ciliaris) which are non-striated. The fibres of the main muscle mass are also termed **extrafusal** to distinguish them from the **intrafusal** fibres of the sensory muscle spindles which provide feedback to the central oculomotor regulatory centres.

4.1 GROSS STRUCTURE

The extrinsic muscles include superior, inferior, medial, and lateral recti and superior and inferior obliques. The superior and lateral recti have posterior ends which are U-shaped, the inferior and medial having linear and dentate osseous attachments.

Scleral insertions are by tendons whose fibres are almost entirely parallel to the long axis of the muscle. These fibres consist of collagen, supported by thick elastic fibres. They resemble scleral fibres, being of the same tissue, but differ in size and, whereas tendon fibres are mostly longitudinal, the scleral fibres run in many directions (Figs 7.5 and 10.10). This imparts a glistening silky appearance to the tendon while the sclera is dull white.

The tendon fibres enter the superficial sclera and quickly merge into it (Fig. 10.10). Only the cessation of the thick elastic fibres marks the junction of tendon with sclera. Occasionally slips leave the main tendons near their scleral attachments, to be attached farther back. These recurrent slips may be missed at squint surgery.

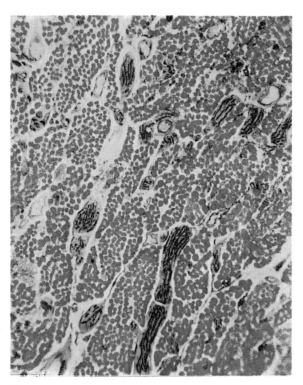

Fig. 4.1 Transverse section of fibres of a human rectus muscle (Masson's stain). Note the abundant nerve supply, visible in fascicles between the muscle fibres.

Extraocular muscles, like branchial muscles, differ in several respects from somatic muscles. They are not fasciculated with dense connective tissue, their fine fibres being loosely united and easily separated. Between them are unusually numerous nerve fibres, each muscle receiving a nerve which, relative to the muscle's size, is very large (Fig. 4.1). Ratios of one nerve fibre to 100 or more muscle fibres are usual in skeletal muscles, but in extraocular muscles the ratio is about 1:5 to 1:10 (Porter *et al.*, 1995).

4.2 ORBITAL AND GLOBAL ZONES

Although at birth fibre size is generally uniform (Kato, 1938), an outer shell of smaller-diameter fibres is later distinguished from a core of larger fibres and this pattern is retained into adult life (Schiefferdecker, 1904; Wohlfart, 1935; Ringel *et al.*, 1978b). These zones are referred to as **orbital** (i.e. outer; facing the orbit) and **global** (i.e. inner; facing the globe and contents of the muscle cone) (Fig. 4.2). Orbital fibre diameter ranges between 5 and 15 μm, while global fibres range between 10 and 40 μm. Within these zones different muscle subtypes have been identified, varying in structure, metabolism and contractile properties and in distribution at different ages (Lyness, 1986).

The global layer of superior oblique is totally enclosed by the orbital layer, while in the recti orbital zones are deficient on their internal surfaces, so that the global layer is exposed to adjacent adipose tissue around the optic nerve at a 'hilum'.

The recti are strap-like, with maximum width at their global insertion (5 mm behind it in the lateral rectus). Although fibres extend from end to end of the muscle belly, from osseous to tendinous attachment (Lockhart and Brandt, 1938; Cooper and Daniel, 1949), the global fibres are longer than the orbital (see below) and only the global tonic fibres appear to run the full length of the muscle belly (Mayr *et al.*, 1975). This maximizes the possible change in length of the muscle in contraction, and contrasts with most skeletal muscles. Shorter fibres are uncommon and therefore myomyous junctions (such as exist between levator oculi and superior palpebral (Müller's) muscle) are unusual. Although size of fibre varies along the muscle's length (Voss, 1957; Alvarado and van Horn, 1975; Davidowitz, Philips and Breinin, 1977), the widths of orbital and global

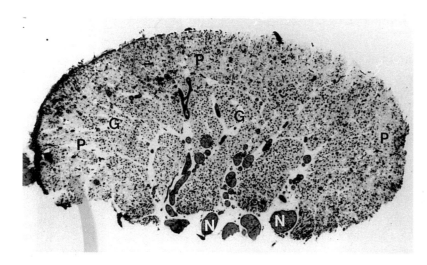

Fig. 4.2 Histological cross-section of an extraocular muscle, stained by myofibrillar ATPase method, preincubation at pH 4.3 and showing nerves (N) entering the global layer (G) at the hylum. Note the speckled pattern of the type I fibres (black), compared with the type II fibres (white) and the difference in diameter of the muscle fibres in the global layer compared with those in the orbital layer or peripheral layer (P). (From Liness, 1986, with permission.)

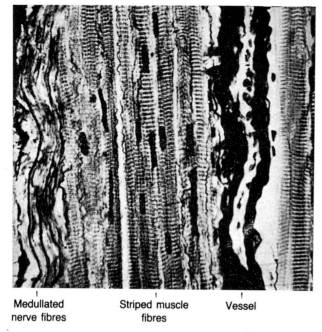

Medullated   Striped muscle   Vessel
nerve fibres   fibres

Fig. 4.3 Structure of the human rectus muscle (Bielchowsky stain).

fibres are similar at each end of the muscle (Locket, 1968). Splitting and tapering of fibres is a feature of muscle in non-primate species.

4.3 GENERAL FEATURES

Each fibre has a diameter of 5–40 μm (cf. 10–100 μm in skeletal muscles), and consists of a **sarcolemma** surrounding a granular **sarcoplasm** in which many **myofibrils**, 1–2 μm in diameter, lie in parallel. The fibres have a punctiform appearance in transverse section and a striated appearance in longitudinal section (Fig. 4.3). Each fibre is, of course, multinucleate, with nuclei internal to the sarcolemma.

Fibres of larger diameter are rapid **'twitch' fibres** with a 'fibrillenstruktur' (Dietert, 1965), having a regular distribution of myofibrils and abundant sarcoplasm. Innervation is by single, 'en plaque' endings (i.e. motor end plates) and in this respect these fibres resemble somatic striated fibres elsewhere (Locket, 1968). Two types of striated twitch fibres are described in lower vertebrates, and representatives of these occur in human and other mammalian extraocular muscles. Other fibres are slow or **'tonic'** in action and have a so-called 'felderstruktur', with ill-defined and myofibrillar arrangements and little sarcoplasm. Their respiratory metabolism is chiefly aerobic and they are innervated by diffuse ('en grappe') myoneural endings. Mitochondria are in general fewer in skeletal than in extraocular muscle

fibres (Miller, 1971). (It is not possible to be dogmatic about this; for instance avian tonic fibres are moderately aerobic, while frog tonic fibres have a low aerobic capacity.)

Although fibres are smaller in the orbital zones than in global zones, both contain mixtures in size of fibre.

4.4 CONNECTIVE TISSUE AND BLOOD SUPPLY

Vessels and nerves enter each muscle belly at its hilum.

The blood supply of the rectus muscles is greater than that of the myocardium, primarily due to the richness of the capillary network in the orbital layer (Wilcox *et al.*, 1981). Capillaries are of the closed type, showing bidirectional vesicular transport (Mwasi and Raviola, 1985).

This blood supply is required by the larger numbers of singly innervated fast twitch muscle fibres in the orbital layer, which have a highly aerobic metabolism. The morphology of these fibres differs greatly between species, particularly in mitochondrial content, which is highest in primates. The proportion of such fibres also differs between extraocular muscles (e.g. in the cat it is highest in medial rectus, lowest in lateral). Blood flow varies roughly in proportion to this and is thought to be highest in the medial rectus, although that in superior rectus may be higher (Wooten and Reis, 1972). Blood flow is highest in those species with the greatest ocular motility (Wilcox *et al.*, 1981).

Fibres in the orbital layer are arranged in discrete fascicles, which are less evident in the global layer. A **perimysium** of collagen, large elastic fibres, vessels and nerves, surrounds muscular fascicles and extends between individual fibres as an **endomysium**. The perimysium is continuous with **epimysium**, which surrounds the entire muscle. Epimysial sheaths of extraocular muscles are negligible near their osseous attachments but are well developed near the globe; their collagen fibres are largely longitudinal on juxtaocular aspects and circular or transverse on their outer aspects.

The unusual amount of elastic tissue in extraocular muscle must have a mechanical effect, perhaps contributing to fine gradation of contraction, though the main factor in this is their profuse innervation, small size of motor unit, and thus the very high 'twitch frequency' before tetanus ensues (i.e. a high frequency of neural impulses is required to achieve a smooth contractile response).

The extraocular muscles possess a resident population of immunocompetent cells including numerous macrophages and a smaller number of HLA-DR positive cells and T cells; B cells are absent. This population is assumed to be of importance in certain orbital immune disorders such as endocrine ophthalmopathy. The majority of the T cells are CD8 (suppressor/cytotoxic) positive, whereas in skeletal muscle, CD4-positive (helper) cells predominate (Schmidt *et al.*, 1993). The medial and inferior recti contain about twice as many macrophages as the lateral rectus and superior oblique muscles.

4.5 NERVE SUPPLY

Each rectus muscle receives its motor supply from a nerve entering its global aspect near the junction of middle and posterior thirds. The abducent nerve enters just posterior to the middle of the lateral rectus. The trochlear nerve enters the orbital surface of the anterior half of the posterior third of the superior oblique, while the branch of the inferior division of the oculomotor nerve supplying the inferior obliques enters at the middle of its posterior border. After entering the muscle belly, each nerve divides and sends branches towards both ends of its muscle.

4.6 MOTOR APPARATUS

Certain generalizations about extraocular muscle fibre structure and classification derive from studies of skeletal muscle.

FINE STRUCTURE OF SKELETAL MUSCLE

The skeletal muscle fibre is elongated, polygonal in cross section, fusiform in shape and about 30–90 μm in diameter (the range in women is consistently less than in men). Fibres may be up to 10 cm in length. Each multinucleate fibre contains many ovoid, peripherally located nuclei (up to 11 μm long), obvious under light microscopy, with adjacent Golgi bodies. The characteristic transverse cross-bandings are the basis of the term 'striated muscle' (Fig. 4.4).

The plasma membrane or **sarcolemma** is bilamellar, 7.5–10 nm thick, surrounded by a basal lamina 36–50 nm in width (the term 'sarcolemma' is sometimes more loosely used to imply the combined layer). Outside this is a layer of delicate reticular connective tissue. Satellite cells, at the interface of sarcolemma and basal lamina, may be capable of myoblastic differentiation (Dubowitz, 1985). The sarcolemmal-associated protein dystrophin is absent from extraocular muscle in the condition of Duchenne

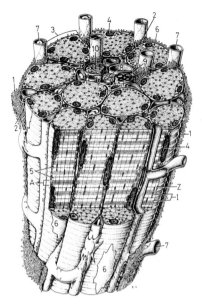

Fig. 4.4 The organization of skeletal muscle. The small fascicle of myofibres is bounded externally at the perimysium (1), a feltwork of collagen fibres which is continuous with a mesh of finer collagen fibrils, the endomysium (2) between the individual myofibres (3). The myofibres themselves contain elongated nuclei (4) and contractile myofibrils (5); small myosatellite cells (6) are closely applied to their external surfaces. Also shown are the numerous longitudinal running capillaries (7) with short transverse interconnections. (From Krstic, 1978, with permission of the author and publishers.)

muscular dystrophy but, contrary to the situation in skeletal muscle, no extraocular muscle degeneration results. The cytoplasm (or **sarcoplasm**) shows several specializations, the most obvious being cylindrical myofibrils composed of contractile protein and occupying 85–90% of the fibre's volume. Hundreds or thousands of myofibrils may be present in a single fibre. The intermyofibrillar sarcoplasm contains, in addition to nuclei, other organelles and membranous systems including the T-system, sarcoplasmic reticulum, mitochondria, Golgi apparatus, glycogen granules and lipid bodies (Fig. 4.4).

Myofibrils

The myofibrils are polygonal in cross-section and extend in parallel bundles along the full length of the fibre. They are composed of linearly arranged **myofilaments**, which form the fibre's repeating unit, the **sarcomere** (Fig. 4.5).

Myofilaments

The myofilaments, chief elements of the sarcomere, are demonstrable by electron microscopy. A series of thick (myosin) myofilaments is found, interdigitating

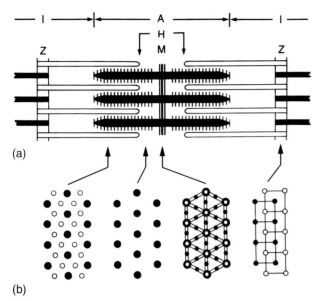

(b)

Fig. 4.5 (a) The structure of the sarcomere. The A band (A) is composed of a hexagonal lattice of thick filaments bearing projections, linked at their mid point by the M-line bridges (M). The I filaments of each half I band (I) arise from the Z discs (Z) as a regular square array and interdigitate with the A filaments to form a second hexagonal lattice. The interval between the central ends of the two sets of I filaments constitutes the H zone (H). The appearances of representative cross-sections through the sarcomere at the points indicated are illustrated in (b).

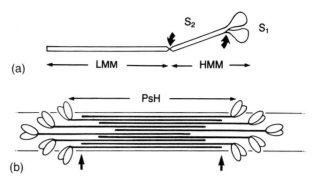

(a)

(b)

Fig. 4.6 (a) The components of the myosin molecule. The rod-shaped shaft of light meromyosin (LMM) is joined by a flexible link to the heavy meromyosin (HMM), which consists of two pear-shaped heads (the S_1 subunits) and the straight shaft (the S_2 subunit). The sites on the molecule susceptible to enzyme attack are indicated by curved arrows. (b) A schematic view of the central region of a thick filament to illustrate the antiparallel packing of the myosin molecules, with the head projecting from the surface of the filament. The region between the most central sets of heads is the 'bear' or 'pseudo H' zone (PsH); arrows mark the somewhat shorter region of overlap of the shafts of the myosin molecules from the two halves of the thick filament. (Courtesy of D. N. Landon.)

and overlapping with a series of thin (actin) filaments. The latter are attached to an electron-dense Z-disc. This overlap and repeating elements along the filaments give rise to the banding pattern. The thick filaments are 10–11 nm wide and 45 nm apart. Thin filaments are 4–5 nm wide. An isotropic (I) band contains only thin filaments and the dense Z-disc to which they are attached. The anisotropic (A) band (dark, because of birefringence), contains the full extent of the thick filaments plus some thin filaments. The gap containing thick filaments alone exhibits the electron-lucent H (Henson) stripe divided by the M (Mittlescheibe) line, which exhibits up to five 'bridge lines' (Sjöstrom *et al.*, 1982).

Myofilament structure

The thick filaments (0.15×11 nm) contain the protein myosin. Each myosin molecule is like a golf club whose 'head' is composed of the globular protein heavy meromyosin (HMM), which has a short tail (Fig. 4.5), and whose shaft consists of a double helix (2 nm wide, 100 nm long) of light meromyosin (LMM). The HMM head bears two active sites: a binding site for actin, and a myosin ATPase site. This molecular region is intimately involved in the

contractile process, the heads representing 'cross-bridges', which interact with binding sites on the actin of thin filaments. The histochemical differentiation of muscle fibres on the basis of ATPase staining reflects the presence of different isomeric forms of myosin which confer differing speeds of fibre shortening.

The arrangement of myosin molecules within thick filaments is depicted in Fig. 4.6, showing that each filament is composed of two mirror-image halves, within each of which the myosin molecules lie in staggered register. The molecules of one half have an opposite polarity to those in the other half (i.e. the 'golf clubs' are stacked end to end).

The thin filaments ($5–6 \times 0.1$ nm) are of fibrous actin (F-actin 60 K; 5.5 nm wide) attached structurally to the Z-discs. F-actin is in the form of a double helix, with the protein tropomyosin (also in the form of a double helix) lying within the actin grooves and shielding the myosin binding sites on the actin molecules. The protein troponin is distributed along the tropomyosin molecules at 40–41 nm intervals (Fig. 4.7). Each thick filament is surrounded by six thin ones. The major proteins of the Z-disc are actinin and actin.

Contraction is caused by the sliding of thin filaments across thick filaments, by forming and re-forming cross-bridges between them. Sarcomeric dimensions thus vary with contractile state: 0.1–0.5 μm in width and 1.5–3.5 μm in length. The A-band (thick filaments) does not change length

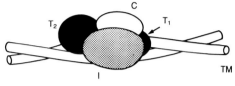

(a)

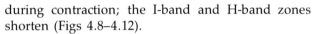

(b)

Fig. 4.7 (a) Diagrammatic view of a section of a monofilament. A double chain of globular actin monomers (A) is wound in a right-handed helix, the grooves between the two chains containing a second double helix of the filamentous protein tropomyosin (TM), to which they are attached. A third protein, troponin (TP), is situated as a series of globular complexes at regular intervals along the filament, attached to a single specific binding site on each tropomyosin molecule. Arrows indicate the junctions between adjacent tropomyosin molecules. (b) The components of a troponin complex attached to the tropomyosin double helix (TM). The calcium-binding properties of the complexes are contained in the C subunit. (Courtesy of D. N. Landon.)

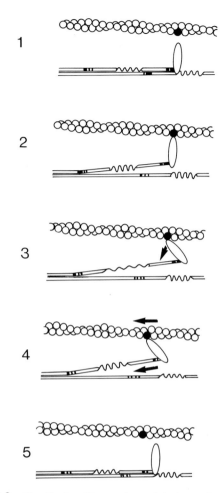

Fig. 4.8 The Huxley–Simmonds model of muscle contraction. (1) Resting state; (2) attachment of S_1 to actin (thin) filament; (3) rotation of S_1 while it is attached to the actin filament, and simultaneous stretching of the elastic component in S_2; (4) movement resulting from retraction of the elastic component; (5) return of cross-bridge to the resting state. (From Best and Taylor, after Harrington (1979).)

during contraction; the I-band and H-band zones shorten (Figs 4.8–4.12).

Between myofibrils are two membranous systems involved in excitation and contraction (Fig. 4.9): the transverse tubular system and the sarcoplasmic reticulum.

Transverse tubular system

The transverse tubular or T system is a tubular extension of the plasmalemma at the level of the junction of the A and I bands in human muscle and is connected to the Z-disc by intermediate filaments of desmin and other proteins (vinculin and a spectrin-like protein). Vinculin is arranged as an orthogonal lattice whose transverse costameres overlie the I-bands but are not present in the Z region. Huxley (1971) showed by tracer studies with ferritin that the lumina of the T system communicate with the extracellular space.

The T system penetrates between myofibrils, almost always encircling them to form a transverse reticulum; longitudinal connections between adjacent nets are a minor component. It is a conducting system intimately concerned with the process of contraction.

Sarcoplasmic reticulum

The sarcoplasmic reticulum is a fenestrated membranous development of the endoplasmic reticulum distributed between and around the myofibrils. It forms sac-like terminal cisternae at the level of the A/I interface which abut the T system: two cisternae, with their associated T tubule, form a triad. In mammalian muscle there are two triads in each sarcomere.

Additional cytoskeletal filaments link myofibrils, keeping them in register, and are attached also to the plasmalemma and nuclear membrane.

The mitochondria are responsible for aerobic generation of high-energy phosphate (ATP), and their number and size vary according to muscle subtype. Other organelles include glycogen granules

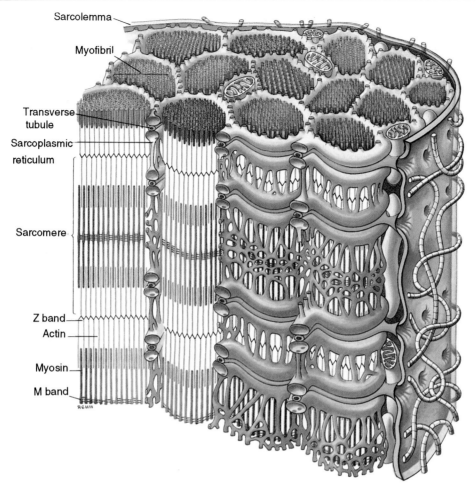

Sarcolemma

Myofibril

Transverse tubule

Sarcoplasmic reticulum

Sarcomere

Z band

Actin

Myosin

M band

Fig. 4.9 Three-dimensional reconstruction of skeletal muscle to show organization of myofibrils, mitochondria and membrane systems. (From Williams, P. L. (ed.) (1995) *Gray's Anatomy*, 38th edition, published by Churchill Livingstone.)

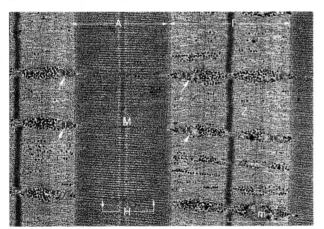

Fig. 4.10 Longitudinal section of human muscle fibre, showing four myofibrils. Dark A bands alternate with pale I bands (I), which are bisected at their mid-points by narrow dense Z lines (Z). In the A filaments the A band is bisected by the fine transverse cross-striations of the M line (M). The thin filaments of the A band and their central ends delimit the H zone (H). Triads, junctions between the sarcoplasmic reticulum and the transverse tubules are marked with arrows. The dense granules between myofibrils and within the I band are glycoprotein; one mitochondrion is shown (m). Scale shows 1 μm. Original magnification ×28 000. (Courtesy of D. N. Landon.)

(15–30 nm), lipid bodies (0.5–1 μm) and a few ribosomes.

INNERVATION OF SKELETAL MUSCLE

Skeletal muscle is supplied by somatic efferent neurones. The cell bodies of nerves supplying muscles in limbs are in the anterior grey column of the spinal cord. Their axons divide to supply a number of muscle fibres, each receiving a single terminal (i.e. they are singly innervated). The group of muscle fibres with their axon of supply is termed a 'motor unit'. A specialized 'en plaque' neuromuscular junction is formed (the motor end plate) (Figs 4.13–4.15).

HISTOCHEMICAL CLASSIFICATION OF SKELETAL MUSCLE (Table 4.1)

The earliest classification of skeletal muscle was based on colour. Later, 'red' and 'white' muscles were noted to have 'slow' or 'fast' contractile properties. The dark

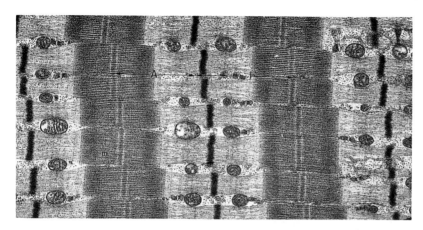

Fig. 4.11 Human skeletal muscle type I, showing the A band (A), I band (I) and a mitochondrion (m). Original magnification ×24 000. (Courtesy of D. N. Landon.)

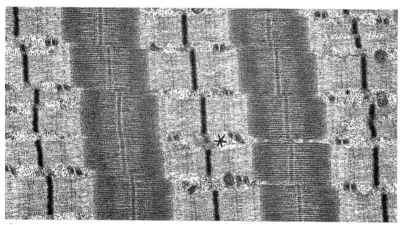

Fig. 4.12 Human skeletal muscle fibre type II. Note the abundant intermyofibrillar glycogen (*). Original magnification ×24 000. (Courtesy of D. N. Landon.)

Table 4.1 Histochemical and immunocytological fibre typing

Feature	Stain
Morphology	Haematoxylin and eosin
	Gomori trichrome
	van Gieson
Myosin	Myosin ATPase without preincubation at pH 9.4
	ATPase with preincubation at pH 4.6
	ATPase with preincubation at pH 4.3
	Anti-embryonic/neonatal myosin
	Anti-slow myosin*
	Anti-tonic myosin
	Anti-fast extraocular myosin*†
Oxidative metabolism (mitochondrial, tricarboxylic acid cycle)	Succinate dehydrogenase
	NADH–tetrazolium reductase
	Menadione-linked alpha-glycerophosphate→ dehydrogenase
Glycolytic metabolism	Periodic acid–Schiff (for glycogen)
	Phosphorylase (glycogen synthesis and breakdown)
Anaerobic glycolysis	Lactate dehydrogenase
Neutral lipids	Sudan black B
Lysozomes	Acid phosphatase
Neuromuscular junctions	Non-specific esterase
Cholinergic receptors	Alpha bungarotoxin–immunoperoxidase

*Cross-reacts with tonic myosin.
†No cross-reaction with fast skeletal myosins.
From Eggers, 1982.

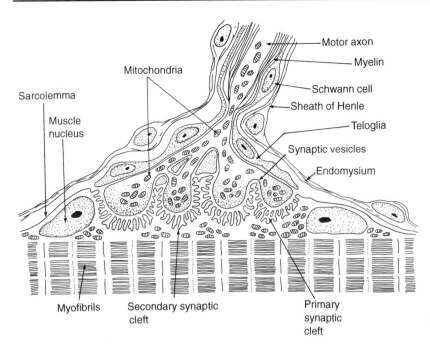

Sarcolemma

Muscle
nucleus

Mitochondria

Motor axon

Myelin

Schwann cell

Sheath of Henle

Teloglia

Synaptic vesicles

Endomysium

Myofibrils

Secondary synaptic
cleft

Primary
synaptic
cleft

Fig. 4.13 Diagram of the motor endplate of mammalian skeletal muscle. (From Coers, 1967.)

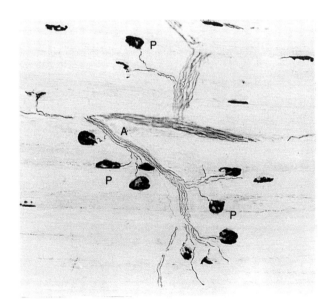

(a)

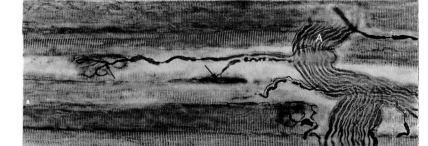

(b)

Fig. 4.14 (a) The endplate zone of mouse soleus muscle. Axons (A) provide an individual supply to compact sole-plates (P). Original magnification ×450.
(b) Neuromuscular junction in a rat soleus muscle. The silver-stained axons (A) break up into a number of fine branches (arrows) within the endplate regions, which are delimited by finely granular anticholinesterase stain. The endplate on the ring, which is viewed in profile, is raised above the general level of the muscle fibre (Doyere's eminence). Original magnification ×1200. (Both figures courtesy of D. N. Landon.)

Table 4.2 Skeletal muscle fibre types

Terminologies

	I	IIA	IIB	IIC
Brooke and Kaiser (1970)	I	IIA	IIB	IIC
Peter et al. (1972)	Slow-twitch–oxidative	Fast-twitch–oxidative glycolytic	Fast-twitch–glycolytic	
Burke et al. (1973)	S	FR	FF	F (intermediate) Intermediate
Gauthier and Lowey (1979)	Red(slow) oxidative	Red (fast) oxidative glycolytic	White glycolytic	

Histochemical profiles

	I	IIA	IIB	IIC
Myosin ATPase (pH 9.4)	Low	High	High	High
Myosin ATPase (pH 4.6)	High	Low	Intermediate	Intermediate
Myosin ATPase (pH 4.3)	High	Low	Low	Intermediate
SDH (mitochondrial aerobic)	High	Intermediate–high	Low	Intermediate
NADH-TR (aerobic)	High	Intermediate–high	Low	Intermediate
LDH (sarcoplasm)	High	Intermediate–high	Low	Intermediate
Men-α-GPD (anaerobic)	Low	High	High	Intermediate
PAS (glycogen)	Low	High	Intermediate–high	Intermediate
Phosphorylase (glycogenolysis)	Low	High	High	High
Oil Red O (lipid)	High	Low	Low	Low
Alkaline phosphatase (capillaries)	High	High	Low	Low

Immunocytochemical profiles (Gauthier, 1979; Gauthier and Lowey, 1979; Pierobon-Bormioli et al., 1980, 1981)

	I	IIA	IIB	IIC
Anti-white myosin (PEC)	Negative	Positive	Positive	Positive
Anti-fast-white myosin (TFL)	Negative	Negative	Positive	Negative
Anti-slow-white myosin (MAS)	Negative	Positive	Negative	Positive
Anti-red myosin (SOL, ALD)	Positive	Negative	Negative	Negative

Ultrastructural profiles (Gauthier, 1969; Padykula and Gauthier, 1970; Schiaffino et al., 1970)

	I	IIA	IIB	IIC
Z-line	Wide	Wide	Narrow	Narrow
Mitochondria	Many, small	Many, large	Few, small	Moderate, small
Sarcoplasmic reticulum T tubules	Elaborate, narrow	Elaborate, narrow	Compact, broad, parallel	Moderate, small
Neuromuscular junctions	Large, widely spaced, deep folds	Discrete, separate, small, elliptical, shallow, sparse folds	Long and flat; long, branching, closely spaced folds	

Physiological profiles (Burke, 1967; Close, 1967; Burke et al., 1973, 1974)

	I	IIA	IIB	IIC
Twitch contraction time (ms)	Slow	Intermediate	Fast	Fast
Twitch tension (g)	Very low	Low	High	Intermediate
Relative fatigue resistance	Resistant (very)	Resistant (moderate)	Sensitive	Intermediate

From Spencer and Porter, 1988.

or red colour is related not only to vascularity, but also to myoglobin content. Myoglobin is a carrier of oxygen in muscle fibres. Dark fibres were found to be rich in intermyofibrillar protoplasm. In higher animals colour seemed related to activity – constantly active muscles being dark. Thus in the domestic fowl, breast muscle is white, leg muscle dark but in birds of flight the opposite is true.

Physiological studies and the development of enzyme histochemistry have permitted the biochemical features of skeletal muscle fibres to be correlated to some extent with functional properties. These are summarized in Table 4.2.

'Slow' and 'fast twitch' fibres are distinguished in skeletal muscle on the basis of the duration of twitch responses. Fibres which are rich in mitochondria

(sometimes referred to as 'red') derive their energy chiefly from aerobic metabolism. They are resistant to fatigue on repeated stimulation. An aerobic metabolism is suggested by strong positive staining for oxidative enzymes, e.g. succinic acid dehydrogenase (SDH) and NADH-tetrazolium reductase (NADH-TR).

Some skeletal muscle fibres show primarily a glycolytic metabolism, suggested histochemically by abundant glycogen stores and strongly positive staining for the enzyme phosphorylase. Such fibres, low in mitochondria, are also referred to as 'white' and are relatively fatiguable on repeated stimulation. Some fibres show both aerobic and glycolytic features.

On the basis of such histochemical features, and

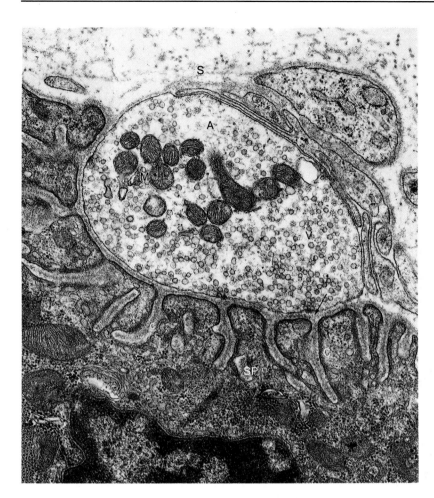

Fig. 4.15 Section through the motor endplate of a rat soleus muscle. The axon terminal (A) is covered externally by Schwann cell processes (S). It contains numerous clear synaptic vesicles and mitochondria (M). It is separated on the myofibril sole-plate (SP) by a layer of basal lamina (extensions of which fill the postsynaptic clefts (C)). An arrow indicates the increased density on the presynaptic membrane associated with vesicle release. Original magnification ×50 000. (Courtesy of D. N. Landon.)

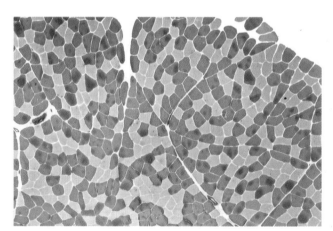

Fig. 4.16 Transverse section of human skeletal muscle stained for myosin ATPase, preincubated at pH 9.4. (Courtesy of W. Squiers.)

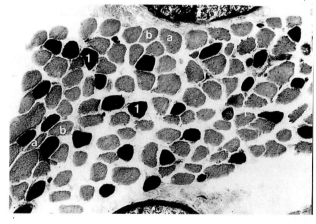

Fig. 4.17 A histological section of an extraocular muscle, stained for myofibrillar ATPase following preincubation at pH 4.3, showing type I muscle fibres (1, stained black) and type IIa and IIb (a and b, lighter stain). Original magnification ×200. (Courtesy of R. Liness.)

Table 4.3 Histochemical profiles of extraocular muscle fibre types

	Orbital		Global			
Fibre type	1	2	3	4	5	6
Trichrome	Coarse/granular	Granular/fine	Coarse/granular	Granular	Granular/fine	Fine
Mean diameter (μm)	24.8 ± 3.8	19.3 ± 3.2	27.2 ± 4.7	34.5 ± 4.6	46.7 ± 6.2	35.7 ± 4.1
Percentage	80	20	33	25	32	10
Myosin ATPase pH 9.4	+++	+++	+++	+++	+++	+/−
Myosin ATPase pH 4.6	+/−	+++	+/−	+/−	+/−	++++
Succinic dehydrogenase	+++/++++	++	++++	+++	++	+
Nicotinamide adenine nucleotide dehydrogenase-tetrazolium reductase	+++	++	++++	+++	++	+
Lactate dehydrogenase	++/+++	++	++++	+++	++	+
Menadione-linked α-glycerophosphate dehydrogenase	++/+++	+	++	+++	++++	+
Sudan black	++/+++	+	+++	++	++	+
Periodic acid–Schiff	++/+++	+/−	++	+	+	+/−
Phosphorylase	++/+++	+	+++	+	+	+
Oil Red O	++/+++	+	+++	++	+	+
Alkaline phosphatase	++++	++	+++	++	+	+
Acetylcholinesterase	Focal, encircle	Multiple	Focal	Focal	Focal	Multiple

+/−, very low; +, low; ++, intermediate; +++, high; ++++, very high
From Spencer and Porter, 1988.

also staining for myosin ATPase at differential pH, two types of muscle fibres have been described (Figs 4.16 and 4.17). The histochemical profile of extraocular muscle is shown in Table 4.3.

Type I muscle fibres

Type I fibres are 'slow twitch', stain weakly for myosin ATPase at pH 9.4 but strongly at acid pH, strongly for oxidative enzymes but weakly for glycolytic enzymes. Such fibres are sometimes termed 'slow, oxidative and fatigue resistant' (Dubowitz and Pearse, 1960a,b; Engel, 1962; Brooke and Kaiser, 1970).

Type II muscle fibres

Type II fibres are 'fast twitch' and stain strongly for ATPase at pH 9.4. They are subdivided into IIA fibres, which stain poorly on preincubation at pH 4.6 and pH 4.3, and IIB which stain poorly at only pH 4.3. Type IIA fibres have oxidative and glycolytic features and are resistant to fatigue on repeated stimulation; type IIB fibres have glycolytic features and are fatiguable. A third subtype, type IIC, is found chiefly in infancy and differs from that shown in adult muscle.

4.7 CLASSIFICATION OF EXTRAOCULAR MUSCLE FIBRES

The earliest studies of extraocular muscle made a distinction between dark-staining fibres with many nuclei and abundant sarcoplasm and 'clear' fibres with few nuclei and little cytoplasm (Cilimbaris, 1910). Thulin (1910) noted that those fibres with plentiful sarcoplasm had a regular myofibril arrangement (fibrillenstruktur) while others had an irregular myofibril arrangement (felderstruktur).

The nomenclature of primate extraocular muscle is becoming more firmly established. Extraocular muscle fibres are narrower than their skeletal counterparts and form much smaller motor units. Most are singly innervated, 'twitch' muscle fibres with a contraction time considerably shorter than that of skeletal muscle, but a substantial proportion are 'tonic' muscle fibres with slow contractile properties and pharmacological responses peculiar to extraocular muscles (and to tensor tympani in the middle ear). This tonic muscle fibre is not present in mammalian skeletal muscle, but resembles the tonic muscle fibre of amphibia and birds. It is multiply innervated, with nerve terminals scattered over the whole fibre surface.

The histochemical approach employed for skeletal muscle has also been used to classify extraocular muscle, but there has been considerable disagreement

Table 4.4 Comparison of mammalian extraocular muscle type classifications

Species	Orbital subtypes		Global subtypes				Reference
Human	IIA, IIC*	I	IIB		IIA, IIC*		Hoogenrad, 1979
Monkey	Granular (IIB)	Coarse†	Granular and fine		Coarse†		Ringel et al., 1978
Monkey	(s.i.)	(m.i.)	red	intermediate	pale	global	Pachter, 1982
			(s.i.)	(s.i.)	(s.i.)	(m.i.)	
Monkey	1	2	3	4	5	6	Spencer and Porter, 1988
Cat, rabbit	1	2	5	4	3	6	Asmussen et al., 1971
Cat	II	IIC		II	II	IIC, I	Hanson, 1977
Cat SR	Small granulated	Large fibril granulated	Small fibril granulated	Lightly granulated	Fibrillar white	Fibrillar white	Peachey et al., 1974
Cat SO	3	5	3	2	1	4	Alvarado and van Horn, 1975
Mammalian vertebrate	Immature twitch	Tonic Slow twitch	Extraocular specific fast twitch			Slow twitch	Rowlerson, 1987
Rabbit	II	I		II		I	Reichmann and Srihari, 1983
Rabbit	Twitch (s.i.)	Tonic (m.i.)	Small, dark	Intermediate	Large, white	Large, fibril	Davidowitz, Phillips and Breinin, 1977
Sheep	Small C	Small G	Small C	Intermediate C	Large A	Large G	Harker, 1972
Rat	Dark	Pale	Dark	Intermediate	Pale	Clear	Mayr, 1971
Mouse	Twitch (s.i.)	Tonic (m.i.)	Small Dark		Large, light (s.i.)	Tonic (m.i.)	Pachter, 1976

Compiled from Eggers, 1982; Rowlerson, 1987; Spencer and Porter, 1988.
Roman numerals imply histochemical assignment to a skeletal fibre subtype.
*Rowlerson (1987) believes the authors' IIC to be more like IIA because the neonatal IIC should show *acid* as well as alkali-stable myosin-ATPase.
†The authors' coarse fibre is histochemically similar to IIA or IIC (Hoogenrad's assignment). However, later studies in human muscle assign coarse Type I granular to type II (Carry, Ringel and Starcevich, 1986).
s.i. = singly innervated; m.i. = multiply innervated.

as to the relative proportions of type I (slow twitch) and type II (fast twitch) fibres present (Tables 4.3 and 4.4) and the characterization of tonic fibres is uncertain, despite the use of *myoneural-junctional stains*. Fibres which are histochemically type II appear to be singly innervated and served by single motor end plates. However, the pattern of innervation of at least some type I fibres (slow twitch) has been multiple, which is a characteristic of tonic fibres. Skeletal muscle types IIA, IIB and IIC do not appear to correspond to those identified in ocular muscle, because ocular muscle fibres contain specific myosins which are different from those of limb muscle.

CURRENT CLASSIFICATIONS OF EXTRAOCULAR MUSCLE

It is apparent that the nomenclature of skeletal muscle, based on histochemical details, refers only to singly innervated twitch fibres, and cannot completely describe the subtypes of extraocular muscle which also include tonic fibres. Asmussen *et al.* (1971) have provided a comprehensive classification of muscle fibres in the cat and other species, similar to that demonstrated in the monkey by Spencer and Porter (1981) and Porter *et al.* (1995) in excellent reviews.

Spencer and Porter nomenclature

Using a numeric classification, independent of that applied to skeletal muscle, the nomenclature of Spencer and Porter (1981) is described below (Table 4.4).

Orbital zone (Table 4.5)

Type 1: Orbital singly innervated   Type 1 fibres are small and make up 80% of the orbital layer, probably accounting for most of the sustained force generated by the muscle. Mitochondria occur in abundant clusters, and individual fibres are ringed by capillaries. In the higher species, the mitochondrial content is greater in this fibre (and the global red singly innervated counterpart) than in the lower species, perhaps reflecting the significant demands of high visual acuity (Porter *et al.*, 1995). There is an abundant and well-delineated sarcoplasmic reticulum and T-system and a regular myofibrillar arrangement. Histochemically, these are coarse, fast-twitch fibres, rich in oxidative enzymes (e.g. SDH) but also capable of anaerobic metabolism. They correspond to skeletal type II. Myosin isoforms vary along the length of the fibre: in the mid-portion of the muscle a fast myosin is found,

Table 4.5 Properties and classification of mammalian sub-primate extraocular muscle

Features	Orbital zone		Global zone			
	Type 1, fast twitch	Type 2 'avian' tonic	Type 3 fast	Type 4 twitch	Type 5	Type 6 'amphibian' tonic
Succinate dehydrogenase activity	+++	++	+	++	+++	(+)
Alkali ATPase	++	(++)**	++	++	++	0**
Acid ATPase	++	+++	(+)	++	++	+++
Relative diameter	+	+	+++	++	+	++
Myofibrillar arrangement	Fibrillenstruktur	Felderstruktur	Fibrillenstruktur			Felderstruktur
Sarcoplasmic reticulum and transverse tubular systems	++	+	+++	+++	++	(+)
Innervation	Single	Multiple	Single	Single	Single	Multiple

Relative reaction or degree: from 0 (negative or very low) through (+), +, ++, to +++ (highest).
*In some species alkali stable myosin ATPase activity may be as high as in twitch fibres (Hanson and Lennerstrand found that unlike the cat, the rat fibres all have alkali-stable ATPase, while 20–40% have acid-stable ATPase).
Modified after Asmussen et al., 1971, from Rowlerson, 1987.

whereas away from the mid-zone there are several myosins and a longitudinal variation in structure. The myosins include a generic fast myosin, IIA, embryonic/neonatal myosin and a myosin specific to eye muscle (Jacoby, Chiarindini and Stefani, 1989a). This fibre type differs from skeletal IIA by its high fatigue resistance and unique myosin profile. It is singly innervated and the elaborate arrangement of motor end plates, which literally encircle the muscle fibres, may have led to their confusion with spiral sensory endings (Ruskell and Wilson, 1983).

Type 2: Orbital multiply innervated fibres   Type 2 is a slow fibre resembling 'amphibian tonic' fibres and comprising 20% of the orbital zone. It stains strongly for myosin ATPase after acid preincubation, but variably with alkaline ATPase and shows moderate oxidative activity. The staining properties for myosin ATPase activity are not uniform along the length of the muscle fibre; thus acid-stable myosin ATPase is found only in the proximal and distal thirds of the fibre. It has sparse membranous systems and an irregular myofibrillar arrangement by electron microscopy. Centrally the fibres resemble skeletal fast twitch fibres (IIC) (but with a lower oxidative capacity), on the basis of ATPase, ultrastructure and a fast myosin isoform. At either end they show the ultrastructural features and slow ATPase of slow contracting fibres and contain an embryonic/neonatal myosin.

Although they are multiply innervated, they show a twitch capability near their centre and a slow contractility proximally and distally (Jacoby, 1989) associated with a structural variation along their length (Davidowitz, 1980; 1982).

Global zone

Types 3–5   These are designated as fast-twitch fibres and, like skeletal type II fibres, show positive staining for ATPase in alkaline conditions. Staining is variable at acid pH.

Type 3: Global red singly innervated   This makes up 30% of the global layer. It stains coarsely and, histochemically, resembles the orbital singly innervated fibre. It is highly oxidative and glycolytic and is regarded as fatigue resistant. It does not show longitudinal structural variation and contains no coexpressed fast or embryonic/neonatal myosins (Bruekner et al., 1994). The fibre does express the myosin IIA isoform along its length, but differs from skeletal IIA by its high mitochondrial content. Functionally, it is assumed to be a fast-twitch and fatigue-resistant fibre.

Type 4: Global intermediate singly innervated   This fibre makes up 25% of the global layer. Ultrastructure and ATPase content suggest that it is a fast-twitch fibre and myosin reactivity suggests a resemblance to skeletal type IIB (Bruekner et al., 1994). Histochemically, the fibre is granular and there are moderate levels of oxidative and aerobic enzymes. There are numerous small mitochondria, singly or in clusters. Myofibril size and sarcoplasmic reticulum content are intermediate between that of the other two singly innervated fibres.

Type 5: Global pale singly innervated   This fibre comprises 30% of the global layer. It resembles type IIB skeletal with respect to modest levels of oxidative

Table 4.6 Generalized mammalian extraocular muscle fibre classification

	Orbital zone			Global zone	
	Immature twitch	Tonic	Slow twitch	Extraocular specific fast twitch	Slow twitch
Succinate dehydrogenase activity	Generally high		−	Low to high	Low
Fibre size	Small to medium			Small to large	Large
Alkali ATPase	++	+*	+*	++	−*
Acid ATPase	−/+	++	++	−	++
Anti-slow myosin	−	+	++	−	++
Anti-tonic myosin	−	++	−	−	−
Anti-embryonic neonatal myosin	most ++ some −	−	−	−	−
Anti-fast EOM	++	−	−	++†	−
Equivalent histochemical limb type (ATPase)	II		I	II	I

Reactivity: ++ (high); + (moderate); − (low or absent).
*In some species (e.g. rat, guinea pig) myosin ATPase is relatively stable.
†A few fibres react strongly for limb myosin (IIA) and occasionally for embryonic/neonatal myosins.
From Rowlerson, 1987.

enzymes, high anaerobic metabolic capacity and fast type, myosin ATPase. Staining for AcCh shows the single locus of large end-plates. Mitochondria are small and few and arranged singly between myofibrils. Overall profile suggests a fast twitch fibre used infrequently because of low fatigue resistance.

Fibre diameter increases from types 3 to 5. All show a regular myofibrillar arrangement on electron microscopy with well-developed sarcoplasmic reticulum and T systems in types 3 and 4 and slightly less so in type 5. They are singly innervated.

Type 6: Global multiply innervated fibres   Type 6 is a slow fibre resembling 'amphibian tonic', with strong acid-stable ATPase features and weak oxidative properties. It makes up 10% of the global layer. Ultrastructurally, it shows a felderstruktur with very large myofibrils, sparse membranous systems and occasional mitochondria in single file. It is multiply innervated, with numerous en-grappe endings along its length. Unlike the type 2 tonic fibre, the staining pattern in type 6 fibres is homogeneous. Myosin expression includes: slow-twitch (type I), slow tonic and (in the rabbit), alpha cardiac myosin (Pierobon-Bormioli *et al.*, 1979, 1980; Jacoby *et al.*, 1990; Roll *et al.*, 1990). The proportions of each type in the global zone are shown in Table 4.4.

As noted above, a clearer picture of the specificity and diversity of extraocular muscle subtypes has emerged from immunohistochemical studies of myosin isoforms (Bormioli *et al.*, 1980; Rowlerson, 1987; Sartore *et al.*, 1987; Jacoby, 1989, 1990; Moll, 1990; Porter *et al.*, 1995). There are as many as ten

heavy myosin isoforms, each with different contractile properties and encoded by distinct mammalian genes (Wieczorall *et al.*, 1981; Storm and Johnson, 1993).

The classification proposed by Rowlerson (1987) is summarized in Table 4.6.

Orbital zone (Table 4.7)

Many orbital zone fibres contain embryonic or neonatal myosins coexpressed with a specific, 'fast' extraocular myosin. The proportion of embryonic and neonatal myosin declines with age but it does not disappear entirely (Wieczorek *et al.*, 1985). The small calibre and less well-organized ultrastructure of these fibres are also consistent with immaturity and it has been suggested that the persistence of immature myosins may relate to the limited load bearing of extraocular muscles (Sartore *et al.*, 1987). In limb muscles, the transition from adult to mature myosins coincides with the onset of load bearing; however, as Rowlerson (1987) points out, this does not explain why these fibres are confined to the orbital layer. There is evidence that the maturation of the extraocular muscles is a response to environmental pressures during development. Postnatal maturation of the extraocular muscles parallels the maturation of retinal circuitry and the establishment of interocular alignment. The most significant development is the increase in mitochondrial content. Thus the development of eye movements parallels the acquisition of fatigue resistance.

Antibodies against 'slow fibre' myosins identify two further ocular fibre types, a slow-twitch and a

Table 4.7 Correlation of primate and non-primate extraocular muscle fibre types

	Orbital zone		Global zone	
Species	Fibre type	M-line	Fibre type	M-line
Rhesus monkey (Miller, 1967)	Peripheral 2	Absent	Large white	Present
	Peripheral 1	Absent	Large red	Absent
			Medium-sized cell	
			with felderstructure	
Rhesus monkey (Cheng and Breinin, 1966)	–	–	Large white	Present
			Large red	Absent
			Slow fibre	Absent
Cat (Alvarado and Van Horn, 1975)	3	Thin	1	40 nm
	5	60 nm	2	Absent
			3	Thin
			4	60 nm
Cat (and other) (Asmussen et al., 1971)	1		1	
	2		2	
			3	
			4	
Mammalian (Rowlerson, 1987)	Immature twitch		Fast fibres with	
	Tonic		specific fast	
	Slow twitch		extraocular myosin	
			slow twitch	

tonic fibre. One antibody which labels slow-twitch fibres also reacts with tonic myosin, but the two fibres are distinguished from each other by an antibody specific for vertebrate tonic fibres and does not react with slow-twitch fibres (Rowlerson, 1987). These fibre types have a (skeletal muscle) type I histochemical profile but only the tonic fibre would correspond to Asmussen's multiply innervated type 2 (tonic fibre).

Global zone

The majority of extraocular muscle fibres contain a myosin specific to extraocular muscle fibres with ATPase properties corresponding to the family of fast myosins. There is no cross-reaction with skeletal muscle. This is the predominant myosin in the global zone twitch fibres and is also present in orbital fibres, as mentioned above. That this vertebrate extraocular muscle myosin is distinct from skeletal muscle myosins may explain the differences in twitch contraction times of extraocular muscle and its very low specific tension output, i.e. the maximum isometric tetanic tension per unit of cross-sectional area. (Rat inferior rectus is about one-third to one-half the value for rat limb muscle.)

A further population of global fibres (amphibian tonic) are immunologically slow twitch but ultrastructurally multiply innervated fibres; their histochemical profile is in keeping with skeletal type I.

A summary of the light microscopic, histochemical and ultrastructural features of the fibre types dis-

cussed above now follows, with reference chiefly to primate and human studies. Areas of debate have been dealt with earlier and the findings of various authors are compared in Tables 4.4 and 4.7.

4.8 FEATURES OF EXTRAOCULAR MUSCLE FIBRES

Fibre diameters are given in Table 4.3.

The change in fibre diameter with age is reported by Engel and Brooke (1966).

TWITCH FIBRES

Slow-twitch fibres

The extent to which muscle fibres corresponding to the slow-twitch (type I) fibres of skeletal muscle are present in extraocular muscle is unclear. Type I-like fibres show a fine stippling with trichrome stains, low to moderate myosin-ATPase activity at pH 9.4 but high activity at low pH. Oxidative activity is low using succinate dehydrogenase stain and moderate with nicotinic acid dehydrogenase–tetrazolium reductase. Glycolytic metabolism as assessed by phosphorylase is limited, and lipid content is low (Hess, 1967; Ringel et al., 1978b). As mentioned earlier, a proportion of fibres with this histochemical profile in the orbital layer contain tonic myosins. These tonic fibres and the type I staining fibres in the global zone are probably multiply innervated with a felderstruktur.

Fast-twitch fibres (singly innervated, fibrillenstruktur)

Type IIA-like fibres

These fibres stain coarsely with trichrome stains, are rich in oxidative activity and are high in ATPase at pH 9.4. The ATPase activity is acid labile. The capability for anaerobic glycolysis is also high, while phosphorylase activity is moderate. Thus these fibres meet the definition for fast, oxidative/glycolytic fibres (Peter *et al.*, 1972) whose high mitochondrial content render them fatigue resistant (Burke, 1981) (Table 4.2). They are also rich in lipid droplets.

Such fibres can utilize energy (ATP) generated in mitochondria through the tricarboxylic acid cycle and from lipid breakdown. They correspond to type 3 (Spencer and Porter, 1981) fibres in extraocular muscle and have some features of type I.

Type IIB-like fibres

These fibres appear granular with trichrome stain, the regular stippling suggesting a regular spacing of myofibrils typical of fibrillenstruktur. Fibres are high in ATPase, which is stable at pH 9.4, moderately stable at pH 4.6 and labile at pH 4.3. Oxidative enzyme activity is low and phosphorylase activity high. It is inferred that these fast-twitch fibres derive energy primarily from glycolysis and that energy is restored more slowly by mitochondrial activity in aerobic conditions. These fibres are fast, glycolytic and fatiguable in the nomenclature of Burke (1981) and Peter *et al.* (1972), and correspond to Spencer and Porter (1981) type 5 in extraocular muscle.

These fibres are 13–35 μm wide, have mainly peripheral nuclei and sparse mitochondria.

Ultrastructure

Fast-twitch fibres, and presumably a proportion of histochemically type I (i.e. slow twitch) fibres, have the regular myofibrillar arrangement and rich membranous systems typical of the fibrillenstruktur. The sarcoplasmic reticulum and T system are essential to the excitation–contraction mechanism of twitch fibres, whose sarcomeres are stimulated by the spread of an action potential from a single end plate. Such membranous systems are ill-developed in tonic fibres whose surfaces are excited at multiple 'en grappe' endings.

Cheng and Breinin (1966) described two large fibre types (25–50 μm wide) in the lateral rectus of rhesus monkeys. Both types showed a regular arrangement of myofibrils, well-delineated sarcoplasmic reticulum, plentiful T systems and numerous triads typical of fibrillenstruktur and twitch fibres. Z-lines were well defined and straight. These were subclassified into a 'red' fibre rich in mitochondria, and a 'white' fibre poor in mitochondria.

'Red' fibres

The numerous mitochondria of the red fibres are distributed in a peripheral rim and also in chains between myofibrils, sometimes extending the length of ten sarcomers; lipid droplets are closely associated. No M-line is present.

This description is similar to that of the large red fibre of Miller (1967) in both the intermediate layer of fibres (between global and orbital layers) and in the global layer itself. Miller speaks of broad and irregular sarcoplasmic columns forming a fine reticular network about the myofibrils, which are confluent in places in longitudinal section. Glycogen particles, less dense than in orbital fibres, are deposited along the sarcoplasmic reticulum and between mitochondria. The ovoid, subsarcoplasmic, perinuclear and intermyofibrillar mitochondria are packed two or three deep. A and I bands are well defined and an M-line is absent.

Cheng and Breinin (1966) equated the red fibre with the slow fibres of soleus or diaphragm. The relative mitochondrial volume of these fibres compared to gastrocnemius is 5.7 (Miller, 1971) (Table 4.8).

'White' fibres

The large 'white' fibre of Cheng and Breinin (1966) shows far fewer mitochondria, concentrated near the Z-line, and limited subsarcolemmal or intermyofibrillar aggregation. The mitochondria are smaller, thinner and with fewer cristae. Lipid droplets are infrequent. These fibres have a distinct M-line.

Cheng and Breinin regarded this as a typical white fibre resembling interosseous muscle and gastrocnemius. A similar large fibre, also possessing an M-line, is described by Miller (1967) as the most frequent type encountered in the global layer. Broad expanses of myofibrils are surrounded by sarcoplasmic sleeves with extensive longitudinal tubules and triads. Nuclei are oval and subsarcolemmal. Thin layers of glycogen granules separate the masses of globular, intermyofibrillar mitochondria. The relative mitochondrial volume compared with gastrocnemius is 2.3 (Miller, 1971), despite the general resemblance of this type of fibre to the 'white' fibres of gastrocnemius. (This emphasizes the difficulty in

Table 4.8 Innervation of mammalian extraocular muscle

Species	Zone	Single innervation	Multiple innervation	Reference
Human				
Child		86	14	Muhlendyk, 1978
Adult		80–90	10–20	Namba *et al.*, 1968
Adult	Orbital	8	92	Ringel *et al.*, 1978
Adult	Global	67	33	
Monkey		85	15	Mayr, 1966
Baboon	Orbital	20	80	Durston, 1974
	Global	88	12	
Cat		70	30	Alvarado and Van Horn, 1975
Sheep		84	16	Harker, 1972
Rat		86	14	Mayr, 1971

All values are percentages.

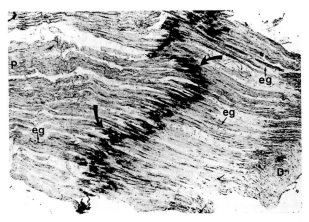

Fig. 4.18 Longitudinal section of human extraocular muscle stained for cholinesterase, showing the innervation band of *en plaque* motor endplates in the middle third of the muscle (arrowed). Note the multiple *en grappe* motor nerve endings (eg) throughout the proximal (P) and distal (D) thirds of the muscle. (Courtesy of R. Liness.)

comparing fibre types between different muscle masses.)

Miller (1967) described a small red fibre in the orbital layer of rhesus monkey extraocular muscle (his peripheral type 2), which resembles the type 3 twitch fibre of the cat (Alvarado and Van Horn, 1975); however, the former had no M-line whereas the latter did. Both are small-diameter fibres with large mitochondria (drumstick or cylindrical in the rhesus monkey muscle) and less sarcoplasmic reticulum than other twitch fibres. In monkey fibres, sarcoplasmic tubules are related primarily to the I-band and longitudinal tubules are deficient in the A-band, but transverse tubules and triads are frequent on either side of the A-band. In the cat, these are singly innervated twitch fibres.

Considering the fibre types described by Spencer and Porter (1981) in the monkey, type 1 fibres show the greatest variation in mitochondrial content near the end plate zone. Mitochondria are numerous and large, especially between myofibrils at the muscle centre and occur as massive subsarcolemmal accumulations. Type 3 fibres are similar, but show fewer mitochondria. The myofibrils are well delineated by the internal membrane system. The mitochondrial content, myofibrillar size and sarcoplasmic reticulum of type 4 fibres are intermediate between that of types 3 and 5. Mitochondria lie singly between the myofibrils or in subsarcolemmal clusters close to the end plates. Type 5 fibres exhibit the largest myofibrils, while the mitochondria which lie between them are sparse (Table 4.5).

Innervation (Table 4.8)

Twitch fibres are innervated by the branches of single motor nerve axons, supplying a small number of muscle fibres and terminating as 'en plaque' endings (Zenker and Anzenbacher, 1964; Pilar and Hess, 1966; Mayr, Stockinger and Zenker, 1966; Namba, Nakamura and Grob, 1968a,b) (Figs 4.18, 4.19 and 4.20). These resemble the motor end plates of striated muscle elsewhere and the endings are rich in cholinesterase (Hess, 1962; Cheng, 1963; Dietert, 1965; Teravainen, 1968). There is an accumulation of nuclei underlying each end plate. The synaptic membrane shows prominent fine junctional folds and there are numerous synaptic vesicles in the terminal axon (Cheng and Breinin, 1966.)

The motor end plates are distributed over a region 1–2 mm wide in the middle third of the muscle's belly, just distal to the union of nerve trunk and muscle (Dietert, 1965) (Fig. 4.21). (The levator muscle is not divided into orbital and global zones, and is innervated entirely with 'en plaque' endings as is about 85% of human extraocular muscle.)

There is a bimodal distribution of axonal diameters in the ocular motor nerves, with peaks at 5 and 11 μm. The larger axons innervate twitch fibres and

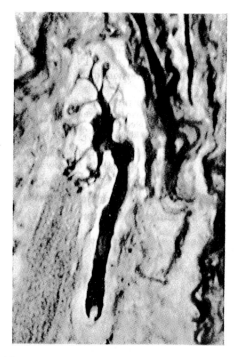

Fig. 4.19   Motor nerve ending in human rectus muscle (Bielchowsky stain).

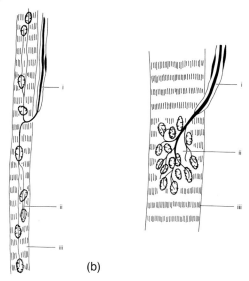

(a)   (b)

Fig. 4.21   (a) Diagram of motor ending on a small peripheral muscle fibre. i = Nerve fibre approaching muscle fibre (the myelin sheath is lost just before the nerve reaches the muscle fibre); ii = fine terminal nerve branch in relation to muscle nuclei; iii = small-diameter muscle fibre. (b) Diagram of motor endplate on large muscle fibre. a = Nerve fibre (the myelin sheath is lost just before it meets the muscle); b = endplate area with nerve branches overlying the muscle nuclei — the oval stuctures; c = cross-striations of muscle fibre. (From Locket, N. A. (1978) *British Orthop. Journal*, **26**, 2, with permission.)

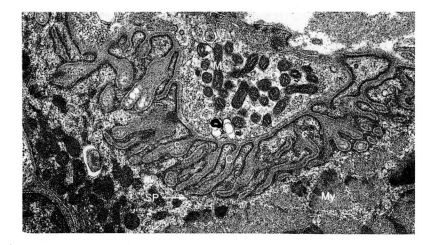

Fig. 4.20   Part of a motor endplate from human skeletal muscle. M = Mitochondria; V = site of vesicle release; C = synaptic cleft; My = myofibril; SP = sole-plate. (Courtesy of D. N. Landon.)

the smaller, tonic fibres. There is evidence for limited division of motor axons after exit from the brain stem. Bors (1926) found an 11% increase in axons of the third and fourth nerve at entry into the muscle, and Torre (1953) reported similar findings for the sixth nerve.

Stimulation and contraction

The characteristic response of skeletal muscle fibres to neural stimulation is the twitch. A train of impulses of sufficient frequency produces a smooth fusion of responses or tetanus.

When a propagated nerve action potential arrives at the motor end plate, packages of acetylcholine stored in the axon terminal are released across the synaptic cleft (Fig. 4.13), a 40–50 nm gap, and bind to receptors on the crests of the postjunctional sarcolemmal folds. Depolarization occurs, with a leakage of both sodium and calcium ions across the membrane. The resting potential of the muscle fibre is about -65 to -90 mV, and depolarization occurs when the potential reaches -60 to -55 mV. In resting muscle the spontaneous quantal release of acetylcholine produces the miniature end-plate potential (mepp), which can be recorded in this region. Contraction is initiated by the development of an end-plate potential (epp).

The epp generates a propagated muscle action potential which spreads across the surface of the fibre. Sarcolemmal depolarization is conducted to the sarcoplasmic reticulum via the T system, possibly as a propagated action potential, and stimulates the release of calcium ions from the reticulum (Ridgway and Gordon, 1975). Within a certain concentration range, binding of calcium determines the level of ATPase activity and the level of tension reached by the fibre during the twitch response. The tension output of the twitch response is lower than during a tetanus.

Excitation–contraction coupling

Binding of calcium to the troponin of the thin filaments causes a conformational change, which exposes the myosin binding sites along the actin molecule (Fig. 4.7).

The interaction of the myosin cross-bridges with the actin molecules causes the thin filaments (containing actin) to slide over the thick filaments (containing myosin). The opposite polarity of the myosin molecules in the two halves of the thick filaments results in the thin filaments and their attached Z-discs moving towards the centre of the sarcomere (Fig. 4.8). The energy for this process derives from the hydrolysis of ATP by the myosin ATPase located in the globular heads of the myosin molecules, which also house the actin binding site. This important HMM region of the myosin molecules contains the means for producing the mechanical event, and the fuel required for it. The muscle twitch is terminated rapidly by the rapid restoration of free calcium to normal by Ca^{2+}-dependent ATPase pumps.

There are two developmentally regulated isoforms of acetylcholine receptors in skeletal muscle, with five subunits (α–ε). In the embryonic receptor they are found as $\alpha_2\beta\gamma\delta$ and in the adult as $\alpha_2\beta\varepsilon\delta$. The embryonic isoform is thought to be retained by multiply innervated fibres. The advanced and sometimes exclusive involvement of extraocular muscles in myasthenia gravis has been attributed to differences in the acetylcholine receptor types expressed in extraocular versus skeletal muscle (Horton et al., 1993; Oda, 1993). It is not clear how this influences the pathogenesis of myasthenia since the antibodies preferentially bind to the neuromuscular junctions of multiply and singly innervated fibres.

Extraocular muscle twitch-fibre contraction

The activation of extraocular twitch fibres is comparable to that of skeletal twitch muscle and makes the extraocular muscles the fastest contracting muscles in the body (e.g. 7.5–10 ms for medial rectus compared with 40 ms for gastrocnemius). The stimulation frequency to induce fusion of extraocular muscle responses is 350–450 Hz (Lennerstrand, 1986) compared with 100 Hz for gastrocnemius. The fusion frequency for extraocular muscle is about ten times that required to induce the twitch responses (Cooper and Eccles, 1930; Bach-y-Rita and Ito, 1966; Lennerstrand, 1974): for skeletal muscle the ratio is about two times greater. Increasing the nerve stimulation frequency above 350 Hz increases the rate of rise in tension but not the level achieved (Barmack et al., 1971; Fuchs and Luschei, 1971).

TONIC FIBRES

As noted earlier, orbital and to a lesser extent global muscle fibres containing tonic myosin may have a histochemical profile resembling skeletal type I fibres. The orbital fibres are type 2 and the global, type 6; they are both multiply innervated (Asmussen et al., 1971; Spencer and Porter, 1981) (Tables 4.6 and 4.7).

Ultrastructure

Tonic fibres are multinucleated, with both central and peripheral nuclei. Mitochondria are plentiful in orbital fibres but sparse in global fibres, for example in cat inferior oblique (Alvarado and Van Horn, 1975).

There appears to be good correspondence between feline and primate subtypes. Tonic fibres have a felderstruktur, characterized by an irregular arrangement of myofibrils and a deficiency of membranous systems.

In the **orbital layer**, the small red 'type 1' fibre described in the rhesus monkey by Miller (1967) is probably equivalent to the tonic fibre described by Alvarado and Van Horn (1975) in the cat, but an M-line is absent in the former and present in the

Table 4.9 Mammalian extraocular muscle fibre diameters and innervation

Species	Orbital zone fibre diameter (μm)		Global zone fibre diameter (μm)				
	Innervation		Innervation				
	Single	Multiple	Single	Single	Single	Multiple	Multiple
Sheep (Harker, 1972)	Small C, 15	Small G, 13	Small C, 15	Intermediate C, 25	Large A, 29	Large G, 32	
Cat superior rectus (Peachey, 1971)	Small, 15	Large, 15	Small granulated, 15	Lightly granulated, 25	Fibrillar white, 35	Fibrillar white	Large granulated, 15
Cat superior oblique (Alvarado and Van Horn, 1975)	Type 3, 12	Type 5, 12	Type 3, 12	Type 2, 22	Type 1, 31	Type 4, 23	Type 5, 12
Rabbit (Davidowitz, Phillips and Breinin, 1975)	10–15	10	Small dark, 10–15	Intermediate, 15–25	Large white, 25–35	Large, 15–20	Pseudorbital, 10–15
Rat (Mayr, 1971)	Dark, 10–25	Clear, 5–10	Dark, 10–20	Intermediate, 20–30	Pale, 30–40	Clear, 15–25	
Mouse (Patcher, 1976)	5–10	3–7	Small dark, 10–15		Large light, 20–25	5–7	

latter. Both have a poorly developed sarcoplasmic reticulum. In the monkey the reticulum is located chiefly around the thin filaments of the I-band, with an incomplete sheath around the fibrils of the A-band. A T system with numerous triads is present at the margins of the A-band. Glycogen granules are localized mostly around the tubules and between the hypolemmal, perinuclear and intermyofibrillar mitochondria and some scattered lipid droplets. The mitochondrial volume compared with gastrocnemius is 5.3 (Miller, 1971). These fibres have prominent Z-lines and H-zones. The cat fibres are multiply innervated and regarded as tonic.

Myofibrils are large and poorly separated by sarcoplasm and have sparse and irregular reticular elements. Respiratory metabolism is aerobic; mitochondria are small, relatively sparse and arranged in peripheral areas of sarcoplasm devoid of myofibrils. Z-lines and H-bands are wide, and tubular networks elaborate (Gauthier, 1969, 1979). Nuclei are both centrally and peripherally disposed within the sarcoplasm.

These fibres, corresponding to type 2 of Spencer and Porter (1981), are wider proximally and distally (where their ultrastructural features are those of a multiply innervated fibre) than centrally, where their features suggest the ability to propagate an action potential (Lennerstrand and Bach-y-Rita, 1975).

Cheng and Breinin (1966) described a small fibre, 8–15 μm wide, in the simian lateral rectus which has

large and ill-defined myofibrils incompletely surrounded by a network of sarcoplasmic reticulum. Transverse tubules are rare and there are no triads. The myofilaments of the A-band (thick and thin) have a regular array as in interosseus twitch fibres, but thin filaments in the I-band, close to the Z-line, are irregularly disposed. This fibre, lacking an M-line, was equated with the slow fibre (i.e. tonic) of lower vertebrates.

This appears to be the same cell as that described by Miller (1967) in the extraocular muscle **global layer** of rhesus monkey. In addition to those features noted above, small clusters of ovoid or globular mitochondria are found on either side of the Z-line, or as parallel doublets astride interruptions in the Z-lines (Z-lines are straight in 'relaxed' muscle or jagged in muscle fixed at original length). Nuclei are elongated and peripheral, or occasionally oval and central. M-lines are poorly defined. The mitochondrial volume compared with gastrocnemius is 0.8 (Miller, 1967). These fibres correspond to type 6.

Studies in primates and other species suggest that these muscles are relatively fatigue resistant (Hoogenraad, Jennekens and Tan, 1979).

Innervation (Tables 4.8 and 4.9)

Tonic fibres are innervated by multiple 'en grappe' endings (Fig. 4.21) (Kupfer, 1960; Hess, 1961;

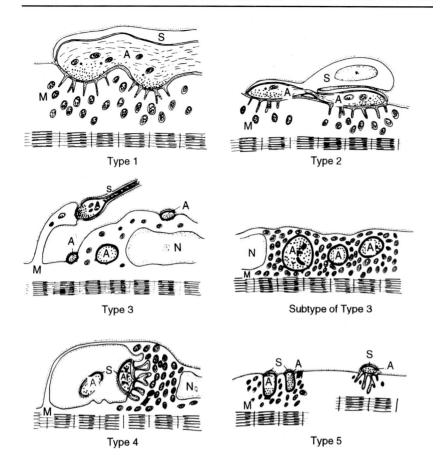

Type 1

Type 2

Type 3

Subtype of Type 3

Type 4

Type 5

Fig. 4.22 Six types of neuromuscular junction in human extraocular muscle, based on electron-microscopic findings. N = nucleus; A = axon; S = Schwann cell; M = mitochondrion. (From Mukuno, K. (1968), *Acta Soc. Ophthal. Jap.*, **72**, 104, with permission.)

Bormioli *et al.*, 1980). Their motor fibres are of finer calibre than those supplying type 2 muscles and they run for some distance parallel with and closely apposed to the muscle fibres. At intervals small swellings commonly overlie the muscle nuclei. Staining for cholinesterase is most marked at these sites. Nerve endings show only rudimentary junctional folds in the synaptic membrane. Well-developed junctional folds are a constant feature of motor end plates in twitch fibres. Granular vesicles, similar to those found in autonomic nerve endings, occur, in addition to typical synaptic vesicles. There is said to be fusion of nerve and muscle plasmalemmas without an intervening basement membrane, a structure known as a nexus, found in muscle spindles and autonomic nerve endings (Cheng and Breinin, 1966). However, this view is not universally accepted. 'En grappe' endings are concentrated over the distal third of the muscle belly (Cheng, 1963).

Many 'en grappe' endings occur on a single tonic fibre, with clusters separated by 10 μm to 2–3 mm.

Studies in monkeys (Zenker and Anzenbacher, 1964; Cheng and Breinin, 1966) and rats (Cheng, 1963) have shown that 'en grappe' endings have postsynaptic folds different from those exhibited by tonic fibres in amphibia.

Teravainen (1969) found two types of multiply innervated muscle fibres in the extraocular muscles of rats: type 1 showed 2–5 small junctions per muscle fibre with a subneural fold, resembling similar junctions in the cat; type 2 showed a greater number of smaller junctions, without such folds.

'En grappe' endings are smaller and lighter staining than end plates. The endings are bead-like, round or oval structures arranged in chains or clusters, sometimes spiralling around a muscle cell. Cholinesterase stains demonstrate endings as a diffuse speckle along the entire muscle belly, but concentrated in its distal third (Cheng, 1963; Dietert, 1965).

Although the individual area occupied by a single 'en grappe' ending is much smaller than that of a motor end plate, the total junctional area offered is probably 12–48% greater. The axons of supply are smaller than those to twitch fibres.

At 'en plaque' and at 'en grappe' endings, an epithelial extension of the perineural sheath forms a fine cellular cuff around both the terminal and its related muscle fibre. These sheaths bear a superficial resemblance to the structure of a muscle spindle, but differ in that the space within the enveloping sheath is open at each end, whereas the capsular space of the muscle spindle is closed. Some such sheaths envelop a muscle fibre and related nerve axons in the absence of a terminal (Ruskell, 1984a).

Mukuno (1968) described six types of junction in human extraocular muscles, but was not able to specify the muscle type supplied (Fig. 4.22).

Physiology of tonic fibre contraction

Stimulation of these multiply innervated muscle fibres produces a slowly graded contraction (Hofmann and Lembeck, 1969; Eakins and Katz, 1971). Fusion frequency is 200 Hz or lower; stimulation at up to 400 Hz increases the force of contraction but neither rate nor force is increased at frequencies above this.

The spontaneous discharges at 'en grappe' endings (miniature small nerve junctional potentials) can be recorded anywhere on the muscle, reflecting the diffuse distribution of these endings. Junctional depolarization is signalled by small nerve junctional potentials (Hess and Pilar, 1963; Kuffler and Gerard, 1974). Unlike twitch fibres, tonic fibres do not exhibit a propagated action potential; instead there is a passive electrotonic spread of depolarization from multiple sites across the fibre surface. The 'en grappe' potentials are smaller than motor end-plate potentials because of the smaller junctional area and lesser quantity of transmitter released. The resting potential of the tonic fibre is lower than that of the twitch fibre, and its membrane resistance is about six times greater.

OTHER MORPHOLOGICAL AND PHARMACOLOGICAL FEATURES OF EXTRAOCULAR MUSCLE

In addition to the presence of the twitch and tonic muscle fibres described above, normal human extraocular muscle commonly shows changes which, if seen in skeletal muscle, would be interpreted as myopathic or degenerative. These include whorled fibres, vacuoles within myofibrillar bundles, hypolemmal inclusions, sarcomere disruption, nemaline rods, smeared Z-lines, mitochondrial clumping and Zebra and Hirano bodies (Martinez et al., 1976). A further type, with circular or hypolemmal myofibrils, has also been noted and termed 'Ringbinden' fibres. Other features suggestive of myopathy are variability in shape and size of fibre, higher proportion of smaller fibres, a larger number of nuclei, and the presence of a mild mononuclear infiltrate (Ringel et al., 1978). The reason for these changes is obscure and may hinder interpretation of extraocular muscle specimens by people who usually interpret biopsies of skeletal muscle.

Extraocular muscle shows signs of ageing from early adult life, with a differential loss of type II fibres (IIa according to Lyness (1986)) from the orbital and then global layer and a later loss of global 'type I' fibres (Lyness, 1986). Also, although mean fibre width of all fibre types is maintained with age, the variance increases.

It is generally assumed that the differences in muscle fibre type, distribution, innervation and physiology reflect in some way differences in function of the extraocular muscles as an oculomotor unit. The singly innervated, fast, oxidative muscle fibres of the orbital layer show the greatest differences phylogenetically and are particularly well developed in the primate, indicating an adaptation to changes in organization and connections within the cerebral cortex related to the fusional requirements of binocular vision and the emergence of vergence and smooth pursuit subsystems (Walls, 1962). A potential role for this fatigue-resistant fibre type may be to maintain stability of fixation over a wide range of gaze.

The global, multiply innervated muscle fibres associated with the palisade endings at the myotendinous junction may contribute a significant part of the holding tension in the primary position, and may smooth and dampen the action of antagonistic muscles during fixation (Browne, 1976).

The action of the muscle relaxant succinylcholine is different in skeletal and extraocular muscles. In skeletal muscle, it is a depolarizing blocker of neuromuscular transmission. In extraocular muscle it selectively activates the multiply innervated fibres, certainly the global, possibly the orbital. This causes ocular alignment during general anaesthesia approximating the primary position and has been interpreted to indicate a role for multiply innervated fibres in achieving ocular alignment.

The aminoacyl class of local anaesthetics (lidocaine, mepivacaine and bupivacaine) used in the region of the orbit, are myotoxic and may cause extraocular muscle palsies. On injection into muscle they induce the release of calcium from intracellular stores and sarcolemmal disruption. Thus unanticipated ptosis or diplopia may follow ocular surgery under local anaesthesia. The toxicity appears to result from direct injection of the affected muscles, and, in the monkey, it appears that a severe response occurs only in the global, pale singly innervated muscle fibres. Botulinum toxin acts by blocking the calcium-dependent release of acetylcholine at the neuromuscular junction (Cull-Candy, 1976). The A serotype is used clinically to induce transient weakening of extraocular muscles in the management of squint, transient relaxation of the levator muscle to protect the ocular surface, and relaxation of facial and other muscles recruited in dystonic muscular disorders (Scott *et al.*, 1973; Scott, 1980).

Injection of botulinum toxin into skeletal muscle, including orbicularis, causes a paralysis secondary to denervation atrophy of the injected muscles. Recovery of skeletal muscle, including the levator, is due to motor neuron sprouting and functional reinnervation (Duchen, 1974; Boothe *et al.*, 1990; Harris *et al.*, 1991; Porter *et al.*, 1991; Horn *et al.*, 1993) and is responsible for its reversibility (Manning *et al.*, 1990; Porter *et al.*, 1993; Bonner *et al.*, 1994). However, in extraocular muscles there are permanent effects. In the monkey there is specific loss of orbital singly innervated muscle (Spender and McNeer, 1987). The effects are more profound in infantile and juvenile monkeys, perhaps because their muscles are still developing (McNeer *et al.*, 1991; Spencer *et al.*, 1992).

4.9 SENSORY APPARATUS OF EXTRAOCULAR MUSCLE

Early studies suggested that sensory fibres from the extraocular muscles pass in the third, fourth and sixth cranial nerves (Tozer and Sherrington, 1910), with cell bodies in the mesencephalic nucleus of the trigeminal nerve. Those in the oculomotor nerve pass ventrally in the tectospinal tract to join the nerve just ventral to its motor nuclei (Tarkhan, 1934). Cooper, Daniel and Whitteridge (1951, 1955) recorded sensory impulses from extraocular muscles. More recent studies suggest that only small numbers of afferent fibres are present in the oculomotor nerves (Porter and Spencer, 1982; Porter, Guthrie and Sparks, 1983). Section of the ophthalmic nerve in the monkey leads to degeneration of 0.9–2.7% of axons in the nerve to the inferior oblique; most of these axons are 1–3 μm in diameter (Ruskell, 1983). Manni, Bortolami and Desole (1966) recorded responses to stretch in sheep and pigs, in a neuronal pool in the medial dorsolateral part of the trigeminal ganglion, with a somatotopic organization reflecting spatial relations in the orbit (Manni, Bortolami and Desole, 1966; Manni, Bortolami and Derck, 1970a; Manni, Bortolami and Deriu, 1970b; Manni, Palmieri and Marini, 1971a,b; Manni *et al.*, 1970c; Manni, Palmieri and Marini, 1971a,b; 1974; Manni and Pettorossi, 1976). This has been confirmed in cats and monkeys (Porter and Spencer, 1982; Porter *et al.*, 1983). First-order neurons end in the trigeminal main sensory and spinal nuclei. In the monkey, terminations are in the pars interpolaris of the spinal trigeminal nucleus and

in the cuneate nucleus of the caudal medulla, overlapping the afferent termination from the dorsal neck muscles (Edney and Porter, 1983; Porter, 1986). Second-order neurons pass to tectum and tegmentum and project to the ventral basal nucleus of the thalamus.

These fibres innervate the following structures (Fig. 4.23):

1. muscle spindles;
2. Golgi tendon organs;
3. palisade endings;
4. spiral nerve endings.

Table 4.10 contains a more extensive listing of sensory endings.

As in the description of extrafusal fibres, it is convenient here to detail the form and function of these sensory structures as they occur in skeletal muscle, where they have been studied in greatest detail, as a model for conditions in extraocular muscles.

MUSCLE SPINDLES

Muscle spindles signal both change and rate of change in length of muscles. A spindle is a structure with a thin torpedo-shaped connective tissue capsule enclosing a number of small intrafusal muscle fibres, arranged in parallel with the extrafusal muscle mass (Fig. 4.23). Nuclei of intrafusal fibres may be grouped centrally to produce a nuclear bag, or may be arranged linearly as a nuclear chain. There are two types of afferent sensory endings on intrafusal fibres: primary endings innervate both nuclear chain and nuclear bag fibres (morphologically annulospiral endings); secondary endings (of group II type afferents) innervate nuclear chain fibres almost exclusively (flower spray endings). Contraction of extrafusal muscle fibres shortens the spindle and reduces the signal. Group II afferents signal mainly length, group Ia, mainly from nuclear bag fibres, both length and rate of change in length. Gamma-efferent fibres to intrafusal fibres control the sensitivity of length detection (Carew and Ghez, 1985).

Muscle spindles in extraocular muscles

Siemmerling (1888) and Buzzard (1908) described muscle spindles in human extraocular muscles (Fig. 4.24) and Cilimbaris (1910) detected them in cows, goats, boars and stags. For many years these observations were not corroborated, until Daniel (1946), Cooper and Daniel (1949) and Cooper *et al.* (1951) described them in human extraocular muscles using

Table 4.10 The sensory apparatus of human extraocular muscle

Muscle receptor	Comment
A: Classical muscle spindle (Cooper and Daniel, 1959)	Principally in anterior and posterior thirds of muscle
B: Atypical muscle spindle Capsulated nerve endings (Sas and Appeltauer, 1963; Spiro and Balm, 1969)	Two nerve fibres encapsulated on extrafusal fibre anterior to motor innervation zone
Muscle capsulated nerve endings (Sas and Appeltauer, 1963; Spiro and Balm, 1969)	One nerve encapsulated on extrafusal fibre three fusiform enlargements, generally anterior to motor innervation zone
C: Golgi tendon organs (Ciaccio, 1891)	Similar to skeletal muscle tendon organs, located entirely on tendon
D: Palisade endings (Ruskell, 1978; Richmond et al., 1984)	Encapsulated nerve endings at the myotendinous junction of global, multiply innervated muscle fibres
E: Spiral endings*	All on extrafusal fibre
Single spiral endings (Daniel, 1946; Gruner, 1961)	Non-encapsulated, in middle third of muscle, medullated nerve fibre
Double spiral endings (Daniel, 1946; Gruner, 1961; Sas and Appeltauer, 1963)	Non-encapsulated medullated nerve fibre, sometimes multiply branched
Multiple spiral endings (Sas and Appeltauer, 1963; Spiro and Balm, 1969)	Anterior to motor innervation zone, several spirals from several nerves on adjacent fibres, large terminal expansions away from spirals
F: Miscellaneous (Sas and Appeltauer, 1963; Spiro and Balm, 1969)	Uncommon and less well described
G: Other receptors Flower-budlike end plates Arboreal sensory termination Brushlike sensory end structures Sensory spools Sensory end bulbs	Occur in intestinal connective tissue

Adapted from Eggers, 1982.
*Spiral endings are now regarded as motor in function.

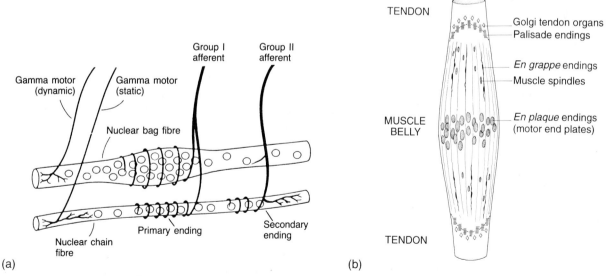

Fig. 4.23 (a) A muscle spindle showing the nuclear bag and nuclear chain intrafusal fibres. Group I (primary) afferents innervate both the nuclear bag and chain fibres, whereas group II (secondary) afferents usually innervate only the nuclear chain fibres. However, they occasionally innervate bag fibres. (From Kandel and Schwarz (eds) (1985) *Principles of Neuroscience*, published by Elsevier Science Publishers.) (b) Schematic diagram to show the disposition of motor and sensory endings on a rectus muscle.

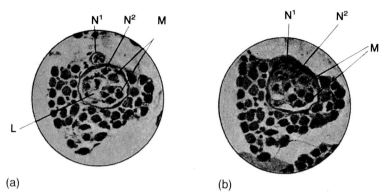

(a) (b)

Fig. 4.24 Reproduction of Farquhar Buzzard's illustration of 1908. The original description is as follows. 'Photographs of the same spindle at levels a short distance from one another in an ocular muscle. N^1 is an extrafusal nerve bundle, which in (b) is being incorporated within the spindle sheath. N^2 Intrafusal nerve fibres. M Intrafusal muscle fibres. L Lymphatic space. Note the equality in size between the intra- and extrafusal muscle fibres and the thick sheath, with spindle-shaped nuclei.'

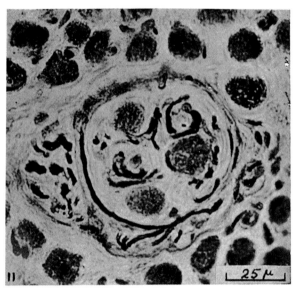

Fig. 4.25 Transverse section of a muscle spindle in a human medial rectus muscle. A well-defined capsule is seen with a nerve trunk incorporated in its wall (left). Within the capsule there are three intrafusal muscle fibres, capillaries and intricate arrangementof nervefibres. One nerve fibre partly encircles the spindle, either just inside or within the walls of the capsule. (Paraffin section, Holmes' 'silver on the slide' method.)

silver methods, confirmed by Merillees, Sunderland and Hayhow (1950) (Figs 4.24 and 4.25). Muscle spindles are concentrated away from the middle third of the muscle belly containing the motor end-plate zone, and are found proximally (inferior rectus; Cooper and Daniel, 1949), distally (superior rectus and oblique; Merillees, Sunderland and Hayhow, 1950) or in both zones (Merillees, Sunderland and Hayhow, 1950) of the muscle belly (Table 4.9b). They occur only among the narrower fibres characteristic of the periphery of these muscles (Locket, 1968) and there may be 22–71 per muscle. Lukas *et al.* (1995) found spindles in all rectus and oblique muscles studied, as follows: medial rectus, 18.8 ± 3.0 SD; lateral rectus, 19.3 ± 1.9; inferior rectus, 34.0 ± 4.4; superior oblique, 27.3 ± 8.2; inferior oblique 4.3 ± 1.8. The numbers were as frequent as those in some skeletal muscles. Their haphazard appearance in different species is not explained. They have been found in humans, chimpanzees, macaques, mice, pigs, sheep, goats, cattle, deer, giraffes and gnus, but not in baboons, cats, dogs, rabbits, rats, foxes or birds.

Each spindle has 1–15 intrafusal fibres in its capsule

Table 4.11 Number of muscle spindles in human extraocular muscles

	Cooper and Daniel, 1949		Merillees, Sunderland and Hayhow, 1950		Voss, 1957	Inoue, 1958
	Proximal	Distal	Proximal third	Distal third		
Medial rectus			37	34	11	47
Inferior rectus	41	6			31	48
Lateral rectus					3	31
Superior rectus			18	33	0	67
Inferior oblique					0	26
Superior oblique			17	54	35	41
			19	40		
			11	40		
			3	19		
			9	26		
			18	32		

From Eggers, 1982.

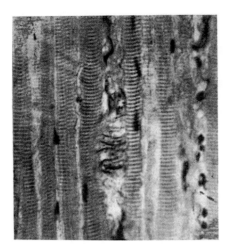

Fig. 4.26 Spiral nerve ending in human rectus muscle (Bielchowsky stain). These are now thought to be motor in nature. See text.

Table 4.12 Morphology of spindles in human extraocular tissue

Length (μm)	900 (100–2600)*
Diameter (μm)	35–65 (20–100)†
Number of intrafusal fibres	4 (1–15)‡
Diameter of intrafusal fibres (μm)	10 (5–30)

All values are average (range).
*30% exceed 1000 μm; †majority of fibres; ‡most 3–7 μm.
From Merrillees, Sunderland and Hayhow, 1950 (but see text).

(four on average), which receive a rich nerve supply (Merillees, Sunderland and Hayhow, 1950) (Table 4.11). They are more delicate and smaller than comparable structures in somatic muscles. There is a small periaxial space and an irregular and divided inner capsule which probably accounts for the difficulty in identification in human muscle (Fig. 4.25). Delicate end plates are present at each pole, and a complex array of myelinated and non-myelinated nerve fibres at the equator encircle the intrafusal fibre. Histochemistry shows positive staining for oxidative enzymes, and intrafusal muscle spindles are rich in acid-labile ATPase and non-specific esterase. They are deficient in glycogen, phosphorylase, lipids, and glycerophosphate dehydrogenase (Spiro and Beilin, 1969).

In a study of human extraocular muscle by Ruskell (1984b), about half of the intrafusal fibres that received no nerve terminals were indistinguishable from extrafusal fibres and had a substantially larger diameter than other intrafusal fibres. Most of the remainder were typical nuclear chain fibres with a single row of centrally placed nuclei, tightly packed myofibrils and distinct H- and M-lines. Nuclear bag fibres were uncommon (four out of ten spindles) but

typical, with two or three nuclei occupying nearly the full width of the fibre at one locus, an indistinct H-line and no M-line. Sensory terminals spiralled equatorially around both fibre types. Not all spindles are enclosed in a connective tissue sheath. Some are invested by perineural epithelial extensions (Ruskell, 1984b). Locket (1968) described large-calibre nerve fibres forming simple and complex spirals around large extrafusal muscle fibres in a well-defined region of the muscle core, just distal to the band of end plates (Fig. 4.26).

Intrafusal fibres vary in width between 5 and 30 μm (average 10 μm); spindles may be 50–900 μm long, with an average width of 20–200 μm. Ruskell (1984b) gives length as 350–725 μm, with a mean of 500 μm.

Separate small γ efferents innervate both the nuclear bag fibres (γ dynamic) and chain fibres (γ static) which regulate the sensitivity of the spindle afferents either to dynamic or static phases of stretch (Fig. 4.27). Gamma-efferents are probably active during contraction of the muscle mass, maintaining sensitivity in the spindle. There is evidence of small-diameter motor fibre innervation of gamma type in extraocular muscle. Donaldson (1960) estimates 8–11 γ efferent fibres in the inferior oblique for each muscle spindle.

Spindles do not mediate an awareness of position; eye position is not appreciated consciously in the absence of visual cues (Brindley and Merton, 1960). Fuchs and Kornhuber (1969) suggested that spindles provide information to the cerebellum concerning size and end points of saccades. Christman and

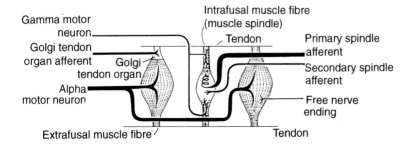

Fig. 4.27 Schematic diagram of the muscle spindle and Golgi tendon organ of skeletal muscle. (From Kandel and Schwarz (eds), (1985) *Principles of Neuroscience*, published by Elsevier Science Publishers.)

Kupfer (1963) proposed a role in fixation nystagmus. Sasaki (1983) and Sears *et al.* (1959) found evidence of extraocular motor neuronal inhibition by stretch receptors while Gernandt (1968) suggested that such receptors may dampen and correct overshoot of ocular movements.

GOLGI TENDON ORGANS

Tendon organs were described by Golgi in 1880, though he did not find them in extraocular muscles. They signal muscle tension in somatic muscles, where they are found in the muscle tendon. Tendon organs consist of a capsule about 1 mm long and 0.1 mm wide, into which 15–20 extrafusal muscle fibres enter through a tight collar. The capsule terminates in braided collagen fibrils, which interweave with large-diameter group 1b afferent axons. Contraction of the muscle compresses the axons and signals an increase in muscle tension (Fig. 4.27). Tendon organs vary in size from 70 to 400 μm long and from 100 to 80 μm wide. In skeletal muscle one end of the organ is in muscle and the other is tendon, while in human extraocular muscle they are completely embedded in tendon.

Golgi tendon organs were described by Marchi (1882) in human extraocular muscle and were confirmed by Sherrington (1897), and Tozer and Sherrington (1910) in the cat. They are found in the anterior musculotendinous junctions, but are rarely observed in extraocular muscles, and may represent an anomalous development of the palisade ending (Ruskell, 1979).

Tendon organs are innervated by one or more myelinated nerve fibres, whose peripheral divisions form plaques in the tendon. Axon enlargements or plates lie between loose tendon fascicles. Small tendon bundles are surrounded by spirals or rings of axon terminals, whose naked, mitochondria-rich processes, surrounded by Schwann cell cytoplasm, indent the collagen bundles. A few vesicles are found in these terminals.

PALISADE ENDINGS

The palisade endings (myotendinous cylinders) are probably the principal sensory apparatus of mammalian extraocular muscle. They consist of encapsulated nerve endings lying at the myotendinous junction which interdigitate with longitudinal fingers of the global, multiply innervated muscle fibres. Richmond *et al.* (1984), using silver stains in human muscle, described them as interwoven networks of fine neural filaments cupped to receive attachments

of a single extrafusal muscle fibre tip. One myelinated axon may branch to supply several neighbouring muscle fibres. They are found in significant numbers in extraocular muscle; more in the horizontal recti than in the vertical recti or obliques (Ruskell, 1978, 1979; Alvarado-Mallart and Pincon-Raymond, 1979).

A sensory function for these structures is suggested by the absence of a basal lamina at the contact zone between muscle and nerve (the intervening cleft is 20–40 nm) (Ruskell, 1978), and the intimate association between the distal expansion of the muscle fibre and the nerve terminal which may isolate the receptor from displacement by passive stretch. Neural stimulation probably results from compression of terminals during contraction of the muscle fibre with which the palisade ending is associated.

SPIRAL NERVE ENDINGS (Fig. 4.26)

Various endings, in the middle third of extraocular muscles, wrap around an extrafusal muscle fibre and are innervated by myelinated fibres. It is now thought that these spiral endings in extraocular muscle are motor endings to singly innervated fibres (Ruskell and Wilson, 1983). Single spiral endings are least numerous and make 3–8 turns around the muscle fibre, terminating in a structure like an end plate. Multiple spirals, winding around in opposite directions, are more frequent (Daniel, 1946; Spiro and Beilin, 1961), and other variants are described. Bach-y-Rita and Ito (1966) proposed a protective role for such endings in cats, preventing overstretch, like Golgi tendon organs in somatic muscles.

4.10 ACTIONS OF THE EYE MUSCLES

Ocular movements take place round a centre corresponding approximately to that of the eye, which is therefore not significantly displaced (Figs 4.28–4.33).

The movements may be resolved and defined relative to three primary axes which pass through the centre of movement at right-angles to each other (Fig. 4.29):

1. The vertical axis, around which the centre of the cornea and visual axis moves laterally (abduction) or medially (adduction).
2. The *transverse axis* is mediolateral, and around it the centre of the cornea ascends (elevation) or descends (depression).
3. The *sagittal axis* is anteroposterior. Around it, so-called wheel rotation takes place, better

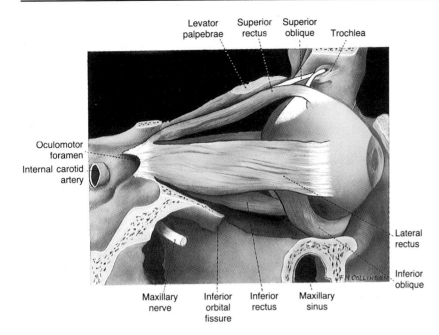

Levator palpebrae
Superior rectus
Superior oblique
Trochlea
Oculomotor foramen
Internal carotid artery
Lateral rectus
Inferior oblique
Maxillary nerve
Inferior orbital fissure
Inferior rectus
Maxillary sinus

Fig. 4.28 Dissection to show the ocular muscles from the lateral aspect. Note especially the oculomotor foramen. From the Anatomy Museum of University College, London.

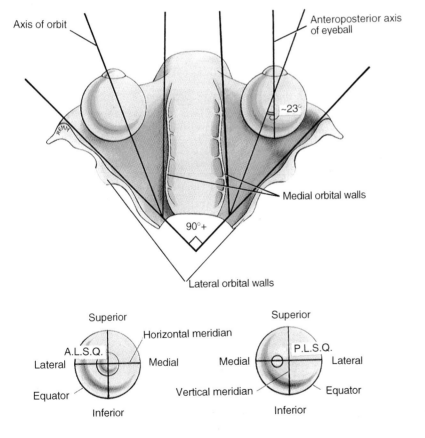

Axis of orbit
Anteroposterior axis of eyeball
~23°
Medial orbital walls
90°+
Lateral orbital walls

Superior
Horizontal meridian
A.L.S.Q.
Lateral
Medial
Equator
Inferior

Superior
P.L.S.Q.
Medial
Lateral
Vertical meridian
Equator
Inferior

Anterior quadrants
Posterior quadrants

Fig. 4.29 The geometry of the orbits and eyes. In the upper diagram note the disparity between the orbital axis and the anteroposterior axis of the eyeball. See text for the significance of this in explaining the actions of individual muscles.

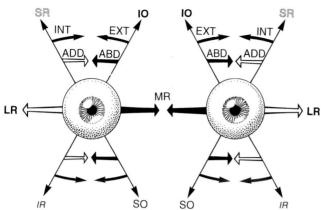

Fig. 4.30 The actions of the extraocular muscles. The long straight arrows show the primary actions of muscle. Note that the primary actions of the vertical recti are elicited in abduction, and of the oblique muscles in adduction. The short straight arrows show the secondary horizontal actions of the vertical recti (adduction) and obliques (abduction). Curved arrows show the tortional actions about an anteroposterior axis. Superior muscles are *intorters*; inferior muscles are *extorters*.

primary action. Only the medial and lateral recti exert their primary actions in the primary position of the eyeball, with the visual axis projected straight forward; for each of the others there is a position in which the primary action is maximal. However, the visual axes only occasionally coincide with these arbitrary directions.

At all times the effect of any muscle can be analysed in relation to the global axes, into **primary**, **secondary** and **tertiary** actions. Thus, for example, the primary action of superior rectus is elevation, which is greatest when the eye is abducted, so that the muscle axis and the global anteroposterior axis are in the same plane. When the eye is adducted a tendency to adduction and intorsion appears, and these secondary and tertiary components of the muscle's effect on the eyeball increase as the visual axis is turned medially. These effects are considered below in connection with each muscle (Fig. 4.30).

defined as intorsion or extorsion as the 'twelve o'clock' on the cornea moves nasally or temporally.

These are necessary conventions, and obviously the posterior pole of the eye moves in an opposite direction, except in torsional movements. It is more important to note that, despite their formalized terms, all movements are rotations, and are not necessarily confined to the above arbitrary axes, the movements of which are sometimes called cardinal. Because of the geometric relations between the orbital and global attachments of each muscle, each acts to greatest effect in one plane, and this is known as its

SYNERGIC ACTION

As elsewhere, extraocular muscles are grouped as synergists. Thus the visual axis can be elevated by the synergic action of the superior rectus and inferior oblique, and depressed by the inferior rectus and superior oblique. But this often-quoted pairing of the muscles is over-simplified.

4.11 THE FOUR RECTI

The four recti are attached posteriorly by a short tendinous ring (annulus tendineus communis). This is oval on cross-section and encloses the optic foramen and the inferomedial end of the superior

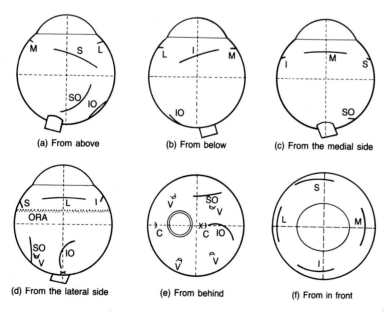

(a) From above

(b) From below

(c) From the medial side

(d) From the lateral side

(e) From behind

(f) From in front

Fig. 4.31 (a–f) The insertions of the eye muscles (right eye). X = Position of the macula; C = long ciliaries; V = venae vorticosae; SO = superior oblique; IO = inferior oblique; M = medial rectus; L = lateral rectus; I = inferior rectus; S = superior rectus. Note the position of the optic nerve. Its centre is just above the horizontal meridian. Note also that many authorities place the attachment of the inferior oblique clearly within the posterior inferior lateral quadrant.

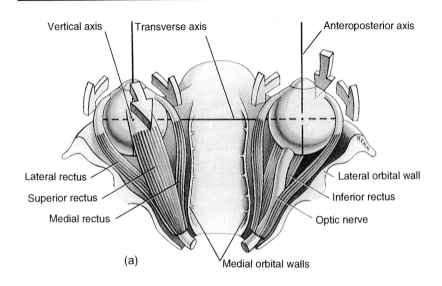

(a)

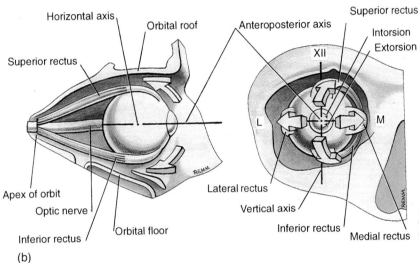

(b)

Fig. 4.32 Diagrams in three dimensions to explain the actions of the recti. See text for details.

Table 4.13 Dimensions of the four recti

	Distance from cornea (mm)	Length of tendon (mm)	Width of tendon (mm)	Width of muscle (mm)
Superior rectus	7.7	5.8	10.8	9.0
Lateral rectus	6.9	8.8	9.2	9.0
Inferior rectus	6.5	5.5	9.8	9.0
Medial rectus	5.5	3.7	10.3	9.0

orbital fissure. The annulus is thickened above and below by two strong common tendons.

The lower tendon is attached to the lesser wing of the sphenoid between the optic foramen and superior orbital fissure, sometimes marked by the infraoptic tubercle (Fig. 1.2). The lower tendon serves part of the medial and lateral recti and the whole of the inferior rectus.

The upper tendon arises from the body of the sphenoid, and serves part of the medial and lateral recti and the whole of the superior rectus (Fig. 5.24).

Because of the slope of the orbital roof the superior and medial recti are attached on a plane anterior to the others. These muscles are also much more closely attached to the dural sheath of the optic nerve (Fig.

1.15). It is this attachment of the superior and medial recti to the nerve sheath which is responsible for the characteristic pain which accompanies extreme movements of the globe in retrobulbar neuritis.

The average length of the recti is 40 mm, the superior being the longest, followed by the medial, lateral and inferior. Extending anteriorly close to the orbital walls they become tendinous and blend with the sclera at varying distances from the cornea, as shown in Table 4.13. (See also Gottrau *et al.*, 1994.)

4.12 SUPERIOR RECTUS

Superior rectus arises from the upper part of the annular tendon superolateral to the optic foramen and the sheath of the optic nerve, in the angle where the dura splits in the optic canal to become orbital periosteum and dural optic sheath. Below the attachment of the levator, it is continuous with the attachments of the medial and lateral recti.

Passing anterolaterally beneath the levator, at 23–25° with the globe's anteroposterior axis, the superior rectus pierces Tenon's capsule and is attached to sclera 7.7 mm from the cornea by a tendon 5.8 mm long along an oblique line, 10.8 mm long and slightly convex forwards (Fig. 4.31). The muscle is about 42 mm in length and 9 mm in width.

RELATIONS

Superior

Superiorly lie the levator and frontal nerve, which separate the superior rectus from the roof of the orbit (Figs 1.15, 5.17 and 5.18).

Inferior

Separated by orbital fat are the ophthalmic artery and nasociliary artery and nerves (Fig. 5.18). The reflected tendon of the superior oblique passes between the superior rectus and globe to its attachment (Fig. 7.2).

Lateral

Between the superior and lateral recti are the lacrimal artery and nerve.

Medial

Between the superior rectus above and medial rectus and oblique below are the ophthalmic artery and nasociliary nerve (Figs 5.18 and 5.21).

NERVES

The superior division of the oculomotor nerve, entering the ocular surface at the junction of its middle and posterior thirds (Fig. 5.24).

BLOOD SUPPLY

The lateral muscular branch of the ophthalmic artery.

ACTIONS

Acting alone, the muscle would rotate the eye from the primary position of forward gaze as to elevate, adduct and intort along the visual axis. What it accomplishes in reality depends upon the position of the eyeball and activity of other extraocular muscles.

The **primary action** is elevation, which increases with abduction and becomes nil in full adduction.

The superior rectus is the only elevator in full abduction because the inferior oblique is ineffective. Hence, when the superior rectus is paralysed, the abducted eye cannot be elevated.

Subsidiary actions are adduction and intorsion.

4.13 INFERIOR RECTUS

Inferior rectus, the shortest of the recti, is attached below the optic foramen by the middle part of the lower common tendon.

Passing anterolaterally along the floor of the orbit at an angle of 23–25°, it is attached to the sclera 6.5 mm from the cornea by a tendon 5.5 mm long. The muscle is about 40 mm long and 9 mm wide. Its line of attachment, 9.8 mm long, is oblique and markedly convex forwards (Fig. 4.31). It is also attached to the lower lid by its fascial sheath (Fig. 5.23).

RELATIONS

Superior

Superiorly lie the eyeball and, separated by fat, the optic nerve and inferior division of the oculomotor nerve (Fig. 5.23).

Lateral

Laterally, the nerve to the inferior oblique runs in front of the lateral border or between it and the lateral rectus.

Inferior

Inferiorly is the floor of the orbit, roofing the maxillary sinus. The muscle is close to the orbital palatine process but is separated by fat from the orbital plate of the maxilla. The infraorbital vessels and nerve in their canal are also inferior.

The inferior oblique crosses below the inferior rectus, their sheaths being united here.

NERVES

By a branch of the inferior division of the oculomotor nerve, entering on its ocular surface about 15 mm from its posterior end (Figs 5.23 and 5.24).

BLOOD SUPPLY

The medial muscular branch of the ophthalmic artery.

ACTIONS

The inferior rectus, acting alone, would depress the visual axis inferomedially with a slight degree of extorsion. It also depresses the lower eyelid.

The **primary action** is depression, which increases in abduction and becomes nil in full adduction. Inferior rectus is the only depressor in abduction.

The **subsidiary actions** are adduction and extorsion, which increase with adduction.

4.14 MEDIAL RECTUS

Medial rectus is the largest ocular muscle and is stronger than the lateral. It is widely attached medial and inferior to the optic foramen by both parts of the common tendon and the sheath of the optic nerve. It is 40 mm long and thicker than the other extraocular muscles, although similar in width and length.

Passing along the medial wall of the orbit medial rectus inserts into the sclera 5.5 mm from the cornea by a tendon 3.7 mm in length. The line of insertion is 10.3 mm, straight, and symmetrically across the horizontal meridian (Fig. 4.31). Visibility of the muscle insertion through the conjunctiva allows swelling to be detected in endocrine exophthalmos.

RELATIONS

Superior

Superiorly is the superior oblique, and between the two muscles are the ophthalmic artery and its eth-

moidal branch and the ethmoidal and infratrochlear nerves (Figs 5.21 and 5.24).

Inferior

The floor of the orbit.

Medial

Medially are peripheral fat, orbital plate of the ethmoid and ethmoidal sinuses.

Lateral

Laterally is the central orbital fat and optic nerve.

NERVES

A branch from the inferior division of the oculomotor nerve enters the lateral surface about 15 mm from the orbital attachment of the muscle.

BLOOD SUPPLY

The medial muscular branch of the ophthalmic artery.

ACTIONS

Medial rectus is regarded as a pure adductor. However, this is true only in the primary position, i.e. with one geometrical anteroposterior axis directed straight forward. If this axis is elevated or depressed by other muscles, medial and lateral recti no longer exert a turning force purely around the vertical axis, but then also exert slight elevator or depressor movements. Such movements may be small and their influence is uncertain, but use is made of this fact when displacing the insertions of the horizontal recti for vertically incomitant squint.

4.15 LATERAL RECTUS

Lateral rectus is attached to both parts of the annular tendon where they cross the superior orbital fissure. It is about 48 mm in length, which is longer than the medial rectus, but only two-thirds of its cross-sectional area. This attachment is continuous, includes the spina recti lateralis on the greater wing of the sphenoid, and is U-shaped and concave towards the optic foramen, the limbs of the U forming the upper and lower heads of the muscle (Figs 4.28 and 5.6).

The muscle at first adjoins the lateral orbital wall separated by a small amount of fat. More anteriorly it passes medially, pierces Tenon's capsule, and reaches the sclera 6.9 mm from the cornea by a tendon 8.8 mm long, at a line of attachment 9.2 mm in length, vertical or slightly convex forwards, and usually symmetrical (Fig. 4.31).

The lateral rectus is often visible through the conjunctiva and Tenon's capsule.

RELATIONS

At the apex of the orbit

Here the two 'heads' of the lateral rectus and the rest of the annular tendon enclose part of the superior orbital fissure, often called the oculomotor foramen (Fig. 4.28). Structures passing through this opening, separated by a thin bar of bone from the optic foramen and nerve, are often said to pass between the two heads of the lateral rectus. They are, from above downwards, the superior oculomotor division, nasociliary nerve, a branch from the internal carotid sympathetic plexus, inferior oculomotor division, ophthalmic veins, and also the abducent nerve here passing from below the inferior oculomotor division to become lateral to both at a level between the two divisions (Fig. 5.6).

Above the upper head of lateral rectus (and hence above the annulus) are the trochlear, frontal and lacrimal nerves, recurrent lacrimal artery, and superior ophthalmic vein. As Hovelacque (1927) stated, these structures do not traverse the narrow superolateral part of the superior orbital fissure, because this is closed by dense fibrous tissue, but pass just above the annulus. Below the annulus is the inferior ophthalmic vein only.

Superior

In the orbit superior to lateral rectus are the lacrimal artery and nerve. The lacrimal gland is anterior. The lacrimal nerve adjoins the whole of its upper border, the artery only the anterior two-thirds (Fig. 5.18).

Inferior

Inferiorly is the floor of the orbit, and anteriorly the tendon of the inferior oblique passing inferior and then medial to the lateral rectus to its attachment (Fig. 4.28).

Medial

Medially, near the apex, between lateral rectus and the optic nerve, are the abducent nerve, ciliary ganglion and ophthalmic artery. Between the muscle and inferior rectus is the nerve to the inferior oblique (Figs 5.24 and 5.26).

Lateral

Laterally the periorbita is posterior (Figs 1.15 and 1.16), perimuscular fat anterior, and most anteriorly is the lacrimal gland between it and bone.

NERVES

The abducent nerve enters lateral rectus on its ocular aspect, just posterior to its midpoint.

BLOOD SUPPLY

The muscle is supplied by the lacrimal artery and lateral muscular branch of the ophthalmic artery.

ACTIONS

The lateral rectus abducts the visual axis in the horizontal plane. (See, however, remarks on actions of medial rectus.)

4.16 SUPERIOR OBLIQUE

Superior oblique, the longest and thinnest extraocular muscle, is attached superomedially to the optic foramen by a narrow tendon partially overlapping the levator. Its length is due to that of its deflected tendon as much as to its belly, which is fusiform and more rounded than that of the other muscles and passes forwards between the roof and medial wall of the orbit to its trochlea or pulley (Figs 5.18 and 5.22).

RELATIONS

The muscle becomes a rounded tendon about 1 cm posterior to the trochlea, beyond which it turns posterolaterally at an angle of about 55° (the trochlear angle), pierces Tenon's capsule, descends slightly inferior to the superior rectus, and spreads out in a fan-shaped attachment in the posterosuperior quadrant along a line of insertion about 10.7 mm long, and convex posterolaterally. Its anterior end lies on about the same meridian as the temporal end of the superior rectus and it makes an angle of about 45° with the anteroposterior plane (Figs 4.28 and 4.34).

The trochlea is a loop of fibrocartilage closed above by fibrous tissue and attached to the fovea or spina trochlearis on the inferior surface of the frontal bone a few millimetres behind the orbital margin. Within

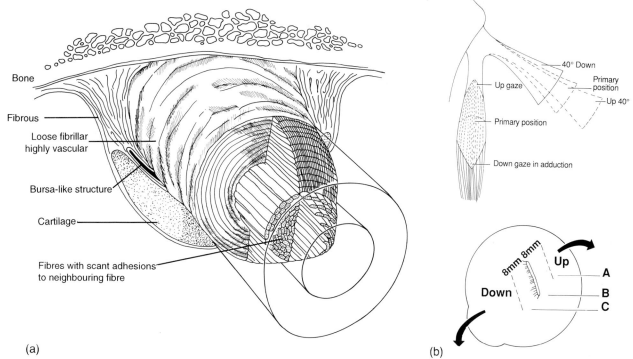

Fig. 4.33   (a) Architecture of the trochlea; (b) change in relative position of the superior oblique insertion, up and down gaze in adduction. (From Helveston, E. M. *et al*. (1982) *Ophthalmology*, **89**, 124, with permission.)

it the tendon is usually described as enclosed in a synovial sheath, and a strong fibrous sheath accompanies it to the eyeball. Studies by Helveston *et al.* (1982) have elucidated the structure of the trochlea, and suggested novel functional features in relation to movement of the superior oblique tendon (see below).

The trochlea is in the form of a grooved cartilaginous saddle whose concave medial surface is directed towards the floor of the trochlear fossa (Fig. 4.33a). The long axis of the saddle is anteroposterior. The trochlea is 5.5 mm long, 4 mm high and 4 mm deep. The intratrochlear part of the tendon, 1.5 mm wide, is received into the concavity of the trochlea. It is surrounded by loose fibrovascular tissue 0.5 mm thick, which is separated from the trochlea by a bursa-like space lined on each side by flattened cells and connective tissue. This highly vascular tissue is thought to permit repair of the working elements of the trochlea. This is the only extraocular muscle with such a rich vascular tunic. The whole trochlea is surrounded by a thick fibrous sheath which secures the trochlear saddle and its contents to the bony medial orbital wall.

Helveston *et al.* (1982) have calculated that in adduction, full excursion of the tendon insertion between maximum elevation (40°) and depression (40°) is 16 mm (i.e. in elevation the insertion moves

8 mm posteriorly, 8 mm anteriorly). In the past, it was conceived that this entire movement was achieved by movement of the tendon as a whole through the trochlear 'pulley'. Helveston's studies have suggested that this is a minor contribution, and that movement is achieved by a sliding of concentric tendinous bundles over one another in a telescopic fashion. Thus in elevation, the V-shaped insertion of muscle into tendon has a forward-directed apex, while in depression (contraction) the apex is directed backwards. In this view, it is only the central tendinous bundles which complete the full excursion (Fig. 4.33b).

Helveston *et al.* (1982) suggest that this anatomy may explain the mechanism of Brown's syndrome in which failure of the tendon to run through the pulley restricts upgaze in adduction on the affected side.

TROCHLEA

The cartilaginal trochlear saddle is 5.5 mm long, with its axis anteroposterior. It is 4 mm wide and 4 mm deep with its groove facing the ethmoidal wall.

The trochlear tendon is composed of 275 loosely interconnected fascicles/bundles. The tendon is 1.5 mm wide.

A loose fibrovascular sheath invests the tendon and

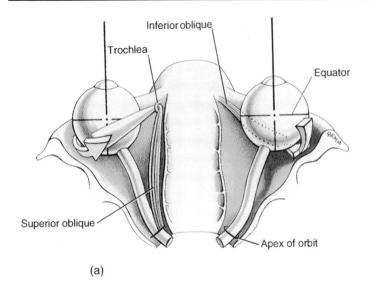

(a)

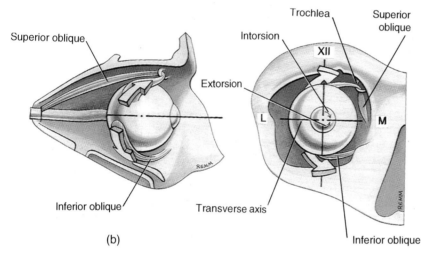

(b)

Fig. 4.34 Diagrams in three dimensions to explain the actions of the oblique muscles.

is separated from the saddle by a **bursa** lined by flattended non-endothelial cells.

The trochlea is surrounded by a thick fibrous sheath 1 mm thick which attaches the trochlea to the **trochlear fossa** medially.

Movement of the tendon through the trochlea is thought to be achieved by a telescoping of concentric rings of tendinous fasciculi upon one another (i.e. the tendon doesn't slide as a single piece through a lubricated pulley, but its component parts telescope over each other). During relaxation the muscle is thought to insert into the tendinous cup; during contraction the situation is reversed, and the tendinous fibres are drawn into the muscle (Helveston *et al.*, 1982).

ACTIONS

Superior oblique elevates the back (and hence depresses the front) of the eyeball. It would also abduct and intort the eyeball if acting in isolation.

The **primary action** is *depression* which increases with adduction, becoming less in progressive abduction. It is the only depressor in adduction.

Subsidiary actions are *abduction* and *intorsion*, increasing with abduction.

Superior oblique and inferior rectus combine as depressors. The abductor action of the oblique muscles is due to their line of pull being posterior to the vertical axis (Figs 4.33 and 4.34).

NERVES

The trochlear nerve, after dividing into three or four branches, enters the muscle superiorly and near its lateral border in the posterior half of its belly (Fig. 5.18).

BLOOD SUPPLY

Superior oblique is served by the superior muscular branch of the ophthalmic artery.

4.17   INFERIOR OBLIQUE

Inferior oblique is the only extraocular muscle attached near the front of the orbit and also has the shortest tendon of insertion (Figs 5.20 and 5.23). This is inevitable if it is to match the belly of superior oblique. Some of its muscle fibres are attached directly to sclera.

Its rounded tendon is attached to a small depression on the orbital plate of the maxilla a little behind the orbital margin and just lateral to the orifice of the nasolacrimal duct. Some of its fibres may, in fact, arise from the fascia covering the lacrimal sac (Figs 4.33, 5.20 and 5.22).

It is inclined posterolaterally at an angle of about 45° with the anteroposterior plane, almost parallel with the tendon of superior oblique, between inferior rectus and orbital floor. Near lateral rectus, it is attached by a very short tendon to the inferior posterolateral quadrant of the globe, largely below the horizontal meridian (Fig. 11.2). The line of attachment is oblique, 9.4 mm long, and convex upwards. As Figs 4.20 and 4.25 show, this attachment (variably sited by different observers) is higher in its quadrant than would be expected if it were a perfect reciprocal to superior oblique. Its posterior or nasal end is about 5 mm from the optic nerve, and thus lies practically over the macula (only 2.2 mm from it) (Poirier, 1911) (Fig. 4.31e). The anterior temporal end lies in about the same meridian as the lower end of the insertion of the lateral rectus.

Although the average angle of the plane of action of the superior and inferior oblique muscles with the vertical anteroposterior plane is 45° the variations in the planes of muscle action are enormous. Narrowing this angle will reduce the torsional action of the muscle and increase its vertical action, while widening the angle will achieve the reverse. (Extremes of these variations result in anomalous, 'A' and 'V' patterns of movement in vertical gaze (see Fells, 1975).)

RELATIONS

The inferior surface of inferior oblique is in contact with periosteum of the orbital floor, to which it is sometimes described as sending a fibrous extension (arcuate expansion) (see Fig. 4.47), but laterally separated from it by fat. As the muscle twists slightly to its global attachment, its inferior surface becomes lateral and covered by lateral rectus and the fascia bulbi. Above, it is in contact with fat and inferior rectus, finally spreading out as it reaches the globe.

NERVES

The inferior division of the oculomotor, which crosses near the mid point of its posterior border to enter the muscle on its superior surface.

BLOOD SUPPLY

Inferior oblique is served by the infraorbital and medial muscular branch of the ophthalmic arteries.

ACTIONS

Inferior oblique elevates the visual axis because it depresses the posterior aspect of the globe. Like superior oblique, it attaches below the anteroposterior axis and thus extorts it.

The **primary action**, elevation, increases as the eye is adducted and is nil in abduction. It is the only elevator in adduction.

The **subsidiary actions**, abduction and extorsion, increase with abduction and decrease with adduction.

4.18   LEVATOR PALPEBRAE SUPERIORIS AND SUPERIOR PALPEBRAL MUSCLE

These muscles are together concerned with elevation of the lid. Levator palpebrae superioris consists of striated muscle innervated by the third cranial nerve, while the superior palpebral muscle of Müller is non-striated and innervated by the sympathetic system.

Although the levator muscle is not separated into orbital and global layers, its muscle fibres correspond to the three singly innervated global types (Spencer and Porter, 1981; Porter et al., 1995). Histochemical and other studies suggest the presence of another fibre type exhibiting an alkali-labile, acid-stable myosin ATPase with features of the skeletal single-innervated slow twitch fibre (type I; e.g. soleus).

LEVATOR PALPEBRAE SUPERIORIS

This muscle arises from the lesser wing of the sphenoid, above and in front of the optic foramen, by a short tendon which blends with the underlying origin of the superior rectus (Fig. 4.36).

The muscle belly, approximately 40 mm in length, passes forwards below the roof of the orbit and superficial to superior rectus. It widens, to become flat and ribbon-like, and at about 1 cm behind the septum orbitale, more or less at the upper fornix and

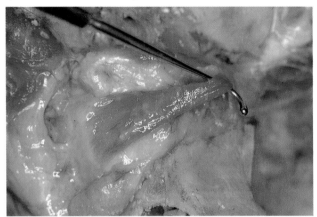

Fig. 4.35 Dissection to show the aponeurosis of the elevator palpebrae muscle from above. (Courtesy of A. Werb.)

a few millimetres in front of the equator of the globe, it ends in a distinct membranous expansion, the **levator aponeurosis**. This spreads out in a fan-shaped manner occupying the whole width of the orbit to give the muscle the form of an isosceles triangle (Fig. 4.35). The origin of the aponeurosis, the musculo tendinous junction, is an important surgical landmark, the '**white line**' which is shiny and quite distinct from the fibres of Müller's muscle that lie deep to it. It is easily identified during surgery for ptosis, particularly by the posterior route. The fleshy part of the levator is horizontal, while its tendinous part is obliquely vertical, moulding itself over the globe of the eye as indeed does the whole of the upper eyelid. The change of direction takes place above the reflected tendon of the superior oblique.

The aponeurosis spreads out into the structures of the lid.

Attachments of the levator aponeurosis (Figs 4.37 and 4.38)

Extremities

The two extremities of the levator aponeurosis are its '*horns*' (cornua).

(a)

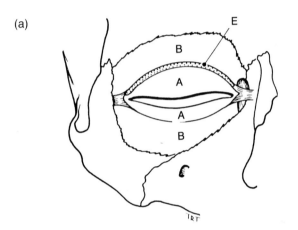

(b)

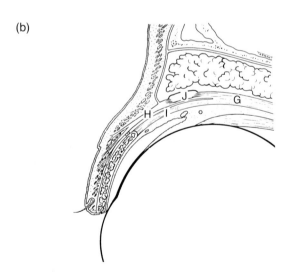

Fig. 4.36 (a) The orbital septum. A = Tarsal plate; B = orbital septum; E = tarsal insertion of the upper lid retractor. (b) Longitudinal section to show the upper lid retractors. G = Levator palpebrae; H = levator aponeurosis; I = superior tarsal (Müller's) muscle. (From Collin, J. R. O. (1989) *A Manual of Systematic Eyelid Surgery*, published by Churchill Livingstone.)

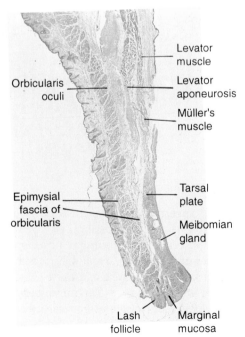

Fig. 4.37 Longitudinal section through the upper lid. (Courtesy of A. Werb.)

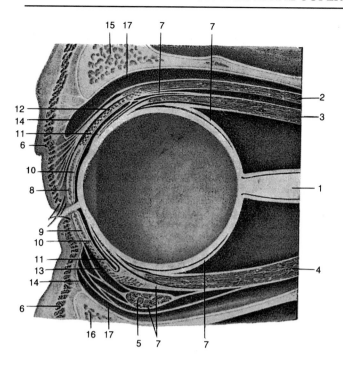

Fig. 4.38 Schematic sagittal section of the eye and its surroundings. 1 = Optic nerve; 2 = levator; 3 = superior rectus; 4 = inferior rectus; 5 = inferior oblique; 6 = orbicularis; 7 = fascia bulbi; 8 = superior tarsus; 9 = inferior tarsus; 10 = palpebral conjunctiva; 11 = bulbar conjunctiva; 12 = superior capsulopalpebral muscle; 13 = superior capsulopalpebral muscle, inferior portion; 14 = septum orbitale; 15 = frontal bone; 16 = maxilla; 17 = periorbita.

The **lateral horn** passes between the orbital and palpebral parts of the lacrimal gland (Fig. 5.23) which is folded around it, and plays a part in supporting the gland against the orbital roof. The lateral horn is attached to the orbital tubercle and to the upper aspect of the lateral palpebral ligament (Fig. 5.20).

The **medial horn** is much weaker than the lateral. It is attached somewhat below the frontolacrimal suture and to the medial palpebral ligament.

In view of these attachments, it must be assumed that the aponeurosis is drawn into a bow shape, concave forwards, on contraction of the levator.

Insertion into lid

The precise insertion of the tendinous aponeurotic sheet as it passes forwards into the substance of the lid has been a matter of controversy. It is generally agreed that the aponeurosis passes downwards towards the lid margin, anterior to the tarsal plate, and is directly apposed to the palpebral portion of the orbicularis muscle. Earlier authors have stated that tendinous extensions of the aponeurosis pass through the muscle bundles of orbicularis, to be inserted into the skin. Such an insertion has been

invoked to explain the location of the superior lid crease, or sulcus, an important cosmetic feature of the lid (Wolff, 1954; Collin, 1983) (Fig. 4.36).

However, Werb's (1984) studies have suggested that the aponeurosis is firmly attached to the fibrous covering on the deep surface of orbicularis, but does not provide tendinous extensions into the skin (Fig. 4.37). In this view the skin of the upper lid is not tethered at the superior lid sulcus. The sulcus is thought to be formed at the upper border of the attachment of the aponeurosis to orbicularis. As the lid elevates, the sulcus is formed and the redundant skin above the aponeurosis attachment simultaneously forms the superior palpebral fold. The absence of tethering of the skin at the site of the superior palpebral sulcus is readily demonstrated when injecting local anaesthetic solution subcutaneously in the upper lid, or by the presence of an upper lid haematoma or oedema; in both situations the sulcus is obliterated (Werb, 1984).

Although many standard accounts of the insertion of the aponeurosis suggest that a proportion of its fibres insert into the anterior surface of the tarsal plate, this has not been confirmed by Werb, who believes that only Müller's muscle is attached directly to the tarsal plate. This must still be regarded as an area of controversy but the epymysium of the orbicularis is intimately associated with the connective tissue at the surface of the tarsal plate; so the argument may be irrelevant.

Sheath of the levator

The sheath of the levator has several points of interest. Below, it is attached to that of superior rectus, and the tissue between the two muscles gains attachment to the upper conjunctival fornix (Fig. 2.49). On the upper aspect of the junction of aponeurosis and muscle the sheath is thickened to form a band (Whitnall, 1921), the medial end of which passes up to the trochlea of superior oblique and to the neighbouring bone and sends a slip to bridge over the supraorbital notch. The lateral end of the band passes above the aponeurosis, and is in part joined to it. Part of it passes into the lacrimal gland and part reaches the lateral orbital wall. Whitnall considers these to be the true check ligaments of the levator (see, however, Nutt, 1955).

THE SUPERIOR PALPEBRAL MUSCLE

The superior palpebral muscle (Müller's muscle) arises from the inferior aspect of the levator palpebrae, to which it is well apposed, just posterior to the fornix. Striated muscle fibres give rise to smooth muscle fibres, with a minimum of connective tissue intervening. It is a flat, sheet-like muscle some 15–20 mm wide at its origin, which widens a little towards its insertion after an almost vertical course of 10 mm (Figs 2.10 and 4.38). The orbital conjunctiva is in contact with the posterior surface of Müller's muscle. Thus pharmacological agents instilled into the conjunctival sac have access to Müller's muscle, and either stimulate contraction and elevation of the lid (e.g. phenylephrine) or inhibit contraction and induce ptosis (e.g. guanethidine).

Attachments

1. The main (and possibly sole) insertion of the superior palpebral muscle is into the upper border of the tarsal plate (Figs 2.10, 4.34b). The muscle is said to control approximately 3 mm of lid elevation.
2. Although many accounts suggest that some fibres of the levator insert into the superior fornix of the conjunctiva, Werb (1984) was unable to demonstrate such attachments.

It follows that a surgical plane can be identified between the tarsal plate and superior palpebral muscle posteriorly on the one hand, and the aponeurosis and levator muscle anteriorly, on the other. Followed upwards this plane meets the origin of the superior palpebral muscle from the levator muscle; followed downwards, it is in the plane of the grey line of the lid margin.

RELATIONS

Above the levator and between it and the roof of the orbit are the trochlear and frontal nerves and the supraorbital vessels. The trochlear nerve crosses the muscle close to its origin from lateral to medial to reach the superior oblique (Figs 1.15 and 5.18).

The supraorbital artery is above the muscle in its anterior half only.

The frontal nerve crosses the muscle obliquely from the lateral to the medial side.

Below the levator is the medial part of superior rectus (which, being the larger muscle, has its lateral edge exposed) and the globe of the eye (Fig. 5.18).

In front of the tendon at its commencement is the retroseptal mass of fat, which is continuous with the upper and medial orbital lobe of fat. Below this the front of the tendon of the levator is in contact with the septum. Behind is the pretarsal space, containing

the peripheral palpebral arcade (Fig. 2.10), and the palpebral portion of the lacrimal gland. The pretarsal space, situated behind the insertion of the tendon, is prolonged laterally behind the lateral horn of the levator and contains the palpebral portion of the lacrimal gland.

NERVES

The superior oculomotor division reaches the muscle either by piercing the medial edge of the superior rectus (and thus forming another bond between the two muscles) or by winding round its medial border.

Sympathetic fibres lead to the unstriated superior palpebral muscle. These autonomic fibres are probably the axons of neurons whose perikarya are situated in the superior cervical sympathetic ganglia of that side. The axons reach the orbit along the internal carotid artery, pass to the oculomotor nerve in the vicinity of the cavernous sinus (i.e. branch off the cavernous sympathetic plexus), and are distributed to the superior and inferior palpebral muscles along the respective divisions of the oculomotor nerve.

BLOOD SUPPLY

This is from the lateral muscular branch of the ophthalmic artery.

ACTIONS

Levator

The levator raises the upper eyelid, uncovering the cornea and sclera, and deepens the superior palpebral fold. Elevation is adjusted to the vertical gaze position of the eyes so that it is greatest in upgaze and least in downgaze. Its antagonist is the palpebral portion of the orbicularis.

Superior palpebral muscle

The superior palpebral muscle adjusts the height of the lid around a level determined primarily by the levator. It also widens the palpebral aperture in surprise or while staring. Sympathetic nerve palsy (Horner's syndrome) causes a ptosis of 3–4 mm, the amount of elevation of which Müller's muscle is capable. A total oculomotor nerve palsy causes a complete ptosis: the intact Müller's muscle, arising from the paralysed levator muscle, is unable to elevate the upper lid in this situation.

4.19 ANOMALOUS EXTRAOCULAR MUSCLES

Certain anomalous muscles have been reported occasionally in the orbit:

- **Gracilis orbitis** or **comes obliqui superioris** originates from the proximal dorsal surface of the superior oblique and inserts on the trochlea or its surrounding connective tissue. It is supplied by the trochlear nerve (Whitnall, 1921).
- The **accessory lateral rectus muscle** is a single slip, sometimes found in the monkey and homologous to the nictating membrane. It is supplied by the abducent nerve (Schnyder, 1984; Spencer and Porter, 1981).

Two anomalous muscles may occasionally be associated with the levator palpebrae superioris:

- **Tensor trochleae** arises from the medial border of the levator muscle and inserts into the trochlea or its environs.
- **Transversus orbitus** attaches between the medial and lateral walls of the orbit, connecting with the levator muscle en route.

Both muscles are supplied by the superior division of the oculomotor nerve (Whitnall, 1921; Isomura, 1977; Sacks, 1985).

4.20 THE CONNECTIVE TISSUE SEPTA OF THE ORBIT

The connective tissue septa of the orbit comprise an orderly and continuous architecture of which the fascia bulbi, fascial sheaths of the muscles, the periorbital membrane and the condensations of the check ligaments and ligament of Lockwood are a part. It has been studied in detail by Koornneef (1977) using thick histological sections. As a whole, the orbital connective tissue can be considered a supporting framework for the eyeball together with the orbital fat. The orbital floor can be removed without depression of the eyeball. This connective tissue apparatus becomes important in orbital blow-out fracture when the septa can become incarcerated in the fracture region, e.g. into the maxillary sinus, and can limit muscle action (Fig. 4.39).

High-resolution CT and MRI have shown that the extraocular muscles move in towards the globe on contraction and outwards on relaxation, over distances ranging from 1.5 to 3.7 mm (Miller and Robins, 1987; Miller, 1989). Otherwise, the disposition of the muscles during eye movement is extremely stable relative to the orbit and is in keeping with the predictions of biomechanical modelling (Robinson, 1975; Miller and Robinson, 1984) and confirmed by CT (Simonz et al., 1985) and by MRI studies before and after muscle transposition (Miller et al., 1993). This stability is due in part to the presence, in the region of the equator of the globe, of connective tissue pulleys, suspended from the orbital walls through which the rectus muscles pass. These connective tissue sheaths couple the extraocular muscles to the globe and orbit and offer constraints which influence the effects of eye muscle surgery (Koornneef, 1986; Demer et al., 1994). They effectively modify the direction of pull of the rectus muscles so that the pulleys become the functional origin of the muscles (Fig. 4.43b) (Demer et al., 1995a,b; Porter et al., 1995).

THE FASCIA BULBI

The fascia bulbi (capsule of Tenon) is a thin fibrous sheath which envelops the globe from the margin of the cornea to the optic nerve. Its inner surface is well defined and in contact with the sclera, connected to it by fine trabeculae. Moreover, the fascia is attached to the globe in front so that, while slight movements may occur between the globe and fascia, in more extensive movements of the globe they probably move together in surrounding fat (Figs 4.40 and 4.41).

Posteriorly the external surface of the fascia is in contact with orbital fat, from which it is separated with difficulty. Anteriorly it is thinner, merging gradually into the subconjunctival connective tissue. It is separated from the conjunctiva by loose connective tissue and can be distinguished from it during surgery. Around the optic nerve (Fig. 4.41), where it is pierced by the ciliary vessels and nerves, the fascia is very thin and difficult to trace to the dural sheath of the optic nerve, with which it is held to be continuous. It is also pierced by the venae vorticosae.

Inferiorly, the fascia bulbi is thickened to form a sling or hammock which supports the globe as the **suspensory ligament of Lockwood** where it is pierced by the tendons of the muscles. It invests them with tubular reflections continuous with their perimysial sheaths, also sending expansions to surrounding structures. The expansion from the lateral rectus is attached to the orbital tubercle of the zygomatic bone, that of the medial rectus to the lacrimal bone. These expansions are strong and have been said to limit muscular action, therefore receiving the name of 'check' ligaments. (Formalin fixation encouraged the discovery of fascial planes in the body. 'Check'

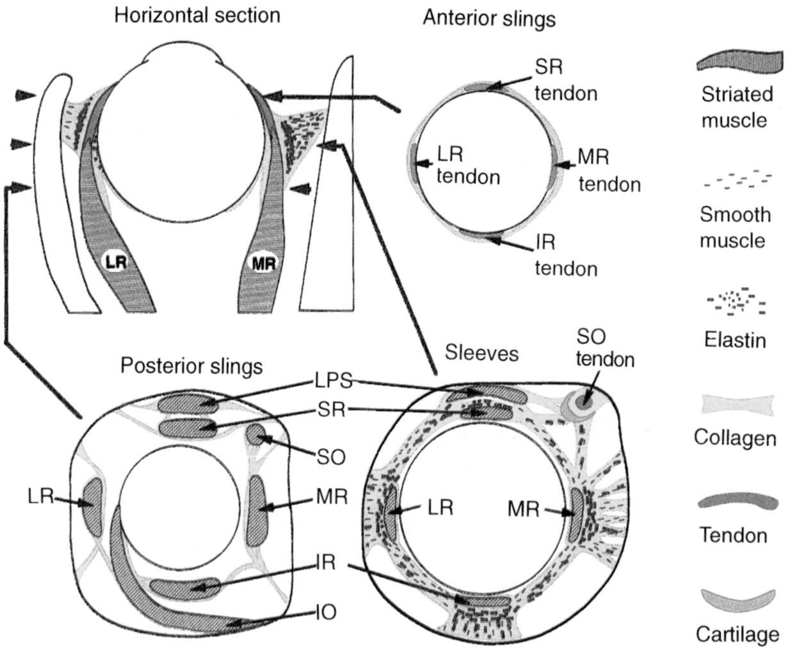

Horizontal section

Anterior slings

SR tendon

LR tendon

MR tendon

IR tendon

LR

MR

Posterior slings

Sleeves

SO tendon

LPS

SR

SO

LR

MR

LR

MR

IR

IO

Striated muscle

Smooth muscle

Elastin

Collagen

Tendon

Cartilage

Fig. 4.39 Diagrammatic representation of structure of orbital connective tissues. IR = inferior rectus; LPS = levator palpebrae superioris; LR = lateral rectus; MR = medial rectus; SO = superior oblique; SR = superior rectus. The three coronal views are represented at the levels indicated by the arrow in the horizontal section. (From Demer, J. L. et al. (1995b) Invest. Ophthalmol. Vis. Sci., **36**, 1125, with permission.)

ligaments are legion, but their functional significance is uncertain – consult Nutt, 1955.) (Fig. 4.42.)

The rectus muscle pulleys

Recently it has been recognized that the rectus muscles pass through connective tissue sleeves or pulleys, located close to the equator of the globe, which stabilize the position of the recti relative to the orbit during the eye movements (Demer et al., 1995). Their effective anteroposterior extent is 13–19 mm. The rectus tendons slide through the pulleys inside thin collagenous sheaths. The pulleys are rich in collagen, elastic tissue and smooth muscle and are most developed around the horizontal recti and particularly the medial rectus. They are stabilized by fibromuscular septa which extend from the pulleys and adjacent sleeves of Tenon's fascia to the orbital walls and to the adjacent muscles and Tenon's capsule (see below). These attachments are incomplete more anteriorly and posteriorly.

The medial rectus pulley consists of a complete ring of collagen which encircles the muscle near the equator, in the posterior part of Tenon's fascia. It is strengthened by an arrangement of collagen in perpendicular bands whose layers show alternating fibre directions (Porter et al., 1995b). It contains smooth muscle, although most of the smooth muscle of Tenon's capsule is anterior to the globe equator.

The circularly arranged posterior Tenon's fascia supports the globe and is attached peripherally to the periorbita, especially at the orbital rim. The periphery

of the fascia is a tough fibromuscular structure composed of dense collagen, elastic tissue and circumferentially arranged smooth muscle.

The expansion from the superior rectus is attached to levator palpebrae by a band in which a bursa may be found (Motais). This is said to facilitate synergistic action between the two muscles: thus, when the eye is elevated, the upper lid also is raised. The expansion from the inferior rectus (Fig. 5.23) passes between it and inferior oblique, then deep to the inferior fornix and palpebral conjunctiva, separated by the unstriated inferior palpebral muscle, and finally becomes attached between the tarsal plate and orbicularis. Thus, inferior rectus may act on the lower lid as the levator acts on the upper. The lid is lowered 2 mm by its action and the lashes everted, a movement aided by contact with the globe.

The fascia bulbi is thought to be derived from perimysial connective tissue, forming an intermuscular membrane which represents an extension of the insertion of the extraocular muscles into the limbus and lids (Neiger, 1960). It develops from periscleral mesenchymal condensations at the third month of intrauterine life (Fink, 1956), exhibits distinct elastic and collagenous fibre layers at the 90-mm stage, and is complete by the 150-mm stage.

SUSPENSORY LIGAMENTS OF THE FORNICES

The fibrous tissue between superior rectus and levator muscles continues forward to the upper fornix

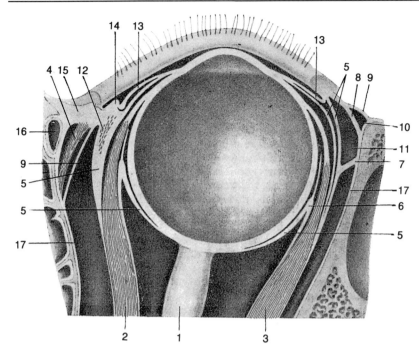

Fig. 4.40 Schematic horizontal section of the eye and its surroundings. 1, optic nerve; 2, medial rectus; 3, lateral rectus; 4, Horner's muscle; 5, fascia bulbi; 6, fascia bulbi; 7, lateral check ligament; 8, aponeurosis of levator; 9, septum orbitale; 10, superior recess; 11, recess for lacrimal gland; 12, medial capsulopalpebral muscle; 13, bulbar conjunctival; 14, caruncle; 15, medial palpebral ligament; 16, lacrimal sac; 17, periorbita. (From Eisler, after Hesser.)

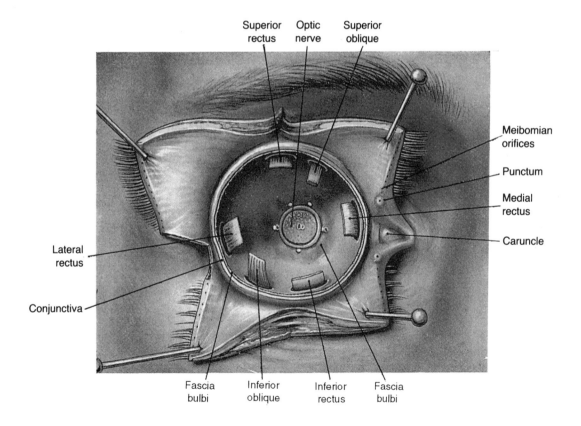

Fig. 4.41 Dissection to show the fascia bulbi (Tenon's capsule). Details visible after removal of the right eyeball.

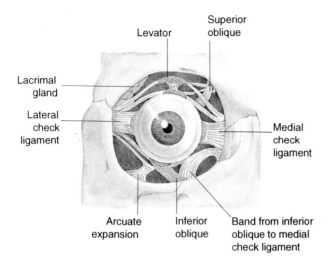

Fig. 4.42 Orbital expansions of the ocular muscles, slightly schematized. The recti sectioned with their sheaths surround the globe and are united by the capsule of Tenon, orbital extensions of levator and superior rectus. Expansion of superior rectus to levator. Arcuate expansion of inferior oblique to floor of orbit. Check ligament from medial and lateral recti, strengthened above and below by superior and inferior expansions.

as the **superior suspensory ligament of the fornix**. If it is cut during ptosis surgery the conjunctiva can prolapse (Collin, 1983). Similarly, the **inferior suspensory ligament of the fornix** in the lower lid is an extension of the fibrous tissue of the lid retractors. If these retractors are lax, as an involutional process, the lower fornix is shallowed (Figs 4.37 and 4.43).

The expansion from superior oblique ascends to the trochlea, that of inferior oblique reaches the lateral orbital floor (Fig. 4.42).

ORBITAL SEPTA

The orbital septa develop later than the extraocular muscle masses and their capillary beds even later still. Fat cells are laid down between the septa after this. The orbital septa start to develop at 3.5 months after conception. It is suggested that they are induced by the onset of eye movements. Welt and Zacharias (1970) described the development of elastic and collagenous septa passing inwards from the periorbita to reach the fascia bulbi. The septa also pass to and between the extraocular muscles and provide specific supportive channels for the ophthalmic veins. The density of the septa varies in different parts of the orbit; in general it is better developed anteriorly and less well developed towards the apex where adipose tissue is increased in amount. The intermuscular membrane (Fig. 4.44) is a condensation of connective tissue between the recti blending

anteriorly with the fascia bulbi (Poirier, 1911). Behind the globe the connective tissue 'sheath' between the four recti is absent, so that distinct intra- and extraconal spaces are lacking (Koornneef, 1977). The intraconal space may, however, occasionally accumulate pus.

At the apex of the orbit, for about 7.1 mm forwards, there are septa from the levator and superior rectus to the periorbita of the roof (Fig. 4.45). Septa passing between the muscle cone and floor are intimately related to the orbital veins and contain smooth muscle. Müller's orbital muscle (unstriated) covers the inferior orbital fissure and is connected to the inferior and lateral rectus by three connective tissue septa. Two are connected to the inferior ophthalmic vein. Further forwards, septa between the lateral, medial and inferior recti and orbital floor contain less smooth muscle. Anteriorly in the orbit septa spread from the levator superioris and superior rectus towards the roof, and between the superior rectus and lateral rectus. More anteriorly, levator superioris forms the lateral aponeurosis, while the smaller medial aponeurosis tangles medially with connective tissue of the superior oblique muscle.

4.21 THE SMOOTH MUSCLE OF THE ORBIT

The so-called capsulopalpebral muscle (of Hesser) is the peribulbar part of the non-striated muscle of the orbit. It consists of superior, inferior and medial palpebral parts, being deficient laterally. Only its superior palpebral part displays definable attachments. The central region of this is the **superior palpebral muscle** (Müller's), which passes from the bulbar aspect of levator palpebrae just behind the fornix to the superior border of the tarsal plate (Figs 2.10 and 4.38). It is 15–20 mm wide and 10 mm in length. It is better defined than other parts of the capsulopalpebral muscle, and lies in fatty connective tissue between the tendon of the levator in front and fascia bulbi and conjunctiva behind, thus helping to limit the pretarsal space.

Extending laterally from the superior palpebral muscles, a slip of non-striated muscle splits to surround the palpebral lobe of the lacrimal gland. A much slighter slip extends from the fascia bulbi to the medial end of the superior tarsal border.

INFERIOR PALPEBRAL MUSCLE

The inferior palpebral muscle (inferior lid retractor) forms the central part of the capsulopalpebral muscle below, passing from the ocular surface of inferior rectus to the lower border of the tarsal plate (Fig.

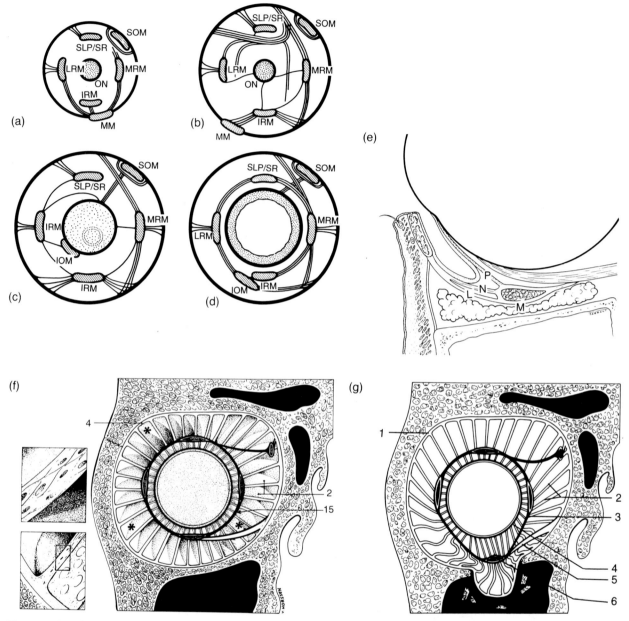

Fig. 4.43(a–d)   Schematic drawings to show the connective tissue septa of the different eye muscles in the orbit. (a) An area near the orbital apex; (b) an area just behind the posterior surface of the globe; (c) just anterior to the posterior surface of the globe; (d) close to the equator of the globe. SLP/SR = Superior levator palpebrae/superior rectus muscle complex; LRM = lateral rectus muscle; IOM = inferior oblique muscle; MM = Müller's muscle; MRM = medial rectus muscle; SOM = superior oblique muscle; ON = optic nerve. (From Koornneef, L. in Duane, T. D. and Jaeger, E. A. (eds), (1987) *Biomedical Foundations of Ophthalmology*, Vol. 1, published by Harper & Row.) (e) The lower lid retractors (L). M = Inferior suspensory (Lockwood's) ligament blending with the sheet of fibrous tissue of the retractor as it splits to enclose the inferior oblique muscle; N = inferior tarsal muscle; P = inferior suspensory ligament of the lower fornix, a part of the fibrous tissue of the lid retractor. (From Collin, J. R. O. (1989) *A Manual of Systematic Eyelid Surgery*, published by Churchill Livingstone.) (f) Schematic representation of the arrangement of connective tissue septa in the anterior orbit in the region of the globe. The septa are shown on the stretch which occurs when the globe is placed on forward traction. 1, periorbita; 2, connective tissue septa; 3, common sheath of the recti; 4, Tenon's capsule. Asterisks (*) denote the sites where smooth muscle cells are found. (g) Schematic drawing to show how the entire motility system is trapped near the orbital floor in an inferior orbital blowout fracture. 1, periorbita; 2, connective tissue septa; 3, common muscle sheath; 4, Tenon's capsule; 5, inferior oblique muscle; 6, inferior rectus muscle.

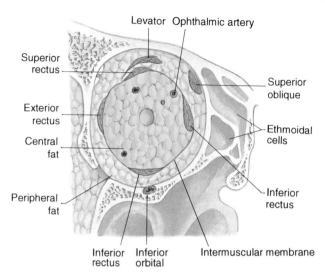

Fig. 4.44 The intermuscular membrane. Right side, posterior segment. The intermuscular membrane joins the recti and divides the orbital fat into central and peripheral regions. There is a recess containing fat under the levator.

4.43). Anteriorly its fibres lie between the palpebral conjunctiva and the inferior part of the septum orbitale in the palpebral extension of the fascia bulbi. The rest of the non-striated muscle here is poorly developed in humans. Medially the capsulopalpebral muscle is represented only by scattered fibres in the fascia bulbi and do not reach the eyelid or fornix (Fig. 4.41).

MUSCULUS ORBITALIS OF MÜLLER

For details see p. 14.

SMOOTH MUSCLE OF THE RECTUS PULLEYS

The smooth muscle supporting the rectus pulleys has a rich sympathetic and parasympathetic innervation, the latter including both cholinergic and nitrergic neurons (Demer, 1995b,c). Sympathetic stimulation is thought to cause smooth muscle contraction and nitrergic stimulation to cause relaxation. The smooth muscle may maintain tension in Tenon's fascia during ageing and fine-tune the position of the pulleys (Bergen, 1982). The greater degree of development of the smooth muscle running medially from the medial rectus pulley has suggested to some that it may play a role in vergence eye movements (Demer *et al.*, 1995b).

4.22 SURGICAL CONSIDERATIONS

From a practical point of view, there are several spaces in the region of the orbit which may be opened up by surgical intrusion, or accumulate fluid or pus:

1. The region bounded by the orbital walls, and anteriorly, the eye, septum orbitale, tarsal plates and palpebral ligaments (preseptal space).

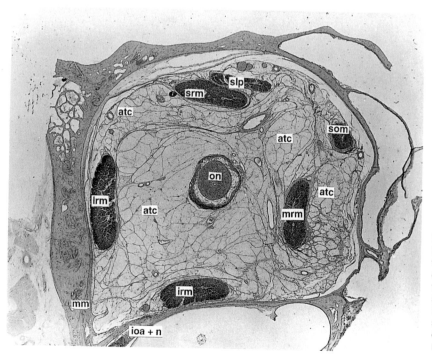

Fig. 4.45 Section 1.4 mm posterior to the back surface of the globe. Diameter vertically is 2.4 cm and transversely 2.7 cm. on = optic nerve; sov = superior ophthalmic vein; slp = superior levator palpebrae; srm = superior rectus; lrm = lateral rectus; irm = inferior rectus; mrm = medial rectus; som = superior oblique; atc = adipose tissue compartment; ioa + n = infraorbital artery and nerve; mm = Müller's muscle.

2. The space immediately behind the orbital septum and in front of the levator aponeurosis is *the preaponeurotic space*. It contains the preaponeurotic fat pads.
3. There is potentially a space between the periorbita and bone.
4. An inner region bounded by the *cone of muscles*, the intermuscular membrane and the fascia bulbi (intraconal space).
5. There is a potential space between the eyeball and fascia bulbi.

4.23 THE ORBITAL FAT

The orbital fat occupies space not occupied by other structures. Formalin fixation artificially hardens it; but in life it is soft, though incompressible, and limited in displacement by the fibrous strands, bands and ligaments which permeate it.

The fat extends from the optic nerve to the orbital walls and from the apex to the septum orbitale. It may cause the septum to bulge but never normally enters the eyelids except in old age. It varies in consistency with the amount of connective tissue it contains.

The fat consists of yellow lobules of fat cells encapsulated in connective tissue, which thus demarcates the lobules. The interlobular septa are soft, vascular and easily distended by oedema fluid.

The orbital fat is divided by the intermuscular membrane into a central or interconal part and a peripheral or extraconal part (Fig. 4.44). Posteriorly where the intermuscular membrane is weak the two are continuous.

CENTRAL ORBITAL FAT

The central fat around the optic nerve is loose and allows movements of the optic nerve and the ciliary vessels and nerves. It is finely lobulated and the septa are thin, as would be expected in such a mobile region. The septa blend with the fascia bulbi. There is thus no space between the fat and fascia, so that in excursions of any extent the fat moves with the eye.

At the surface of the optic nerve the central adipose connective tissue condenses into a limiting membrane which separates it from the dural sheath of the nerve. The space between them (the 'supravaginal space' of Schwalbe) is crossed by fibre strands, an arrangement probably produced by, and certainly facilitating, movement of the optic nerve.

PERIPHERAL ORBITAL FAT

The peripheral fat is between the periorbita and cone of muscles. It is limited anteriorly by the septum orbitale and enclosed by a thin membrane united to the periorbita by weak processes. Blood vessels may pass between it and the periorbita into the eyelids, but not the conjunctiva; however, rupture of the septum may cause subconjunctival ecchymosis. Posteriorly the fat covers the recti near their attachments. Between these muscles it forms four lobes, the posterior parts of which become continuous with the central fat, united by numerous connective tissue septa. Anteriorly it is in contact with the intermuscular membrane and fascia bulbi. Superficially each lobe partially covers the muscles between which it lies. The connective tissue of the lobes blends with the sheaths of muscles and their prolongations, periorbita, and septum orbitale.

Superolateral lobe

The superolateral lobe lies between the superior and lateral recti, overlaps superior rectus and is separated from the superomedial lobe by the frontal nerve. It covers the lateral rectus, but the lacrimal gland separates it from the septum.

Inferolateral lobe

The inferolateral lobe is between the lateral and inferior recti. At its lower border is the nerve to the inferior oblique. It broadens anteriorly and reaches the septum around the inferior oblique. The remainder is behind the expansion of the medial rectus to the septum; it lies posterior to the lacrimal sac and lacrimal part of the orbicularis oculi.

Inferomedial lobe

The inferomedial lobe lies between the inferior and medial recti. It also enlarges anteriorly and sends a prolongation to the septum on either side of the inferior oblique muscle. The remainder of the lobe lies behind the expansion of medial rectus on the posterior aspect of the septum, that is, posterior to Horner's muscle and the lacrimal sac.

Superomedial lobe

The superomedial lobe lies between superior rectus and levator laterally and medial rectus, and is partly separated from the periorbita by the superior oblique. Anteriorly to the septum orbitale, and also above the trochlea through the superior aperture, it forms a retroseptal mass along the anterior margin of the check ligament of the levator muscle.

PRE-APONEUROTIC FAT PADS

In the upper lid these lie immediately behind the orbital septum on the levator aponeurosis (Figs 4.38 and 4.46): there is a small **medial** and a large **central** compartment, with the lacrimal gland lying laterally. This is an important relationship to recall when excising fat from the upper lid for a blepharoplasty (Collin, 1983). The lower lid fat pads also lie in front of the lid retractors and behind the septum (Figs 4.43 and 4.46): there is a small **lateral** and a large **central** pad. The fat pads provide a useful landmark for the levator aponeurosis and lower lid retractor. Traction on the fat pads during blepharoplasty may cause deep orbital haemorrhage and blindness (Collin, 1983).

Although the disposition of orbital fascia and adipose tissue may be involved in extension of infections and surgical operations, there is another, wider aspect of these arrangements. Collectively these tissues provide a flexible and incompressible suspension for the orbital structures, in particular for the eyeball. This must preserve an accurate relationship to its fellow eye if binocular vision is to be maintained (see Koornneef, 1977).

4.24 APERTURES ADJOINING THE ORBITAL OPENING THROUGH WHICH FAT MAY HERNIATE

When the septum orbitale is removed the 'base' or aperture of the orbit is seen to be partially closed by the globe and its muscles and the fibroelastic expansions to the walls of the orbit close to its margin.

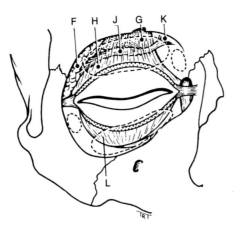

Fig. 4.46 The preaponeurotic fat pad. F = Lacrimal gland; G = levator palpebrae; H = levator aponeurosis; J = superior suspensory (Whitnall's) ligament; K = trochlea, L = inferior lid retractor. (From Collin, J. R. O. (1989) *A Manual of Systematic Eyelid Surgery*, published by Churchill Livingstone.)

These expansions and the oblique muscles bound five orifices between the orbital margin and globe, through which fat may herniate towards the orbital septum (Fig. 4.47).

SUPERIOR APERTURE

The superior aperture, like a comma, lies between the orbital roof and upper surface of the levator. Its 'head' is medial and near the trochlea of the superior oblique; its tail reaches the lacrimal gland. Through this aperture herniation from the superomedial lobe may form a retroseptal mass.

SUPEROMEDIAL APERTURE

The superomedial aperture is a vertical oval between the tendon of superior oblique and the medial check ligament. It may transmit a process of the superomedial lobe, forming a common prominence in the elderly. The infratrochlear nerve, dorsal nasal artery and angular vein also pass through it.

INFEROMEDIAL APERTURE

Also oval, this lies between the medial check ligament, inferior oblique, and the lacrimal sac.

INFERIOR APERTURE

The inferior aperture is triangular and between the inferior oblique, its arcuate expansion (Fig. 4.47), and orbital floor.

INFEROLATERAL APERTURE

The inferolateral aperture is small and lies between the arcuate expansion and lateral check ligament.

In general, these apertures form communications between the orbital cavity and deep strata of the eyelids. Through them blood and pus may also pass out from the space between the periorbita and peripheral fat to the septum orbitale.

4.25 OCULAR MOVEMENTS

An extensive literature exists on the topic of ocular movements (Cogan, 1956; Bach-y-Rita, Collin and Hyde, 1971; Baker and Berthoz, 1977; Henn, Hepp and Buttner-ennever, 1982; Henn, Buttner-ennever and Hepp, 1982; Pedersen, Abel and Troost, 1982; Eggers, 1982; Leigh and Zee, 1983; 1991) and this section draws heavily on these sources. The function of the individual muscles has been dealt with earlier.

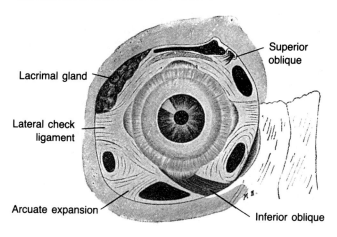

Fig. 4.47 The hernial orifices at the base of the orbit. The eyelids and the septum orbitale have been removed, together with the fat which had herniated through the orifices.

For practical purposes the movements of each eyeball can be regarded as rotations about three primary axes: vertical, horizontal and anteroposterior. The globe is prevented from visually significant displacement during contraction by the resistance of the incompressible soft tissues which surround it and a stability in the orbit brought about by the presence of supportive connective tissue sheaths, bands, septa and capsules. The isolated action of each muscle is depicted in Fig. 4.30. If we disregard for a moment the binocular movements, it is at once apparent that any rotation must alter the distance between the orbital and ocular attachments of all its six muscles; some shorten and some lengthen, and there is abundant evidence to show that such adjustments occur in all six muscles (Sherrington, 1905; Szentagothai, 1943).

No extraocular muscle normally acts alone. The muscles of each eye act in concert to produce a specific eye movement; contraction of one muscle (the **agonist**), is accompanied by a graded relaxation of its **antagonist**. Thus, the six muscles attached to one globe may be regarded as three pairs of muscles, each member of a pair acting reciprocally as ipsilateral agonist or antagonist in a particular eye movement: medial and lateral rectus, superior and inferior rectus and the obliques of each eye are antagonistic pairs and excitation of one member of a pair is associated with reciprocal inhibition of the other. The pair of muscles which move the eyes in the same direction, in conjugate gaze (often referred to as 'yoke' muscles), behave as **synergists**. These are designated **ipsilateral** and **contralateral**, according to context (e.g. left lateral rectus is the contralateral synergist of right medial rectus). By the same token, the terms ipsilateral and contralateral **antagonist** are also used.

If we consider the actions of individual muscles and how they modify each other, a comparatively simple concept of uniocular and binocular activities will emerge.

The medial and lateral recti are natural opponents, whose reciprocal contractions and relaxations move the visual axes in a horizontal plane, but both oblique muscles can also act as abductors and the superior and inferior recti as adductors. Moreover, if both muscles in a pair contract to an equal extent, their tendencies to elevate or depress the visual axis and to intort or extort it are opposed and cancelled out. Thus, the medial, superior and inferior recti act as an adductor group, their abductor opponents being the lateral rectus and both oblique muscles.

Two important categories of eye movement which may be identified in the binocular state are **versions**, in which the visual axes are moved in parallel (conjugate gaze), and **vergence** movements, in which the eyes converge or diverge.

Whether in conjugate gaze (parallel movements of the visual axes, as in scanning relatively distant objects) or in convergent (or divergent) inclination to transfer attention from a distant to a proximate focus of regard (or vice versa) such movements are, of course, not always in a horizontal plane. Consequently, the contributions of synergistic medial and lateral recti (and for that matter the synergistic vertical recti or obliques) are not always equal, but must be so adjusted that each visual axis can, for example, be inclined downwards and medially, as in the common act of transferring the gaze from distant objects to objects held in the hands. (Head and neck movements are, of course, also involved.) The reverse movement can be carried out to an equal extent, while preserving binocular vision, a reminder that divergence of the visual axes must be as precise as convergence. Moreover, convergence from distant gaze to a near point on one side or the other brings one medial rectus and the opposite lateral rectus into an integration as precise as in convergence towards the mid field, carried out by synergy of both medial recti. By such complex and yet flexible integration between the 12 extraocular muscles, binocular vision can be maintained without lapse into diplopia over almost a hemisphere in the visual environment, the gaze being transferred in any direction to objects near and far, often with great rapidity.

In assessing a patient with paralytic squint the palsied muscle may be more readily identified (e.g. lateral rectus or superior oblique) if the eye movements are tested in the horizontal and oblique meridia (i.e. to the right or left, or up or down to the right or left). In this way the yoke muscles (synergists) of the two eyes may be assessed in tandem and underaction of the paralysed muscle (or overaction of its yoke muscle) detected. This allows the primary vertical actions of the vertical recti and obliques to be paired. The yoke muscle pairs are thus medial rectus and contralateral lateral rectus (horizontal versions); superior rectus and contralateral inferior oblique (dextro- or laevoelevation); inferior rectus and contralateral superior oblique (dextro- or laevodepression) (Fig. 4.30).

Humans, like other animals with frontal vision and overlapping visual fields, possess the basis for binocular vision, and with it the need to perform vergence movements which ensure that both foveas are trained on the same visual target, however near, by a simultaneous and opposite movement of each eye.

In order to maintain surveillance over the visual world and adjust attention to fresh objects of interest, eye movements are modified by a variety of sensory inputs which signal from proprioceptors in head, neck, trunk and limbs, and indicate the body's position in space and the target's position in the visual world. Effective use of foveal vision demands that the line of sight be directed independently of head position. Reflex adjustments in response to proprioceptive, vestibular and visual afferents are combined and further modified at higher brain stem cerebral level.

TYPES OF EYE MOVEMENT

There are several different types of eye movement. **Rapid** movements include voluntary and spontaneous saccades, the fast phases of vestibular and optokinetic nystagmus, and rapid eye movements (REM) of sleep. **Slow** movements include voluntary pursuit and vergence movements, as well as reflex optokinetic and vestibularly induced slow phases.

The premotor 'command' for horizontal movements arises in the paramedian pontine reticular formation (PPRF), that for vertical movement in the rostral mesencephalic reticular formation including the rostral interstitial nucleus of the medial longitudinal fasciculus (riMLF), and perhaps the interstitial nucleus of Cajal (INC). Activity in these regions is precisely coordinated by interconnections, and there are projections to the nuclear subgroups concerned with eye movements. In turn, the riMLF and INC receive afferents from the vestibular system and cerebellum, the superior colliculi, accessory optic system and cortex (Fig. 4.48).

Experimental evidence suggesting the localization of function in the central nervous system is

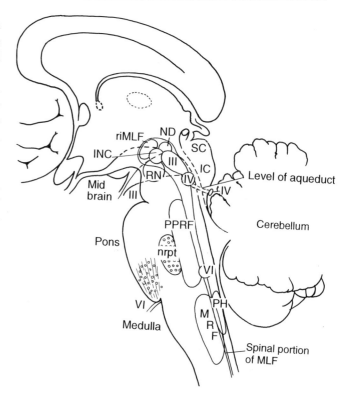

Fig. 4.48 Parasagittal section through the brain stem. IC = Inferior colliculus; INC = interstitial nucleus of Cajal; MLF = medial longitudinal fasciculus; MRF = medullary reticular formation; ND = nucleus of Darkschewitsch; PH = perihypoglossal nucleus; riMLF = rostral interstitial medial longitudinal fasciculus; SC = superior colliculus; PPRF = paramedian pontine reticular formation; III, IV, VI = cranial nerve nuclei or nerves. (From Leigh, R. J. and Zee, D. S. (1991) *The Neurology of Eye Movements*; 2nd edition, published by F. A. Davis.)

sometimes corroborated by clinical observation. Thus, lesions in the PPRF or rostral mesencephalic reticular formation lead to loss of horizontal or vertical conjugate movements. Lesions in certain afferent pathways impair the generation of nystagmus; mesencephalic lesions impair vergence movements. Lesions of coordinating structures, such as the cerebellum, impair the velocity and precision of eye movements.

All eye movements occur against the viscous drag of orbital tissues, including the muscles. Any eye position must be maintained against the elastic restoring forces of orbital structures. These mechanical forces influence all ocular movement.

The functional properties of human and monkey muscles have been studied by imaging techniques, length-tension measurements and single motor unit recording techniques. The extraocular muscles are among the fastest and the most fatigue resistant of the mammalian muscles, with an isometric contraction rate about twice as fast as limb muscle, and a blood flow, and hence potential oxidative capacity, higher than in any skeletal muscle. The twitch contraction rates of extraocular muscles are also characterized by a low tension output, related perhaps to their unique myosin content and relevant to their low load-bearing function. Thus the relationship between the rate of sarcomere shortening and relative load borne by extraocular muscles and skeletal muscle is similar (see Porter *et al.*, 1995, for references).

The concept that the small, tonic muscles are involved with fixation and slow eye movements, and that the twitch system supplies the basis for rapid eye movements, is no longer tenable. Instead, the different types of motor unit are now regarded as a final common pathway for all forms of eye movement. Intraoperative electromyography studies, recording activity simultaneously in multiple motor units, have shown that the sustained discharge associated with a given eye position, is independent of the type of movement employed to reach that position and that all types of fibre participate in every type of movement whether conjugate or dysjunctive.

In the saccades it is conceived that all motor units are recruited synchronously. However, at the end of a discharge, or for slow movements, there is differential recruitment which is position dependent. The orbital singly innervated and global red singly innervated are recruited first, well in the off-direction of the muscle, then the multiply innervated units, probably near the primary position, and then very fast but fatigable muscle fibres, well into the on-direction of the muscle. Thus the orbital singly innervated and global red singly innervated would be recruited in practically all saccades, but only in extreme to intermediate gaze. Motor neurone size may be a determinant of the sequence of recruitment; the orbital layer of the monkey medial rectus muscle is innervated by a distinct population of small motor neurones which might be recruited early.

The extraocular muscles show a significant degree of activity, even when the eye is directed well into the off-direction of the muscle. Collins (1975) argues that this sustained activity eliminates slack and allows the eye movement system to operate in the linear region of the length–tension curve. The resting tension of innervated extraocular muscles always exceeds 10 g, a tension at or above which the length–tension curves become straight lines.

4.26 NEURAL BASIS FOR EYE MOVEMENTS

The neural basis for the movements outlined above may now be examined in detail.

CORTICAL REGIONS

Several widely separated regions of the cerebral cortex are involved in ocular movements. On the criterion of excitation of eye movements these include the **occipital cortex**, the **frontal eye field** and the **parietal cortex**.

Area striata of the occipital cortex (area 17)

The striate cortex is the primary cortical reception area for visual information, with important connections to visuomotor areas (Fig. 4.49):

Afferents

These include a few connections from the pontine reticular formation. There are reciprocal connections with the inferior and lateral pulvinar (Ogren and Henderson, 1976).

Efferents

These comprise pretectal, superior collicular and posterior thalamic projections.

The occipital centre may be concerned with the fixation reflex, that is, with bringing on to the fovea the image of an object which has gained interest at the periphery of the retina. Stimulation of the visual area (areas 17 and 18) causes conjugate deviation in various directions, especially contralateral. Area 19 also responds. Accommodation can be elicited from area 18.

Clinical studies suggest a pathway from an oculomotor 'centre' in the parieto-occipital region to the tectum (Daroff, Troost and Leigh, 1978), running in the internal sagittal stratum parallel to the optic radiation. Although this is questioned (Sharpe and Deck, 1978), parieto-occipital lesions do affect ipsilateral smooth pursuit (Garey, Jones and Powell, 1968; Sharp and Deck, 1978).

The frontal eye fields

The frontal oculomotor area (Brodman 8, with parts of 6 and 9) or frontal eye field occupies the posterior part of the middle frontal gyrus (the prearcuate gyrus). In monkeys stimulation of area 8 results in contralateral conjugate deviation of the eyes, and also head movements (Ferrier, 1874) (Fig. 4.50); pupillary dilatation may also be elicited. Both voluntary and reflex ocular movements may be mediated by this area. The movements are simple. Descending projection fibres have been traced to the mid brain, but

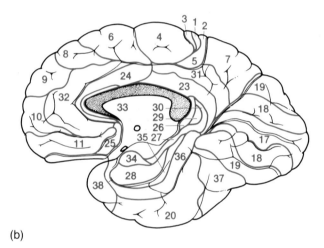

(a)

(b)

Fig. 4.49 Cytoarchitectural map of the human brain. (a) Lateral and (b) medial surfaces.

not to individual nuclei. Occipital association and thalamic afferents (dorsomedial nucleus) reach the area. (For a review of earlier work see Crosby, Humphrey and Laver, 1962.)

Afferents

These include connections with the thalamus and several cortical regions, including superior temporal, peristriate and parietal (area 7), where visual and eye movement-related neurons have been identified.

Efferents

Efferents project to basal ganglia, thalamus, pretectal region (including the nucleus of the optic tract), superior colliculus and portions of mid brain and

pontine reticular formations (see also Kunzle and Akert, 1977).

Each frontal eye field projects to the contralateral frontal eye field and to ipsilateral cortical areas concerned with visual perception, for example parietal 7 and peristriate cortex (formerly area 19, now subdivided). Descending projections of the prefrontal cortex traverse the anterior limb of the internal capsule and divide into dorsal and ventral tracts in the rostral diencephalon (Leichnetz, 1981; Leigh and Zee, 1983) (Fig. 4.51).

The dorsal transthalamic tract

This traverses and partially synapses in the dorsomedial and intralaminar thalamic nuclei and medial pulvinar. It then synapses in the pretectal nuclei and deep superior colliculus.

The ventral pedunculotegmental tract

This descends in the most ventral zone of the cerebral peduncle, supplying some fibres to the subthalamic nucleus and deeper colliculus, but ending chiefly in the PPRF. (Kunzle and Akert (1977) found no projections to the PPRF in their radioautographic studies.)

Third prefrontal bundle

A third prefrontal oculomotor bundle may arise at the diencephalic-mesencephalic junction dorsomedial to the tractus retroflexus and rostral pole of the red nucleus. It projects unilaterally to the RiMLF and INC and bilaterally to the nucleus of Darkschewitsch and the rostral portion of oculomotor nucleus. The functions of these connections are not established.

The frontal eye fields encode neural activity topographically, as in the superior colliculus (Robinson and Fuchs, 1969). Activity at different sites relates to saccades of different size and direction. In alert monkeys trained to look towards targets, neurons in a restricted portion of the frontal eye field exhibiting visual receptive fields discharge before, and specifically in relation to, the saccades elicited by a visual target lying within those fields (Goldberg and Bushnell, 1981). Stimulation of the frontal eye field shows a latency before a saccade of 30–40 ms, which slightly exceeds the latency prior to saccades elicited via the colliculus.

Purely vertical saccades are elicited by simultaneous stimulation of corresponding sites in the horizontal eye fields, the horizontal saccades

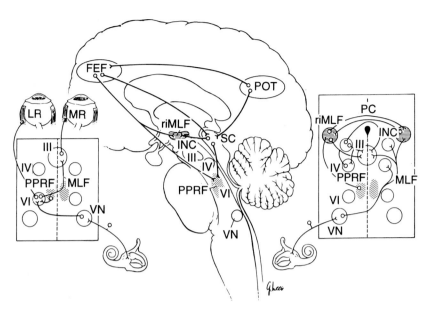

Fig. 4.50 Summary of eye movement control. The centre figure shows supranuclear connections from the frontal eye fields (FEF) and the parieto-occipital temporal junctional region (POT) to the superior colliculus (SC), rostral interstitial nucleus of the medial longitudinal fasciculus (riMLF) and the paramedian pontine reticular formation (PPRF). The FEF and SC are involved in saccade production and the POT is thought to be involved in pursuit movement. The schematic drawing on the left shows brain stem pathways for horizontal gaze. Axons from cell bodies in the PPRF travel to the ipsilateral abducens nucleus (VI) to synapse with abducens motor neurons whose axons travel to the ipsilateral rectus muscle (LR) and with internuclear neurons whose axons cross the mid-line and travel in the medial longitudinal fasciculus (MLF) to portions of the oculomotor nucleus (III) concerned with contralateral medial rectus (MR) function. The drawing on the right shows brain stem pathways for vertical gaze. Important structures include the riMLF, PPRF, the interstitial nucleus of Cajal (INC) and the posterior commissure (PC). Note that axons from cell bodies in the vestibular nuclei (VN) travel directly to the abducens nuclei and mostly via the MLF to the oculomotor nuclei. IV = Trochlea nucleus. (From Miller, N. (1985) *Clinical Neuro-Ophthalmology*, 4th edition, published by Williams and Wilkins.)

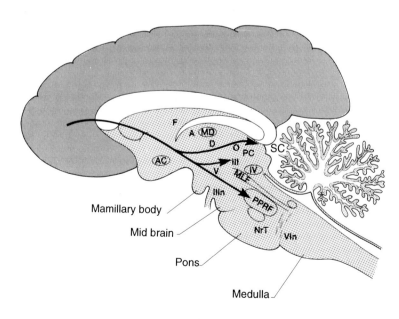

Fig. 4.51 Prefrontal cortical projections to ocular motor structures in the monkey. D = 'Transthalamic' pathways; V = classic 'pedunculotegmental' pathway; MD = dorsomedial nuclei; SC = superior colliculus; PPRF = paramedian pontine reticular formation; O = oculomotor nucleus; A = anterior thalamic nucleus; AC = anterior commissure; F = fornix; III, IV = third and fourth cranial nerves; MLF = medial longitudinal fasciculus; PC = posterior commissure. (Modified from Leigh, R. J. and Zee, D. S. (1991) *The Neurology of Eye Movements*, 2nd edition, published by F. A. Davis, After Leichnetz, 1981.)

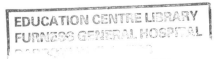

cancelling out. The frontal eye fields may be concerned with maintaining visual attention, directing the eyes to objects of interest while other images are ignored. Human frontal lobe lesions cause a transient loss of contralateral saccades (Daroff and Hoyt, 1971).

Parietal cortex

A role has been suggested for parietal area 7 related to attention to visual targets (Mountcastle *et al.*, 1975; Bushnell, Goldbere and Robinson, 1981).

Afferents

Area 7 has afferents from the cingulate gyrus and basal forebrain and an indirect representation of the visual world from the pretectal region and superior colliculus, via thalamic nuclei (Jones and Powell, 1970). There are also afferents from the frontal eye field and prestriate cortex.

Efferents

Efferents project to the pretectal region and superior colliculus, to the circumaqueductal grey matter, and to ipsilateral and contralateral parietal lobes (Petras, 1971).

Neurons in primate inferior parietal lobes are active before and during certain ocular movements (Lynch *et al.*, 1977). **Fixation** neurons fire during fixation or smooth pursuit, **tracking** neurons during pursuit only, and **saccadic** neurons before and during visually evoked, but not spontaneous, saccades. Activity is related to volition, and is associated with maintaining or shifting attention, rather than to amplitude or direction of movement (Lynch *et al.*, 1977). Bushnell, Goldbere and Robinson (1981) have shown that area 7 cells are not 'saccade-specific'; although they are activated during non-ocular movements (e.g. reaching towards a visual stimulus), activity is not enhanced during spontaneous saccades unrelated to a visual stimulus.

Conjugate deviation has been produced in experimental animals by stimulation of the angular gyrus. This occupies parts of areas 38 and 39, and curves round the posterior end of the middle temporal gyrus; it is part of the inferior parietal lobule and contains some small pyramidal neurons. Operative removal of the area has not resulted in any oculomotor defect.

Biparietal lesions may produce an ocular motor apraxia (Cogan, 1965).

SUB-CORTICAL REGIONS

There are connections between the frontal eye fields and basal ganglia (Kunzle and Akert, 1977), and between substantia nigra and superior colliculus (Jayarman, Batton and Carpenter, 1977). The discharge of neurons in the pars reticulata of the substantia is modulated in relation to saccades to both actual and remembered targets. They project to (and probably inhibit) neurons in the deeper layers of the superior colliculus. Patients with extrapyramidal disease frequently show saccadic abnormalities.

The **pulvinar** receives afferents from the visual cortex and superior colliculus (Mathers, 1971; Benevento and Rezak, 1976).

Stimulation of the **thalamus** in primates induces saccades, while lesions may disturb visual discriminatory tasks (Carpenter, 1977; Ungerleider and Christensen, 1979), and impair saccadic accuracy and the ability to match ocular to target position (Optican, 1982).

THE CEREBELLUM

The cerebellum is a major coordinator of movements involving striated muscle, including eye movements. This control requires afferents from the visual and vestibular apparatus, the neck and other proprioceptors, and projections to supranuclear zones concerned in ocular movements, both smooth pursuit and saccades.

It comprises the phylogenetically ancient **archaeocerebellum** (flocculonodular node), the **palaeocerebellum** (anterior lobe, excluding lingula, and including pyramid and uvula of the middle lobe), and the **neocerebellum** (middle lobe excluding pyramid and uvula but including vermis) (Fig. 4.52). The **mossy fibres** of the cerebellum carry the main afferent input from the olive, spinocerebellar, pontocerebellar and primary and secondary vestibulocerebellar sources. The climbing fibres, which have a remarkable one-to-one relationship with cerebellar Purkinje fibres, arise from pontine nuclei, inferior olive and the medial reticular formation (Figs 4.53 and 4.54).

Flocculonodular lobe (vestibulocerebellum)

This includes the flocculi, nodulus, ventral uvula and paraflocculi, all receiving direct projections from vestibular nuclei.

Afferents

Afferents come from the inferior olivary nuclei (climbing fibres), reticular formation (mossy fibres),

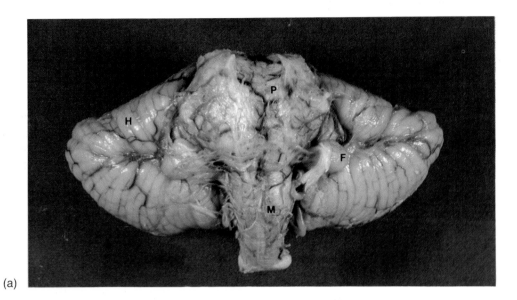

(a)

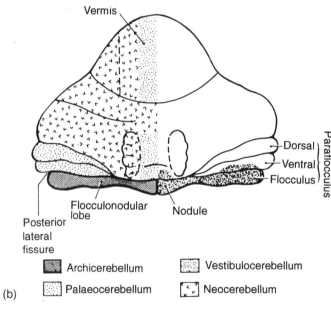

(b)

Archicerebellum

Palaeocerebellum

Vestibulocerebellum

Neocerebellum

Fig. 4.52 Human cerebellum. (a) Ventral view. F = Flocculus; H = hemisphere; M = medulla; P = pons. (Courtesy of B. McDonald.) (b) Schematic drawing of the subdivisions of the human cerebellum. The left half of the drawing shows the three main subdivisions: the archicerebellum, the flocculonodular node; the paleocerebellum; anterior vermis, the pyramids, the uvula, the paraflocculus and the neocerebellum. The right half of the diagram shows the structures of the vestibulocerebellum: the flocculonodular lobe, the dorsal and ventral paraflocculi. (From Miller, N. (1985) *Clinical Neuro-Ophthalmology*, 4th edition, published by Williams and Wilkins.)

vestibular and perihypoglossal nuclei (Fig. 4.55). Reciprocal projections reach the vestibular nuclei and nuclei prepositi hypoglossi (Alley, 1977).

Visual information reaches each flocculus via connections involving the retina, contralateral pretectum and inferior olivary nucleus (Scalia, 1972). A visual cortical projection to pontine nuclei also relays to each paraflocculus (mossy fibres) (Burne, Mihailoff and Woodward, 1978). The nucleus of the optic tract and some floccular neurons encode information about direction and velocity of visual targets (Simpson and Alley, 1974; Collewijn, 1977).

The vestibulocerebellum modulates smooth pursuit and the vestibulo-ocular reflex (Lisberger and Fuchs, 1978a,b). It is concerned with adjustments matching head and eye movements with target

movements ('gain control') (Gonshor and Melvill Jones, 1976).

Dorsal lesions of the human vestibulocerebellum lead to loss of coordination of eye movements with overshoot of saccades.

Vermis

The dorsal cerebellar vermis, especially lobules V, VI and VII, and subjacent fastigial nuclei are concerned in saccadic control.

Afferents

These include projections from the vestibular and basal pontine nuclei. The latter receive visual

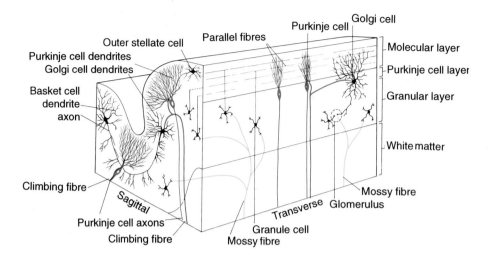

Fig. 4.53 Schematic diagram of the cerebellar cortex in sagittal and transverse planes to show cell and fibre arrangements. Pürkinje cells and cell processes (axons and dendrites) are shown in blue. Mossy fibres are in yellow; climbing fibres are in red. Golgi cells, basket cells and outer stellate cells are in black, while the dendritic arborizations of Pürkinje cells are oriented in a sagittal plane. Dendrites of the Goigi cells show no similar arrangement. Layers of the cerebellar cortex are indicated. (Redrawn from Carpenter, M. B. (1976) *Human Neuroanatomy*, published by Williams and Wilkins.)

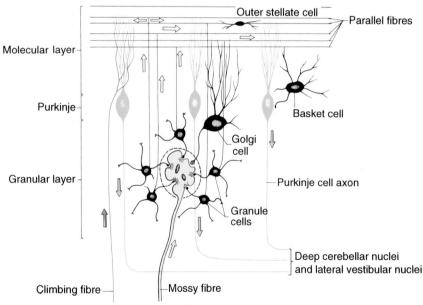

Fig. 4.54 Schematic diagram of the cellular and fibre elements of the cerebellar cortex between the longitudinal axis of a folium. Excitatory inputs are conveyed by the mossy fibres (yellow) and the climbing fibres (red). The broken line represents a glia lamella ensheathing glomerulus containing: a mossy fibre rosette, several granule cell dendrites and one Golgi cell axon. Axons of granule cells ascend to the molecular layer, bifurcate and form an extensive system of parallel fibres, which synapse on the spiny processes of the Pürkinje cells (blue). Climbing fibres traverse the granular layer and ascend the dendrites of the Pürkinje cells, where they synapse on smooth branchlets. Arrows indicate the direction of impulse conduction. Outer stellate and basket cells are shown in the molecular layer but axons of the basket cells which ramify about Pürkinje cell somata are not shown. (Redrawn from Carpenter, M. B. (1976) *Human Neuroanatomy*, published by Williams and Wilkins.)

afferents from superior colliculus (Hoddevik *et al.*, 1977), lateral geniculate body, and striate cortex (Fig. 4.55). There are also cervical and ocular proprioceptive afferents.

Efferents

These project indirectly to oculomotor nuclei via vestibular or fastigial–vestibular connections (Walberg, 1961).

Purkinje cells in the vermis discharge 25 ms before a saccade (Llinas and Wolfe, 1977) or at the time of a saccade (Kase, Miller and Noda, 1980; Hepp, Henn and Jaeger, 1982; Keller, 1982).

Stimulation induces conjugate saccades with an ipsilateral horizontal component (Ron and Robinson, 1973): lobule V, up-gaze to horizontal positions; VI and VII, horizontal to down-gaze positions. Saccadic direction is encoded topographically as in the frontal eye fields and superior colliculi, but amplitude is

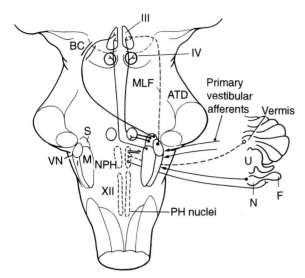

Fig. 4.55 Vestibulocerebellar connections concerned with eye movements. ATD = ascending tract of Deiters; BC = brachium conjunctivum; F = flocculus; MLF = medial longitudinal fasciculus; N = nodulus; NPH = nucleus prepositus hypoglossi; PH = perihypoglossal nucleus; VN = vestibular nuclei (I = inferior; L = lateral; M = medial; S = superior; U = uvula).

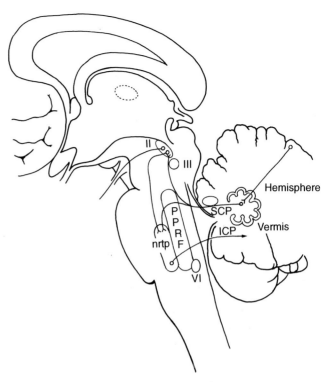

Fig. 4.56 Sagittal section of the brain stem to show cerebellar connections. ICP = inferior cerebellar peduncle; nrtp = nucleus reticularis tegmenti pontis; PPRF = pontine paramedial reticular formation; SCP = superior cerebellar peduncle; II, III, VI = cranial nerve nuclei.

dependent on stimulus intensity. A given stimulus always takes the eye to the same orbital location, with the saccade being 'goal directed' (Leigh and Zee, 1983).

THE CEREBELLAR HEMISPHERES

Projections from the hemispheres leave the dentate nuclei via each brachium conjunctivum to reach the ocular motor nuclei, either directly (Carpenter and Strominger, 1964; Ron and Robinson, 1973) or via a relay in the nucleus reticularis tegmenti pontis. This nucleus is just ventral to the pontine paramedium reticular formation and has reciprocal connections with ocular motor neurons (Maciewicz and Spencer, 1977) (Fig. 4.56).

Stimulation of the hemispheres may produce saccades or smooth pursuit (Carpenter and Strominger, 1964; Ron and Robinson, 1973).

VESTIBULAR APPARATUS (Fig. 4.57)

The organs of balance provide information about movement and position of the head which is used in the synthesis of any eye movement and adjustment of trunk and limb posture (see Leigh and Zee, 1983). Vestibulo-ocular reflexes prevent image slip during eye movements.

The membranous labyrinth in the temporal bone contains the **cristae** of the semicircular canals, which respond to head rotation, and the **maculae** of the utricle and saccule which sense head position (gravity). All possess specialized hair cells, with projections into the endolymph, which generate a neural impulse on stimulation. The processes of each hair cell contain many **stereocilia** and a single **kinocilium**. Deflection of stereocilia towards the kinocilium stimulates the cell, deflection away inhibits it.

Semicircular canals

The stereocilia of the cristae are embedded in a gelatinous **cupula**, one in each **ampulla** of the three canals. With any head movement, a flow of endolymph in each semicircular canal bends the cupula and alters the neural signal from the hair cell at its base. Flow of endolymph in the horizontal canals towards the ampulla or utricle is excitatory; in vertical canals (anterior and posterior) flow away from the ampulla or utricle is excitatory.

The canals are paired in a similar plane bilaterally (e.g. right and left horizontal; each anterior with the

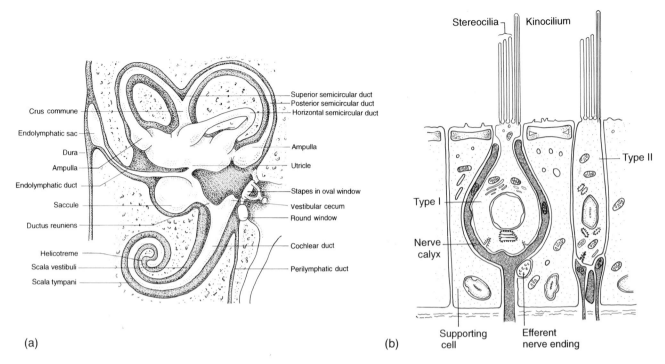

(a)

(b)

Fig. 4.57 (a) Membranous labyrinth, showing auditory structures (cochlear duct) and vestibular structures (utricle, saccule and semicircular ducts). (From Kandel, E. R. and Schwarz (eds) (1985) *Principles of Neural Science* 2nd Edition, published by Elsevier Scientific Publishers.) (b) Schematic drawing of the two types of hair cells in the vestibular apparatus of mammals. Note the different kinds of nerve endings in contact with the cells, the symmetric arrangement of the bundles of sensory hairs and the many stereocilia with a single kinocilium in the periphery. (From Miller, N. R. (1985) *Clinical Neuro-Ophthalmology*, 4th Edition, published by Williams & Wilkins.)

contralateral posterior). Thus, for example, a head movement inducing flow of endolymph away from the ampulla of the right anterior canal (excitatory) coincides with flow towards that of the left posterior canal (inhibitory), and an excitatory stimulus from one side is reinforced by a contralateral inhibitory stimulus. Each canal induces ocular movements approximately in its own plane (Floren's Law), and influences the yoke pair of extraocular muscles which are prime movers in that plane, regardless of the initial orbital position of the eyes. These relationships are summarized in Table 4.11 and illustrated in Fig. 4.58.

The utricle and saccule

The maculae of the utricle and saccule respond to linear acceleration, particularly gravity, and are mainly concerned with static, tilted positions of the head. They lie in planes approximately at right-angles. Hair cells have processes embedded in a gelatinous matrix, containing calcium carbonate crystals called **otoconia**. The arrangement of the macular hair cells allows detection of any linear motion permitted in three-dimensional space.

The vestibular nerves

Nerve fibres from the cristae and maculae traverse perforations of each lamina cribrosa to reach the vestibular ganglion at the lateral end of the internal auditory meatus. The vestibular nerve formed by its centripetal fibres then passes medially across the *cerebellopontine angle* inferior to the facial and posterior to the cochlear nerves, to enter the brain stem between the inferior cerebellar peduncle and trigeminal spinal tract (Fig. 4.59). These primary vestibular axons project mainly to the vestibular nuclei and the flocculonodular lobe.

Vestibular nuclei

The vestibular nuclei (superior, medial, lateral and inferior) are clustered under the floor of the fourth ventricle. This complex reaches caudally into the pons near the angle between floor and lateral wall of the ventricle (Fig. 4.60) (Carpenter, 1976).

Efferents

1. Substantial projections enter the medial longitudinal fasciculus, and are distributed thus to the oculomotor and other brain stem nuclei.

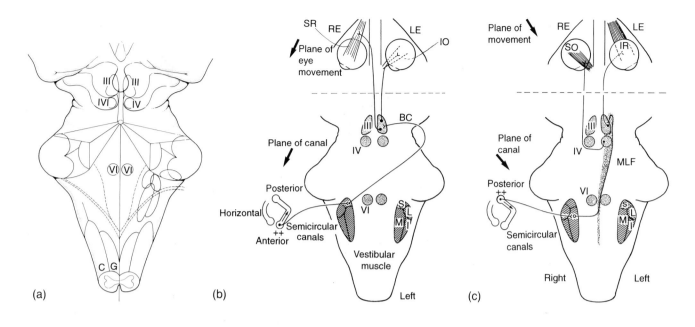

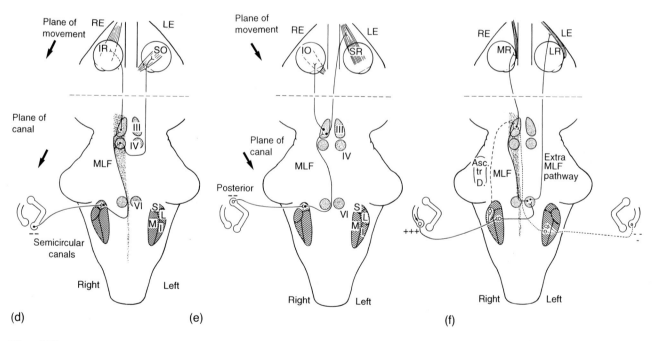

Fig. 4.58 Schematic representation of the oculomotor nuclei in the brain stem (a) and the pathways activated during stimulation of eye movement by the vestibular apparatus (semicircular canals). (b) Dextroelevation; excitation of the right anterior canal (an inhibition of the paired left posterior canal) stimulates gaze up to the right. Note the double decussation involved in excitation of the ipsilateral superior rectus muscle (i.e. superior vestibular nucleus to contralateral brachium conjunctivum to contralateral third nucleus; activation of superior rectus motor neurons to stimulate the ipsilateral superior rectus). Note that flow, *away* from the ampulla, is excitatory in the vertical canals and flow *towards* the ampulla is excitatory in the horizontal canal. (c) Laevodepression. Excitation of right posterior canal (inhibition of left anterior canal) stimulates down gaze left. (d) Dextrodepression. Inhibition of right anterior canal (excitation of left posterior canal) stimulates down gaze right. (e) Laevoelevation. Inhibition of right posterior canal (excitation of left anterior canal) stimulates up gaze left. (f) Laevoversion. Head turn to the right excites the right horizontal canal (inhibits the left horizontal canal) and stimulates gaze to the left. There is a slow movement to the left and a nystagmus with a rapid phase to the right, i.e. 'right nystagmus'.

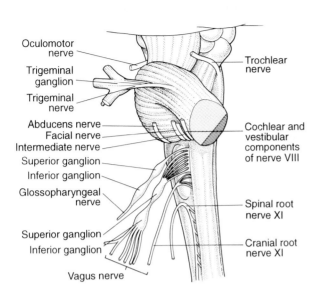

Fig. 4.59 The brain stem and cranial nerves, showing the peripheral ganglia. (From Carpenter, M. B. (1976) *Human Neuroanatomy*, published by Williams and Wilkins.)

2. Vestibulocerebellar efferents from inferior and medial vestibular nuclei to vestibulocerebellum and vermis are also substantial, and are described on page 160.
3. Vestibulospinal efferents descend from the lateral vestibular nucleus.

Vestibular connections

Mossy fibres of the vestibular nerve project directly to the vestibulocerebellum (flocculus, nodulus, ventral uvula and paraflocculus), which also receives mossy fibre projections from the vestibular, peri-hypoglossal and pontine nuclei, and climbing fibres from the contralateral inferior olive (Fig. 4.53).

Purkinje cells of the flocculus project in part directly back to ipsilateral vestibular nuclei, peri-hypoglossal and deep cerebellar nuclei. Purkinje cells of the flocculus may project bilaterally via the fastigial nucleus to the vestibular nuclei.

There are also vestibulothalamic and parietal connections.

Vestibulocerebellar lesions have little effect on the vestibulo-ocular reflex and maintenance of eye position. Flocculectomy impairs adaptation of the vestibulo-ocular reflex to altered sensory circumstances such as altered refraction (Optican *et al.*, 1980): flocculectomy also causes 'post-saccadic' drift (Zee *et al.*, 1981), whereas ablation of vermis and subjacent fastigial nuclei causes saccadic 'overshoot' (Optican and Robinson, 1980).

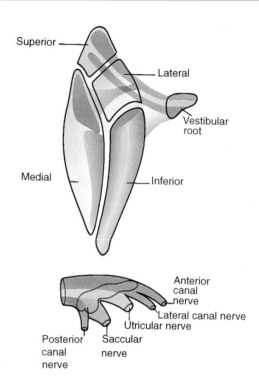

Fig. 4.60 Diagrammatic representation of the relationships between portions of the vestibular ganglia and central fibres projecting to parts of the vestibular nuclear complex. The vestibular ganglia are shown in a modified transverse plane, while the vestibular nerve root and the vestibular nuclear complex are drawn in a stylised fashion, as they would appear in horizontal sections of the brain stem. Only the principal central projections of distinctive parts of the vestibular ganglia are shown. Portions of the vestibular ganglia innervating the cristae of the semicircular canals (*green*) project primarily to the superior vestibular nucleus and rostral parts of the medial vestibular nucleus. Portions of the superior vestibular ganglion (*yellow*) innervating the macula of the utricle project central fibres primarily to parts of the inferior and medial vestibular nuclei. Fibres from portions of the inferior vestibular ganglion innervating the macula of the saccule (*pink*) project mainly to dorsolateral parts of the inferior vestibular nucleus. Some cells in the vestibular ganglia project fibres to parts of all vestibular nuclei, so that each part of the labyrinth has a unique as well as common projection, within the vestibular nuclear complex (Redrawn from Stein, B. M. and Carpenter, M. B. (1967) *Am. J. Anat.*, **120**, 281.)

SUPERIOR COLLICULI

The superior colliculi are two rounded elevations situated on the dorsal aspect of the mid brain, separated from each other by a vertical sulcus containing the pineal gland. A transverse sulcus separates the superior and inferior colliculi (Fig. 5.13). Above each superior colliculus is the thalamus. Superiorly in the mid line is the great cerebral vein, entering the straight sinus (Fig. 4.61). Postero-superior to the whole tectum, which comprises all four col-

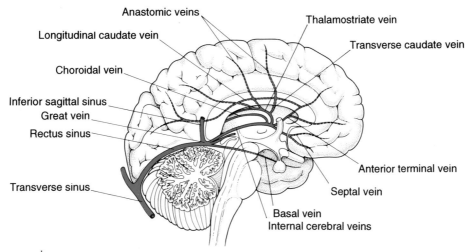

Fig. 4.61 Mid-sagittal view of the internal cerebral veins, showing the relationship of the great vein of Galen to the straight sinus (sinus rectus). (From Carpenter, M. B. (1976) *Human Neuroanatomy*, published by Williams & Wilkins.)

liculi, is the cerebellum. Both structures are covered by pia and arachnoid maters, between which is the cisterna of the great cerebral vein, a local dilatation of the subarachnoid space (Fig. 15.90).

The superior colliculi have a laminated structure (Carpenter, 1976) (Fig. 4.62):

1. stratum zonale;
2. stratum cinereum (outer grey layer);
3. stratum opticum (superficial white layer);
4. stratum lemnisci (middle and deep grey and white layers) (Fig. 4.62).

Afferents

The ipsilateral striate cortex projects to layer 3 of the rostral third of the colliculus via the optic radiation, lateral geniculate body, and brachium of the superior colliculus. These afferents end in the superficial and middle grey layers (2 and 4). The contralateral hemifield including the macular field is topographically represented (Fig. 4.63) (Wilson and Toyne, 1970).

Retinal ganglion cell axons project to layer 3 of the caudal two-thirds of the colliculus and terminate in the superficial and middle grey layers. The contralateral hemifield, excluding the macular field, is topographically represented, with the inferior quadrant lateral and superior medial. The central 30° of the field occupy the rostral three-quarters of the reception area, the peripheral 60° the caudal quarter (Brouwer and Zeeeman, 1926a,b).

Corticotectal tracts come from frontal eye field, parietal and temporal cortex. The frontotectal pathway is transtegmental (Kuypers and Lawrence, 1967).

Spinotectal tracts connect the spinal cord and

medulla to the optic tectum. There are also afferents from the inferior colliculus.

Efferents

Tectoreticular fibres project profusely and bilaterally to the supraoptic nuclei dorsal in the mid brain reticular formation: Interstitial nucleus of Cajal and posterior commissural nucleus of Darkschewitsch (Fig. 4.48). There are no direct projections to the oculomotor nuclei (Szentagothai, 1950; Altman and Carpenter, 1961). **Tectopontine fibres** pass deep to the inferior colliculus to reach the dorsolateral pontine nuclei.

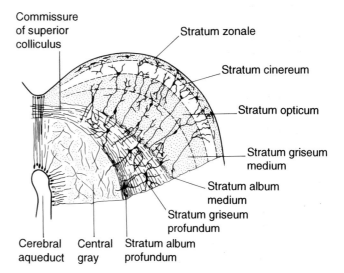

Fig. 4.62 Cellular lamination and organization of the superior colliculus based on reconstruction from Golgi preparations taken from an 8-month human fetus. (From Carpenter, M. B. (1976) *Human Neuroanatomy*, published by Williams & Wilkins.)

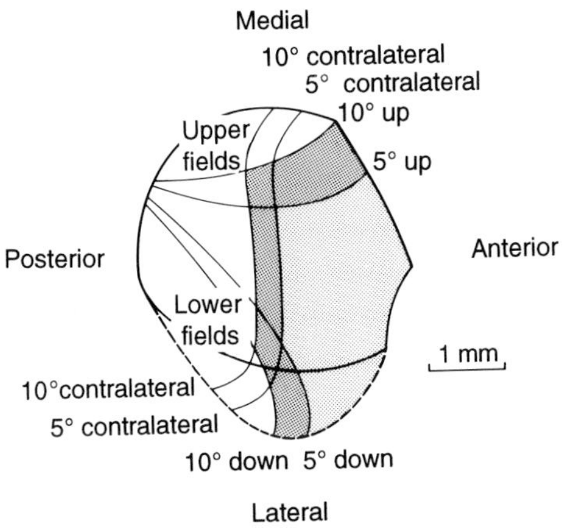

Fig. 4.63 Topographic representation of the visual field on the superior colliculus. The stippled area represents the part of the contralateral visual field within 5° of the fovea. Striped and stippled areas combined represent the part of the contralateral field within 10° of the fovea. (From Leigh, R. J. and Zee, D. S. (1991) *The Neurology of Eye Movements*, 2nd edition, published by F. A. Davis.)

Projections from the deep grey layer reach the **contralateral** colliculus. Also, via the dorsal supraoptic decussation (Fountain decussation of Meynert), tectospinal and tectobulbar fibres pass into the medial longitudinal fasciculus in the medulla, mainly to cervical spinal neurons.

Tectothalamic projections end in the pulvinar, dorsal and ventral lateral geniculate nuclei and possibly pretectum, to connect with the extrageniculate visual pathway (Harting *et al.*, 1973). There are no cortical projections.

Functions of the superior colliculi

Each superior colliculus receives an orderly topographical retinal projection (Fig. 4.63). Point stimulation causes a saccade to a point in the visual field corresponding to its retinal projection. Sensory and motor maps lie in register in the colliculus. The dorsal colliculus is primarily sensory and receives direct retinal input. It projects to the lateral geniculate body and pulvinar; the ventral portion appears to be motor, receiving visual input from the striate cortex and projecting to motor areas in the subthalmus and brain stem (Wurtz and Albano, 1980). The superficial colliculus may be concerned with visual processing and the deep colliculus with orientation movements of head and eyes in response to novel stimuli (Harting *et al.*, 1973). Superficial and deep layers of the colliculus may project to an outflow from the intermediate strata. Mohler and Wurtz (1976) identified neurons at the junction of superficial and deep strata whose responses were enhanced before a visually evoked saccade, but not before spontaneous saccades ('visually triggered movement cells').

Stimulation of the superior colliculus in an alert monkey elicits saccades whose amplitude and direction depend on the location of the stimulus. Smallest saccades are elicited anterolaterally, largest posteriorly (Fig. 4.50). Purely vertical saccades occur with bilateral stimulation of corresponding points (Robinson, 1972; Schiller and Stryker, 1972).

Superficial cells may respond to stationary and moving visual stimuli. **Deep** cells usually discharge before saccades to a specific area in the visual field. Other cells combine eye position information with a retinal error signal to compute target position in relation to the head. This signal might be used by movement cells of the deep layers to produce saccades to a target in space (Mays and Sparks, 1980a,b).

Superficial and deep strata may function independently: visually evoked activity in the superficial strata does not always lead to eye-movement-related activity in the deeper strata; movement-related activity in the deeper strata is not always associated with visually evoked activity in the superficial strata (Wurtz and Albano, 1980).

THE PERIHYPOGLOSSAL NUCLEI

The perihypoglossal nuclei, medial to the vestibular nucleus, are thought to be involved in neural integration of vertical and horizontal eye movements (Baker *et al.*, 1978) (Figs 4.64 and 4.65). The most prominent is the **nucleus prepositus hypoglossi**, extending from the rostral pole of the hypoglossal nucleus almost to the abducent nucleus. Caudally it continues into the **nucleus intercalatus**, between the hypoglossal and dorsal vagal nuclei (Fig. 5.1). Another member, the **sublingual nucleus** (of Roller), lies ventral to the rostral hypoglossal pole, near to its radicular fibres (Carpenter, 1976).

Afferents

Afferents to the perihypoglossal complex include RiMLF, and the INC representing a visual input. There are afferents from the PPRF and flocculus and from the vermis via the fastigial nucleus (Alley, Baker and Simpson, 1975) and all the ocular motor nuclei (Nyberg-Hansen, 1966; Baker, Berthoz and Delgardo-Garcia, 1977; Evinger *et al.*, 1975).

Intracellular recordings in the perihypoglossal nuclei resemble those from vestibular nuclei, including ipsilateral inhibition and contralateral excitation of ocular motor neurons (Baker and Berthoz, 1975).

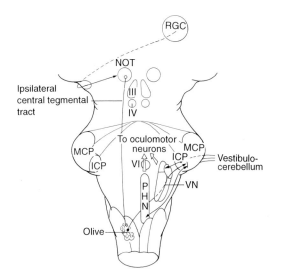

Fig. 4.64 Vestibulocerebellar and perihypoglossal connections. ICP = Inferior cerebellar peduncle; MCP = middle cerebellar peduncle; PHN = perihypoglossal nucleus; NOT = nucleus of the optic tract; RGC = retinal ganglion cell; VN = vestibular nucleus; III, IV, VI = cranial nerve nuclei.

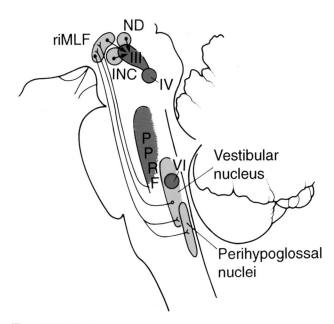

Fig. 4.65 Sagittal section of the brain stem illustrating connections of the rostral interstitial medial longitudinal fasciculus (riMLF). INC = Interstitial nucleus of Cajal; ND = nucleus of Darkschewitsch; PPRF = pontine paramedian reticular formation; III, IV, VI = cranial nerve nuclei.

This may represent an additional vestibulocerebello-ocular pathway, concerned with the modulation of vertical and horizontal eye movements (Baker *et al.*, 1978), which would explain their pontine and mesencephalic connections. Studies in primates demonstrate numerous perihypoglossal neurons which

encode eye position (Miles, 1974; Keller and Daniels, 1975; Lopez-Barnes *et al.*, 1982).

MEDIAL LONGITUDINAL FASCICULUS

This fasciculus, composed of myelinated fibres from nuclei at various levels, extends from rostral mid brain to spinal cord. At all levels, it is situated close to the mid line, and ventral to the aqueduct, fourth ventricle and central canal. Below the abducent level most fibres are descending; above this level, ascending fibres predominate (Carpenter, 1976). It is in intimate relation with many motor and other nuclei, including those of the ocular motor nerves.

At its cranial end, lateral to the third ventricle, the fasciculus is connected to the interstitial posterior commissural and other nuclei. In the mid brain it is ventral to the central grey matter and to the floor of the fourth ventricle in the pons. It connects the oculomotor and trochlear nuclei and abducent nuclei.

The fasciculus mediates correlation between these motor nuclei, and all four vestibular nuclei (Mc-Masters, Weiss and Carpenter, 1966). It is a constant feature of vertebrate brain stems, providing an 'intersegmental' integration of movements associated with vision and hearing. It has extensive connections with the flocculonodular lobe of the cerebellum through the vestibular nuclei (see Brodal, Pompeinano and Walberg, 1962; Macilewicz and Spencer, 1977; Yamamoto, Shimoyama and Highstein, 1978). In these highly complex activities at least eight cranial nerves (optic, oculomotor, trochlear, trigeminal, abducent, facial, vestibulocochlear and accessory) are involved, together with many spinal nerves, especially at cervical levels.

Descending fibres

Descending fibres originate mainly in the medial vestibular nucleus, but also in the reticular formation, superior colliculi and nucleus of Cajal. Descending fibres from the medial vestibular nucleus, both crossed and uncrossed, provide mono-synaptic inhibition to upper cervical motor neurons in the labyrinthine regulation of head position (Wilson and Yoshida, 1969).

Ascending fibres

Arising from vestibular nuclei, these have differential and overlapping projections to the oculomotor nuclei (McMasters, Weiss and Carpenter, 1966; Carpenter, 1971) (Fig. 4.66). Projections from the superior ves-

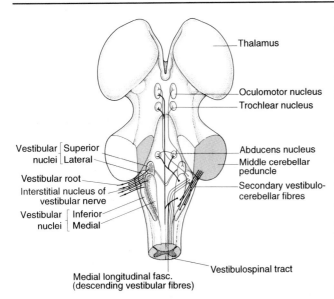

Fig. 4.66 Schematic diagram of some of the principal fibre projections of the vestibular system. (From Carpenter, M. B. (1976) *Human Neuroanatomy*, published by Williams and Wilkins.)

tibular nucleus rostral to the abducent nuclei ascend in the ipsilateral fasciculus, to the trochlear and dorsal oculomotor nucleus (inferior rectus motor neurons).

Ventral parts of the lateral vestibular nucleus project to the contralateral abducent and trochlear nuclei and parts of the oculomotor complex.

Projections from the inferior vestibular nucleus in the fasciculus are sparse; none is known to reach neurons innervating levator palpebrae.

Reciprocal fascicular connections represent the axons of internuclear neurons in the oculomotor and abducent nuclei. The rostral projection is contralateral, crossing at the abducent level. There is a bilateral projection from the oculomotor to the abducent nucleus (Graybiel, 1977). Approximately half of the cells in the abducent nucleus and about 3% in the oculomotor nucleus are internuclear neurons (Steiger and Büttner-Ennever, 1978). There is thus a predominance of ascending projections.

A discrete area of the reticular formation receives a projection from internuclear oculomotor neurons and superior colliculus, and projects to the cerebellar vermis (Kawamura, Brodal and Hoddevik, 1974; Harting *et al.*, 1975). The reticular formation also relays from other supranuclear structures to cerebellar cortex.

Abducent internuclear neurons project mainly to contralateral oculomotor neurons for medial rectus and inferior recti (Baker and Highstein, 1975; Büttner-Ennever, 1977). The medial rectus projection is excitatory, probably conducting signals for all

saccades (Delgado-Garcia, Baker and Highstein, 1977), and possibly also for pursuit and fixational movements (King, Lisberger and Fuchs, 1976). (Medial rectus motor neurons receive no vestibular or reticular projections.)

4.27 GENERATION OF EYE MOVEMENTS

VESTIBULAR AND OPTOKINETIC REFLEXES

Vestibular and optokinetic systems combine to maintain visual direction despite head movement. The angular acceleration of even brief head movements stimulates the semicircular canals; the visual system responds to movement in the visual world.

THE VESTIBULO-OCULAR REFLEX

This reflex generates a slow following response in a direction opposite to the head movement, followed by a rapid phase in the same direction (towards the approaching visual scene). The otoliths in the labyrinth generate ocular counter-rolling in response to head tilt. The reflex is mediated by a three-neuron arc (vestibular nerve, vestibular and oculomotor nuclei) and a parallel polysynaptic accessory optic route (reticular formation, perihypoglossal nuclei), and interstitial nucleus (Precht, 1978; 1979).

The spontaneous discharge of the vestibular apparatus is modulated in response to head rotations, tilting and tipping of the head. Connections between the vestibular and oculomotor neurons receive an indirect excitatory vestibular projection via the medial longitudinal fasciculus (and to a lesser extent in primates, the lateral vestibular tract of Deiter). Vestibular neurons project to the contralateral abducent nucleus, to abducent motor neurons and to internuclear neurons, the last carrying the signal via the medial longitudinal fasciculus to the ipsilateral medial rectus motor neurons which receive no direct inhibitory projection (Leigh and Zee, 1983) (Figs 4.48 and 4.60).

For vertical eye movements, vestibular neurons project via the medial longitudinal fasciculus (and possibly brachium conjunctivum) to oculomotor and trochlear nuclei (Fig. 4.48).

Two additional vestibular neuronal groups reinforce the vestibulo-ocular reflexes: type I vestibular neurons are excited by ipsilateral horizontal rotations, and inhibited by contralateral rotations. Type II neurons show the reverse responses. An intervestibular commissure allows type I neurons to activate contralateral type II neurons receiving input from the ipsilateral horizontal canal. A similar reciprocal innervation exists for vertical rotations (Precht, 1979; Wilson and Melvill Jones, 1979) (Table 4.11).

THE OPTOKINETIC SYSTEM

The optokinetic response evoked by rotation of the visual field before the eyes consists of a movement following the moving scene, succeeded by a rapid saccade in the opposite direction. The response is to peripheral retinal stimulation (Henn, Hepp and Büttner-Ennever, 1982). Visual afferents project to vestibular nuclei by several routes, facilitating integration of the vestibulo-ocular and optokinetic reflexes. Transient head rotation thus stimulates both reflexes as follows: the vestibulo-ocular reflex with a latency of only 10 ms occurs first (Optican and Robinson, 1980) and is reinforced by the optokinetic reflex with a latency of at least 70 ms (representing the retinobulbar response time). During sustained rotation with the eyes open vestibular drive decreases as endolymph movement ceases. However, the optokinetic system maintains a steady discharge from the vestibular nuclei to sustain the compensatory optokinetic nystagmus.

Optokinetic nystagmus is induced by moving, full-field, visual stimuli. The eyes reach stimulus velocity within 2 ms of stimulus onset, mainly via a smooth pursuit response. The response is then sustained by stored neural activity within the vestibular nuclei. This velocity storage mechanism is responsible for an optokinetic after-nystagmus which is evident in darkness (Waespe and Henn, 1977a).

In monkeys, these same vestibular nuclei respond to head rotation (Henn, Young and Finley, 1974; Waespe and Henn, 1977b). Thus, during combined vestibular and optokinetic stimulation (which occurs for instance during self rotation), as the vestibular drive declines the optokinetic input persists, maintains a steady vestibular discharge and continues to generate compensatory eye movements (Leigh and Zee, 1991).

Anatomy

Visual input from the retina reaches the vestibular nucleus via an accessory optic path which includes pretectal nuclei such as the **nucleus of the optic tract** (NOT) (Collewijn, 1975), **reticular nucleus** of the pontine tegmentum (Keller and Crandall, 1981a), and the **medial pontine nuclei** (Keller and Crandall, 1981b). The perihypoglossal nuclei (Vemura and Cohen, 1973) and vestibular commissure are also involved (Dejong et al., 1980).

THE ACCESSORY OPTIC SYSTEM

In the rabbit, the pathway involved in the optokinetic response consists of retinofugal projections to the nucleus of the optic tract and accessory optic system, which are relayed to the medial vestibular nucleus via the nucleus prepositus hypoglossi and the medullary reticular formation (Collewijn, 1981). The morphology of these is well described in the pigeon, chicken, rabbit, rat and cat. In the primate, the nuclei of the accessory optic system are much reduced in size (Mai, 1978; Simpson, 1984), reflecting the increased role of transcortical projections in the optokinetic response, the increased telencephalization of vision in primates with the development of foveal vision (Weber and Giolli, 1986), and the change in optic flow during locomotion with the evolution of frontal vision (Leigh and Zee, 1991).

There is a significant retinofugal projection to the accessory optic system in monkeys, where studies by anterograde and retrograde tracers using a post-mortem paraphenyline diamine technique have confirmed the human anatomy (Cooper, 1986; Cooper and Magnin, 1987; Fredericks et al., 1988). In both species the accessory optic pathway may project to the pontine nuclei (Keller and Crandall, 1983) and vestibular system; it also relays, via the inferior olive, to the vestibulocerebellum (Hoffman et al., 1988).

It has been suggested that the main function of this system is to correct for the 'retinal slip' of images during self movement. The outflow to the vestibular system assists in stabilizing the eyes, neck, trunk and limbs during rotation (Fredericks et al., 1988). Connections with the preoculomotor and prebrain stem nuclei probably assist this reflex process (Giolli et al., 1984).

The accessory optic system generally consists of two sets of retinofugal optic fibres, the **inferior** and **superior fasciculi**, and three target nuclei in the mid brain, the **dorsal**, **lateral** and **medial terminal nuclei**. There is also a nucleus whose neurons are intercalated between the posterior fibres of the superior fasciculus (the inSFp). The location of these nuclei in the rostral mid brain is depicted in Fig. 4.67 (Fredericks et al., 1988).

In the primate there is a cortical contribution to the optokinetic nystagmus (OKN) response. In the monkey, neurons in the middle temporal (MT), medial superior temporal (MST) and posterior parietal (PP) visual areas respond to large, moving visual stimuli, with a short latency. The medial superior temporal area projects to the accessory optic system, and to dorsolateral pontine nuclei thought to lie in the smooth pursuit pathway (Tusa, 1988;

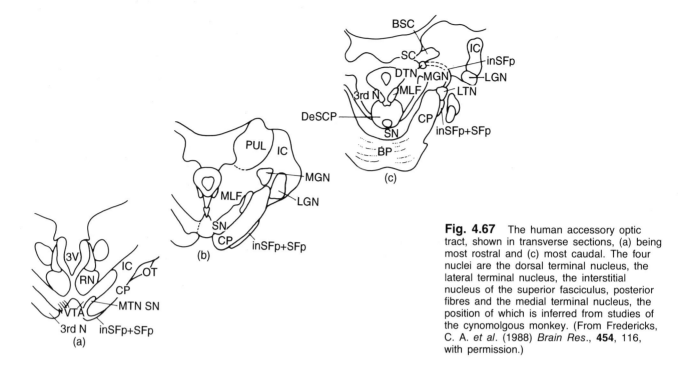

Fig. 4.67 The human accessory optic tract, shown in transverse sections, (a) being most rostral and (c) most caudal. The four nuclei are the dorsal terminal nucleus, the lateral terminal nucleus, the interstitial nucleus of the superior fasciculus, posterior fibres and the medial terminal nucleus, the position of which is inferred from studies of the cynomolgous monkey. (From Fredericks, C. A. *et al.* (1988) *Brain Res.*, **454**, 116, with permission.)

Maioli, Squatrito and Domeniconi, 1989; Tusa and Zee, 1989).

In lower mammals, neurons of the accessory optic system have large receptive fields and their responses are speed- and direction-selective to slow, whole-field movement of the visual world. In the monkey, neurons in the nucleus of the optic tract and dorsal terminal nucleus encode the speed of movement of images on the retina during optokinetic nystagmus. Experimental lesions in these regions in the monkey abolish the velocity storage component of optokinetic nystagmus responsible for the optokinetic after-discharge (Hoffman *et al.*, 1988; Hoffmann and Distler, 1989), but leave smooth pursuit intact. Neurons in the lateral terminal nucleus respond to upward-moving visual stimuli.

Optokinetic nystagmus of the newborn human infant is mediated entirely by brain stem accessory optic system pathways and resembles the response of species such as the rabbit, which show nasotemporal asymmetry with a more developed monocular response to targets approaching from the temporal side. This immature response is retained in amblyopes (Westall and Schorr, 1985). In the normal infant, a symmetrical response is achieved by the age of 2 months, with the maturation of the transcortical pathway.

The cortical contribution to primate optokinetic nystagmus is supported by experimental studies. Bilateral occipital lobectomy in monkeys causes loss of the smooth pursuit component of optokinetic nystagmus and induces a nasotemporal asymmetry of response; unilateral lobectomy does not induce asymmetry. Lesions at the temporo – occipital–parietal junction, such as area MT in the monkey, impair saccades to targets in the contralateral hemifield and also smooth pursuit.

Lesions of the medial superior temporal area (equivalent to Brodmann areas 19 and 39) lead to impaired smooth pursuit towards the side of the lesion (Thurston *et al.*, 1988; Leigh, 1989) and impaired full field (Dursteler and Wurtz, 1988).

In humans, unilateral parietal lesions (especially of the inferior parietal lobule and underlying white matter) cause asymmetry of smooth pursuit, and an impairment of the optokinetic nucleus with stimuli moving towards the side of the lesion (Fox and Holmes, 1926; Cogan and Loeb, 1949; Kjallman and Frisen, 1986; Heide *et al.*, 1990). Patients with bilateral occipital lobe lesions usually lack the optokinetic nucleus, although the amount of extrastriate cortex affected may be important (Brindley, Gautier-Smith and Lewin, 1969).

4.28 TYPES OF EYE MOVEMENT

SACCADES

A saccade is a rapid eye movement changing fixation to a new object of interest. Saccades also occur in the fast phase of nystagmus and in REM sleep. A typical saccade accelerates to peak velocity about half-way through the movement, gently decelerates and then stops abruptly at a new eye position. A fixed relation exists between peak velocity (maximum 700°/s) and amplitude of movement (Dell'Osso and Daroff, 1990). Saccadic reaction time (between target appearance and onset of movement) is about 200 ms. A saccade is 'programmed' on the basis of 'retinal error' (the distance between retinal target image and fovea). Within the time taken for this visual signal to traverse retinal and central visual pathways to reach the brain stem ocular motor mechanisms (about 70 ms), the saccadic response can be modified by visual information (Becker and Jurgens, 1979). Beyond this point, response is (relatively) immutable. Retinal blurring is not appreciated during the saccades due to an elevation of the visual threshold by approximately 0.5 log units (Chase and Kalill, 1972).

There are two components to a saccade: the **rapid phase** is brought about by a pulse of neural impulses which overcome orbital viscous drag to move the eye rapidly from one point to another; the new position is maintained against orbital elastic restoring forces by a **tonic step of impulses** characteristic for that eye position. The pulse and step are combined to produce a smooth movement (Fig. 4.53).

'Pulse' component

The neural substrate for horizontal saccades lies in the caudal pons and for vertical saccades in the rostral mid brain. Saccadic size is encoded in these premotor centres by the duration of firing, and therefore the spatial information provided by topographical sensory maps of the striate cortex, frontal eye field and superior colliculus must be converted into a temporal series of impulses at these sites. The central nervous system converts a visual signal about target position on the retina into information about target location in space using eye, head, and body position signals (Leigh and Zee, 1983).

'Burst' neurons

The premotor command for the pulse of a horizontal saccade arises in neurons in the PPRF which project to the ipsilateral abducent nucleus. They discharge shortly before and during the saccadic motor neuron pulse ('medium lead' burst neurons). The firing rate is correlated with eye velocity. These burst neurons also project to internuclear neurons in the abducent nucleus whose axons pass to the contralateral medial rectus motor neurons and bring gaze to the same

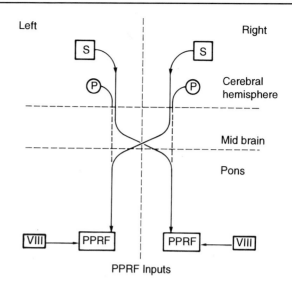

Fig. 4.68 Inputs to PPRF (VIII = vestibular input; S = saccadic path; P = pursuit path). (From Dell'Osso L. F. and Daroff, R. B. (1990) *Doc. Ophthalmol.*, **19**, 155.)

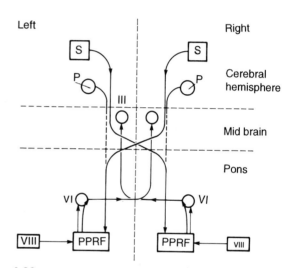

Fig. 4.69 Ocular motor control system. This indicates saccadic (S), pursuit (P) and vestibular (VIII) inputs to PPRF and its output to the abducens nucleus (VI) and the oculomotor nucleus (III). (From Dell'Osso, L. F. and Daroff, R. B. (1990) *Doc. Ophthalmol.*, **19**, 155.)

side. Inhibitory 'burst' neurons lie just caudal to the abducent nucleus in the rostral medulla, and provide a reciprocal innervation, sending inhibitory signals to the contralateral abducent nucleus (Hikosaka, Igusa and Imai, 1978; Hepp and Henn, 1979; Grantyn, Baker and Grantyn, 1980; Igusa, Sasaki and Shimazu, 1980).

Higher control for the vertical pulse is mediated in the riMLF at the ventral mid brain–thalamus junction (Fig. 4.70). These neurons project to the ocular motor

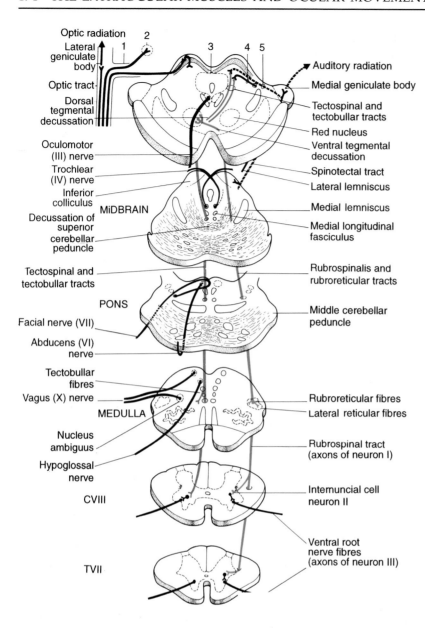

Optic radiation
Lateral geniculate body
Optic tract
Dorsal tegmental decussation
Oculomotor (III) nerve
Trochlear (IV) nerve
Inferior colliculus
MIDBRAIN
Decussation of superior cerebellar peduncle
Tectospinal and tectobullar tracts
PONS
Facial nerve (VII)
Abducens (VI) nerve
Tectobullar fibres
Vagus (X) nerve
MEDULLA
Nucleus ambiguus
Hypoglossal nerve
CVIII
TVII

Auditory radiation
Medial geniculate body
Tectospinal and tectobullar tracts
Red nucleus
Ventral tegmental decussation
Spinotectal tract
Lateral lemniscus
Medial lemniscus
Medial longitudinal fasciculus
Rubrospinalis and rubroreticular tracts
Middle cerebellar peduncle
Rubroreticular fibres
Lateral reticular fibres
Rubrospinal tract (axons of neuron I)
Internuncial cell neuron II
Ventral root nerve fibres (axons of neuron III)

Fig. 4.70 Diagram of the rubrospinal (*red*) and tectospinal (*blue*) tracts. Rubrospinal fibres arise somatotopically from the red nucleus, cross in the ventral tegmental decussation and descend to spinal levels where the fibres terminate in parts of laminae V, VI and VII of Rexed. Crossed rubrobulbar fibres project to parts of the facial nucleus (not shown) and to the lateral reticular nucleus of the medulla (rubroreticular fibres). Uncrossed rubrobulbar fibres (not shown) descend in the central tegmental tract and terminate in the dorsal lamella of the ipsilateral principal olivary nucleus. Tectospinal fibres arise from deep layers of the superior colliculus, cross in the dorsal tegmental decussation and descend initially ventral to the medial longitudinal fasciculus. At medullary levels these fibres become incorporated in the medial longitudinal fasciculus. Fibres of the tectospinal tract descend only to lower cervical spinal segments. Numbers of midbrain structures include: 1, the brachium of the superior colliculus; 2, the pretectal area; 3, commissure of the superior colliculus; 4, spinotectal tract; and 5, collicular fibres from the lateral lemniscus. (From Carpenter, M. B. (1976) *Human Neuroanatomy*, published by Williams and Wilkins.)

nuclei concerned with vertical movement and to the interstitial nucleus (Büttner-Ennever and Büttner, 1978). Neurons in the more rostral PPRF fire several hundred milliseconds before horizontal and vertical saccades ('long lead' burst neurons) and may encode saccadic direction. They receive projections from the superior colliculus, frontal eye fields and nucleus cuneiformis (lateral to mid brain reticular region) (Cohen *et al.*, 1981; Waitzman and Cohen, 1981).

Lesions in the prerubral fields cause vertical saccadic palsies in primates (Büttner-Ennever *et al.*, 1982), while lesions to the interstitial nucleus of Cajal disturb visually guided but not vestibularly induced contralateral saccades.

Cells near the abducent nucleus in the middle raphe complex tonically inhibit 'burst' cells between saccades, and it may be that their function is to suppress 'burst' cell activity during maintained fixation. However, their activity pauses just before, and for the duration of, a saccade and permits the burst cells to discharge. If such 'pause' cells are stimulated during saccades, movement is aborted (Keller, 1977).

Step component

The new position at the end of a saccade is maintained by a train of impulses arising from tonic neurons of the PPRF which may be part of a neural integrator. Every position is specified by a unique pattern of activity in the ocular motor neurons (Robinson, 1975).

SMOOTH PURSUIT

The neural mechanism for smooth pursuit (tracking) must be considered separately from optokinetic slow phases. Smooth pursuit maintains a target image on the fovea throughout a tracking movement: latency for the response is 130 ms (Robinson, 1965).

The stimulus for smooth pursuit is movement of an image in the region of the fovea; the system is primarily sensitive to retinal slip velocity (displacement of the target image from or towards the fovea) and adjusts eye velocity to match that of the target by negative feedback control (Fig. 4.54). Retinal image position may also be a factor (Pola and Wyatt, 1980).

The neural substrate for smooth pursuit movements is uncertain; but signals related to pursuit movements have been recorded from:

1. accessory optic system;
2. brain stem reticular formation;
3. cerebellar flocculi;
4. occipitoparietal region and other cortical areas.

The accessory optic system

This comprises regions outside the primary visual cortex which receive retinal projections via the optic tract. In the primate they include:

- The pretectal nuclei of the mid brain which project to the nucleus of the transpeduncular tract (Giolli, 1963) (ventromedial to red nucleus and medial to the substantia nigra). The latter shows increased activity during tracking.
- The medial pontine and vestibular nuclei and the recticular nucleus of the pontine tegmentum (Waespe and Henn, 1977; Keller and Crandall, 1981b). The system may relay information to the vestibular nuclei, a final common pathway for the optokinetic response.

The brain stem reticular formation

This contains neurons which encode eye position, some of which modulate their discharge during ipsilateral pursuit or during vestibular slow phases. Other units lying below the abducens nucleus may generate the premotor command. They discharge at rates related to pursuit velocity and are not modulated by vestibular signals (Keller, 1974).

Cerebellar flocculi

The cerebellar flocculus receives visual input via mossy and possibly climbing fibres and vestibular input via mossy fibres. The 'gaze velocity' Purkinje cells of the flocculus discharge at a rate which relates to eye velocity during tracking, and are thought to sum the vestibular and eye velocity signals to generate a pursuit gaze velocity in space. Gaze velocity Purkinje cells may project to the perihypoglossal nuclei or PPRF, structures thought to be important in the final synthesis of the gaze command (Miles and Fuller, 1975; Lisberger and Fuchs, 1978a,b; Miles, Braitman and Dow, 1980).

The dentate nucleus and nearby Y-group of vestibular nuclei (probably receiving a floccular projection) have been implicated in the control of vertical smooth pursuit and cancellation of the vestibulo-ocular reflex in combined head and eye tracing. In primates, there is some evidence that the pursuit signal and cancellation of the vestibulo-ocular reflex are subserved by different mechanisms (Robinson, 1982).

Higher control of smooth pursuit

The higher control of smooth pursuit is poorly understood, although a number of pathways have received attention.

A potential role has been suggested for a region of the parieto-occipital cortex in the generation of voluntary pursuit movements. The parietotemporal cortex projects to ipsilateral pontine nuclei and thereby gains indirect access to the cerebellum. This may be important for the performance of pursuit movements, but parietal lobe activity during smooth pursuit movements is generally thought to be related to attention, rather than the neural coding of eye movements.

Projections from the frontal eye fields and superior colliculi may carry pursuit drives, and Darrof and Hoyt (1971) have postulated double decussation of a pursuit pathway:

- at the mid brain decussation of Meynert (Fig. 4.55); and
- at the mid brain pontine junction.

Although a projection from the striate cortex to the ipsilateral superior colliculus has been suggested to play a role in smooth pursuit, lesions do not impair pursuit movements. However, where polysynaptic pathways are involved in the synthesis and control of eye movements, isolated lesions to single pathways often have only minor or transient effects.

VERGENCE MOVEMENTS

The role of vergence in maintaining precise alignment of the eyes on a near target is dealt with by Leigh and Zee (1983; 1991).

Perception of 'single vision' requires that the images of an object of interest fall on corresponding points of each retina (e.g. the foveae) so that fusion may take place. If the images of an object fall on non-corresponding points then the object is simultaneously perceived in separate visual directions, and diplopia is experienced. This disparity of retinal images stimulates **fusional vergence** movements which achieve a relatively precise correspondence of images on the retina. A certain degree of horizontal disparity is accepted over which single vision is still achieved (Panum's area) and the slight dissimilarities of the retinal image resulting from the different viewpoint of each eye are responsible for stereoscopic vision.

Fusional vergence movements are linked synkinetically to accommodation and miosis. Accommodation is stimulated by retinal blur and itself stimulates a convergent movement. The amount of convergence induced by an accommodative effort is a relatively fixed ratio in an individual (accommodative convergence/accommodation or AC/A ratio) and the deficiency of accommodative convergence to a near target is taken up by the fusional vergence mechanism to achieve mutual alignment of the visual axes.

Vergence movements are slow and result from a sudden step change in tonic innervation of the horizontal eye muscles acting against the viscous drag of the orbital contents. They may take up to a second to complete. The reaction time for fusional vergence is under 20 ms and for accommodative vergence is about 200 ms. During convergence, the medial rectus receives a step increase and the lateral rectus a step decrease in innervation.

The neural substrate for vergence movements is not fully known. The premotor command passes directly to the medial rectus portion of the oculomotor nucleus. Neurons at several sites may be concerned with vergence movements (Fig. 4.70).

Mid brain

Mid brain units lateral to the oculomotor nucleus discharge in relation to the convergence angle and are not activated by conjugate eye movement. Stimulation of other units within the oculomotor nucleus may induce vergence movements.

Pons

Pontine stimulation between the medial longitudinal fasciculus (MLF) produces vergence movements, but the vergence system does not use the MLF.

Cerebellum

In monkeys, cerebellar ablation transiently impairs vergence.

Cortex

Cortical involvement in vergence movements has been detected. Such movements occur in relation to stimulation of areas 19 and 22 of the occipital cortex. Certain cells of the visual cortex which respond to a 'retinal disparity' stimulus could provide a sensory input to fusional vergence movements. Neurons in area 7 of the parietal cortex may be activated during sagittal tracking.

Reciprocal modulation of abducens motor neuron activity occurs during vergence movements. The pathway may include a projection from the oculomotor internuclear neurons dorsal to the caudal oculomotor complex projecting to the ipsilateral and contralateral abducens nuclei.

It has been suggested that the outer orbital muscle fibre layer of the medial rectus muscle may be concerned with vergence movements. They are supplied by the dorsomedial group of small motor neurons (group C).

4.29 BLOOD SUPPLY OF MID BRAIN CENTRES

The tectum of the mid brain is supplied by a pial plexus which arises from the posterior cerebral and superior cerebellar arteries, the former providing the main supply to the superior colliculi. According to Alexais and D'Astros (1982), the oculomotor and trochlear nuclei are supplied by specific end arteries from the posterior cerebral artery which enter the mid brain through the posterior perforated substance (Fig. 15.79). Stopford, however, stated that the supply is from the basilar artery. The abducent nuclei are supplied by a specific end artery from the basilar (Stopford, 1916, 1917). Further details on mesencephalic vessels have been recorded (Lazorthes et al., 1958; Khan, 1969; and especially Duvernoy, 1978).

Duvernoy's monograph is the most extensive study to date. He confirms the end arterial nature of penetrating vessels. He describes in detail such arteries as the collicular (quadrigeminal) of Kahn, 1969.

The venous return is partly by the cortical veins and partly by the basal vein which runs close to the posterior cerebral artery. (For a recent account of the veins draining the brain stem consult the monograph of Duvernoy, 1978.)

CHAPTER FIVE

Innervation and nerves of the orbit

5.1   THE OCULOMOTOR (THIRD CRANIAL) NERVE

SUPERFICIAL EMERGENCE

The oculomotor nerve emerges as 10–15 rootlets from the sulcus oculomotorius medial to the basis pedunculi, but a small lateral root may emerge through the adjacent ventral peduncular surface. The most inferior rootlets are near the superior border of the pons and termination of the basilar artery (Figs 5.1, 15.30 and 15.68). Between the two nerves is the posterior perforated substance.

The posterior cerebral artery is first medial to the emerging nerve and then curves round its highest rootlets, often sending twigs between them. The superior cerebellar artery, at the upper border of the pons, is inferior to the oculomotor nerve (Figs 5.2 and 5.5).

COURSE AND RELATIONS

In the posterior cranial fossa

Surrounded by pia and cerebrospinal fluid, the nerve descends anteriorly in the cisterna interpeduncularis (Fig. 5.3), between the posterior cerebral and superior cerebellar arteries (Figs 5.3 and 5.4). The cisterna is a trapezoid dilatation of the subarachnoid space completed below by an arachnoid expansion between the temporal lobes; it is limited anteriorly by the optic tracts and chiasma, posteriorly by the peduncles. In its floor are the mamillary bodies, tuber cinereum, infundibulum and hypophysis cerebri, with the circulus arteriosus inferior to them.

At first somewhat flattened, the nerve spirals to bring inferior fibres superior. Leaving the arteries, it becomes a rounded cord and runs superomedial to the margin of the tentorium cerebelli and trochlear nerve, inferolateral to the posterior communicating artery (Fig. 5.2). It crosses laterally inferior to the optic tract (Figs 5.5 and 15.57). Superolateral is the uncus (Fig. 15.71). For about 1 cm, i.e. from the posterior clinoid process to where it pierces the dura, the nerve is in contact with arachnoid.

In the middle cranial fossa

Here the nerve lies lateral to the posterior clinoid process, above the tentorium cerebelli, lateral to the hypophyseal fossa and above the cavernous sinus. It pierces the arachnoid between the anterior and posterior clinoid processes to enter the dura near the forward prolongation of the unattached margin of the tentorium cerebelli, and traverses the roof of the sinus to reach its lateral wall (Figs 5.4, 5.15 and 5.16). Here the trochlear nerve and first and second divisions of the trigeminal nerve are inferolateral to it; inferomedial are the abducent nerve and internal carotid artery actually in the sinus (Fig. 3.16). In the lateral wall the oculomotor nerve communicates with the ophthalmic division and the internal carotid sympathetic plexus of the sympathetic around the carotid artery. At the anterior end of the sinus, near the optic foramen, the oculomotor and trochlear nerves may become inferior to the ophthalmic

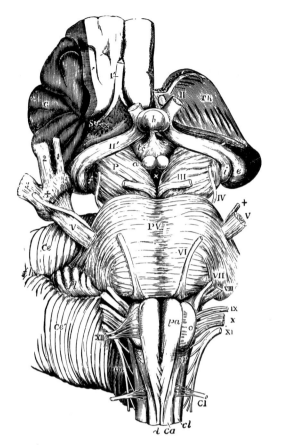

Fig. 5.1 Ventral aspect of the brain stem, showing the attachments of the cranial nerves. The following references apply to the roots of the nerves. I' = right olfactory tract, divided near its middle; II = left optic nerve springing from the chiasma, which is concealed by the pituitary body; II' = right optic tract; the left tract is seen passing back into *i* and *e*, the medial and lateral roots; III = left oculomotor nerve; IV = trochlear; V, V = sensory roots of the trigeminal nerves; +, + = motor roots, the + of the right side is placed on the trigeminal ganglion; 1 = ophthalmic division; 2 = maxillary division; 3 = mandibular division; VI = left abducent nerve; VII = facial nerve; VIII = eighth nerve; IX = glossopharyngeal nerve; X = vagus nerve; XI = accessory nerve; XII = right hypoglossal nerve; at *o*, on the left side, the rootlets are seen cut short; C1 = suboccipital or first cervical nerve. (From *Quain's Anatomy*)

division, here dividing into terminal branches (Figs 5.4 and 5.25).

The oculomotor nerve now enters the superior orbital fissure, dividing into a small superior and larger inferior branch. Here the nerve is crossed by the trochlear nerve, which becomes superomedial to it.

In the superior orbital fissure

The two divisions of the oculomotor nerve traverse the fissure within the annular tendon, between the two heads of the lateral rectus (Fig. 5.6); the

nasociliary nerve passes them and the abducent nerve lies at first inferior then lateral to them. The trochlear, frontal and lacrimal nerves traverse the wide region of the fissure above the tendon.

In the orbit

The **superior division** diverges medially above the optic nerve and behind the nasociliary nerve to supply the superior rectus on its undersurface at the junction of middle and posterior thirds (Figs 5.21, 5.23 and 5.24). A branch to the levator palpebrae superioris pierces the superior rectus or skirts its medial border.

The **inferior division**, much the larger, divides immediately into branches to the medial rectus, inferior rectus, and inferior oblique muscles. The branch to medial rectus passes under the optic nerve to enter the muscle on its ocular aspect near the junction of middle and posterior thirds (Fig. 5.24); that to the inferior rectus enters the muscle from above near the junction of middle and posterior thirds. The branch to the inferior oblique runs along the floor of the orbit near the lateral border of the inferior rectus or between this and the lateral rectus. It crosses above the posterior border of the inferior oblique at about its middle, and enters the upper surface of the muscle as two or three branches. It also supplies a ramus to the ciliary ganglion (Fig. 5.22).

COMMUNICATIONS AND VARIETIES

For variations in this and other nerves consult Quain (1900) and Hovelacque (1927). Communications in the cavernous sinus between the three ocular motor nerves are frequent (Sunderland and Hughes, 1946). The superior oculomotor division sometimes communicates with the nasociliary nerve, and it may partly supply the superior oblique muscle, and even the lateral rectus when the abducent nerve is absent. Its branch to the ciliary ganglion may be so short that the ganglion is sessile upon the nerve to the inferior oblique muscle.

SUMMARY OF THE OCULOMOTOR NERVE (Fig. 5.23)

The superior branch supplies superior rectus and levator palpebrae superioris. The inferior branch suplies medial rectus, inferior rectus, inferior oblique and the motor root of the ciliary ganglion.

Thus, the oculomotor nerve supplies all the extrinsic muscles of the eye except the lateral rectus and superior oblique, and also innervates the sphincter

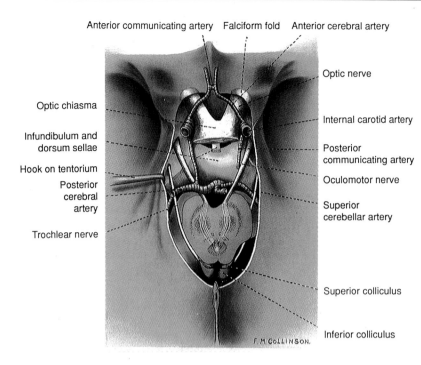

Anterior communicating artery   Falciform fold   Anterior cerebral artery

Optic nerve

Optic chiasma

Internal carotid artery

Infundibulum and dorsum sellae

Posterior communicating artery

Hook on tentorium

Oculomotor nerve

Posterior cerebral artery

Superior cerebellar artery

Trochlear nerve

Superior colliculus

Inferior colliculus

F. M. COLLINSON.

Fig. 5.2 The oculomotor and trochlear nerves and the relation of the arterial circle of Willis to the pituitary fossa. The mid brain is divided in the aperture of the tentorium, and the cerebrum removed. On the right side, the posterior cerebral and posterior communicating arteries are cut short to expose the origin of the oculomotor nerve. On the left side the tentorium and cerebral peduncle are slightly separated to show the trochlear nerve more fully.

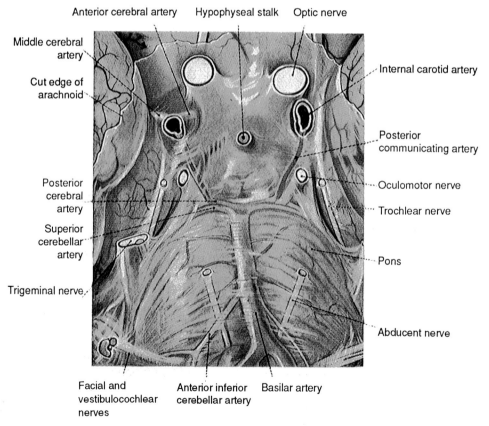

Anterior cerebral artery   Hypophyseal stalk   Optic nerve

Middle cerebral artery

Internal carotid artery

Cut edge of arachnoid

Posterior communicating artery

Posterior cerebral artery

Oculomotor nerve

Trochlear nerve

Superior cerebellar artery

Pons

Trigeminal nerve

Abducent nerve

Facial and vestibulocochlear nerves

Anterior inferior cerebellar artery

Basilar artery

Fig. 5.3 The cisterna interpeduncularis and cisterna pontis. A portion of the base of the brain with the arachnoid in situ showing the relation of this membrane to the cranial nerves (II to VIII) and to the circle of Willis.

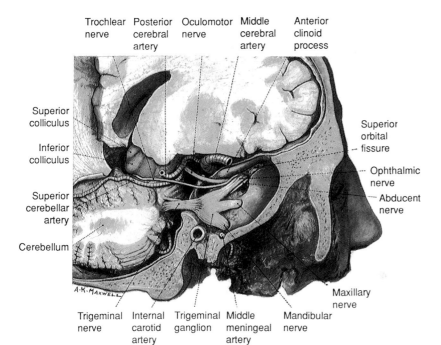

Trochlear nerve   Posterior cerebral artery   Oculomotor nerve   Middle cerebral artery   Anterior clinoid process

Superior colliculus

Inferior colliculus

Superior cerebellar artery

Cerebellum

A·K·MAXWELL

Superior orbital fissure

Ophthalmic nerve

Abducent nerve

Maxillary nerve

Trigeminal nerve   Internal carotid artery   Trigeminal ganglion   Middle meningeal artery   Mandibular nerve

Fig. 5.4 Dissection to show the intracranial course of the oculomotor nerves. (Wolff's dissection.)

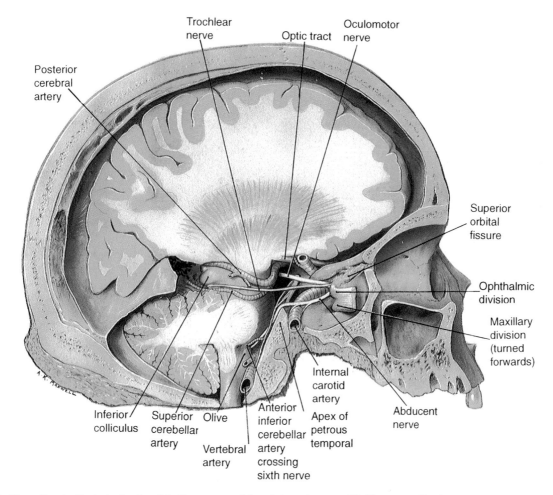

Trochlear nerve   Optic tract   Oculomotor nerve

Posterior cerebral artery

Superior orbital fissure

Ophthalmic division

Maxillary division (turned forwards)

Internal carotid artery

Apex of petrous temporal

Abducent nerve

A.K. MAXWELL

Inferior colliculus   Superior cerebellar artery   Olive   Vertebral artery   Anterior inferior cerebellar artery crossing sixth nerve

Fig. 5.5 Dissection to illustrate the bend in the course of the abducent nerve. (Wolff's preparation.)

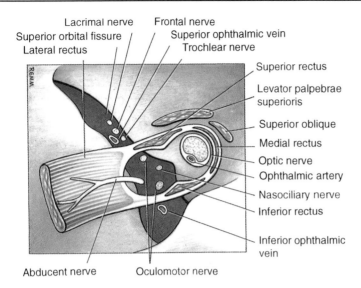

Fig. 5.6 Diagram of the structures passing through the superior orbital fissure and optic foramen. Note that nothing passes through the narrow portion of the fissure.

pupillae and the ciliary muscle through its parasympathetic nerve fibres.

NUCLEUS AND CONNECTIONS

The nuclei of the ocular motor nerves, except the part of the oculomotor innervating intrinsic muscles, belong to the somatic efferent nuclear column (Fig. 5.7) and are composed of large multipolar cells like those of the anterior grey column in the spinal cord. Each oculomotor nucleus is a small column of multi-

polar nerve cells extending for about 10 mm in the floor of the cerebral aqueduct at the level of the superior colliculus. Superiorly it approaches the floor of the third ventricle; below, it ends level with the lower border of the superior colliculus. Dorsomedial to each oculomotor nucleus is the adjacent circuma-queductal grey zone; ventrolateral to each is the corresponding medial longitudinal fasciculus (Fig. 5.8). Inferiorly, or caudally, the oculomotor nucleus is continuous with the trochlear.

LOCALIZATION WITHIN THE NUCLEI

Punctate lesions within these small nuclei are rare; localized vascular lesions are more common, but neither have provided reliable evidence of functional

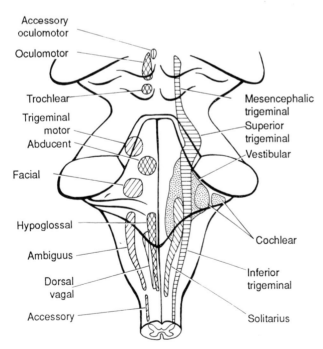

Fig. 5.7 Dorsal projection of cranial nerve nuclei. Somatic and branchial nerve nuclei are left of the mid line, general and special sensory nuclei to the right.

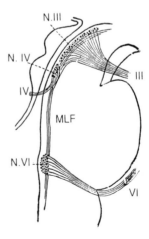

Fig. 5.8 The oculomotor, trochlear and abducent nuclei. Sagittal section showing the nerves (III, IV and VI) and their nuclei (N.III, N.IV and N.VI). MLF = medial longitudinal fasciculus.

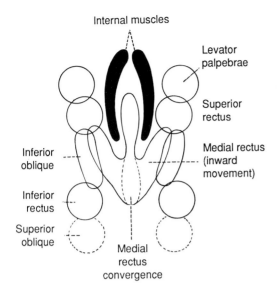

Fig. 5.9 Ventral (anterior) view of the oculomotor nuclei, showing muscle representation. The accessory (Edinger–Westphal) nuclei are in solid block.

organization. Exact localization within the human oculomotor complex of nuclei is uncertain, despite the evidence of partial ophthalmoplegias. However, it is unlikely to differ much in arrangement from other primates. The evidence of experimentation is conflicting, but there is nevertheless some accord in the results of many studies. The twentieth-century workers in this field are Abd-el-Malek (1938), Szentágothai (1942), Bender and Weinstein (1943), Danis (1948), Warwick (1953; 1956; 1964), Tarlov and Tarlov (1971, 1972, 1975), and Büttner-Ennever *et al.* (1982); their papers should be consulted for details. For topographical accounts of the primate oculomotor complex consult Tsuchida (1906), Le Gros Clark (1926) and Crosby and Woodburne (1943). The formerly accepted scheme of Brouwer (1918) (Fig. 5.9) was shown by Warwick (1953) to be very different in the monkey although it cannot be equated even with modern work on the mere topography of the human oculomotor complex.

Former ideas

The oculomotor nuclei, taken as a whole, were regarded as consisting of five parts: two **main lateral** nuclei, an unpaired central **nucleus of Perlia** uniting the main nuclei, and paired small-celled **nuclei of Edinger-Westphal** cranial to the others (Fig. 5.9). But modern topographical observations divide the **lateral nucleus** into ventral and dorsal columns, arranged rostrocaudally in the long axis of the mid brain. The **central nucleus** is absent from some primates,

marked in others, variable and unimpressive in mankind. Its development is not related to binocular vision and convergence (Warwick, 1955). The accessory (Edinger-Westphal) nuclei fuse into a median mass at their (rostral) extremities as the **anteromedian nucleus**. At caudal levels there is another mid line entity, the **caudal central nucleus**, which is a much better developed mass of neurons than the highly variable intermediate group, Perlia's central nucleus.

Despite these topographical views, which have been accumulated and refined over many decades and epitomized in Fig. 5.10, a concept of motor pools (chiefly due to Bernheimer, 1897, and Brouwer, 1918) has been repeated from textbook to textbook (Fig. 5.9). This concept, repeated once more here for historical interest, is patently out of accord with the topographical picture. It has received little support and much disagreement from either Bernheimer's own contemporary experimenters or those of recent years quoted above. These outdated views may be stated briefly as follows.

The **main lateral nuclei** contain centres for motor nerves to the eye muscles, each being innervated by a well-defined group of neurons, the groups being rostrocaudally for levator palpebrae superioris (probably), superior rectus, inferior oblique, and inferior rectus. The centre for the medial rectus (medial movement) was put next to the median nucleus of Perlia. The **central nucleus of Perlia** was regarded as concerned with convergence. Thus convergence and medial movement, whose centres adjoin, might be separately affected. The **nucleus of Edinger-Westphal** paired, interposed between the two lateral nuclei, and composed of small multipolar cells of preganglionic autonomic type, was reasonably regarded as a pupillomotor centre.

The fibres from the cranial part of the oculomotor nucleus were described as ipsilateral, those from the caudal part some were held to be direct and crossed.

Modern views

The foregoing description, though curiously vague (particularly as to the central nucleus), was representative of textbook accounts until recent years, and was based primarily on Bernheimer's experiments on monkeys and Brouwer's speculations upon median control of convergence. Modern experimenters have substantiated little of these views, differing among themselves in some respects. All those quoted above agree that few if any radicular fibres cross before entering the oculomotor nerve. All agree in assigning

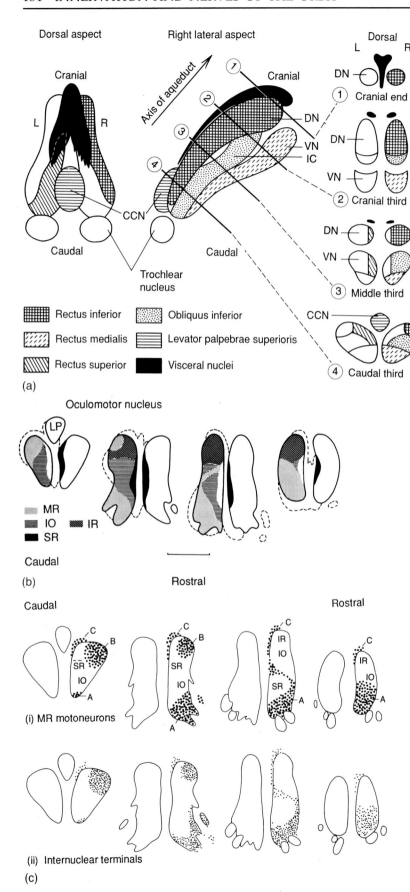

(a)

Fig. 5.10 (a) Localization in the oculomotor nuclear complex of the Rhesus macaque (after Warwick, 1953). The entire complex, including right and left and median somatic nuclei and accessory (autonomic) nuclei, is shown in dorsal and right lateral views, with representative sections as indicated. DN = Dorsal nucleus; VN = ventral nucleus; IC = intermediate column; CCN = caudal central nucleus.

(b) Transverse sections to show the arrangement of the oculomotor nucleus of monkey. From left to right the sections are taken from caudal to rostral. Coloured areas outline the root of motor neurons innervating the extraocular muscles of one orbit. The upper figures indicate the location of large motor neurons. The lower figures indicate the small motor neurons supplying these muscles, which lie mainly peripheral to the large cell motor neurons. (Courtesy of J.A. Büttner-Ennever.)

(c) Schematic representation of the termination of the abducens internuclear pathway of the oculomotor nucleus, drawn in transverse sections in the stereotaxic plane. (i) The stippled areas indicate the location of medial rectus motor neurons in the oculomotor nucleus (left to right: caudal to rostral); (ii) stippled areas indicate the pattern of termination of the abducens internuclear fibres. Note that the internuclear fibres terminate directly only on those parts of the oculomotor nucleus containing medial rectus motor neurons. SR = Superior rectus motor neurons; IO = inferior rectus motor neurons. (From Büttner-Ennever, J.A. and Akert, A. (1981) *J. Comp. Neurol.*, **197**, 17, with permission.)

little importance to the central nucleus in structural or functional terms. All agree that the accessory nuclei (Edinger-Westphal columns) are the parasympathetic component of the oculomotor complex. A study using a retrograde degeneration technique in the cat (Tarlov and Tarlov, 1971), yielded results partly confirming the findings of Warwick (1953), but with interesting differences which suggest that the dorsoventral arrangement of motor pools may exhibit species peculiarities. These results necessarily differ from the diagram of Brouwer and Bernheimer because they accord with the topography of the oculomotor complex. Using other techniques Büttner-Ennever *et al.* (1982) and Spencer *et al.* (1982) have deduced further modifications (see also Porter, 1984).

OCULOMOTOR COMPLEX OF THE MONKEY

Warwick (1953) showed that a dorsoventral rather than a craniocaudal organization exists (Fig. 5.10). This has been modified by the studies of Büttner-Ennever. Humans have a relatively broader oculomotor complex than monkeys, but it is unlikely that the functional pattern is much different, as the topographical arrangement is basically similar. Levator palpebrae superioris is supplied bilaterally from the central caudal nucleus. The superior rectus is supplied from the opposite lateral nucleus (intermediate column). The remaining muscles are supplied ipsilaterally as indicated in Fig. 5.10. The anteromedian and Edinger-Westphal nuclei are parasympathetic and supply the sphincter pupillae and ciliary muscles, but further details remain uncertain.

CENTRAL COURSE

The oculomotor fibres curve with a lateral convexity through the medial longitudinal bundle, tegmentum, red nucleus, and medial margin of the substantia nigra, to emerge from the sulcus oculomotorius on the medial aspect of the basis pedunculi (Figs 5.2 and 5.11)

STRUCTURE

Like the abducent and trochlear nerves the oculomotor nerve is large compared with the muscles it supplies. It contains about 24 000 fibres. Most fibres are large and motor in function, but there are many fine fibres, some of which are probably afferent, and a few reach the ciliary ganglion. Some of the finer

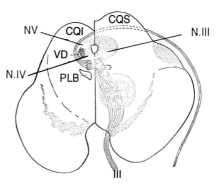

Fig. 5.11 Oculomotor and trochlear nuclei. The mid brain is divided transversely at different levels on the two sides, the section on the right side of the figure passing through the superior, and on the left side through the inferior, colliculus. VD = Mesencephalic root of the trigeminal nerve; NV = its nucleus; CQS = superior colliculus; CQI = inferior colliculus; PLB = medial longitudinal fasciculus; N.III = nucleus of nerve III; N.IV = nucleus of nerve IV.

fibres have long been considered proprioceptive and, because they appeared more prominent in the orbital part of the oculomotor nerve (Tozer and Sherrington, 1910), many subsequent workers have favoured the view that proprioceptive fibres of the ocular motor nerves are transferred peripherally into the ophthalmic trigeminal division to enter the pons. Bortolami *et al.* (1977) and Manni *et al.* (1978) claim that some peripheral oculomotor fibres belong to neurons of the trigeminal ganglion. Boeke (1927) regarded the unmyelinated fibres as sympathetic, but they are not affected by cervical sympathectomy (Hines, 1931). Woollard (1931) believed these axons to be proprioceptive. A voluminous and controversial literature has accumulated on this topic. Recent reviews and experimental studies (unfortunately not easy to access) are in the PhD theses of Foster (1973) and Sivanandasingham (1973). The work of Winckler (1937), Cooper and her collaborators, Daniel and Whitteridge (1955), Manni, Bertolami and De Sole (1967) and Batini and Buisseret (1974) suggests that species differences exist. The most recent studies cited above and those of Bach-y-Rita *et al.* (1971) indicate that, in primates at least, some ocular proprioceptive fibres enter the brain in the motor nerves of the ocular muscles.

In cross-section the oculomotor nerve is seen to be surrounded by a thin perineurium and well-marked pial sheath (Fig. 5.12). The sheath contains a few small blood vessels and is intersected by numerous thick irregular septa from the pia, which, however, are not related to branching. In the cavernous sinus the superior division has been described as forming an area like a cap on the rest of the nerve, but no clear

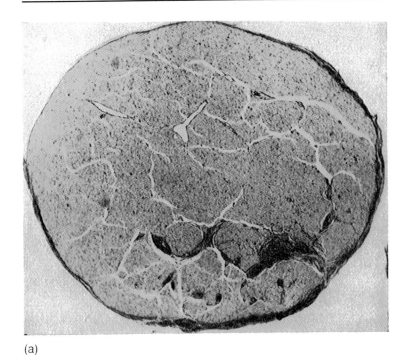

(a)

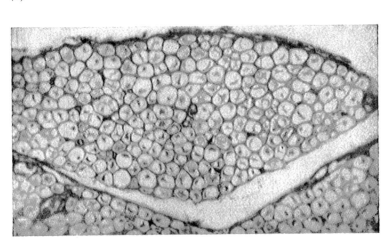

(b)

Fig. 5.12 (a) Transverse section of the oculomotor nerve near its emergence; (b) partial transverse section of the oculomotor nerve.

indication of the branches of the inferior division is apparent (Sunderland and Hughes, 1946). Fuchs (1917) placed the pupillary fibres centrally, and this explained escape of the intrinsic eye muscles in fractures involving the oculomotor nerve: Sunderland and Hughes (1946), however, held that pupilloconstrictor fibres, varying in diameter from 3 to 5 μm, are concentrated in a superior arc in the nerve from cavernous sinus to mid brain and may, therefore, be affected alone in pressure from above. However, fine medullated fibres are scattered throughout the nerve and also occur in the trochlear and abducens.

THE BLOOD SUPPLY OF THE OCULAR MOTOR NERVES

All nerves are supplied with blood from adjacent vessels, which are usually small and variable. Such a nutrient artery divides into ascending and descending branches which anastomose in the epineurium with similar branches from others. From these epineural vessels fine branches penetrate into the perineurium, with further anastomoses, and their terminal arterioles enter fasciculi to form rich longitudinal capillary plexuses along the full length of the nerve. These are reinforced by other nutrient arteries, but no part of the intrafascicular plexus is dominated by any one artery.

The blood supply of the oculomotor, trochlear and abducent nerves is similarly arranged, the nutrient arteries being derived from any adjacent smaller arteries. Though not often noted, it is obvious that deprivation of this blood supply by spasm, thrombosis or embolism may produce paralysis or paresis of the muscles supplied.

PRACTICAL CONSIDERATIONS

Interruption

Interruption of the oculomotor nerve results in:

- ptosis, from paralysis of the levator;
- lateral deviation due to unopposed action of the lateral rectus and superior oblique. Because the eye is in abduction, depression due to the superior oblique is nil or minimal. There is inability to look upwards, downwards or medially beyond the mid line;
- intorsion whenever the eye is directed inferomedially (action of superior oblique);
- semi-dilation of the pupil, from unopposed sympathetic innervation, and does not react to light or accommodation;
- inability of the eye to accommodate.

Syndrome of Weber

The syndrome of Weber is oculomotor paralysis associated with facial paralysis and contralateral hemiplegia. The former is of upper motor neuron type, and the upper part of the face is spared. The syndrome is due to a mid brain lesion, involving corticospinal fibres above their decussation. The **syndrome of Benedikt** is similar, but the hemiplegia is associated with tremors, which may be due to involvement of the red nucleus.

The oculomotor and trochlear nerves are more commonly affected by pressure from hypophyseal enlargement than the abducent, perhaps because of the latter's relation to the internal carotid artery (Fig. 5.5).

The oculomotor nerve may be compressed by an aneurysm of the posterior cerebral, superior cerebellar, basilar, posterior communicating, or internal carotid arteries.

5.2 THE TROCHLEAR (FOURTH CRANIAL) NERVE

The trochlear, the most slender of the cranial nerves, has the longest intracranial course (75 mm). Its name is derived from the trochlea of the superior oblique muscle, which it innervates.

SUPERFICIAL EMERGENCE (Fig. 5.13)

Crossing in the superior medullary velum, a part of the roof of the fourth ventricle, the trochlear nerve emerges from the upper part of this as two or three rootlets medial to the superior cerebellar peduncle and below the inferior colliculus. (Nathan and Goldhammer, 1973, have published a special

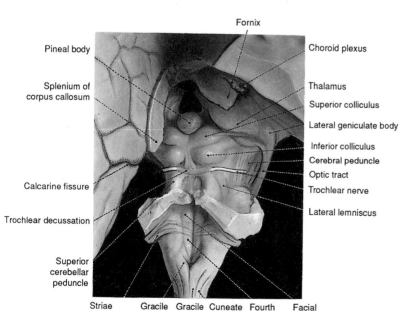

Fornix
Pineal body
Choroid plexus
Splenium of corpus callosum
Thalamus
Superior colliculus
Lateral geniculate body
Inferior colliculus
Cerebral peduncle
Optic tract
Calcarine fissure
Trochlear nerve
Lateral lemniscus
Trochlear decussation
Superior cerebellar peduncle
Striae medullares   Gracile tubercle   Gracile bundle   Cuneate bundle   Fourth ventricle   Facial colliculus

Fig. 5.13 Dissection to show the emergence of the trochlear nerves (Wolff's preparation).

study of the radicles of the trochlear nerve.) Its attachment to the velum is very fragile. It is the only cranial nerve to issue from the dorsal aspect of the central nervous system.

RELATIONS

In the posterior cranial fossa

Here the nerve is in the subarachnoid space, immersed in cerebrospinal fluid. It is at first posterior to the superior cerebellar peduncle, where it is crossed by a branch of the superior cerebellar artery ascending to the inferior colliculus. It curves round the peduncle at the upper border of the pons between and parallel to the posterior cerebral and superior cerebellar arteries (Figs 5.4 and 5.5). It appears ventrally between the temporal lobe and pons (Fig. 5.3). At first inferomedial to the margin of the tentorium cerebelli, it soon disappears beneath it (Figs 5.3 and 15.58). The trigeminal nerve, emerging from the lateral aspect of the pons, is inferolateral to the trochlear (Fig. 5.4). The oculomotor nerve is superomedial, but because it slopes down and forwards the two nerves converge as they proceed anteriorly and eventually cross (Figs 5.2, 5.4 and 5.5).

Where the nerve enters the middle cranial fossa, lateral to the dorsum sellae and still below the unattached margin of the tentorium cerebelli, it acquires a short sleeve of arachnoid which it loses where it pierces the dura. In its subarachnoid course it is at first covered by pial tissue, which quickly becomes adventitial.

In the middle cranial fossa

The nerve pierces the dura in the angle between the 'free' margin and attached border of the tentorium cerebelli to enter the lateral wall of the cavernous sinus superomedial to the trigeminal ganglion and lateral to the hypophyseal fossa (Figs 5.4, 5.5 and 5.16). Here the oculomotor nerve is at first superomedial but just before it enters the superior orbital (sphenoidal) fissure the trochlear crosses over it to become medial. The first and second divisions of the trigeminal are inferolateral and, in the sinus itself, the abducent nerve and internal carotid artery are inferomedial.

In the superior orbital (sphenoidal) fissure

The trochlear nerve enters the orbit through the wide region of the fissure above the annular tendon. The frontal and lacrimal nerves are lateral to it and the ophthalmic vein is inferior (Figs 5.6 and 5.16).

In the orbit

The trochlear leaves the frontal nerve at an acute angle, inclining anteromedially below the orbital roof (Fig. 5.17) and above the levator and superior rectus (Fig. 5.18). It fans out into three or four branches which supply the superior oblique on its superior surface near the lateral border, the most anterior branch at the junction of posterior and middle thirds and the most posterior about 8 mm beyond its origin.

NUCLEUS AND CONNECTIONS

The two trochlear nuclei are situated dorsally in the tegmentum of the mid brain, ventrolateral to the cerebral aqueduct, dorsal to the medial longitudinal bundles (in which they are partially embedded), and at a level corresponding to the superior part of the inferior colliculus (Figs 5.8 and 5.11). Like the oculomotor nuclei, with which they are continuous above, the trochlear nuclei belong to the somatic efferent column.

From each nucleus, nerve fibres run first laterally to the medial aspect of the mesencephalic nucleus of the trigeminal nerve, then caudally parallel to the aqueduct. At the lower border of the inferior colliculus they turn medially to decussate in the superior medullary velum. Hence each superior oblique is supplied from the contralateral trochlear nucleus. The fibres emerge on the medial aspect of the superior cerebral peduncle.

Trochlear neurons are densely staining cells, multipolar, with average dimensions of 40–50 μm. The existence of other cells, possibly interneurons, within or near the trochlear nucleus is a matter of debate. Extrinsic connections are corticobulbar, tectobulbar, and (via the medial longitudinal fasciculus) with various other brain stem nuclei, such as the oculomotor, abducent, vestibular, and possibly others.

There is frequently a small **accessory trochlear nucleus**, caudal to the main one.

A proprioceptor component has long been ascribed to the trochlear nerve (see Crosby et al., 1962, for discussion of the evidence).

COMMUNICATIONS AND VARIATIONS

In the lateral wall of the cavernous sinus the trochlear nerve is connected with the internal carotid sympathetic plexus and with the ophthalmic division by a filament which possibly contains proprioceptive nerve fibres.

Rarely, the trochlear nerve may pierce the levator and has been observed occasionally to send a branch forward to orbicularis oculi, or to join the supratrochlear, the infratrochlear, the nasociliary or frontal nerves (Thane). Consult Quain (1900) and Hovelacque (1927) for further details.

STRUCTURE

The trochlear nerve consists of about 3400 fibres, mostly of large size (Björkman and Wohlfart, 1936), but in fetal life the number is larger, as many as 6000 according to Mustafa and Gamble (1979), who gave an adult count of 2400. One investigation of human trochlear nerve (Zaki, 1960) showed it to contain 2400 fibres proximal to, and 3500 distal to, the cavernous sinus, suggesting that a population of fibres of large diameter and possibly of proprioceptive function, may leave the nerve peripherally perhaps to join the trigeminal. Such communications in the vicinity of the cavernous sinus were denied by Sunderland and Hughes (1946).

PRACTICAL CONSIDERATIONS

Interruption of the trochlear nerve, anatomical or physiological, paralyses the superior oblique muscle:

- greatest limitation of movement occurs when, in full adduction, the patient attempts to look downwards, because the superior oblique is then normally most effective as a depressor;
- the face is often turned downwards and towards the normal side to counteract this;
- diplopia occurs on looking downwards, and is homonymous. The false image is below, and its upper end is tilted towards the true image, i.e. in the direction of action of the paralysed muscle.

5.3   THE ABDUCENT (SIXTH CRANIAL) NERVE

SUPERFICIAL EMERGENCE

The abducent nerve emerges between the lower border of the pons and lateral part of the pyramid as seven or eight rootlets, some of which may emerge through the pons (Figs 5.1 and 5.4). Unlike the rootlets of the oculomotor and trochlear nerves, which soon join up, the abducent rootlets join at varying and greater distances from emergence and some may remain separate (Fig. 5.16) until the nerve pierces the dura.

COURSE

The nerve passes upwards and anterolaterally in the subarachnoid space of the posterior cranial fossa to pierce the arachnoid and dura lateral to the dorsum sellae. It ascends between the layers of dura on the posterior surface of the petrous bone near its apex, turning anteriorly to traverse the cavernous sinus. It enters the orbit through the superior orbital fissure within the annular tendon to supply the lateral rectus muscle. (For variations, consult Nathan, Ovaknine and Kosary, 1974.)

RELATIONS

At emergence

The abducent nerves are about 1 cm apart, and between them is the basilar artery at its formation from the two vertebrals. Sometimes an asymmetric vertebral artery may curve up to lie under the nerve. Lateral to each abducent is the emergence of the facial nerve at the lateral side of the olive (Figs 5.1, 15.30 and 15.68).

In the posterior cranial fossa

The nerve, at first flat and visibly fasciculated, becomes rounder and firmer. Sleeved by pia mater it ascends anterolaterally in the cisterna pontis of the subarachnoid space (Fig. 5.3) between the pons and occipital bone (Fig. 5.4). A course of 15 mm takes it to its entry into dura mater covering the basoccipital bone about 2 cm inferolateral to the posterior clinoid process, and posteromedial to the inferior petrosal sinus in the petrobasilar suture (Fig. 5.15). The spheno-occipital suture is about 1.5 cm from the dorsum sellae and therefore the nerve pierces the dura opposite the occipital bone. It is held to the pons by arachnoid (Fig. 5.3), but is not completely covered by it until near to the dura. Just after its emergence the nerve is crossed by the anterior inferior cerebellar artery (Figs 5.5 and 5.14). Usually the artery is ventral, but it may be dorsal or pass between the abducent rootlets (Stopford, 1916, 1917). The oculomotor, trochlear and trigeminal nerves are at a higher level, but gradually approach the abducent as they pass towards the middle cranial fossa. The abducent nerve passes inferior to the inferior petrosal

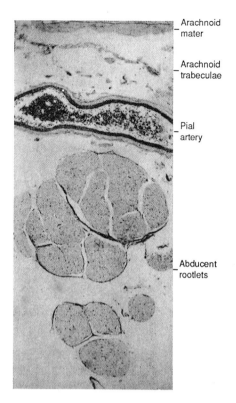

Fig. 5.14 Relation of the sixth nerve to the arachnoid and anterior inferior cerebellar arteries. The abducent rootlets are unlimited here.

sinus in an anterolateral direction, and ascends the petrous temporal near its apex. It here occupies a variable groove (Hovelacque, 1927). At the upper border of the bone, it turns forward at a right-angle under the petrosphenoidal ligament and superior petrosal sinus to enter the cavernous sinus (Figs 5.5

and 5.15) with the inferior petrosal sinus by a common opening (Fig. 5.15). Often the nerve pierces the inferior sinus, entering the cavernous sinus within the inferior petrosal sinus.

In the cavernous sinus

The nerve here runs forwards almost horizontally. Posteriorly it spirals round the lateral aspect of the ascending part of the internal carotid artery (Fig. 5.15). This second bend varies: it may be a mere lateral displacement by the ascending part of the internal carotid, or (more rarely) approach a right-angle. Beyond this the nerve is inferolateral to the horizontal portion of the artery (Figs 3.16 and 5.5) with its sympathetic plexus, which may communicate with the nerve. In the lateral wall of the sinus, in descending order, are the oculomotor, trochlear, ophthalmic, and maxillary nerves. The abducent nerve is usually in the sinus, with a separate sheath, but may adhere to the lateral wall directly or by a septum of dura mater. Lateral to the sinus is the trigeminal ganglion (Figs 5.15 and 5.16).

In the superior orbital fissure

The abducent nerve traverses the fissure within the annulus of Zinn, at first below the divisions of the oculomotor nerve, then between them and lateral to the nasociliary nerve (Fig. 5.6).

In the orbit

The nerve divides into three or four filaments which enter the ocular surface of the lateral rectus muscle behind its mid point.

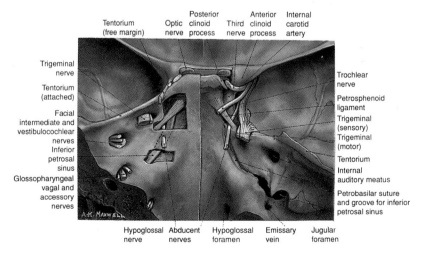

Fig. 5.15 Dissection to show relations of the abducent nerve to the petrous temporal nerve, inferior petrosal sinus, etc. On the right side the dura mater has been removed to show osseus relations. (Wolff's dissection.)

COMMUNICATIONS

The abducent nerve receives a sympathetic branch in the cavernous sinus, and communicates with the ophthalmic nerve before entering the orbit.

VARIATIONS

The nerve may arise by two roots which pass separately to the superior orbital fissure. It may pass above the petroclinoid ligament or give rise to a branch to the ciliary ganglion. The nasociliary nerve may be a branch of the abducent. The abducent nerve may be absent, being replaced by the oculomotor.

NUCLEUS AND CENTRAL CONNECTIONS

The abducent nucleus is a small mass of large multipolar cells, round in section and near the mid line in the tegmentum of the pons ventral to the colliculus facialis. The colliculus facialis is an elevation in the floor of the fourth ventricle, produced by the genu of the facial nerve (Figs 5.13 and 5.15). The medial longitudinal bundle is ventromedial. Partly intermingled with these larger neurons are more numerous small multipolar cells which form the so-called nucleus para-abducens. The total number of both types of neuron is about 22 000 (Konigsmark *et al.*, 1969); most cannot therefore be sources of abducent axons (see below). Evidence suggests that some may ascend through the medial longitudinal fasciculus to the oculomotor complex. The radicular fibres pass anteriorly through much of the pons, at first medial to the corpus trapezoideum, then lateral to the pyramid, some fibres traversing it (Figs 5.8 and 5.15).

Connections

Some axons pass from the abducent (and para-abducent) nucleus into the medial longitudinal bundle to the oculomotor, trochlear and vestibular nuclei; they are likely to be concerned with muscle integration; the projection to the vestibular complex of nuclei (which is balanced by an inhibitory vestibulotrochlear path – see Tarlov and Tarlov, 1975) must mediate oculovestibular coordination in orientational activity. Like the other motor nuclei for the ocular muscles, the abducens receives corticonuclear, colliculonuclear, tectobulbar, and possibly other connections, which subserve influences from the visual cortex and superior colliculus.

STRUCTURE

The nerve contains 6000–7000 fibres as it leaves the brain stem (Björkman and Wohlfart, 1936): the most recent estimate is 6600 (Konigsmark *et al.*, 1969). The contrast between these figures and the nuclear counts cited above remains unexplained, and the problem is not eased by findings in kittens that 50–90% of abducent neurons are radicular. A clear definition of the nucleus has not yet been made, and the problem is even exacerbated by demonstration of neurons immediately rostral to the abducent nucleus (Büttner-Ennever, 1977) which may belong to the same complex; however, these are not considered radicular but part of a projection to the oculomotor nuclei.

PRACTICAL CONSIDERATIONS

Abducent nerve damage results in paralysis of the lateral rectus muscle, with internal strabismus. The eye cannot be directed laterally beyond the mid point. Diplopia is homonymous, and is worse on looking towards the affected side.

Fractures of the base of the skull often involve the abducent nerve, owing to its contact with the basi-occipital and petrous bones.

Abducent nerve damage has little diagnostic value as a localizing sign. The abducent is the most vulnerable cranial nerve; almost any type of intracranial lesion may involve it. Many theories have been evoked to account for this (see Walsh, Hoyt and Miller, 1969; Ashworth, 1973).

5.4   THE TRIGEMINAL (FIFTH CRANIAL) NERVE

The trigeminal, largest of the cranial nerves, resembles a spinal nerve in having motor and sensory roots with a ganglion on the latter.

SUPERFICIAL EMERGENCE

The two roots emerge together, slightly above the mid level of the lateral surface of the pons. The sensory trunk is much the larger and inferolateral to the motor trunk (Figs 5.1 and 5.4).

COURSE AND RELATIONS

The two roots pass forwards, ascending slightly through the pontine cistern in the posterior cranial fossa for about 1 cm to reach a groove on the upper border of the petrous bone. They have separate pial and arachnoid sheaths blending with their epineurial sheaths. The arachnoid and pial sheaths are continuous through 'adventitious' connective tissue (Fig. 5.1).

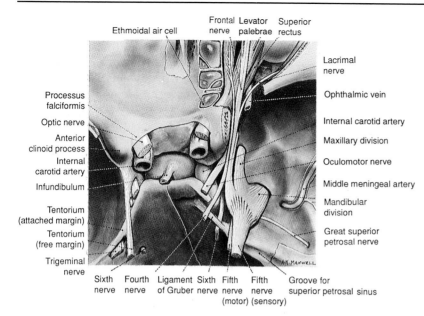

Fig. 5.16 Dissection to show nerves passing from the middle cranial fossa into the orbit. (Wolff's preparation.)

Inferior to the trigeminal nerve, the facial and vestibulocochlear nerves diverge towards the internal acoustic meatus. Above is the cerebellum, the margin of the tentorium cerebelli and the trochlear nerve.

The abducent nerve, emerging about 1.5 cm inferomedial to the trigeminal, approaches it and lies close to its medial side at the apex of the petrous bone (Fig. 5.15). The trigeminal pierces the dura under its attached tentorial border which contains the superior petrosal sinus. Now in the middle cranial fossa, it spreads out in a plexiform manner and joins the posterior concave aspect of the trigeminal ganglion (Figs 5.15 and 5.16). The nerve thus enters the middle fossa by an aperture formed by the petrous notch and tentorial dura mater.

THE TRIGEMINAL GANGLION

This is a sensory ganglion, analogous to those of the dorsal roots of spinal nerves (it may thus harbour herpes virus). It is crescentic, with its concavity posteromedial, and is sited in a fossa lateral to the apex of the petrous temporal bone, separated from the horizontal part of the internal carotid artery by a thin shelf of bone roofing the foramen lacerum. The ganglion is enclosed in dura mater prolonged from the posterior cranial fossa, which encloses both roots and fuses with the anterior half of the ganglion thus forming the cavum trigeminale which is lined with arachnoid. Thus both roots and the posterior half of the ganglion are bathed by cerebrospinal fluid. The 'cave' is said to be between the two layers (meningeal and endosteal) of the dura mater (like venous sinuses), but the arrangement is really more complex.

Lateral to the ganglion is the foramen spinosum, transmitting the middle meningeal artery (an obstruction in approaching it by the temporal route). Medial are the cavernous sinus, internal carotid artery, and ocular motor nerves (Figs 5.4 and 5.5), and beyond these the hypophysis cerebri. Superior are the uncus and temporal lobe, and inferior the greater and lesser (superficial) petrosal nerves, motor trigeminal root and internal carotid artery.

The trigeminal ganglion lies about 4 cm medial to a point just above the articular tubercle palpable at the root of the zygoma. Consequently, an extradural approach to the ganglion across the middle fossa may cause facial paralysis due to traction on the greater petrosal nerve, producing trauma at the geniculate ganglion of the facial nerve.

The motor root has no connection with the ganglion, passing anterolaterally below it to join the mandibular division.

The concave posterior aspect of the ganglion is continuous with the sensory root. From its anterior convex border emerge the ophthalmic, maxillary and mandibular divisions. The ganglion receives communications from the internal carotid sympathetic plexus; from its posterior part a few filaments pass to the tentorial dura mater.

Small accessory ganglia may occur along the concave border of the trigeminal ganglion; they correspond to the accessory ganglia which are present between the posterior root ganglion and the spinal cord. The ganglion contains neurons similar to those in the latter. Most are large unipolar neurons, with peripheral processes in the three divisions of the nerve and central axons passing to the trigeminal nuclei in the brain stem. Proprioceptor axons pass through the ganglion to nerve cells in the mesencephalic trigeminal nucleus. Some degree of functional or somatotopic localization has been described in the ganglion (Kerr and Lysak, 1964; Lende and Poulos, 1970).

5.5 THE OPHTHALMIC NERVE (V₁)

The ophthalmic nerve, smallest of the trigeminal divisions, enters the convex anterior border of the trigeminal ganglion superomedially. It extends in the lateral wall of the cavernous sinus, separately enclosed by dura mater, and is hence covered laterally by two layers of dura (Hovelacque, 1927). Superior are the oculomotor and trochlear nerves, medially the abducent nerve and internal carotid artery, and inferolaterally the maxillary nerve. After a course of about 2.5 cm in the sinus it divides, posterior to the superior orbital fissure, into lacrimal, frontal and nasociliary branches, which enter the orbit through the fissure (Figs 5.6, 5.17, 5.18, 5.21 and 5.24).

In the cavernous sinus, the ophthalmic nerve is said to be joined by branches of communication from the ocular motor nerves (probably proprioceptive) and from the internal carotid sympathetic plexus. The former communications are controversial. A recurrent branch, the nervus tentorii, innervates the dura mater (Figs 5.27 and 15.58), leaving the division near its origin and crossing the trochlear nerve, to which it is usually adherent and may indeed traverse (hence sometimes being described as a trochlear branch).

The branches of the ophthalmic nerve are:

1. lacrimal;
2. frontal
   (a) supratrochlear;
   (b) supraorbital;
3. nasociliary
   (a) sensory root of ciliary ganglion;
   (b) long ciliary nerves;
   (c) posterior ethmoidal;
   (d) infratrochlear;
   (e) anterior ethmoidal
      (i) medial nasal;
      (ii) lateral nasal;
      (iii) external nasal.

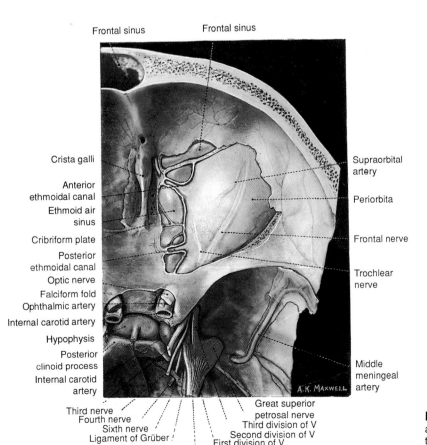

Fig. 5.17 Dissection of the orbit from above. Various structures are visible through the periorbita after removal of the orbital 'roof'. (Wolff's dissection.)

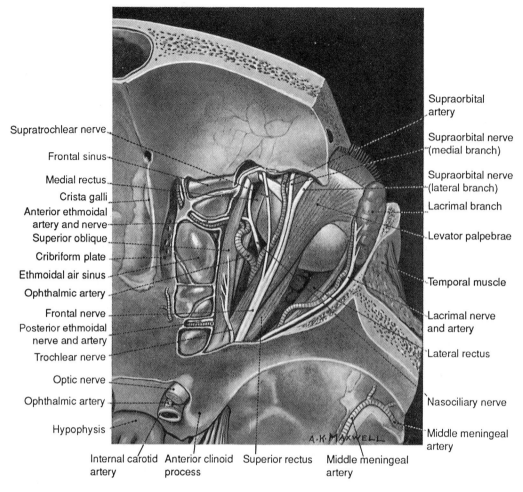

Supratrochlear nerve

Frontal sinus

Medial rectus

Crista galli

Anterior ethmoidal artery and nerve

Superior oblique

Cribriform plate

Ethmoidal air sinus

Ophthalmic artery

Frontal nerve

Posterior ethmoidal nerve and artery

Trochlear nerve

Optic nerve

Ophthalmic artery

Hypophysis

Internal carotid artery   Anterior clinoid process   Superior rectus   Middle meningeal artery

Supraorbital artery

Supraorbital nerve (medial branch)

Supraorbital nerve (lateral branch)

Lacrimal branch

Levator palpebrae

Temporal muscle

Lacrimal nerve and artery

Lateral rectus

Nasociliary nerve

Middle meningeal artery

A.K. MAXWELL

Fig. 5.18 Dissection of the orbit from above, periorbita removed. (Wolff's dissection.)

The lacrimal nerve

Smallest of the terminal branches of the division and arising well forwards in the middle cranial fossa, this nerve passes through the wide region of the superior orbital fissure above the annular tendon, lateral to the frontal and trochlear nerves, and superomedial to the ophthalmic vein. In the orbit the nerve runs laterally and parallel to the narrow part of the fissure, then forwards near the upper border of the lateral rectus muscle to reach the lacrimal gland. In the distal two-thirds of its course above the lateral rectus, it is accompanied by the lacrimal artery (Fig. 5.18). Its orbital course is sinuous like a fixed bayonet (Fig. 5.27) (Hovelacque and Reinhold, 1917). Before reaching the gland the nerve communicates with the zygomatic nerve (Fig. 5.24); traversing the gland, which it supplies, it ramifies in the conjunctiva and skin of the lateral part of the upper lid, which it reaches through the septum orbitale.

The frontal nerve

This is the largest ophthalmic branch, and starts in the cavernous sinus behind the superior orbital fissure, by which it enters the orbit. Here, it lies above the annular tendon between the lacrimal and the trochlear nerves. It runs forwards between the periosteum (periorbita) and levator palpebrae superioris. Near the orbital margin the frontal nerve divides into supratrochlear and supraorbital branches. In the specimen shown in Fig. 5.18 the division is unusually posterior.

The supratrochlear nerve (Fig. 5.18)

Smaller than the supraorbital nerve, the supratrochlear nerve runs forwards above the trochlea of the superior oblique muscle near which it communicates with the infratrochlear branch of the nasociliary nerve.

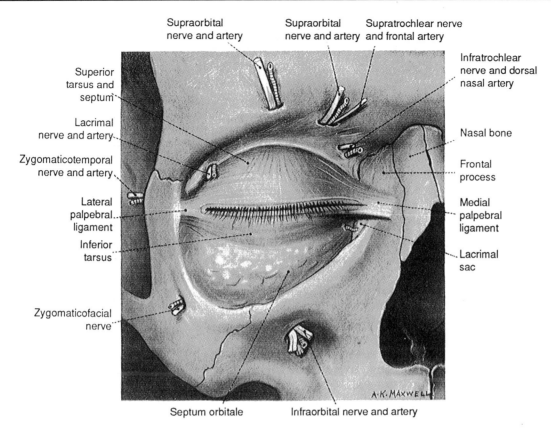

Fig. 5.19 Dissection of the orbit from in front. Orbicularis removed to show septum orbitale. (Wolff's dissection.)

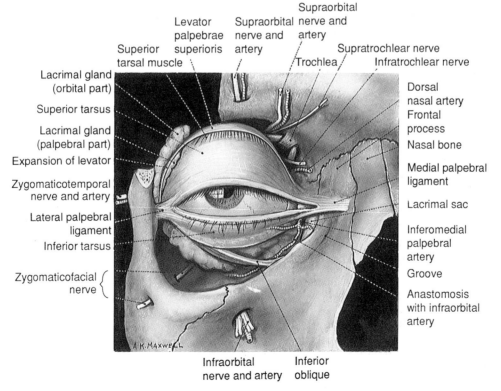

Fig. 5.20 Dissection of the orbit from in front, septum removed. (Wolff's dissection.)

In company with the supratrochlear artery the nerve ascends over the orbital margin about 1.25 cm from the mid line and deep to the orbicularis and corrugator supercilii. It sends branches of supply to the skin of the forehead and to the upper lid and conjunctiva.

The supraorbital nerve

This is the larger terminal branch of the frontal nerve, continuing the former's direction; it passes above the levator with the supraorbital artery medial to it, both leaving the orbit by the supraorbital notch or foramen (Figs 5.19 and 5.20). Occasionally the supraorbital nerve divides into medial and lateral branches in the orbit (Fig. 5.18), the lateral then occupying the supraorbital notch and the medial crossing the orbital margin between the trochlea and supraorbital notch. Usually the medial branch occupies a separate notch (of Henle) or rarely a foramen. The supraorbital nerve supplies the forehead and scalp to the vertex, and also the upper eyelid, and the conjunctiva, its branches usually intercommunicating. Those in the scalp are between periosteum and the orbicular and frontal muscles, through which they reach the skin. They frequently groove the bone. Rami to the upper lid pass through orbicularis. The nerve also sends a ramus to the frontal sinus and diploë through a small aperture in the supraorbital notch.

The nasociliary nerve

Derived from the inferomedial aspect of the ophthalmic, this nerve is commonly the first of the terminal branches. Intermediate in size between the lacrimal and frontal nerves, it lies first in the lateral wall of the cavernous sinus. It passes through the superior orbital fissure within the annular tendon, between the oculomotor divisions close to the sympathetic root of the ciliary ganglion, which is inferomedial. In the orbit it turns medially, with the ophthalmic artery, above the optic nerve in front of the superior oculomotor division (Fig. 5.21), and below the superior rectus. Near the anterior ethmoidal foramen it divides into the anterior ethmoidal and infratrochlear nerves.

Branches

Sensory root of ciliary ganglion   The long or sensory root of the ciliary ganglion leaves the nasociliary nerve near the superior orbital fissure. It is slender, 5–12 mm long, and passes lateral to the optic nerve to the posterosuperior angle of the ganglion (Figs 5.21–5.23).

The long ciliary nerves   These arise as a pair where the nasociliary crosses the optic nerve, to which they

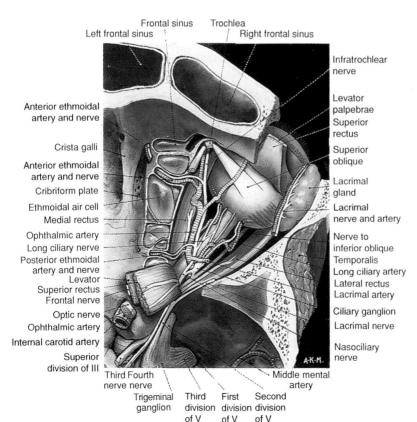

Fig. 5.21 Dissection of the orbit from above. The levator and superior rectus have been reflected. (Wolff's dissection.)

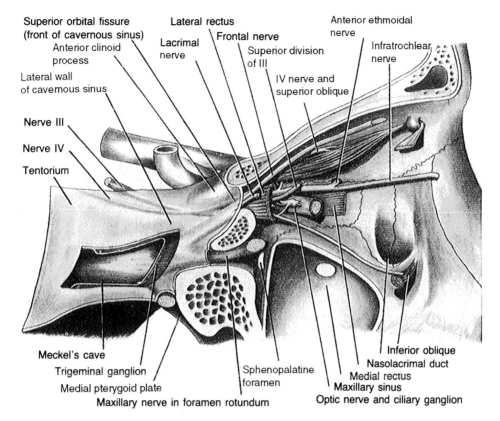

Fig. 5.22 Longitudinal section through the right orbit and middle cranial fossa, viewed from the lateral side.

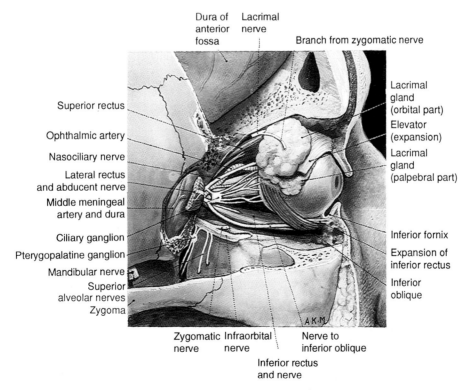

Fig. 5.23 Dissection of the right orbit from the lateral side. (Wolff's preparation.)

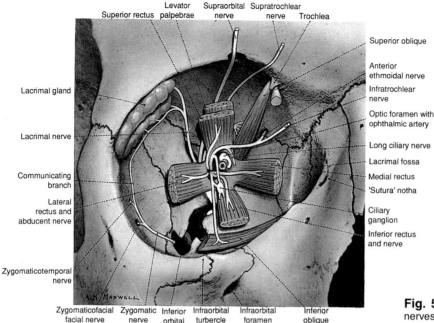

Superior rectus · Levator palpebrae · Supraorbital nerve · Supratrochlear nerve · Trochlea

Lacrimal gland

Lacrimal nerve

Communicating branch

Lateral rectus and abducent nerve

Zygomaticotemporal nerve

Superior oblique

Anterior ethmoidal nerve

Infratrochlear nerve

Optic foramen with ophthalmic artery

Long ciliary nerve

Lacrimal fossa

Medial rectus

'Sutura' notha

Ciliary ganglion

Inferior rectus and nerve

Zygomaticofacial facial nerve · Zygomatic nerve · Inferior orbital fissure · Infraorbital turbercle · Infraorbital foramen · Inferior oblique

Fig. 5.24 Dissection to show the orbital nerves from in front. (Based on Wolff's dissections.)

are medial. With the short ciliary nerves they pierce the sclera (Fig. 11.2), passing between this and the choroid (Fig. 7.58) to supply sensory fibres to the iris, cornea and ciliary muscle and sympathetic fibres to the dilatator pupillae.

The posterior ethmoidal nerve   The posterior ethmoidal nerve enters the posterior ethmoidal foramen between the superior oblique and medial rectus and, with its accompanying artery, supplies the sphenoidal and posterior ethmoidal sinuses.

The infratrochlear nerve (Figs 5.20, 5.21)   A terminal branch of the nasociliary, this nerve skirts the lower border of the superior oblique and passes below its trochlea. Near the trochlear it is connected to the supratrochlear, to appear on the face. Its branches supply the skin and conjunctiva round the medial angle of the eye, the root of the nose, lacrimal sac and canaliculi and the caruncle. It communicates with the supraorbital and infraorbital nerves.

The anterior ethmoidal nerve   Passing between the superior oblique and medial rectus, this nerve leaves the orbit with the anterior ethmoidal artery by the anterior ethmoidal canal, between the frontal and ethmoid bones, to supply the middle and anterior ethmoidal sinuses and frontal infundibulum. It enters the anterior cranial fossa at the side of the cribriform plate. Inclining medially it passes in dura mater to the 'nasal slit' in the cribriform plate, being here close

to the anterior pole of the olfactory bulb (Fig. 5.25) but separated from it by dura. The slit conducts the nerve to the roof of the nose, where its lateral nasal branches innervate the anterosuperior region of the lateral wall and medial nasal branches supply the anterior part of the septum. The nerve then occupies a groove (Figs 1.13 and 5.32) on the posterior surface of the nasal bone, which it notches to appear on the face as the external nasal nerve, to skin over the cartilaginous part of the nose, down to its tip.

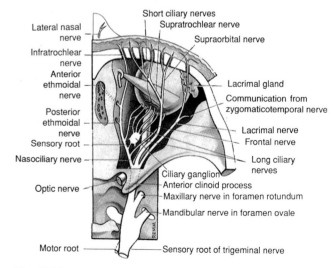

Lateral nasal nerve

Infratrochlear nerve

Anterior ethmoidal nerve

Posterior ethmoidal nerve

Sensory root

Nasociliary nerve

Optic nerve

Motor root

Short ciliary nerves

Supratrochlear nerve

Supraorbital nerve

Lacrimal gland

Communication from zygomaticotemporal nerve

Lacrimal nerve

Frontal nerve

Long ciliary nerves

Ciliary ganglion

Anterior clinoid process

Maxillary nerve in foramen rotundum

Mandibular nerve in foramen ovale

Sensory root of trigeminal nerve

Fig. 5.25 The ophthalmic division of the trigeminal nerve. Note: the ciliary ganglion normally lies *lateral* to the optic nerve.

Variations

The infratrochlear nerve may be replaced by the supratrochlear. Branches may pass from the anterior ethmoidal to the levator, the oculomotor and abducent nerves, and frontal sinus. For details consult Le Double (1897) and Quain (1900).

5.6   THE CILIARY GANGLION

The ciliary ganglion is easily found by locating the nerve to the inferior oblique. With the muscle exposed from the front, the nerve is identified as it crosses the middle of its posterior border (Fig. 5.23).

The ciliary ganglion is a small, somewhat polygonal body about 2 mm in anteroposterior and 1 mm in vertical dimensions, situated posteriorly in the orbit about 1 cm anterior to the optic foramen between the optic nerve and lateral rectus muscle, in contact with the nerve, but separated from the muscle by fat. Usually it lies close to the ophthalmic artery (Figs 5.21, 5.22, 5.25 and 5.26). Three roots or rami enter it posteriorly (Fig. 5.28): the long or sensory root; the short or parasympathetic root; the sympathetic root.

The sensory and sympathetic fibres pass through without interruption, and in some vertebrates actually bypass the ganglion, whose only essential 'root' is parasympathetic. (For comparative anatomy see Grimes and Sallmann, 1960.)

SENSORY ROOT

The long or sensory root branches from the nasociliary nerve just after the nerve has entered the orbit. It is slender, 6–12 mm long, and passes along

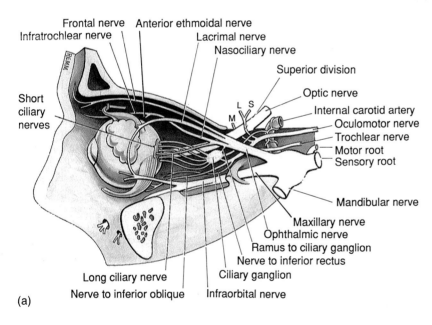

Frontal nerve   Anterior ethmoidal nerve
Infratrochlear nerve
Lacrimal nerve
Nasociliary nerve
Superior division
Optic nerve
Short ciliary nerves
Internal carotid artery
L S
M
Oculomotor nerve
Trochlear nerve
Motor root
Sensory root
Mandibular nerve
Maxillary nerve
Ophthalmic nerve
Ramus to ciliary ganglion
Nerve to inferior rectus
Long ciliary nerve
Ciliary ganglion
Nerve to inferior oblique
Infraorbital nerve
(a)

Fig. 5.26 (a) The ciliary ganglion and oculomotor nerve. S = Nerve to the superior rectus; L = nerve to the levator; M = nerve to the medial rectus. (The sympathetic ramus from the carotid plexus to the ciliary ganglion is not labelled, but is easy to identify.)

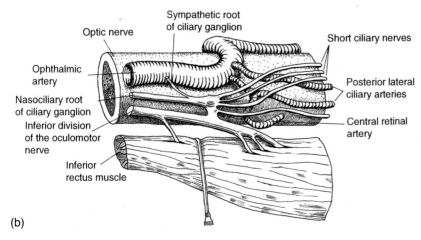

Sympathetic root of ciliary ganglion
Optic nerve
Short ciliary nerves
Ophthalmic artery
Nasociliary root of ciliary ganglion
Inferior division of the oculomotor nerve
Posterior lateral ciliary arteries
Central retinal artery
Inferior rectus muscle
(b)

(b) The ciliary ganglion and its relationship to the arteries, viewed from the lateral side of the orbit. (From Eliškova, M. (1973) *Br. J. Ophthalmol.*, **57**, 766, with permission.)

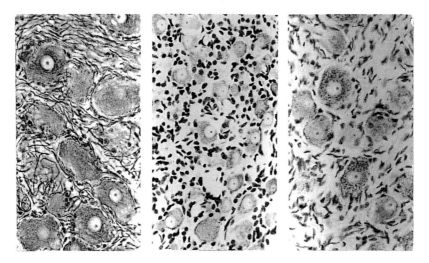

Fig. 5.27 Photomicrographs of the ciliary ganglion neurons (right and left) and the superior cervical sympathetic ganglion neurons (centre), all at the same magnification, stained by cresyl violet (left and centre) and Romanes' technique (right). Contrast the size and granule features of the ciliary and sympathetic neurons. The relatively large diameter of the ciliary ganglion neurons, in both mammals and birds, has not been widely recognized. They are not typical autonomic neurons.

the lateral side of the optic nerve to the postero-superior part of the ganglion. It contains sensory fibres from the cornea, iris and ciliary body, and possibly sympathetic fibres to the dilatator pupillae.

SHORT ROOT

The short or motor root leaves the nerve to innervate the inferior oblique a few millimetres beyond its origin from the inferior division of the oculomotor nerve. It is thicker than the sensory root and only 1–2 mm long, and passes up and forwards to the posteroinferior angle of the ganglion. It carries parasympathetic fibres to the sphincter pupillae and ciliary muscle which synapse in the ganglion.

SYMPATHETIC ROOT

The sympathetic root is derived from the internal carotid plexus and traverses the superior orbital fissure within the annular tendon inferomedial to the nasociliary nerve. It is close below the long root, with which it may be blended, and enters the ganglion between the other roots. It carries constrictor fibres to the blood vessels of the eye, and possibly fibres to dilatator pupillae.

BLOOD SUPPLY

The blood supply of the ciliary ganglion, despite the otherwise voluminous literature on this small structure, has attracted little study. Kuzetsova (1963) recorded observations on its vascularization in human fetal and neonatal material; more recently, Elišková (1969, 1973) has studied India ink preparations (in rhesus and in human fetal and postnatal material) and reports the supply to be from the posterior ciliary, muscular, ophthalmic and central retinal arteries (Fig. 5.29).

BRANCHES

The preganglionic parasympathetic neurons whose axons reach the ciliary ganglion are in the accessory oculomotor nuclei (of Edinger-Westphal). They are myelinated, and in the ganglion they synapse with the dendrites and perikarya of the postganglionic neurons (Fig. 5.27), whose thinly myelinated axons form the short ciliary nerves which usually contain small groups of displaced ganglion cells (Fig. 5.28). Their postganglionic axons are most unusual, possibly unique, in being non-myelinated.

The short ciliary nerves, 6–10 in number, are delicate, sinuous branches which emerge from the anterior end of the ganglion in two groups. They accompany the short ciliary arteries above and below the optic nerve, the lower group being larger. They connect with each other and the long ciliary nerves, supply branches to the optic nerve and ophthalmic artery, and pierce the sclera around the optic nerve. They run anteriorly between the choroid and sclera, grooving the latter, to the ciliary muscle on whose surface they form the ciliary plexus, innervating the iris, ciliary body, and cornea.

VARIATIONS

The parasympathetic 'root' may be so short that the ganglion is sessile on the nerve to the inferior oblique muscle. Connections with the trochlear and abducent nerves have been described. Consult Quain (1900) and Hovelacque (1927).

The ciliary ganglion contains multipolar neurons, mostly of unusually large size (about 45 μm in

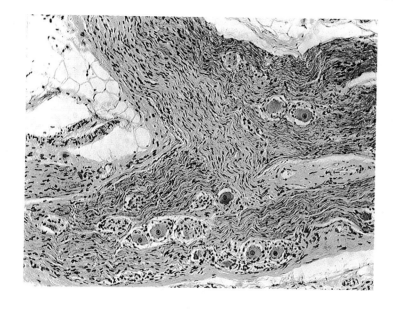

Fig. 5.28 Ganglion cells in the short ciliary nerves. (Wolff's preparation.)

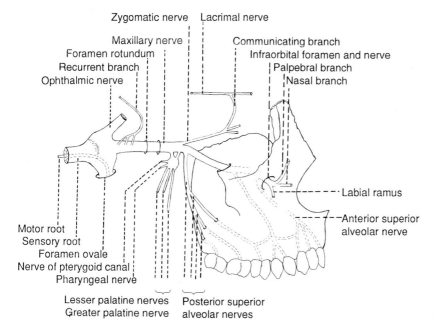

Zygomatic nerve   Lacrimal nerve

Maxillary nerve

Foramen rotundum

Recurrent branch

Ophthalmic nerve

Communicating branch

Infraorbital foramen and nerve

Palpebral branch

Nasal branch

Labial ramus

Anterior superior alveolar nerve

Motor root

Sensory root

Foramen ovale

Nerve of pterygoid canal

Pharyngeal nerve

Lesser palatine nerves

Greater palatine nerve

Posterior superior alveolar nerves

Fig. 5.29 Diagram of the maxillary nerve (lateral wall).

diameter) for autonomic postganglion cells. Some observers distinguished many classes of cells in the ganglion, but these views have not been sustained. They form a largely uniform population (Warwick, 1954). Small numbers of smaller neurons, typical of those in sympathetic ganglia, also occur and may be interneurons or aberrant postganglionic sympathetic neurons. Experiments show that most of the ganglion cells (about 97%) innervate the ciliaris muscle, a small number only innervating the sphincter pupillae (Warwick, 1954), which accords with the great difference in the size of the two muscles. The ciliary ganglia may not be the **only** source of parasympathetic fibres for the eyeball. The episcleral ganglia of Axenfeld (1907) have long been suspected to provide a secondary route. (See Stotler, 1937; Morgan and Harrigan, 1951.) In primates (including humans) (Phillips, 1972) the numbers of episcleral ganglia are small and inconstant, which suggests an insignificant role in miosis (Consult Givner, 1939; Nathan and Turner, 1942.)

5.7 THE MAXILLARY NERVE (V₂) (Fig. 5.29)

The maxillary nerve, intermediate in size between the ophthalmic and mandibular nerves, issues between them from the anterior border of the trigeminal ganglion. It is inferolateral in the cavernous sinus and grooves (Figs 3.16 and 5.4) the greater wing of the sphenoid as it approaches the foramen rotundum, through which it enters the pterygopalatine fossa. Turning laterally behind the palatine bone it divides, at the inferior orbital fissure, into the infraorbital and zygomatic nerves.

RELATIONS

In the cranial cavity

The maxillary nerve is inferolateral in the wall of the cavernous sinus. Superior to it is the ophthalmic division and laterally the temporal lobe. When the sphenoidal sinus is large the nerve may extend into the great wing of the sphenoid between the foramina ovale and rotundum, which may account for involvement of the nerve in sinus disease.

In the pterygopalatine fossa

Here the nerve lies near the end of the maxillary artery, a plexus of veins, and ethmoidal sinuses in the orbital process of the palatine bone, with the danger of involvement with sinusitis.

BRANCHES

Middle meningeal nerve

In the cranial cavity a recurrent branch (middle meningeal nerve) supplies dura mater in the anterior part of the middle cranial fossa.

Pterygopalatine nerves

In the pterygopalatine fossa two short pterygopalatine nerves provide the sensory root of the pterygopalatine (sphenopalatine) ganglion.

Posterior superior alveolar nerves

The posterior superior alveolar (dental) nerves, usually three, leave before the maxillary nerve divides in the inferior orbital fissure. These nerves enter canals in the maxilla through small foramina on its infratemporal surface, supplying molar teeth, adjoining gingival tissues, periodontal ligaments, and mucous membrane of the maxillary sinus.

Infraorbital nerve

The infraorbital nerve runs forwards from the inferior orbital fissure on the orbital plate of the maxilla, first in a groove, then in a canal with the infraorbital artery, emerging on the face through the infraorbital foramen. The **middle superior alveolar** (dental) **nerve** branches off in the infraorbital groove and descends in the lateral wall of the maxilla to upper premolar teeth and adjoining sinus mucosa. It is occasionally absent, sometimes multiple (Wood Jones, 1939; Fitzgerald, 1956). The **anterior superior alveolar** (dental) **nerve** arises in the infraorbital canal, curves laterally and then inferomedially below the infraorbital foramen to supply the canine and incisor teeth, mucosa of the maxillary sinus, and anteroinferior area of the lateral wall and floor of the nose.

The infraorbital nerve emerges between levator labii superioris and levator anguli oris, dividing into many branches, some of which join those of the facial nerve. These branches radiate to supply skin: **labial branches** supply the upper lip and mucous membrane of the vestibule (including the labial gum) from the mid line to the second bicuspid tooth; **nasal branches** supply the side of the lower part of the nose; **palpebral branches** supply the skin and conjunctiva of the lower lid.

Zygomatic nerve

The zygomatic nerve turns laterally from the inferior orbital fissure, dividing into zygomaticotemporal and zygomaticofacial branches.

The **zygomaticotemporal nerve** ascends in a groove on the lateral orbital wall, communicates with the lacrimal nerve, a suggested autonomic route to the lacrimal gland, and enters a canal in the zygomatic bone, which leads it to the temporal fossa. Here it ascends, pierces the temporal fascia behind the zygomatic tubercle, and, connecting with branches of the facial nerve, supplies skin over the anterior temporal region to the orbital margin. The supposed lacrimal secretomotor route has been criticized by Ruskell (1971), whose studies suggest a direct path.

The **zygomaticofacial nerve** also enters a canal in the zygomatic bone, which leads it to the face. Here, communicating with the facial nerve, it traverses orbicularis to supply skin over the cheek.

Variations

The zygomatic nerve may enter one canal and then divide in bone. The lacrimal communication may replace the zygomaticotemporal nerve; a twig from the infraorbital may replace the zygomaticofacial nerve, which may issue onto the face as two or more branches.

5.8   THE PTERYGOPALATINE (SPHENOPALATINE) GANGLION

The pterygopalatine ganglion (of Meckel) is located in the upper part of the pterygopalatine fossa, lateral to the sphenopalatine foramen and dependent from the maxillary nerve by its two pterygopalatine branches or 'roots' (Figs 5.23, 5.29 and 5.30).

THE PTERYGOPALATINE ROOTS

Sensory

The pterygopalatine ganglion receives a contingent of sensory fibres from the maxillary nerve by the posterior pterygopalatine nerve, most of whose fibres leave the ganglion by various branches to innervate sensitive tissues in the orbit, nose, and pharynx (see below). A few fibres return to the maxillary nerve through the anterior 'root'. None of these fibres is interrupted in the ganglion, being merely passengers through a ganglion which is basically autonomic.

Autonomic motor

The nerve of the pterygoid canal is formed in the foramen lacerum by union of the greater petrosal nerve (parasympathetic), from the geniculate ganglion, with the deep petrosal nerve from the internal carotid sympathetic plexus (Fig. 5.30). The nerve is thus a mixed autonomic nerve. It passes through a canal in the sphenoid bone to the pterygopalatine fossa, where it joins the ganglion. The deep petrosal nerve comes from neurons in the superior cervical sympathetic ganglion by way of the carotid plexus. These postganglionic fibres traverse the pterygopalatine ganglion without relay to enter its branches of distribution, some probably to the maxillary nerve through the anterior root. All sympathetic fibres thus pass through the ganglion. They are mostly vasoconstrictor in function to arterioles in the territory of the maxillary division.

The greater petrosal nerve carries parasympathetic preganglionic fibres, which are considered to form synapses with postganglionic neurons in the pterygopalatine ganglion, the evidence for this being largely physiological; they were said to innervate the lacrimal gland, reaching it via the zygomatic nerve and its communication with the lacrimal nerve. Other parasympathetic fibres probably supply mucous glands in the nose, nasopharynx, paranasal sinuses and palate. These alone relay in the ganglion; their preganglionic neurons are ascribed to the superior salivatory nucleus of the pons, the fibres leaving the brain stem in the nervus intermedius (Fig. 16.2). The identity of this nucleus is not as certain as the term implies; it is probably near the caudal end of the facial motor nucleus. The result of stimulation of this pathway is not only lacrimation, but secretion from a wide area of nasal and palatal mucosa – hence the name 'ganglion of hay fever' commonly given to the pterygopalatine ganglion. Its neurons have received little attention, but appear to be similar to those in

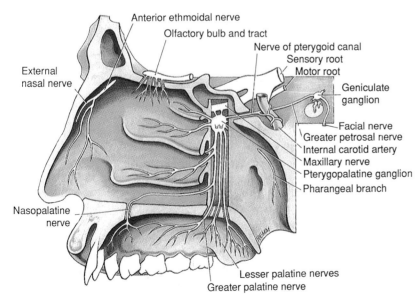

Fig. 5.30 Nerves of the lateral wall of the nose.

other antonomic ganglia (Warwick, 1954). In an unpublished doctoral thesis (City University of London, 1982) Wilson described the cells to be ultrastructurally like other autonomic neurons, but more closely packed than in other ganglia. She estimated the population of a single macaque ganglion at 17 000.

BRANCHES

Each of the branches of the ganglion may (and usually does) include all three components – somatic sensory, parasympathetic secretomotor and sympathetic vasomotor. Orbital branches supply the periosteum at the apex of the floor of the orbit. Ruskell (1970, 1971) has drawn attention to experimental evidence indicating that in monkeys these rami provide a route for parasympathetic fibres to the lacrimal gland.

The nasopalatine nerve

This nerve enters the nose by the sphenopalatine foramen, crosses its roof, descends in a groove on the vomer, and supplies mucous membrane all along this course. It traverses the incisive canal to supply the mucoperiosteum behind the incisor teeth. (It is sometimes regarded as the largest of the posterior superior nasal group.)

The posterior superior nasal nerves

These nerves also enter the nose through the sphenopalatine foramen, and turn forwards to supply the posterosuperior part of the lateral nasal wall and part of the septum. They are hence divisible into lateral and medial groups.

The greater palatine nerve

This nerve descends in a canal formed between the maxilla and vertical palatine plate, producing multiple twigs which pierce both bones to supply the mucosa of the maxillary sinus and of the posteroinferior part of the lateral nasal wall. Emerging through the greater palatine foramen the nerve turns to supply the mucoperiosteum of the hard palate as far as the incisive canal.

The lesser palatine nerves

Often branches of the greater palatine nerves, these nerves traverse the lesser palatine canals and, behind the crest of the palatine bone, turn posteriorly to supply mucous membrane on both surfaces of the soft palate.

Pharyngeal branch

The pharyngeal branch passes through the palatinovaginal canal to supply the mucosa of the nasopharynx.

Orbitociliary nerve

By dissection, microscopy and electron microscopy Ruskell (1973) has demonstrated an almost constant branch of the maxillary nerve, just beyond its emergence from the foramen rotundum in the pterygopalatine fossa, which passes into the orbit through the inferior orbital fissure to join the ciliary ganglion. He calls this the orbitociliary nerve, considering it sensory, its fibres passing to the eyeball with those of the ophthalmic division in the short ciliary nerves. This nerve also sends small rami to a retro-orbital plexus described by the same worker.

5.9 THE MANDIBULAR NERVE (V₃)

The mandibular division of the trigeminal nerve is the union of a large sensory branch from the trigeminal ganglion and the trigeminal motor root, the whole of which thus enters this division. The two nerves pass separately through the foramen ovale, and unite into one trunk, which has the tensor palati and auditory tube medial to it and laterally the lateral pterygoid and middle meningeal artery. (For further details see standard texts such as *Gray's Anatomy*).

5.10 NUCLEI AND CENTRAL CONNECTIONS OF THE TRIGEMINAL NERVE

THE TRIGEMINAL SENSORY NUCLEI

These nuclei extend throughout the brain stem. The **mesencephalic nucleus** is slender (Fig. 5.31). The **principal sensory nucleus** is situated dorsolaterally in the pons ventral to the superior cerebellar peduncle. The medullary **nucleus of the spinal tract** is continuous with the principal nucleus above and the substantia gelatinosa at the level of the second cervical segment (Fig. 5.7).

Axons from the neurons in the trigeminal ganglion pass dorsally through the pons to synapse with interneurons in the main nucleus; others descend to

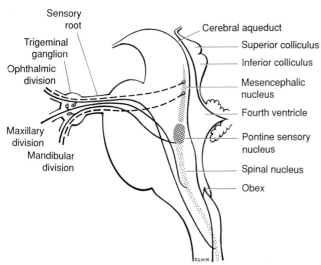

Fig. 5.31 Scheme of the sensory nuclei of V. Note that the ophthalmic fibres go to the lowest part of the spinal nucleus at the level of the second cervical nerve, i.e. the face is represented upside down in the long spinal nucleus of the trigeminal nerve. Interrupted lines indicate proprioceptive fibres.

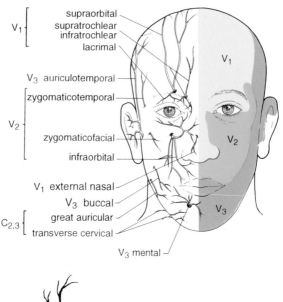

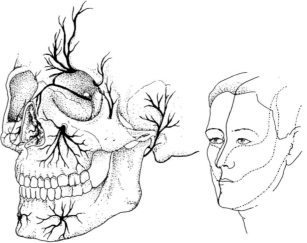

Fig. 5.32 Sensory innervation of the face.

the spinal nucleus, as the so-called spinal tract. About half of these entering fibres themselves divide into ascending and descending branches; the rest spread out to their destinations without division.

The main sensory nucleus is probably concerned with fine discriminative touch. The spinal nucleus mediates thermal and tactile sensibility; fibres from the ophthalmic division go to the lowest part of this nucleus, those from the maxillary division are intermediate, while those from the mandibular division end highest.

The mesencephalic nucleus is located in the grey matter lateral to the aqueduct. It consists of 'primary' sensory neurons, whose axons, probably derived from all three divisions of the trigeminal nerve, pass directly through the ganglion, a unique arrangement in the central nervous system of mammals (Johnston, 1909).

MOTOR NUCLEUS

The motor nucleus is located in the lateral tegmental region of the pons medial to the main sensory nucleus and nearer the floor of the fourth ventricle. It is in line with the nucleus ambiguus and facial nucleus (Fig. 5.11), all three being branchial or special visceral efferent in morphological terms.

CONNECTIONS

Since the trigeminal nerve serves so much of the head in sensory functions, as well as the whole mas-

ticatory musculature, its central connections with other cranial nerves, especially those of the orbit, tongue, and face, are extensive. The sensory nuclei project to the postcentral gyrus via the trigeminal lemniscus, the central posterior medial nucleus of the thalamus, and to nuclei of motor cranial nerves and tectum, cerebellum, reticular system, subthalamic nucleus, etc.

Figure 5.32 illustrates the sensory innervation of the face by the three divisions of the trigeminal nerve.

5.11 THE FACIAL (SEVENTH CRANIAL) NERVE

The facial nerve is branchial in origin, and should contain special visceral efferent (branchiomotor) and afferent (gustatory) nerve fibres, and general visceral

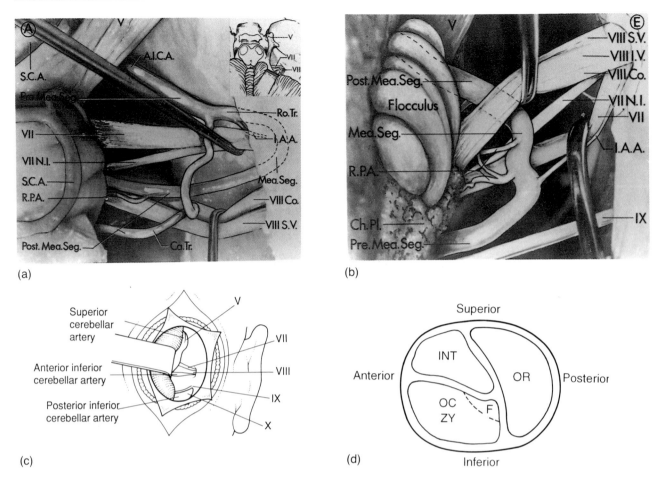

Fig. 5.33 Relationships of the nervus intermedius, facial and vestibulocochlear nerve trunks and the superior and anterior inferior cerebellar arteries. (a) Nervus intermedius (VII N.I.) exits from the brainstem between the facial nerve trunk (VII) and the vestibulocochlear (VIII Co.) and superior vestibular (VIII S.V.) nerve trunks. Note relationships of the rostral (Ro.Tr.) and caudal (Ca.Tr.) branches of the anterior inferior cerebellar artery (A.I.C.A.) to the facial–vestibulocochlear nerve complex. (b) The facial nerve (VII) and branches of the vestibulocochlear nerve (VII S.V., VII I.V., VII Co.) have been separated to show the nervus intermedius (VII N.I.). The premeatal and postmeatal segments (Mea. Seg.) of the anterior inferior cerebellar artery can be shown passing between the nerve trunks. V, trigeminal nerve; IX, glossopharyngeal nerve; Ch.Pl., choroid plexus; I.A.A. internal auditory artery; Mea. Seg., meatal segment; R.P.A., recurrent perforating branches of the anterior inferior cerebellar artery; S.C.A., superior cerebellar artery. (c) Relationships of the cerebellar arteries and the trigeminal (V), facial (VII), vestibulocochlear (VIII), glossopharyngeal (IX) and vagus (X) nerves. (From Martin, R. G. *et al.* (1980), *Neurosurg.* **6**, 483). (d) Location of the nervus intermedius within the facial nerve trunk just before it reaches the geniculate ganglion. The nervus intermedius (INT) occupies an anterior, superior position in the segment and makes up about 25% of the volume of the nerve at this point. Other branches of the facial nerve include the frontal (F), ocular (OC), oral (OR), and zygomatic (ZY). (Podvinec, M. and Pfaltz, C. R. (1976), *Acta Otolaryngol.* **81**, 173).

efferent fibres (parasympathetic). Certain of these issue as a separate trunk, the nervus intermedius, sometimes considered to be a cranial nerve 'in its own right'. This is misleading. The gustatory and parasympathetic components simply enter or leave the brain stem as a separate trunk (in 20% of 73 dissections it was not even a separate nerve – see Rhoton, Obayashi and Hollinshead, 1968.) Some prefer to consider the two parts or roots of the nerve as the intermediofacial nerve or facial complex. The usual description of the intermediate nerve as the 'sensory root' is equally misleading, since many of

its fibres are efferent parasympathetic, supplying the submandibular and sublingual salivary glands, lacrimal gland, palatine and nasal mucosal glands, and glandular cells in paranasal sinuses.

The facial nerve emerges at the lower border of the pons in the recess between the olive and inferior cerebellar peduncle (Fig. 5.1), lateral to the abducent and medial to the vestibulocochlear nerves. The intermediate nerve is lateral to the main facial trunk. The two nerves run anterolaterally in the posterior cranial fossa to the internal acoustic meatus. The nervus intermedius is here between the facial trunk

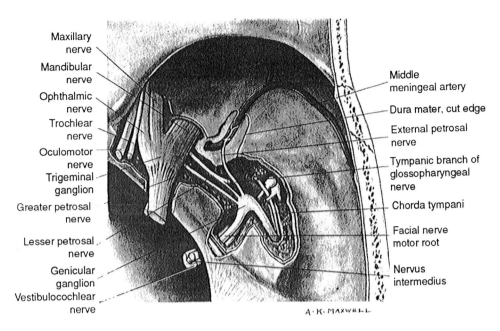

Fig. 5.34 Dissection of the right middle cranial fossa to show the course and some connections of the facial nerve within the temporal bone. (From Williams, P.L. *et al.* (eds) (1995) *Gray's Anatomy*, 38th edition, published by Churchill Livingstone.)

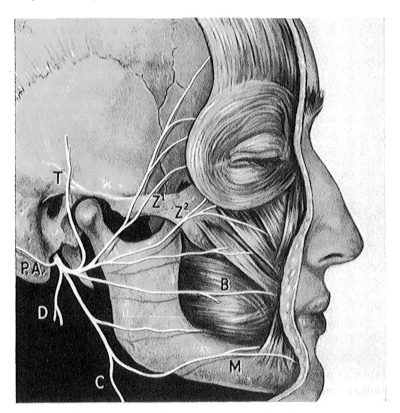

Fig. 5.35 The extracranial distribution of the facial nerve. PA = Posterior auricular; D = branch to posterior belly of the digastric and stylohyoid; T = temporal branch; Z¹ = upper zygomatic branches; Z² = lower zygomatic branches; B = buccal branch; M = mandibular branch; C = cervical branch.

and the vestibulocochlear nerve, the latter being grooved by it (Fig. 5.33). These structures, with the labyrinthine artery, enter the meatus, the bottom of which is the lamina cribosa, divided into four parts by a horizontal and vertical partitions. The facial nerve, including the nervus intermedius, traverses the anterosuperior quadrant, into the facial canal. Continuing laterally for 4 mm, the nerve turns posteriorly above the vestibule in the direction of the internal auditory meatus, to reach the middle ear. The geniculate ganglion is at the bend (geniculum) of the nerve, where the nervus intermedius fuses with it. Adjacent to the tympanic cavity the nerve is in the facial canal, between its roof and medial wall, above the promontory and fenestra vestibuli (ovalis). The bone may be partly absent, and then the nerve, separated by little more than mucoperiosteum from the cavity, may be affected by tympanic infections (Fig. 5.34).

Near the junction of medial and posterior walls of the tympanic cavity the nerve curves down and backwards to issue from the stylomastoid foramen. The descending part of this second bend ridges the medial wall of the aditus, and above it is the bulge of the lateral semicircular canal. Emerging, the nerve gives off two branches (Fig. 5.35) and divides into a larger upper and a lower division (temporozygomatic and cervicofacial). These turn anteriorly in the parotid gland, superficial to the retromandibular (posterior facial) vein and external carotid artery, and divide, within the gland, into somewhat variable temporal, zygomatic, buccal, mandibular and cervical rami, distributed to the facial musculature. (For variations see Hovelacque, 1927.) In infants, with as yet no mastoid process, the facial nerve, being more lateral than inferior at its exit, is more easily damaged by injuries or at operation (mastoidectomy). Regional blockade of the facial nerve can be achieved by injecting the nerve with local anaesthetic as it leaves the stylomastoid foramen (O'Brien technique).

BRANCHES

In the temporal bone

- Greater petrosal nerve;
- tympanic branches;
- nerve to stapedius;
- chorda tympani.

At exit from the stylomastoid foramen

- Posterior auricular, supplying occipitalis and some auricular muscles;
- digastric;
- stylohyoid.

On the face

- Temporal to orbicularis, etc.;
- zygomatic, also to orbicularis;

- buccal, to muscles of nose and upper lip;
- mandibular, to muscles of lower lip;
- cervical, to platysma.

The greater petrosal nerve and the chorda tympani contain fibres which enter or leave the brain stem only in the nervus intermedius; they are gustatory fibres from the tongue and soft palate and parasympathetic secretomotor fibres. The tympanic rami contain fibres which travel in both parts of the facial nerve. All the fibres travelling in the intermediate nerve leave either the geniculate ganglion or the intrapetrous part of the facial nerve, which hence contains no 'intermediate' fibres in its extracranial course.

The greater petrosal nerve

This nerve branches from the geniculate ganglion. It passes through a canal, which opens at a groove on the anterior surface of the petrous bone (Fig. 5.16). The canal carries the nerve under the trigeminal ganglion to the foramen lacerum, where it unites with the deep petrosal, from the internal carotid sympathetic plexus. Together, they form the nerve of the pterygoid canal, which joins the pterygopalatine ganglion via the pterygoid canal (Fig. 5.30). The greater petrosal nerve contains taste fibres for the mucous membrane of the soft palate and secretory fibres to the palatal, nasal and lacrimal glands.

The tympanic branches

The tympanic branches join the lesser petrosal nerve as it emerges from the tympanic plexus. These facial fibres thus join glossopharyngeal fibres, and are secretomotor, via the lesser petrosal nerve and otic ganglion relay, to the parotid gland. Some facial fibres, reaching the tympanic cavity through the tympanic rami, may supply the tympanic membrane and part of the pinna. (The secretomotor fibres mentioned above may be derived from the vagus nerve – see Vidić, 1968.) The sensory fibres commonly encroach on the external surface of the tympanic membrane and skin of the external auditory meatus and pinna. This may explain the presence here of vesicles in some cases of facial herpes (for further details, see Brodal, 1969).

The temporal branch

The temporal branch supplies the auriculares anterior and superior, and part of frontalis (Fig. 5.36).

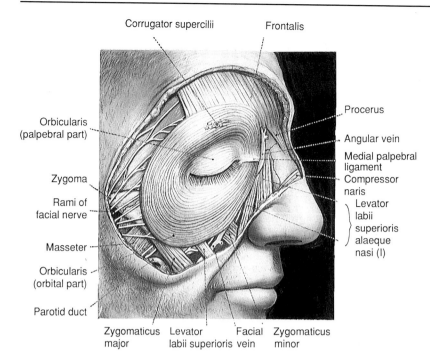

Fig. 5.36 Dissection of the orbit from in front. Orbicularis oculi (Wolff's dissection).

Zygomatic branches

The zygomatic branches form two groups, the upper of which (Fig. 5.35, Z^1) runs subcutaneously across the zygomatic arch to supply frontalis, orbicularis oculi, corrugator supercilii, and procerus (Fig. 5.6). Interruption of these nerves prevents full closure of the eyelids, and leads to corneal exposure and desiccation. The lower zygomatic branches (Fig. 5.3, Z^2) cross the zygomatic bone to supply orbicularis in the lower lid and in part the elevators of the upper lip.

The buccal branch

This branch runs forwards below the parotid duct to supply buccinator, zygomaticus major et minor, risorius, levator anguli oris and levator labii superioris alaeque nasi.

The mandibular branch

This branch commonly descends into the neck and crosses the lower border of the mandible with the facial artery at the anterior border of masseter. Here it is vulnerable to trauma. It supplies depressor anguli oris, depressor labii inferioris, and mentalis.

Cervical branch

The cervical branch descends to supply platysma.

NUCLEI AND CENTRAL CONNECTIONS

The sensory fibres issuing in the nervus intermedius have their nerve cells in the geniculate ganglion. They are unipolar neurons, with peripheral processes distributed as above. Their central axons reach cranial levels of the nucleus solitarius, which projects to the ventral nuclei of the dorsal thalamus and thence to the postcentral gyrus. The somatic sensory fibres of the facial nucleus (from the tympanic membrane and pinna) have unknown connections.

The branchial motor nucleus of the nerve consists of large multipolar neurons like those of the nucleus ambiguus, both being components of the branchial column. The facial nucleus is near its point of exit, but its fibres first run posteromedially to the floor of the fourth ventricle, where they almost encircle the abducent nucleus, forming the colliculus facilialis in the floor of the ventricle before turning anterolaterally between their own nucleus and the spinal root of the trigeminal nerve, to emerge between the olive and inferior cerebella peduncle (Figs 5.1, 5.35 and 5.37).

COMMUNICATIONS

Like other cranial nerves, the facial nerve has numerous peripheral connections with others, including those with the vestibulocochlear, vagal, glossopharyngeal, lesser occipital, trigeminal and transverse cervical cutaneous nerves. It has been stated that the facial nerve supplies orbicularis oculi

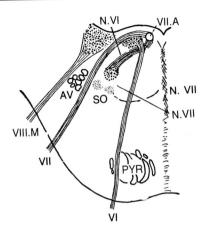

Fig. 5.37 The abducent and facial nerves and their nuclei. The outline represents a transverse section of the lower part of the pons, on to which the course of the facial nerve is projected. VI, N.VI = Abducent nerve and nucleus; VII = facial nerve; VII.A = ascending portion of the root of the facial nerve, supposed to be seen in optical section; N.VII = facial nucleus; SO = trapezoid body; AV = mesencephalic tract of the trigeminal nerve; VIII.M = medial root of the vestibulocochlear nerve.

via the oculomotor nerve (and other facial muscles via this and other cranial nerves), in an effort to explain 'sparing' of upper facial muscles in supranuclear facial nerve paralysis. These speculations are unfounded, and the explanation is to be found in central connections.

5.12 THE VESTIBULOCOCHLEAR (EIGHTH CRANIAL) NERVE

The vestibulocochlear (statoacoustic or auditory) nerve is well named. Its vestibular component serves the phylogenetically older part of the labyrinth, the semicircular canals, the cochlea being less developed in earlier vertebrates. The nerve appears immediately inferior to the pons and close to the facial nerve, the nervus intermedius issuing between them. The inferior cerebellar peduncle is here posterior and the cochlear division skirts its lateral side to reach the cochlear nuclei, whereas the vestibular division passes into the brainstem medial to the peduncle. The nerve runs anterolaterally to the internal acoustic

(auditory) meatus, its two portions forming a groove below the facial nerve, the nervus intermedius lying between them. Accompanied by the labyrinthine branch of the basilar artery, these structures enter the meatus, at the bottom of which the vestibulocochlear nerve divides into branches which pass through the lamina cribrosa. The cochlear division passes through the anteroinferior quadrant to reach the cochlea. The branches of the vestibular division pass through the two posterior quadrants, the nerves to the utricle and superior and lateral semicircular canals being above, the nerves to the sacculus and posterior semicircular canal below. (For work on the topography and components of the nerve consult the papers of Bergström, 1973, and the monographs of Rasmussen, 1960; Brodal, 1969.)

NUCLEI AND CENTRAL CONNECTIONS

The spiral ganglion of the cochlear division is in the cochlear modiolus. Its peripheral fibres come from the spiral organ of Corti. The ganglion of the vestibular division is in the internal auditory meatus. Its peripheral fibres come from the maculae and cristae of the utricle, saccule and semicircular canals. The two nerves unite in the internal auditory meatus. The cochlear ends in two nuclei, dorsal and ventral to the inferior cerebellar peduncle. From the dorsal cochlear nucleus second-order neurons traverse the peduncle to join the contralateral lateral lemniscus. Axons from the neurons in the ventral nucleus also join the lateral lemniscus to connect with the inferior colliculus. Fibres from the lateral lemniscus synapse in the medial geniculate nucleus, whence fibres traverse the posterior limb of the internal capsule to reach the anterior transverse gyrus of the temporal lobe. The vestibular fibres are distributed to all the vestibular nuclei, which partly underlie the area acoustica of the fourth ventricle and are partly anterior to the inferior cerebellar peduncle. Some fibres also pass directly into the cerebellum. (For details of the central cochlear and vestibular connections see Rasmussen and Windle, 1960; Crosby, Humphrey and Lauer, 1962; Whitfield, 1967; Brodal, 1969; Williams and Warwick, 1980.)

CHAPTER SIX

The eyeball and its dimensions

This chapter summarizes the gross anatomy and topography of the eyeball. Further details are given within specific chapters.

6.1　ORBITAL LOCATION

Each eyeball is located in the anterior orbit, nearer to the roof and lateral wall than to the other walls (Fig. 6.1), and occupies only one-fifth of the orbital cavity. In forward gaze the corneal summit is equidistant from the superior and inferior orbital margins. A straight line running across the superior and inferior orbital margins would rarely touch the cornea, while a line joining the medial and lateral margins would leave almost one-third of the globe anterior to it. The eyeball is thus least protected on its lateral side. Here surgical approach is easiest; and

blows from the lower lateral side may damage or even rupture the globe (Fig. 6.2).

The interpupillary distance is 58–60 mm; the distance between medial canthi is approximately half this in the adult. These distances are altered in certain dysmorphic cranial disorders. The interpupillary distance is increased in hypertelorism and the intercanthal distance increases in Waardenberg's syndrome (telecanthus).

The eyeball is not spherical, but consists of two modified spheres fused together. The anterior, the **cornea**, is of smaller radius (7.8 mm) than the posterior, the **sclera** (12 mm). Their junction, the **limbus**, is marked at the surface by the **external scleral sulcus** (Fig. 6.3).

The globe is widest at its anteroposterior diameter (24 mm), and is flattened in its vertical (23 mm), as

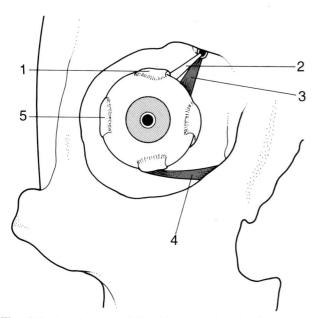

Fig. 6.1 Anterior view of the oblique muscles. 1 = Superior rectus; 2 = reflected tendon of the superior oblique; 3 = muscle body of the superior oblique; 4 = inferior oblique muscle; 5 = lateral rectus muscle. (From Renard, G., Lemasson, C. and Saraux, H. (1965) *Anatomie de l'oeil et de ses Annexes*, published by Paul Masson.)

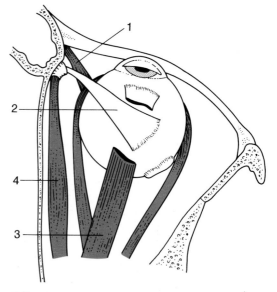

Fig. 6.2 View of the oblique muscles from above. 1 = Inferior oblique; 2 = reflected tendon of the superior oblique; 3 = superior rectus muscle (sectioned to reveal the superior oblique tendon); 4 = the muscle belly of the superior oblique. (From Renard, G., Lemasson, C. and Saraux, H. (1965) *Anatomie de l'oeil et de ses Annexes*, published by Paul Masson.)

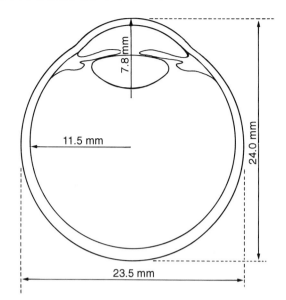

Fig. 6.3 Sagittal section of the globe.

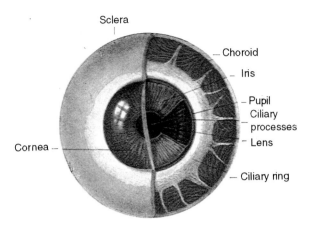

Fig. 6.4 Anterior aspect of the eye. Parts of the cornea, sclera and iris have been removed to show the internal structures.

compared with its horizontal, diameter (23.5 mm) (Fig. 6.3).

6.2 LAYERS AND COMPARTMENTS OF THE EYEBALL

The eyeball consists of three concentric layers surrounding the transparent media (Figs 6.4 and 6.5).

CORNEOSCLERAL ENVELOPE

The external layer is the tough, inelastic, corneoscleral envelope. The **cornea**, its anterior sixth, is perfectly transparent, while its posterior five-sixths, the **sclera**, is white and opaque.

UVEA

The middle layer, the uvea, is highly vascular and hence nutritive. It consists from behind forwards of the **choroid** and **ciliary body**, and the **iris**, which is perforated by the pupil.

The iris, located in the plane of the limbus, separates the anterior chamber in front from the lens and its suspensory ligament behind. Behind the iris and surrounding the equatorial region of the lens is the smaller posterior chamber, continuous through the pupil with the anterior chamber. Aqueous humour, secreted by the ciliary body, flows into the posterior chamber, through the pupil and out of the globe through a drainage apparatus at the angle of the anterior chamber. The space behind the lens and ciliary body, and within the concavity of the retina, is filled with the vitreous.

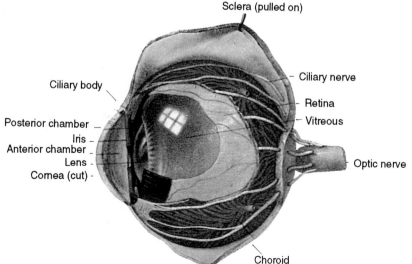

Fig. 6.5 Preparation to show the coats and contents of the eye. Parts of the sclera, cornea, choroid, ciliary body, iris and retina have been removed.

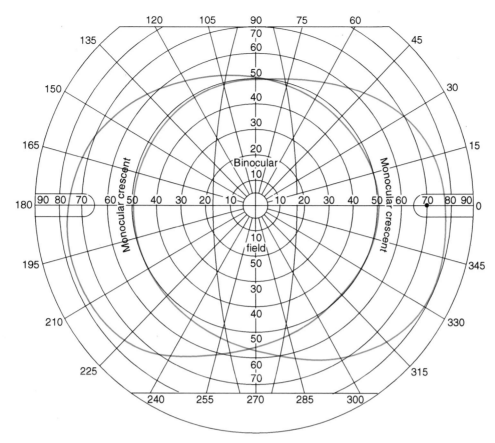

Fig. 6.6 The superimposed binocular fields of a normal adult male, to demonstrate the central region of binocular overlap and the peripheral, monocular crescents.

RETINA

The internal photosensitive layer is the retina, consisting of receptors and neurons and concerned with initial processing of visual information. Visual fixation is achieved by the **fovea**, a specialized retinal area that contains cones exclusively.

The corneoscleral coat confines the intraocular pressure and preserves the eye's dimensions. The uveal circulation is not only the source of the intraocular fluid but also nourishes the outer, non-vascularized retinal layers.

The construction of the globe, its motility and location in the orbit, are specifically adapted to create, maintain and conserve the visual process.

The forward-looking eyes of primates provide almost total overlap of the visual fields (Fig. 6.6). This overlap is the basis for stereopsis, maintained over a wide field of gaze and while tracking objects moving towards or away from an observer or across the visual field. Coincidence of visual direction of the two eyes is achieved by their stable suspension in the orbits and is modified as necessary by the coordinated activity of the extraocular muscles.

6.3 DESCRIPTIVE TERMINOLOGY

The summit of the corneal curvature is its **anterior pole**; the centre of the scleral curve is its **posterior pole**, slightly nasal to the fovea (Fig. 6.7). A line joining these points is the **geometric axis**. Anteroposterior planes passing through the poles are meridia, and are conveniently numbered as the hours of a clock: the **sagittal meridian** divides the globe vertically from 12 to 6 o'clock into nasal and temporal halves; the **horizontal meridian** passes from 9 o'clock (temporally) to 3 o'clock (nasally) and divides the globe into upper and lower halves. A coronal or frontal plane passing through the equator of the globe divides it into anterior and posterior halves.

The **geometric equator** of the eye is a circle around its external surface equidistant from the two poles. If the globe were a perfect sphere, this would be a perfect circle in a coronal plane at right-angles to the geometric axis, but the sclera bulges temporally, so that the **anatomical equator**, equidistant from the poles of the *actual*, not the theoretical, eye is tilted backwards on the temporal side (1–15 mm) and forwards nasally (Salzmann, 1912) (Fig. 6.8). Its plane

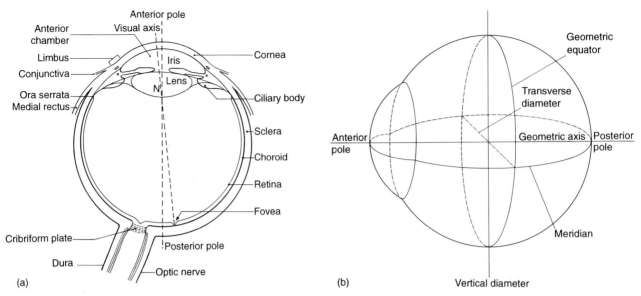

Fig. 6.7 The principal coordinates and planes of the human globe.

is not, therefore, quite perpendicular to the geometric axis (Kestenbaum, 1963). The elongation of the globe in axial myopia shifts the posterior pole and hence the geometric equator backwards, but has little influence on features anterior to the equator, e.g. distances from limbus to ora serrata or, to a lesser extent, the vortex veins. Kestenbaum (1963) introduced the term **surgical equator** to describe the greatest circumference of the globe approximately in the coronal plane. This will not be materially influenced by prolongation of the poles in axial myopia

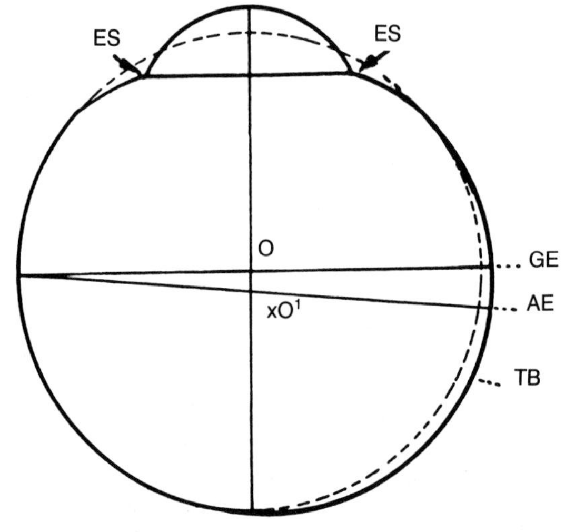

or corneal ectasia, but is increased in congenital glaucoma (where the globe is enlarged) while decreased in microphthalmos (where it is smaller).

The **geometric centre** of the eyeball (actually the centre of the scleral sphere) is about 12 mm behind the anterior pole. Of the 'scleral circle' 300° is occupied by sclera, the rest being cornea (Fig. 6.7b). The corneal radius is 7.8 mm. The corneal surface (arc) occupies 95.5° of the 'corneal circle' (about 13 mm). The **centre of rotation** of the eye is behind its geometric centre (13.1 mm, not 12 mm). It lies close to, but not on, the optic axis.

OPTIC LINES AND AXES

The dioptric apparatus of the eye, chiefly the interfaces of the air and tear film, and the lens with the aqueous and vitreous, focuses an inverted image of the visual scene on the retina (Fig. 6.9). The extent of this image on the retina, is the **visual field**. Points in the visual field may be connected to retinal points by 'visual lines', each passing through the eye's **nodal point**. This point lies on the **geometric axis** near the posterior pole of the lens, 7.2 mm behind the corneal apex (there are actually two nodal points, one 7.08 and one 7.33 mm behind the lens). The nodal point is about 17.2 mm anterior to the central retina (Gullstrand, 1912).

The **visual axis** is a line connecting the fovea to a fixation point in the visual field. The **optic axis** is a line passing through the centres of the anterior and posterior curves of the cornea and lens and the principal, focal and nodal points. (Actually the line does not pass precisely through all of these; the lens

Fig. 6.8 Deviations of the globe from the scleral sphere. −−−−−Theoretical scleral circle; ——— actual deviation from the ideal; AE = anatomic equator; ES = external sulcus sclerae; GE = geometric equator; O = geometric centre of the scleral sphere; O' = the approximate centre of the scleral bulge; TB = temporal bulge. (From Kestenbaum, A. (1963) *Applied Anatomy of the Eye*, published by Grune & Stratton.)

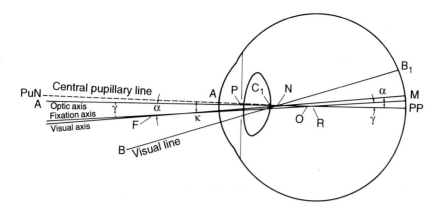

Fig. 6.9 Axis and angles of the eye. A = Anterior pole (intersection of optic axis and cornea); B = a target in the visual field; B_1 = the corresponding retinal point; BNB = the visual line; C_1 = centre of curvature of the cornea; F = fixation point; FNM = visual axis; M = centre of the macula; N = nodal point (intersection of all visual lines); O = geometric centre of the scleral sphere (the *optic axis* is a line approximately containing O, C_1 and the centre of curvature of the surfaces of the lens); P = centre of the corneal base close to the centre of the pupil; PP = posterior pole (the intersection of optic axis and sclera); PuN = perpendicular corneal line (almost coincident with the optic axis). Note that angle α = FNA and is the same as the angle in N between the visual axis and the optic axis. Angle γ = FRA, the angle in R between the fixation axis and optic axis. Angle κ = PuNF, and is the same as the angle in N between the central pupillary line and visual axis. (From Kestenbaum, A. (1963) *Applied Anatomy of the Eye*, published by Grune & Stratton.)

is slightly tilted, with its temporal edge more posterior – Fig. 6.8.) The optic axis intersects the corneal surface about 0.25 mm nasal to its centre. It intersects the visual axis at the nodal point but is more nasal posteriorly, because the posterior pole is slightly nasal to the fovea. The angle between the optic and visual axis is the **angle alpha**. This angle is large in the infant but decreases with age, because of differences in the relative rates of retinal growth between fovea and disc compared with the rest of the retina.

The **fixation axis** connects the centre of rotation to the point of fixation. It lies near to the visual axis but does not pass through the nodal point. The **central pupillary line** is erected perpendicular to the cornea at its centre, and approximates with the optic axis. The angle between this pupillary line and visual axis is **angle kappa**, and approximates to angle alpha.

In shape the eyeball is asymmetric, the curves of its layers being shorter nasally than temporally (Hogan, Alvarado and Weddell, 1971), with the ora serrata about 1 mm more anterior on the nasal side. The pupil and lens are displaced slightly to the nasal side, making the anterior chamber narrower there (Hogan, Alvarado and Weddell, 1971). The lens is tilted, with its nasal edge more anterior. The optic nerve is about 4 mm nasal to the fovea.

The sclera's temporal bulge causes a deviation of the theoretical horopter, which assumes the posterior globe to be perfectly spherical. The **horopter** is that locus of points in visual space which are seen singly and in the same frontal plane as the fixation point (i.e. their images fall on corresponding retinal points

of the two eyes (Fig. 6.10)). Points to the right or left of fixation are imaged on the temporal hemiretina of one eye and the nasal hemiretina of the other. As the

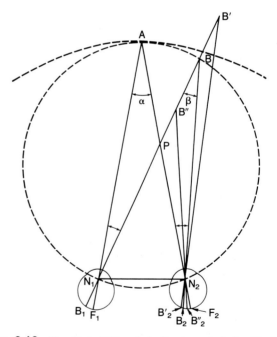

Fig. 6.10 The Vieth–Müller circle (the horopter). A = Fixation point; AF = visual axis of the two eyes convergent on A (circle AN_1N_2 is the Vieth–Müller circle); B = a point on the circle passing through the point fixated and the nodal points of the eyes (B′ and B″ are two points on the N_1B, outside and inside the circle); B_1 = the retinal point in the left eye corresponding with B, B′ and B″; B_2, B_2', B_2'' = retinal point in the right eye corresponding with B, B′ and B″; F_1, F_2 = foveal centres of the two eyes. α, β are the periphery angles above the cord N_1 N_2 at A and B. (From Kestenbaum, A. (1963) *Applied Anatomy of the Eye*, published by Grune & Stratton.)

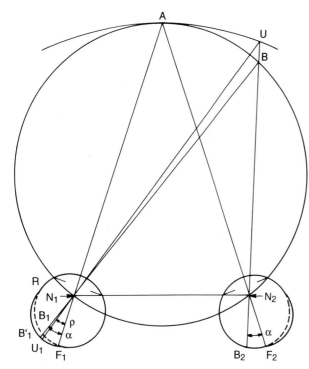

Fig. 6.11 The Herring–Hillebrand deviation and temporal bulge of the sclera. A = Fixation point; B = a point on the Vieth–Müller theoretical 'horopter'; B_1 = point where B would be imaged if the left retina were part of a real sphere; B'_1 = the image of B on the real left retina; B_2 = image of B on the right retina; F_1 and F_2 = centres of the foveas; N_1 and N_2 = nodal points; U_1 = point on the left retina which is as far from F_1 as B_2 is from F_2; U = point that is imaged on U_1 and B_2.

curves of the nasal and temporal retinas are not the same (because of the temporal bulge), the horopter itself is less curved, and for a distance of about 2 m the horopter is almost a straight line (Kestenbaum, 1963) (Fig. 6.11).

6.4   TOPOGRAPHIC ANATOMY (Table 6.1)

CONJUNCTIVAL SAC

The conjunctival sac is formed by the continuous, non-keratinized epithelium which lines the ocular surface and merges with the corneal epithelium. The tarsal conjunctiva lines the lids, extends into the fornices and then reflects onto the globe as its bulbar part. The distances from the lid margins or the limbus are given in Fig. 6.12.

At the corneoscleral limbus above and below are the **palisades of Vogt**, a series of radially oriented finger-like processes consisting of vascular, connective tissue palisades alternating with intervening zones of thickened epithelium (up to ten cell layers). The limbus is the location of the stem cells of the cornea which give rise to new corneal epithelial cells

by a process of division and centripetal migration. (Bron, 1973; Thoft and Friend, 1983). In pigmented eyes, the interpalisades are strikingly outlined by pigment located in the basal cells; in such eyes the centripetal flow of cells is visible as 'pigment slide'.

The **conjunctival epithelium** is rich in goblet cells which secrete mucus, except at the limbus. Inflammatory cells concerned with ocular defence are found both in the epithelium and subepithelially. The stem cells of the conjunctiva are located in the fornices.

CORNEA

The cornea is ellipsoid and shortest in its vertical diameter because of the scleral overlap above and below: its horizontal diameter is 11.75 mm and its vertical 10.6 mm (Fig. 6.13). The anterior radius of curvature is about 7.8 mm on the optic axis. The refractive index of the cornea is 1.376: it is the most transparent tissue of the eye. The interface between air and precorneal tear film contributes 45 dioptres to the total 60 dioptric power of the non-accommodated eye. The cornea has several layers:

1. a non-keratinizing surface **epithelium**;
2. a tough connective tissue **stroma**, rich in ground substance, accounting for 90% of its thickness. The narrow separation and fine diameter of its collagen fibrils account for its near-perfect transparency;
3. the **endothelium** – a single posterior cellular layer in contact with the aqueous humour seated on a thick basal lamina (Descemet's membrane). It actively removes water from the stroma, thereby maintaining deturgescence and clarity. At birth, cell density ranges from 3500 to 4000 cells/mm^2. The adult endothelial density is from 1500 to 2500 cells/mm^3 with a total number of about 300 000 to 500 000. Mitosis is unusual in the absence of injury.

SCLERA

The sclera is a tough coat of connective tissue whose collagen fibrils vary widely in diameter and are intricately interwoven. This accounts for its light-scattering properties, which render it opaque. The sclera is thinnest beneath the attachments of rectus muscles (0.3 mm) and at the equator (0.4 mm), thicker near the limbus (0.8 mm) and thickest around the optic nerve (1.0–1.35 mm). The direction of the collagen bundles reinforces the strength of the sclera at the limbus and at its forward continuity with the tendons of muscles, but the sclera is more pliable

Table 6.1 Dimensions and related measurements concerning the globe

	Adult	Infant	
Globe			
Weight (gm)	7.14[T]; **7.45**[Ws]; 7.5[H]	Neonate 1 year 13–15 years	2.29[Wh] 4.05 5.87–6.5[Ws]
Specific gravity	**1.077**[Sch]		
Volume (ml)	6.5[Ws]; **7.2**[Ws]		
Surface area (cm^2)	**22.86**[Br]		
Diameter A–P (mm)	24.15[Me]	Birth	16.4[Ws]
	24.2 (22.9–26.4)[Sa]	Birth	16–17[So]
	24.26[Sa]		17.1[Sa]
	21–26[Ste]	3 years	22.5–23[So]
	29 (myopia)[Ste]		
	20 (hypermetropia)[Ste]		
Transverse (mm)		Infant	16.00[Ws,Me]
	24.13[Me]		
	23.6 (22.2–26.4)[Sa]		
Vertical (mm)		Infant	15.4[Ws]
	23.2 (22.2–25.8)[Sa]		
	23.5[Ste,Me]		
	23.7[Sa]		

Transverse and vertical diameters are less variable than sagittal.
Male eyes are slightly larger than female[Sa], e.g.:

		Male	Female
A–P		24.6	23.9
Transverse		23.5	23.0
Vertical		23.9	23.4
Inter-pupillary distance:		58–60 mm	
Inter-canthal distance:	(mode)	33–34[Wa]	32–33
	range	24–39	
	(mean)	31.7[Fr]	30.8
	range	26–38	

In the **reduced eye** of Donders, the two principal points and two nodal points of the schematic eye are reduced each to a single principal and nodal point. Some dimensions of the reduced eye are: Refractive Index: 1.336 Nodal Point: 7.08 behind the anterior corneal surface (i.e. in posterior lens). The anterior focal distance is 17.05 mm anterior to the nodal point (15.7 mm in front of the anterior cornea). Its posterior focal distance is 22.78 mm (or 24.13 mm behind the anterior cornea), i.e., in an average eye, it lies in the retinal plane.

Conjunctiva			
Conjunctival sac; depth (lid margin to fornix) (mm)	Temporal Superior Inferior	5[Ba] 13 9	
Limbus to fornix distance (mm)	Nasal Temporal Superior Inferior	7[Wh,T] 14 8–10 8–10	
Limbal palisades (μm)	Palisade width Interpalisade width Length	30–50[Vo]; 40[G] 100–150[Vo]; 70[G] 70–90[Vo]; 36[G]	

Cornea			
Area			
Anterior (mm^2)	106[Br]		
Posterior (mm^2)	110		
Diameter			
Horizontal (mm)	11.75	10[MG]	
Vertical (mm)	10.6		
Height (mm)	2.6[H]	7.1[Me,Man]	
Radius of curvature			
Anterior – central (mm)	7.8[H]		
Posterior – central (mm)	6.5[H] (6.2–6.8)	7[Wl]	

	Adult	Infant
Cornea (contd)		
Anterior arc length (mm)	11.6[Br]; 13.0[K]	
Thickness – central (mm)	0.52[M]	
Thickness – peripheral (mm)	0.67 (fourth decade); 0.63 (sixth decade)[Ma]	
Endothelial cell density	500 000/mm^2; 3000–3500/mm^2 young adult[Yere]	
Corneal refractive index	1.376	
Power (dioptres)	42; 45[TT]	48.4[Mo]
Sclera		
Thickness (mm)[H]		
Sub-rectus		
Pre-rectus	0.3	
Equator	0.6	
Limbus	0.4–0.6	
Peri-papillary	0.8	
Radius of curvature (mm)	1.0	
External	12.0	
Internal	11.5	
Limbus		
Meridional width (mm)		
Superior/inferior	2.0	
Medial/lateral	1.5	
Marginal vascular arcades (mm)	0.5	

The limbus is not of equal width around its circumference. Because of the greater scleral overlap above and below, a hypertrophied Schwalbe's line (posterior embryotoxon) is more likely to be visible on biomicroscopy in the horizontal meridian.

	Adult	Infant
Anterior chamber		
Depth (mm)	3.15 (2.6–4.4)	
Volume (μl)	250; 186 ± 37[Br] Regression 7.5% per decade	
Surface area (mm^2)	323[Br]	
Diameter (mm)	11.3–12.4	
Posterior chamber		
Volume (μl)	65[Br]	
Drainage angle		
Circumference (mm)	35.5–38	
Trabecular width (mm)	0.8 (anteroposterior)	
Diameter of Schlemm's canal (μm)	200–400 long axis; 10–25 short axis	
Number of collector veins	25–35	
Width of collector veins at origin (μm)	20–90	
Number of aqueous veins	2–8	
Iris		
Area (mm^2)	110[Br]	
Diameter (mm)	12.0	
Circumference (mm)	38.0	
Thickness Root (mm)	0.5	
Collarette (mm)	0.6	
Pupillary zone width (mm)	1.6	3.1
Ciliary zone width (mm)	2.4	4.1 (dark adapted)
Pupil diameter (mm)	1.5–8.0	

	Adult	Infant

Ciliary body

The ciliary body is narrower medially and above.

	Adult	Infant
Total width (mm)		
Temporal (mm)	7.5–8[H]	
Nasal (mm)	6.5–7.0	
Superior (mm)	7.0	
Inferior (mm)	7.0	
Medial/superior	5.5–6.3[TT]	
Temporal/inferior	4.5–5.2[TT]	
Ciliaris width (mm)	Average 2.0	
Ciliaris area (mm^2)	600[B]	
Pars plana width all zones (mm)	3.5–4.5[TT]	
Pars plana area (mm^2)	245[Br]	
Number of ciliary processes	70–80	

Aqueous

	Adult	Infant
Bulk flow (μl/min)	2.26	
(monkey)	(1.5–2.0)[Br]	
Uveoscleral flow (monkey) (μl/min)	0.5	
% of A/C volume	1–2%	

Intraocular pressure (mm Hg)   15 (10–21)

Suprachoroidal space

	Adult	Infant
Outer surface area (cm^2)	16[H]	

Choroid

	Adult	Infant
Surface area (m^2)	1180	
Thickness:		
sub foveal (mm)	0.3	
elsewhere (mm)	0.1–10.15[JE]	
Volume (μl)	100	
Ora thickness (μm)	3–18	
Bruch's membrane thickness:		
general (μm)	2	
peripapillary (μm)	2–4	
periphery (μm)	1–2	

Ciliary arteries/nerves

	Adult	Infant
Short posterior ciliary arteries/nerves	20	
Long posterior ciliary arteries/nerves	1 nasal, 1 temporal; (the arteries split into two in scleral canals)	

Lens

The slight tilt of the lens about a vertical axis places its nasal edge posterior to its temporal edge

	Adult	Infant
Area Anterior (mm^2)	83[Br]	
Posterior (mm^2)	87[Br]	
Volume (μl)	140[Br]	
	163 age 20–40 years[He]	
	240 age 80–90 years[He]	
Weight (mg)	180 at 25 years	85 at birth
	250 at 90 years	65–130 at birth[H]
Sagittal width (mm)	4–5	Neonate 3.8[Ge]
	3–8	3.5–4.0 newborn[H]
	4.0 up to 50 years[H]	
	4.75–5.75 by 90 years[H]	

	Adult	Infant
Lens (contd)		
Equatorial diameter (mm)	9; 9–10	6.5 neonate[Wf,H]
Circumference (mm)	31.4 (with 10.0 mm diameter)	
Anterior radius of curvature (mm)	10 (8–14)[Wf]	5 neonate[Pf]
Posterior radius of curvature (mm)	6 (4–7.5)[Wf]	4 neonate[Pf]
Distance: posterior lens to retina (mm)	17.3[K]	
Refractive Index: cortex	1.386	1.433[Wo]
nuclear	1.41	1.477[Wl]
'overall'	1.42	
Lens power (dioptres)	16–20	38.4[Lu]

Zonule		
Origin (mm)	1.5 anterior to ora	
Lens insertion (mm)	2.55 band over equator of the lens	
	1.5 on anterior lens surface[TT]	
	1.0 on posterior lens surface[TT]	

Vitreous		
Area (mm^2)	1330[Br]	
Volume (mm^3)	5900[Br]	

Retina[TT,O,H]		
Foveola width (mm)	0.35	
Fovea centralis (mm)	1.85	
Rod-free zone (mm)	0.57	
Parafoveal band (mm)	0.5	
Perifoveal band (mm)	1.5	
Macula lutea (mm)	5 in the horizontal	
Area centralis (mm)	5–6 in the horizontal:	
	subtends 18°20' of the visual field	

Rods		
Rod number	(110–125) × 10^6	
Maximum density per mm^2	160 000 (2.5–3.0 mm from foveal centre,	
	at the edge of the area centralis)	
Peripheral density per mm^2	23 000–50 000	

Cones		
Cone number	(6.3–6.8) × 10^6	
Maximum density per mm^2	147 300 (at the foveola)	
Peripheral density per mm^2	5000	
Cones of the foveola	2500	
Cones in the rod-free fovea	35 000	
Total foveal cones	100 000	

Pigment epithelium		
Pigment epithelial number	(4.2–6.5) × 10^6	

Key to references

Ba Baker (1900)
Br Brubacker and Pedersen (1983)
Fr Freihofer (1980)
Ge Gernet (1964a)
G Goldberg and Bron (1982)
H Hogan, Alvarado and Weddell (1971)
He Heine (1898)
JE J. Ernest cited by Brubacker and Pederson (1982)
K Kestenbaum (1963)

Lu Luyckx (1966)
M Maurice (1969)
Ma Martola and Baum (1968)
Man Mandell (1967)
Me Merkel and Orr (1892)
MG Marshall and Grindle (1978)
Mo Molnár (1970)
O Østerberg (1935)
Pf von Pflugk (1909)
Sa Salzmann (1912)
So Sorsby and Sheridan (1960)

Ste Stenstrom (1946)
T Testut or Testut and Merkel (1905)
TT Tripathi and Tripathi (1984)
Vo Vogt (1921)
Wa Waardenburg (1951)
Wf Wolff (1976)
Wh Whitnall (1921)
Wl Weale (1982)
Wo Woinow (1874)
Ws Weiss (1897)

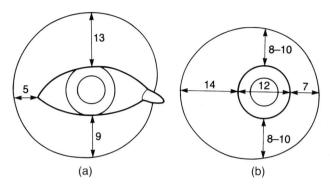

Fig. 6.12 (a) Dimensions (in mm) of the human conjunctival sac, measured from the lid margins with the eye open; (b) dimensions (in mm) of the human conjunctival sac, measured from the limbus with an assumed corneal diameter of 12 mm. (From Tripathi, R. C. and Tripathi, B. J. in Davson, H. (ed) (1984) *The Eye*, published by Academic Press.)

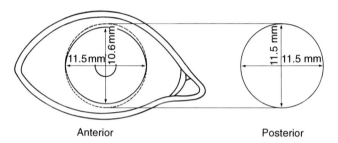

Fig. 6.13 The elliptical shape of the anterior and round shape of the posterior corneal edges; also the vertical and horizontal diameters of the anterior and posterior cornea. (From Hogan, M.J., Alvardo, J.A. and Weddell, J.E. (1971) *Histology of the Human Eye*, published by W.B. Saunders.)

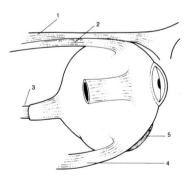

Fig. 6.14 General view of Tenon's capsule on the globe. 1 = Sheath of superior oblique; 2 = superior rectus; 3 = optic nerve; 4 = inferior rectus; 5 = inferior oblique. (From Renard, G., Lemasson, C. and Saraux, H. (1965) *Anatomie de l'oeil et de ses Annexes*, published by Paul Masson.)

near the optic foramen, where its fibrils are continuous with its dural sheath (Jakobiec and Ozanics, 1982). There is less ground substance associated with the sclera than with the cornea.

The loose vascular connective tissue layer over the sclera's outer surface is the **episclera**, which anteriorly separates sclera from the bulbar conjunctiva.

The globe is invested with a thin fascia of connective tissue (Tenon's capsule), which is fused anteriorly with the episclera at the limbus, but is prolonged around the muscle sheaths, and posteriorly over the distal part of the optic nerve (Fig. 6.14).

LIMBUS

The limbus is a specialized transitional zone at the external scleral sulcus, where sclera merges with cornea, the convex corneal edge being accommodated by a reciprocal concavity at the anterior scleral margin. The scleral overlap is greater above than below (Fig. 6.15); here the corneal epithelium

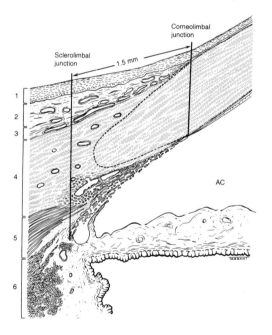

Fig. 6.15 Diagrammatic representation of the limbus showing various structures from superficial to deep regions.
1 = Conjunctiva; 2 = conjunctival stroma; 3 = Tenon's and episclera; 4 = limbal or cornea sclera stroma containing intrascleral plexus of veins and collector channels from Schlemm's canal; 5 = meridional portion of ciliary muscle; 6 = radial and circular portions of ciliary muscle. The pathologist's limbus is about 1.5 mm wide and extends posteriorly from a line joining the peripheral termination of Bowman's zone of the cornea and Descemet's membrane. This histologist's limbus (dotted line) is represented by a cone-shaped termination of the corneal lamellae into the sclera. (From Tripathi, R. C. and Tripathi, B. J. in Davson, H. (ed.) (1984) *The Eye*, published by Academic Press.)

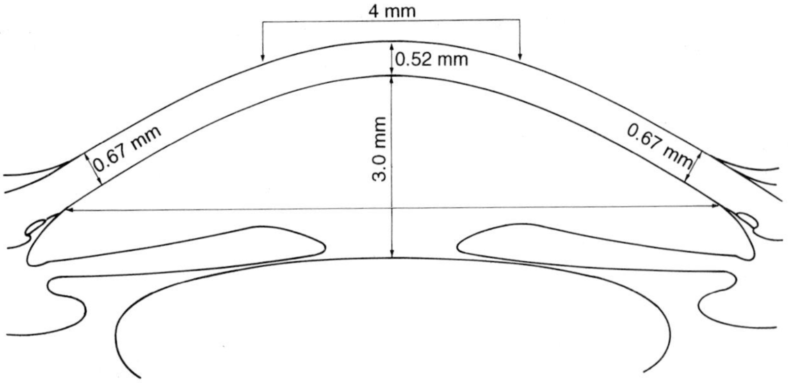

Fig. 6.16 Sagittal view of the anterior segment showing the corneal height and the central 4 mm of the cornea (which is optically important), also the comparative thickness of the central and peripheral cornea. (From Hogan, M.J., Alvarado, J.A. and Weddell, J.E. (1971) *History of the Human Eye*, published by W.B. Saunders.)

becomes conjunctival, though lacking the goblet cells of bulbar conjunctiva. Superiorly and inferiorly a papillary arrangement appears, giving rise to a distinct palisade pattern.

The superficial width of the limbus is 2 mm in the vertical meridian and 1.5 mm in the horizontal. Its corneal limit is the termination of Bowman's layer anteriorly and of Descemet's layer posteriorly; its scleral limit is the tip of the scleral spur. Anteroexternal to the scleral spur is the internal scleral sulcus, which contains the trabecular meshwork and canal of Schlemm. At the limbus, the collagen lamellae lose their regular fibril width and separation in the cornea and blend with the interwoven networks of the sclera.

ANTERIOR CHAMBER

The anterior chamber is a compartment filled with aqueous humour, lying behind the cornea and in front of the iris and the lens in the pupillary space. It is shallower in hypermetropes and deeper in myopes, but is almost equal in the two eyes of the same individual. The axial depth of the chamber is about 3.0 mm (range 2.6–4.4 mm) and its volume in the emmetrope is about 250 µl. (The posterior chamber's volume is about 60 µl (Fig. 6.16).)

The **angle** of the chamber is its most peripheral part and gives access to the drainage structures by which aqueous leaves the eye (hence the term **drainage angle**) (Fig. 6.17). Its features are, in sequence:

1. the trabecular meshwork, 0.8–1 mm wide in meridional section and the main site of resistance to outflow of aqueous;
2. the canal of Schlemm, a circumferential channel 30–45 µm in diameter, located in the internal scleral sulcus;
3. 25–35 collector channels 20–90 µm wide, which empty into deep scleral plexuses and into;
4. about 2–8 aqueous veins, which deliver aqueous directly into the episcleral venous plexuses.

IRIS

The iris is a diaphragm whose periphery is attached to the anteromedial aspect of the ciliary muscle. It forms the posterior boundary of the anterior chamber, is about 12 mm in diameter, 0.6 mm thick at the collarette (its thickest point) and 0.5 mm at its periphery. It is perforated by the **pupil**, which is displaced slightly nasal to centre, and its pupillary margin rests posteriorly on the anterior surface of the lens. The degree of contact varies with pupil size and is greatest in mid-dilatation. Pupil size also regulates the entry of light into the eye.

In cross-section the iris shows a stromal layer anteriorly and a double epithelial layer posteriorly. The stroma is continuous with that in the ciliary body at the iridial periphery.

The anterior iridial surface is divided into a **pupillary zone**, from pupil margin to collarette (1.6 mm), and a **ciliary zone** peripheral to this (2.4 mm). The anterior leaf of mesenchyme is lacking in the pupillary zone, which exhibits numerous crypts. The ciliary zone exhibits circular contraction ridges, and also radial ridges that correspond to the location of the iris vessels.

Layers of the iris

The layers of the iris are:

1. the **anterior border** layer, a network of fibroblasts and pigment cells. The degree of pigmentation determines iridial colour;
2. the **anterior leaf** of stroma;
3. the **posterior leaf**, containing nerves and blood vessels;
4. the **sphincter muscle** (1 mm wide) in the pupillary zone, readily visible in blue irides. Contraction, induced by parasympathetic stimulation, causes pupil constriction;
5. the **dilator muscle**, chiefly in the ciliary zone, consists of processes of the anterior

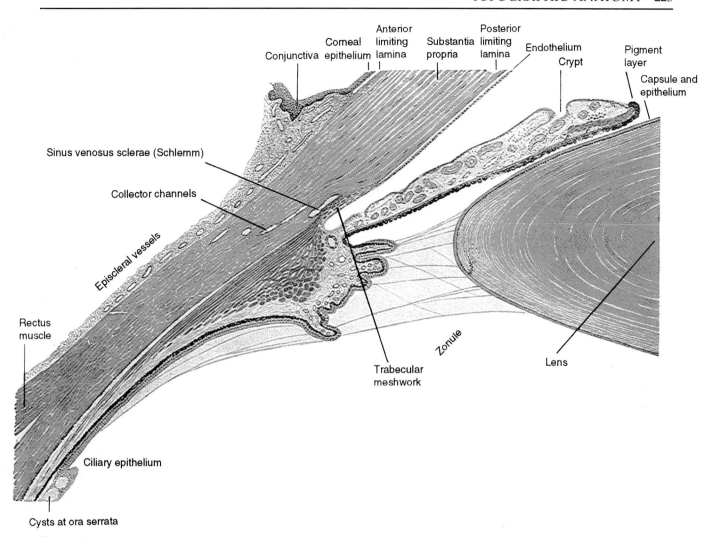

Conjunctiva Corneal epithelium Anterior limiting lamina Substantia propria Posterior limiting lamina Endothelium Crypt Pigment layer Capsule and epithelium

Sinus venosus sclerae (Schlemm)

Collector channels

Episcleral vessels

Rectus muscle

Ciliary epithelium

Trabecular meshwork

Zonule

Lens

Cysts at ora serrata

Fig. 6.17 Meridional section through the limbic region of the eye.

myoepithelium extending as a sheet central to the sphincter's margin. Contraction, induced by sympathetic innervation, causes pupil dilatation;

6. the **anterior myoepithelium**, pigmented;
7. the **posterior pigmented epithelium**;
8. a **basal lamina**.

The major arterial circle of the iris, located in the anterior face of the ciliary body, gives off numerous radial branches supplying iridial tissues. It is reinforced by an inconstant minor arterial circle within the collarette.

CILIARY BODY

The ciliary body extends from the scleral spur to the ora serrata, a scalloped anterior margin of the retina (Fig. 6.18). In meridional section it is divided into a posterior **pars plana** (3.5–4.5 mm wide) and an

anterior **pars plicata** (about 2 mm wide), which bears 70–80 mm radial ciliary processes and encloses most of the ciliary muscle.

The width of the ciliary body is 4.5–5.2 mm nasally, 5.6–6.3 mm temporally (Hogan, Alvarado and Weddell, 1971).

Layers of the ciliary body

From within outwards these are:

1. an internal **limiting membrane**;
2. a non-pigmented **epithelium** which, in the region of the ciliary processes, is specialized for secretion of aqueous humour, which is under autonomic and humoral control;
3. a pigmented **epithelium**;
4. a **stroma** of connective tissue containing vessels and nerves and non-striated muscle; the meridional part of the ciliary muscle is chiefly in

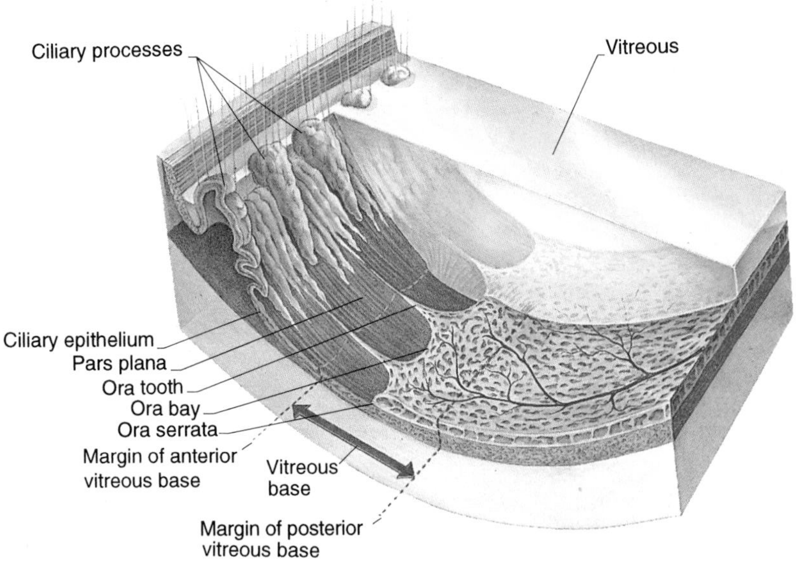

Ciliary processes

Vitreous

Ciliary epithelium
Pars plana
Ora tooth
Ora bay
Ora serrata
Margin of anterior
vitreous base
Vitreous
base
Margin of posterior
vitreous base

Fig. 6.18 Drawing of the vitreous base to show the pars plana and dentate processes of the ora serrata.

the pars plana, its radial and circular parts in the pars ciliaris.

A **supraciliary zone**, filled with pigmented cells and loose connective tissue, lies outside the ciliary body.

AQUEOUS HUMOUR

This clear fluid is secreted at a rate of about 2.5 μl/min and drains from the anterior chamber chiefly by bulk flow through the conventional drainage pathway, but also via a uveoscleral route from the anterior chamber into the supraciliary space. Secretion is under autonomic and humoral control. The rate of secretion and drainage maintains the intraocular pressure within the narrow range of 10–21 mmHg.

The aqueous humour supplies nutrients to the cornea and lens and exchanges gases and metabolites with these avascular tissues, serving the role of a vascular supply. This avascularity makes a major contribution to the transparency of these structures.

CHOROID

The choroid is chiefly a vascular layer nutritive to outer retinal layers. Its anterior boundary is the ora serrata and posteriorly it ends around the optic nerve head. The choroid is thickest beneath the fovea (0.3 mm) and thinnest at the ora (0.1–0.15 mm). It is supplied chiefly by the short posterior ciliary arteries, but also by the long posterior vessels, which traverse it in the nasal and temporal horizontal meridians. Rutnin (1967) has studied the visibility of choroidal structures ophthalmoscopically. Venous blood drains by multiple tributaries into several venae vorticosae

(vortex veins) whose formation is visible on fundoscopy in almost 90% of cases (Fig. 6.19). About half of these show an ampulliform dilatation prior to formation. The vortex veins traverse a scleral canal and, because of confluence, fewer veins exit at the scleral surface than are visible internally: fundus examination shows that about eight vortex veins (range 4–15) enter the canals (two per quadrant) while six (range 5–8; average 5.82) leave them. Internally, there are fewer veins nasally than temporally, externally the case is reversed. The intrascleral course averages 4.53 mm (1.25–8.5 mm), is longest superotemporally and shortest inferonasally (Rutnin, 1967). The vortex veins drain into the orbital veins, of which the chief is the superior ophthalmic, which enters the cavernous sinus through the superior orbital fissure. The long ciliary nerves and arteries pass forwards together in the horizontal meridian. Before reaching the suprachoroidal space they occupy discrete scleral canals separated by a thin septum. The nerve usually splits into two within its canal and the artery lies between the divisions, above the larger part on the nasal side, and above

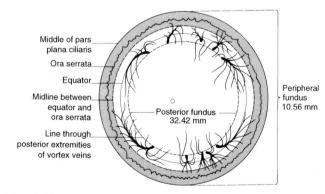

Middle of pars
plana ciliaris
Ora serrata
Equator
Midline between
equator and
ora serrata
Line through
posterior extremities
of vortex veins

Peripheral
fundus
10.56 mm

Posterior fundus
32.42 mm

Fig. 6.19 The vortex veins. (Redrawn from Rutnin, 1967)

the smaller on the temporal side. Nerve and artery become visible ophthalmoscopically about one-quarter to one-half the distance from disc to equator, inferior to the disc.

One or more short ciliary nerves are visible in 85% of eyes. They are most often seen close to the vertical meridian and below, where they are larger than above. Away from the vertical meridian the nerves are more numerous on the temporal side. Short ciliary arteries are less visible and appear 3–4.5 mm anterior to the disc.

Layers of the choroid

The layers of the choroid coat are:

1. an external layer of large vessels (**Haller's layer**);
2. a middle layer of vessels intermediate in size (**Sattler's layer**);
3. an internal layer of fenestrated capillaries, the **choriocapillaris**, intimately related to Bruch's membrane.

All these vessels lie in a loose matrix of connective tissue rich in melanocytes, and permeated by nerve fibres.

4. **Bruch's membrane**, about 2 μm thick, is formed by the basal laminae of the choriocapillaris and retinal pigment epithelium with an intervening zone of collagen and elastic tissue. It provides a barrier restricting movement of large molecules from the choroid. It is about 2 μm thick, rich in collagen, but also contains a middle elastic zone.

LENS

The lens is biconvex and centred behind the pupil (Fig. 6.17). It is the second most transparent tissue of the eye (the most transparent being the cornea). Its refractive index is high, effectively 1.42 because of the high protein content of its fibres. The lens grows throughout life, and in the adult its axial thickness is 4–5 mm and its equatorial diameter 9–10 mm. The anterior radius of curvature is 9–10 mm and the posterior 5.5–6 mm. The lens is suspended from the ciliary body by a system of suspensory ligaments or zonules. In distant gaze the lens is held under tension by the zonule; during accommodation the contraction of the ciliary muscle relaxes this and allows the lens to take up a more convex shape, thus increasing its optical power and focusing for near vision.

The lens is confined within a thick, somewhat elastic, collagenous **capsule** which is the basal lamina of the lenticular epithelium, a single cellular layer under its anterior aspect. The lens otherwise consists of regular, fusiform fibre cells packed closely in layers. Their long axes are meridional and they arch over the coronal plane to interdigitate with one another anteriorly and posteriorly at well-defined sutures. The fibres at the **core** or **nucleus** of the lens lack organelles, and those of the **cortex** or **outer lens** contain them only in their superficial part. Pre-equatorial mitosis of the lens epithelium adds new generations of fibres to the cortex, by which the lens grows throughout life.

ZONULE

The zonule consists of fine fibrils of glycoprotein, which arise from the epithelium of the pars plana and lateral walls and valleys of the pars plicata and insert into the zonular lamella of the lental capsule on both sides of the equator. When the ciliary muscle contracts during accommodation the distance between origin and insertion is reduced and the lens takes up a more curved shape. As the lens ages and grows, its capacity to change shape is gradually lost, as is the youthful ability to focus for near objects.

VITREOUS HUMOUR

This forms more than two-thirds of the ocular volume and occupies the retinal cup or vitreous cavity (Fig. 6.20). It is composed of a transparent gel (which is 98% water) of hyaluronic acid, embedded in which are fine embryonic collagenous fibrils, different from those in cornea and sclera. In places these serve to attach the vitreous to structures at its surface – including the retina at the discal margin, macula, vessels, the posterior lental capsule just central to the zonular attachments, and, most importantly, across a band 3–4 mm wide overlapping pars plana and peripheral retina (the 'vitreous base'). In the infant this is a narrow band just posterior to the ora serrata. In the outer layer (cortex) of the vitreous are a few cells (hyalocytes) which have synthetic functions.

The outer aspect of the vitreous is its hyaloid face. This invaginates between the ciliary processes as it extends from the vitreous base to its lenticular attachment. The postlenticular space separates the lens from a cup-shaped depression in the anterior vitreous face, the **patellar fossa**. The margin of the latter adheres to the lens over a circular zone, the **ligamentum hyaloidocapsulare** which is strong in youth but weakens with age. The hyaloid canal runs a sinuous

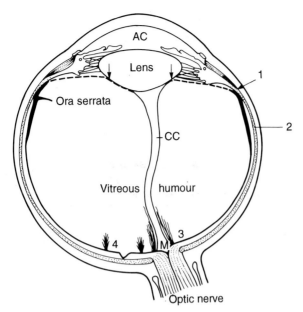

Fig. 6.20 Schematic view of the vitreous compartment. The vitreous body is traversed by Cloquet's canal (CC) containing hyaloidean vitreous that extends in an S-shaped fashion from a funnel-shaped expansion on the posterior aspect of the lens to the optic nerve head, where there is a smaller expansion, the so-called area of Martegiani (M). Anteriorly the vitreous face is in contact with the posterior lens surface, separated only by the capillary space of Berger which extends peripherally into the retrozonular space of the posterior chamber, the so-called canal of Petit. In young eyes the vitreous face is adherent to the posterior lens capsule in the region of the so-called hyaloideocapsular ligament (arrows). The vitreous body is firmly attached (solid line) to about a 2 mm zone of the pars plana (1), and is continuous posteriorly to about a 4 mm span of the peripheral retina (2). The dotted line anteriorly represents the anterior vitreous face which in places is in contact with the posterior zonular fibres. Posteriorly the vitreous face is attached at the edge of the optic disc (3) although not as firmly as at the vitreous base. A similar annual attachment 3–4 mm in diameter is seen in young eyes at the macular region (4). ACD = Anterior chamber. (From Tripathi, R. C. and Tripathi, B. J. in Davson, H. (ed.) (1984) *The Eye*, published by Academic Press.)

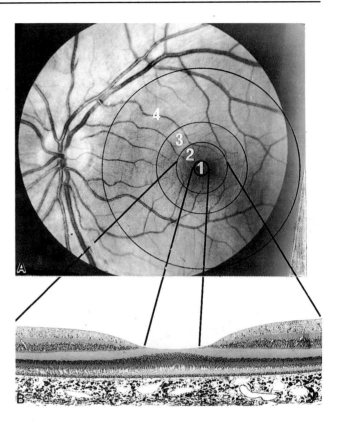

Fig. 6.21 (a) Fundus photograph of left human eye showing topographic demarcation of the area centralis measuring 5.5–6 mm in diameter (outermost circle) and its subdivision (inner circles). From an anatomic standpoint, the zones demarcated are in fact horizontal elliptical, rather than circular, as shown diagrammatically here. The central area of the macular region is represented by the fovea centralis (2), approximately 1.85 mm in diameter, which has a central pit, the foveola (1) 0.35 mm in diameter. The anatomically distinguishable retinal belts surrounding the fovea centralis are the parafovea (3), 0.55 mm wide, and the perifovea (4), 1.5 mm wide. (b) Transverse section of foveal retina matched to the fundus photograph shown in (a). (From Tripathi, R. C. and Tripathi, B. J. in Davson, H. (ed.) (1984) *The Eye*, published by Academic Press.)

course from the postlenticular space to a funnel-shaped expansion at the optic disc. In infancy the structure of the vitreous is relatively homogeneous. With age the density falls (more in the central than the cortical vitreous) and radiating condensations spread out as *tracts* from the ciliary and retinal surface.

RETINA

The retina develops from the optic cup, an outgrowth of the brain. The outer wall becomes retinal pigment epithelium, the inner, the neural retina, includes the light-sensitive photoreceptors (the rods and cones). Except at the ora serrata and margin of the optic disc, adhesion between these layers is weak and depends on pigment epithelial cell invaginations which form

sheaths around the outer segments of photoreceptors, the presence of an interphotoreceptor matrix, and the high osmotic pressure of the choroidal extracellular compartment compared with that in retinal compartment, opposed across the pigment epithelium.

The retina extends from the scalloped margin of the ora serrata anteriorly to the **optic nerve head**, the collection point for the axons of its ganglion cells. The centre of the optic disc is about 4 mm nasal to the fovea. At the centre of the rod-free fovea centralis (1.85 mm wide) is the **foveola** (0.35 mm wide). The 0.5 mm wide band outside this defines the **parafovea**, and the 1.5 mm band beyond this is the **perifovea**. These zones together make up the **macula** (area centralis) (Fig. 6.21).

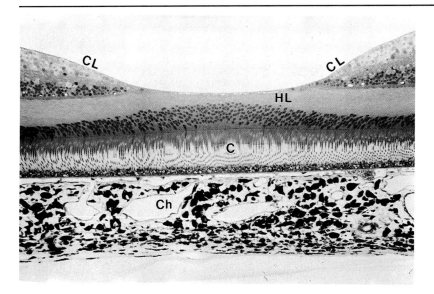

Fig. 6.22 Transverse section of the human retina passing through the foveola. In this region, the photoreceptors are exclusively cones (C) which have long, slender, rod-like inner and outer segments. Because of this external limiting membrane (arrows) is bowed forward and derives the name 'fovea externa'. The outer nuclear layer (ON) is thickened and the photoreceptor axons (Henle's fibres) or outer plexiform layer (HL) radiate to synapse with the dendrites of the inner nuclear layer (INL) which terminates at the edge of the foveola with the slope of the clivus (CL). The extreme thinness of the retina at the foveola is due to absence of inner retinal layers (nerve fibres), ganglion cells, inner plexiform and nuclear layers. PE = Pigment epithelium. (Original magnification ×300.) (From Tripathi, R. C. and Tripathi, B. J. in Davson, H. (ed.) (1984) *The Eye*, published by Academic Press.)

The retina proper has a surface area of 266 mm². It is thickest near the disc margins (0.56 mm) and thinnest at the ora serrata (0.1 mm).

Each retina has $77.9-107.3 \times 10^6$ rods and $4.08-5.29 \times 10^6$ cones, the density varying across it. Density of cones is highest at the rod-free foveola (199 000/mm²; total 3500) and decreases towards the periphery (5000/mm²). The fovea centralis contains approximately 100 000 cones. Rods first appear 130 μm from the foveal centre and reach maximum density (160 000/mm²) 2.5–3.0 mm from the fovea (at the edge of the area centralis): peripheral density is 23–50 000/mm². Cones are concerned with daylight colour vision; they have a relatively high luminance threshold (Fig. 6.22); rods are sensitive to shorter wavelengths (at the blue end of the spectrum) and have much lower thresholds than the cones.

Layers of the retina

Because of the uniform organization of its cellular elements, the retina has an apparent layering, as follows:

1. pigment epithelium;
2. photoreceptor layer (outer and inner segments);
3. the outer limiting membrane;
4. the outer nuclear layer, containing nuclei of photoreceptors;
5. the outer plexiform layer;
6. the inner nuclear layer, containing nuclei of bipolar cells, horizontal cells, amacrine cells, and Müller cells;
7. the inner plexiform layer;
8. the layer of ganglion cells, containing their somas;
9. the layer of nerve fibre axons of ganglion cells, which are non-myelinated;
10. the inner limiting membrane.

Pigment epithelium

The pigment epithelium contains about $4.2-6.5 \times 10^6$ cells with attachment structures in the apical region tight junctions, which provide an external blood–retinal barrier. This limits entry of material from choroid into retina. Specialized apical processes form sheaths around the photoreceptor outer segments and facilitate interchanges between these cells. The pigment epithelium ingests and removes the tips of the growing outer segments with a diurnal rhythm. Functions include the delivery and recycling of vitamin A, required for production of rhodopsin and iodopsin. Cells are laden with pigment granules, which, like the chroidal pigment, reduce disturbance of retinal images by back-scatter from the sclera.

Neuroretina

The layers of the neuroretina are organized around three major neural elements, synapsing in sequence. Photoreceptors synapse with bipolar cells in the **external plexiform layer**; the bipolar cells synapse with ganglion cells in the inner plexiform layer. The bipolar cells synapse with amacrine and horizontal cells in their own layer, and also participate in synapses with receptors and ganglion cells in the plexiform layers. These neurons are involved in processing the visual signal before transmission along ganglion cell axons to the lateral geniculate body. The glial cells of the retina are astrocytes and Müller's cells; Müller's cell processes invest most neural elements in the retina and extend across the retinal thickness. At the inner surface of the retina they interlace. Their basal lamina is the **inner limiting 'membrane'**. In the outer retina they form junctions with each other and with the photoreceptors, and at a level external to the receptor nuclei they form an extensive series of junctional complexes, the **outer limiting 'membrane'**. Their microvillous processes extend beyond this, around outer photoreceptor segments and into the subretinal space. Their function is more than nutrition and mechanical support: they may regulate retinal pH, take up certain neurotransmitters, possess retinoid-binding proteins and contribute to retinal electrical responses.

The **rod** and **cone cells** are concerned with transduction of light impulses into outer and inner segments, connected by a cilium. The stacked discs of the outer segments contain a photopigment, which absorbs photons incident on them. The inner segments are rich in mitochondria, Golgi bodies and ribosomes. An interphotoreceptor matrix intervenes between the outer segments.

The photoreceptor cells terminate in synaptic specializations, called spherules (in rods) and pedicles (in cones). Both photoreceptors make contact with bipolar cells and the interaction is modulated by horizontal cells in a sequence of synaptic interactions called triads. The bipolar cells transmit the modified signals from the photoreceptor cells to the ganglion cells but again the signal is modulated this time by the action of amacrine cells.

The retinal axons converge to the optic nerve head, maintaining their retinoptic array, so that peripheral fibres enter the periphery of the nerve and peripapillary fibres more centrally. Nerve fibres temporal to the fovea are said to start from a horizontal raphe. Ganglion cells are displaced away from the foveal cones, so that the retina here is half the thickness of retina elsewhere. This displacement reduces light scattering at the fovea and facilitates resolution of fine detail.

The retinal arteries and veins form superior and inferior nasal and temporal arches spreading from the optic disc head. They are internal to the layer of nerve fibres. The retinal capillaries supply only the inner layers of the retina.

The ratio of choroidal to retinal blood flow is about 10:1.

The **optic nerve head** receives about 1.2 million retinal axons, which turn at about a right-angle to enter the optic nerve. Its centre is 3.42 (± 0.34) mm medial and 0.1 mm inferior to the fovea. Its vertical diameter is 1.86 (± 0.21) mm and its horizontal diameter 1.75 (± 0.19) mm (Straatsma, Foos and Spencer, 1969), and it lies 27 mm from the nasal and 31 mm from the temporal limbus. The axons pass through the multilamellar fenestrations of the collagenous lamina cribrosa, which occupies the posterior scleral foramen. The bundles of axons here and in the nerve itself are separated from all other structures by astrocytes; thus the axons do not make contact with the lamina's collagen bundles or septa of the optic nerve. Astrocytes cover the nerve's periphery, intervening between axons and retina or choroid anterior to the lamina, and the collagenous pial sheath posterior to it. Astrocytes also occur in a central depression at the vitreal surface of the disc (the **optic cup**), and their processes continue into the Müllerian processes of the internal limiting membrane at the disc's margin; some of these are remnants of glial tissues surrounding the embryonic hyaloid artery.

Trabeculae of the lamina cribrosa and septa of the retrolaminar nerve carry vessels into the nerve's substance. The **optic disc head** is supplied by branches of the short ciliary arteries, except for its layer of nerve fibres which is supplied by the central retinal artery's prelaminar part.

Axons immediately behind the lamina cribrosa and in the optic nerve are myelinated, and in keeping with this, oligodendrocytes, which maintain the myelin sheath, accompany the astrocytes.

6.5 SURFACE ANATOMY

The sites of structures entering or leaving the eyeball are important surgically, as are surface projections of internal structures.

THE LIMBUS

The conjunctival epithelium ends at the periphery of Bowman's layer of the cornea, which is an elliptical surface and marker for the corneal limbus. This is indicated by slit-lamp as the axial limit of the corneal marginal arcades of the cornea. The deepest recess of the anterior chamber lies 2.0 mm behind the corneal limbus above and below.

The corneal limbus is defined internally by the end of Descemet's membrane which, as Schwalbe's line, is readily seen on gonioscopy, and forms the circular inner rim of the cornea (Fig. 6.23). Because of the elliptical contour of the cornea's outer rim, the plane joining the two, and representing the central face of the corneal limbus, is angulated more towards the optic axis in the vertical meridian than in the horizontal. An incision at the corneal limbus, directed anteroposteriorly or towards the angle, is more likely

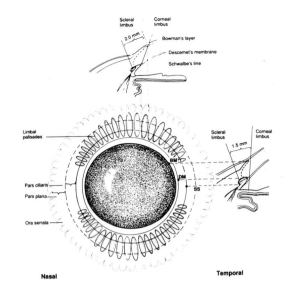

(a)

to encounter and damage the trabecular meshwork than if directed from the temporal side. The scleral spur, the posterior or sclerocorneal limit of the limbus, runs in a circle, parallel to Schwalbe's line.

The distance of various structures from the limbus is shown in Table 6.1.

CILIARY BODY LANDMARKS

The anterior margin of the ciliary body corresponds precisely to the tip of the scleral spur, and is therefore 2 mm behind the corneal limbus in the vertical meridian and 1.5 mm in the horizontal. The pars plicata is 2 mm wide, so that its posterior border is 2 mm behind this point in all meridia. The width of the pars plana varies with meridian (4.0–4.5 mm): thus the ora serrata is 6.5–7.0 mm behind the corneal limbus nasally, 7.5–8.0 mm temporally, 7 mm above

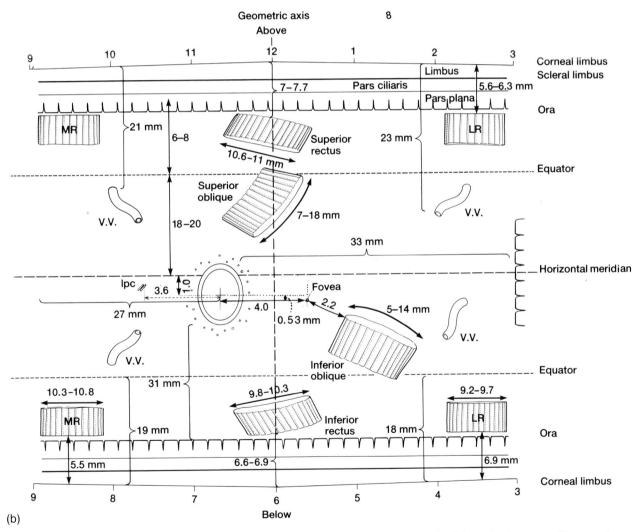

(b)

Fig. 6.23 (a) Schematic diagram of the limbus in vertical and horizontal cross-section (b) Schematic diagram to illustrate the distances of various structures entering or leaving the globe from the limbus. The right globe is viewed from behind.

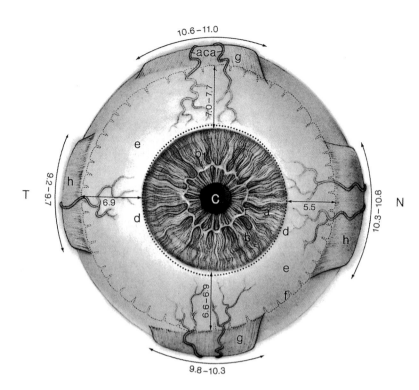

Fig. 6.24 Anterior aspect of the normal human eye. The cornea (A) is anterior to the iris (B) and pupil (C). The elliptical shape of the anterior corneal margin (arrows) is compared to the round shape of its posterior one (dotted line). The collarette of the iris is evident at B_1. The pupil is displaced slightly nasally. The limbal area and external scleral sulcus surround the margin of the cornea (D). Sclera (E) is peripheral to the limbus. The ora serrata (F) is shown as a lightly dotted line. It is more posterior on the temporal than nasal side. Superior and inferior rectus tendons (G) are curved and inserted obliquely to the axis of the eye. The tendons of the medial and latera recti (H) also have curved insertions which are not oblique to the horizontal meridian. Each rectus muscle has two anterior ciliary arteries (ACA) except the lateral rectus, which has one. N = Nasal; T = temporal. The measurements of the structures are given in the illustration. (From Hogan, M.J., Alvarado, J.A. and Weddell, J.E. (1971) *Histology of the Human Eye*, published by W.B. Saunders.)

and below (Fig. 6.24). As mentioned earlier, the ora is therefore tilted about the vertical, and closer to the limbus nasally than temporally. These measurements influence the site selected at the surface of the sclera to enter the eye via the pars plana: too anterior an approach will risk haemorrhage and damage to the ciliary body, too posterior will risk retinal damage and subsequent retinal detachment. The infant pars plana width is less than that in the adult, and this influences the choice of entry site for intraocular procedures via this route.

Intrascleral nerve loops, representing the recursive course of branches of posterior ciliary nerves, are sometimes encountered at the level of the pars plana.

In the living eye, particularly when lightly pigmented, the position of the ora and the junction between pars ciliaris and pars plana can be shown by transillumination through the dilated pupil. The pars ciliaris is then very dark, the pars plana of intermediate density, and the ora a dark line. (This technique also identifies the locations of long posterior ciliary nerves and arteries in the horizontal meridian, and the location and solid or cystic nature of choroidal or retinal tumours.)

Distances of structures from the ora serrata appear in Table 6.1.

The anterior ciliary arteries emerge from attach-ments of the rectus muscles (one for each lateral rectus, two for the others) and pass anteriorly in the episclera. At a variable distance from the limbus they branch, a deep ramus penetrating the sclera to join the posterior ciliary and the major arterial circle of the iris. The superficial ramus continues as an episcleral artery. Global attachments of extraocular muscles are important surgical landmarks, particularly in surgical treatment of squint. They vary considerably.

RECTUS MUSCLE INSERTIONS (Fig. 6.24)

Those of the horizontal recti are vertical and of the vertical recti slightly oblique, with the nasal ends closer to the limbus than the temporal. Muscle widths and distances from the limbus are given in Table 6.1.

OBLIQUE MUSCLE INSERTIONS

These are largely behind the equator (Figs 6.25 and 6.26).

Superior oblique

That of the superior oblique is long (7–18 mm) and curved, with its concavity anterior. Its obliquity places the posterior end 17–19 mm from the limbus,

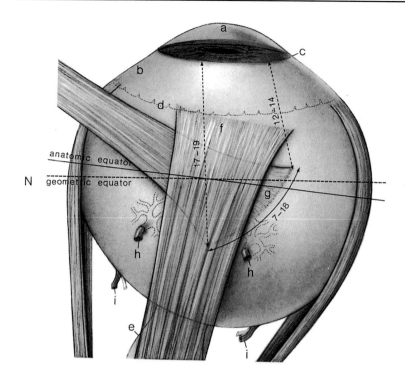

Fig. 6.25 Drawing of the upper half of the eye. The contrasting degree of curvature of the cornea (A) and sclera (B) are evident. At the limbus (C), where they join, is the external scleral sulcus. The relation of the ora serrata (D) to the surface is shown. The nasal displacement of the optic nerve (E) with respect to the posterior pole of the eye makes the three layers of the temporal eye longer than those on the nasal side. The slightly curved oblique insertion of the superior rectus muscle is at (F), and the tendinous oblique insertion of the superior oblique muscle is at (G). Two vortex veins are seen (H), and the long posterior ciliary arteries and nerves are at (I). T = Temporal; N = nasal. (From Hogan, M.J., Alvardo, J.A. and Weddell, J.E. (1971) *Histology of the Human Eye*, published by W.B. Saunders.)

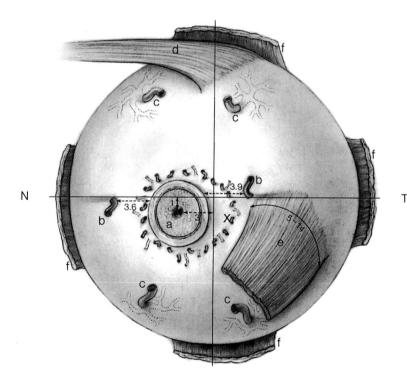

Fig. 6.26 Drawing of the posterior aspect of the eye. The optic nerve (A) with its central vessels and surrounding meningeal sheaths is seen. Its centre is located 3 mm nasal and 1 mm inferior to the posterior pole of the eye. Surrounding it are the short posterior ciliary arteries and nerves. The approximate position of the macula is at (X). Along the horizontal meridian which bisects the eye are the long posterior ciliary arteries and nerves (B). The exits of four vortex veins are shown, one for each quadrant (C). The curved, oblique insertions of the superior oblique (D) and inferior oblique (E) muscles are seen. The cut ends of the four rectus muscles are at (F). T = Temporal; N = nasal. (From Hogan, M.J., Alvardo, J.A. and Weddell, J.E. (1971) *Histology of the Human Eye*, published by W.B. Saunders.)

the anterior end 12–14 mm and hence near the lateral end of the superior rectus insertion. (Its posterior edge may be as far as 14 mm from the medial end of the superior rectus (Hogan, Alvarado and Weddell, 1971).)

Inferior oblique

The inferior oblique attachment is shorter (5–14 mm) and is also curved, with its concavity directed inferiorly. Its obliquity places the temporal margin anterior to its nasal margin. The posterior margin is thus 3–6 mm anterior to the edge of the optic nerve, 1 mm below its lower limit (Fig. 6.18) and 1–2 mm from the fovea (Fig. 6.22). Also the posterior muscle margin is close to the lower temporal vortex vein. This is an important relationship to remember during surgery on the inferior oblique muscle.

VORTEX VEINS

Classically, four vortex veins are described on the scleral surface, one in each quadrant: Rutnin (1967), however, found about six vortex vein exits per eye, with more nasally (3.36) than temporally (2.46). They are closer to the vertical meridian temporally than nasally. The arc distance from the limbus averages 19.86 mm (range 13.75–25 mm) with the inferotemporal veins most anterior and most variable in both horizontal and vertical meridia. The superotemporal are the most posterior and least variable (Fig. 6.26); most lie about 3.0 mm behind the equator.

The optic nerve emerges from the globe a little medial and below the posterior pole, the centre of the nerve lying 3 mm medial to the vertical meridian and 1 mm below the horizontal meridian (Whitnall, 1932).

THE POSTERIOR CILIARY NERVES AND ARTERIES

These perforate the sclera around the optic nerve. About 20 short posterior ciliary arteries and 10 short posterior ciliary nerves traverse the sclera in a ring which is nearer to the nerve on the nasal side. The two long posterior ciliary arteries and nerves enter the sclera approximately in the horizontal meridian, 3.6 mm nasal or 3.9 mm temporal to the nerve. Their course in the suprachoroid may be visible through the sclera anteriorly, under the muscle attachments where the sclera is thin, and may be demonstrated by transillumination through the dilated pupil. Additional long ciliary arteries and nerves may occur, especially below, piercing the sclera more anteriorly (Hogan, Alvarado and Weddell, 1971).

CHAPTER SEVEN
The cornea and sclera

7.1   THE CORNEA

The cornea is a transparent avascular tissue with a smooth, convex surface and concave inner surface, which resembles a small watch-glass. Its structure gives some indication of the diverse functional demands upon the tissue. The cornea must be transparent, refract light, contain the intraocular pressure and provide a protective interface with the environment. Each of these functions is provided by a highly specialized substructural organization, and in an absence of vessels.

The main function of the cornea is optical; it forms the principal refractive surface, accounting for some 70% (40–45 dioptres) of the total refractive power. Refractive requirements are met by the regular anterior curvature of the cornea and the optically smooth quality of the overlying tear film. The resistance of the cornea, which provides a protective layer and resists the ocular pressure, is due to the collagenous components of the stroma. Most of the refraction of the eye occurs not in the lens but at the front surface of the cornea at the tear/air interface. Transparency of the corneal stroma is achieved by the regularity and fineness of its collagen fibrils and the closeness and homogeneity of their packing. Water is constantly pumped out of the cornea by its posterior layer, the endothelium. This maintains the optical homogeneity of the corneal layers and prevents swelling and clouding. The cornea is thus an evolutionary compromise, being a multicomponent, thick, tough avascular tissue with a smooth surface and uniform curvature.

The curvature of the cornea is greater than that of the sclera so that a slight external furrow (the sulcus sclerae) separates it from the sclera. This furrow may be demonstrated in the living eye by specular reflection from the overlying tear film. The line of junction is most obvious when an eye is divided by meridional section: in the living subject it corresponds roughly to the periphery of the visible iris.

DIMENSIONS

In front the cornea appears elliptical, being 11.7 mm wide in the horizontal meridian and 10.6 mm in the vertical. The posterior surface of the cornea appears circular, about 11.7 mm in diameter. This difference is due to the greater overlap of sclera and conjunctiva above and below than laterally (Fig. 7.1). The cornea is 1% wider in males (Priestley-Smith, 1890). The axial thickness of the cornea is 0.52 mm (Donaldson, 1966; Maurice, 1969) with a peripheral thickness of 0.67 mm. Topographic measurements have been made by Rapuano, Fishbaugh and Strike (1993). At birth the cornea is slightly thicker than that in children, perhaps reflecting the onset of endothelial function close to the time of birth (Smelser, 1960). Its surface area is about 1.3 cm^2, one-sixth of the surface area of the globe (Table 7.1).

The cornea forms part of what is almost a sphere, but it is usually more curved in the vertical than the horizontal meridian, giving rise to astigmatism 'with the rule'. In its central third, the **optical zone**, the radius of curvature of the anterior surface is about 7.8 mm and that of the posterior 6.5 mm, in adult males. Peripheral cornea is more flattened.

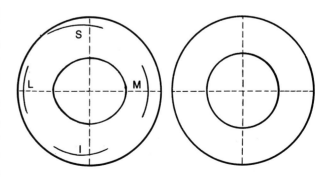

Fig. 7.1 In the anterior aspect the cornea is transversely ellipsoid, whereas its posterior aspect is circular. S, M, I and L indicate the points of attachment of the recti.

Table 7.1 Composition of human cornea and sclera†

Cornea		%
Water		78
Collagen		15
of which:		
Type I	50–55%	
Type III	≤1%	
Type IV	8–10%	
Type VI	25–30%	
Other protein		5
Keratan sulphate		0.7
Chondroitin/dermatan sulphate		0.3
Hyaluronic acid		+
Salts		1.0

Sclera	
Collagen	
Type I	(mainly)
Type III	6
Type V	
Type VI	
Type VIII	
Chondroitin/dermatan sulphate	
Hyaluronic acid	
Keratan sulphate	
Salts	

†From Maurice (1969); Berman (1991) Marshall 1993; Kucharz 1992

The glycosaminoglycans (GAGs) are high molecular weight carbohydrate polymers covalently linked, except in the case of hyaluronic acid, to a protein core. The complex is termed a proteoglycan (PG). Keratan sulphate PG is termed lumican and has a molecular weight of about 3–20 K (Axelsson and Heingärd, 1978); chondroitin/dermatan sulphate PG, known as decarin, has a molecular weight of about 10–50 K (Scott, 1988). Keratan sulphate GAG contains glucosamine and galactose; chondroitin sulphate, galactosamine and glucuronic acid. Dermatain sulphate contains galactosamine with iduronic/glucuronic acid and hyaluronic acid contains glucosamine with glucuronic acid.

In the cornea, sulphation of chondroitin/dermatan increases towards the periphery. The dermatan component of this molecule is more prevalent in sclera than cornea. There is a greater amount of hyaluronic acid in the sclera than in the cornea, while the keratan sulphate content of the sclera is low.

TOPOGRAPHY

Corneal shape is important to the fitting of contact lenses. As measured by keratometry the average anterior radius of curvature 7.2–8.4 mm in Caucasians, and steeper in Asiatics. The cornea is flatter in men than in women, and is broader in races with brachycephalic skulls (e.g. 14 mm for Celts) with flatter curves (Ruben, 1975). The anterior curvature of the cornea is spherical over a small zone 2–4 mm in diameter which is decentred upwards and outwards relative to the visual axis, but correctly

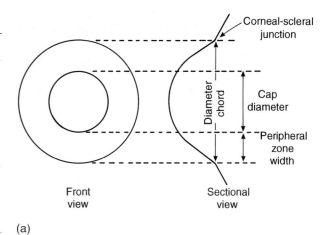

(a)

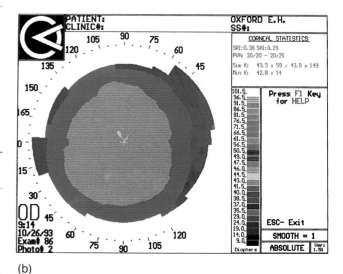

(b)

Fig. 7.2 (a) Drawing to show the location of the 'corneal cap'; (b) topography of a cornea with low asphericity.

centred for the pupillary aperture (which lies 0.4 mm temporally). This is sometimes termed the **corneal apex** or **cap** (Fig. 7.2a). The corneal curvature varies from apex to limbus. There is greater flattening nasally than temporally, and above than below, although variations occur (Mandell, 1967). The corneal curvature is steeper in the infant eye (Mandell, 1967). Near the limbus, corneal curvature increases before entering the trough-like contour of the limbal zone (Fig. 7.2b). These features influence the fitting of contact lenses. The cornea flattens slightly on convergence (Lopping and Weale, 1965).

The apical radius of the posterior corneal surface is 5.8 mm; the radius flattens in the periphery, faster than the anterior radius (Patel, Marshall and Fitzke, 1993).

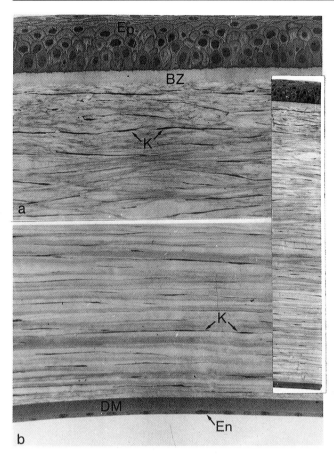

Fig. 7.3 Meridional section of the human cornea, stained with haematoxylin and eosin. (a) Epithelium and anterior stroma; (b) endothelium and posterior stroma. Inset shows full corneal thickness. BZ = Bowman's zone; DM = Descemet's membrane; En = endothelium; Ep = epithelium; K = keratocytes.

STRUCTURE

Behind the precorneal film are five tissue layers (Fig. 7.3):

1. epithelium;
2. Bowman's layer;
3. stroma;
4. Descemet's membrane;
5. endothelium.

Epithelium

The corneal epithelium is stratified, squamous and non-keratinized (Fig. 7.4). It is continuous with that of the conjunctiva at the corneal limbus, but differs strikingly in possessing no goblet cells. The epithelium is 50–90 μm thick and consists of five or six layers of nucleated cells (Fig. 7.5). Thickness has been measured accurately by high-frequency ultrasound at 50.7 μm (Reinstein *et al.*, 1994). The deepest of these, the **basal cells**, stand in a palisade-like manner in perfect alignment on a basal lamina (Fig. 7.6). They form the germinative layer of the epithelium, continuous peripherally with that of the limbus. These basal cells are columnar (10 μm wide and 15 μm tall) with rounded heads and flat bases. Each nucleus is oval and oriented parallel to the cell's long axis.

The second epithelial layer (the **'wing'** or **'umbrella' cells**) consists of polyhedral cells, convex anteriorly, which cap the basal cells, and send processes between them. The long axes of their oval nuclei are parallel to the corneal surface.

The next two or three layers are also polyhedral and become wider and increasingly flattened towards the surface. The surface cells have the largest surface area and this is greater in the periphery (e.g. 850 μm² above) compared to centrally (560 μm) (Mathers and Lemp, 1992; see also Tsŭbota, 1992; Tomii and Kinoshita, 1994). The most superficial cells may be as wide as 50 μm and 4 μm in depth; they retain their nuclei, and do not show keratinization. Their flattened nuclei project backwards, leaving the surface perfectly smooth.

Ultrastructural features

The epithelial cells contain the usual organelles of actively metabolizing cells. Mitochondria are small and scarce in the basal cells but are moderately abundant in the wing and middle cell layers. There is a high glycogen content in the form of large (20–30 nm) and small (10 nm) granules, especially in the wing and superficial cells. The amount of glycogen falls in hypoxic conditions, or during wound healing (Kuwabara, Perkins and Cogan, 1976). The cells contain a cytoplasmic meshwork of electron-dense **tonofibrils** (intermediate filaments), similar to those found in other epithelia composed of cytokeratins (Sun and Vidrich, 1981) (Fig. 7.7). Occasional slender basal cells with electron-dense cytoplasm may represent recently divided cells. The plasma membranes of contiguous cells interdigitate with their neighbours with an intervening space of no more than 20 nm. Adhesion is achieved by numerous **desmosomes** (Fawcett, 1966). These structures are presumably sufficiently labile to allow movement over a period of time as cells migrate to the surface. They are sparse between the superficial and wing cells. The basal cells are connected to one another by desmosomes and to the underlying basal lamina by hemidesmosomes.

Both the wing and basal cells possess numerous tonofibrils about 8 nm in diameter, and in basal cells so-called anchoring filaments pass through the

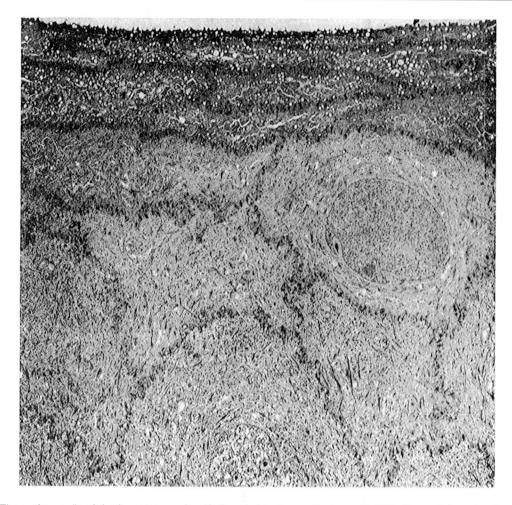

Fig. 7.4 The surface cells of the human corneal epithelium (original magnification ×69 000). These flattened cells are vital and show no sign of keratinization. Microvilli project from the free surface. Note reciprocal folding of adjoining surfaces of the cells at all levels. (Courtesy of Dr John Marshall and Mr P. L. Ansell, Institute of Ophthalmology, London.)

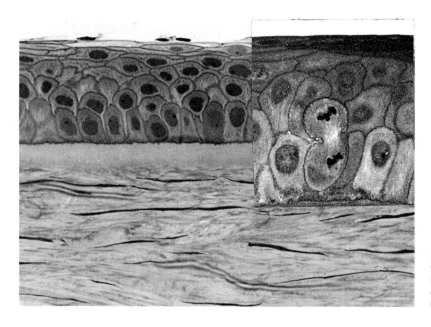

Fig. 7.5 Section to show the typical architecture of the corneal epithelium. Note the pyknotic nuclei of exfoliating surface squamous cells. The inset shows a mitosing epithelial cell in the peripheral cornea. Original magnification × 800; inset × 1000.

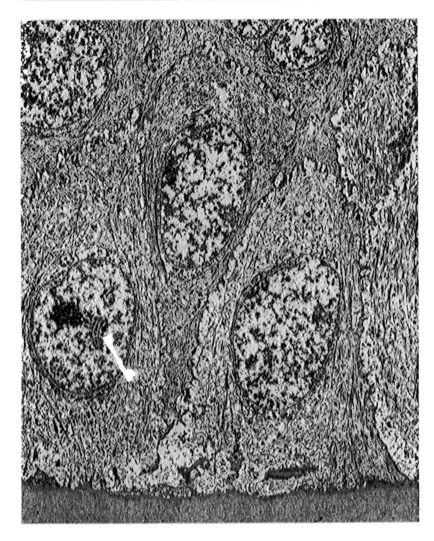

Fig. 7.6 The basal cells of the human cornea (original magnification ×7500). The basal cells adjoin a basement membrane contiguous with the limiting layer of Bowman's membrane (below). (Courtesy of Dr John Marshall and Mr P. L. Ansell, Institute of Ophthalmology, London.)

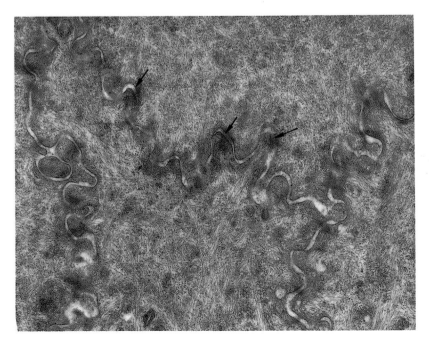

Fig. 7.7 Tortuous, parallel intercellular borders of corneal epithelial cells, joined in places by hemidesmosomes (arrows). The cells contain abundant tonofilaments. Original magnification × 38 000.

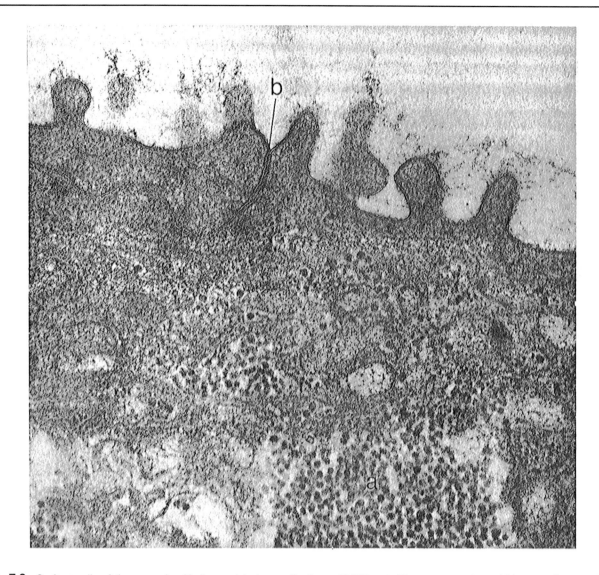

Fig. 7.8 Surface cells of the corneal epithelium, original magnification ×90 000. a = Glycogen granules, which are a feature of the surface cells; b = a zonula occludens. Zonulae occludentae are encountered exclusively along the lateral intercellular space of surface cells. (From Hogan, M. J., Alvarado, J. A. and Weddell, J. E., (1971) *Histology of the Eye. An Atlas and Textbook*, published by W. B. Saunders.)

hemidesmosomal structures to be inserted into the underlying basal lamina. This is a strong attachment and if the corneal surface is scraped by a scalpel blade, fragments of the ruptured basal cells remain attached to the basal lamina (Khodadoust *et al.*, 1968). The mode of attachment between contiguous epithelial cells at the surface differs from that of deeper cells: in addition to the desmosomal connections, **tight junctions** (zonulae occludentes) run circumferentially between contiguous surface cells (Fig. 7.8) (Tonjum, 1974). These tight junctions are relatively impermeable to small molecules such as sodium ions and confer on the epithelium as a whole the properties of a semipermeable membrane in respect of the bathing precorneal tear film. The entry

of water and small molecules from the stroma is not restricted, which permits the occurrence of epithelial oedema, with widening of the intercellular space, for instance when the endothelial pump fails (Goldman and Kuwabara, 1968).

The most superficial cells of the epithelium are mostly hexagonal and firmly attached to each other at relatively straight cell boundaries. They exhibit surface microvilli or microplicae (Pfister, 1973; Pfister and Burstein, 1976), sometimes regarded as an exaggeration of the plasma membrane infoldings which exist between all contiguous epithelial cells (Fig. 7.9). Microvilli are about 0.5 μm high, 0.3 μm wide and 0.5 μm apart. It is likely that the microvilli serve a physical function in stabilizing the deep precorneal

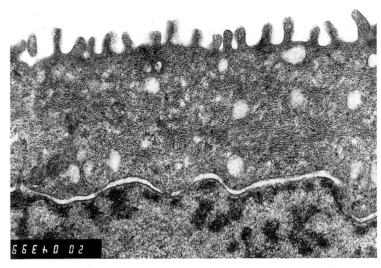

(a)

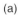

Fig. 7.9   (a) Superficial cells of the corneal epithelium showing conspicuous finger-like projections of microvilli. The vesicular structures are probably derived from Golgi apparatus and may have a role in secretion of the glycoprotein that coats the cell surface as its glycocalyx. Original magnification ×4500.

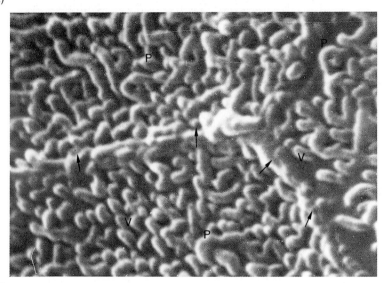

(b)

(b) Scanning electron micrograph of human corneal epithelium, showing microvilli (V) and microplicae (P). At the cell junctions microplicae predominate, causing a ridge-like appearance of the border (arrows). Original magnification ×150 000.

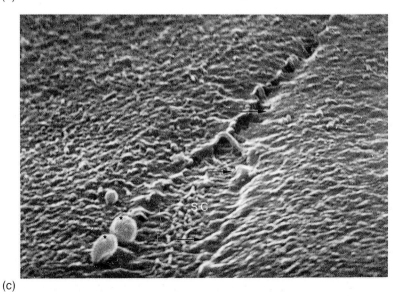

(c)

(c) An exfoliating cell of the corneal epithelium. Note the lifting of the cell edges along the intercellular border (arrows) exposing the underlying squamous cell (SC) with its pre-existing microvilli. The asterisks denote bleb-like structures, probably resulting from oedematous surface projections. Original magnification ×6000.

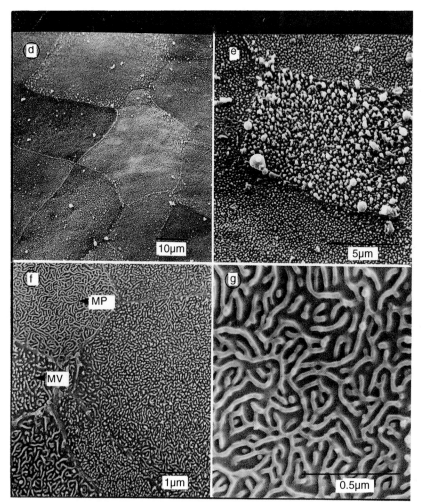

Fig. 7.9 **(contd)** (d–g) Normal human corneal epithelial surface is shown in a specimen removed for central traumatic scarring. (d) and (e) are from one button and (f) and (g) are from another. (d) Epithelial cells form a polygonal mosaic on the surface of the cornea. (e) Surface cells presenting only a small portion of their surface are covered with microvilli. Adjacent large cells are covered primarily by stubby microvilli. (f) A wide variety of microvilli (MV) and microplicae (MP) is present in adjacent cells in this specimen. (g) Interlacing microplicae are found in a single older cell. Occasional microvilli are present between ridges.

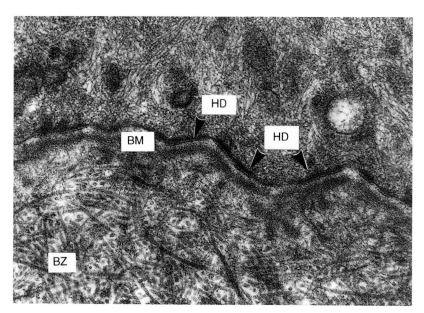

Fig. 7.10 Attachment of basal cells to the basement membrane (BM) is mediated by hemidesmosomes (HD). Note the abundant keratin fibrils within the basal cells, and the extension of basement membrane into Bowman's zone of the stroma (BZ). TEM, original magnification ×34 000.

tear film. The glycoprotein coat of the surface plasma membrane is described in the section on tears. Scanning microscopy also demonstrates 'light' and 'dark' cells with varying density and type of microvilli present. It has been suggested that the dark cells are older and about to desquamate (Hoffman, 1972).

Dendritic cells have been identified in the corneal epithelium (Segawa, 1964; Smelser and Ozanics,

1965) and it seems likely that some of these are Langerhans cells, important members of the immune recognition system, responsible for the processing and presentation of foreign antigens to lymphocytes. These cells, and DR positive macrophages, are present in fetal corneal epithelium and stroma, but disappear in the mature corneal except in peripheral epithelium (Diaz-Araya et al. 1995). They are almost

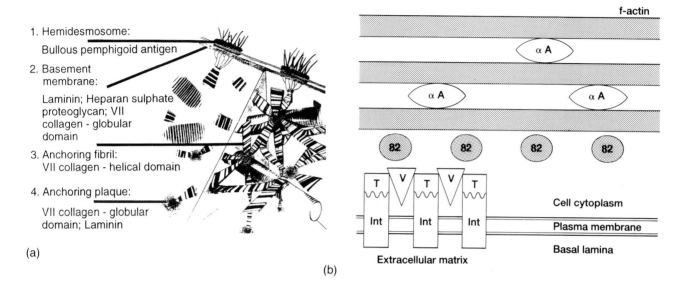

(a)

1. Hemidesmosome:
   Bullous pemphigoid antigen
2. Basement membrane:
   Laminin; Heparan sulphate proteoglycan; VII collagen - globular domain
3. Anchoring fibril:
   VII collagen - helical domain
4. Anchoring plaque:
   VII collagen - globular domain; Laminin

(b)

Extracellular matrix

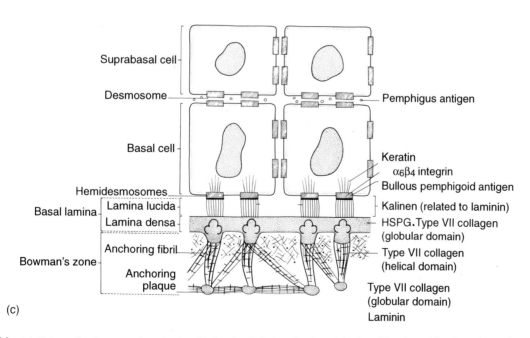

(c)

Suprabasal cell
Desmosome
Basal cell
Hemidesmosomes
Basal lamina — Lamina lucida / Lamina densa
Anchoring fibril
Bowman's zone — Anchoring plaque

Pemphigus antigen
Keratin
α6β4 integrin
Bullous pemphigoid antigen
Kalinen (related to laminin)
HSPG.Type VII collagen (globular domain)
Type VII collagen (helical domain)
Type VII collagen (globular domain)
Laminin

Fig. 7.11 (a) Schematic diagram of anchoring fibril network below the basal lamina. Top: branching insertions of anchoring fibrils into basal lamina below hemidesmosomes are depicted. Branching and anastomosing cross-banded fibrils spray out among type I collagen fibrils, some inserting into dense, anchoring plaques, composed of the non-helical domains of type VII collagen. (b) Schematic diagram of the interface between a basal epithelial cell and the subjacent basal lamina. αA = Alpha actinin; Int = integrin; T = talin; V = vinculin; 82 = K protein. (c) Schematic diagram depicting the attachment of the epithelial cells to the subjacent lamina and corneal stroma. HPSG = heparan sulphate proteoglycan.

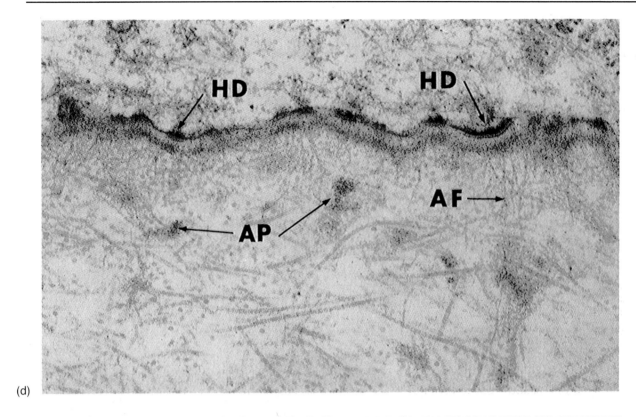

(d)

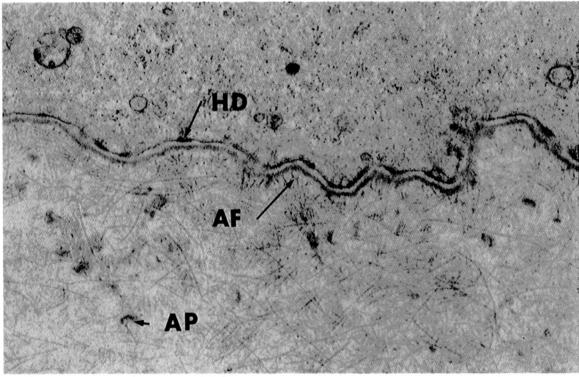

(e)

Fig. 7.11 **(contd)** (d, e) Cross-sections through the adhesion zone of the cornea of a 27-week fetus and a 9-month-old infant (original magnifications (a) ×51 000; (b) ×21 000). Note numerous mature hemidesmosomes (HD) and cross-banded anchoring fibrils (AF), as well as anchoring plaques (AP).

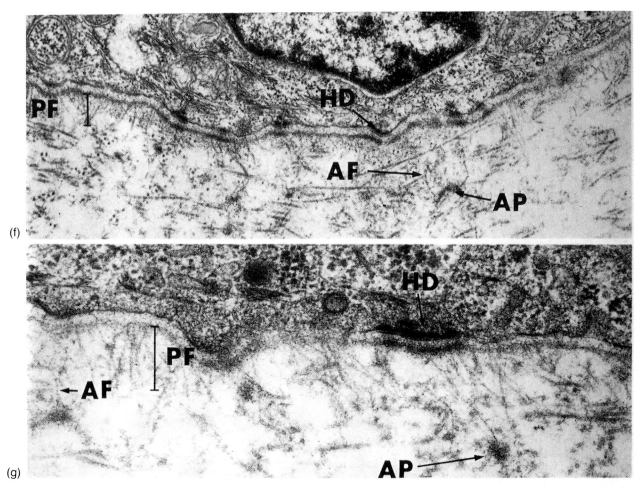

Fig. 7.11 **(contd)** (f, g) Cross-sections through the basement membrane zone in developing human cornea of 15 and 17 weeks, respectively (original magnifications (f) ×31 000; (g) × 51 000). Note hemidesmosomes (HD), cross-banded anchoring fibrils (AF) and anchoring plaques (AP), as well as the palisade of filaments (PF) at all stages of development.

totally absent from the central cornea (Vantrappen *et al.*, 1985) but will populate this region in response to infection.

Basal lamina

The basal lamina is secreted by the basal cells, which also synthesize the hemidesmosomal structures concerned in attachment of epithelium to the lamina (Kenyon, 1969) (Fig. 7.10). The basal lamina is an irregular zone (0.5–1 μm wide) of granuloamorphous and filamentary materials. A deep osmiophilic **lamina densa** (30–60 nm) and a superficial **lamina lucida** (24 nm) are distinguished ultrastructurally. It is thicker peripherally and is thickened in diabetes (Snip, Thoft and Tolentino, 1979) and certain corneal disorders (Kenyon, 1969). The lamina consists of collagen and glycoprotein constituents integrated structurally with the underlying Bowman's layer, to

which it is firmly attached by an array of short anchoring filaments. It stains a deep pink with periodic acid–Schiff reagent.

The detailed molecular organization of the dermo-epidermal junction of the skin has been clarified in recent years by immuno- and electrohistochemical studies (Briggaman, 1982), and many of these features are shared by the cornea and conjunctiva. In the skin, the hemidesmosome consists of an electron-dense attachment plaque on the cytoplasmic face of the inner leaflet of the basal epithelial cell (Fig. 7.11). α_6 Integrin is localized along the lateral and basal membranes of the basal cells but is found in combination with β_4 within the hemidesmosome. With age the distribution of α_6 becomes less continuous, but the density of hemidesmosomes does not change (Trinkaus-Randall *et al.* 1993). Tonofilaments course towards the plaque but terminate in a relatively electron-dense zone separated from the

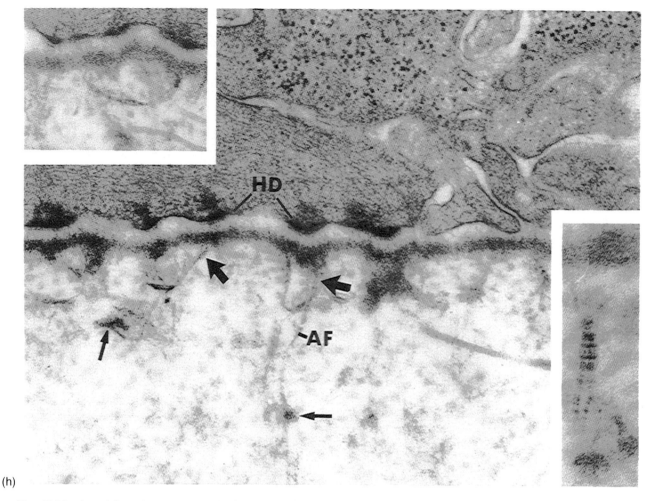

(h)

Fig. 7.11 (**contd** (h) Cross-sections of rabbit cornea demonstrating anchoring fibrils (AF) below the basal lamina. Main micrograph shows the anchoring fibril (large arrows – original magnification ×73 900). Insertion into basal lamina is particularly evident opposite hemidesmosomes (HD). Anchoring plaques are indicated by small arrows. The upper inset (original magnification ×73 900) shows an anchoring fibril inserting at each end into basal lamina, which is an infrequent finding. In the lower inset (original magnification ×93 000) a cross-banded fibril may be seen splaying out at its insertion into the basal lamina above and into the electron-dense anchoring plaque below. 24-hour tissue cultured specimen. (a, h from Gipson, I. K., Spurr-Michaud, S. J. and Tisdale, A. S. (1987) *Invest. Ophthalmol. Vis. Sci.*, **28**, 212–20, with permission; c, modified from Gipson, I. K. and Wojnarowska, F.; d–g from Tisdale, A. S., Spurr-Michaud, S. J. and Gipson, I. K. (1988) *Invest. Ophthalmol. Vis. Sci.*, **29**, 727–36, with permission.)

plaque by a narrow electron-lucent zone. The lamina lucida is relatively amorphous, and exhibits a fine electron-dense seam, the **sub-basal dense plaque**. Fine **anchoring filaments** traverse this zone and mesh with the lamina densa which has a granuloamorphous structure. It is traversed by electron-dense **anchoring fibrils** which in the cornea form narrow bundles which insert into the subjacent stroma or Bowman's layer, terminating in **anchoring plaques** (Gipson, Spurr-Michaud and Tisdale, 1987). These structures are composed of type VII collagen. This arrangement accounts for the tight adherence of the basal epithelium to subjacent cornea. The lamina lucida contains the glycoprotein laminin, and at the basal plasmalemma bullous pemphigoid antigen. The lamina densa contains type IV collagen but in the primate only in the peripheral cornea. Many other glycoproteins, including fibronectin, have been localized to the basal lamina, chiefly to the lamina lucida. The cohesion between the basal lamina and Bowman's zone may be loosened by lipid solvents, stromal oedema and inflammation but it remains attached to the basal cells. The basal lamina may be destroyed by proteolytic enzymes such as trypsin and chymotrypsin. With old age, and in diabetes, it becomes thickened and multilamellar. Patches of oxytalan fibres and calcific spherules may appear especially at the periphery of the cornea.

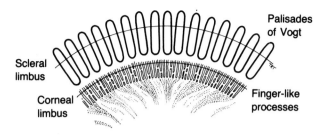

Fig. 7.12 Schematic drawing of the upper limbus in a pigmented subject to show the relation between the limbus, the palisades of Vogt and the finger-like radial epithelial processes of the peripheral cornea. (From Bron, A. J., *Trans. Ophthalmol. Soc. UK*, (1973) **93**, 455, with permission.)

Physiology

Metabolism   The corneal epithelium is rich in glycogen, which serves as an energy store in the aerobic conditions which normally obtain at the corneal epithelial surface. (With the eyes open, the tear P_{O_2} is 155 mmHg; with the eyes closed this drops to about 55 mmHg.) In hypoxic conditions, such as those induced by a tight contact lens, the epithelial glycogen level falls. Hypoxia also produces a profound fall in corneal sensitivity, and Millodot and O'Leary (1979) have adduced a role for a cholinergic sensory system from this, because prolonged lid closure causes a profound fall in the normally high level of choline acetylase in rabbit epithelium (Mindel and Millag, 1978). The concentrations of acetylcholine and acetylcholinesterase in the corneal epithelium are as high as in brain tissue. This is not entirely explained by the presence of corneal nerves, and substantial quantities of the acetylcholinesterase (over 50% of the normal level) remain in the epithelium after trigeminal section (Petersen, Lee and Donn, 1965; V. Brucke *et al.*, 1949). A role for acetylcholine in transport processes has been postulated (Klyce, Neufeld and Zadunaisky, 1973) or in regulating epithelial cell mitosis, because acetylcholine may stimulate cyclic GMP (cGMP) production, and cGMP stimulates epithelial cell mitosis (Cavanagh and Colley, 1979).

Turnover   Early studies using tritiated thymidine suggested that the epithelium was replaced approximately weekly by the division of basal epithelial cells (Hannah, Bicknell and O'Brien 1961). It was conceived that one daughter cell from a division remained in the basal layer while the other was displaced to the surface, from where it was ultimately shed. It is now recognized that the germinative region of the corneal epithelium, represented by the presence of **stem cells**, lies at the limbus (Davenger

and Evenson, 1971; Bron, 1973). Cells migrate from the limbus towards the centre of the cornea at a much slower rate, which may be as long as a year (Kaye, 1980). The high turnover suggested by early studies may reflect divisions of the stem cell progeny (see below).

Cotsarelis *et al.* (1986) indicated that certain slow-cycling cells located in the basal region of the limbus were stem cells. This is supported by studies which demonstrate that limbal basal cells can be distinguished from corneal epithelial cells and from other limbal epithelial cells by their expression of cytokeratins. In the rabbit, cytokeratins typical of differentiated cells (e.g. CK3) are expressed by *corneal epithelial cells* and *suprabasal* limbal epithelial cells (Schermer *et al.*, 1986; Rodriguez *et al.*, 1987), while *basal* limbal cells are negative for these cytokeratins and positive for a group of acidic cytokeratins staining with the antibody AE1 (Wiley *et al.*, 1991). Thoft and Friend (1983) proposed, on the basis of experimental evidence, that there was both a limbal basal and a corneal basal epithelial source for corneal epithelial cells (the so called XYZ hypothesis). The sequence of events from proliferation of stem cells to desquamation of superficial corneal epithelial cells is thought to involve cell division by the slow-cycling stem cells, whose daughter cells, the **transient amplifying cells**, migrate centripetally. They undergo a limited series of cell divisions prior to terminal differentiation and ultimate shedding (Tseng *et al.*, 1989). It seems likely that the basally dividing corneal epithelial cells are transient amplifying cells rather than a separate set of stem cells. This concept is in keeping with the observation that epithelial cells from the corneal periphery, especially above, show a higher proliferative rate *in vitro* than those from the central cornea. It also explains the presence of perilimbal wedges of pigment migration seen biomicroscopically in pigmented eyes by Hendkind (1967) (Fig. 7.12) and other clinical evidence of centripetal migration, such as the epithelial vortex patterns encountered in chloroquine toxicity and Fabry disease (Bron, 1973).

Lauweryns *et al.*, (1991; 1993a,b) have identified a distinct population of basal cells, lying in clusters at the junction between the limbus and the peripheral cornea, which they call transitional cells (TC). Clusters of these cells are invariably present in the superior cornea, less so in the inferior cornea and only occasionally in the nasal and temporal regions. They are considerably smaller than surrounding epithelial cells and their nuclei contain prominent nucleoli. Ultrastructurally, they show large nucleoli, marginated nuclear chromatin, prominent bundles of intermediate filaments (IFs) and many desmosomes and hemidesmosomes. These cells do not express CK3 (characteristic of the differentiated suprabasal limbal cell and mature corneal epithelium), but, like the limbal basal cells, they stain positively with the antibody AE1, which recognizes a 48 kDa keratin expressed in hyperproliferative states (Weiss, 1984). They also coexpress CK19 and vimentin (Vi), a profile typical of other regenerative regions. In the non-keratinizing stratified squamous epithelia of the exocervix, vagina, tongue, oral mucosa and oesophagus, the basal region occupied by stem cells and transient amplifying cells contains cells which express CK19 (Bartek et al., 1986; Franke et al., 1986; Kaspar et al., 1987; Morgan et al., 1987; Lindberg et al., 1989). Lauweryns et al. (1993a,b) have mooted that the mosaic suprabasal expression of CK19 in the peripheral corneal epithelium and occasionally the central corneal epithelium could be a marker for retained proliferative capacity by centrally migrating corneal epithelial cells. However, it should be noted that bulbar conjunctival epithelium also expresses CK19 although its stem cell population is thought to be confined to the fornices. Coexpression of cytokeratins with vimentin is more frequently observed in fetal than adult tissues and may correlate with changes in shape characteristic of migrating epithelial cells (Bukusoglu and Zieske, 1988; Paranko et al., 1986).

Transitional cells have many features in common with limbal basal cells. Like the limbal basal cells, they show a granular staining for $\alpha_6\beta_4$ integrin, a marker for the hemidesmosome, the limbal density of which is lower than in cornea (Gipson, 1989). They also both stain positively with AE1, strongly for metallothionein, but negatively for CK3 and transferrin receptor. It has been argued that many of these characteristics are those of cells residing in proliferating compartments (Lauweryns, 1993a,b). If it is accepted that stem cells are housed in the basal region of the limbus, then it would seem that the cell type described by Lauweryns, lying central to the limbus, is likely to represent a transient amplifying cell. It resembles the cell described by Zieske and Wasson (1992) as expressing alpha enolase, an enzyme which is inducible by epidermal growth factor (EGF). The expression of EGF receptor (EGFR) in the limbus is said to be three times that in the central cornea, which suggests that the limbal region may be equipped to respond to a proliferative message. It is also topographically relevant that the distribution of TC clusters in the peripheral cornea mirrors that of type IV collagen of the basement membrane. Type IV collagen is present in the basement membrane

throughout the limbus, but only in the superior, peripheral cornea (Cleutjens, 1990; Kolega et al., 1989).

Repair Mitosis is inhibited by injury, adrenergic agents and surface anaesthetics (Friedenwald and Buschke, 1944a,b) and is associated with an elevation of cAMP (Butterfield and Neufeld, 1977). Epithelial cell loss is followed by a distinctive sequence of reparative events. Injury leads to an abrupt cessation of local mitosis, and repair of the defect occurs by a process of centripetal slide. It appears that the rearrangement of actin fibrils (Gipson and Anderson, 1977; Gipson, Westcott and Brooksby, 1982) within fine filopodial extensions of cells at the margin of an erosion are essential for the process of migration (Pfister, 1975). These cells must detach themselves from the underlying basal lamina and travel in an amoeboid manner across the cornea until their progress is halted by contact inhibition. They then anchor, and mitosis resumes until epithelial thickness is re-established. Before this process is complete, surface tight junctions are re-established to restore the permeability characteristics of the epithelium (Thoft and Friend, 1977). A further and critical feature of the normal healing process is re-establishment of adhesion between the basal epithelial cells and the underlying Bowman's layer. Khodadoust et al. (1968) showed that tight adhesion was established in 7 days after abrading rabbit cornea when the basal lamina was intact, but that after keratectomy (in which the basal lamina and some underlying stroma is removed) adhesion is delayed for 6 weeks while fresh basal laminar material and hemidesmosomal attachments are laid down.

After total epithelial loss including the total limbus the adjacent conjunctival epithelium is capable of resurfacing the cornea, though at a reduced rate. The cornea becomes covered with a vascularized, conjunctival type of epithelium containing goblet cells. If a small part of the limbus is retained, including surviving stem cells, then there is an initial resurfacing with an epithelium which contains goblet cells, but these later disappear and the epithelium gradually takes on the appearance and metabolic behaviour of corneal epithelial cells. This process was formerly thought to be due to a process of transdifferentiation (Thoft and Friend, 1977), i.e. conversion of cells from conjunctival to corneal type. However, it now appears that it represents the slow restoration of cells to corneal type by migrating residual limbal stem cells (Tseng et al., 1982).

Attachment The basal epithelial cells are firmly attached to basal lamina by hemidesmosomes and anchoring filaments (Kenyon, 1969; Gipson, Spurr-Michaud and Tisdale, 1987). These attachments become less firm in epithelial corneal oedema and in this circumstance the epithelium may be readily detached spontaneously or by trivial injury such as lid rubbing or insertion and removal of a contact lens.

Epithelial–stromal interaction   There is some co-operation between the corneal epithelium and stroma in the healing process after injury. Weimar (1960) showed that stromal wound strength was greater after corneal incision if the epithelium was intact during healing. Also, the modification of stromal ground substance after stromal injury is modified by the presence of the epithelium. After penetrating injury epithelial cells migrate into, and may remain within, the stromal defect.

Collagen synthesis   Each of the cell types of the cornea is capable of secreting collagen. The epithelium is concerned with the turnover of basal laminar collagen and this turnover is increased after injury. In certain diseases excessive amounts of basal laminar material, including its glycoprotein constituents, are laid down as an abnormal response.

Bowman's layer (anterior limiting lamina)

Before electron microscopy was developed, Bowman's layer was thought to be a specialized corneal membrane, but it is now described as a modified region of the anterior stroma. Some observers believe that the epithelium has a role in the laying down and maintenance of Bowman's layer (Kuwabara, 1978).

Bowman's layer is a narrow, acellular homogeneous zone, 8–14 μm thick, immediately subjacent to the basal lamina of the cornea epithelium (Fig. 7.13). In pathological conditions (such as corneal oedema or certain corneal dystrophies) and after death, the epithelium separates readily from this limiting layer. The anterior surface is smooth and parallel to that of the cornea; though sharply defined from the overlying epithelium anteriorly it is infiltrated by the lamina densa and merges into the stroma behind. The perimeter of Bowman's layer, which has a rounded border, delineates the anterior junction between cornea and limbus and is marked clinically by summits of the marginal arcades of the limbal capillaries.

An analogous Bowman's layer is encountered in non-human primates, but not in other mammals, in some avian species and reptiles and also in elasmobranchs.

Ultrastructural features

Ultrastructurally Bowman's layer consists of a felted meshwork of fine collagen fibrils of uniform size, lying in a ground substance (Fig. 7.14). Fibril diameter (24–27 nm) is less than that of substantia propria. In the posterior region of this layer the fibrils become progressively more orderly in their orientation, blending and interweaving with the fibrils of the anterior stroma. Here and there anteriorly, bundles of the stromal lamella insert into the Bowman's layer. The compacted arrangement of the collagen confers great strength to this zone. Bowman's layer is relatively resistant to trauma, both mechanical and infective; once destroyed it is not renewed (Duke-Elder and Wybar, 1961) but is replaced by coarse scar tissue. It is perforated in many places by unmyelinated nerves in transit to the corneal epithelium (Tripathi and Tripathi, 1984).

Although at normal or raised intraocular pressure Bowman's layer is under tension and appears smooth, a series of convex ridges can be generated at its surface when tension is relaxed, as during corneal indentation applanation tonometry, hypotony, manipulation of the cornea during surgery (when the cornea may become concave forwards), or during application of a pressure bandage. These ridges correspond to an arrangement of strap-like stromal bundles which insert into Bowman's layer and when the cornea is relaxed define a polygonal or chicken-wire pattern (Fig. 7.15). They are responsible for the **anterior corneal mosaic** which may be induced at the surface of all normal corneae by massage through the lid. The pattern is then revealed in the epithelium by fluorescein (Bron, 1968; Bron and Tripathi, 1969) (Fig. 7.16). In prolonged hypotony and atrophia bulbi, the degenerative changes in the ridges contribute to secondary anterior crocodile shagreen (Tripathi and Bron, 1972).

Stroma (substantia propria)

The stroma, about 500 μm thick, consists of regularly arranged lamellae of collagen bundles (200–300 centrally and 500 in the periphery: Hamada, 1974). These vary between 9 and 260 μm in width and 1.15 and 2 μm in height (Hogan, Alvarado and Weddell, 1971), and lie in a proteoglycan ground substance together with a relatively small population of cells, the **keratocytes**. The lamellae are arranged in layers parallel with each other and with the corneal surfaces (Fig. 7.18). They are thought to run generally from limbus to limbus (Hogan, Alvarado and Weddell,

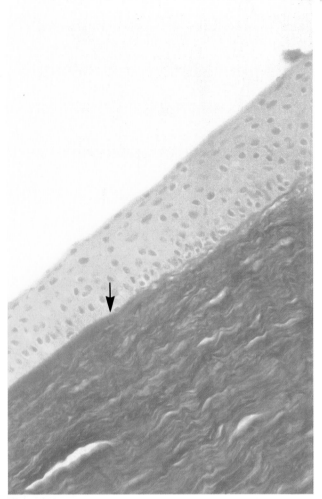

Fig. 7.13 Micrograph of the corneal limbus, showing the junction between the sclera and Bowman's layer (arrowed).

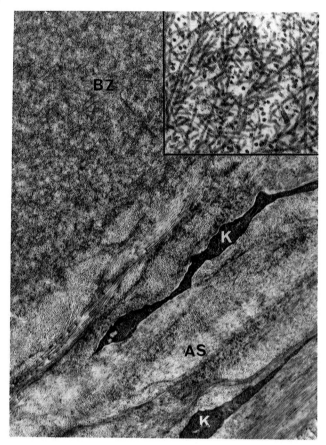

Fig. 7.14 Electron micrograph of Bowman's zone (BZ) and the anterior stroma (AS) in the human cornea, showing collagen fibrils mingling in at the interface. K = Keratocytes. Original magnification ×80 000. Inset (original magnification ×40 000) shows the felt-like arrangement of collagen in Bowman's zone.

1971; Maurice, 1984) although this arrangement is less precise in the anterior third of the stroma (McTigue, 1967) and has yet to be convincingly demonstrated. Here there is greater interweave and some lamellae pass forwards obliquely to be inserted into Bowman's layer (Polack, 1961; Tripathi and Bron, 1975).

In the deeper stroma the lamellae form strap-like ribbons which run approximately at right-angles to those in consecutive layers. Kokott (1938) studied their organization by multiple insertions of fine needles at various depths in the stroma. He has depicted the straps as running at varying angles to one another, at different levels and, in the more peripheral layers, as receiving insertions from the scleral bundles and reflecting the insertions of the rectus muscles (Fig. 7.54). At the limbus, the bundles appeared to take a circular course. This anatomy may influence the different effects of corneal or limbal incision during cataract surgery on postoperative corneal shape. A slight waviness in the plane of the

cornea gives rise to coarse cross-striations on specular microscopy in the living eye (Gallagher and Maurice, 1977) (Fig. 7.18). Occasionally, the lamellae branch and hence, in histologic section, appear to be cut in different directions in any section. The union between neighbouring bands slightly hinders separation of the cornea into lamellae, anteriorly more than posteriorly; even so, lamellar separation is readily achieved by blunt dissection and is the basis for lamellar corneal grafting. This is in contrast to the interweaving of collagen bundles in the sclera which is more complex and precludes ready separation. The arrangement of the lamellae is poorly shown with wax embedding and thick sections for light microscopy: a better impression is obtained from epoxy-resin embedded tissue and semi-thin sections stained with toluidine blue (Fig. 7.3), or by electron microscopy. Similarly the keratocytes of the stroma are poorly seen on light microscopy, only their flattened nuclei being visible readily in haematoxylin and eosin preparations.

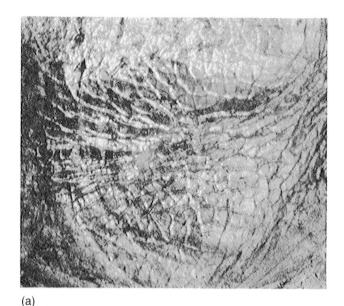

(a)

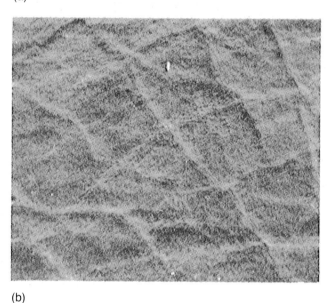

(b)

Fig. 7.15 (a) Polygonal ridge pattern seen in a fixed dehydrated and gold-coated cornea. The ridge pattern was created by inducing hypotony of the globe before fixation. These ridges are readily observed during cataract surgery, when the cornea is rendered relatively concave by manipulation. (b) SEM of Bowman's layer after removal of the corneal epithelium, showing the polygonal ridge pattern of the anterior corneal mosaic. Original magnification ×114. (From Bron, A. J. and Tripathi, R. C. (1970) *Br. J. Physiol. Optics*, **25**, 8, with permission.)

Ultrastructural features

Each stromal lamella comprises a band of collagen fibrils arranged in parallel (Fig. 7.20). Fibrils show the typical 64-nm periodicity of connective tissue collagens with a microperiod of 6 nm. The banding pattern is best shown by negative staining after

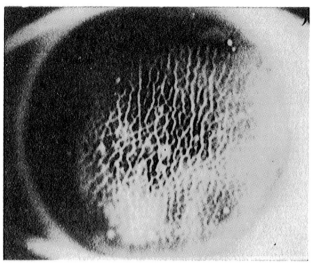

Fig. 7.16 Demonstration of the anterior corneal mosaic with fluorescein in the tear film. The cornea is gently massaged, through the lids, for a number of seconds. Fluorescein in the tear film demonstrates a transient 'chicken-wire' network of interlacing grooves (lid massage induces a network of ridges at the surface of the cornea, which compress and thin the overlying epithelium. When the pressure is released the areas of thinning persist transiently as grooves, which are demonstrated by fluorescein). (From Bron, A. J. and Tripathi, R. C. (1970) *Br. J. Physiol. Optics*, **25**, 8, with permission.)

removal of proteoglycan. The alternating bands of varying electron density within the 64-nm 'D-period' are designated a to e (Fig 7.21). There is a unique uniformity of fibril diameter: although there is a slight increase in fibril diameter passing from the front to the back of the cornea (27 nm opposed to 35 nm), there is no general agreement (for example Pouliquen, 1987 quotes anterior and posterior to be the same, at 22 (±1) nm). Variation within lamellae is minimal and there is remarkable regularity of separation both within and between lamellae. (The interfibrillar separation is said to be approximately equal to fibril diameter: however, Pouliquen (1980) gives a value of 43.2 (±1.7) nm, and 45.6 nm in the pre-Descemet's region.) Interfibrillar distance is said to fall slightly with age (Kanai and Kaufman, 1973). This precise ordering of collagen fibrils is responsible for the transparency of the corneal stroma.

The keratocytes of the corneal stroma occupy 2.5–5% of its volume (Langham and Taylor, 1956; Maurice and Riley, 1968) and are responsible for synthesis of the stromal collagen and proteoglycan during development and maintaining it thereafter. In transverse sections of the cornea (Fig. 7.22) they appear as long, thin, flattened cells (maximally 2 μm thick) running parallel to the corneal surface, and viewed from either corneal surface as stellate cells with many processes in tangential sections or in

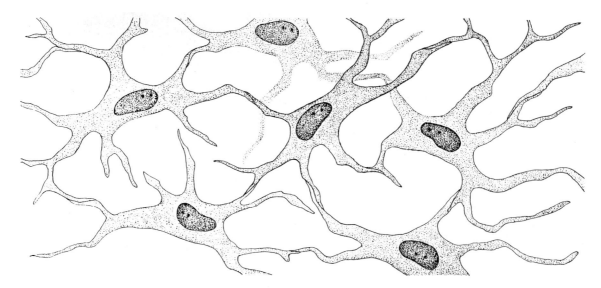

Fig. 7.17 Schematic diagram to show contact between fibroblasts lying between the stromal lamellae. The cells are thin and flat, with long processes that contact those of other cells in the same plane. Occasionally they may be joined by a macula occludens. (From Hogan, M. J., Alvarado, J. A. and Weddell, J. E. (1971) *Histology of the Eye. An Atlas and Textbook*, published by W. B. Saunders.)

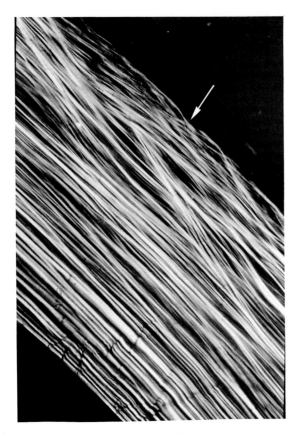

Fig. 7.18 Transverse section of the cornea viewed by polarized light reveals its superimposed pattern of collagen lamellae. Note the criss-crossing and oblique orientation of the collagen lamellae in the superficial stroma, which eventually terminate in Bowman's zone (arrowed). In the deeper stroma the lamellae are regularly organized. Original magnification ×245.

silver preparations (Duke-Elder and Wybar, 1961). Keratocytes occur throughout the cornea; and only in humans are they found predominantly between lamellae (Fig. 7.23); occasionally within lamellae (Fig. 7.24). Their stellate processes extend for great distances and frequent contacts are made with other keratocytes in the same horizontal plane, usually with a 20 nm gap between and sometimes with the formation of maculae occludentes, adhaerentes or gap junctions (Fig. 7.17). Anteroposterior connections between keratocytes in adjacent planes do not occur. An electron-lucent zone intervenes between the keratocytes and neighbouring collagen fibrils. Keratocytes have long flattened nuclei and, while their sparse cytoplasm contains a full complement of organelles, they are few in number. In normal cornea there is a limited rough endoplasmic reticulum but it becomes extensively developed in activated keratocytes of injured or inflamed cornea (Kuwabara, 1978). Around many keratocytes an amorphous or fine fibrillar electron-dense material is observed, which may be a precursor of proteoglycan or collagen fibrils and is found in relation to membrane pits, some of which may be coated, or to thickened zones in the cell membrane which show a hemidesmosome-like appearance (Kuwabara, 1978).

Three other types of cells occasionally occur in normal corneal stroma: lymphocytes, macrophages and (very rarely) polymorphonuclear leucocytes.

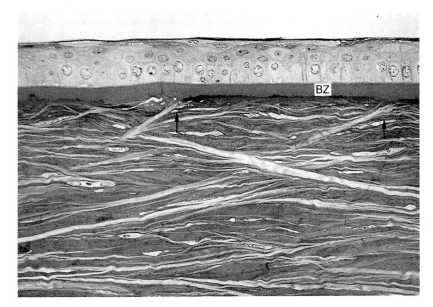

Fig. 7.19 Section of anterior corneal stroma seen by semi-polarized light, revealing irregular coarse, branching and interlacing pattern of collagen lamellae. Arrows denote insertion of prominent collagen lamellae into the acellular Bowman's zone (BZ).

Stromal repair

Repair of the stroma after small central injuries involves keratocyte activation, migration and transformation into fibroblasts and the production of scar tissue. Before closure of the surface defect by an epithelial plug, some polymorphonuclear leucocytes may enter the stroma from the tear fluid. Larger wounds provoke a rapid vascular response in addition, with an invasion by polymorphonuclear leucocytes and monocytes. Transformation of the monocytes into fibroblasts requires the presence of an overlying epithelium. (Consult Maurice (1984) for further details; the subject of corneal neovascularization is discussed by Garner, 1986.)

Collagen fibrils are initially laid down without regularity, and are larger than in normal cornea (Schwarz, 1953b). Remodelling of the scar tissue ensues, with thinning of fibrils, reformation of lamellae over many months and an increase in transparency (Cintron and Kublin, 1977). Lymphatic channels, normally absent from the cornea, appear in vascularized scars and persist after injury (Collin, 1970a,b).

Descemet's membrane (posterior limiting layer)

Descemet's membrane is the basal lamina of the corneal endothelium and first appears at the second month of gestation. Its synthesis continues throughout adult life, so that while it is only 3–4 μm thick at birth it is 5 μm thick in childhood and reaches a thickness of 10–12 μm in the adult (Tripathi, 1972b; Wulle, 1972) (Fig. 7.25). Although it appears homogeneous under light microscopy,

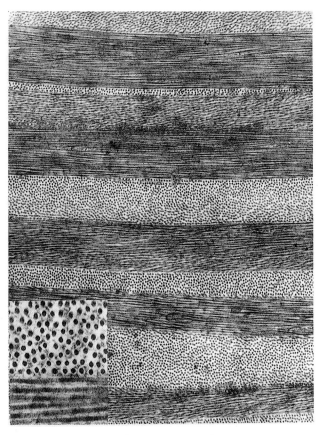

Fig. 7.20 Electron micrograph of mid-corneal stroma, showing similar width of lamellae, which cross each other approximately at right-angles (original magnification ×32 500). The inset shows fine web-like material interspersed among the regularly spaced collagen fibrils cut transversely (original magnification ×90 000).

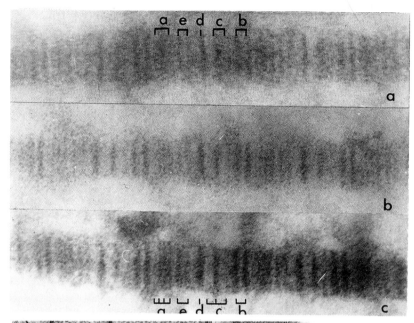

Fig. 7.21 The banding pattern of human corneal collagen (a) stained with PTA only, (b) stained with uranyl acetate only and (c) stained with PTA followed by uranyl acetate. All original magnification ×750 000. (Courtesy of K. Meek.)

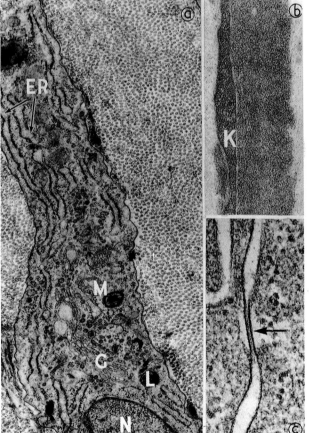

Fig. 7.22 (a) Electron micrograph of a young keratocyte, showing various intracellular organelles. ER = Well-developed rough-surfaced endoplasmic reticulum; G = Golgi apparatus; L = lysosomes; M = mitochondrion; N = nucleus. Original magnification ×28 150. (b) Granulofibrillar material adjacent to a keratocyte process (K). Original magnification ×48 500. (c) An occluding zonule (arrow) between juxtaposed cell processes of keratocytes, probably indicative of the embryonic character of these corneal fibroblasts. Original magnification ×121 300.

it has a laminated structure which may be demonstrated by polarization (Kohler and Tobgy, 1929; Baud and Balvoine, 1953), dark field (Peschell, 1905; Grignolo, 1954) or electron microscopy. This reflects a structural difference between its fetal and postnatal components.

Descemet's membrane is a strong resistant sheet, closely applied to the back of the corneal stroma, from which, unlike Bowman's layer, it is sharply defined (Fig. 7.26) and the plane of separation is used at lamellar keratoplasty. Bowman's and Descemet's layers are not homologous; the former is a modified zone of the anterior stroma, and not a basal lamina. Descemet's membrane thickens with age and in degenerative conditions of the corneal epithelium such as congenital endothelial dystrophy or posterior polymorphous dystrophy.

The major protein of Descemet's layer is type IV collagen. Its glycoprotein and proteoglycan content are responsible for the brilliant pink staining with periodic acid–Schiff reagent as is common with other basal laminae. Otherwise its appearance is undistinguished by light microscopy and it stains poorly with haematoxylin and eosin.

Ultrastructural features

The laminated structure of Descemet's membrane has been demonstrated by several workers (Grignolo, 1954; Feeney and Garron, 1961; Jakus, 1961; Kaye and Pappas, 1962; Hogan, Alvarado and Weddell, 1971). The anterior third of the adult Descemet's membrane corresponds to that part produced in fetal life and is therefore oldest (Fig. 7.27). It shows an

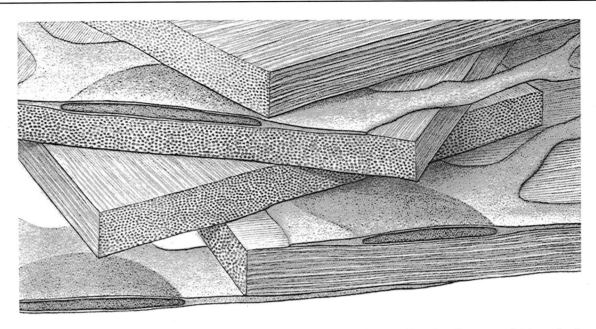

Fig. 7.23 Schematic diagram of the corneal stromal lamellae. The collagen fibrils within a lamella are parallel to each other. Successive lamellae run approximately at right-angles to each other. Keratocytes are located between the lamellae. (From Hogan, M. J., Alvarado, J. A. and Weddell, J. E. (1971) *Histology of the Eye. An Atlas and Textbook*, published by W. B. Saunders.)

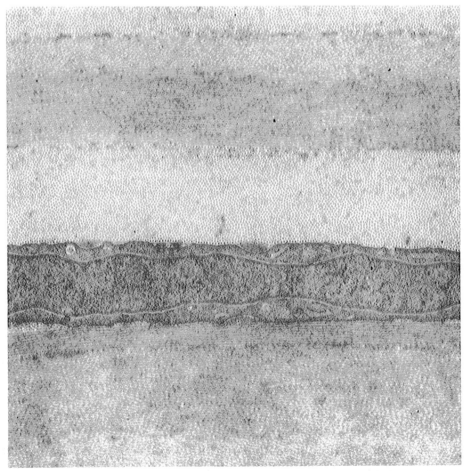

Fig. 7.24 A human corneal corpuscle (electron micrograph, original magnification ×30 000). A corneal corpuscle is visible in part, within a lamella of transversely divided fibres, but very close to a thin stratum of fibres divided longitudinally. (Courtesy of Dr John Marshall and Mr P. L. Ansell, Institute of Ophthalmology, London. Preparation by Mrs B. Tilly.)

Fig. 7.25 TEM of Descemet's membrane in meridional section. The fetal part of Descemet's membrane (f) shows a periodic, banded structure while the older portion of the membrane in the adult eye shows a more homogeneous granular structure. Original magnification ×19 400. (Courtesy of Y. Pouliquen.)

irregular banded pattern in cross-section quite unlike that of type I collagen, and ranging between 100 and 110 nm (type I, 64 nm). In tangential section the membrane appears to consist of superimposed flat plates forming a lamellar pattern of equilateral triangles with sides of about 110 nm. The triangles are interconnected by electron-dense nodes and internodes (Fig. 7.28) (Tripathi and Tripathi, 1984). The banding develops in about the fifth month of intrauterine life, when the layer has a thickness of about 3.1 μm (range 2.2–4.5 μm).

The posterior two-thirds of the membrane is formed after birth, and consists of a homogeneous fibrillogranular material. The zone adjoining the endothelium is the most recently formed. In diseases of the corneal endothelium where thickness and morphology of Descemet's layer is altered, the presence of a normal anterior banded layer can be taken to signify onset of the disorder after birth (Waring, Laibson and Rodrigues, 1974). Posteriorly, Descemet's membrane and the endothelial sheet are attached by modified hemidesmosomes.

In the ageing cornea, bands of long-spacing collagen may be found in Descemet's membrane. This is more likely to represent polymerization of the collagen rather than newly secreted material given its distance from the endothelial cells. Also, in the ageing cornea, focal overproduction of basal lamina-like material produces peripheral excrescences called Hassal–Henle warts (Fig. 7.29). These are fissured and show receding cytoplasmic invaginations on their endothelial faces. Although they have been deemed a part of a 'physiological ageing process' by some, they resemble Descemet's warts of the central cornea (cornea guttata). The relationship of these latter to more profound abnormalities of Descemet's membrane and the corneal endothelium in Fuchs' dystrophy signifies that they result from a functional abnormality of their parent endothelial cells. The presence of Hassal–Henle warts is not associated

with any clinical abnormality in corneal function but cornea guttata are associated with an increase in endothelial permeability. The excrescences of cornea guttata increase in number with age (Lorenzetti and Kaufman, 1968).

The peripheral rim of Descemet's membrane is the internal landmark of the corneal limbus and marks the anterior limit of the drainage angle (Schwalbe's line). It is prominent in 15–20% of individuals and is hypertrophied in congenital anomalies in which

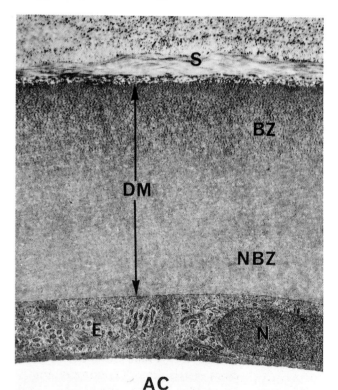

Fig. 7.26 Electron micrograph of the Descemet's membrane (DM) of a 55-year-old human in anteroposterior section, showing a banded zone (BZ) and non-banded zone (NBZ). AC = Anterior chamber; E = endothelium; N = nucleus of an endothelial cell; S = stroma. Original magnification approx. ×6300.

Fig. 7.27 An oblique section through the anterior banded region of Descemet's membrane at the junction with the posterior lamella of the corneal stroma. Note the interdigitation between the fine filaments of Descemet's membrane and the collagen fibrils of the stroma. The posterior part of Descemet's membrane in the adult has a more granular appearance. Original magnification ×49 250. (Courtesy of Y. Pouliquen.)

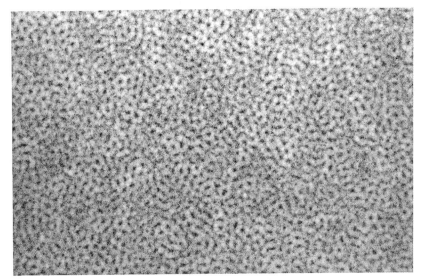

Fig. 7.28 TEM: tangential section of the anterior part of Descemet's membrane, showing a three-dimensional lattice pattern. The fine collagenous filaments form a regular polygonal pattern, with each polygon showing a central nodular densification. Original magnification ×26 950. (Courtesy of Y. Pouliquen.)

it may appear as a visible shelf on gonioscopy (posterior embryotoxon). Despite the absence of elastic tissue in Descemet's membrane, the layer has an unusual property; when stripped by injury, as at surgery, it will form into a coil which may be seen by biomicroscopy as a highly refractile cigar-shaped roll curling towards the stroma. (The lens capsule, also a thickened basal lamina, has similar properties but curls outwards.) After traumatic interruption of Descemet's membrane and the endothelial layer (which may result from penetrating injury, birth trauma, stretching of the cornea in infantile glaucoma, or rupture in the acute hydrops of keratoconus), the endothelial layer will resurface the defect by spread of its cells and synthesis of fresh basal lamina structurally identical to normal Descemet's layer. This contrasts again with Bowman's

layer, which is replaced by disorganized coarse fibrillar scar tissue after injury.

Endothelium

The endothelium is a single layer of hexagonal, cuboidal cells applied to the posterior aspect of Descemet's membrane (Fig. 7.30). These cells differentiate from cells that migrate from the limbal area at the earliest developmental stage. The origins of these cells have recently been reappraised. They are not vascular in origin, and unlike vascular endothelial cells, fail to stain with antibody against factor VIII-related antigen. In avian eyes they derive from neural crest (Johnstone, Bhakdinaronk and Reid, 1973, 1978; Noden, 1978) and there is some evidence in human cornea that they are of

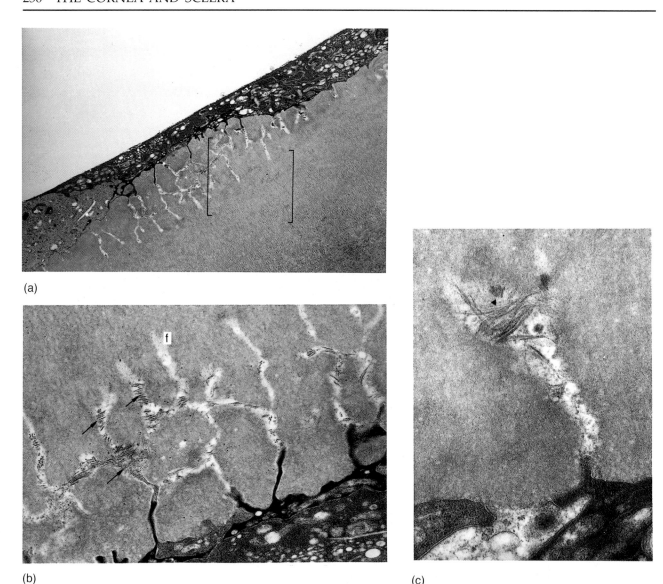

(a)

(b)   (c)

Fig. 7.29 (a) TEM of the peripheral cornea in the normal adult to show an extended Hassal–Henle wart. Descemet's membrane is thickened and fissured in this region and the overlying endothelium is thinned. There are duplications of the inner plasma membranes of the endothelium with membranous and cytoplasmic extensions into the fissured regions. Original magnification ×7350. (b) High-power view of the bracketed zone in (a). The fissured regions of the 'wart' contain fibril-granular material (arrows). F = Fissure. Original magnification ×20 520. (c) Enlargement to show banded collagen fibrils (arrowhead) within a fissure. Original magnification ×41 050. (Courtesy of Y. Pouliquen.)

neuroectodermal origin. Thus Adamis *et al.* (1985) showed staining of human endothelium with antibody against neuron-specific enolase; staining of posterior keratocytes was also demonstrated showing their origin from neural crest.

While mitosis may occur in young human endothelial cells, it is infrequent in the adult and it appears that cornea is supplied with a relatively fixed population of about 500 000 cells which are replaced in a limited way after injury. There is great individual variation in cell counts. A gradual decrease in density and increase in shape variation

(polymegathism) occur with age (Shaw *et al.*, 1978): in youth, the cells are predominantly hexagonal in shape in the plane of the cornea but with age become increasingly polymorphic (Fig. 7.31). Sherrand, Novakovic and Speedwell (1987) suggested (on the basis of various reports and their own experience with specular microscopy) that endothelial density is about 6000 cells/mm^2 at birth and falls by about 26% in the first year. A further 26% is lost over the next 11 years but the rate of loss slows and possibly stabilizes around middle age, especially in polymegathous endothelium (Blatt, Rao and Ac-

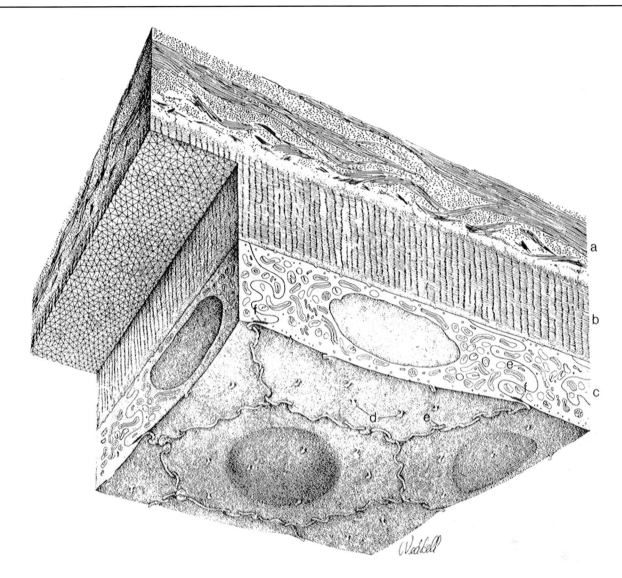

Fig. 7.30   Three-dimensional drawing of the deep cornea showing (a) deepest corneal lamellae, (b) Descemet's membrane and (c) the epithelium. Some branches of the deeper stromal lamellae split posteriorly to merge with Descemet's membrane. Descemet's membrane is seen in the meridional and tangential planes. The collagenous lattice with this membrane has intersecting filaments which form nodes separated from each other by 110 nm. They are exactly registered on each other to form a linear pattern in meridional sections. The polygonal endothelial cells show (d) microvilli, which protrude into the anterior chamber at intercellular junctions. The intercellular space near the anterior chamber is closed by a zonula occludens (f). The cytoplasm contains abundant mitochondria. The nucleus is flattened in the anteroposterior axis. (From Hogan, M. J., Alvarado, J. A. and Weddell, J. E. (1971) *Histology of the Eye. An Atlas and Textbook*, published by W. B. Saunders.)

quavella, 1979) (Figs 7.32 and 7.33). After injury of any kind, damaged cells are replaced by a spreading of cells from adjacent zones, the cells increasing in area (up to three times their span) but decreasing in height (Fig. 7.34).

At birth the cells are 10 μm in height, but become extremely flat (3–5 μm) with age (Kuwabara, 1978). The width of the adult cell is 18–20 μm. The endothelial cell has an oval nucleus located centrally and about 7 μm in width.

Ultrastructural features

The lateral borders of the cells are markedly convoluted to produce a complex interdigitation with neighbouring cells (Fig. 7.35). The anterior (basal) and the posterior (apical) cell membranes are relatively flat. The **anterior cell membrane** is in contact with Descemet's membrane, and attached to it by modified hemidesmosomes. There are numerous focal areas of increased density along its length

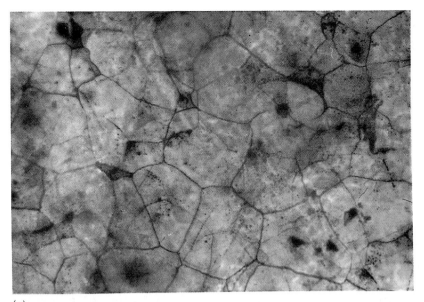

(a)

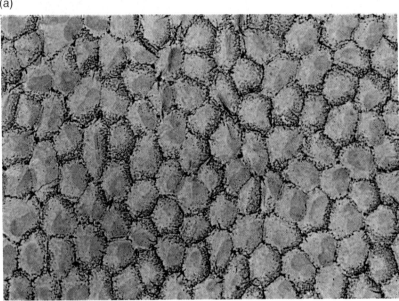

(b)

Fig. 7.31 (a) Silver preparation of the surface layer of the corneal epithelium reveals the size and outline of the surface squamous cells. Photomicrograph: original magnification ×480. (b) Flat preparation of corneal endothelium stained with silver to reveal the typical hexagonal arrangement of cells with tortuous intercellular borders. Photomicrograph: original magnification ×580.

which are said to be derived from the absorption of pinocytotic vesicles (Hogan, Alvarado and Weddell, 1971). The lateral cell membranes of contiguous cells run an extremely sinuous course in the anteroposterior plane, and these interdigitations fold over one another at the apical aspect of the cell to form a **marginal fold** at the apicolateral interface (Kaye, Pappas and Donn, 1961). On scanning microscopy these folds can be seen to interdigitate with each other at the cell borders (Fig. 7.36). The lateral intercellular space is about 20 nm for the greater part of its length (Burstein and Maurice, 1978; Hirsch *et al.*, 1982) but the width measured is dependent on the fixative used (Hodson and Mayes, 1979). The

cells are firmly bound together by cell junctions (including maculae adhaerentes and, less commonly, maculae occludentes along the anterior two-thirds of the membrane) and junctional complexes, comprising maculae occludentes and gap junctions in relation to the posterior third and the apicolateral interface (Fig. 7.37). Membrane separation is about 2 nm in the region of the gap junction (Kreutzinger, 1976; Leuenberger, 1973), and there is membrane fusion at the maculae occludentes (Hirsch *et al.*, 1977; Ottersen and Vegge, 1977). (Earlier studies suggested the presence of zonulae occludentes running around the contiguous borders of the cells but their presence has not been confirmed.)

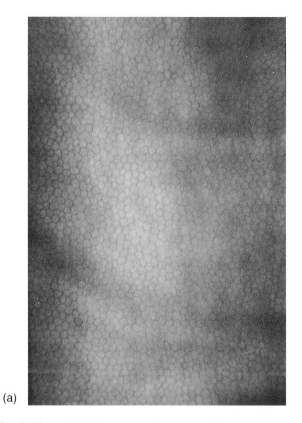

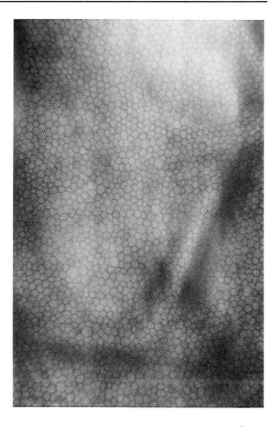

(a)

(b)

Fig. 7.32 Wide-field specular microscopy of human corneal endothelium in (a) a 24-year-old man (cell count 2593 cells/mm^2) and (b) an 83-year-old woman (cell count 2134 cells/mm^2). (Courtesy of E. Sherrard.)

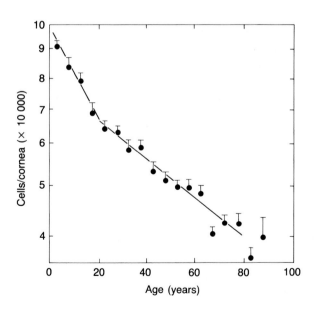

Fig. 7.33 Graph showing the decline in mean endothelial cell population with age in the human cornea. There is a steep decline for ages from 3 to 25 years and a more gradual decline from 25 to 88 years. The two lines were best-fit curves using the method of least squares. (From Laule *et al.* (1978) *Arch. Ophthalmol.* **36**, 2031, with permission.)

Wulle (1972) observed immature cell junctions in developing human eyes loosely connecting mesenchymal cells, which form the corneal endothelium between the seventh and eighth weeks of gestation. Occluding junctions, resembling maculae occludentes, appear in the eighth week. In the middle of the fourth month, coinciding with the commencement of aqueous humour formation, junctions (then termed zonulae occludentes) appear between endothelial cells and come to resemble those of the adult after the fifth month. Desmosomes are rare on the lateral cell membrane, but both maculae adhaerentes and maculae occludentes occur along the anterior two-thirds of the membranes, though they are uncommon (Fig. 7.38).

The surface of the posterior cell membrane shows 20–30 microvilli per cell, 0.1–0.2 μm in width and 0.5–0.6 μm in height. Other than to increase absorptive surface area, their function is unknown (Blumcke and Morgenroth, 1967). Rarely cilia occur, directed into the anterior chamber and related to a pair of centrioles in the posterior aspect of the cytoplasm. They are more frequent towards the periphery (Svedberg and Bill, 1972; Renard *et al.*, 1976). On the basis of this, Hogan, Alvarado and Weddell (1971) have suggested an origin for these cells common with those of the corneotrabecular sheets and cells on the anterior surface of the iris. Gallagher (1980) believes

that all endothelial cells possess cilia and this was supported by the studies of Wolf (1968a) using casts.

The endothelial cell membranes are typical unit membranes and show pinocytic vesicles along the inner surfaces of all membrane faces (Fig. 7.39). Kuwabara (1978) has found these to be infrequent, but experimental studies using tracer materials (Maurice, 1953; Kaye, Pappas and Donn, 1961; Kaye and Pappas, 1962; Iwamoto and Smelser, 1965) demonstrated the transfer of particulate material (e.g. Thorotrast) from anterior chamber into the intercellular space anteriorly and to the inner surface of Descemet's membrane. The possibility of increased pinocytotic activity in response to the particulate matter does arise.

The subcellular organization reflects that the endothelium is extremely active metabolically. Large numbers of mitochondria are distributed throughout the cell, particularly around the nucleus. Of the cells of the eye, only the retinal pigment epithelium and the ellipsoids of the retinal photoreceptors show a greater density of mitochondria. Both rough and smooth endoplasmic reticulum are present, in addition to free ribosomes. The Golgi apparatus is perinuclear in location, facing the anterior chamber. A condensation of cytoplasm rich in actin, the **terminal web**, lies close to the posterior membrane (Rahi and Ashton, 1978; Gallagher, 1980). It is about 2 nm in thickness, and in other cells is associated with the location of tight junctions (Iwamoto and Smelser, 1965).

In man, the existence of a coating over the outer surface of the posterior membrane (Sperling and Jacobson, 1980) is uncertain.

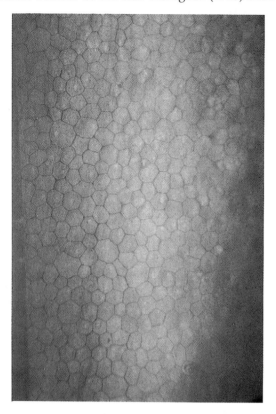

Fig. 7.34 Specular micrograph of the endothelium of a human corneal graft patient. There is marked variation in endothelial cell size and shape and the cell borders are more easy to see than in a normal young cornea (cell density 587 cells/mm^2). (Courtesy of E. Sherrard.)

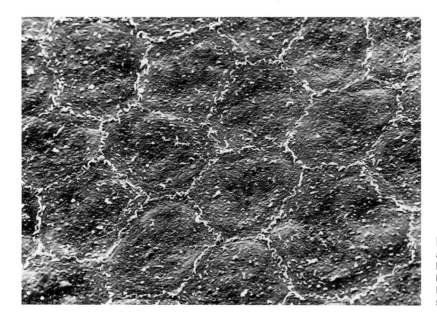

Fig. 7.35 Scanning electron micrograph of a human corneal endothelium, showing hexagonal pattern with tortuous intercellular borders marked by microvillous projections. Note also a few microvilli on the cell surface. Original magnification × 1840.

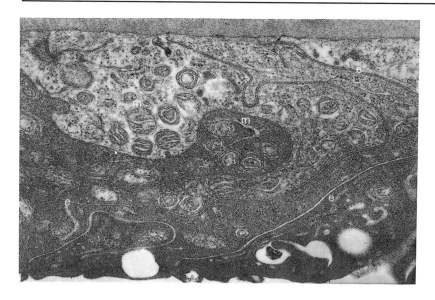

Fig. 7.36 TEM of the corneal endothelium. Meridional section showing marked undulation of the lateral walls of adjacent endothelial cells. The intercellular space can be traced for long distances up to a point close to the anterior chamber below. The cells are liberally supplied with mitochondria (m) and the cisternae of rough-surfaced endoplasmic reticulum (e) are scattered through the cytoplasm. Original magnification ×33 516. (Courtesy of Y. Pouliquen.)

Physiology

Nutrition   The endothelium plays a major role in maintaining corneal transparency. Essential nutrients (such as glucose and amino acids) must pass across its surface to supply the cellular needs of all of the corneal layers; oxygen derived from the aqueous supplies the requirements of the endothelium and posterior stroma (Po_2 55 mmHg).

Fluid regulation   Physiological studies have shown that this delicate monolayer of cells is responsible for maintaining the corneal stroma free of oedema, in a state of relative deturgescence. This it does in two ways: first it provides a barrier function to the ingress of salt and metabolites into the stroma, which has a spontaneous tendency to take up salt and consequently, by osmosis, water; second, it actively reduces the osmotic pressure of the stroma by metabolically pumping the bicarbonate ions out of the stroma and back into the aqueous humour (Fig. 7.40).

The barrier properties of the corneal endothelium, which have recently been shown to be relatively simple, need a little explanation. On their lateral walls, posteriorly, the cells exhibit apparent tight junctions (part of a junctional complex). The term 'tight junctions' is misleading, for it seems clear that they do not impede the diffusion of ions to any great extent. Most of the barrier function is provided by the geometry of the intercellular space, and all passive movement of ions and metabolites across the monolayer takes place through the intercellular spaces between the cells. Compared to most monolayers of cells, corneal endothelium is rela-

tively 'leaky', mainly because of the shortness of the interdigitating intercellular space and the absence of a physiologically functional tight junction. Nevertheless, the barrier function is well balanced and matched to the activity of the outward-directed bicarbonate ion pump (Hodson and Miller, 1976). In contrast to its solvents, the water molecules of aqueous humour and stroma pass with greater freedom directly through the cells of the monolayer (Hodson and Lawton, 1987; Hodson and Wigham, 1987) ensuring that the water potential of both stromal fluid and aqueous humour is equal. Changes in corneal hydration are, therefore, rate-limited by the balance between the net passive diffusion of ions between the cells and into the stroma and the active bicarbonate pump which works through the cells, in the opposite direction, out of the stroma.

In this way it can be seen that stromal hydration is regulated by a system of pump-leak of ions, chiefly under the control of the corneal endothelium. The epithelium plays a minor role in regulating corneal hydration although it has a major barrier function.

The gap junctions found between corneal endothelial cells serve to facilitate cell-to-cell transport of ions and result in electrical coupling of endothelial cells.

Injury and repair   Great interest has been focused on the endothelial response to injury because of its dual role as barrier and fluid pump of the cornea. The pumping activity of the corneal endothelium may be inhibited experimentally by drugs such as ouabain, and permeability of the endothelium increased by destruction of the endothelial gap junctions. Physical and chemical damage to the human corneal

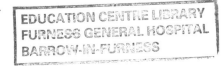

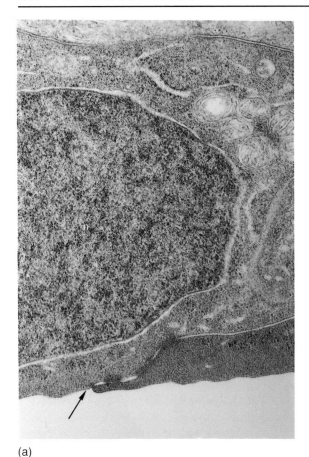

(a)

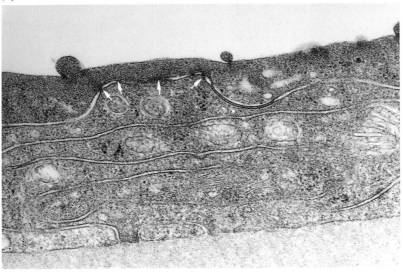

(b)

Fig. 7.37 (a) TEM of the endothelium, showing the apicolateral overlap of the membranes of adjoining cells and closure of the intercellular space by a junctional complex which includes an incomplete tight junction (arrow). n = Nucleus. Original magnification ×44 800. (b) The apicolateral junctional region between neighbouring endothelial cells, showing tight junctions (arrows) and a macula occludens (*). Original magnification ×62 100. (Courtesy of Y. Pouliquen.)

endothelium result in loss of endothelial cells, and because of the poor reparative power of human endothelium the loss in continuity of the endothelial sheet is made up by a sliding process in which neighbouring cells move over to fill the gap. This is accompanied by enlargement of the cells to cover the original area. Thus, after injury, the endothelial cell density falls, the cell area increases and the cell height decreases. This sliding phenomenon is not distributed equally across the whole of the corneal surface and after a localized injury will be confined to the immediate neighbourhood of the injury. Although the healed endothelium may exhibit a regular hexagonal endothelial pattern, some endothelial polymorphism is common. Endothelial injury produces corneal oedema due to loss of

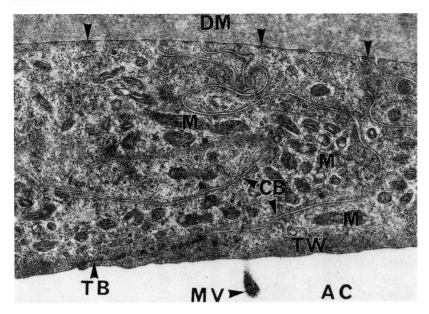

Fig. 7.38 The corneal endothelium is attached to Descemet's membrane (DM) by modified desmosomes (arrowed). Note the condensed and fibrillar cytoplasm forming a 'terminal web' (TW), a microvillus (MV) projecting into the anterior chamber (AC), an attachment body or 'terminal bar' (TB), the convoluted cell borders (CB) and an abundance of filamentous mitochondria (M). Electron micrograph, original magnification ×17 500.

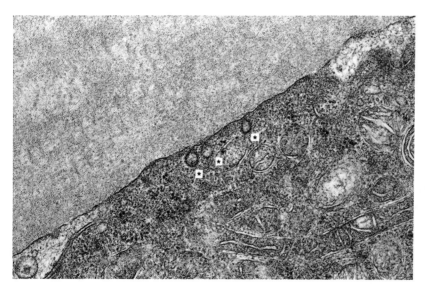

Fig. 7.39 TEM of the junction between Descemet's membrane and the endothelium. Three pinocytotic vesicles are shown at the interface (*). Original magnification ×62 100. (Courtesy of Y. Pouliquen.)

the specialized junctions between endothelial cells and of the pumping function of the cells at the site of injury. With re-establishment of the endothelial sheet, these specialized junctions and the normal pumping and permeability characteristics of the endothelium return, with the disappearance of corneal oedema. The process of sliding of cells and decreased endothelial cell density is a normal ageing phenomenon, which accounts for the fall in endothelial density which occurs with age. Adult human endothelial cells rarely undergo cell division spontaneously. It appears that the cornea receives its full complement of cells at or about birth (about 5 000 000 cells). Although occasional mitotic figures are found in human corneal endothelium (Kauf-

man, Capella and Robbins, 1966) and experimental studies in primates have demonstrated incorporation of thymidine into endothelial cells after endothelial injury (Gloor *et al.*, 1980), repair of endothelial damage is generally by slide rather than mitosis. This behaviour of human endothelial cells is of major clinical importance.

STRUCTURAL PROTEINS OF THE CORNEA

Collagen is the major structural component of the cornea, while proteoglycan accounts for most of the 'ground substance' material. Some glycoprotein is present.

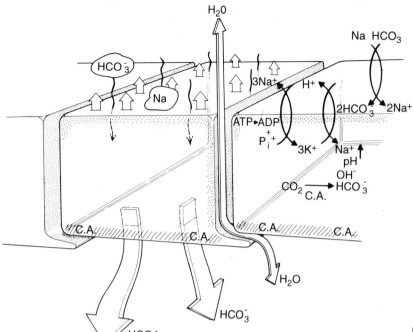

Fig. 7.40 Diagram illustrating the endothelium pump of the cornea.

Collagen

The cornea is unusual in the variety of molecular collagen types which it contains (Fig. 7.41). There is also significant species variation. The ocular collagen types are well summarized by Bailey (1987) and include the **fibrous collagens** types I, II, III and V, **non-fibrous collagen** type IV and **filamentous collagens** types VI, VIII, IX and X.

The basal lamina of the epithelium contains type IV collagen in its periphery. The predominant collagen (about 90%) of the stroma is type I and thus resembles the collagen of sclera and muscle tendon. The proportion of other types has been variously estimated: type III has been found to comprise 2% in the rabbit embryo and under 1% in the adult by Lee and Davison (1981), or up to 20% in the adult by Freeman (1982); type II is found in the embryonic cornea; type V increases with maturation from 5 to 10% and may be the predominant collagen of Bowman's layer. Linsenmayer et al. (1985) found type V collagen to be present in avian cornea in masked form, revealed by immunohistochemical staining only after treatment with acetic acid to swell the fibres. The occurrence of hybrid fibrils of type I and type V collagen may be a determinant of the narrow fibril size of stromal collagen. Alternatively, the relative lack of type III, which normally co-distributes with type I (e.g. in skin and tendon) may contribute

to the ability to form narrow fibres. Recently, type VI collagen has been identified as a major constituent of extracellular matrix of the human cornea (Zimmerman et al., 1986).

Descemet's membrane contains predominantly type IV collagen, with about 10% type V (Kefalides, 1978). Recently a high proportion of type VIII collagen has been noted (Labermeier et al., 1983; Kapoor et al., 1986; Benya and Padilla, 1986).

Stromal collagen shows a high order of specialization with its fine and uniform fibril size, uniform fibril separation and high level of fibrillar organization. Stromal fibril diameter resembles that of embryonic collagen. Various explanations for the fine fibril size have been offered, and the role of molecular hybrids has been mentioned above. Stromal collagen is highly glycosylated (about five times that of tendon collagen) and glycosylation occurs within the 'gap' region of the fibril (which axially separates each collagen molecule within a fibril) and the 'overlap' region (which arises because of the staggered relationship between the molecules within the fibril). Glycosylation within the overlap region probably hinders the orderly packing of fibrils and thus this too may prevent the formation of fibrils of large size (Fig. 7.42).

Proteoglycan distribution in the extrafibrillar matrix probably influences fibril diameter and the orderly packing of stromal fibrils. Non-fibrillar, type IV

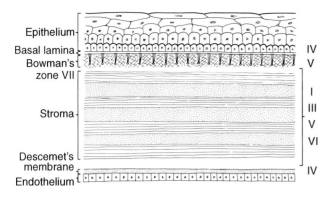

Epithelium
Basal lamina
Bowman's zone VII
Stroma
Descemet's membrane
Endothelium

IV
V
I
III
V
VI
IV

Fig. 7.41 Schematic diagram illustrating the distribution of collagen types at different levels in the cornea.

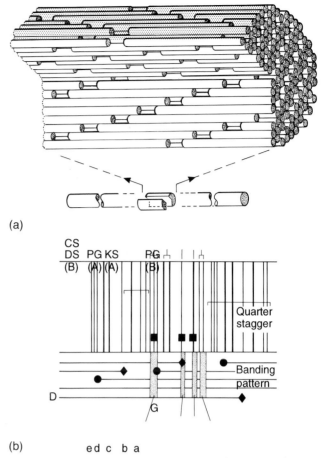

(a)

(b)

CS
DS PG KS
(B) (A)(A)

PG
(B)

Quarter stagger

Banding pattern

D

G

e d c b a

Fig. 7.42 The packaging of collagen in quarter-stagger array. This gives rise to the typical 64-nm banding pattern of collagen in stained specimens. ((a) Courtesy of J. Ibrahim.)

collagen of Descemet's membrane is more highly glycosylated than type I collagen, but its amorphous ultrastructural appearance may owe much to the platelike tertiary structure of the type IV collagen molecule itself.

Proteoglycans

Proteoglycans constitute most of the ground substance material between the stromal fibrils, of which keratan sulphate represents 50% and chondroitin and chondroitin sulphate the remainder. Borcherding *et al.* (1975) found keratan sulphate to be the major constituent in central stroma with chondroitin the minor constituent, while chondroitin sulphate replaced chondroitin in peripheral cornea. In the peripheral cornea there is an increasing proportion of dermatan sulphate and a fall in keratan sulphate.

Proteoglycan interacts with the collagen fibrils in a precise way in relation to its banding pattern (Fig. 7.43). This banding pattern reflects the charge distribution along the amino acids of the collagen molecule, and the ordering of the collagen fibrils in a staggered array within the fibril (Meek and Holmes, 1983). X-ray diffraction (Meek, Elliott and Nave, 1986) and electrohistochemical staining (Scott, 1980; Scott and Haigh, 1985) have demonstrated dermatan sulphate to be located in the gap region as well as at several sites outside it, while keratan sulphate is located in the overlap region. It has been suggested by Scott (1985) that dermatan sulphate in the gap region may play a role in inhibiting calcification in normally non-calcifying tissues such as tendon and cornea and skin. Proteoglycan is found in fixed ratio to collagen in the cornea across the species. Where the collagen fibrils are narrower, the fibrils are closer and there is less proteoglycan (Meek and Leonard, 1993).

Electrohistochemistry reveals that proteoglycan is attached in a ladderlike arrangement along the collagen fibrils, and also between them. Much of the stromal proteoglycan can be extracted from the cornea with weak salt solutions suggesting non-covalent attachment to collagen, therefore (although it is certain that this matrix material plays a role in resisting compressive forces on the cornea) its contribution to the tensile and shear strength of the cornea is uncertain. The proteoglycans provide the colloidal osmotic force responsible for the tendency of the cornea to swell. This is counteracted normally by the endothelial (and less epithelial) water pumps which maintain the cornea at its normal level of deturgescence and transparency.

Stromal oedema is accompanied by altered biosynthesis of ground substance and appearance of dermatan sulphate centrally, normally confined to the limbal region. A similar modification, with loss of keratan sulphate and increased heparan sulphate and hyaluronate, is associated with corneal scarring (Anseth, 1961b).

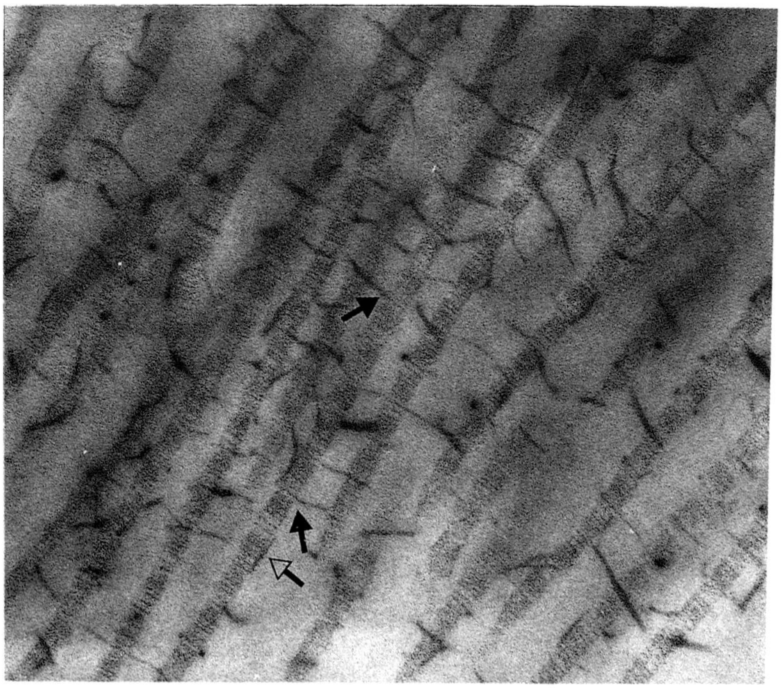

Fig. 7.43 Human stromal corneal collagen stained with Cupromeronic blue to show the organization of proteoglycan molecules along and between the collagen fibrils. (Courtesy of John Scott.)

CORNEAL TRANSPARENCY

The cornea transmits nearly 100% of the light that enters it, despite the changes in refractive index between its elements, the collagen fibrils and ground substance of the stroma. Maurice (1957) explained the transparency of the stroma on the basis of a lattice arrangement of the collagen fibrils. He argued that, because of their small diameter and regularity of separation, back-scattered light would be almost completely suppressed by destructive interference. This theory was modified slightly by Goldman (Goldman and Benedek, 1967; Goldman *et al.*, 1968) who suggested that a perfect crystalline lattice periodicity is not necessary for sufficient destructive interference to occur. Thus, if fibril separation and diameter is less than a third of the wavelength of the incident light, almost perfect transparency will ensue (Farrell *et al.*, 1983). This is the situation which obtains in the normal cornea. Transparency is lost when this regular ordering of corneal elements is destroyed, such as in corneal scarring when new collagen fibrils are laid down which have a wide variation in separation and fibril diameter and an irregular interweaving. In stromal corneal oedema, increased separation of collagen fibrils is due to formation of 'fluid lakes', and results in stromal clouding. Collagen fibril thickness probably also increases. However, in contrast to oedema of the corneal epithelium, the accumulated fluid results in an irregular epithelial surface and the irregular astigmatism produced at the air–tear interface degrades retinal image formation in a more potent manner (Miller and Benedek, 1973). In milder degrees of epithelial oedema, which may occur when wearing ill-fitting contact lenses or as a result of markedly raised intraocular pressure, the basal epithelial cells, which are regularly arranged, become separated by oedema fluid of differing refractive index to the cells themselves. This creates a diffraction grating effect so that the patient sees rainbows round white lights. This is an important symptom in subacute angle-closure glaucoma where the rise in intraocular pressure leads to epithelial oedema.

NERVES OF THE CORNEA

The cornea is supplied by the ophthalmic division of the trigeminal nerve via the anterior ciliary nerves and those of the surrounding conjunctiva (Figs 7.44 and 7.45). There is also a supply from the cervical sympathetic providing adrenergic fibres to the limbus. This division supplies almost the whole of the eye and its appendages, giving warning of injury for instance by a foreign body, and can be regarded as the 'sentinel of the eye'. The anterior ciliary nerves enter the sclera from the perichoroidal space a short distance behind the limbus. They connect with each other and with the conjunctival nerves, forming **pericorneal plexuses** at various levels.

The nerves pass into the cornea as 60–80 flattened,

mainly myelinated branches about 8 μm wide and surrounded by perineurium (Matsuda, 1968). After about 1–2 mm they usually lose their myelin sheaths (Fig. 7.46) and divide into two groups – anterior and posterior. (In rabbit and mouse some thinly myelinated nerves may be found in the deeper stroma up to the stromal centre.) The **anterior nerves** (40–50) pass through the substance of the corneal stroma and form a plexus subjacent to the anterior limiting membrane. Some controversy exists as to whether they then traverse Bowman's layer to reach the corneal epithelium: Lim and Ruskell (1978) failed to demonstrate nerve axons penetrating this layer from the stroma in monkey corneas but examples of penetrating fibres have been shown in the human eye and presumably supply the subepithelial plexus of nerve fibres (Figs 7.47 and 7.48) (Engelbrecht, 1953; Duke-Elder and Wybar, 1961; Matsuda, 1968; Schimmelpfennig, 1982). The density of this supply is not established. Ruskell's studies in the primate suggest that there is also a rich additional contribution to the subepithelial plexus from conjunctival neurons, a finding confirmed by Schimmelpfennig (1982). Clinically, dichotomously branching nerve filaments may be seen with the slit-lamp, entering the subepithelial zone.

It is not entirely clear whether the 'subepithelial' plexus is truly under the basal layer (Attias, 1912), within it (Wolter, 1956), or just superficial to it (as depicted by Schimmelpfennig, 1982). Nevertheless, the nerves which contribute to it enter as a series of leashes which divide dichotomously to form a parallel network of fibres which run for up to 2 mm, interconnected by multiple beaded fibres of smaller diameter. These give rise to fine free nerve terminals, also beaded, which branch dichotomously in the superficial epithelial layers. Some beaded nerves of the plexus make contact with Langerhans cells (Schimmelpfennig, 1982). The beaded regions contain mitochondria (Matsuda, 1968). Confocal microscopy suggests that there is a slow centripetal movement of basal cells and nerve terminals over time (Auran *et al.*, 1995).

The **posterior** group of nerves (40 or 50) pass to the posterior part of the cornea to innervate the posterior stroma excluding Descemet's membrane. Axons have been shown to terminate in the stroma in prepared whole mounts (Attias, 1912; Boeke, 1925; Zander and Weddell, 1951), but the question remains whether staining was complete. Such terminal filaments could function as tension 'receptors' for the corneoscleral envelope.

Autonomic and peptidergic innervation is described in Chapter 16.

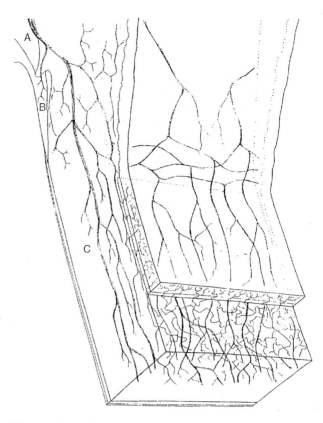

Fig. 7.44 Schematic representation of the innervation of the limbus and cornea. A long ciliary nerve (A) supplies the limbal region and then sends branches into the cornea. Nerves also supply the trabecular meshwork (B) in the region of the canal of Schlemm. Note the paucity of nerves in the deep cornea (C) and their absence in the region of Descemet's membrane. (From Hogan, M. J., Alvarado, J. A. and Weddell, J. E. (1971) *Histology of the Eye. An Atlas and Textbook*, published by W. B. Saunders.)

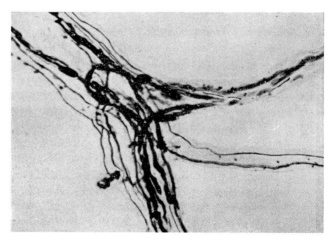

Fig. 7.45 Flat section of nerves at the limbus (Bielchowsky stain).

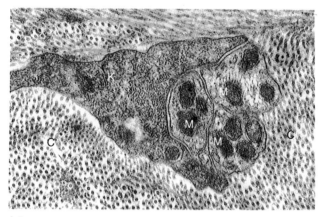

(a)

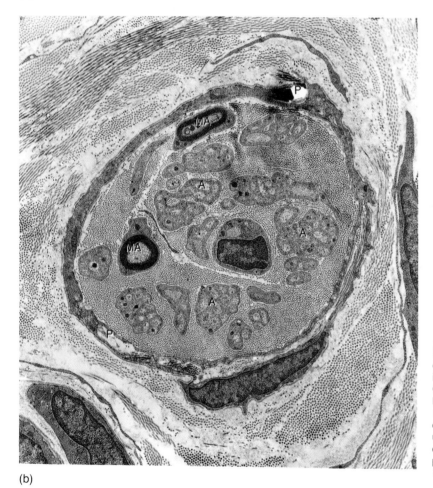

(b)

Fig. 7.46 (a) Electron micrograph of corneal stroma to show unmyelinated axons indenting a stromal keratocyte. C = Collagen fibrils; K = keratocyte; M = mitochondria. Original magnification ×45 000. (b) A nerve bundle at the corneoscleral limbus. Myelinated (MA) and unmyelinated (A) bundles of axons in a collagenous matrix are enclosed by a perineum (P). Original magnification ×15 000.

7.2 THE LIMBAL TRANSITION ZONE

The limbus is the junctional zone, about 1.5 mm wide in the horizontal plane and 2 mm in the vertical, between the cornea and the sclera, its internal edge being called the **corneal limbus** and its external edge the **scleral limbus**.

The corneal limbus is demonstrated by a line joining the termination of Bowman's layer to the termination of Descemet's membrane. The termination of Bowman's layer is indicated on biomicroscopy by the internal limit of the marginal arcade of corneal vessels, seen best at the upper and lower limbus. The termination of Descemet's layer is visible on gonioscopy as the most anterior landmark of the drainage angle, Schwalbe's line, which may at times be

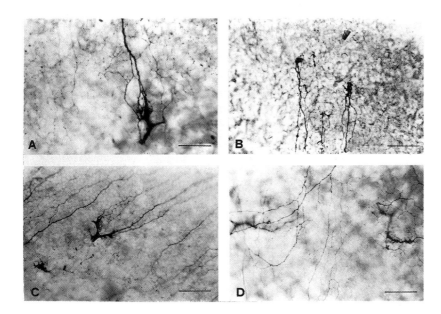

Fig. 7.47 Termination of the nerve terminals in the corneal epithelium. (Courtesy of B. H. Schimmelpfennig.)

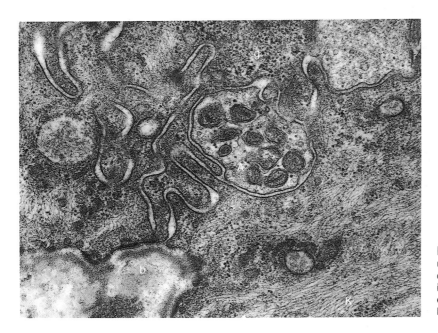

Fig. 7.48 Electron micrograph of an unmyelinated nerve terminal within the corneal epithelium lying within the intercellular space between two basal epithelial cells. A = Nerve axon; b = basal lamina; g = glycogen; K = keratin.

hypertrophied (anterior embryotoxon) as a congenital anomaly and is then visible on gonioscopy as a fine internal ridge.

The scleral limbus is less clearly defined by a line perpendicular to the surface, passing through the scleral spur.

Within the limbal zone, the orderly packing of the corneal collagen gives way to the coarse interweaving of scleral fibres, and the fibril diameter increases markedly from the narrow range of fine fibril diameters in the cornea to the broad range found in the sclera. The interfibrillar distance is also less

constant in the sclera (Fig. 7.49). The diminished ordering of these fibrils, together with the water content of its ground substance, results in the lack of transparency of the sclera. Collagen fibrils are said to run a circular course at the limbus, which is the weakest region in the corneoscleral envelope as assessed by bursting pressure (Maurice, 1962). Traumatic rupture of the globe is equally common at the limbus or under a rectus muscle at the equator because the sclera is thinnest at these positions (Cherry, 1972).

There is also a transition in type of ground

substance on passing from cornea to the sclera. In the central cornea keratan sulphate predominates, with chondroitin as the other proteoglycan. In the peripheral cornea chondroitin sulphate appears, and at the limbus itself there is a marked fall in keratan sulphate, with the appearance of dermatan sulphate and hyaluronic acid, which are also found in the sclera (Borcherding *et al.*, 1975). These authors correlated the degree of fibre organization with proteoglycan content and concluded that the precisely ordered spacing of corneal collagen fibres is determined by specific constraints imposed by the conformation of keratan sulphate. It is also likely that the fineness and regularity of fibril size is determined by the level of glycosylation of the collagen molecules that makes up the fibrils.

For further details of the limbus see Chapter 8.

7.3   THE EPISCLERA

The episclera is the loose connective tissue outside the sclera, anteriorly connecting sclera and conjunctiva. It lies beneath the avascular fascia bulbi (Tenon's capsule) and is connected to the capsule by fibrous bands. For the most part, the episclera is continuous with the loose tissue of Tenon's capsule, while its deeper layers are more compact as they give

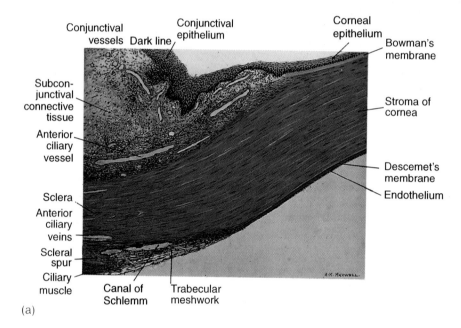

(a)

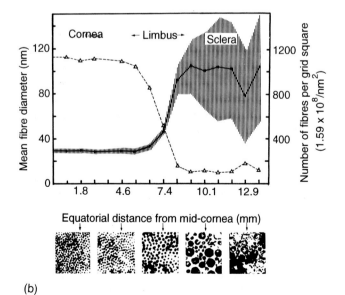

(b)

Fig. 7.49 (a) Section at the corneoscleral junction. (b) Comparison of the average number of collagen fibres per unit area (Δ—Δ) with the mean fibre diameter (●—●) ±1s.d. (shaded area) as a function of distance from the mid-cornea. Arrows indicate location of electron micrographs along the central vertical axis from mid-cornea to sclera (original magnification × 40 000). (From Borcherding, M. S. *et al.* (1975) *Exp. Eye Res.*, **21**, with permission.)

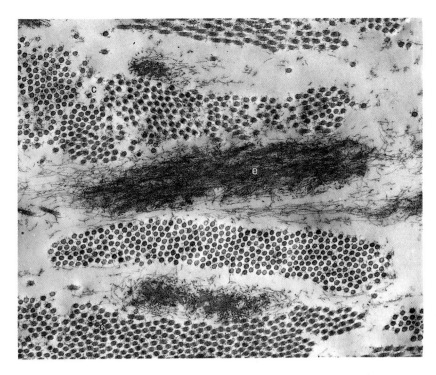

Fig. 7.50 TEM of deep conjunctival stroma consisting of loosely arranged bundles of regular collagen fibrils (c) cut transversely and obliquely and elastic fibres (e) with their microfibrillar and dense amorphous elements. Original magnification ×40 000.

way to sclera proper. It is thickest anterior to the rectus muscle because it blends with Tenon's capsule and the vascular tissues around these muscles. This vascularity distinguishes the episclera from Tenon's capsule and the sclera itself. Behind the ocular attachments of the recti episclera is thin.

The fibrils of episcleral collagen are finer than those of the sclera and more widely spaced, forming bundles which are less compact. Ground substance is more abundant. Elastin fibrils are also present (Fig. 7.50). Cells include typical fibroblasts, melanocytes, some macrophages and a few lymphocytes.

The posterior ciliary arteries supply a wide-meshed rete of vessels behind the rectus insertions, two venules to each arteriole, while a denser meshwork of vessels anterior to the insertions is supplied by episcleral branches of the anterior ciliary arteries. A capillary plexus exists only in this anterior episcleral zone. Vascular dilatation here, in keratitis or iritis, is called ciliary injection. Hogan, Alvarado and Weddell (1971) regard these capillaries as unfenestrated, unlike those of the conjunctiva.

Myelinated and unmyelinated nerves traverse the episclera, some ending there without specialization.

7.4 THE SCLERA

The sclera is the main part of the outer coat of the eye, is roughly spherical and forms just under five-sixths of the fibrous external tunic. It consists almost entirely of collagen, within a lesser amount of ground substance material than in the cornea, contains scanty fibrocytes (sclerocytes) and is relatively avascular. Like the cornea it is comparatively tough and protects the intraocular contents from injury and mechanical displacement. Its mechanical strength also serves to contain the intraocular pressure and at the same time prevents deformations of the globe by resisting the stresses and strains induced by contractions of the extraocular muscles.

MECHANICAL PROPERTIES

The intraocular pressure causes a stretching of the scleral collagen and thus this tissue is always under slight tension. Although the distensibility of the sclera is poor it is often described as viscoelastic, because it exhibits the typical biphasic response of such materials when suddenly deformed. Scleral deformation is thus accompanied by an elastic component, which results in a rapid but very brief lengthening, followed by a viscid component which results in a slow stretching (St Helen and McEwan, 1961). In children with infantile glaucoma this slow scleral stretching in response to a sustained increase in intraocular pressure results in the buphthalmic globe. In later life the amount that the sclera stretches in response to changes in intraocular pressure is not in direct proportion to pressure rise, because rigidity of sclera increases with stretch. However, expansion and thinning of the sclera (but not the cornea) is a feature of progressive myopia.

TRANSPARENCY

In adults the sclera is normally white, and its visible anterior portion is referred to as the 'white' of the eye. It is also usually opaque, although some diffuse light does enter the globe through the sclera. This relative translucency allows the location of intraocular tumours by transillumination through the globe, when the dense tumour casts a dark shadow. The opacity of the sclera is related in part to its water content of about 68%: if the water content falls below 40% or rises above 80% then the sclera becomes lucent. This is in contrast to the cornea where increased hydration invariably leads to a loss of transparency.

If, as in childhood, the sclera is thin, or if there is a pathological alteration in scleral hydration, then the resultant changes in optical qualities result in the sclera appearing blue or blue-grey. The coloration may be generalized (as in the eyes of the newborn), focal (for instance beneath the bulbar insertions of the rectus muscles where the sclera is thinnest), or as a transient effect of drying and thinning of the sclera during surgery. In each case there is an increase in the amount of light falling on, and therefore absorbed by, the underlying uvea. The blue hue is imparted by the greater scattering of shorter wavelengths by the scleral collagen.

DIMENSIONS

The dimensions of the scleral sphere vary in the adult human eye but on average the coronal diameter lies between 22 and 24 mm, with that in males being 0.5 mm larger than in females. At birth the anteroposterior diameter is 16–17 mm, increasing to 22.5 mm by the age of 3 years and reaching full adult dimension by the age of 13 years (Sorsby and Sheridan, 1960).

Scleral thickness varies, being thickest (1 mm) near the optic nerve, thinning progressively to 0.6 mm at the equator, and thinnest (0.3 mm) at the rectus muscle insertions. However, the tendons of these muscles effectively increase scleral thickness to 0.6 mm, and from this point to the limbus there is a gradual increase in thickness to 0.8 mm. It is generally thought that the sclera thins with increasing age (Vannas and Teir, 1960), but some authorities dispute this and relate apparent changes in thickness to age-related differences in distension and water content (Weale, 1982).

APERTURES

The sclera is pierced by two potential openings: the **anterior scleral foramen**, filled by the cornea, and the **posterior scleral foramen** occupied by optic nerve. The sclera is also traversed by a number of channels or **emissaria** which provide passage for arteries, veins and nerves. These emissaria are usually classified in relation to their position on the globe and fall into three groups: **anterior, middle** and **posterior** (Figs 7.51 and 7.52).

Anterior scleral foramen

The sclera meets and anatomically merges with the cornea at the so-called anterior scleral foramen. Both the internal and external margins of the scleral aspect of the sclerocorneal junction extend more anteriorly than the main body of the sclera. This creates a concave circumferential groove called the **internal scleral sulcus** that is occupied by the trabecular meshwork. The external margin of the anterior scleral foramen is oval, with its long axis (11.7 mm) oriented horizontally and its short axis (10.6 mm) vertically; hence the disparity in the width of the limbus from vertical to horizontal planes. Internally the foramen is circular, with a diameter of 11.7 mm that corresponds to the internal diameter of the cornea.

Externally the sclera bears a shallow groove, called the **external scleral sulcus** (sulcus sclerae), which forms an annulus just posterior to the corneoscleral junction. In the living eye, it is not readily apparent because the sulcus is filled with conjunctival tissue and vessels.

Posterior scleral foramen

The posterior aperture in the sclera provides an exit from the globe for the optic nerve. This short canal is located 3 mm medial to the mid line and 1 mm below the horizontal meridian. The canal has the form of a truncated cone with an internal opening 1.5–2.0 mm in diameter and an external one 3.0–3.5 mm across.

Unlike the anterior scleral foramen, scleral fibres extend across the posterior opening on its choroidal aspect as a specialized network of bands or bundles termed the **lamina cribrosa** or **cribriform plate**. This structure provides support and anchorage for the optic nerve fibres passing through it, and also reinforces the globe at its weakest point. The major part of the lamina is formed by collagen and elastin fibres extending from the innermost third of the

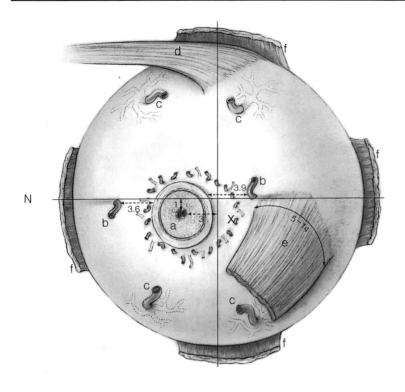

Fig. 7.51 Drawing of the posterior globe. T = Temporal; N = nasal. The optic nerve (a), with its central vessels and surrounding meningeal sheaths, is seen. Its centre is located 3 mm nasal and 1 mm inferior to the posterior pole of the eye. Surrounding it are the short posterior ciliary arteries and nerves. The approximate position of the macula is at **X**. Along the horizontal meridian which bisects the eye are the long posterior ciliary arteries and nerves (b). The exits of four vortex veins are shown, one for each quadrant (c). The curved, oblique insertions of the superior oblique (d) and inferior oblique (e) muscles are seen. The cut ends of the four rectus muscles are at (f). (From Hogan, M. J., Alvarado, J. A. and Weddell, J. E. (1971) *Histology of the Eye. An Atlas and Textbook*, published by W. B. Saunders.)

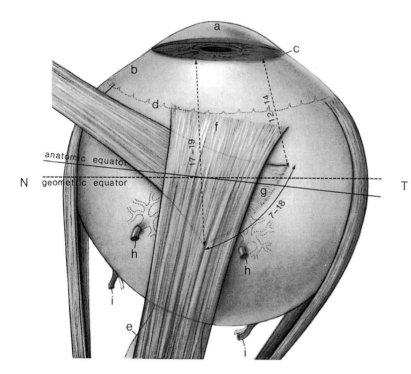

Fig. 7.52 Drawing of the upper half of the eye. T = Temporal; N = nasal. The contrasting degree of curvature of the cornea (a) and sclera (b) are evident. At the limbus (c), where they join, is the external scleral sulcus. The relation of the ora serrata (d) to the surface is shown. The nasal displacement of the optic nerve (e) with respect to the posterior pole of the eye makes the three layers of the temporal eye longer than those on the nasal side. The slightly curved oblique insertion of the superior rectus muscle is at (f) and the tendinous oblique insertion of the superior oblique muscle is at (g). Two vortex veins are seen at (h) and the long posterior ciliary arteries and nerves are at (i). (From Hogan, M.J., Alvarado, J.A. and Weddell, J.E. (1971) *Histology of the Eye. An Atlas and Textbook*, published by W.B. Saunders.)

sclera. Not all the fibre bundles traverse the canal from side to side; some insert into the connective tissue surrounding the central retinal vessels. Each layer of collagen fibres within the lamina cribrosa is like a loosely woven cloth or net, and while the 'weft' and 'warp' in adjacent layers intersect at a variety of angles the holes within the net remain relatively aligned with each hole providing unobstructed passage for the bundles of nerve fibres. The perforations within the lamina cribrosa are thin short canals formed by a series of superimposed, congruent openings.

The intraocular aspect of the lamina cribrosa is concave (Wolter, 1957; Hayreh and Vrabec, 1966). In chronic glaucoma, in response to a sustained rise in intraocular pressure and in ischaemic optic neuropathy, the lamina cribrosa is displaced further posteriorly, leading to the enlargement of the optic cup in these diseases.

The fibres from the outer two-thirds of the sclera do not traverse the foramen, but turn through a right-angle and run outwards to blend with the dural covering of the optic nerve.

For a detailed discussion of the lamina cribrosa in relation to the optic nerve see Chapter 15.

Emissaria

The channels through which vessels and nerves pass through the sclera are lined by a layer of loose connective tissue with collagen fibres parallel to the direction of these structures.

Anterior emissaria

The anterior apertures provide passage for anterior ciliary arteries, anterior ciliary veins, aqueous veins and the ciliary nerves; most of the channels are near to the limbus.

There are two anterior ciliary arteries in each rectus muscle, with the exception of the lateral rectus which has only one. These vessels leave the muscles and enter the sclera obliquely just anterior to their tendinous insertions. The largest branch of these vessels passes through the sclera to enter the ciliary body to form the major arterial circle of the iris. Although the anterior ciliary arteries do not give rise to a capillary bed within the sclera, some small branches bend anteriorly and, in conjunction with the subconjunctival vascular plexus, fan out to form the episcleral plexus.

For each anterior ciliary artery there are two anterior ciliary veins emerging over the ciliary body. They often share a channel with a branch of a posterior ciliary nerve which passes almost to the surface before looping back to enter the ciliary body (nerve loop of Axenfeld) present in 12% of eyes, sometimes bilateral (1%), and occasionally multiple (Stevenson, 1963). They appear within an emissarium in company with blood vessels, or between the rectus muscle insertions. Clinically they present a smooth, glistening grey dome-shaped appearance, are 1–2 mm across, and are often associated with some pigment.

Aqueous veins from the canal of Schlemm may leave through the sclera or may form deep and superficial plexuses within it, just posterior to the limbus. For a detailed discussion of these in relation to aqueous outflow see Chapter 8.

Middle emissaria

The middle apertures lie behind the equator and transmit the vortex veins (vena vorticosae) of the choroid. Some authorities group these veins with the posterior group of apertures (Hogan, Alvarado and Weddell, 1971).

There are four main vortex veins, although accessory veins occur, so that the average eye may seem to have six or seven such structures. The apertures for accessory veins are always located within 1 to 2 mm of those of the main veins. The distances of the internal and external apertures of the vortex veins from the limbus have been summarized by Salzmann (1912): each channel runs obliquely and is about 4 mm long (Table 7.2).

Thus the superior vortex veins always lie further posterior (7–8 mm) to the equator than do the inferior pair (5–6 mm) (see Chapter 11).

Posterior emissaria

The posterior apertures transmit the ciliary arteries and nerves.

The long posterior arteries and nerves (two of each) pierce the sclera about 3–4 mm from the optic nerve, in the horizontal meridian. They pass obliquely forward for 3–5 mm to the suprachoroidal space and then to the ciliary body. In their canals they are surrounded by loose connective tissue and separated by a small amount of pigmented tissue. Occasional smaller, additional long ciliary nerves enter above, or more often below.

About 20 short ciliary arteries and nerves penetrate the sclera around the optic nerve and supply the posterior sclera and choroid. The blood supply to the optic disc is described in Chapter 15.

Table 7.2

	External orifice (mm)	Internal orifice (mm)
Superoexternal	22	18
Superointernal	20	16
Inferoexternal	19	15
Inferointernal	18	14.5

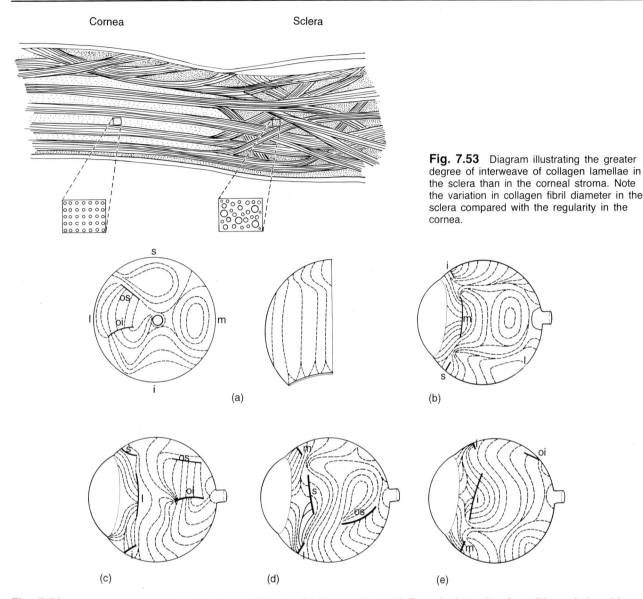

Fig. 7.53 Diagram illustrating the greater degree of interweave of collagen lamellae in the sclera than in the corneal stroma. Note the variation in collagen fibril diameter in the sclera compared with the regularity in the cornea.

Fig. 7.54 Illustration of the direction of collagen fibres in the human sclera. (a) From the internal surface; (b) nasal view; (c) lateral view; (d) from above; (e) from below. i = Inferior rectus; l = lateral rectus; m = medial rectus; oi = inferior oblique; os = superior oblique; s = superior rectus. (From Kokott, W. (1938) *A. von Graefes Arch. Ophthalmol.*, **138**, 424.

SCLERAL ORGANIZATION

The sclera is composed of compact interlacing bundles of collagen, some elastic tissue, and a smaller quantity of ground substance than found in the cornea (Table 7.1). Elastic fibres interlace with the collagen bundles and are largely in the *lamina fusca*, next to the choroid. They are found at the limbus, lamina cribrosa and are sparse at the equator (Krekeler, 1923).

The collagen bundles are 10–16 μm thick and 100–140 μm wide, while those that form the scleral spur are 30–50 μm wide and up to 10 μm thick (Salzmann, 1912). The bands are mostly parallel to the surface, but they cross each other in all directions and may divide dichotomously and reunite (Fig. 7.53). The imbrication is so dense, especially anteriorly, that blunt dissection of its layers may be difficult.

Kokott (1934, 1938) interpreted the organization of the scleral collagen bundles in terms of the forces acting on its different parts. Just as the direction and strength of bony trabeculae in the neck of the femur are determined by the stresses to which it is subjected (Woodhead-Galloway, 1981), so the array of scleral fibres is determined by the intraocular tension and the pull of the various muscles acting on the globe (Fig. 7.54). The inner aspect of the sclera shows a simple meridional pattern of bundle directions. The tendinous bundles of the recti penetrate into the sclera as parallel fibres which then spread out in a fan-shaped manner to blend with the meridional fibres of the sclera. The tendons of the obliques behave similarly but blend with the oblique or equatorial fibres of the sclera or form gently sinuous bundles running between the lines of their insertion. At the limbus, especially near the scleral spur, deep bundles run coronally, parallel to the limbus; while more superficial fibres form loops concave posteriorly, which become progressively more meridional, especially near the rectus muscle insertions. The peripapillary bundles are coronally circular for a distance beyond the posterior apertures of about 4 mm. Equatorial bundles are also circular in the coronal plane, with loops forming a posterior convexity. Between these zones, the posterior bundles are arranged like the net around a balloon, while the internal fibres are more meridional (Weale, 1982).

Within each bundle the collagen fibrils are parallel and show wide variation in diameter and spacing. Widths ranging from 28 to 280 nm are given by Schwarz (1953a,b) with larger diameters (166 nm) in the superficial layers and smaller in the deeper ones (100 nm) (Spitznas, Luciano and Reale, 1970). This variation and large diameter of the fibrils are distinctly different from that of the cornea and account for the opacity of the sclera. Tapered ends on some fibrils have been reported by Rohen (1964).

The 64 nm banding pattern of collagen fibrils is more readily demonstrated in sclera than cornea, perhaps because of the lesser coating with ground substance material (Fig. 7.55). Scleral collagen is chiefly type I, with a moderate amount of type III. The ground substance includes chondroitin sulphate, dermatan sulphate and hyaluronic acid.

Numerous elastic fibres occur throughout the sclera (Aurell and Holmgren, 1941), arranged parallel to the collagenous bands (Virchow, 1910) (Fig. 7.56). They are most numerous in the second decade of life. With age the amount of elastic tissue falls and between 20 and 60 years the reduction is more pronounced in the anterior than posterior sclera. The lamina cribrosa is particularly rich in elastin.

CELLS

Scattered fibroblasts are located between the collagen bundles of the sclera, flattened cells with small nuclei and long branching processes which do not make intimate contact though they approach closely.

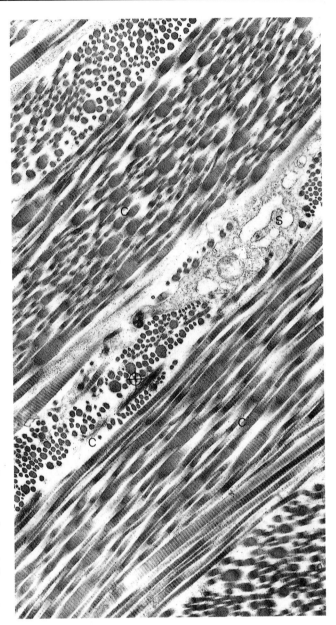

Fig. 7.55 Typical high-power electron micrograph of the mid-anterior stroma of a 40-year-old human sclera. Collagen bundles (C) are cut longitudinally, obliquely and in transverse section. Note the well-marked banding pattern and the marked variation in fibril diameter (○), which is clearly visible in those fibrils cut transversely. S = Scleral fibrocyte. Original magnification ×26 250. (Courtesy of R. Young.)

The deeper scleral lamellae contain a large number of melanocytes and pigmented macrophages, which derive from the lamina fusca of the choroid and supraciliary region (see Chapter 11).

BLOOD SUPPLY

The sclera is relatively avascular. Anteriorly the anterior ciliary arteries send branches to the deep

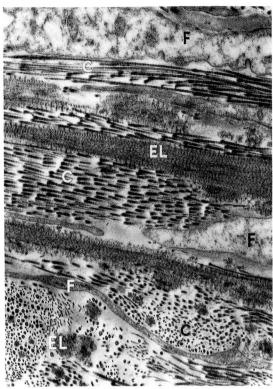

Fig. 7.56 Electron micrograph of the anترioscleral stroma from a senile eye, showing collagen fibrils (C) cut in various planes: longitudinal, oblique and transverse. Note also the elastic fibres (EL) cut longitudinally and transversely, the former showing a serrated edge, and the fibroblast processes (F). Original magnification ×25 000.

Fig. 7.57 Section of choroid (above) and sclera (original magnification ×260). A long ciliary nerve appears between the two strata. (Courtesy of Dr John Marshall, Institute of Ophthalmology, London.)

sclera in the region of Schlemm's canal, while posteriorly the short ciliary arteries supply scleral short posterior ciliary branches to the disc and peripapillary sclera, their role being supplemented by the circle of Zinn (if present). The episcleral plexus of vessels sends fine twigs to the sclera, but at the equator such vessels are infrequent. It is likely that the choroid, closely apposed to the deep surface of the sclera, provides it with some nourishment; the choroidal capillaries are fenestrated, and the sclera does not present a major barrier to the diffusion even of large molecules, such as albumin (Bill, 1966a,b; 1968). Hence subtenon or subconjunctivally injected drugs can reach the internal tunics of the eye.

NERVES

The short ciliary nerves supply some fibres to the scleral surface before they enter the emissaria and some to the stroma while within them. The remainder of the sclera is supplied by branches from the long posterior ciliary nerves (Fig. 7.57). At the limbus, branches are given to the trabecular meshwork and neighbouring sclera, before proceeding to the cornea.

AGEING OF THE SCLERA

As age progresses the sclera becomes more rigid and the diameter of its collagen and occasionally elastin fibrils increases (Schwartz, 1953). Friedenwald (1952) and Vannas and Teir (1960) noted thinning, but Melanowski and Stachow (1958) did not. Histochemical staining is reduced, particularly near Schlemm's canal. In some older eyes a patch of scleral translucency appears, oval in shape (6 × 1 mm), parallel

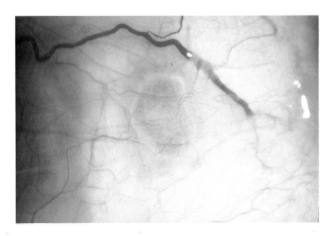

Fig. 7.58 Scleral plaque in a senile patient.

to and just anterior to the insertions of the horizontal recti. These are termed scleral plaques, and are associated with a deposition of calcium sulphate (Cogan and Kuwabara, 1959a) (Fig. 7.58). A more finely distributed accumulation of calcium salts also occurs. The yellowish hue of older sclerae is attributed to the deposition of lipids. Like other dense collagenous tissues, it acts as a trap for esterified cholesterol (Broekhuyse, 1975). Yellowing of the sclera is also a diagnostic feature of jaundice.

CHAPTER EIGHT

Anterior chamber and drainage angle

Because of the significance of the chamber angle in the disease glaucoma, the anatomy of this region has received considerable attention from many authors. This chapter draws heavily on material from Garron *et al.* (1959), Hogan, Alvarado and Weddell (1971), Tripathi (1971, 1974, 1977a), Tripathi and Tripathi (1982), Grierson and Lee (1974, 1975), Lee, Grierson and McMenamin (1982), Bill (1975, 1977), Bill and Svedbergh (1972) and Gong, Tripathi and Tripathi (1996).

8.1   ANTERIOR CHAMBER

The anterior chamber is bounded anteriorly by the inner surface of the cornea, except at its far periphery where it is related to trabecular meshwork. Posteriorly it is bounded by the lens within the pupillary aperture, by the anterior surface of the iris, and peripherally by the anterior face of the ciliary body. The anterior and posterior boundaries meet at the **drainage angle** of the chamber (Fig. 8.1). The anterior chamber communicates with the extracellular spaces of the iris, ciliary body and trabecular meshwork and, through the pupillary aperture, with the posterior chamber of the eye.

Anterior chamber volume is in the region of 220 μl, and the average depth is 3.15 (range 2.6–4.4) mm. Chamber diameter varies from 11.3 to 12.4 mm (Tripathi and Tripathi, 1982). Depth has been studied optically by Weekers and Grieten (1961), Weekers, Grieten and Lavergne (1961), Weekers *et al.* (1963), Aizawa (1958) and others (Brown, 1973a; Johnson, Passmore and Brubaker, 1977; Johnson, Coates and Brubaker, 1978). Chamber depth decreases by 0.01 mm per year of life, and is shallower in the hypermetropic than the myopic eye. (The chamber deepens by 0.06 mm for each dioptre of myopia.) Anterior chamber volume decreases by 0.11 μl per year of life, but is 0.69 μl larger per dioptre of myopia (Brubaker *et al.*, 1981). Chamber depth is diminished slightly during accommodation, partly by increased anterior lens curvature, and partly by forward translocation of the lens (Brown, 1973a).

8.2   CORNEOSCLERAL LIMBUS

The corneoscleral limbus is a translucent transitional zone, approximately 1.5 mm in diameter, between clear cornea and opaque sclera but wider in the vertical plane (~2 mm). Centrally, the corneolimbal junction is demarcated by a line joining the termination of Bowman's layer to the termination of Descemet's membrane. Peripherally, the **sclerolimbal junction** is demarcated by a parallel line passing through the scleral spur (Figs 8.1 and 8.2).

The limbus can be divided into three zones:

1. The deep limbus, which contains the **trabecular meshwork** and **Schlemm's canal**.
2. The mid limbus containing the transitional **corneoscleral stroma** which projects, with a conoid profile, into the scleral limbus. It also contains the **intrascleral venous plexus**.
3. The superficial limbus, which consists of the **episclera**, Tenon's capsule, the conjunctival stroma and the limbal conjunctival epithelium with its specialized anatomical features.

8.3   CLINICAL FEATURES OF THE DRAINAGE ANGLE

The anterior chamber accommodates the aqueous drainage mechanism of the eye. The bulk of the aqueous flows through the trabecular meshwork into the canal of Schlemm and drains into the intra- and episcleral venous systems. This is the 'conventional'

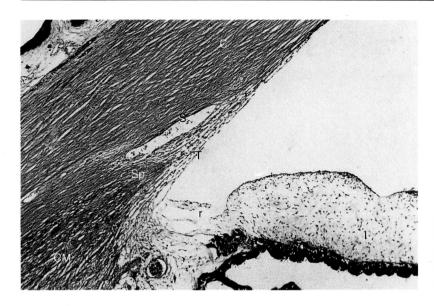

Fig. 8.1 Light micrograph of the anterior chamber angle. C = cornea; CM = ciliary muscle; I = iris stroma; S = Schlemm's canal; r = angle recess; Sp = scleral spur; T = trabecular meshwork. (Courtesy of Dr D. Lucas.)

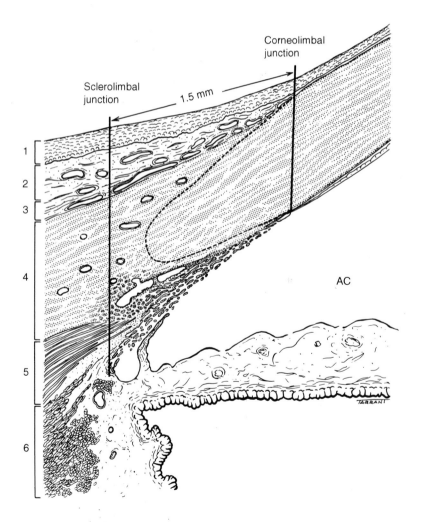

Fig. 8.2 The limbal region in a human eye. 1 = conjunctival epithelium; 2 = conjunctival stroma; 3 = Tenon's capsule and episclera; 4 = limbal or corneoscleral stroma; 5 = longitudinal portion of ciliary muscle; 6 = circular and radial portions of ciliary muscle. AC = anterior chamber. The histologist's limbus is denoted by a dotted line, the pathologist's and clinician's limbus by solid lines. The corneolimbal junction is demarcated by the most central extent of the marginal arcade of vessels. The landmark for the sclerolimbal junction is not visible clinically but corresponds to the tip of the scleral spur. (From Tripathi, R. C. and Tripathi, B. J., in Davson H. (ed.) (1984) The Eye, vol 1A, published by Academic Press.)

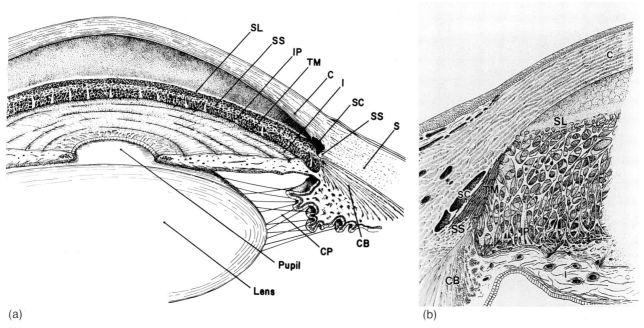

(a)

(b)

Fig. 8.3 Semidiagrammatic representation of the structures of the angle of the anterior chamber. (a) Composite gonioscopic and crosssectional view of the anterior segment of the eye. (b) Enlarged view. Note the superimposed trabecular sheets with intra- and intertrabecular spaces through which aqueous humour flows to reach the canal of Schlemm. SL = Schwalbe's line; SS = scleral spur; IP = iris process; TM = trabecular meshwork; C = cornea; I = iris; SC = Schlemm's canal; S = sclera; CB = ciliary body; Z = zonules. (From Tripathi, R. C. and Tripathi, B. J. in Duane, T. A. and Jaeger, E. W. (eds) (1982) *Biomedical Foundations of Ophthalmology*, *Vol. 1*, published by Harper and Row.)

outflow pathway. Obstruction of this pathway leads to a rise in intraocular pressure, a condition termed glaucoma. If the anterior chamber is shallow then it is possible for the peripheral iris to come into contact with the peripheral cornea and prevent aqueous drainage in this way. This is **primary angle closure glaucoma** and may be precipitated by pupil dilatation.

In another form of glaucoma, **primary open angle glaucoma**, aqueous outflow is obstructed chiefly by a rise in resistance to the passage of aqueous across the meshwork and into Schlemm's canal. In this case the iris tissue does not obstruct drainage of aqueous, and the angle is designated as 'open'. The width of the angle, and whether it is open or closed, can be assessed clinically by means of the gonioscope, a contact lens and mirror which optically permits direct viewing of the angle landmarks unobstructed by the translucent limbal tissue (Fig. 8.3).

The gonioscopic features of the limbus are usually observed with magnification, at the slit-lamp. They are as follows (Tripathi and Tripathi, 1982).

CILIARY BAND

In the angle recess, the most posterior landmark is the dark ciliary band, which represents the anterior face of the ciliary body including the insertion of the ciliary muscle into the scleral spur. This lies at the apex of the chamber angle.

SCLERAL SPUR

The scleral spur is a pale, translucent narrow strip of scleral tissue which is located anterior to the ciliary band and marks the posterior boundary of the corneoscleral meshwork.

TRABECULAR MESHWORK

Anterior to the scleral spur is a broad band of tissue approximately 750 μm in width, which is relatively featureless in the unpigmented eye and extends from scleral spur to Schwalbe's ring. The trabecular band covers the internal aspect of the canal of Schlemm. The canal may sometimes be made visible during gonioscopy, when blood refluxes retrogradely into the canal, and appears as a pink strip visible through the meshwork. (Usually the canal is free of blood; reflux occurs because the gonioscope, when applied to the surface of the eye, obstructs episcleral venous drainage and reverses blood flow (Busacca, 1945).) At other times, when the meshwork is pigmented, the pigment is concentrated over the region of the canal, and delineates it in this way.

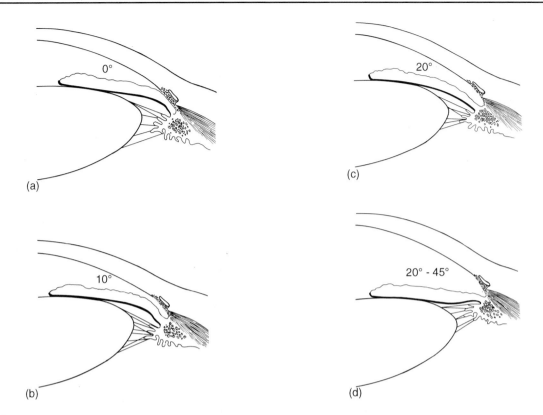

Fig. 8.4 Different grades of anterior chamber angle width. (a) Grade 0, closure imminent or present; (b) grade 1, approximately 10° open, narrow angle susceptible to closure; (c) grade 2, approximately 20° open, moderately narrow angle, less occludable although closure possible; (d) grades 3–4, wide open angle (20–45°). Such angles are usually associated with a deep anterior chamber and relatively flat iris profile. Angle closure is not possible. This is the most common anatomical finding in normal young subjects. (From Tripathi, R. C. and Tripathi, B. J. in Duane, T. A. and Jaeger, E. W. (eds) (1982) *Biomedical Foundations of Ophthalmology*, *Vol. 1*, published by Harper and Row.)

SCHWALBE'S RING

The anterior limit of the drainage angle is termed Schwalbe's ring or line. This is a fine scalloped border at the termination of Descemet's membrane which usually lies in the plane of the posterior corneal surface but in 15–20% of normal subjects may be variably hypertrophied and project as a delicate, glistening ridge into the anterior chamber (**posterior embryotoxon**). It is sometimes lightly pigmented.

ANGLE RECESS

The apex of the angle lies in a plane 0.6–1.0 mm behind the most anterior aspect of the lens capsule. The iris therefore curves backwards peripherally at the iris root to a variable extent to form the angle recess. The width of this recess varies according to the size of the eye, depth of the chamber, state of the pupil and other factors, so that different angle widths are referred to clinically, from the widest (encountered in the aphakic or pseudophakic eye) to the narrowest (encountered in the small, hypermetropic or microphthalmic eye, Fig. 8.4).

The anatomical basis for these clinical landmarks is discussed in more detail below.

8.4 THE OUTFLOW APPARATUS

The features of the outflow apparatus are as follows:

1. internal scleral sulcus
   (a) sulcus;
   (b) Schwalbe's ring;
   (c) scleral spur;
2. trabecular meshwork
   (a) uveal meshwork;
   (b) corneoscleral meshwork;
   (c) trabecular structure;
   (d) iris processes;
   (e) pericanalicular connective tissue;
   (f) extracellular matrix;

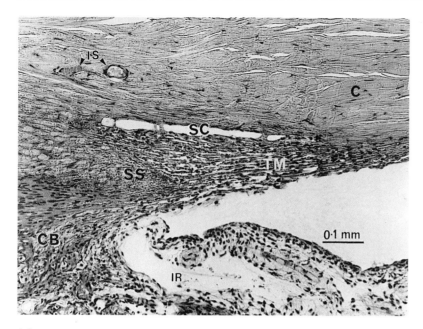

(a)

Fig. 8.5 Meridional section of the scleral spur (SS) in a human eye. (a) The scleral roll forms the posterior boundary of Schlemm's canal (SC) while the sloping anteromedial border of the spur provides attachment for the corneoscleral trabecular sheets (TM). The meridional muscle fibres of the ciliary body (CB) are inserted into the posterior edge of the spur. The uveal trabecular sheets pass below the spur. C = peripheral cornea.

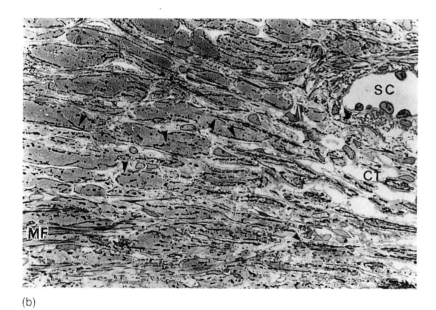

(b)

(b) The elastic element of the spur, seen as dense dots and lines (arrowheads) depending on the plane of section, is distributed predominantly around irregularly-shaped bundles of collagen fibres. These extracellular elements are continuous with those of the corneoscleral trabeculae (CT). The ciliary muscle fibres (MF) terminate into the spur. SC = Schlemm's canal. Original magnification ×880. (From Tripathi, R. C. and Tripathi, B. J. in Duane, T. A. and Jaeger, E. W. (eds) (1982) *Biomedical Foundations of Ophthalmology*, *Vol. 1*, published by Harper and Row.)

3. canal of Schlemm and collector channels
   (a) Schlemm's canal;
   (b) endothelial lining;
   (c) giant vacuoles;
   (d) collector channels;
4. intrascleral arteries of the limbus;
5. innervation of the outflow apparatus;
6. uveoscleral drainage pathway;
7. location of the resistance to outflow;
8. regulation of ocular pressure;
9. ageing, and the outflow apparatus in primary open angle glaucoma.

INTERNAL SCLERAL SULCUS

The sulcus

The sulcus is a circular groove on the inner aspect of the corneoscleral limbus, extending from the termination of Descemet's membrane, anteriorly demarcated by Schwalbe's ring, to the scleral spur posteriorly (Figs 8.1 and 8.5). The portion of the spur which forms the posterior boundary of the sulcus is sometimes called the scleral roll. The sulcus completely accommodates the canal of Schlemm externally, and

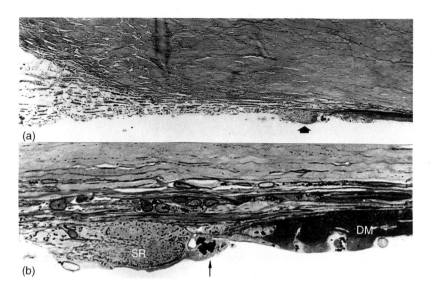

Fig. 8.6 (a) Anterior terminal of trabecular meshwork into deep corneal lamellae and anterior ring of Schwalbe (arrow) as seen in the light micrograph of a meridional section of the human eye. Original magnification ×220; (b) higher magnification of the ring of Schwalbe (SR); dot-like structures represent transversely cut elastic fibres. Descemet's membrane (DM) shows nodular profiles of Hassal–Henle warts. Note the termination of trabecular sheets into deep corneal lamellae and transition of corneal endothelium. The transitional endothelium (arrow) contains trapped pigment granules. Original magnification ×895. (From Tripathi, R. C. and Tripathi, B. J. in Duane, T. A. and Jaeger, E. W. (eds) (1982) *Biomedical Foundations of Ophthalmology, Vol. 1*, published by Harper and Row.)

the corneoscleral portion of the trabecular meshwork internally (Fig. 8.1).

Schwalbe's ring

Schwalbe's ring is the anterior border ring of the trabecular region (Schwalbe, 1870) and contains circularly arranged collagen fibres (periodicity 64 nm) intermixed with elastic fibres. With age there are also patches of long-spacing or 'curly' collagen. The ring marks the transition between the corneal endothelium and the trabecular cells and also the termination of Descemet's membrane (Fig. 8.6) which, however, may split at times to enclose the inner and outer aspects of Schwalbe's ring and may show fine extensions into the cortical zone of the uveal trabeculae.

Scleral spur

The scleral spur is a wedge-shaped circular ridge which marks the deep aspect of the sclerolimbal junction. It receives the insertion of the anterior tendons of the longitudinal ciliary muscle on its inner aspect (Schwalbe, 1870; Salzmann, 1912; Rohen, 1956; Kupfer, 1962; Iwamoto, 1964; Rohen *et al.*, 1967; Tripathi and Tripathi, 1982). Its anteromedial base forms the posterior margin of the scleral sulcus and receives the posterior attachment of the corneoscleral meshwork (Fig. 8.5).

The scleral spur contains collagen and elastic tissue with a circular arrangement like that of the trabecular beams of the corneoscleral and cribriform or juxtacanicular meshwork with which it blends. The collagen fibrils vary in diameter from 35 to 80 nm, and widen towards the sclera (Tripathi and Tripathi, 1982). The connective tissue components are continuous with those of the corneoscleral trabeculae where they become covered by trabecular cells. Contraction of the ciliary muscle pulls the spur posteriorly and opens up the trabecular spaces. This is a likely mode of action for miotics to reduce outflow resistance (Unger and Rohen, 1958; Rohen and Unger, 1959; Moses and Arnzen, 1980; Grierson, Lee and McMenamin, 1981).

Recently it has been shown that there are contractile, **myofibroblast-like cells** oriented circumferentially within the scleral spur, which have sparse mitochondria and are rich in smooth muscle alpha-actin and myosin (Tamm *et al.*, 1992b). They have an interrupted basal lamina and lack the desmin and intermediate filaments characteristic of the adjacent ciliary smooth muscle cells (Tamm *et al.*, 1991, 1992b). These **scleral spur cells** (SSC) form tendon-like contacts with the elastic fibres of the scleral spur which are continuous with those of the adjacent trabecular meshwork. Thus changes in SSC tone might modulate outflow resistance by altering trabecular architecture. Some trabecular meshwork cells also stain positively for smooth muscle alpha actinin and smooth muscle actin (de Kater *et al.*, 1990, 1992; Flugel *et al.*, 1992).

Individual SSC are innervated by unmyelinated axons which derive exclusively from neurons that run forwards in the supraciliary space. They contrast with the myelinated axons which supply the mechanoreceptors of the scleral spur (Tamm *et al.*, 1994). The axons run circumferentially in the scleral spur, parallel to the arrangement of the connective tissue elements and their terminals contact the cell membranes closely, without an intervening basal lamina. The nerve endings contain granular and agranular vesicles, generally regarded to be characteristic of adrenergic nerves, but this is not confirmed by immunohistochemistry. An adrenergic innervation of the monkey scleral spur has been reported, and is in keeping with our knowledge of anterior chamber innervation in this species (Laties and Jacobowitz, 1966; Ehinger, 1966b, 1971). However, Tamm *et al.* (1995b), note that similar vesicles have been observed in non-adrenergic terminals in the enteric nervous system (Gordon-Weeks and Hobbs, 1979; Gordon-Weeks, 1988).

The ciliary muscle cells receive a dense cholinergic innervation (Bozler, 1948; Barany *et al.*, 1982; Erickson-Lamy *et al.*, 1987), whereas the varicose axons which innervate the human SSC are immunoreactive for NPY, SP, CGRP, VIP and NO, and are negative for acetylcholinesterase. The posterior trabecular meshwork receives a similar innervation (Stone, Kuwayama and Laties, 1989; Tamm *et al.*, 1995b). A parasympathetic origin for the VIP- and nitrergic fibres of the scleral spur from the pterygopalatine ganglion is quite likely, given that such fibres contribute to ocular innervation in the human and primate eye (Ruskell, 1970a,b). There is also the possibility that some of these fibres may arise in the human eye from the intrinsic VIP- and nitrergic fibres of the choroid, in which region these transmitters are also coexpressed (Flugel *et al.*, 1994). It is of interest that in the monkey, where the intrinsic plexus of the choroid is much smaller than in the human, no VIP- or nitrergic fibres are present in the scleral spur.

Although most NPY positive neurons are localized in sympathetic fibres, some neurons coexpress NPY and VIP, and are thought to have their origin in the parasympathetic pathway via the pterygopalatine ganglion. Most, but not all, SP-positive fibres innervating the SSC were also positive for CGRP, but all CGRP-positive fibres colocalized with SP. The precise origin of these fibres is not known. Most of the fibres exhibiting colocalization are likely to be sensory fibres that derive from the trigeminal ganglion (Stone and Kuwayama, 1987; Stone, Kuwayama and Laties, 1989). Of those fibres which are positive for SP but negative for CGRP, it may be noted that a similar coexpression has been demonstrated in the pterygopalatine and ciliary ganglia in cynomolgous monkeys (van der Werf, 1993; Zhang *et al.*, 1994).

The complex peptidergic and nitrergic innervation of the SSC is thought to provide a basis for modulating the resistance of the outflow pathway through the tendon-like contacts of the SSC with the elastic fibres of the trabecular meshwork. In the cynomolgous monkey, injection of VIP (Nilsson *et al.*, 1986), CGRP (Almegard and Andersson, 1990) or of various nitrovasodilators, causes an increase in outflow facility.

TRABECULAR MESHWORK

The trabecular meshwork is a spongework of connective tissue beams which are arranged as superimposed perforated sheets. The beams are disposed circularly in the chamber angle and extend from Schwalbe's ring anteriorly to the scleral spur and junction of iris and ciliary body posteriorly (Figs 8.1 and 8.7). The inner portion of the trabecular meshwork is referred to as the **uveal meshwork** and the outer portion, connected to the spur and closer to Schlemm's canal, is the **corneoscleral meshwork**. In meridional section they are arbitrarily divided from

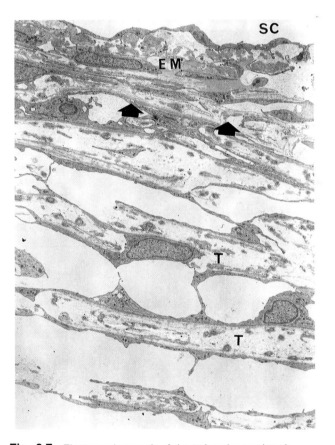

Fig. 8.7 Electron micrograph of the trabecular meshwork. Trabeculae (T) of the corneoscleral meshwork are evident. The arrows demarcate the transition between the corneoscleral meshwork and the juxtacanalicular region (JCT) of the inner wall of Schlemm's canal (SC). Original magnification ×3000. (Courtesy of Dr I. Grierson.)

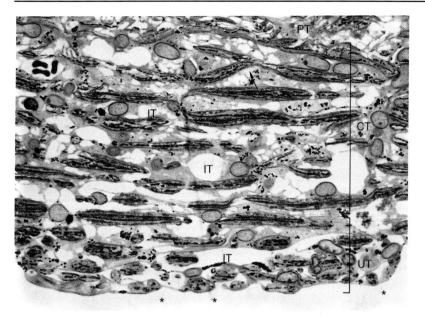

Fig. 8.8 Light micrograph of anterior trabecular meshwork in a 70-year-old human. This meridional section shows the morphology of uveal trabeculae (UT) and corneoscleral trabeculae (CT). Note the rounded profile of the inner uveal trabecular sheets (*) compared with the flattened profile of the outer uveal and corneoscleral sheets, and a progressive narrowing of inter-trabecular spaces (IT) in the latter region. PT = pericanalicular connective tissue. The arrow denotes branching of a trabecular sheet. Original magnification ×760. (From Tripathi, R. C. and Tripathi, B. J. in Duane, T. A. and Jaeger, E. W. (eds) (1982) *Biomedical Foundations of Ophthalmology, Vol. 1*, published by Harper and Row.)

one another by a line joining Schwalbe's ring to the innermost margin of the scleral spur, so that anterior to the scleral spur the uveal meshwork is related to corneoscleral meshwork on its outer surface and beneath the scleral spur it spreads over the anterior tip of the ciliary body (Figs 8.1 and 8.5). The spaces of the trabecular meshwork decrease in size progressively from within outwards. The meridional width of the trabecular meshwork posteriorly, near the scleral spur, is 120–180 μm. The dimensions are wider in the myopic than the hypermetropic eye.

Between the outermost corneoscleral trabecular sheet and the endothelial lining of Schlemm's canal is a cell-rich zone, the peri- or juxta-canalicular–connective tissue zone (or endothelial or cribriform meshwork). The extracellular spaces of the trabecular meshwork contain hydrophilic glycosaminoglycans and collagenous material which must influence the resistance to aqueous flow accorded by the meshwork spaces.

Uveal meshwork

The inner uveal meshwork (1–2 layers) is made up of cord-like trabeculae which interlace, and taper anteriorly. The innermost trabeculae may pass from the ciliary muscle almost to the region of Schwalbe's ring. Posteriorly, there are two to five layers and the outer layers have a more circular orientation and a more flattened profile concentric with the limbus, resembling that of the corneoscleral sheets (Figs 8.5 and 8.8) (Spencer, Alvarado and Hayes, 1968; Anderson, 1969a; Tripathi, 1969, 1974).

Posteriorly, the trabeculae may be connected either with the circular and radial muscle fibres of the ciliary

body, or with the meridional ciliary muscle fibres, but this distinction may be difficult to show histologically (Ashton, Brini and Smith, 1956). Henderson suggested that the uveal trabeculae represented a tendinous extension of the ciliary muscle cells (the so-called pectinate ligament), which in humans generally terminates behind the scleral spur (Henderson, 1908). Anteriorly, the uveal trabeculae converge, to end by joining the periphery of Descemet's membrane, the inner part of Schwalbe's ring, the corneal lamellae, or the corneoscleral trabeculae (Fig. 8.9). The cellular lining of the uveal trabeculae is contiguous anteriorly with the kerocytes in the deeper region of the cornea and its endothelium.

The individual cords of the uveal trabeculae have a diameter of 4–6 μm in the mid region, being thicker posteriorly and narrower anteriorly. The inter-trabecular spaces range in size from 20 to 75 μm.

The corneoscleral meshwork

This is made up of flattened, perforated sheets, each about 5–12 μm in thickness in the mid portion and separated from each other by 5–20 μm (the intertrabecular space) (Figs 8.5, 8.7 and 8.8). Anastomosing bands between superficial and deep layers ranging from 2 to 5 μm in thickness, delineate the intratrabecular spaces.

There are approximately 8 to 15 trabecular layers with a total width of 120–150 μm. Anteriorly the sheets converge, obliterate the intertrabecular spaces and merge with the inner corneal lamellae and the trabecular cells interface with the keratocytes. Posteriorly they are inserted into the scleral roll (Tripathi and Tripathi, 1982). The intratrabecular spaces of the

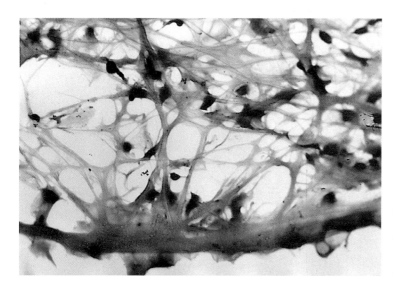

(a)

Fig. 8.9 Flat preparations of the trabecular meshwork as viewed from the anterior chamber aspect. (a) The attachment of some uveal trabeculae with a prominent line of Schwalbe (SL). Brightfield microscopy, teased preparation stained with methylene blue, original magnification ×240.

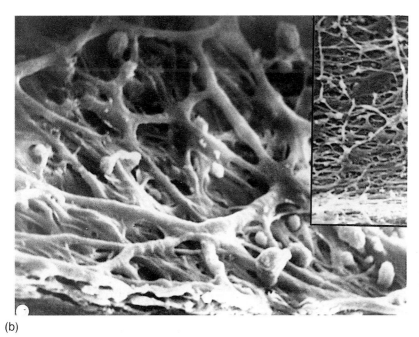

(b)

(b) Scanning electron micrograph showing netlike arrangement of uveal trabeculae. The long axes of the deeper trabecular sheets are oriented circumferentially. Original magnification ×1350; inset ×315. (From Tripathi, R. C. and Tripathi, B. J. in Duane, T. A. and Jaeger, E. W. (eds) (1982) *Biomedical Foundations of Ophthalmology*, *Vol. 1*, published by Harper and Row.)

outer layers of the corneoscleral sheets vary between 2 and 20 μm, and are therefore narrower than the uveoscleral meshes. Spaces decrease in size from within outwards.

Trabecular structure

The basic structure of the uveal and corneoscleral beams is as follows. Each sheet has a covering of trabecular cells, occasionally incomplete, a subcellular cortex (the 'glass membrane' of earlier histologists; Salzmann, 1912) and an inner collagenous core exhibiting randomly distributed elastic tissue.

The collagen is oriented in the long axis of the trabecular beam.

Trabecular cells

The trabecular cells are elongated in the long axis of the trabecular sheet and are 4–8 μm in thickness centrally, and about 120 μm in length. A nuclear bulge is frequently present and occasionally a cilium. Neighbouring cells make contact by long cytoplasmic processes and apposed surfaces are attached by maculae adherentes and gap junctions. The cells show the usual organelles including a central

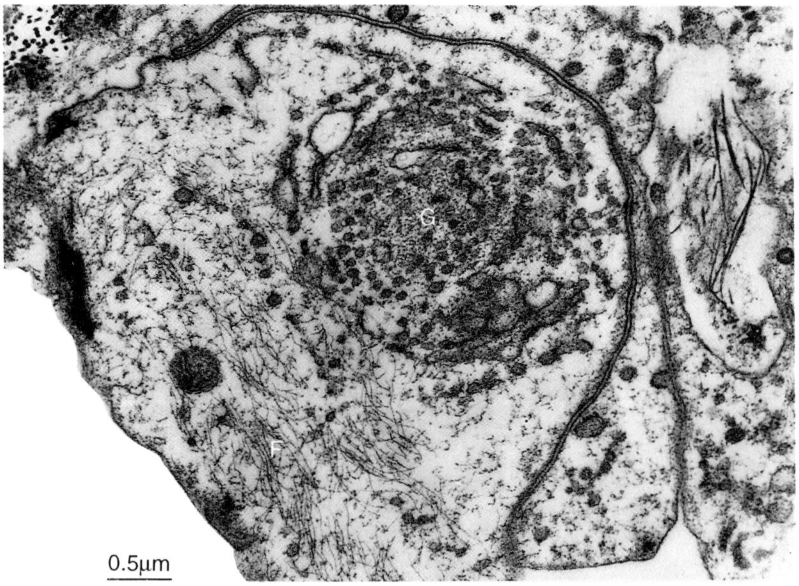

Fig. 8.10 Electron micrograph of the trabecular cells in an adult human eye. Note the prominent Golgi apparatus (G) and many fine cytoplasmic filaments (F). PTA stain, original magnification ×39 000. (From Tripathi, R. C. in Davson, H. and Graham, L.T. (eds) (1974) *The Eye*, published by Academic Press.)

nucleus, moderate amount of mitochondria, rough and smooth endoplasmic reticulum, well-developed Golgi apparatus, lysozomes, pinocytotic vesices and vesicular bodies (Hogan, Alvarado and Weddell, 1971; Tripathi, 1974). They also contain cytoskeletal filamentous proteins which may play a role in altering the meshwork configuration (Fig. 8.10). The trabecular cells are thought to perform various synthetic activities including the secretion of basal laminar material, collagen and glycosaminoglycans (Gong, Tripathi and Tripathi, 1996). The cells are actively phagocytic and may contain pigment and other inclusion materials which increases with age. A number of authors believe that these cells are involved in a self-cleansing mechanism which keeps the trabecular 'filter' clean.

The trabecular cells provide a lining for the inter- and intratrabecular spaces. Although the cellular surface is coated with macromolecules which are rich in terminal sialic acid residues (Tripathi, 1977a; Tripathi and Tripathi, 1982; Tripathi, Millard and Triparthi, 1990), there is no evidence for the presence of a hyaluronate gel filling the open spaces of the uveal and corneoscleral meshworks (Gong, Underhill and Freddo, 1994).

Cortical zone

The cortical zone consists of a periodic acid–Schiff positive basal laminar material which is attached to the trabecular cells by poorly defined hemidesmosomes and is otherwise separated by a lamina lucida (Fig. 8.11). Its inner limit is not well defined

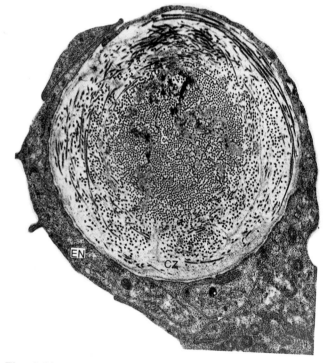

Fig. 8.11 Electron micrograph of a 2-year-old human eye from which the inner uveal beam has been cut transversely. The core is occupied by compactly arranged collagen fibrils (C) intermixed with elastic elements. Towards the periphery collagen fibrils are circumferential and intermixed in places with basement membrane material. EN = cellular covering of the beam; CZ = cortical zone. PTA stained, original magnification ×20 000. (From Tripathi, R. C. and Tripathi, B. J. in Duane, T. A. and Jaeger, E. W. (eds) (1982) *Biomedical Foundations of Ophthalmology, Vol. 1*, published by Harper and Row.)

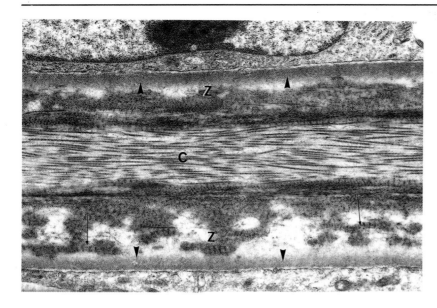

Fig. 8.12 TEM of trabecular meshwork: corneoscleral trabecula showing the basement membrane beneath the endothelial cover (arrowheads), the cortical zone (Z) and the collagen core (C). The wide-spacing collagen is also evident (arrows). Original magnification ×30 000. (Courtesy of Dr I. Grierson.)

and infiltrates the connective tissue elements of the core. The basal laminar material in the uveal trabeculae extends into the peripheral portion of Descemet's membrane. Within the basal lamina are found clumps of fusiform, long-spacing ('curly') collagen, with a periodicity ranging from 30–40 to 80–120 nm (Rohen and Lütjen-Drecoll, 1971; Tripathi and Tripathi, 1982; Tawara, Varner and Hollyfield, 1989; Marshall, Konstas and Lee, 1990; Gong, Freddo and Johnson, 1992).

Core

The core of each trabecular sheet is formed by collagen types I, II, and IV, fibronectin, thrombospondin, elastic tissue, chondroitin sulphate, dermatan sulphate, and 'curly' collagen (Rohen and Lütjen-Drecoll, 1971; Tripathi and Tripathi, 1982; Floyd, Cleveland and Worthen, 1985; Tawara, Varner and Hollyfield, 1989; Gong, Trinkaus-Randall and Freddo, 1989; Gong, Freddo and Johnson, 1992; Gong, Tripathi and Tripathi, 1996; Marshall, Konstas and Lee, 1991; Tripathi et al. 1991). The regular collagen fibrils (30–50 nm wide) are oriented along the long axis of the trabecular sheets of the corneoscleral trabeculae. In the uveal trabeculae, this compact core is often surrounded by a circular arrangement of regular collagen fibrils just deep to the cortical zone (Fig. 8.11). The orientation of collagen fibrils in the trabecular sheets is probably determined by the direction of pull exerted by the ciliary muscle on the uveal beams and through the scleral spur on the corneoscleral beams (Tripathi and Tripathi, 1982).

In the uveal trabeculae, elastic fibres are mainly central in the core. In the corneoscleral sheets, however, they are more prominent and may show a major distribution around the core, and are orientated along the long axis of the collagen fibrils. By electron microscopy the elastic tissue shows the usual fibrillar and amorphous components, separated into identifiable central amorphous and peripheral fibrillar zones (Tripathi and Tripathi, 1982). The elastic tissue imparts a recoil to the elements of the meshwork, permitting recovery after deformation. Thus widening of the trabecular spaces on ciliary muscle contraction would be followed by a resumption of meshwork spacing on relaxation of the muscle.

The iris processes

These are broad-based flat triangular bands which taper anteriorly and bridge the angle recess from the iris root to the uveal trabeculae into which they merge. Sometimes, they reach the level of the scleral spur, and occasionally to Schwalbe's line (Fig. 8.13). They are usually sparse in number and are found in about one-third of the normal population. In brown eyes, the processes are pigmented, but are grey in eyes with blue irides. Their structure resembles that of the iris tissue with which they are continuous. Broad iris processes partially obscure the angle recess. They are phylogenetically homologous with the pectinate ligaments of ungulates and other animals, but do not perform the same supportive function to the iris root (Tripathi, 1974).

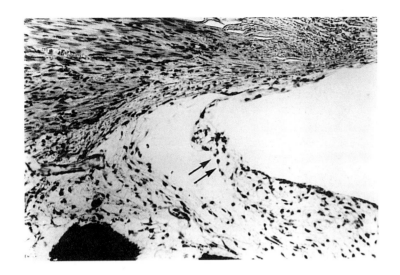

(a)

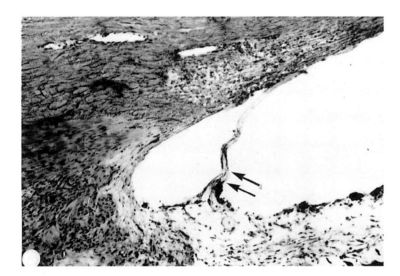

(b)

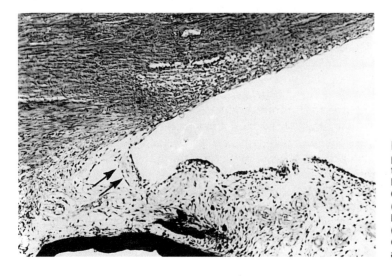

(c)

Fig. 8.13 Varying profiles of iris processes (arrows) of meridional sections of the angle of the anterior chamber of the human eyes as seen by light microscopy. Original magnifications: (a) ×360, (b) ×190, (c) ×170. (From Tripathi, R. C. and Tripathi, B. J. in Duane, T. A. and Jaeger, W. E. (eds) (1982) *Biomedical Foundations of Ophthalmology, Vol. 1,* published by Harper and Row.)

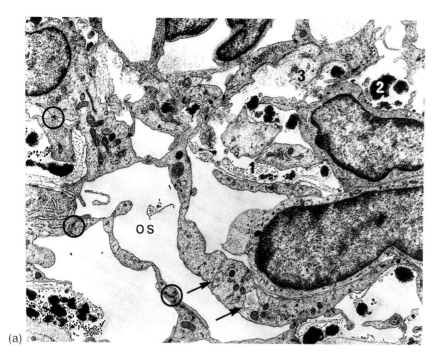

(a)

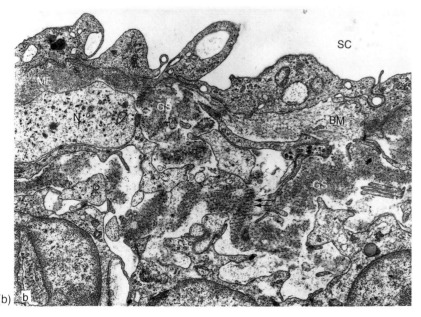

(b)

Fig. 8.14   Electron micrographs of an 80-year-old normotensive human eye. (a) Pericanalicular connective tissue zone (juxtacanicular meshwork), showing its cellular component with the usual intracellular organelles, some dilated cisternae of rough-surfaced endoplasmic reticulum (arrows), and long interlacing cytoplasmic processes of the cells joined infrequently by maculae occludentae and desmosomes (circled). In the open intercommunicating intercellular spaces (OS), the fibrous elements seen are collagen fibrils (1), elastic tissue (2), and basal lamina material (3). The basal lamina immediately beneath the lining membrane of Schlemm's canal is tenuous, interrupted and irregular. Original magnification ×18 900. (From Tripathi, R. C. (1977) *Experimental Eye Research* **25**, 65.)

(b) Pericanalicular region in the same eye in a different area of the canal (SC). Note the variations in morphology, the extracellular elements consisting of granuloamorphous substance (GS), microfibrillar elements (MF), basement membrane material (BM), and banded structures ('curly' collagen with variable periodicity – arrows). N = nerve terminal. Original magnification ×18 000. (From Tripathi, R. C. in Duane, T. A. and Jaeger, E. W. (eds) (1982) *Biomedical Foundations of Ophthalmology, Vol. 1,* published by Harper and Row.)

Peri- or juxtacanalicular connective tissue

The peri- or juxtacanalicular connective tissue zone invests Schlemm's canal in its entire extent.

On the trabecular aspect it has been termed variously as the endothelial meshwork (Speakman, 1960) or area cribriforme (Unger and Rohen, 1959). It has a thickness of 2–20 µm and is interposed between the endothelial lining of the canal and the outermost corneoscleral trabecular sheet. This region consists of 2–5 layers of loosely arranged cells,

embedded in an extracellular matrix. The cells exhibit long slender processes, and attach to one another irregularly by maculae occludentes, desmosomes and gap junctions. Spaces exist between the cells, up to 10 µm in width, through which aqueous humour can percolate to reach the lining endothelium of Schlemm's canal (Fig. 8.14) (Tripathi and Tripathi, 1982). The outermost of these cells share a basal lamina with the endothelial cells of Schlemm's canal.

The pericanalicular cells have important phagocytic

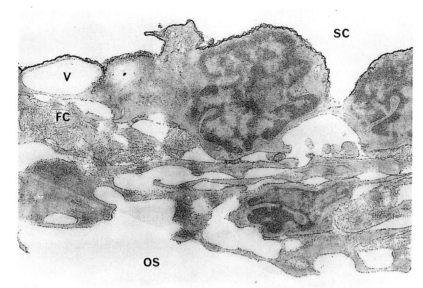

Fig. 8.15 Transmission electron micrograph of the pericanalicular region and Schlemm's canal after treatment with colloidal iron at pH 1.3 to demonstrate the presence of macromolecules rich in terminal sialic acid residues. The reaction product is present diffusely in the fibrous component (FC) of the extracellular matrix and decorates with plasma membranes of the pericanalicular cells and the endothelial cells of Schlemm's canal. The reaction product is dense along the luminal surface of Schlemm's canal (SC). OS = open space in pericanalicular region; V = vacuolar structure. Original magnification ×19 000. (From Tripathi, R. C. (1977) *Experimental Eye Research* **25**, 65.)

and secretory properties related to the self-cleansing role of the meshwork and to the production of the extracellular matrix, respectively. This portion of the drainage system is thought to make a major contribution to outflow resistance, not only because the pathways are narrow and tortuous, but because of the presence of the extracellular proteoglycans and glycoproteins (Vegge, 1967; Inomata, Bill and Smelser, 1972; Bill, 1975; Grierson and Lee, 1975; Lutjen-Drecoll, Futa and Rohen, 1981).

The pericanalicular zone adjacent to the outer wall of Schlemm's canal is less cellular than its trabecular counterpart and shows a compact arrangement of fibrocytic cells, 4–8 cells deep. The zone is 5–15 μm thick and occupied mainly by an irregular but dense arrangement of collagen as well as elastic tissue and granular amorphous material. There is a transitional zone 20–30 μm thick between this zone and the sclera outside it. It is composed of up to ten lamellae of collagen fibrils which increasingly resemble those of the sclera.

Extracellular matrix

The major components of the extracellular matrix, in which the cells of the pericanalicular region are embedded, include collagen types I, III, IV, V, and VI, fibronectin, chondroitin and dermatan sulphates associated with the callogen fibrils, hyaluronic acid, and elastic tissue. Many of these macromolecules (type VI collagen, fibronectin, as well as chondroitin and dermatan sulphates) have sialic acid as their terminal sugar residue and their distribution in the pericanalicular region can be demonstrated electron histochemically (Fig. 8.15). Analysis by serial sections has revealed that the elastic fibres are arranged as a

network, the so-called cribriform plexus (Rohen, Futa and Lütjen-Drecoll, 1981), which forms an integral part of the extracellular matrix in this region. Be-

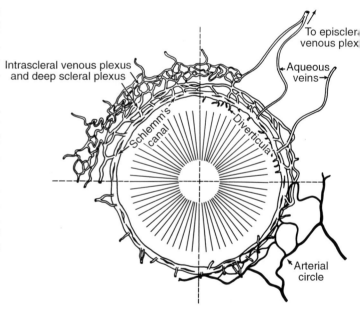

Fig. 8.16 Diagrammatic representation illustrating the canal of Schlemm and its relationships with the arterial and venous vascular supply. For clarity, the various systems have been limited to only parts of the circumference of the canal. Small, tortuous, blind diverticula (so-called Sondermann's channels) extend from the canal into the trabecular meshwork. Externally, the collector channels arising from the canal of Schlemm anastomose to form the intrascleral and deep scleral plexuses. At irregular intervals around the circumference, aqueous veins arise either from the canal or from the intrascleral plexus and connect directly to the episcleral veins. The arterial supply approximates closely the canal, but there is no direct communication between the two. (From Tripathi, R. C. and Tripathi, B. J. in Duane, T. A. and Jaeger, E. W. (eds) (1982) *Biomedical Foundations of Ophthalmology, Vol. 1*, published by Harper and Row.)

cause the elastic fibres are connected to both a sub-class of tendons from the longitudinal ciliary muscle and the basal lamina of the endothelial cells of Schlemm's canal, the plexus has the capability of effecting alterations in the permeability of this region (Rohen, Futa and Lütjen-Drecoll, 1981; Gong, Trinkaus-Randall and Freddo, 1989; Gong, Tripathi and Tripathi, 1996).

Recent morphometric and computational modelling studies suggest that the open spaces in this region of the aqueous outflow pathway may contain a gel-like substance (Ethier *et al.*, 1986) which could contribute to the resistance to aqueous outflow encountered in this region. Glycosaminoglycans and proteoglycans are not retained during processing of tissue for conventional light and transmission electron microscopy. By using special techniques, it has been shown that the electronlucent open spaces in the pericanalicular region are fewer and smaller than has been demonstrated previously (Marshall, Konstas and Lee, 1990).

CANAL OF SCHLEMM AND COLLECTOR CHANNELS

Schlemm's canal

The canal of Schlemm (Schlemm, 1830) is a narrow circular tube some 36 mm in circumference, which is lined by endothelium (McEwen, 1965; Tripathi and Tripathi, 1982) (Figs 8.16 and 8.17). It lies in the outer

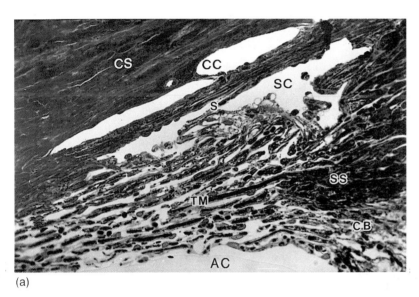

(a)

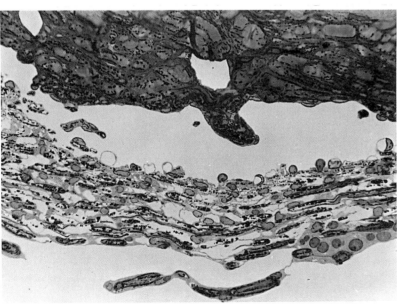

(b)

Fig. 8.17 Varying profiles of the canal of Schlemm in meridional sections of human eyes, as seen by light microscopy. AC = anterior chamber; CB = ciliary body; S = septum; CS = corneoscleral wall; CC = collector channels; TM = trabecular meshwork. Semithin epoxy-resin embedded tissue sections. Original magnifications: (a) ×260, (b) ×880. (From Tripathi, R. C. and Tripathi, B. J. in Duane, T. A. and Jaeger, E. W. (eds) (1982) *Biomedical Foundations of Ophthalmology, Vol. 1*, published by Harper and Row.)

portion of the internal scleral sulcus. It conducts aqueous humour from the trabecular region to the episcleral venous network via the collector channels. A zone of pericanicular connective tissue separates the inner and outer walls of Schlemm's canal from the trabecular meshwork and sclera, respectively. The lumen is elongated and oval, or sometimes triangular in cross-section (Ashton, 1951), or may vary in cross-section, being divided by septa or exhibiting multiple channels. Generally, it is about 200–400 μm long in its meridional axis and 10–25 μm in its shorter axis (Tripathi and Tripathi, 1982).

The endothelial lining of the canal sits on a basal lamina which is of irregular density and merges with that in the interstices of the adjacent pericanalicular connective tissue. On the inner wall of Schlemm's canal, the basal lamina is deficient in places which leaves the basal aspect of the cells bare (Tripathi, 1974). Its interrupted nature suggests that normally it may not provide significant resistance to the flow of aqueous humour. The major components of the basal lamina are collagen type IV, laminin, fibronectin, and heparan sulphate proteoglycan (Murphy et al., 1987; Tawara, Varner and Hollyfield, 1989; Marshall, Konstas and Lee, 1990; Gong, Freddo and Johnson, 1992; Gong, Tripathi and Tripathi, 1996).

Some processes extend from the canal into the pericanalicular tissue and on the trabecular side more developed diverticulae of the lumen are identified (Sondermann's canals; Sondermann, 1933) (Fig. 8.18). Although they increase the available sur-

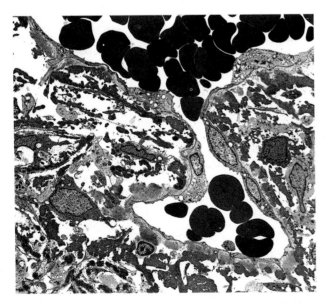

Fig. 8.18 TEM of a blind diverticulum in the inner wall of Schlemm's canal (Sondermann's canal). The canal contains erythrocytes from reflux filling. Original magnification ×1200. (Courtesy of Dr I. Grierson.)

face area of Schlemm's canal, they do not provide any direct communication with the spaces of the pericanalicular zone. The endothelium resembles that lining the inner wall of Schlemm's canal elsewhere (Tripathi and Tripathi, 1982).

Endothelial lining

Inner wall

For many years there was controversy over whether there was (Schwalbe, 1870), or was not (Leber, 1865, 1903), an open communication between the anterior chamber and the canal of Schlemm. It is now generally conceded that the vacuolar configurations of the endothelium provide a mechanism for direct communication between the extracellular spaces of the trabecular zone and the canal of Schlemm, and are probably the major route for the entry of aqueous into the canal. This concept has been developed over a number of years, by studies employing light and electron microscopy, morphometric and tracer techniques (see Tripathi and Tripathi, 1974, 1977, 1982, for review).

Lining

Schlemm's canal is lined by a single layer of spindle-shaped endothelial cells, oriented parallel to its circumference. These are clearly demonstrated by scanning electron microscopy (Fig. 8.19). In the inner wall they are 40–120 μm long, 4–12 μm wide, and are 0.2 μm thick (Holmberg, 1965; Tripathi and Tripathi, 1982). They are connected by poorly defined tight junctions and maculae adherentae, and by occasional gap junctions with cells of the pericanalicular tissue. The junctions occupy only a small area of the cell membrane, and do not prevent the passage of leucocytes or macrophages across the intercellular space. The luminal surface of the cells exhibits sparse microvilli. Their cytoplasm shows numerous free ribosomes and microfilaments and also many pinocytotic vesicles (Fig. 8.20).

Giant vacuoles

The most prominent features of the inner wall of the canal of Schlemm are the 'giant vacuoles'. These are invaginations which are generally globular in profile on meridional sections as revealed by transmission electron microscopy. The vacuoles measure from 4 to 6 μm in width and up to 25 μm in length and usually are oriented along the long axis of the cell (Figs 8.21, 8.22). It is thought that they arise by invagination of

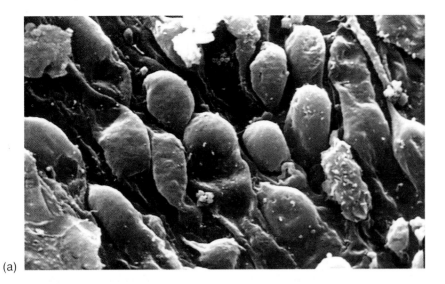

(a)

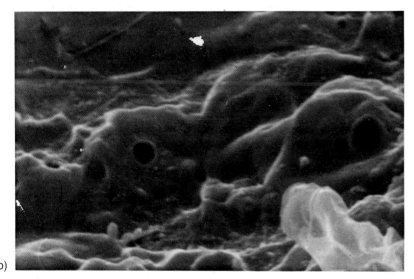

(b)

Fig. 8.19 SEM of the endothelial lining of Schlemm's canal. (a) Original magnification ×2000; (b) original magnification × 10 000. (Courtesy of Dr I. Grierson.)

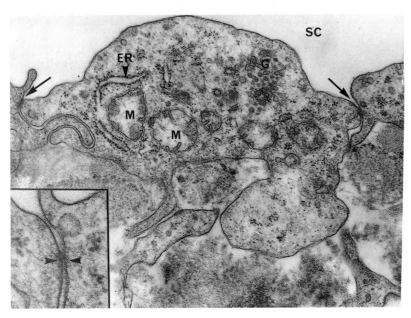

Fig. 8.20 Transmission electron micrograph of endothelial cells lining the trabecular wall of Schlemm's canal (SC) showing various intracellular organelles. Cytoplasmic projections (P) extend from the cell into the subendothelial connective tissue region probably to provide anchorage. Adjacent cell borders show simple end-to-end contact, overlap, and complex interdigitation (arrows). M = mitochondria; ER = endoplasmic retirulum; G = Golgi apparatus. Original magnification ×27 000. Inset: higher magnification of an intercellular contact zone between adjacent cells lining Schlemm's canal showing a poorly defined 'tight' junction (arrowheads). Original magnification ×90 000. (From Tripathi, R. C. (1977) *Experimental Eye Research* **25**, 65.)

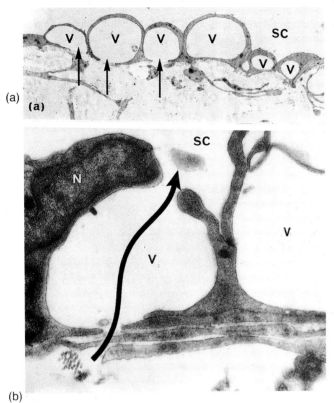

(a)

(b)

Fig. 8.21 (a) Survey electron micrograph of the endothelial lining of Schlemm's canal (SC) in a human eye, showing that most of the vacuolar configurations (V) at this level are in direct communication (arrows) with the subendothelial extracellular spaces, which contain aqueous humour in life. Original magnification ×3970; (b) electronmicrograph of a vacuolar structure, which at this level shows both basal and apical openings, thus constituting a transient vacuolar transcellular channel (arrow). In this way, the fluid-containing extracellular space on the basal aspect of the cell is temporarily connected with the lumen of Schlemm's canal (SC), allowing bulk outflow of aqueous humour. N = indented nucleus of the cell. Original magnification ×23 825. (From Tripathi, R. C. (1977) *Experimental Eye Research*, **25**, 65.)

the basal plasmalemma of the endothelial cells, thus providing access for aqueous humour in the pericanalicular region (Garron *et al.*, 1958; Garron and Feeney, 1959; Holmberg, 1959, 1965; Speakman, 1960; Kayes, 1967; Vegge, 1963, 1967; Tripathi, 1968, 1969, 1971, 1972, 1974, 1977a). A smaller proportion of the vacuoles also communicate with the canal of Schlemm via a luminal opening or pore, by which a **transcellular channel** may be formed (Tripathi, 1968, 1969, 1971, 1972, 1974, 1977a; Tripathi and Tripathi, 1982). The pore aperture may be up to 2.5 μm in diameter, while the basal invagination may be up to 4 μm wide. It has been calculated that, at any given instant, 2% of the total population of vacuoles are at the stage of transcellular channels and this number could account for the observed rate of aqueous outflow in normal eyes. The suggestion that pore frequency is greater in the nasal quadrant of the canal was not borne out by Grierson (1976).

Tracer studies have shown that materials of varying diameter may pass through transcellular channels from the anterior chamber into the canal of Schlemm. This has been demonstrated using thorotrast, ferritin, gold and horseradish peroxidase. Not all vacuoles fill, however. Even structures of cellular size, such as red cells, may pass through these channels by reason of their deformability, though glaucoma following haemorrhage into the vitreous or anterior chamber may be produced by macrophages, red cell ghosts and sickled red cells (Fenton and Zimmerman, 1963; Tripathi, 1977a; Grierson *et al.*, 1978a,b; Campbell, Simmons and Grant, 1976; Goldberg, 1979). Such cells become trapped in the inner portion of the meshwork.

A number of studies have demonstrated the formation of endothelial vacuoles to be pressure depend-

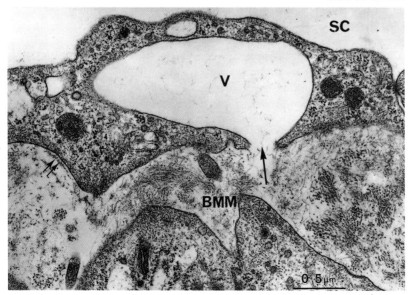

Fig. 8.22 Electron micrograph of the basement membrane material (BMM) beneath the endothelial lining of Schlemm's canal. Note the irregular thickness of the basal lamina in places adhering as an interrupted thin band (small double arrows), while in other places it is loosely organized and consists of both amorphous and microfibrillar elements. The basement membrane is, however, interrupted across the basal invagination in the cell (arrow) that forms macrovacuolar configurations (V), which at times may contain some flocculent material. SC = Schlemm's canal. Original magnification ×44 000. (From Tripathi, R. C. in Davson, H. and Graham, L. T., (eds) (1974) *The Eye*, published by Academic Press.)

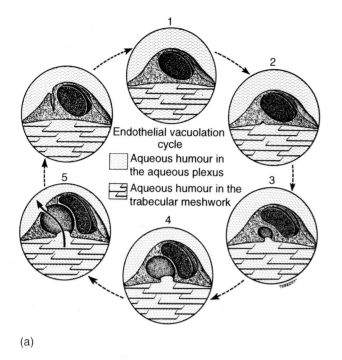

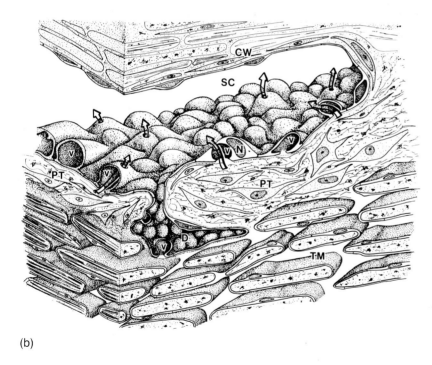

Fig. 8.23 (a) Concept of the cyclical sequence of events in the formation of vacuolar transcellular channels and mechanism of bulk flow of aqueous humour across the endothelial barrier of Schlemm's canal. Initially, vacuoles are formed by a membranous depression or infolding of the basal aspect of the cell surface (stage 2). Progressive enlargement of this infolding leads to formation of a macrovacuolar structure (stages 3 and 4), which eventually opens on the luminal aspect of the cell surface (stage 5) thus forming a transient vacuolar transcellular channel (continuous arrow). Bulk flow of aqueous takes place down a pressure gradient (i.e. from the meshwork into the lumen of Schlemm's canal) through such vacuolar transendothelial channels, which act as one-way valves. After a time, the basal infolding is occluded and the cell returns to its non-vacuolated state (stage 1). On morphological and physiological grounds, this mechanism is postulated to be equally applicable to the bulk flow of cerebrospinal fluid from the subarachnoid space into the dural sinus across the mesothelial barrier of arachnoid villi. (From Tripathi, R. C. (1977) *Experimental Eye Research* **25**, 65.) (b) A composite three-dimensional schematic rendering of the walls of Schlemm's canal (SC) and adjacent trabecular meshwork (TM). The spindle-shaped endothelial cells lining the trabecular wall of Schlemm's canal are characterized by luminal bulges corresponding to unique macrovacuolar configurations (v) and nuclei (N). The macrovacuolar configurations are formed by surface invaginations on the basal aspect of individual cells which gradually enlarge to open eventually on the apical aspect of the cell surface thus forming transcellular channels (arrows) for the bulk flow of aqueous humour down a pressure gradient. The endothelial lining of the trabecular wall is supported by a variable zone of cell-rich pericanalicular tissue (PT) below which lie the organized superimposed trabecular sheets having inter- and intratrabecular spaces that allow the flow of aqueous humour from the anterior chamber to the canal of Schlemm. The compact corneoscleral wall (CW) of Schlemm's canal is formed by lamellar arrangement of collagen and elastic tissue. (From Tripathi, R. C. and Tripathi, B. J. in Duane, T. A. and Jaeger, E. W. (eds) (1982) *Biomedical Foundations of Ophthalmology*, Vol. 1, published by Harper and Row.)

ent, so that their number and size are reduced at low pressures and increased at high pressures (Johnstone and Grant 1973; Tripathi, 1974, 1977b; Grierson and Lee, 1975, 1977, 1978; Kayes, 1975; Svedbergh, 1975). (In the monkey eye, the frequency of giant vacuoles was found to be 1900/mm length (Grierson and Lee, 1977) and 3200/mm (Inomata, Bill and Smelser,

1972).) Tripathi (1971, 1974, 1977a) proposed that the endothelial cells of the inner wall of Schlemm's canal have the ability to transfer aqueous in bulk, by a cyclical, pressure-dependent process involving the formation of vacuoles and transcellular channels (Fig. 8.23). Whether this represents an active process involving a regulatory, homeostatic mechanism, or

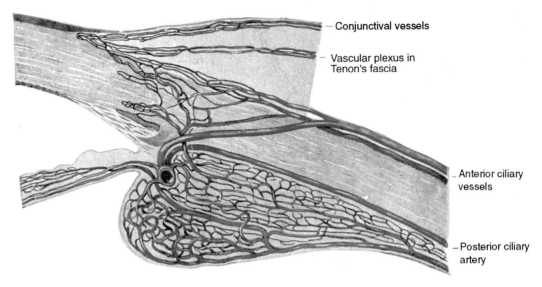

Conjunctival vessels

Vascular plexus in
Tenon's fascia

Anterior ciliary
vessels

Posterior ciliary
artery

Fig. 8.24 The vessels of the anterior segment.

whether it is a passive phenomenon independent of energy remains to be elucidated. Whichever way this argument is resolved, it is accepted that aqueous enters the canal of Schlemm almost entirely by a transcellular route, and only about 1% of the total conductance of the inner wall of the canal can be attributed to the non-vacuolar channels found in the narrow marginal portions of the endothelial cells (Bill, 1975; Grierson and Lee, 1978; Raviola and Raviola, 1981).

Outer wall

The endothelial cells of the outer wall of Schlemm's canal are longer, flatter and smoother in outline than those on the trabecular side. The cells are joined by zonulae occludentes, show rare giant vacuoles on their luminal aspect and rest on a basal lamina which is thicker and more continuous than that on the trabecular side. Although morphologically it would seem that access of aqueous to the outer pericanalicular tissue must be limited, tracer studies have demonstrated that a route exists (Tripathi, 1977a; Tripathi and Tripathi, 1982).

Collector channels

The collector channels arise at irregular intervals from the outer wall of the canal of Schlemm (Figs 8.16 and 8.17). They are 25–35 in number and drain into three interconnecting venous plexuses: the deep and mid scleral and the **episcleral venous plexuses**. Up to eight of these vessels drain directly into the episcleral venous plexus and are known as **aqueous veins**.

They were first recognized by Ascher (1942) and their connection with the canal of Schlemm was confirmed by Ashton (1952). With the slit-lamp microscope, they may be seen subconjunctivally either as clear vessels, or showing a bilaminar flow pattern representing the presence of both blood and aqueous (Goldmann, 1946). The pressure relationships between these aqueous channels and the neighbouring episcleral veins into which they drain were studied by Ascher (1942, 1949). They are found near the limbus (about 2 mm from it), most often inferonasally and often commencing in a hook-shaped bend where they emerge from the sclera. They may run a course of 1–10 mm before joining an episcleral vein. The collector channels are lined by vascular endothelium similar to that of the outer wall of Schlemm's canal. They are relatively wide at their origin (20–90 μm), but taper towards their anastomoses with the venous channels. No valves are present in the system. The channels are surrounded by a thin connective tissue.

The **deep scleral plexus** is made up of fine branches of the anterior ciliary veins and drains into the **mid scleral** plexus which forms a large interconnecting **intrascleral** venous network at the limbus (Fig. 8.24). This receives, in addition, blood from the ciliary venous plexus. Posteriorly the intrascleral plexus drains into the episcleral plexus and thence towards the anterior ciliary veins. The **episcleral venous plexus** in addition to its communication with the intrascleral plexus and the aqueous veins, receives blood from the conjunctival veins draining the perilimbal conjunctiva (Maggiore, 1917, 1924).

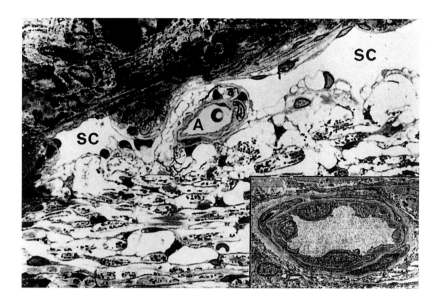

Fig. 8.25 Light micrograph of meridional section of trabecular meshwork tissue showing the location of an arteriolar twig (A) coursing through Schlemm's canal but separated from the latter by its adventitial wall. Original magnification ×1020. Inset: Transmission electron micrograph of an arteriolar twig revealing its continuous endothelial lining (E) and one to two layers of muscle cells (M). An unmyelineated nerve bundle (N) with Schwann cell is present in the vicinity of the arteriole. Original magnification ×12 000. (From Tripathi, R. C. and Tripathi, B. J. in Duane, T. A. and Jaeger, E. W. (eds) (1982) *Biomedical Foundations of Ophthalmology, Vol. 1*, published by Harper and Row.)

INTRASCLERAL ARTERIES OF THE LIMBUS

It has long been known that an incomplete arterial circle accompanies the canal of Schlemm, derived from the superficial and deep terminal branches of the anterior ciliary arteries (Friedenwald, 1936). Occasional arterioles pass through the lumen of the canal separated only by their adventitia, while others lie in its external wall or bridge the septa. No direct openings into the canal of Schlemm have ever been identified, and a role for this arterial system relating to aqueous drainage has not been accepted. The purpose of this rich limbal arteriolar supply is to provide nutrition to the tissues of this region. The arterioles show a non-fenestrated endothelial lining and a 1–2 layer medial coat (Fig. 8.25) (Ashton and Smith, 1953, Tripathi and Tripathi, 1982).

INNERVATION OF THE OUTFLOW APPARATUS (Fig. 8.26)

The innervation of the outflow apparatus derives from the **supraciliary nerve plexus** and the **ciliary plexus** in the region of the scleral spur. Both myelinated and non-myelinated nerve fibres have been demonstrated throughout the trabecular meshwork. Myelinated fibres are most commonly found towards the posterior attachment of the trabecular sheet. Nerve fibres have been observed within the core of the trabecular sheets and crossing the intratrabecular spaces. Nerve endings are more plentiful in the region of the inner portion of the pericanalicular zone. Various workers have identified fibres and terminals in the trabecular meshwork (Vrabec, 1954, 1961; Kurus, 1958; Valu, 1963), and these have been studied more fully by electron microscopy (Feeney, 1962; Chapman and Spelsberg, 1963; Holmberg, 1965; Hogan, Alvarado and Weddell, 1971; Tripathi, 1974; Nomura and Smelser, 1974; Ruskell, 1976; Tripathi and Tripathi, 1982). Nomura and Smelser (1974) reported nerve terminals chiefly in the posterior region of the trabecular meshwork anterior to the insertion of the longitudinal ciliary muscle and considered that about one-third were adrenergic. Ruskell (1976) found unmyelinated nerve fibres throughout the trabecular meshwork and Schlemm's canal system, and most frequently in the pericanalicular tissue, with some fibres adjacent to the endothelial lining of Schlemm's canal. There was a large variation in the numbers of axons. Tripathi found fewer adrenergic terminals than Nomura and Smelser (Tripathi and Tripathi, 1982) and a more diffuse distribution in the meshwork. Various other workers have demonstrated nerves in the meshwork. Holland (Holland, Von Sallman and Collins, 1956, 1957) believes them to be both somatic and autonomic. Lamers (1962) has suggested that they are sensory. Tripathi and Tripathi (1982) believe that both parasympathetic and adrenergic autonomic fibres and sensory fibres are represented. Although it is tempting to designate a role for such innervation in the homeostasis of intraocular pressure, no such function has been established.

NERVE ENDINGS WITH STRUCTURAL CHARACTERISTICS OF MECHANORECEPTORS IN THE HUMAN SCLERAL SPUR (Tamm *et al.*, 1994)

The inner layers of the mammalian eye are innervated by sensory nerves of trigeminal origin. Most of these

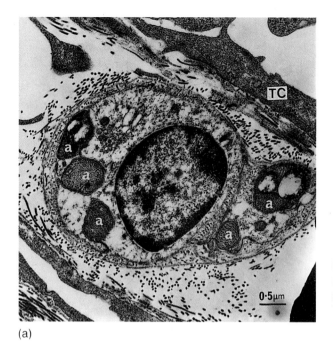

(a)

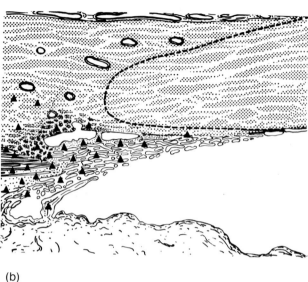

(b)

Fig. 8.26 Innervation of the trabecular meshwork of the human eye. (a) Transmission electron micrograph showing several axons (a) surrounded by a Schwann cell within the core of a trabecular sheet. TC = trabecular cell. Original magnification ×26 000.

(b) Diagrammatic representation of the distribution of nerve terminals (▲) in the region of the trabecular meshwork and Schlemm's canal system. (From Tripathi, R. C. and Tripathi, B. J. in Duane, T. A. and Jaeger, E. W. (eds) (1982) *Biomedical Foundations of Ophthalmology, Vol. 1*, published by Harper and Row.)

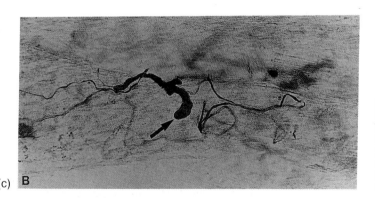

(c) B

(c) Whole-mount preparation of a sector of the scleral spur of a 67-year-old donor, with 0.5 mm circumferential length immunostained with antibodies against neurofilament proteins. The anterior insertion of the ciliary muscle is situated beyond the top of the individual micrographs, the trabecular meshwork beyond the bottom.

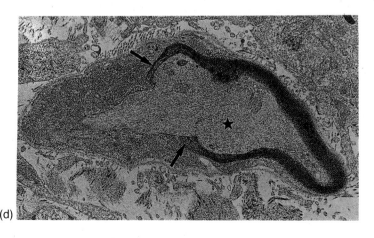

(d)

(d) The club-shaped terminals derive from myelinated axons with a diameter of 3 to 3.5 μm. The axons (asterisked) lose their myelin sheath (arrows) and form distinctive half nodes of Ranvier (electron micrograph, ×7000).

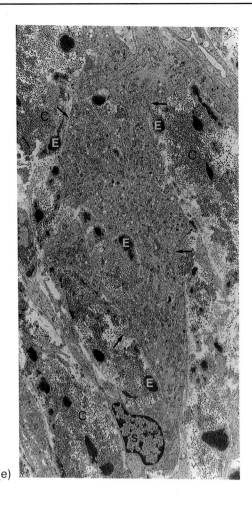

(e)

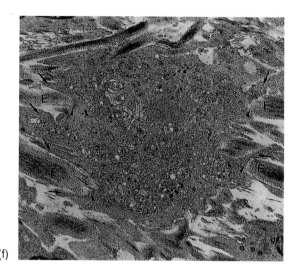

(f)

Fig 8.26 (contd)   (e) Electron micrograph of a club-shaped terminal in the scleral spur (donor aged 38 years). The terminal has a length of approximately 25 μm and is densely surrounded by collagen (C) and elastic fibres (E). The surface of the terminal is partly ensheathed by flat processes of Schwann cells (S). Nonetheless, large parts of the cell membrane are still exposed directly to the extracellular fibrils (arrows, ×6300). (f) Tangential section of a scleral spur terminal. (Electron micrograph ×5000; donor aged 56 years.) The terminal is embedded in a meshwork of numerous, circularly one elastic fibres (E) that are in close contact with the cell membrane of the terminal (arrowheads). In addition the terminal forms protrusions that surround larger parts of the nerve fibres (arrows). ((b)–(f) from Tamm *et al.* (1994) *Invest. Ophthalmol. Vis. Sci.* **35**, 1157, with permission.)

fibres are type C (Holland *et al.*, 1957; Bergmannson, 1977; Ten Tuscher *et al.*, 1989; Beckers *et al.*, 1992). Some of these fibres stain for SP or CGRP, and may participate in the irritative responses of the eye through an axon reflex (Stone, Kuyawama and Laties, 1989; Bill, 1990; Janig and Morrison, 1986).

Numerous axons, which stain positively for neurofilament proteins, run forwards parallel to the muscle bundles in the meridional part of the ciliary muscle, near its insertion into the scleral spur. The axons lie in the interstitial spaces between the muscle bundles. Solitary myelinated fibres, 2–3.5 μm wide, predominate, and give rise to thin **unmyelinated** fibres which terminate between the muscle cells.

Some of the transciliary **myelinated** fibres pass forwards beyond the anterior insertion of the ciliary muscle and give rise to a loose network of circumferentially oriented axons at the level of the scleral spur. They are supplemented by myelinated fibres which have run forwards in the supraciliary space. These **spur axons** are found mainly at the inner aspect of the spur and they give branches to the meshwork. In places, the myelinated spur axons lose their

myelin sheaths, branch profusely and terminate in **club-shaped nerve endings** which have the morphological features of mechanoreceptors found elsewhere in the body (Fig. 8.26c,d,f) (Tamm *et al.*, 1994). Although there has been uncertainty about the existence of such specialized receptors in the past (Bergmannson, 1977; Ruskell, 1982), they are probably identical to structures demonstrated by silver impregnation techniques, and discussed as 'baroreceptors' by Kurus (1955) and Castro-Carreira (1967). They are found throughout the whole circumference of the scleral spur region and are supplied by terminals (about 3 μm wide) from myelinated axons. The receptors stain for neurofilament proteins and synaptophysin, a marker for synaptic vesicles (Wiedenmann and Huttner, 1989). It should be noted that positive staining for synaptophysin is also exhibited by afferent terminals, and probably associated with agranular vesicles (de Camilli *et al.*, 1988).

The intense staining of the axon terminals for neurofilament protein is in keeping with their myelinated status, and they are assumed to be the afferent terminals of trigeminal neurons. In the monkey, 20% of neurons in the spur region are derived from the trigeminal region, and positive staining with one neurofilament antibody suggested that these might be fast-conducting type A sensory neurons (Tamm *et al.*, 1994).

The club-shaped endings, distributed regularly around the circumference of the scleral spur, are larger and more densely arranged in older subjects, which suggests that they probably increase in size with age (Wolter, 1959; Vrabec, 1965; Valu, 1962; Tamm *et al.*, 1994) and also in chronic simple glaucoma (Tamm *et al.*, 1994).

Morphologically, the endings contain abundant neurofilaments (8–10 nm thick), granular and agranular vesicles, mitochondria and lamellated, lysosome-like structures (Fig. 8.26e,f). These are similar to visceral mechanoreceptors in other parts of the body (Halata, 1975; Choukov, 1978; Andres, 1974) such as the carotid sinus (Rees, 1967; Bock and Gorgas, 1976; Knoche and Addicks, 1976; Knoche *et al.*, 1977, 1980), aortic arch (Krauhs, 1979), respiratory system (von During and Andres, 1988) atrial endocardium (Tranum-Jenson, 1975) and oesophagus (Neuhuber and Clerc, 1990) and also in tissues such as the skin, tendons and joint capsules (Halata *et al.*, 1985).

The endings are invested with a continuous basal lamina, but incompletely covered by a Schwann-cell sheath. Where the sheath is absent, the cell membranes of the endings are in contact with the neighbouring connective tissue and in particular with elastic fibres, which merge with the basal lamina and in some places are associated with specialized membrane densities. Contact between the nerve terminals and the extracellular connective tissue fibrils is characteristic of mechanoreceptors elsewhere.

Three potential roles have been proposed for these presumed mechanoreceptors (Tamm *et al.*, 1994). They may act as proprioceptive tendon organs for the ciliary muscle, whose longitudinal fibres insert into the scleral spur. They could also influence the contraction of the myofibroblastic scleral spur cells (Tamm *et al.*, 1992b) which have 'microtendon-like' insertions into the elastic tissue of the scleral spur. Additionally, they could perform a baroreceptor function in reponse to changes in intraocular pressure. Physiological studies suggest that such structures exist in the eye, since sensory discharges have been recorded in relation to the changes in ocular pressure (von Sallmann *et al.*, 1958; Lele and Grimes, 1960; Perkins, 1961; Belmonte, 1971; Zuazo, 1986). Belmonte *et al.* (1971) suggested that the ciliary nerves of the cat eye contain afferent fibres, which

respond tonically within the normal range of intraocular pressure, and originate from slowly adapting mechanoreceptors sensitive to changes in intraocular pressure.

UVEOSCLERAL DRAINAGE PATHWAY

The anterior portion of the ciliary body extends into the chamber angle and is inverted internally by the uveoscleral meshwork, behind the scleral spur. The cellular lining of uveal trabeculae is incomplete, and in any case there is no continuous cellular layer on the anterior iris face, so that aqueous has direct access from the anterior chamber into the ciliary body and thence into the supraciliary and suprachoroidal compartments (Fig. 8.27). These are potential spaces occupied by a loose framework of collagen interspersed with fibrocytes and melanocytes. (They may become occupied by transudate or exudate in the

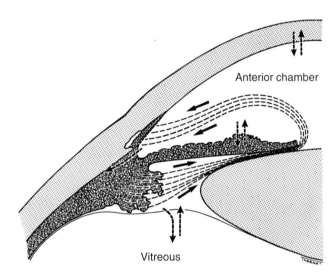

Fig. 8.27 Diagrammatic representation of the drainage pathways of the aqueous humour. The aqueous humour, formed in the posterior chamber (pc) by the ciliary processes, flows into the anterior chamber through the pupil. In normal human eyes, the main drainage route for bulk outflow is the conventional drainage pathway constituted by the trabecular meshwork and Schlemm's canal (SC). Subsidiary drainage routes include (1) the uveoscleral and uveovortex, that is, through the anterior face of the ciliary body into the suprachoroidal space; (2) exchange across the anterior vitreous face; (3) exchange across the iris vessels; and (4) exchange across the corneal endothelium. The role of 2, 3, and 4 in the net removal of aqueous humour appears to be insignificant because the net loss is equivalent to net gain through a two-way exchange. Under pathological conditions, however, these accessory drainage routes may assume greater significance. Drainage by the uveoscleral route is exploited in operations of cyclodialysis. L = lens. (From Tripathi, R. C. and Tripathi, B. J. in Duane, T. A. and Jaeger, E. W. (eds) (1982) *Biomedical Foundations of Ophthalmology, Vol. 1*, published by Harper and Row.)

formation of a choroidal detachment.) The route from the anterior chamber into suprachoroidal space has been demonstrated to provide egress for a small portion of the aqueous humour which does not leave by the conventional pathway. Fluid leaves the suprachoroidal space either by diffusion through the sclera or by absorption into the uveal vascular system including the vortex veins (the uveovortex outflow) (Tripathi and Cole, 1976; Tripathi, 1977b). Although there is some debate as to whether this system is pressure dependent (Lee and Grierson, 1982) or pressure independent (Tripathi and Tripathi, 1982) over the normal ocular pressure range, it is generally agreed that it accounts for about 10% of the total bulk aqueous outflow in the human.

LOCATION OF THE RESISTANCE TO OUTFLOW

The vascular pressure in the episcleral venous system is in the region of 9 mmHg and the intraocular pressure varies between 10 and 21 mmHg, with a mean value in the region of 15 mmHg. The pressure gradient from the anterior chamber to the episcleral veins is explained by a resistance to flow residing somewhere in the conventional outflow pathway. The resistance has been calculated to be 3 mmHg/μl/min (Grant, 1958). The resistance to outflow is often expressed as its reciprocal, the **facility of outflow** (e.g. 0.3 μl mmHg/min). In primary open-angle glaucoma (chronic simple glaucoma) the resistance to outflow increases, due to changes in the outflow structures (and therefore outflow facility falls).

The precise distribution of the outflow resistance along the channels of the outflow pathway is still under debate, despite many studies of the subject (Grant, 1963; Ellingson and Grant, 1971; Cole and Tripathi, 1971; Tripathi, 1971; Bill and Svedbergh, 1972; Tripathi, 1977a; Grierson and Lee, 1978; Erikson and Svedbergh, 1980). Nevertheless, certain generalizations may be made.

The conventional outflow pathway accounts for about 90% of the pressure-dependent outflow resistance, while the uveoscleral pathway accounts for the remainder of the bulk flow. Peterson, Jocson and Sears (1971) estimated that 10–15% of the resistance in the conventional outflow route resided in channels lying in the outer half or two-thirds of the perilimbal sclera, 25% in channels in the deeper sclera and 60–65% in the meshwork system and Schlemm's canal. This approximates to the 75% determined for trabecular meshwork and Schlemm's canal in human studies (Grant, 1963; Ellingson and Grant, 1971). Early theoretical studies by Cole and Tripathi

(1971) suggested that the endothelial monolayer of Schlemm's canal was a site of relatively high resistance to aqueous outflow. Subsequent studies, however, based on ultrastructural analysis of transendothelial channels in the human outflow system suggest that less than 10% of the outflow resistance of the meshwork and inner wall of Schlemm's canal reside in this layer (Bill and Svedbergh, 1972; Grierson, Lee and Abraham, 1979). However, more recent calculations, also based on scanning electron microscopic studies of the distribution of pores on the inner wall of Schlemm's canal, have estimated a 'pore invagination' resistance of 24% of the outflow resistance internal to Schlemm's canal (Moseley, Grierson and Lee, 1983). All such studies are dependent on the accuracy of measurement, the number and dimensions of transcellular channels and this in turn is dependent on the conditions under which specimens are obtained, and techniques of processing and examination. Those who believe that inner wall resistance is high consider the overall resistance of the conventional pathway to be regulated by the numbers and size of transcellular channels formed at a given instant. Those who believe that the inner wall resistance is low consider that the frequency of transcellular channels is a passive phenomenon related to the pressure gradient across the endothelial lining of Schlemm's canal.

The spaces of the trabecular meshwork, both intra-(lying within a single sheet) and inter- (lying between adjacent sheets), decrease in size from within outwards. It is likely that resistance in the system increases in the same direction. The spaces of the uveoscleral system probably offer negligible resistance, while the morphology of the pericanalicular tissue adjacent to the inner wall of Schlemm's canal suggests that it contributes a relatively high resistance to aqueous flow compared to the trabecular meshwork proper.

REGULATION OF INTRAOCULAR PRESSURE

The manner by which intraocular pressure is controlled is not fully understood. It is likely that both aqueous secretion and outflow resistance are regulated. A rise in pressure will eventually inhibit aqueous inflow (Bill and Barany, 1966). Similarly, a rise in ocular pressure should concurrently open out the spaces of the trabecular meshwork and increase the number of transcellular channels found in the inner wall of Schlemm's canal. This also may increase the washout of material from the extracellular space but this is not the case in primary open-angle glaucoma.

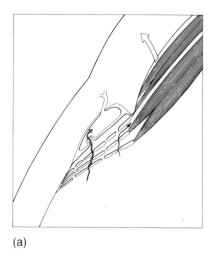
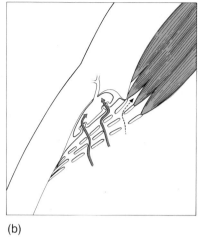

(a)　　　　　　　　　　　　(b)

Fig. 8.28 The effect of ciliary muscle contraction on the outflow pathways. Contraction thickens the muscle bundles, eliminating spaces between them and reducing uveoscleral outflow. At the same time, the action of the muscle on the scleral spur and trabecular meshwork itself opens up the meshwork, reducing resistance across the meshwork, and facilitating flow into Schlemm's canal. (a) Ciliary muscle relaxed; (b) ciliary muscle contracted.

Although cholinergic drugs (such as pilocarpine) and drugs with an alpha-adrenergic action (such as adrenaline) have only a small pressure-lowering effect in normal eyes, their effect in lowering ocular pressure in open-angle glaucoma is well established. In the normal eye their effect on pressure is buffered by homeostatic regulating mechanisms: both lower the resistance of the outflow pathway. Pilocarpine may increase the numbers of transcellular pores within the lining endothelium of Schlemm's canal (Griersen, Lee and Abraham, 1978; Griersen, Lee and McMenamin, 1981). Also, by its action on the ciliary muscle, which is inserted into the scleral spur and uveoscleral meshwork, pilocarpine achieves an opening-out of the spaces of the meshwork (Fig. 8.28). The manner in which adrenaline works is unclear, though some of its action may be a direct one on the trabecular cells (Tripathi and Tripathi, 1981) and some on the vascular networks into which the collector channels drain (Hart, 1972; Langham and Palewicz, 1977). Adrenergic beta-blocking agents and carbonic anhydrase inhibitors used in the treatment of glaucoma reduce the rate of secretion of aqueous humour by the ciliary body (Davson, 1980; Schenker and Jablonski, 1981).

THE AGEING EYE AND OPEN-ANGLE GLAUCOMA

A number of structural changes are observed in the drainage angle with advancing age that may contribute to the increase in resistance which is encountered in ageing eyes. An exaggeration of this process may contribute further to the increased resistance in primary open-angle glaucoma.

With ageing, the thickness of the trabecular sheets increases two- to threefold, mainly due to an accumulation of 'curly' collagen in the cortical zone and core of the beams, as well as basement membrane material (Fig. 8.29). However, the amounts of collagen-associated proteoglycans

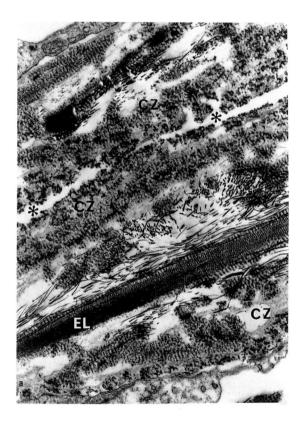

Fig. 8.29 Trabecular meshwork of an 80-year-old normotensive human eye in meridional section. The trabecular sheets have a thickened cortical zone (CZ) which contains abundant 'curly' collagen and basement membrane material. Asterisk denotes lack of trabecular cells between two adjacent sheets. EL = elastic tissue associated with banded structures. Transmission electron micrograph, original magnification ×20 000. (Trom Tripathi, R. C. and Tripathi, B. J. in Duane, T. A. and Jaeger, E. W. (eds) (1982) *Biomedical Foundations of Ophthalmology, Vol. 1*, published by Harper and Row.)

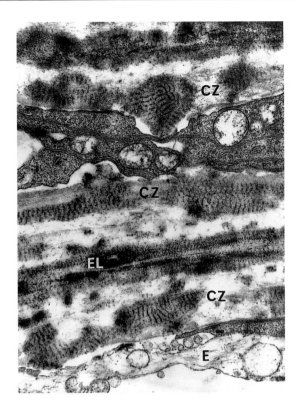

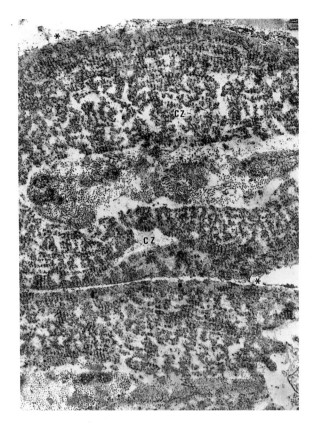

Fig. 8.30 Trabecular meshwork of an 84-year-old patient with advanced primary open-angle glaucoma, in meridional section. The trabecular cells (TC) show degenerative changes and the thickened cortical zone (CZ) contains basement membrane material and 'curly' collagen. EL = elastic tissue. Transmission electron micrography, original magnification ×24 000. (From Tripathi, R. C. and Tripathi, B. J. in Duane, T. A. and Jaeger, E. W. (eds) (1982) *Biomedical Foundations of Ophthalmology, Vol. 1*, published by Harper and Row.)

Fig. 8.31 Trabecular meshwork from a patient with advanced glaucoma, in meridional section. The pronounced thickening of the cortical zone (CZ) of individual sheets as well as the marked degeneration of the trabecular cells (asterisk) has resulted in hyalinization of the meshwork. Transmission electron micrograph, original magnification ×19 000. (From Tripathi, R. T. and Tripathi, B. J. in Duane, T. A. and Jaeger, E. W. (eds) (1982) *Biomedical Foundations of Ophthalmology, Vol. 1*, published by Harper and Row.)

(chondroitin and dermatan sulphates) decrease (Gong, Freddo and Johnson, 1992) and the peripheral microfibrillar component of elastin becomes obscure (Tripathi and Tripathi, 1982). Degenerative changes occur in the trabecular cells and the number of cells is reduced (Fig. 8.29) which results in a depletion of the cellular covering and subsequent fusion of the trabecular beams, a process referred to as hyalinization of the meshwork (Tripathi, 1977b; Rodrigues *et al.*, 1980; Spencer, 1985; Alvarado *et al.*, 1981; McMenamin, Lee and Aitken, 1986; Grierson and Howes, 1987; Yanoff and Fine, 1988; Gong, Tripathi and Tripathi, 1996). The consequent reduction in the open spaces of the meshwork is implicated in the age-related predilection for the development of increased resistance to aqueous outflow and elevated intraocular pressure. Cell loss also occurs in the pericanalicular region, together with an accumulation of the 55 nm banded

component which ensheaths the elastic fibres and other extracellular matrix molecules such as 'curly' collagen and fibronectin. The content of hyaluronic acid in this region of ageing eyes is decreased (Knepper *et al.*, 1989; Gong and Freddo, 1994). Biochemical investigations show an increase in the amounts of fibronectin, type VI collagen, and thrombospondin, and a decrease in laminin (Millard, Tripathi and Tripathi, 1987; Tripathi *et al.*, 1997). However, laminin has been shown to accumulate beneath the endothelial lining of Schlemm's canal in ageing eyes (Marshall, Konstas and Lee, 1990).

Morphologically similar, but exaggerated, changes are observed in eyes with primary open-angle glaucoma (Figs 8.30 and 8.31). Compared to age-matched normal eyes, the amount of 'curly' collagen in the trabecular beams is greatly increased and there is a further reduction in the numbers of trabecular cells (Tripathi, 1972, 1977b; Rodrigues *et*

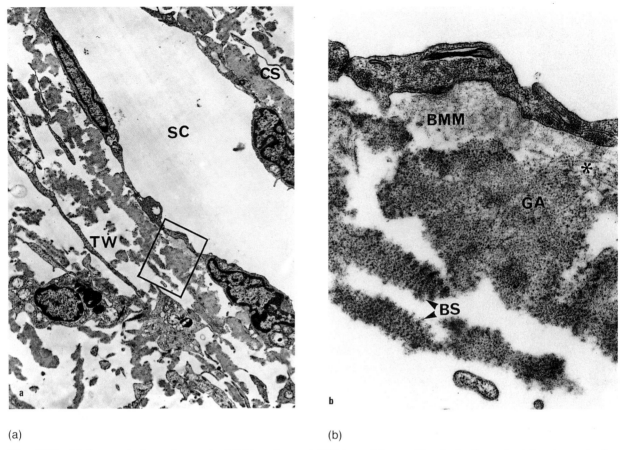

(a)   (b)

Fig. 8.32 (a) Survey electron micrograph of Schlemm's canal (SC) in an 84-year-old patient with moderately advanced primary open-angle glaucoma. Among various changes, there is an accumulation of granuloamorphous material associated with some banded structures (note the presence of similar material in the corneoscleral wall, CS) and hypocellularity of the pericanalicular tissue of the trabecular wall (TW). The enclosed area is shown at higher magnification in (b). Original magnification ×6250. (b) Beneath the endothelial lining, the presence of basement membrane material (BMM), granuloamorphous element (GA) associated with degenerate elastic tissue, banded profiles (BS) and degenerate collagen fibrils (asterisk) is apparent. Original magnification ×48 000. (From Tripathi, R. T. in Leydhecker, W. (ed) (1974) *Glaukom-Symposium Würzburg*, published by Enke Verlag.)

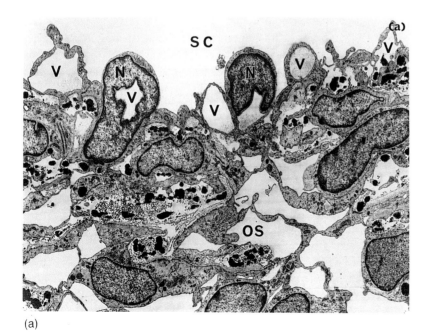

Fig. 8.33 (a) Survey electron micrograph of the trabecular wall of Schlemm's canal (SC) of an 82-year-old normotensive human eye, in meridional section. The endothelial lining (N = cell nuclei) is a single layer of cells, many of which contain vacuolar configurations (V). OS = open extracellular space of the pericanalicular region. Original magnification ×8750.

(a)

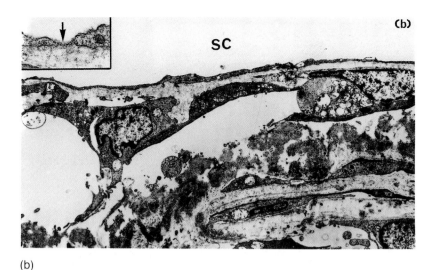

(b)

Fig. 8.33 (contd) (b) Survey electron micrograph of the trabecular wall of Schlemm's canal (SC) in an 84-year-old patient with advanced primary open-angle glaucoma. The endothelial lining is attenuated with a loss of vacuolar structures. Inset shows a markedly attenuated area in the lining of Schlemm's canal and the presence of a 'fenestration' bridged by a membranous diaphragm. Original magnification ×7000; inset ×62 000. (From Tripathi, R. C. (1977) *Experimental Eye Research* **25**, 76.)

al., 1980; Spencer, 1985; Alvarado, Murphy and Juster, 1984; Yanoff and Fine, 1988; Lütjen-Drecoll *et al.*, 1989). In the pericanalicular region, noteworthy changes include increased amounts of fibronectin and elastin as well as its 55 mm sheath component which has the appearance of a granuloamorphous material (Fig. 8.32) and decreased amounts of hyaluronic acid (Lütjen-Drecoll *et al.*, 1986; Babizhayev and Brodskaya, 1989; Knepper *et al.*, 1989;

Gong and Freddo, 1994). The paucity of giant vacuoles in the endothelial lining of Schlemm's canal is usually a significant finding (Fig. 8.33) (Rohen and Witmer, 1972; Tripathi, 1972, 1977c), although some investigators have disputed this (Fink, Felix and Fletcher, 1972, 1978). The attenuation of Schlemm's canal may be an early event (Nesterov, 1970; Moses, 1977) while a decrease in the diameter of the collector channels is not apparent early in the disease.

CHAPTER NINE
The iris

9.1 GROSS APPEARANCE

The iris is the most anterior portion of the uveal tract. It lies in the frontal plane of the eye between the anterior and posterior chamber and is bathed on both surfaces by the aqueous. It is continuous peripherally with the anterior aspect of the mid point of the ciliary body and in this way an anterior band of the ciliary body and the scleral spur into which it is inserted, contribute to the boundaries of the anterior chamber at the drainage angle.

The diameter of the iris is approximately 12 mm, and its circumference 38 mm (Fig. 9.1). It is thickest (0.6 mm) at the collarette and thinnest at the iris 'root'

(0.5 mm), where it is readily torn away from its attachment to the ciliary body by contusion, injury or as a surgical procedure (iridodialysis). The **pupil** pierces the iris diaphragm slightly below and nasal to its centre, but lying on the optical axis behind the optical zone of the cornea. The pupillary margin rests lightly on the anterior surface of the lens, so that it lies in a plane anterior to the iris root. When the lens is removed (aphakia) the iris is flat and often tremulous. Contact between the posterior surface of the iris and the lens creates a relative pupil block to the flow of aqueous humour through the pupil, which is most marked in mid-dilatation. This may encourage a forward bowing of the iris (physiological

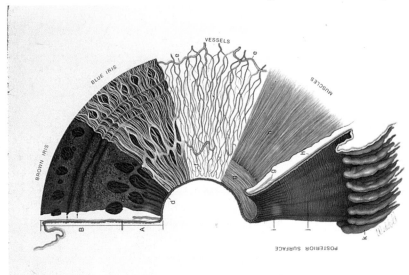

Fig. 9.1 Composite drawing of the surfaces and layers of the iris. Beginning at the upper left and proceeding clockwise the iris cross-section shows the pupillary (A) and ciliary portions (B), and surface view shows a brown iris with its dense, matted anterior border layer. Circular contraction furrows are shown (arrows) in the ciliary portion of the iris. Fuchs' crypts (c) are seen at either side of the collarette in the pupillary and ciliary portion and peripherally near the iris root. The pigment ruff is seen at the pupillary edge (d). The blue iris surface shows a less dense anterior border layer and more prominent trabeculae. The iris vessels are shown beginning at the major arterial circle in the ciliary body (e). Radical branches of the arteries and veins extend towards the pupillary region. The arteries form the incomplete minor arterial circle (f), from which branches extend towards the pupil, forming capillary arcades. The sector below it demonstrates the circular arrangement of the sphincter muscle (g) and the radial processes of the dilator muscle (h). The posterior surface of the iris shows the radial contraction furrows (i) and the structural folds (j) of Schwalbe. Circular contraction folds are also present in the ciliary portion. The pars plicata of the ciliary body is at (k). (From Hogan, M. J., Alvarado, J. A. and Weddell, J. E. (1971) *Histology of the Human Eye*, published by W. B. Saunders.)

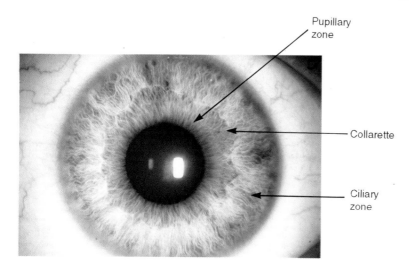

Pupillary zone

Collarette

Ciliary zone

Fig. 9.2 The normal iris.

bombé) which in predisposed narrow angles may precipitate angle closure glaucoma.

Embryologically, the iris can be divided into three layers; two anterior layers and a posterior layer (Fig. 9.2). Originally, the anterior layers were termed 'mesodermal' but in view of the major contribution of neural crest cells to their development, they are more appropriately designated as 'mesenchymal'.

SUPERFICIAL MESENCHYMAL LAYER

The superficial mesenchymal layer is shorter than the deeper layer and extends from the ciliary border to the **collarette**, which forms a dentate fringe, separated to a varying degree from the middle layer.

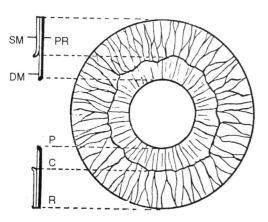

Fig. 9.3 Diagram showing the structure of the iris. The retinal layer appears at the edge of the pupil, where it forms the pigment border (P). The mesodermal layer is separable into a deep layer (DM), running from the root of the iris to the pupil and a superficial layer (SM), the axial limit of which forms the collarette (C). R = periphery of iris; PR = posterior retinal layer. The crypts of the iris situated in the ciliary portion may be considered as openings distributed in the superficial mesodermal layer (anterior).

This superficial layer gives the ciliary portion of the iris its colour. In it are the iris crypts, bounded by the trabeculae of the collarette, which are the remains of obliterated vessels that passed to the pupillary membrane during embryonic life (Lauber, 1908) (Figs 9.3 and 9.4).

DEEP MESENCHYMAL LAYER

The deep mesenchymal layer extends from the ciliary border to the pupillary edge. In lightly pigmented irides it has a radial fibrillary appearance and is transparent, so that the deeply pigmented ectodermal layer is visible through it.

The superficial mesenchymal layer is only loosely attached to the deeper one and glides freely over it. It does not participate greatly in movements of the rest of the iris. Thus, as the pupil dilates the pupillary edge approaches nearer to the collarette, so that the pupillary remnants, when present, may seem to arise from the pupil margin and not the collarette itself.

There are other changes as the pupil dilates. The pupillary ruff becomes thinned and may disappear. There is a more distinct step between collarette and pupil margin. The crypts become oblique, the vessels more tortuous, and the contraction and **peripheral furrows** deepen (see below). The border zone disappears.

The pupil regulates the entry of light into the eye: it is pinpoint in bright sunlight and widely dilated in the dark. The range of pupil diameter lies between 1.5 and 8 mm in youth; in old age the resting pupil size is often smaller because of fibrotic changes in the sphincter and atrophy of the dilator muscle. The pupil can be dilated to over 9 mm with mydriatic drops but dilatation is restricted in diabetics by dysautonomic changes (Yanoff and Fine, 1989).

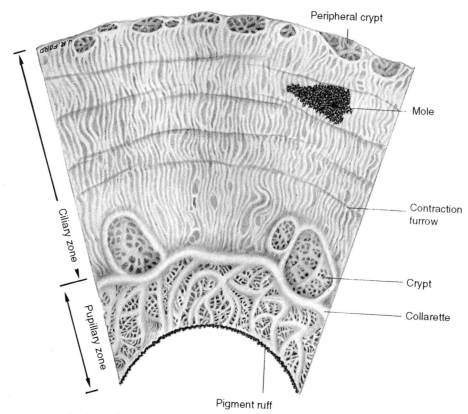

Fig. 9.4 Surface anatomy of the front of the iris.

The sphincter encircles the pupil, is innervated mainly by parasympathetic nerve endings and constricts the pupil on contraction (miosis). The dilator muscle fibres run radially; innervation is chiefly by the sympathetic and contraction dilates the pupil (mydriasis). These muscles show a reciprocal innervation. Pupil constriction occurs during accommodation for near and improves the depth of field while reducing spherical aberration. It also occurs during inflammation or after injury, in response to fifth nerve stimulation and the release of mediator substances such as prostaglandin or substance P.

COLOUR

Iris colour is determined chiefly by the melanocytes in the stroma and anterior border layer (Fig. 9.1). When the iris is brown the melanocytes are profuse and well pigmented. In the blue iris there is a paucity of melanocytes and while the longer wavelengths of light are absorbed, the shorter wavelengths in the blue region of the spectrum are back-scattered or reflected. The stroma of the blue iris contains amelanotic cells whose non-pigmented granules are of unknown composition (Yanoff and Fine, 1989).

The albino iris is a pale, buff colour because of the absence of pigmented melanocytes. With increasing levels of illumination the iris takes on a pinkish colour because light which has traversed the sclera and pupil transilluminates the iris from behind. Iris colour is inherited; brown as a dominant trait, blue as a recessive trait. In Caucasians the iris is blue at birth because of a paucity of stromal melanocytes. By the age of 3–5 months it adopts its adult colouration. In the black and brown races, there is a denser stroma and some pigmented melanocytes, so that at birth the iris appears a slate grey. In some individuals there is a segmental variation of iris colour or the colour may be different between the two eyes (heterochromia).

9.2 MACROSCOPIC APPEARANCE

ANTERIOR SURFACE

The anterior surface of the iris (Figs 9.5, 9.6 and 9.7) is generally richly textured, but in the darker races, where iris pigment is increased, the surface is smooth and velvety and the texture is masked.

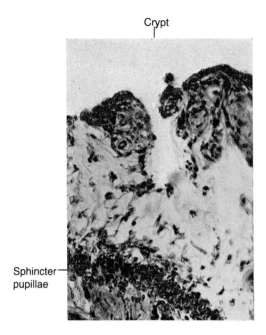

Crypt

Sphincter pupillae

Fig. 9.5 Meridional section of crypt of Fuchs.

Collarette

The collarette consists of a series of trabeculae forming a sometimes interrupted circular ridge. It lies about 1.6 mm from the pupil margin and divides the surface into an outer **ciliary zone** and an inner **pupillary zone**, which often differ in colour (Figs 9.1c, 9.3 and 9.4). The iris is slightly thickened at the collarette (0.6 mm), which overlies an incomplete vascular circle (**circulus vasculosus iridis minor**. The vascular connection between the minor circle and the **tunica vasculosa lentis** disappears before birth, but a remnant ('**pupillary membrane**') may be present at birth, and is frequently seen in premature babies where it is a confirmation of gestational age (Fig. 9.8).

Fuchs' crypts

The iris surface has a trabecular structure which is most exaggerated in the pupillary zone and collarette region where there are deficiencies in the superficial layers. Large, pit-like depressions are termed **Fuchs' crypts**. Similar, smaller crypts occur at the iris periphery and are best seen during examination of the chamber angle by gonioscopy (Fig. 9.9). In blue eyes, especially in children, the peripheral perforated zones are seen as dark rings near the iris root. The collarette and the crypts appear after birth.

Pupillary ruff

The posterior epithelial layers of the iris extend forward at the pupil margin as the **pupillary ruff**, whose crenations result from a forward extension of the radial folds of the posterior iris surface. The crenations are most marked above and in miosis (Fig. 9.10). The ruff marks the anterior limit of the embryonic optic cup.

Iris sphincter

In blue irises or where the stroma is atrophic, the **iris sphincter** is visible as a buff-coloured, flat circular strap-like muscle, 0.75 mm wide, encircling the pupil (Figs 9.1 and 9.11). The central part of the ciliary zone is smooth, but peripherally several **contraction furrows** occur, concentric with the pupil, which deepen as the pupil dilates. There is less pigment at the base of a furrow, which is best seen in a dark iris with a

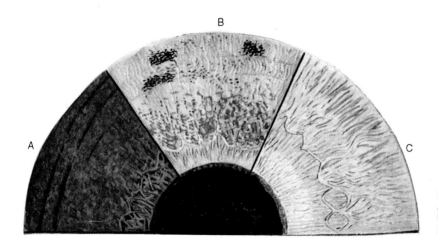

Fig. 9.6 Varieties of human iris. A = deeply pigmented type (Bengali); B = medium European; C = blonde European.

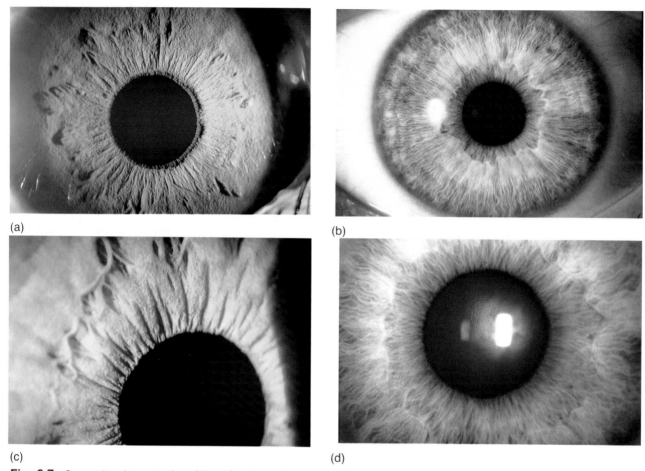

(a)

(b)

(c)

(d)

Fig. 9.7 Composite picture to show irises of various colours and mesodermal texture.

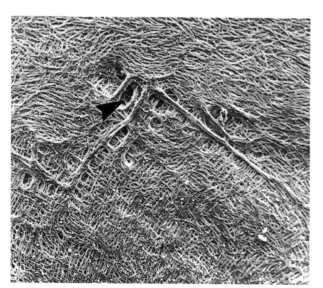

Fig. 9.8 Scanning electron micrograph of the collarette region of the anterior iris surface showing a branching vessel of the minor circle of the iris and small crypts of Fuchs (arrowhead). (Courtesy of T. Freddo.)

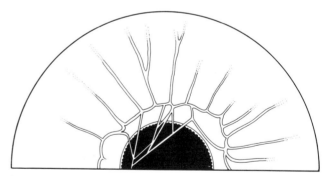

Fig. 9.9 The pupillary membrane at birth. (From Mann (1957) *Developmental Abnormalities of the Eye*, 2nd edition, published by Lippincott, with permission.)

small pupil (Fuchs). In the ciliary zone there are radial streaks which are straight with a small pupil and wavy when it is dilated.

With the slit-lamp microscope, it is possible, in blue irises, to see the epithelial layers of the iris, which appear as a copper-coloured line in the slit-beam,

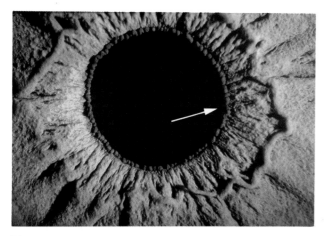

Fig. 9.10 Brown iris showing a prominent pupillary ruff (arrowed).

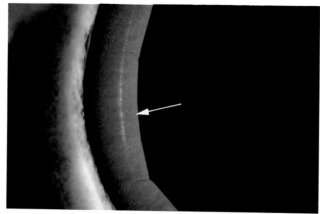

Fig. 9.12 Iris cyst. The two layers of the iris epithelium are separated by fluid so that the posterior surface of the posterior pigmented epithelium is visible at the pupil margin (arrow).

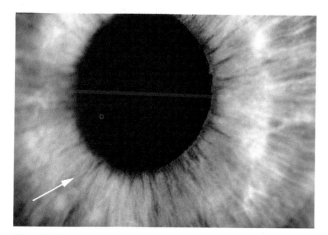

Fig. 9.11 Blue iris to show the sphincter (arrowed) underlying the posterior mesodermal layer.

deep to the stroma. The colour is due mainly to pigment in the posterior epithelial layer. Colour is lacking in albinism, or overlying a cyst of the epithelium, where the posterior epithelium is displaced backwards and separated from the anterior epithelium (Fig. 9.12).

POSTERIOR SURFACE

The posterior surface of the iris is dark brown and smooth and displays the following radial and circular furrows (Figs 9.1, 9.13, 9.14 and 9.15).

Schwalbe's contraction folds

Numerous, small folds extend radially for 1 mm from the edge of the pupil. Because the posterior pigmented layers extend forward around the pupil, these folds are responsible for the crenated appearance of the pupillary margin.

Schwalbe's structural furrows

These involve both epithelial and vascular layers. They begin 1.5 mm from the pupil margin, where they are narrow and deep, but become shallow and broaden towards the peripheral iris. They pass into the valleys of the ciliary processes.

Circular furrows

Fine circular furrows cross the structural furrows at regular intervals and are due to variation in the thickness of the pigment epithelium and the arrangement of the stroma into ridges with the furrows between. The furrows are incomplete. They are least developed behind the sphincter and most developed at the iris root. The high proliferative capacity of the epithelial cells in this region may account for the frequency of pigmentary cysts here (Yanoff and Fine, 1989).

Pits

Distinct pits are found scattered over the pigment epithelium and represent desmosomal structures in the posterior epithelial layer (Rodrigues, Hackett and Donohoo, 1988) (Fig. 9.15).

9.3 STRUCTURE

The layers of the iris from anterior to posterior are:

1. anterior border layer;
2. stroma and sphincter muscle;
3. anterior epithelium and dilator muscle;
4. posterior pigmented epithelium.

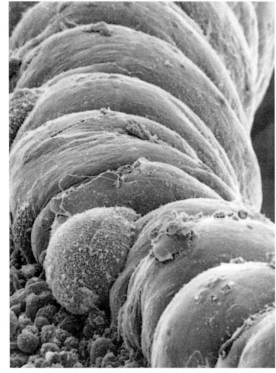

(a)

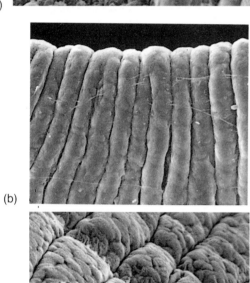

(b)

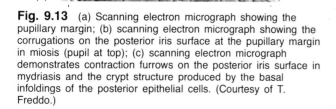

(c)

Fig. 9.13 (a) Scanning electron micrograph showing the pupillary margin; (b) scanning electron micrograph showing the corrugations on the posterior iris surface at the pupillary margin in miosis (pupil at top); (c) scanning electron micrograph demonstrates contraction furrows on the posterior iris surface in mydriasis and the crypt structure produced by the basal infoldings of the posterior epithelial cells. (Courtesy of T. Freddo.)

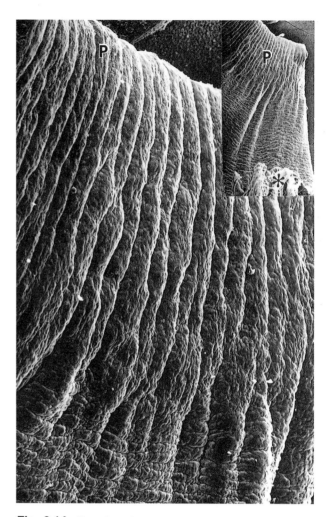

Fig. 9.14 Scanning electron micrograph of the posterior surface of the infant iris showing prominent longitudinal furrows near the pupillary region (P) (original magnification ×80). Inset shows portions of ciliary processes (*) at the periphery of the iris. The pupillary region is indicated by P (original magnification ×10). (From Rodrigues, M. M., Hackett, J. and Donohoo, P. in Duane T. D. and Jaeger, E. A. (eds) (1988) *Biomedical Foundations of Ophthalmology, Vol. 1*, published by J. B. Lippincott, with permission.)

While a complete epithelial covering with endothelial-like cells may occur anteriorly in some mammals (Walls, 1963), electron microscopy has established that no such sheet occurs in human iris (Tousimis and Fine, 1959) except in the first two years of life (Vrabec, 1952).

ANTERIOR BORDER LAYER (Figs 9.16–9.20)

The anterior border layer is a condensation of connective tissue and pigment cells derived from the anterior stroma. **Fibroblasts** form a fairly continuous sheet of flat stellate cells and interlacing processes, stretching from the iris root, where there is continuity with the ciliary body stroma, to the pupil, where they

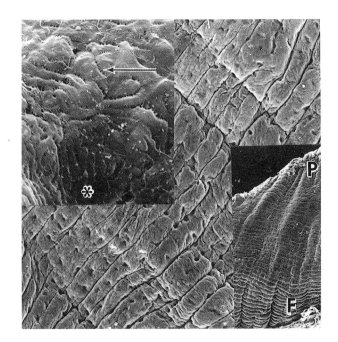

Fig. 9.15 Scanning electron micrograph of the posterior iris surface shows longitudinal furrows and numerous pit-like structures (original magnification ×165). Upper inset shows higher magnification of a pit (*) with flattened epithelial cells connected by desmosomes (arrow) at the edges (original magnification ×6000). Lower inset shows prominent peripheral circumferential folds (F). The pupil is indicated by P (original magnification ×33). (From Rodrigues, M. M., Hackett, J. and Donohoo, P. in Duane, T. D. and Jaeger, E. A. (eds) (1988) *Biomedical Foundations of Ophthalmology, Vol. 1,* published by J. P. Lippincott.)

drainage angle as fine **iris processes** which insert anterior to the scleral spur and sometimes up to Schwalbe's line (Lichter, 1969).

Three types of intercellular junction are reported to join the cells of the anterior border layer, including gap junctions, intermediate junctions and discontinuous tight junctions (Freddo, Townes-Anderson and Raviola, 1980; Raviola, Sagaties and Miller, 1987). All of these junctions occur principally between cells of like type with the exception that gap junctions have been shown to exist between fibroblasts and melanocytes in one species of monkey (Ringvold, 1975). Capillaries and venules are present in this layer as well as numerous nerve endings, which terminate in the subjacent stroma. Naevus-like clusters are probably derived from Schwann cells. Small elevated white or yellowish, **Wölfflin spots** are found in the anterior border layer at the iris periphery, most often in blue or grey irides (Schmidt, 1971). The border layer is absent at crypts and thinned at contraction furrows. It is thickest in the pupillary zone and at the periphery of the ciliary zone. The layer is responsible for the colour of the iris, is thin in the blue iris and thick and densely pigmented in the brown iris. Melanocytes may accumulate locally to form an **iris freckle**, or be distributed more diffusely to produce a patch of hyperheterochromia or heterochromia of one iris in comparison to the other.

reach the epithelium of the pupillary ruff. The fibroblasts exhibit microvilli and cilia which project into the anterior chamber (Fig. 9.10a–d). Pigmented uveal **melanocytes**, also oriented parallel to the surface, lie deep to the fibroblasts (Fig. 9.12). In about 57% of eyes the anterior border layer extends into the

STROMA

The stroma consists of a loose collagenous network containing (Figs 9.21–9.23):

* the sphincter pupillae muscle;

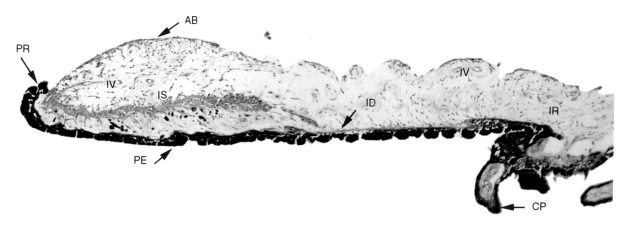

Fig. 9.16 Cross-sectional view of iris and ciliary body. The anterior border layer (AB) forms a distinct zone at the iris surface. The iris dilator muscle (ID), derived from the processes of the anterior myoepithelium, lies deep to the sphincter muscle as it approaches the pupil. IR = iris root (note the continuity between the iris and ciliary body structure); IS = iris sphincter; IV = iris vessels; PE = posterior pigment epithelium; PR = pupillary ruff, curling around the pupil margin; CP = ciliary process.

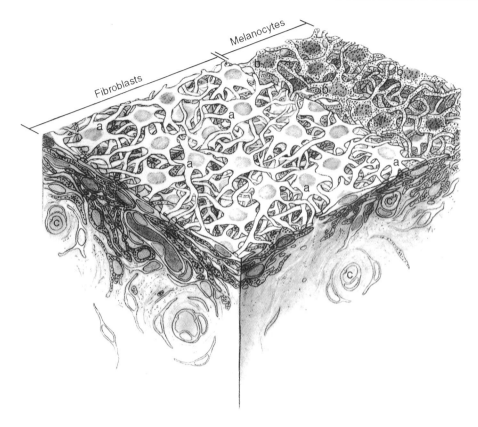

Fig. 9.17 Anterior layers of the iris. The anterior border layer is covered by a single layer of fibroblasts (a) whose long, branching processes interconnect with each other. The branching processes of the fibroblasts form varying-sized openings on the iris surface. Beneath the layer of fibroblasts is a fairly dense aggregation of melanocytes and a few fibroblasts. The superficial layer of fibroblasts has been removed at (b) to show these cells. The number of cells in the anterior border layer is greater than in the underlying stroma. The iris stroma contains a number of capillaries (c) which sometimes are quite close to the surface. (From Hogan, M. J., Alvarado, J. A. and Weddell, J. E. (1971) *Histology of the Human Eye*, published by W. B. Saunders.)

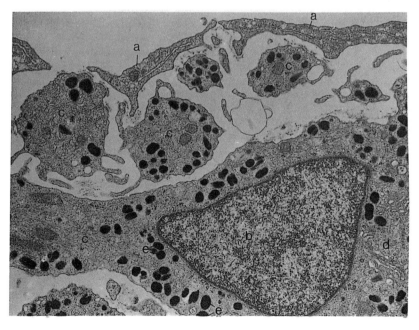

Fig. 9.18 Anterior border layer, electron micrograph. The thin layer of fibroblasts on the anterior iris surface (a) is not continuous. Melanocytes (b) and their processes (c) form part of the anterior border layer. The Golgi apparatus (d) and melanin granules (e) are shown (original magnification ×18 000). (From Hogan, M. J., Alvarado, J. A. and Weddell, J. E. (1971) *Histology of the Human Eye*, published by W. B. Saunders.)

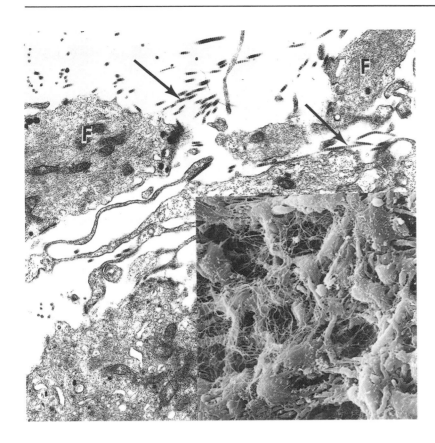

Fig. 9.19 The anterior border of the iris is composed of a discontinuous layer of fibroblasts (F) and interspersed collagen fibrils (arrows) (original magnification ×13 800). Inset shows fibroblasts and a meshwork of collagen connecting fibroblasts (original magnification ×40 500). (From Rodrigues, M. M. Hackett, J. and Donohoo, P. in Duane, T. D. and Jaeger, E. A. (eds) (1988) *Biomedical Foundations of Ophthalmology, Vol. 1*, published by J. P. Lippincott.)

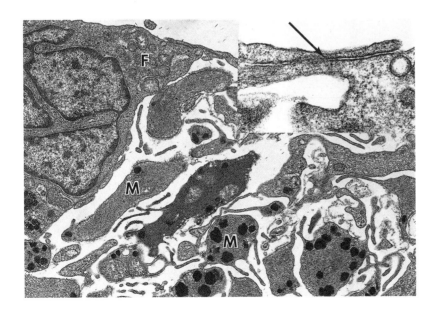

Fig. 9.20 Inset shows a junctional complex (arrow) forming the anterior border layer of the iris. (Scanning electron microscopy, original magnification ×1500) Melanocytes (M) are present beneath the fibroblasts (F) of the anterior border layer (original magnification ×10 500). (From Rodrigues, M. M. Hackett, J. and Donohoo, P. in Duane, T.D. and Jaeger, E.A. (eds) (1988) *Biomedical Foundations of Ophthalmology, Vol. 1*, published by J. P. Lippincott.)

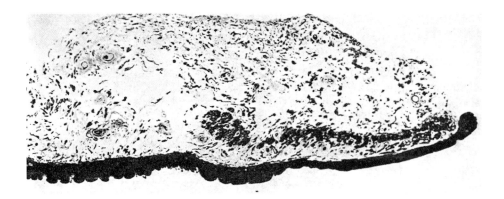

Fig. 9.21 Section of human pupillary margin (original magnification ×285).

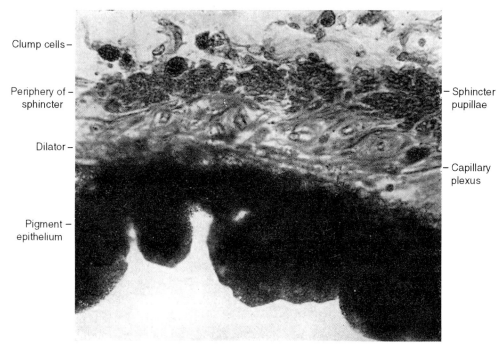

Clump cells —

Periphery of — sphincter

Dilator —

Pigment — epithelium

— Sphincter pupillae

— Capillary plexus

Fig. 9.22 Meridional section of posterior layers of iris.

- the vessels and nerves of the iris;
- cellular elements: fibroblasts, melanocytes, clump cells and mast cells.

The collagen bundles are interlaced and are arranged as curved clockwise and anticlockwise arcades. This arrangement is less regular than in birds, the lower primates and other mammals (Rohen, 1961). The bundles are condensed around vessels and nerves and have an annular orientation near the pupil. The fibres are attached to the iridial muscles, the anterior border layer and the ciliary stroma. There is no elastin. Wide spaces exist in the stroma containing a hyaluronidase-sensitive glycosaminoglycan (Zim-

merman, 1957). This loose arrangement permits a free diffusion of aqueous and large molecules into the stroma (up to 200 μm) and probably facilitates pupil movement.

Sphincter pupillae muscle

The sphincter pupillae is a flat muscular strap 0.75 mm wide and 0.1–0.17 mm thick, which encircles the pupil margin (Figs 9.23 and 9.24). It lies in the stroma deep to the surface and, despite its origin embryologically from the anterior epithelium, is actually separated from this layer by a thin sheet of stromal collagen and dilator fibre processes, to

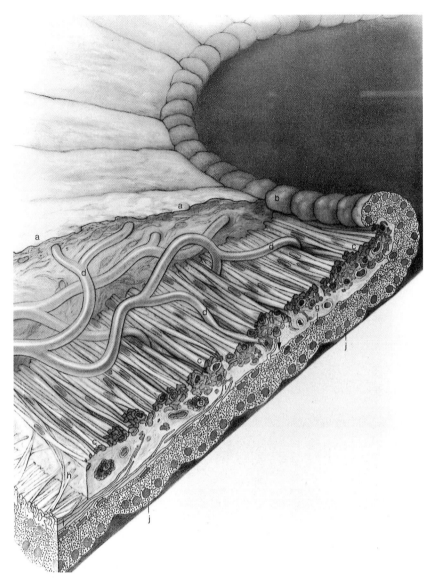

Fig. 9.23 Pupillary portion of the iris. The anterior border layer (a) terminates at the pigment ruff (b). The sphincter muscle is at (c). Vessel arcades (d) from the minor circle extend through the pupil towards the sphincter muscle. The sphincter muscle and iris epithelium are close to each other at the pupil margin. Capillaries, nerves, melanocytes and clump cells (e) are found within and around the muscle. The three to five layers of dilator muscle (f) gradually diminish in number until they terminate behind the mid portion of the sphincter muscle (arrow), leaving lower cuboidal epithelial cells (g) to form the anterior epithelium to the pupillary margin. Spur-like extensions from the dilator muscle form Michel's spur (h) and Fuchs' spur (i), but extend anteriorly to blend with the sphincter muscle. The posterior epithelium (j) is formed by tall columnar cells with basal nuclei. Its apical surface is contiguous with the apical surface of the anterior epithelium. (From Hogan, M. J., Alvarado, J. A. and Weddell, J. E. (1971) *Histology of the Human Eye*, published by W. B. Saunders.)

which it is firmly bound. Thus, even after a broad iridectomy, which removes a sector of iris sphincter, the remaining sphincter can still constrict the remaining pupil margin. The fibres contain some melanin granules of neuroepithelial type.

Each fusiform smooth muscle cell within the sphincter is enveloped in a basal lamina. The cells are grouped in bundles of 5–8, with gap junctions between them, which facilitate the spread of depolarizing current within a muscle grouping. The cytoplasm of each muscle fibre contains myofilaments and scattered densities similar to the Z-bands of striated muscle which may provide attachment for the filaments. All the usual organelles are present, and the nuclei are central within the fibres (Fig. 9.15b).

In the connective tissue which separates the muscle groups, melanocytes and nerve fibres are found (Fig. 9.25). The nerves break up into small bundles of 2–4

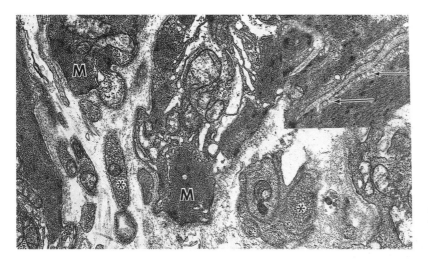

Fig. 9.24 Sphincter muscle (M) cells are surrounded by basement membrane and show patches of electron-dense material and myofilaments. Synaptic vesicles are indicated by asterisks (original magnification ×23 100). Inset shows smooth muscle cell with pinocytotic vesicles (arrows) adjacent to the plasma membrane (original magnification ×23 100). (From Rodrigues, M. M., Hackett, J. and Donohoo, P. in Duane, T. D. and Jaeger, E. A. (eds) (1988) *Biomedical Foundations of Ophthalmology, Vol. 1*, published by J. P. Lippincott.)

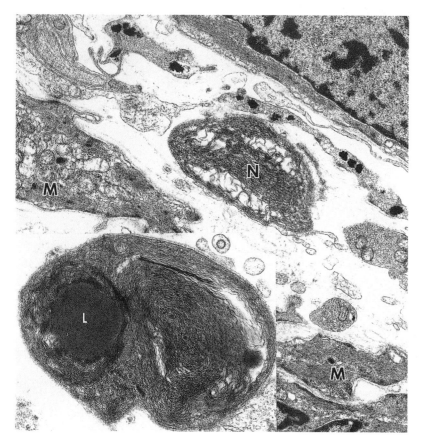

Fig. 9.25 Myelinated nerve (N) in the iris stroma near the sphincter muscle. Smooth muscle cells are indicated by M (original magnification ×18 000). Inset shows myelinated nerve with lipid material (L) (original magnification ×30 000). (From Rodrigues, M. M., Hackett, J. and Donohoo, P. in Duane, T. D. and Jaeger, E. A. (eds) (1988) *Biomedical Foundations of Ophthalmology, Vol. 1*, published by J. P. Lippincott.)

axons, usually surrounded by a Schwann cell. The nerve terminals end close to the periphery of the muscle group, and no closer than 0.1 μm from the cell membranes, in relation to a single muscle fibre of a group.

Blood vessels

The blood vessels of the iris are described here and in further detail in Chapter 11. They are radially oriented with a slightly sinuous course, which allows them to accommodate to the movements of the pupil. In the blue iris they are visible as pale streaks in the stroma and their course can be demonstrated by fluorescein angiography (Fig. 9.26). The arteries arise mainly from the major arterial circle of the iris (an anastomosis which actually lies in the ciliary body, anterior to the ciliary muscle) (Fig. 9.27). Some authors report that the major circle is not always continuous (Fryczkowski, 1978; Greider and Egbert,

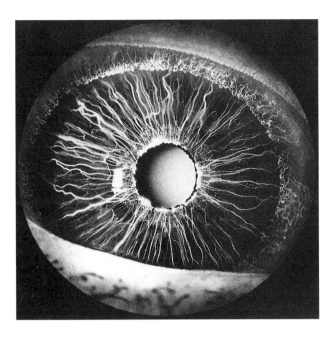

Fig. 9.26 Fluorescein angiogram of the iris. (Courtesy of R. Marsh.)

1980), and the same is true in the macaque monkey (Freddo and Raviola, 1982b). Some arteries also arise directly from the anterior ciliary arteries after they have pierced the sclera to reach the ciliary body (Woodlief, 1980). Their calibre diminishes rapidly, close to their entry into the iris stroma. They then form a series of vascular arcades.

Complete tenotomy in macaques and baboons reduces anterior segment blood flow by 70 to 80%. Angiographic studies of iris ischaemia following rectus muscle tenotomies suggest that the degree of collateral supply from the major circle of the iris is not great (Hayreh and Scott, 1978). (See chapter 10 for further detail.) The iris arteries have been said to resemble those of the major circle, which has a muscularis but no internal elastic lamina. A thin, muscular tunica media was described in human iris vessels by Tousimis and Fine (1959), and Vegge and Ringvold (1969), and Hogan, Alvarado and Weddell (1971a) maintained that smooth muscle cells were present. However, Ikui *et al.* (1960) reported that smooth muscle and elastic tissue were absent from

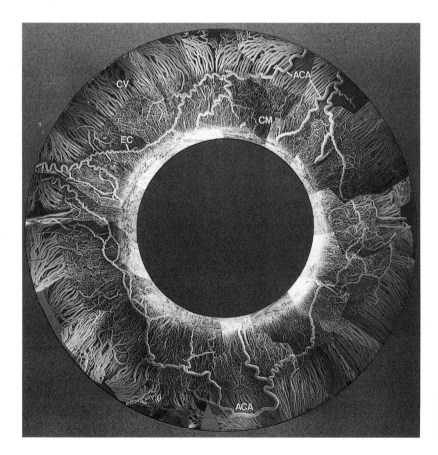

Fig. 9.27 Methyl methacrylate cast of the anterior uveal vessels: montage.
ACA = anterior ciliary arteries; CM = ciliary muscle; CV = ciliary veins.

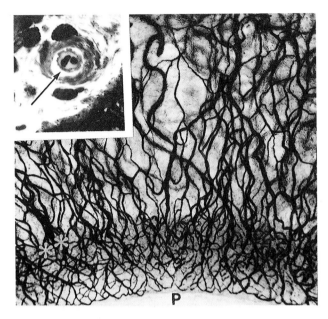

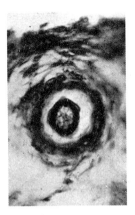

Fig. 9.29 Transverse section of an artery of the iris (Zenker. Mallory's triple stain), to show the two tubes and the loose tissue between them.

Fig. 9.28 Whole-mount preparation of monkey iris injected with horseradish peroxidase. ** = collarette; P = pupil. Inset: light micrograph showing the typical 'tube-within-a-tube' structure of iris blood vessels. By electron microscopy, the open space within the adventitia denoted by the arrow is seen to contain a fine, loosely arranged collagenous matrix. (Courtesy of T. Freddo.)

all iris vessels, and Freddo and Raviola (1982b) found the same in *Macaca mulatta*. Their study demonstrated that iridial vessels in the macaque monkey have a homogeneous structure, regardless of diameter, and lack the usual organization into arteries, capillaries and veins found in other tissues (they possess no ACV units). The entire vascular network is formed instead of vessels of differing diameters but identical fine structure. Freddo and Raviola suggested that this could explain the lack of a clear-cut filling pattern of

arterioles, capillaries and venules in human iris angiograms, and the absence of a distinct venous phase typical of retinal angiograms.

In essence, this difference reflects the absence of smooth muscle cells from vessels of arterial or venous size. Only the capillaries, whose calibres lie between 10 and 15 μm, may be correctly designated as such, while arterioles, postcapillary venules and venules cannot be properly classified. The terms 'arteriole' and 'venule' will continue to be used in this text for the pre- and postcapillary vessels, but with the recognition that the iridial vascular structure differs from that in other parts of the body. The basic structure of the iridial vessel wall in the monkey is thus as follows (Figs 9.28–9.31):

1. A continuous layer of endothelial cells rests on a basal lamina. These cells exhibit blunt luminal protrusions and slender basal lamellae.

Space   Adventitia

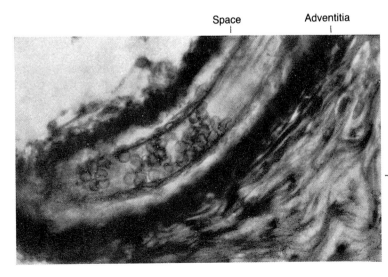

—Iris stroma

Fig. 9.30 Longitudinal section of an artery of the iris to show the 'space' between media and adventitia, which is continuous with the iris stroma.

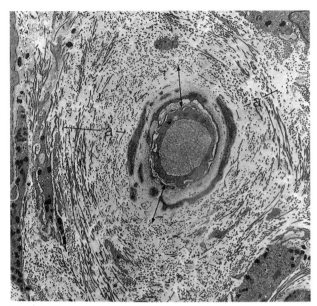

Fig. 9.31 Small iris arteriole. The zone enclosed by arrows is the characteristic clear perivascular space which has been described by light microscopy. This clear zone contains a dense ground substance which is associated with the endothelial basement membrane, a few collagen fibrils and some cell processes. Outside this zone is the dense circular collagenous zone (a) which is so clearly seen with the light microscope (original magnification ×2200). (From Hogan, M.J., Alvarado, J. A. and Weddell, J. E. (1971) *Histology of the Human Eye*, published by W. B. Saunders.)

2. A discontinuous layer of pericytes lies between two thick layers of basal lamina, which derives from both cellular layers. Their processes interdigitate with those of the endothelial cells through fenestrations in the basal lamina.
3. There is no smooth muscle layer. Instead there follows an adventitia of fibroblasts, melanocytes and occasional macrophages arranged in one or two layers. Most vessels in the iris have a particularly well-developed adventitia, containing circularly oriented collagen, within which is a much less dense zone containing fewer fibrils and ground substance (Figs 9.28–9.31). This creates a distinctive tubular arrangement which is said to adapt the vessels to iris movement.

The inner zone is positive for type VI collagen and contains fine fibrils (30–60 nm), which connect the basement membrane with the outer sheath. The outer sheath is structurally different from the inner; it is positive for fibronectin and contains fibrils of varying diameter (30–125 nm).

The arterioles have a heavy tissue adventitia, the venules a thinner one. Larger veins lie in the anterior stroma while those near the dilator are smaller. The venous collector channels traverse the ciliary body to reach the venous system at the ciliary plexus (Saari, 1972; Rodrigues, Hackett and Donohoo, 1987).

The vascular endothelium

The vascular endothelium of the human iris is not fenestrated (Vegge and Ringvold, 1969; Hogan, Alvarado and Weddell, 1971; Ikui *et al.*, 1960; Lai, 1967), like that of the vervet and rhesus monkey (Vegge, 1972; Raviola, 1974), the rabbit, pig, guinea-pig and cat (Saari, 1975). Fenestrations are present in the vascular endothelium of kittens (Schall, Burns and Bellhorn, 1980) but not in rhesus monkeys as young as six months (Freddo and Raviola, 1982a). In the fetal monkey they are regularly found at the root of the iris (Townes-Anderson and Raviola, 1981a). In the rat, both fenestrated and non-fenestrated vessels are observed (Castenholz, 1970, 1971). In the monkey the endothelium is continuous and the intercellular clefts are closed to tracer molecules such as horse-radish peroxidase, by zonulae occludentae. Freeze fracture studies show that the endothelial cells of the iris vessels are joined by two types of intercellular junction: zonular tight junctions and gap junctions (Fig. 9.32).

Zonulae occludentae are represented by a complex network of anastomosing and branching strands that seal the intercellular cleft. They are preferentially associated with the outer leaf (E face) of the plasma membrane. The strands of the E face are in perfect register with complementary grooves on the P face. The numbers of strands vary from one to eight (over half consisting of two to four). The degree of complexity of the junction, represented by the number of strands and the frequency of branching, is higher in these capillaries than in those of other tissues such as dog lung or human placenta. The tight junctions between the endothelial lining cells of Schlemm's canal are also less complex than the junctions of iris vessels.

Gap junctions are rare along the intercellular cleft. They are occasionally seen on freeze-fracture, within the tight junctional network, as aggregates of closely packed particles on the P face, which are complemented by arrays of pits on the E face. No interendothelial junctions of venular type (Simionescu, Simionescu and Palade, 1978) are encountered (Freddo and Raviola, 1982b). The sparsely distributed intramembranous particles, seen on freeze-fracture within the junctional network, probably represent simple intermediate junctions (Townes-Anderson and Raviola, 1981). Plasmalemmal vesicles are encountered in freeze-fracture

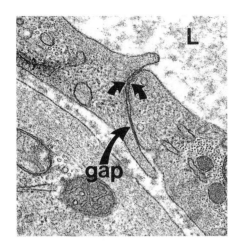

(a)

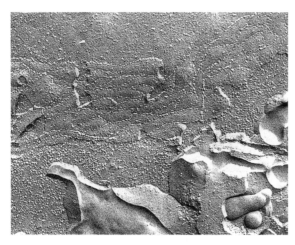

(b)

Fig. 9.32 (a) Transmission electron microscopy demonstrates that iris vessel endothelial cells are joined by tight junctions (paired arrows) and gap junctions. l = lumen; (b) freeze-fracture electron micrograph demonstrates the typical network of branching and anastomosing strands of the tight junctions joining iris vascular endothelial cells. (Courtesy of T. Freddo.)

replicas, and are also found in other vascular endothelia.

The cytoplasm of the endothelial cells is unremarkable, except for the presence of occasional rod-shaped bodies (resembling Weibel Palade bodies), and crystalloid inclusions associated with the rough endoplasmic reticulum. These have also been reported in developing and adult ocular vessels of the macaque (Raviola, 1974). They are increased in iridial vessels of patients with chronic simple glaucoma (Matsuda and Sugiura, 1970; Krstic and Postic, 1978).

The pericytes

The pericytes of the iris vessels are similar to those found elsewhere, including ocular vessels such as

in the retina (Kuwabara and Cogan, 1960, 1963; Cogan, Toussaint and Kuwabara, 1961; Ishikawa, 1963; Hogan and Feeney, 1963a; deOliviera, 1966). They exhibit a variable complement of filaments subjacent to the adluminal plasma membrane (facing the lumen) (Epling, 1966; Rhodin, 1968; Weibel, 1974; Forbes, Rennels and Nelson, 1977; Tilton, Kilo and Williamson, 1979). An asymmetrical distribution of plasmalemmal vesicles is concentrated at the abluminal surface, as seen in the small vessels of the retina (Ishikawa, 1963), corneal limbus (Iwamoto and Smelser, 1965b) and myocardium (Forbes, Rennels and Nelson, 1977).

The endothelial cells and associated pericytes are invested with a basal lamina approximately 0.5–3 μm wide. Outside this zone is a zone of sparse, longitudinally oriented collagen 7 μm wide,

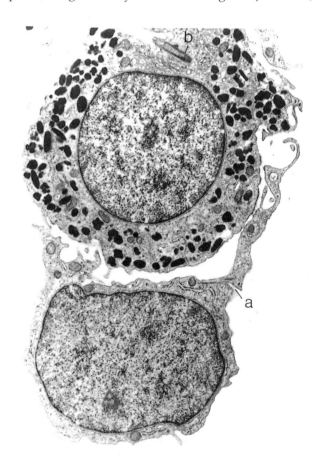

Fig. 9.33 A melanocyte and a fibroblast in the iris stroma. The melanocytes of the stroma have a more abundant cytoplasm than those of the anterior border layer. The two cells shown here are separated from each other by a narrow intercellular space (a). A cilium projects into the iris stroma from the cytoplasm of the melanocyte (b). The melanocyte granules are completely melanized (original magnification ×13 200). (From Hogan, M. J., Alvarado, J. A. and Weddell, J. E. (1971) *Histology of the Human Eye*, published by W. B. Saunders.)

surrounded by a granular ground substance and a further connective tissue layer 10 μm wide (Hogan, Alvarado and Weddell, 1971; Rodrigues, Hackett and Donohoo, 1988; Hutchinson, Rodrigues and Grossniklaus, 1995). Larger capillaries have a more continuous layer of pericytes and a thicker basal lamina. In the monkey, the collagen sheath surrounding the adventitia is composed of circularly arranged collagen fibrils 60–80 nm in diameter, separated from the adventitia by a variable space containing a sparse network of finer fibrils, 20–30 nm in diameter. Vessels located in the more cellular parts of the stroma, for instance the anterior border layer, are invested in a thicker and more cellular adventitia.

Nerves

The iris nerves are derived from the long and short ciliaries, which accompany the corresponding arteries, pierce the sclera around the optic nerve, and run forwards between choroid and sclera to the ciliary plexus. Here, numerous branches arise, largely un-myelinated and showing many gangliform enlargements. Their fibres form plexuses (a) in the anterior border layer (possible sensory), (b) around the larger blood vessels and (c) anterior to the dilator pupillae. They supply nerve filaments to all layers except the posterior pigmented epithelium. From the plexus on the dilator muscle many non-myelinated fibres inner-vate muscle cells through endings which may contain synaptic vesicles and form close contacts (20 nm). The dilator muscle receives a sympathetic innervation and the sphincter muscle a parasympathetic innervation, but adrenergic and cholinergic innervation has been shown in both muscles (Lowenstein and Loewenfeld, 1969). (See chapter 16 for further details of autonomic and peptidergic supply.) Some nerves supply uveal vessels and some the intrinsic muscles of the eye. They display many gangliform enlargements and are myelinated and non-myelinated (see chapter 17). Nerve filaments form plexuses along larger blood vessels and are found in relation to all layers except the posterior pigmented epithelium.

Cellular elements of the stroma

Fibroblasts

The fibroblast, the most common stromal cell, is found around blood vessels, nerves and muscle tissue and throughout the iris substance (Fig. 9.33).

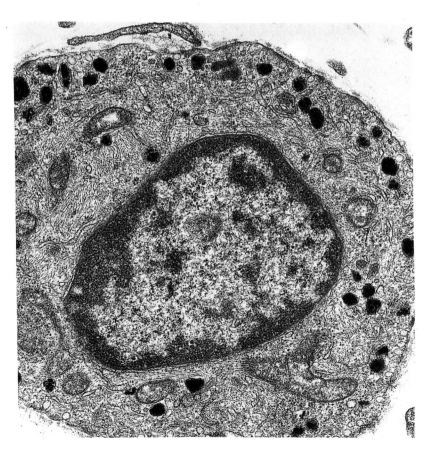

Fig. 9.34 Iris stromal melanocyte with mature melanosomes (original magnification ×37 500). (From Rodrigues, M. M., Hackett, J. and Donohoo, P. in Duane, T. D. and Jaeger, E. A. (eds) (1988) *Biomedical Foundations of Ophthalmology, Vol. 1*, published by J. P. Lippincott.)

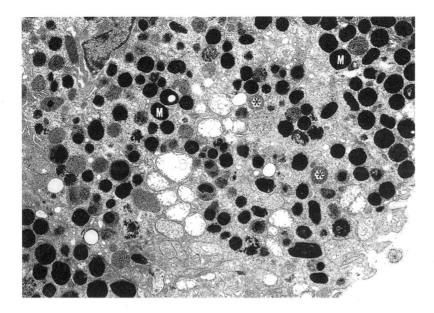

Fig. 9.35 Numerous immature melanosomes (asterisks), interspersed with mature melanosomes (M), are present at the iris root (original magnification ×10 500). (From Rodrigues, M. M., Hackett, J. and Donohoo, P. in Duane, T. D. and Jaeger, E. A. (eds) (1988) *Biomedical Foundations of Ophthalmology, Vol. 1*, published by J. P. Lippincott.)

Melanocytes

Melanocytes, with branching processes up to 100 μm long, form plexuses with each other and are arranged as cuffs around the vessel adventitia. Their melanin granules, up to 0.5 μm in diameter, are round, oval and in various stages of maturation (Figs 9.34 and 9.35).

Clump cells

Clump cells are large round cells up to 100 μm wide, filled with inclusion granules and covered with fine villous processes 1–2 μm long and 0.1 μm wide (Tousimis and Fine, 1959; Iwamoto, 1961) (Figs 9.36–9.38). They are found in the pupillary por-

tion of the iris, especially round the sphincter. The majority of clump cells (type 1) are believed to be pigment-filled macrophages (Wobman and Fine, 1972). Their granules are regarded as residual bodies, containing mainly melanin granules. The large melanin granules in clump cells of the posterior stroma resemble those of the iris epithelium from which they have been said to arise (Elschnig and Lauber, 1907) (Figs 9.36–9.38). Smaller granules are found in clusters of clump cells in the anterior stroma and resemble melanocyte granules. These type 2 clump cells are surrounded by a basal lamina, and are believed to be displaced neuroectoderm cells of similar origin to the iris sphincter. Clump cells are found in all irises, including blue and albinotic irises

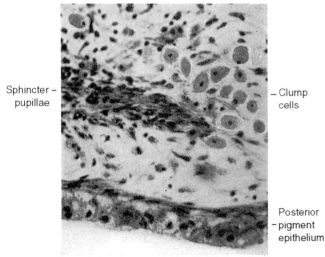

Sphincter pupillae — Clump cells — Posterior pigment epithelium

Fig. 9.36 Bleached section of portion of iris to show clump cells.

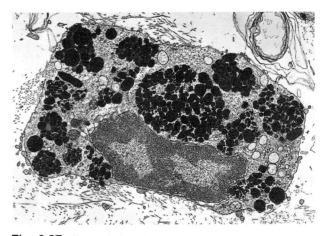

Fig. 9.37 Transmission electron micrograph. A clump cell is seen near the iris sphincter. Note the numerous clusters of melanosomes. (Courtesy of T. Freddo.)

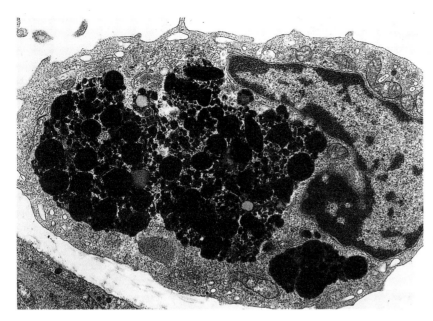

Fig. 9.38 Type I clump cell (macrophage) in the pupillary region (original magnification ×18 000). (From Rodrigues, M. M., Hackett, J. and Donohoo, P. in Duane, T. D. and Jaeger, E. A. (eds) (1988) *Biomedical Foundations of Ophthalmology, Vol. 1*, published by J. P. Lippincott.)

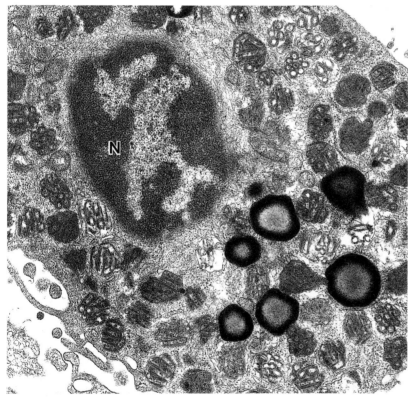

Fig. 9.39 Iris stromal mast cell with myriad scroll-like cytoplasmic structures. The nucleus is indicated by N (original magnification ×30 000). (From Rodrigues, M. M., Hackett, J. and Donohoo, P. in Duane, T. D. and Jaeger, E. A. (eds) (1988) *Biomedical Foundations of Ophthalmology, Vol. 1*, published by J. P. Lippincott.)

where they may be seen with the slit-lamp. Their number increases with age.

Mast cells

Mast cells are found in the stroma. They are round, have villous processes and contain characteristic dense amorphous or 'Swiss roll' inclusions (Hogan, Alvarado and Weddell, 1971) (Figs 9.39 and 9.40).

Extracellular matrix of stroma

Fibrils staining postively for type VI collagen are found around the sphincter and dilator muscle fibres and extending into the nearby stroma. A strand of such fibrils connects the dilator at the iris root with the circular and reticular parts of the ciliary muscle and also stains positive for type IV collagen, as well as for laminin and fibronectin. These strands may perform

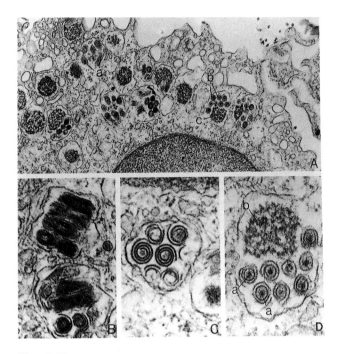

Fig. 9.40 (A) Iris stromal mast cell. This type is less commonly found in the iris, but is abundant in the limbus. This mast cell is distinguished by the fact that many of its granules contain cylindrical structures which are seen in longitudinal section (a) or in cross-section (b). A finely granular material is also contained (c) within the granules (original magnification ×27 000). (B) Higher magnification to show the cylindrical structures within the membrane of the mast cell granules. They are uniformly dense and of equal length (original magnification ×60 000). (C) View of the cross-sections of the cylindrical structures. Each cylinder contains an electron-dense material (original magnification ×90 000). (D) Cylinders in mast cell granules seen in cross-section. The core material (a) and a mass of granular material (b) are found within the granules (original magnification ×99 000). (From Hogan, M. J., Alvarado, J. A. and Weddell, J. E. (1971) *Histology of the Human Eye,* published by W. B. Saunders.)

an anchoring function. There is intense staining for type VI in the inner zone of the the iris vessel sheath, and elsewhere in the stroma a fine fibrillar staining occurs, and there is endoneurial staining of the iris nerves. The disposition of laminin is similar. There is a strong reaction for type IV collagen on the basement membranes of the iris vessels, muscles and the endoneurium of the nerves.

Fibronectin is present throughout the stroma, especially around the iris muscles. It·is present in the basement membranes of the capillaries, and along the endoneuria, and is found in the outer part of the iris vessel sheath.

ANTERIOR EPITHELIUM AND DILATOR MUSCLE (DILATOR PUPILLAE)

The anterior epithelium is about 12.5 μm thick and shows an apical portion which adjoins the posterior epithelium and a basal portion abutting the stroma, whose cellular processes are specialized to form the smooth muscle-dilator pupillae (Figs 9.41–9.43).

Dilator pupillae

The muscular processes of its cells are radially oriented, measure up to 60 μm long and 7 μm wide, are filled with myofilaments and extend from the iris root towards the pupil. Close to the pupil margin, dilator muscle processes fuse with the deep surface of the sphincter; at the mid zone of the sphincter a spur of dilator processes and pigment passes into the sphincter (**Fuchs' spur**) and a similar spur (**von Michels' spur**) is attached to the peripheral border of the sphincter (Fig. 9.44). There is a further insertion into the iris stroma at its root (**Grünert's spur**). Peripherally, the dilator is continued to an attachment in the ciliary body. When the muscle contracts, it pulls the pupillary margin towards the ciliary body, dilating the pupil. At birth the dilator is poorly developed and the pupil responds poorly to mydriatics.

The muscular portion of the anterior epithelium ends opposite the mid point of the sphincter. Central to this, the cells become cuboidal in shape or are irregular.

Electron microscopy shows the dilator muscle processes to be about 3–5 layers thick and to be surrounded by a basal lamina which is not present around the apical epithelium. The cytoplasm is filled with myofilaments about 3 nm in diameter whose densities resemble the Z-bands of skeletal muscle (Fig. 9.45).

The dilator muscle is innervated by the sympathetic via the long ciliary nerves. Their endings come to lie about 20 nm from the cell membrane (Fig. 9.46).

The apical portion of the anterior epithelium is its epithelial portion which interdigitates with that of the posterior epithelium by numerous microvilli, to leave a space of about 20 nm into which some cilia may project (Fig. 9.47). The intercellular junctions of the iris epithelia of *Macaca mulatta* have been studied by Freddo (1984). The lateral cell margins of the anterior iris myoepithelium are joined by puncta adhaerentes, desmosomes and gap junctions (Figs 9.43 and 9.48). The desmosomes and puncta adhaerentes are restricted to the apicolateral region of these cells. The apposed apical surfaces of the anterior and posterior epithelia are also joined by puncta adhaerentes, desmosomes and gap junctions, and the largest complement of gap junctions are in this region. The presence of numerous gap junctions joining the cells within and between the iris epithelial

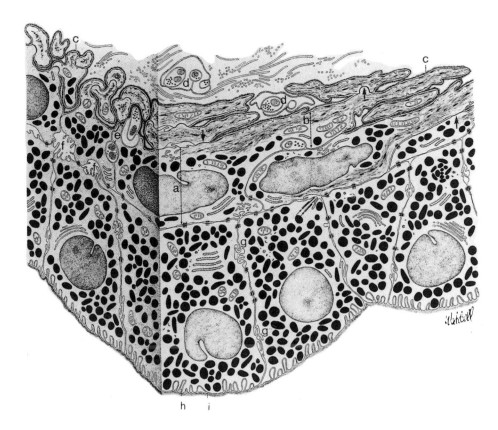

Fig. 9.41 Posterior epithelial layers. The anterior iris epithelium has two morphologically distinct portions: an apical epithelial portion (a) and a basal muscular portion (b). The cytoplasm of the basal portion is filled with myofibrils and a moderate number of mitochondria. The tongue-like muscular processes overlap each other, creating three to five layers. Tight junctions (arrows) like those in the sphincter are found between the dilator muscle cells. A basement membrane (c) surrounds the muscle processes. Unmyelinated nerves and their associated Schwann cells (d) as well as a few naked axons innervate the muscle. The axon at (e) is in close contact with the anterior epithelium, being separated from it by a space measuring 20 nm in width. The cytoplasm of the epithelial portions contains cell organelles, melanin granules, the nucleus and bundles of myofilaments. Most of the intercellular junctions present here are maculae occludentes and only a few desmosomes are present; desmosomes are not found in the muscular portion. The apical surface of the anterior epithelium is found in the muscular portion. The apical surface of the anterior epithelium is contiguous with that of the posterior epithelium. Desmosomes and tight junctions join the two layers, but there are some areas of separation (f) between the cells. The spaces so formed are filled with microvilli, and an occasional cilium is also found here (double arrows). The posterior pigmented iris epithelium shows lateral interdigitations (g) and areas of infolding along its basal surface (h). A typical basement membrane is also found on the basal side (i). Numerous tight junctions and desmosomes occur along the lateral and apical walls. The cytoplasm of this epithelium has numerous melanin granules measuring around 0.8 µm in cross-section and up to 2.5 µm in length. Stacks of cisternae of the rough-surfaced endoplasmic reticulum, clustered unattached ribosomes, mitochondria and a Golgi apparatus are commonly observed. (From Hogan, M. J., Alvarado, J. A. and Weddell, J. E. (1971) *Histology of the Human Eye*, published by W. B. Saunders.)

cell layers allows them to function as a syncytium which facilitates the coordination of reflex and other kinds of pupil movements.

The association between puncta adhaerentes and gap junctions is found in other tissues; for example they join the apices of the pigmented and unpigmented epithelial layers of the ciliary epithelium (Raviola and Raviola, 1978). It has been suggested that punctal junctions may be a prerequisite for gap junction formation, and it has been noted that in folliculogenesis they bear a reciprocal relationship in the membrane, 'adhaerens' junctions reducing in number as gap junctions increase (Albertini, 1980).

The lateral intercellular space is about 20 nm. The nucleus is located in the apical portion of the cell together with a moderate number of mitochondria, pigment granules, free ribosomes, and some myofilaments. Rough and smooth endoplasmic reticulum is present.

POSTERIOR PIGMENT EPITHELIUM

The posterior pigment epithelium is a layer of cells derived from the internal layer of the optic cup. The epithelial cells are heavily pigmented that cytoplasmic details are difficult to make out except in albinotic

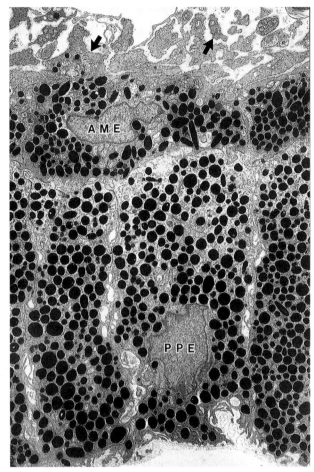

Fig. 9.42 Transmission electron micrograph of the anterior myoepithelium (AME) and posterior pigmented epithelium (PPE) of the iris. Arrows denote basal processes of the anterior myoepithelial cells that constitute the dilator muscle of the iris. (From Freddo, T. (1984) *Invest. Ophthalmol. Vis. Sci.*, **25**, 1094.)

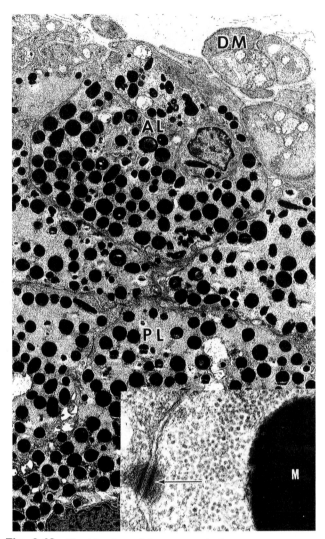

Fig. 9.43 The iris pigment is composed of a narrower anterior layer (AL) continuous with the dilator muscle (DM) and a wider posterior layer (PL) (original magnification ×6450). Inset shows desmosome (arrow) connecting epithelial layers laterally. Portion of a melanosome is indicated by M (original magnification ×82 500). (From Rodrigues, M. M., Hackett, J. and Donohoo, P. in Duane, T. D. and Jaeger, E. A. (eds) (1988) *Biomedical Foundations of Ophthalmology, Vol. 1*, published by J. P. Lippincott.)

or bleached preparations. The cells are columnar, about 36–55 μm high and 16–25 μm wide (Salzmann, 1912a). There is a gradual loss of pigmentation at the iris periphery where the epithelial sheet becomes continuous with that of the ciliary body (Fig. 9.49). The abundant pigment granules are spherical or cigar-shaped, membrane-bound and much larger than those of the melanocytes (Feeney, Grieshaber and Hogan, 1965) (Fig. 9.41). The cytoplasm contains a round nucleus, mitochondria, rough endoplasmic reticulum and Golgi apparatus. Glycogen granules are present and are increased in the eyes of patients with diabetes.

The apical surfaces of the epithelial cells form microvilli which interdigitate with the microvilli of the anterior epithelium (Fig. 9.47). There are scattered 20 nm spaces between them (Tousimis and Fine, 1959; Ueno, 1961). The well-developed des-

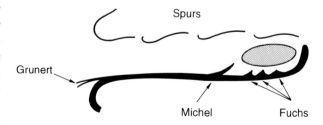

Fig. 9.44 Schematic drawing showing location of often pigmented 'spurs' that project from region of dilator muscle of iris. (From Fine, B. S. and Yanoff, M. (1972) *Ocular Histology: A Text and Atlas*, published by Harper and Row.)

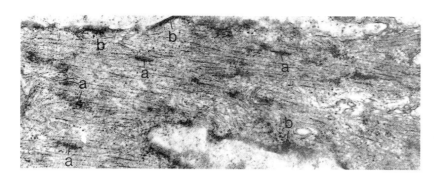

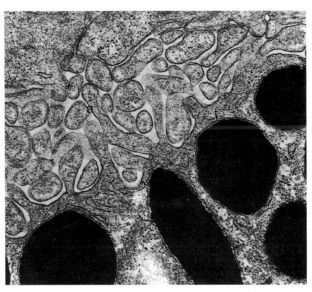

Fig. 9.45 Anterior iris epithelium, to show the details of the myofilaments in the dilator muscle. The filaments appear to be of one type and they form areas (a) which are reminiscent of the Z-discs of skeletal muscle. The characteristic densities of the cell membrane of smooth muscle are also present (b) (original magnification ×27 000). (From Hogan, M. J., Alvarado, J. A. and Weddell, J. E. (1971) *Histology of the Human Eye*, published by W. B. Saunders.)

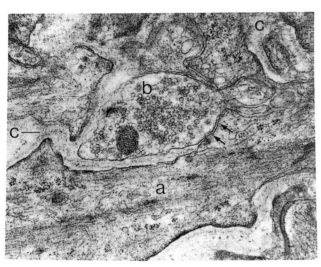

Fig. 9.46 Dilator muscle fibre (a) innervated by a single axon (b) containing numerous synaptic vesicles and a mitochondrion. The nerve comes into close apposition with the muscle (arrows), being separated from it by a space measuring approximately 20 nm; the basement membrane (c) is excluded from this site (original magnification ×21 000). (From Hogan, M.J., Alvarado, J.A. and Weddell, J.E. (1971) *Histology of the Human Eye*, published by W.B. Saunders.)

Fig. 9.47 Posterior pigmented iris epithelium at its junction with the anterior epithelium. At (a) numerous obliquely sectioned microvilli from both epithelial layers fill a space found between the two epithelia. The membrane encircling the melanin granules of the posterior epithelium is clearly shown (arrows) (original magnification ×45 000). (From Hogan, M. J., Alvarado, J. A. and Weddell, J. E. (1971) *Histology of the Human Eye*, published by W. B. Saunders.)

mosomes between the lateral and apical surfaces of the two epithelial layers provide a tight adhesion between the layers and a means by which stresses generated by pupil movement, and in particular by myoepithelial contraction, are distributed evenly across the epithelium. When posterior synechiae (inflammatory adhesions between iris and lens) are ruptured, the epithelial fragment remaining on the lens capsule contains both layers. However, spontaneously occurring primary epithelial cysts of the iris occur in the plane between these two layers and are embryologically homologous with a detachment of the retina (Fig. 9.12).

The lateral surfaces show some interdigitations and an intercellular space of 20 nm. Adjacent posterior pigmented epithelial cells of the iris are joined by an apicolateral junctional complex, consisting of a zonula occludens, zonula adhaerens, and gap junction (Freddo, 1984) (Figs 9.48 and 9.50). These junctions are of similar structure and complexity to the zonulae occludentae of the non-pigmented epithelium of the ciliary body. The posterior epithelial cells are also joined by one or more desmosomes. The basal cell membrane faces the posterior chamber and shows numerous infoldings extending deep into the cell cytoplasm. The basal

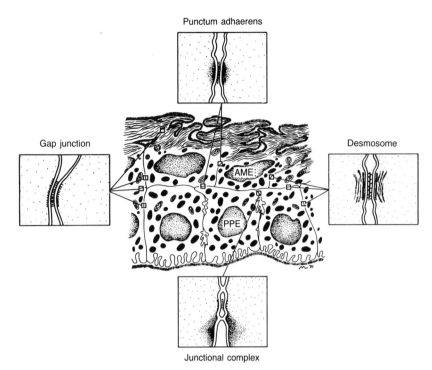

Punctum adhaerens

Gap junction

AME

PPE

Desmosome

Junctional complex

Fig. 9.48 Summary of types and locations of various intercellular junctions present in the iris epithelium. (Courtesy of T. Freddo.)

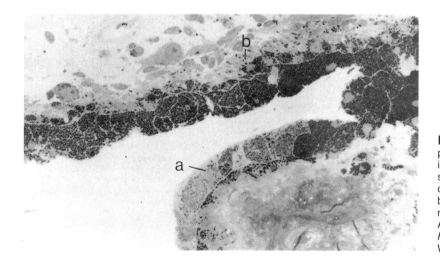

Fig. 9.49 Peripheral iris and anterior pars plicata of the ciliary body. The transition of iris epithelium to that of the ciliary body is shown. The posterior epithelium loses most of its pigment at (a) and the dilator muscle begins to disappear at (b) (original magnification ×640). (From Hogan, M. J., Alvarado, J. A. and Weddell, J. E. (1971) *Histology of the Human Eye*, published by W. B. Saunders.)

lamina follows the basal membrane except at these infoldings and is continuous with the inner limiting membrane of the ciliary body (Lim and Webber, 1975) (Fig 9.51 and 9.52).

9.4 MOVEMENT OF FLUID AND SOLUTE ACROSS THE IRIS

It has already been noted that the anterior surface of the iris and its stroma are freely accessible to the diffusion of fluid and solute from the aqueous humour. In this respect, the anterior and posterior chambers of the eye have different permeability properties. The anterior chamber has leaky walls by which water may leave either by diffusion across the corneal endothelium, the iris or ciliary body stroma, or by pressure-dependent bulk flow via the conventional drainage pathway or uveoscleral system. The posterior chamber is completely secluded by the impermeable epithelia of the iris and ciliary body (Raviola, 1977). The iris pigment epithelium is also able to pump anions out of the posterior chamber (Cunha-Vaz, 1979).

The features of the capillaries of the iris and ciliary body are different, the ciliary capillaries being permeable and the iris capillaries impermeable to tracer

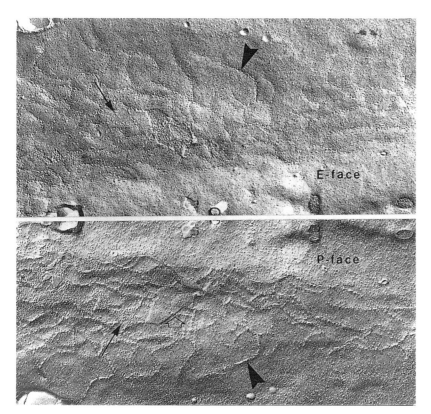

Fig. 9.50 Freeze-fracture electron micrograph demonstrating complimentary replicas of continuous zonulae occludentes joining the apico-lateral surfaces of posterior pigmented epithelial cells. Free spurs are present at the basal surface of these junctions (arrowheads) and gap junctions are occasionally observed intercalated within the tight junctional matrix of branching and anastomosing strands (arrows). (Courtesy of T. Freddo.)

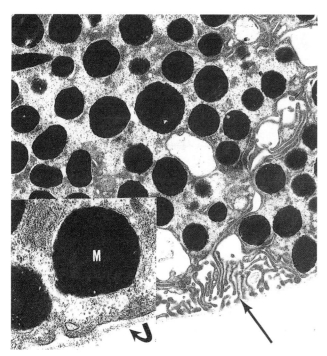

Fig. 9.51 The posterior layer of iris pigment epithelium displays cells with numerous basal infoldings (arrow) (original magnification ×13 800). Inset at higher magnification (original magnification ×37 500) shows a membrane-bound melanosome (M) and basement membrane (arrow). (From Rodrigues, M. M., Hackett, J. and Donohoo, P. in Duane, T. D. and Jaeger, E.A. (eds) (1988) *Biomedical Foundations of Ophthalmology, Vol. 1*, published by J. P. Lippincott.)

materials such as horseradish peroxidase (Vegge, 1971; Raviola, 1974). Furthermore, the few plasma-lemmal vesicles of the endothelial cells of the iris capillaries are incapable of transporting significant amounts of tracer material across the endothelium. Thus, in normal conditions, only tiny amounts of plasma proteins reach the anterior chamber by way of the iris vessels, although protein (which leaks into the ciliary body stroma via the fenestrated ciliary vessels) will have access to the anterior chamber at the iris root. However, although intravenously injected horseradish peroxidase diffuses readily into the stroma of the iris root from the ciliary body stroma, it is prevented from reaching the posterior chamber across the iris epithelia, by the zonulae occludentae of the posterior pigmented epithelium.

The continuous, non-fenestrated vascular endothelium prevents the entry of proteins and tracer molecules from the vessel lumen into the iris stroma in the normal eye (Smith, 1971; Raviola, 1977). With inflammation (e.g. iritis) this barrier breaks down and allows protein to pass into the aqueous, where it becomes visible by slit lamp microscopy as an aqueous flare. Freddo and Sacks-Wilner (1989) observed simplification and disruption of endothelial tight junctions in endotoxin-induced uveitis in rabbits, which resulted in a leakage of tracer primarily through the interendothelial clefts of the vessels. In these

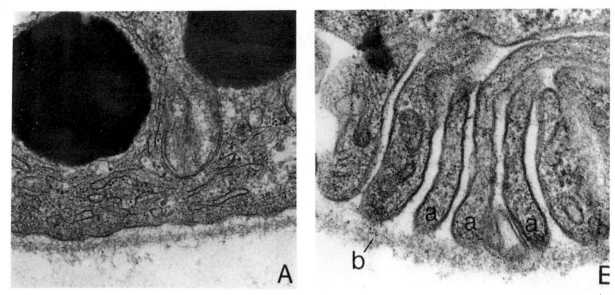

Fig. 9.52 (A) Iris posterior epithelium. The basal surface of the posterior epithelium faces the posterior chamber and the lens. A thin basement membrane is found on this surface (original magnification ×45 000). (B) Numerous infoldings (a) also occur on the basal surface of the posterior epithelium. Note that the basement membrane (b) continues along without entering the infoldings of the cell membrane (original magnification ×60 000). (From Hogan, M. J., Alvarado, J. A. and Weddell, J. E. (1971) *Histology of the Human Eye*, published by W. B. Saunders.)

studies, junctional simplification involved a reduction of junctional strands, and a loss of the ridges and grooves of the P and E faces. These changes were similar to (but possibly less marked than) the changes observed in ciliary epithelium during uveitis (Freddo, 1987). In other tissues which possess a distinct arteriole-capillary-venular unit, the increase in permeability associated with inflammation commonly affects the postcapillary venule, for which there appears to be no parallel in the iridial vessels. Instead, the junctions of the iridial vessels are more characteristic of true arterioles (Simionescu *et al.*, 1975).

Although the retinal vessels have similar permeability characteristics to the iris capillaries, they respond differently to inflammatory mediators. The iridial vessels become leaky to intravenously injected carbon particles or thorotrast after exposure to histamine, whereas the retinal vessels do not (Ashton and Cunha-Vaz, 1965; Shakib and Cunha-Vaz, 1966). It is of interest, however, that while the iris vessels of the cat, rabbit and rat become permeable to tracers after paracentesis, the monkey iris vessels do not (Szalay, Nunziata and Henkind, 1975; Raviola, 1974, 1977).

CHAPTER TEN

The posterior chamber and ciliary body

10.1 THE POSTERIOR CHAMBER

The posterior chamber is a fluid-filled space lying posteromedial to the iris and ciliary body, and anterior to the anterior vitreous face (Fig. 10.1). It is conveniently divided into three compartments by the fibres of the suspensory ligament which pass across the ciliary body to the lens:

1. prezonular compartment (posterior chamber proper);
2. zonular compartment;
3. retrozonular compartment.

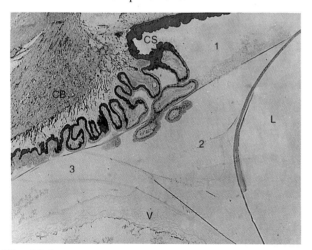

Fig. 10.1 The three subdivisions of the posterior chamber as seen in meridional section of a human globe. 1, Posterior chamber proper or prezonular space; 2, zonular circumlental space of canal of Hanover; 3, retrozonular space or canal of Petit. The canal of Petit widens towards the ciliary body (CB) and narrows towards the lens (L). CS, ciliary sulcus; V, condensed anterior face of vitreous. Original magnification ×56. (From Tripathi, R. C. and Tripathi, B. J. in Davson, H. (ed.) (1974) *The Eye, Vol. 1A*, published by Academic Press).

PREZONULAR COMPARTMENT

The prezonular compartment is triangular in cross-section, with the apex of the triangle at the point of contact between the pupillary margin of the iris and the anterior surface of the lens. The anterior wall is formed by the pigment epithelium of the iris and the posterior by the lens and its zonules. The base is formed by the ciliary processes and valleys between them, in which are the **recesses of Kuhnt**. The junction between the prezonular and zonular compartments at the level of the zonule is represented by the ill-defined plane of the anteromost zonular fibres. However, this boundary may be functionally distinct, because the zonular compartment contains ground substance material similar to that found in the vitreous (hyaluronic acid) which, particularly in the young eye, may restrict the flow of aqueous and the diffusion of solute posteriorly. Aqueous humour, secreted into the anterior compartment by the ciliary processes, follows the pressure gradient and flows through the pupil into the anterior chamber. The shape and volume of the anterior compartment vary with pupil size so that its volume is smallest, and access to the anterior chamber greatest, with the pupil dilated maximally. Contact between the posterior surface of the iris and anterior capsule of the lens is also altered by pupil size, and is said to be greatest with the pupil in mid dilatation so that a state of relative pupil block is created which bulges the iris forwards slightly. In some predisposed eyes with narrow angles this may precipitate angle-closure glaucoma. The composition of the aqueous humour is altered during its passage towards the pupil, by an exchange of materials with the lens and iris.

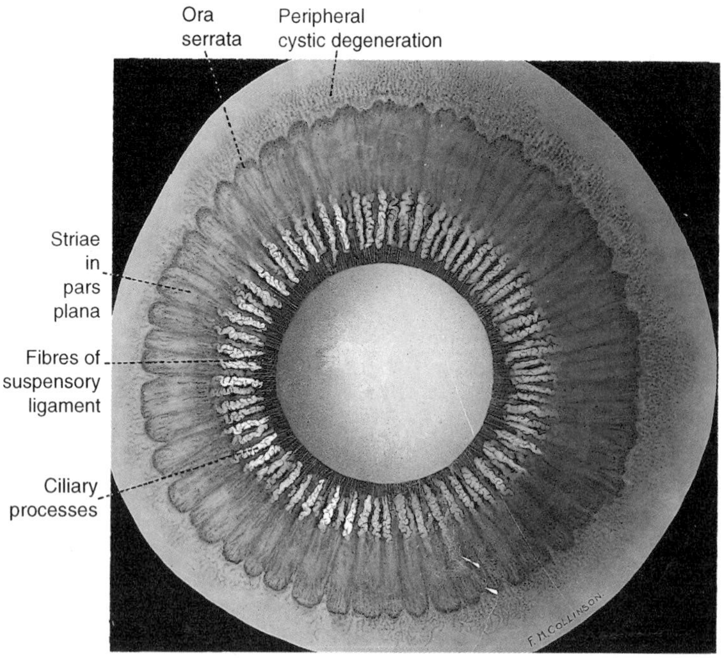

Ora serrata   Peripheral cystic degeneration

Striae in pars plana

Fibres of suspensory ligament

Ciliary processes

Fig. 10.2 The ciliary body, suspensory ligament, lens and ora serrata, seen from behind. Note that the serrations of the ora are less evident temporally, where cystic degeneration (shown by the mottled appearance) is most developed.

The groove formed by the reflection of the peripheral iris epithelium on to the pars ciliaris of the ciliary body is called the ciliary sulcus. It may sometimes offer support to, or be the site of fixation of, the haptic of an intraocular lens implant. The mean sulcus diameter is 11.25 mm (SD ± 0.38 mm) (Orgel *et al.*, 1993; Smith *et al.*, 1987; Davis *et al.*, 1991).

ZONULAR COMPARTMENT

The zonular compartment of the posterior chamber lies within and between the anterior and posterior layers of the zonule. The anatomy of the zonular attachments and spaces is described in Chapters 12 and 13.

RETROZONULAR COMPARTMENT

The retrozonular compartment consists of a slit-like space, the so-called **retrozonular space of Petit**. It lies between the posterior aspect of the zonular fibres and the anterior hyaloid face. It extends laterally to the attachment of the vitreous base in the region of the ora serrata, and centrally to the condensation of the vitreous on the posterior lens capsule (**ligament of Wieger**, *ligamentum hyaloideocapsulare*) which separates it from the **retrolental space (of Berger)**.

10.2 THE CILIARY BODY

If the eyeball is bisected through its anteroposterior axis and the vitreous, lens and retina removed, the

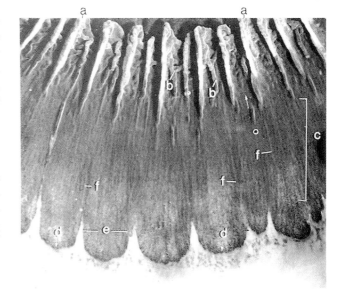

Fig. 10.3 Light micrograph of the ciliary body of a young person. The pars plicata is formed by the major ciliary processes (a) and smaller accessory or intermediate processes (b). The ciliary processes of the young eye are narrow and have smooth contours. The pars plana (c) ends posteriorly at the ora serrata where the scalloped bays (d) are narrow and dentate processes (e) are shown. Striae or linear markings (f) originate from the dentate processes and extend towards the valleys of the pars plicata (arrow). (From Hogan, M. J., Alvarado, J. A. and Weddell, J. E. (1971) *Histology of the Human Eye. An Atlas and Textbook*, published by W. B. Saunders. Original micrograph taken by R. Y. Foos.)

continuity of the choroid, ciliary body and iris is clearly seen.

The choroid extends to the ora serrata, the dentate fringe limit of the retina. Anterior to this is the ciliary

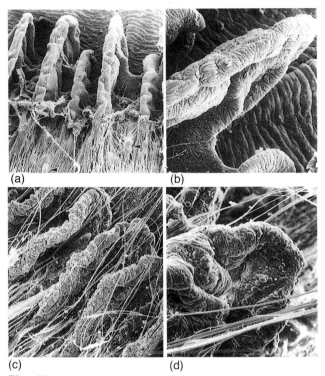

Fig. 10.4 The ciliary processes in infant and adult, visualized by scanning microscopy. (a, b) Age 3 months. The zonules have been rolled back to reveal the simple infantile processes. Several minor plicae (arrowhead) are visible. The peripheral iris folds are seen above (original magnification: a ×60; b ×115); (c, d) age 85 years. The processes are larger, more convoluted, and warty (original magnification: c ×45; d ×110). (From Streeten, B. W. in Duane, T. D. and Jaeger, E. A. (eds) (1992) *Biomedical Foundations of Ophthalmology*, published by Harper and Row.)

body whose black colour easily distinguishes it from the brown choroid. In the coronally sectioned eye the ciliary body can be seen from behind to be a circular body conforming on its outer aspect to the scleral curvature and extending between the ora serrata and scleral spur (Figs 10.1 and 10.2). It presents two main zones, the smooth **pars plana** (orbiculus ciliaris) posteriorly, and the **pars plicata** (corona ciliaris) anteriorly. The ora serrata forms the anterior limit of the retina and choroid further forward (Fig. 10.3). The neuroretina and retinal pigment epithelium derived from the two layers of the optic cup become the non-pigmented and pigmented epithelium of ciliary body, respectively; the vasculature of the choroid is replaced by that of the ciliary body. The ora serrata exhibits forward extensions or dentate processes and intervening bays, which are well marked on the nasal side and less so temporally. The dentate processes may be pointed or blunt and are usually directed towards a minor ciliary process. Giant dentate processes are seen in 16% of cases,

forming a meridional fold of anomalous retinal and ciliary epithelium which passes forwards to a major ciliary complex. This has been called a 'meridional complex' (Straatsma *et al.*, 1968, 1969; Spencer, Foos and Straatsma, 1969).

The anteroposterior width of the ciliary body varies between 6.0 and 6.5 mm, being widest inferotemporally and narrowest superonasally. The width of the pars plicata is about 2.0 mm and that of the pars plana about 4.0–4.5 mm. The limits of the ora serrata measured on the surface of the eye from the corneoscleral limbus (Schwalbe's line, 1.5 mm anterior to the scleral spur) are: temporal 7.5–8.0 mm; nasal 6.5–7.0 mm; and superior and inferior 7.0 mm. (Average values given by Straatsma *et al.* (1968) are: temporal 6.5 mm; nasal 5.73 mm; superior 6.14 mm and inferior 6.20 mm.) These measurements are important surgically in the pars plana approach to the vitreous space. The pars plana is a relatively avascular zone; entry at this site avoids haemorrhage and damage to the retina. In the infant eye, the ciliary body is shorter and the pars plana is more anterior (Fig. 10.4). The ora serrata may be identified at the surface of the globe by transillumination of the sclera via the pupil; the heavy pigmentation in the ciliary body masks transillumination of the globe anterior to the ora.

PARS PLANA

The internal surface of the pars plana is smooth to the naked eye but low magnification shows the ciliary **striae (of Schultze)**, slight, dark ridges which converge anteriorly from the dentate processes of the ora serrata to the valleys between the ciliary processes. Occasional 'teeth' extend forwards as **meridional folds** which merge with the posterior end of a ciliary process (Spencer, Foos and Straatsma, 1969). There is often a dark band just in front of and following the contours of the ora serrata.

The **posterior zonular fibres** take origin from a band of the pars plana 1.5 mm wide, lying 1.5 mm anterior to the ora. They pass along the lateral edges of the striae to the ciliary valleys. The **vitreous base** gains attachment to the epithelium of the pars plana over a band extending 1.5–2.0 mm forward from the ora. A grey line often present behind its anterior limit is visible on gonioscopy.

PARS PLICATA

The pars plicata derives its name from the 70–80 buff-coloured ridges, the **ciliary processes**, which project inwards from the anterior portion of the

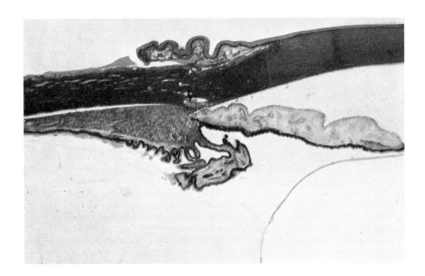

Fig. 10.5 Meridional section of the anterior segment of the eye (Zenker fixation, Mallory's triple stain). This section is from an eye with a small malignant melanoma at the macula. The narrowness of the angle of the anterior chamber is an artefact.

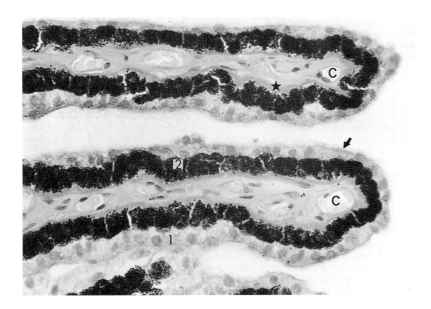

Fig. 10.6 Sectional view of ciliary processes. Each process is covered by a double layer of epithelial cells. The outer, non-pigmented layer (1) is covered on its external surface by basement membrane (arrow) that is a continuation of the internal limiting membrane of the retina over the entire ciliary process. The inner, pigmented layer (2) rests on a cuticular layer (*). The connective tissue of each process contains many capillaries (c). (Original magnification ×448.)

ciliary body (Figs 10.4–10.6). The ciliary epithelium, which is the secretory source of the aqueous humour, forms the internal surface. The intervening valleys are darker and sometimes bear smaller, accessory processes. The processes are roughly symmetrical but vary in size, so that major and minor processes may be identified. They become longer and taller with age (Reese, 1934). The wider anterior end which may fuse with that of neighbouring processes, is termed the **head**. Average dimensions are: length 2.0 mm; width 0.5 mm; height 0.8–1.0 mm (Hogan, Alvarado and Weddell, 1971). Giant processes may be found in the nasal, horizontal meridian (Streeten, 1995). In meridional section (Fig. 10.5) the ciliary body is triangular, with its shortest side anterior. The base of the triangle faces the posterior chamber and posterior aspect of the iris but at the root of the iris it is separated from the anterior chamber angle only by the lamellae of the trabecular meshwork, the ciliary muscle actually inserting into the uveal meshwork (Fig. 10.5). The outer side of the triangle, formed by the ciliary muscle, lies against the sclera with the supraciliary tissue intervening. The inner aspect bears the ciliary processes and is related anteriorly to the fibres of the suspensory ligament (which are bathed in aqueous) and posteriorly to the vitreous. The equator of the lens is about 0.5 mm from the processes.

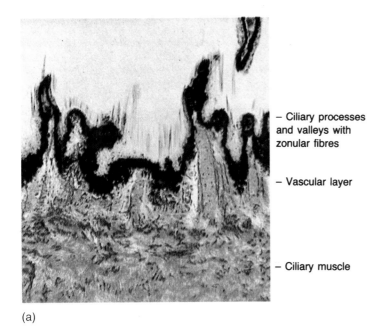

– Ciliary processes and valleys with zonular fibres

– Vascular layer

– Ciliary muscle

(a)

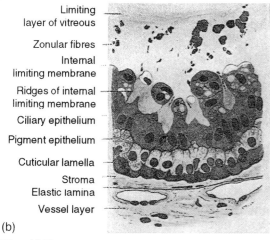

Limiting layer of vitreous
Zonular fibres
Internal limiting membrane
Ridges of internal limiting membrane
Ciliary epithelium
Pigment epithelium
Cuticular lamella
Stroma
Elastic lamina
Vessel layer

(b)

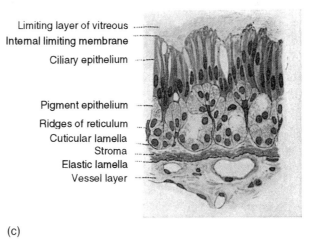

Limiting layer of vitreous
Internal limiting membrane
Ciliary epithelium

Pigment epithelium
Ridges of reticulum
Cuticular lamella
Stroma
Elastic lamella
Vessel layer

(c)

Fig. 10.7 (a) Coronal section of the posterior portion of the corona ciliaris (Zenker fixation, Mallory's triple stain). Artery passing through the ciliary muscle; (b) bleached transverse section of the orbiculus ciliaris near the corona ciliaris (original magnification ×380); (c) bleached transverse section of the orbiculus ciliaris (pars plana) near the ora serrata (original magnification ×320).

STRUCTURE

From without inwards, the ciliary body consists of the following layers (Figs 10.7–10.10):

1. supraciliary layers;
2. ciliary muscle;
3. stroma;
4. epithelial layers:
   (a) external limiting membrane or anterior basement membrane;
   (b) pigmented epithelium;
   (c) non-pigmented epithelium;
   (d) inner basement membrane (internal limiting membrane).

The supraciliary layer

This resembles the suprachoroidea of the choroid and consists of strands of collagen derived partly from the suprachoroid, and also from extensions of the external longitudinal layers of the ciliary muscle. The collagen enters and mingles with the collagen framework of the overlying sclera. Melanocytes and fibroblasts are enmeshed in this tissue. This potential

Pigment cells
| Surface cells
| I

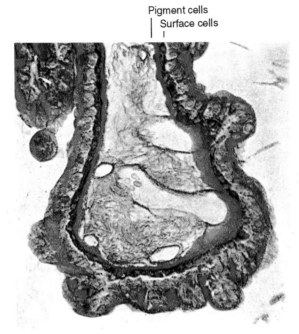

Fig. 10.8 Meridional section of the ciliary process (Zenker fixation, Mallory's triple stain). Note the presence of blue staining, basal lamina and proliferation of clear cells to form papillae.

Epithelium —
Pigment layer —
Stroma —
Ciliary —
muscle
Supraciliaris —

Sclera —

Medial _
rectus

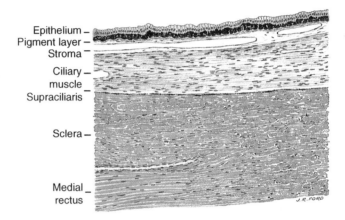

Fig. 10.9 Anteroposterior section of the ciliary body (orbiculus). Wolff's preparation.

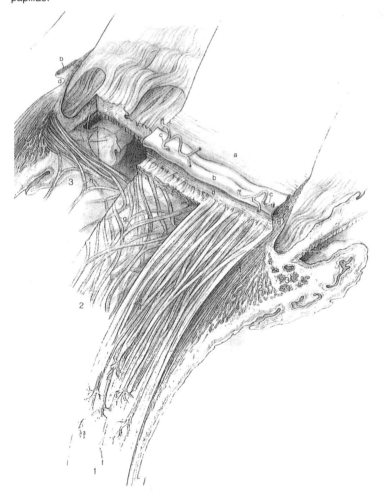

Fig. 10.10 Drawing of the ciliary body showing the ciliary muscle and its components. The cornea and sclera have been dissected away but the trabecular meshwork (a), Schlemm's canal (b), two external collectors (c), and the scleral spur (d) have been left undisturbed. The three components of the ciliary muscle are shown separately, viewed from the outside and sectioned meridionally. Section 1 shows the longitudinal ciliary muscle; in Section 2 the longitudinal ciliary muscle has been dissected away to show the radial ciliary muscle; in Section 3 only the innermost circular ciliary muscle is shown. According to Calasans (1953), the ciliary muscle originates in the ciliary tendon, which includes the scleral spur (d) and the adjacent connective tissue. The cells originate as paired V-shaped bundles. The longitudinal muscle forms long V-shaped trellises (e), which terminate in the epichoroidal stars (f). The arms of the V-shaped bundles formed by the radial muscle meet at wide angles (g) and terminate in the ciliary processes. The V-shaped bundles of the circular muscle originate at such distant points in the ciliary tendon that their arms meet at a very wide angle (h). The iridic portion is shown at (i) joining the circular muscle cells. (From Hogan, M. J., Alvarado, J. A. and Weddell, J. E. (1971) *Histology of the Human Eye. An Atlas and Textbook*, published by W. B. Saunders.)

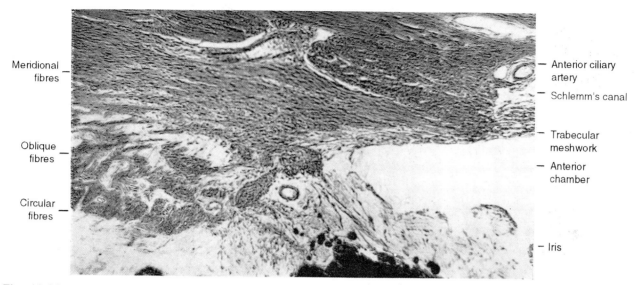

Meridional fibres

Oblique fibres

Circular fibres

Anterior ciliary artery

Schlemm's canal

Trabecular meshwork

Anterior chamber

Iris

Fig. 10.11   Meridional section of the angle of the anterior chamber (Zenker fixation, Mallory's triple stain). Note how the deepest fibres of the trabecular meshwork pass outwards to give attachment to circular fibres and also to some radial fibres of the ciliary muscle. An iris process crosses the angle and merges with the innermost layer of the uveal trabecular sheets.

space, together with that of the suprachoroidea, forms the route of exit for aqueous humour via the 'unconventional' pathway (Inomata, Bill and Smelser, 1972; Bill, 1977; Sherman, Green and Laties, 1978). The space may be expanded pathologically by transudate or exudate associated with ciliary body and choroidal detachment. Detachment of the ciliary body reduces the secretion of aqueous humour (Bill, 1977).

Ciliary muscle

In meridional section, ciliary muscle resembles a right-angled triangle, the right-angle being internal and facing the ciliary processes. The posterior acute angle points to the choroid and the hypotenuse is parallel to the sclera (Figs 10.5 and 10.11). The overall form of the ciliary body depends on that of the muscle, which consists of flat bundles of non-striated fibres, the most external being longitudinal or meridional, the intermediate radial or oblique, and the most internal circular or 'sphincteric'. Calasans (1953) envisaged most of the fibres as arising from the scleral spur by a collagenous **ciliary tendon**, while authors regard this as the point of insertion (Mollier, 1938; Rohen, 1952, 1964).

Calasans also suggested that muscle bundles arise as V-shaped pairs (Fig. 10.10), with the outermost bundles meeting at a narrow angle posteriorly and having a mainly longitudinal orientation, the next deepest fibres at a broader angle running obliquely

to form the **radial** fibres, and the deepest most anterior bundles arising at an extremely wide angle and having a mainly circular orientation. The muscle gains attachment anteriorly by collagenous tendons into the scleral striata and to the iris wall. Posteriorly it is attached by an elastic tendon and elastic fibres in the membrane of Bruch in the pars plana. Although the radial layer is commonly described as a discrete entity (Figs 6.18 and 10.12), all three layers exchange fibres (Rohen, 1952).

The **circular fibres** (Müller) occupy the internal part of the ciliary body. They are nearest to the lens and parallel to the limbus. The fibres are thus cut transversely in meridional section (Fig. 10.11).

The tendinous attachment of the muscle to the corneoscleral limbus is the main union between the corneoscleral coat and the uveal tract. Internal to the spur, but never anterior to it, oblique and circular muscle fibres are inserted into the posterior part of the uveoscleral meshwork (Hogan, Alvarado and Weddell, 1971; Tripathi and Tripathi, 1982). This arrangement has been postulated to increase trabecular pore size during accommodation and after the instillation of miotics (Rohen, Lütjen and Bárány, 1967; Kaufman and Barany, 1976; Grierson, Lee and Abraham, 1978a,b).

The outer longitudinal muscle bundles end posteriorly in the supraciliary lamina and suprachoroidea in so-called **epichoroidal muscle stars** as far back as the anterior third of the choroid. They occur as branched stellate forms on both surfaces of the

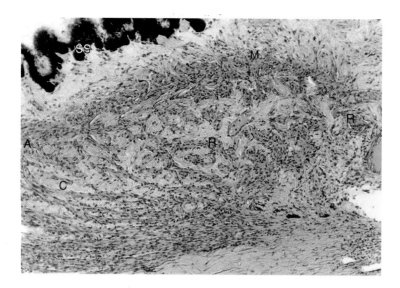

Fig. 10.12 The anterior part of human ciliary muscle to show its three main components: meridional fibres (M), radial fibres (R) and circular fibres (C), poorly developed in this subject. A = Major arterial circle; SS = scleral spur. (Original magnification ×150.)

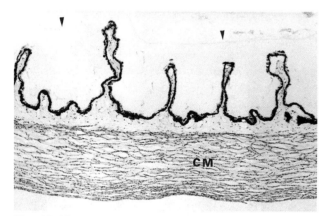

Fig. 10.13 Pars plicata of the ciliary body cut coronally, perpendicular to the usual plane. Ciliary muscle (CM) does not extend into the ciliary processes, but has the same thickness under the processes and valleys. The anterior hyaloid membrane is visible above the processes (arrowheads). (Haematoxylin and eosin, original magnification ×120.) (From Streeten, B. W. in Duane, T. D. and Jaeger, E. A. (eds) (1992) *Biomedical Foundations of Ophthalmology*, published by Harper and Row, with permission.)

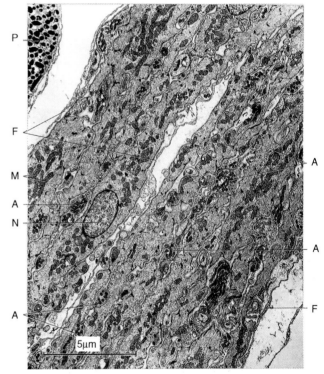

Fig. 10.14 Bundle of smooth muscle fibres in the ciliary body of a catfish. The muscle bundles are ensheathed by fibroblasts. N = Nucleus of a smooth muscle fibre; M = mitochondrion; A = axon; P = pigment cell. Original magnification ×3000. (Courtesy of E. van der Zypen.)

supraciliary lamina, flattened in the plane of the lamellae. Their three to five primary processes and variable number of dichotomous terminal processes are best studied in teased preparations. In meridional section they appear as slender spindles (Salzmann, 1912). These correspond to the elastic tendons described in the monkey eye, and their distribution within the ciliary valleys in an elastic network inserted into the elastic layer of Bruch's membrane, and into the capillaries of the pars plana. The ciliary muscle does not extend into the ciliary processes and is equally thick in the valleys as under the processes (Streeten, 1995) (Figs 10.13 and 10.14).

Ultrastructure

In the primate, the morphology of fetal or neonatal muscle cells differs from that of the mature fibre (Lütjen-Drecoll, Tamm and Kaufmann, 1988). In the early fetus, each ciliary muscle bundle is separated

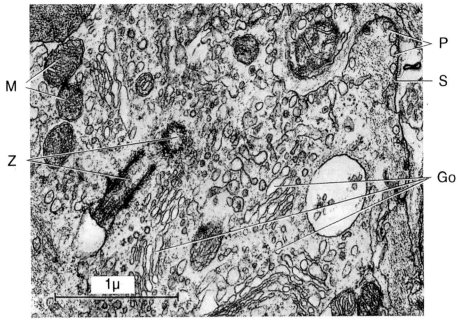

Fig. 10.15 Golgi complex (Go) within the ciliary muscle fibre of a monkey. M = Mitochondrion; S = sarcolemma; P = pinocytotic vesicles; Z = centriole. (Original magnification × 20 000.) (From van der Zypen, E. (1967). *A.v. Graefs Arch Klin Exp Ophthalmol.*, **271**, with permission.)

by numerous fibroblasts, and is not yet attached to the trabecular meshwork. The fibres resemble vascular smooth muscle cells, with densely packed myofibrils and few mitochondria. These muscle cells are sparsely innervated, attached by desmosomes, and their thin basement membranes (containing collagens I, III and IV but no laminin (Noske *et al.*, 1994)), are connected by fine collagen fibres.

The mature ciliary muscle fibre is a multiunit, rather than syncytial, smooth muscle (Bozler, 1948), sparsely supplied with gap junctions between adjacent cells.

Ultrastructurally the ciliary muscle resembles unstriated muscle elsewhere, except for an abundance of mitochondria and endoplasmic reticulum and more well-developed Golgi apparatus (Streeten, 1987) close to the cell nucleus (Figs 10.14 and 10.15) (Ishikawa, 1962) and the fact that the muscle cells are arranged in bundles surrounded by a thin sheath of fibroblasts rather than primarily by collagenous tissue elements (van der Zypen, 1967) (Fig. 10.16). Each fibre is filled by actin filaments showing densities along their length and at the plasma membrane. There are numerous pinocytotic vesicles beneath the membrane. Each muscle cell possesses a basement membrane, separated by a gap of 30 nm. Occasional neighbouring muscle cells adhere by a tight junction or a macula adherens through a breach in this membrane.

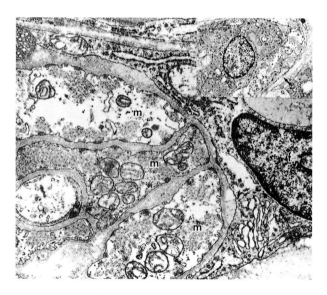

Fig. 10.16 Three muscle fibres (m) enclosed by a fibrocyte (f). Thick basement membrane is visible around each muscle fibre and several synapses. Inset: Thin fingers of fibrocyte cytoplasm (arrow) surround a bundle of ciliary muscle fibres. (Original magnification ×33 800; inset ×8500.) (From Streeten, B. W. in Duane, T. D. and Jaeger, E. A. (eds) (1992) *Biomedical Foundations of Ophthalmology*, published by Harper and Row, with permission.)

The muscle cells exhibit a central core of mitochondria, with myofilaments arranged peripherally. The muscle cells branch, and are connected at discrete points by desmosomes or maculae adhaerentae (Fig.

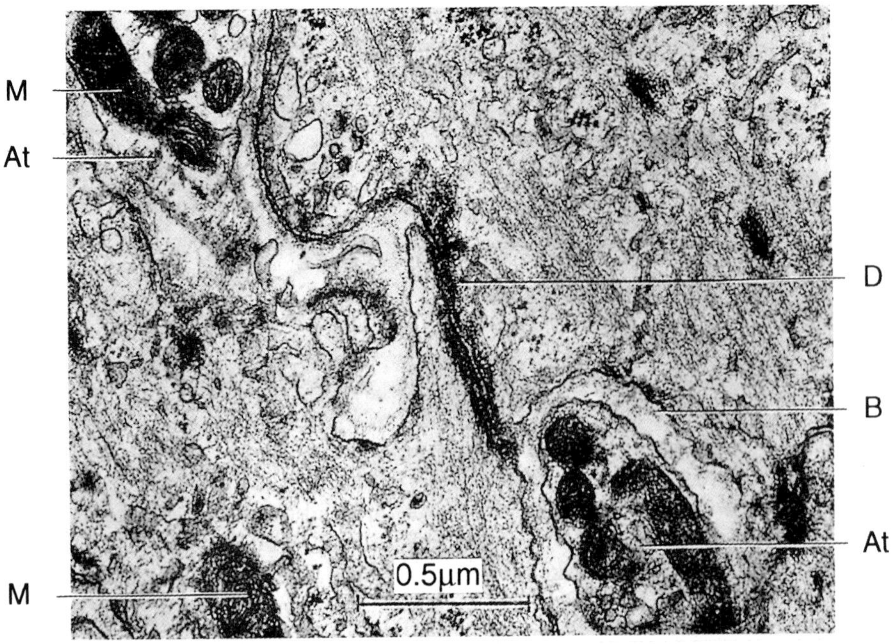

Fig. 10.17 A region of intermuscular contact in a monkey ciliary muscle. D = Desmosome; B = basal membrane; M = mitochondrion; At = axon terminal. (From van der Zypen, E. (1967). *A.v. Graefs Arch Klin Exp Ophthalmol*, **271**, 143–168, with permission.)

10.17). The muscle bundles are surrounded by a thin collagenous sheath and a layer of perimysial cells. Certain structural features resemble those of striated muscle, since they have almost parallel myofibrils, electron-dense structures resembling Z-bands (Ishikawa, 1962; van der Zypen, 1967) (Fig. 10.18), and a rich innervation (Townes-Anderson and Raviola, 1978). The ability of ciliary muscle to contract and relax rapidly is in keeping with this morphology. Histochemically, ciliary muscle can be distinguished from vascular smooth muscle; the circular and inner reticular parts of the muscle resemble tonic extraocular muscle fibres in their staining characteristics, while the anterior tips of the meridional muscle resemble rapid twitch fibres (Asmussen *et al.*, 1971; Flugel *et al.*, 1990). Ultrastructural differences between meridional and circular muscle cells were reported by Ishikawa (1962).

Age-related ciliary muscle degeneration

With age, degenerative changes appear in the primate ciliary muscle, which include the appearance of membranous whorls, or 'fingerprints' within the muscle fibres, similar to those seen in denervated human striate muscle (Miledi and Slater, 1969) or in certain human muscle diseases (Behnke, 1976). Such changes have also been observed in normal guinea-pig iris (Gabella, 1974). Increasing numbers of lysosomes and lipofuscin inclusions are also noted in the muscle fibres with age, and myelin figures are found within the nerve axons and terminals, just as have been described in striated muscle (Miller, 1975). These changes have also been described in human ciliary muscle (van der Zypen, 1970). In older monkeys, the basement membranes are thickened and fused in places and there are 'microvillous' folds of the lateral sarcolemma. Occasional degenerated and hyalinized muscle cells are found. Dense connective tissue appears between the longitudinal and reticular parts of the muscle.

Neuromuscular junctions are mainly indirect, with the synaptic membrane contacting the basement membrane of the muscle cell (Figs 10.19 and 10.20). Direct junctions between synaptic and muscle membranes, unlike other smooth muscle systems, are infrequent, but have been seen more frequently in the region of the scleral spur (Uga, 1968). Occasionally an unusual direct junction with broad synaptic contact over a depression in the cell surface is also found (Ishikawa, 1962) (Fig. 10.21).

Stroma

The stroma of the ciliary body is a collagenous connective tissue containing vessels, nerves and cells, and which separates the bundles of the ciliary muscle superficially and forms a distinct and highly vascular inner connective tissue layer deep to this. The

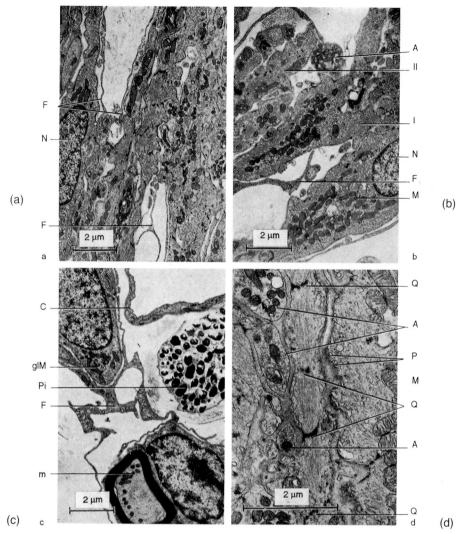

Fig. 10.18 Bundles of ciliary muscle fibre from the catfish. (a) A bridge between muscle bundles; (b) forking of a muscle bundle (I = longitudinal section; II = oblique section); (c) the end of a muscle bundle; (d) oblique (Q) bands between the contractile elements of a smooth muscle fibre. glM = Smooth muscle fibre; N = nucleus of a smooth muscle fibre, F = fibrocyte; m = markhaltiges axon; A = marklose axon terminal, free from a Schwann cell sheath; Pi = pigment cell; M = mitochondrion; P = pinocytotic vesicles; C = capillary endothelium (original magnifications: (a) ×4500; (b) ×6000; (c) ×5000; (d) × 10 000). (From van der Zypen, E. (1967). *A.v. Graefs Arch Klin Exp Ophthalmol,* **271,** 143–168, with permission.)

subepithelial connective tissue increases in amount in the second decade chiefly in the pars placata, which accounts for the expansion of the ciliary processes into their adult form. Capillaries in this layer are fenestrated, but in the outer stroma they are not (Figs 10.22 and 10.23).

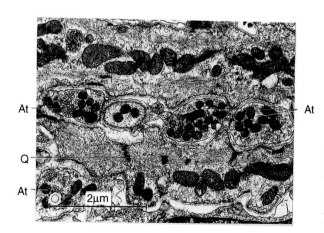

Fig. 10.19 Nerves within the ciliary muscle of the monkey. Nerve bundle near to the fibroblastic sheath. Axon (A) still surrounded by the superficial Schwann cell membrane (Sc). The axon terminal (At) is filled with synaptic vesicles (SV) and mitochondria (M) are relatively free of Schwann cell cytoplasm at the level of the synapse. N = nucleus of a Schwann cell (original magnification ×8000). (From van der Zypen, E. (1967). *A.v. Graefs Arch Klin Exp Ophthalmol,* **271,** 143–168, with permission.)

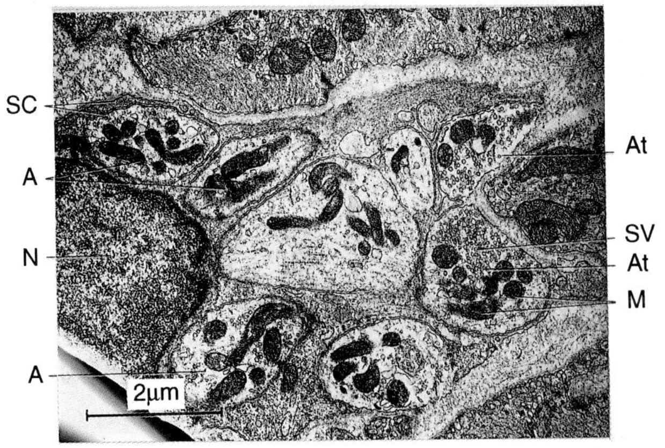

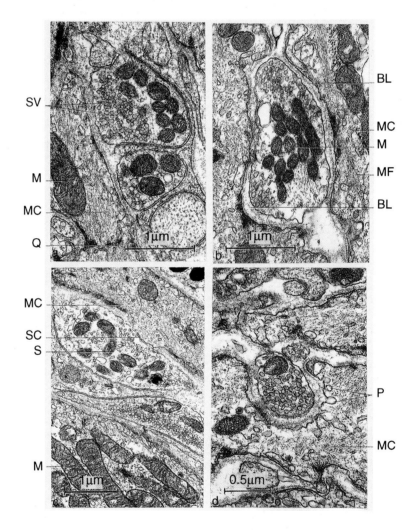

Fig. 10.20 Nerves within the ciliary muscle of the monkey, showing axon terminals (At) lying between the muscle fibres. Note absence of the Schwann cell. Q = Oblique band (original magnification ×12 000). (From van der Zypen, E. (1967). *A.v. Graefs Arch Klin Exp Ophthalmol*, **271**, 143–168, with permission.)

Fig. 10.21 Synapse formation in the monkey ciliary muscle. (a) Axon terminal, partly ensheathed by a Schwann cell. A synaptic cleft of 70 nm is occupied by a basal lamina 40 nm wide; (b) synapse completely lacking a Schwann cell covering, showing synaptic contact between a single nerve terminal with two muscle fibres. One synaptic space is of 60 nm, containing a basal lamina (BL) 20 nm wide. A second synaptic space of 90 nm is also visible, containing two basal laminae (BL) of similar dimensions; (c) a true synapse. Synaptic space is 10 nm and the basal laminae have been interrupted. The pre- and postsynaptic membranes (SC) have thickened; (d) invaginating synapse, synaptic space 90 nm. MC = smooth muscle fibre with mitochondria (M), myofilaments (MF), oblique (Q) band and pinocytotic vesicles (P). The synapse contains synaptic vesicles (SV) and mitochondria. (Original magnifications: a ×12 500; b ×22 000; c ×12 500; d ×20 000. (From van der Zypen, E. (1967). *A.v. Graefs Arch Klin Exp Ophthalmol*, **271**, 143–168, with permission.)

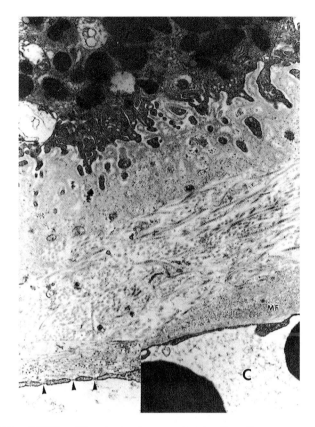

Fig. 10.22 Ciliary body stroma underlying the ciliary processes and anterior pars plicata. Even at the age of 18 years, the basement membrane is thick. Collagen and other fine filaments fill the narrow space between the epithelium and fenestrated capillary wall (C). (Inset) Clumps of tubular microfibrils are closely associated with the wall. (Original magnification ×17 300; inset × 43 000. (From Streeten, B. W. in Duane, T. D. and Jaeger, E. A. (eds) (1992) *Biomedical Foundations of Ophthalmology*, published by Harper and Row, with permission.)

The ciliary muscle stroma is minimal at birth but increases with age, chiefly in the circular and radial portions. It forms thin longitudinal lamellae around the longitudinal muscle fibres, continuous with the supraciliary lamina and, like the lamina, contains pigment cells. The stroma of the radial portion is dense and reticular and contains blood vessels, nerves and, in deeply pigmented eyes, melanocytes (Fig. 10.24). The stroma of the circular portion is loose, as in the root of the iris, with which it is continuous.

The inner connective tissue layer lies between muscle and the basement membrane of the pigmented epithelium. It is thin over the pars plana and thicker over the pars plicata, and particularly condensed along the crests of the ciliary processes. Posteriorly this inner layer is continuous with the choroidal stroma; superficially it mingles with the denser connective tissue of the ciliary muscle. Anteriorly it is continuous with the stroma of the iris and at the iris root, and the loose connective tissue separates ciliary muscle from the anterior chamber. With age an amorphous material accumulates in the deep aspect of the stroma, and thickens the basement membrane (see below). Hyaline degeneration of the stroma also occurs with age. Melanocytes are less plentiful here than in the choroid, and may be absent in the ciliary processes and anterior stroma. Their melanosomes are 0.3–0.8 μm wide.

Stromal extracellular matrix

Laminin, fibronectin, and several collagen types are found within the ciliary body. Type VI collagen is found in various forms (Rittig *et al.*, 1990).

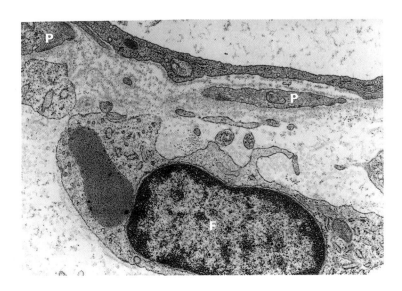

Fig. 10.23 Intermittent pericyte (P) coverage and lack of fenestrae in the endothelial cell wall characterize the capillaries of the deeper stroma in the deeper stroma of the pars plicata. The uveal fibroblast (F) has active rough endoplasmic reticulum, a large cisterna with granular material and clumps of microfibrils close to the wall. (From Streeten, B. W. in Duane, T. D. and Jaeger, E. A. (eds) (1992) *Biomedical Foundations of Ophthalmology*, published by Harper and Row, with permission.)

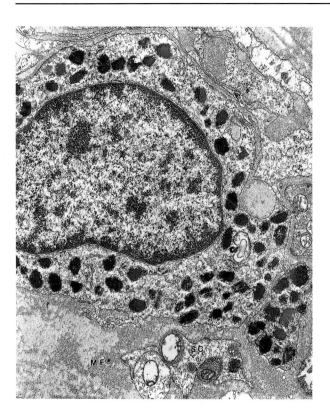

Fig. 10.24 Melanocyte with dense melanosomes in the ciliary stroma surrounded by collagen fibres and microfibrils (MF). A Schwann cell (SC) enveloping small nerve fibres is present below. Original magnification ×26 200. (From Streeten, B. W. in Duane, T. D. and Jaeger, E. A. (eds) (1992) *Biomedical Foundations of Ophthalmology*, published by Harper and Row, with permission.)

Type VI collagen is distributed asymmetrically around the fenestrated capillaries, within connective tissue lying between the epithelium and ciliary muscle (referred to in the monkey as the ground plate). It is more abundant on the side that faces away from the epithelium, and thus provides secure mechanical anchoring for the vessels without interfering with the secretory needs of the ciliary epithelium.

The aggregated form of type VI collagen (curly, or long-spacing collagen) forms the sheaths around the anterior elastic tendons of the ciliary muscle (Lütjen-Drecoll, 1988). The collagen is found at the tips of the oblique and circular muscle bundles, as they insert into the trabecular meshwork. Similar sheaths invest the elastic fibres of the trabecular meshwork and the sulcus sclerae (Lütjen-Drecoll *et al.*, 1981; Rohen and Lütjen-Drecoll, 1981; Lütjen-Drecoll *et al.*, 1989).

Type VI collagen and laminin are seen diffusely in the ciliary muscle, and within the connective tissue ground plate between the muscle and the overlying epithelium. Type VI collagen is found along the basement membrane of the individual muscle cells, and more intensely around the muscle bundles. Fibrils staining positively for both type VI collagen and laminin extend out from the muscle bundles into the adjacent intermuscular connective tissue. These fibrils split up in a brush-like manner, particularly where the inner, reticular part of the muscle faces the ground plate. The fibrils are assumed to play a mechanical role in transmitting force between the muscle cells and the intermuscular connective tissue, allowing each muscle bundle to act as an individual unit. Individual muscle cells are sparsely, if at all, connected to their neighbours by gap junctions (Townes-Anderson and Raviola, 1978).

Type VI collagen is also found along the basement membranes of the ciliary vascular and endothelial basement membranes, but, unlike type IV collagen, is not located along epithelial basement membranes.

Other extracellular matrix proteins are found within the ciliary body (Rittig *et al.*, 1990). There is linear staining for type IV collagen around the ciliary muscle cells, particularly near the scleral spur and in relation to the fenestrated capillaries under the ciliary epithelium. Staining of the epithelial basement membrane and the endoneurium of the ciliary nerves is weaker.

Staining for fibronectin is weak around the muscle cells, but is stronger in the reticular and circular parts than in the longitudinal part. Laminin staining is seen around the muscle cells, but more strongly around the muscle bundles, forming a sheath which spreads into the neighbouring tissue. This is most developed in that part of the muscle facing the ground plate, in much the same way as for type VI collagen. Staining for laminin around the ciliary capillaries, the endoneurium and the epithelial basement membrane resembles that for type IV collagen.

VASCULATURE OF THE CILIARY BODY

The vasculature of the ciliary body runs mainly in the stroma, particularly the inner stromal layer. The pars plana vascular layer is like that of the choroid, with which it is continuous, but it is narrower, and lacks a choriocapillaris. Its vessels consist chiefly of veins running backwards and parallel to each other. The arteries to the ciliary body are branches of the long posterior and anterior ciliary arteries (Fig. 10.25) and pass through the substance of the ciliary muscle. The circulus arteriosus iridis major lies behind the root of the iris, just in front of the circular portion of the ciliary muscle (Fig. 10.11), in the loose connective tissue which separates it from the anterior chamber.

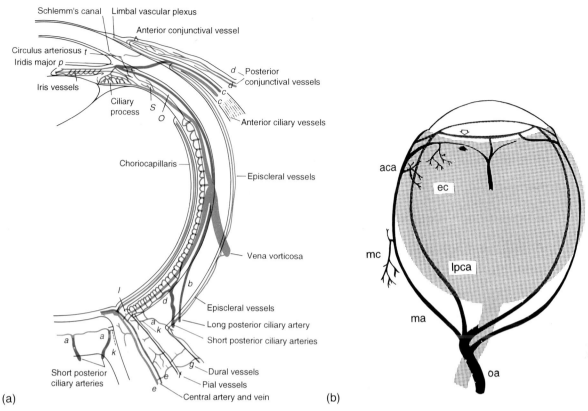

(a)   (b)

Fig. 10.25 (a) The blood supply of the eye. k = Branch of short posterior ciliary to the optic nerve; l = anastomoses between choroidal and central vessels. In the case of the artery this is capillary only; s = vein from ciliary muscle to vena vorticosa; t = branch of anterior ciliary vein from ciliary muscle; o = recurrent artery; (b) delivery of blood to the anterior segment. The arterial circulation of the anterior segment consists of superficial and deep coronal arterial circles (the episcleral arterial circle, the major circle of the iris and the intramuscular circle of the ciliary body). These are supplied by sagittal arterial rings (the long posterior ciliary arteries, the muscular and anterior ciliary arteries and the perforating branches of these systems). oa = Ophthalmic artery; lpca = long posterior ciliary artery; ma = artery of the rectus muscle; ec = episcleral capillaries; mc = capillaries of the rectus muscle; aca = anterior ciliary artery. Note, according to some authors the major arterial circle is supplied predominantly by the long posterior ciliary arteries while the intramuscular circle is supplied chiefly by the perforating branches of the anterior ciliary arteries – see text, and Figure 10.26. (From Meyer, P. A. R. (1989), *Eye*, **3**, 121, with permission.)

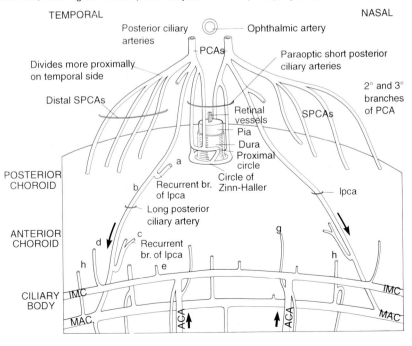

Fig. 10.26 Schematic drawing of the distribution of the ciliary arteries. IMC = intramuscular ciliary arterial circle; MAC = major arterial circle of the iris; PCA = posterior ciliary artery; SPCA = short posterior ciliary arteries; ACA = anterior ciliary arteries; lpca = long posterior ciliary artery; a = recurrent branch of the long posterior ciliary artery; b = long posterior ciliary artery; c = recurrent branch of the long posterior ciliary artery; d = anterior choroidal branch of the ciliary intramuscular circle; e = branch of the IMC; f = iris artery arising from a ciliary process branch of the MAC; g = branch to the anterior choroid from the anterior ciliary artery; h = branch to the anterior choroid from the MAC; i = iris artery arising from the MAC branch to the choroid; j = iris artery arising from the anterior ciliary artery.

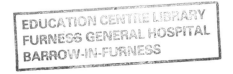

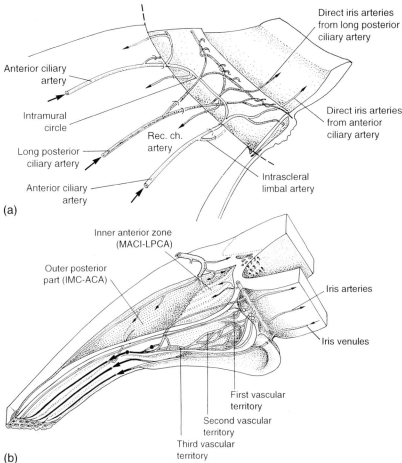

Anterior ciliary artery

Intramural circle

Long posterior ciliary artery

Anterior ciliary artery

Rec. ch. artery

Direct iris arteries from long posterior ciliary artery

Direct iris arteries from anterior ciliary artery

Intrascleral limbal artery

(a)

Inner anterior zone (MACI-LPCA)

Outer posterior part (IMC-ACA)

Iris arteries

Iris venules

First vascular territory

Second vascular territory

Third vascular territory

(b)

Fig. 10.27 (a) Schematic drawing of the architecture of the major vessels in the human anterior segment, outer view, limbal zone and cornea removed to show the vasculature of the ciliary body and iris: long posterior ciliary artery (LPCA), branches of the anterior ciliary arteries (ACA), major arterial circle of the iris (MACI: note the plait-like pattern of the different segments), iris artery coming from the MACI, iris artery coming from the ACA, anastomoses of the perforating branches of the ACA forming an intramuscular circle, recurrent choroidal arteries and branches for the scleral and limbal capillaries;
(b) schematic drawing of the vascular architecture in the human ciliary body in sagittal section to show: perforating branches of the ACA, the MACI, the first vascular territory (open circle), terminal arteriole (afferent segment), the second vascular territory (open circle), terminal arterioles (afferent segment), third vascular territory (located in the posterior portion of the major and minor ciliary processes), arterioles to the inner and anterior parts of the ciliary muscle (dark hatching), arterioles to the outer and posterior parts of the ciliary muscle (dark hatching), recurrent choroidal arteries, venous capillaries from the ciliary muscle, iris artery and the iris venule (dark circle) efferent venous segment of the marginal venule related to the second and third territory. Redrawn from Funk, R. and Rohen, J. W. (1990) *Exp. Eye Res.*, **51**, 651).

This artery is a typical small artery with two or three layers of smooth muscle cells and a loose adventitia. The internal elastic lamina is poorly developed. The endothelial and muscle cells possess a basement membrane. The blood supply of the ciliary muscle and the ciliary processes is described in Chapter 11, but is summarized here.

The ciliary muscle blood supply

The inner and anterior part of the ciliary muscle is supplied by the major arterial circle, while the outer and posterior part is supplied by the intramuscular circle of the ciliary body (Fig. 10.26). This may reflect functional differences between these regions of the muscle. The major circle itself is formed in the human eye predominantly by the long posterior ciliary arteries, while the intramuscular circle is formed by penetrating branches of the anterior ciliary arteries which lie mainly in the vertical plane. Perforating trunks of the anterior ciliary arteries supply 10 to 12 recurrent choroidal arteries to the anterior choroid, and the major circle also gives rise to some recurrent choroidal arteries. In all sectors, anastomoses exist between branches of the anterior and long posterior ciliary arteries (Funk and Rohen, 1990). Venules drain from the ciliary body, and then empty into the ciliary valleys or join those of the pars plana.

The ciliary process blood supply

The vasculature of the ciliary processes is divided into three territories. The first lies anteriorly at the crests of the major processes, a region which appears specialized for the secretion of aqueous humour (Fig. 10.27). These anterior arteries show focal constrictions which may have a functional role in regulating perfusion pressure in the ciliary processes and may influence ultrafiltration (Figs 10.28a,b; 10.29a,b). In the rabbit and monkey, this region is more susceptible to breakdown of the blood–aqueous barrier than are other zones. The ciliary blood flow is autoregulated and the vascular anatomy probably permits the shunting of blood between adjacent major processes. Sympathetic stimulation or adrenaline causes a reduction in ciliary process blood flow (Fig. 10.29c,d).

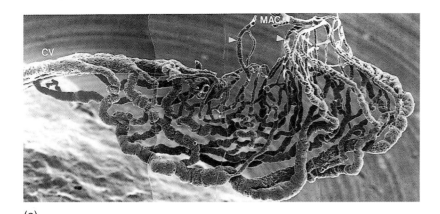

(a)

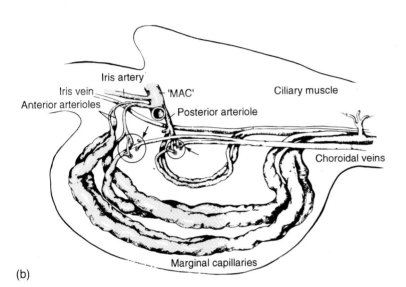

(b)

Fig. 10.28 (a) Profile of a single ciliary process. Constricted anterior arterioles (arrows) enter the anterior part of the process to provide large irregular capillaries resembling the veins that occupy the margins of the process. Posteriorly, large-calibre arterioles (arrowheads) originate and enter the middle of the process to divide into smaller capillaries generally confined to the base of the process. All capillaries travel posteriorly to drain into the choroidal veins (CV). MAC = major arterial circle. Original magnification ×150.
(b) Summary of the angioarchitecture of the primate major ciliary process, profile view. Each process is supplied by anterior and posterior arterioles, radiating from the major arterial circle (MAC). The characteristically constricted anterior arterioles supply the anterior aspect of the ciliary process, forming large, irregularly dilated marginal process capillaries resembling veins, and draining posteriorly into the choroidal veins. The posterior arterioles appear to be less constricted and provide posteriorly draining capillaries generally confined to the base of the process. At both levels, laterally directed arterioles form interprocess capillary networks (circled areas). From here, some capillaries re-enter the ciliary processes, to form interprocess communications anteriorly (not shown) and posteriorly. Other capillaries enter interprocess venous arcades (arrows), which drain directly into the choroidal veins and bypass the ciliary process entirely. The choroidal veins originate in four anterior sources: iris veins, ciliary processes, interprocess arcades, and the ciliary muscle. (From Morrison, J. C. and van Buskirk, E. M. (1984). *Am J Ophthalmol*, **97**, 372–383, with permission.)

The second vascular territory also lies in the anterior part of the major processes, both deep in its central part and superficially, while the third territory supplies the minor processes.

The ciliary processes contain no muscle and are the most vascular region of the whole eye. The vascular core is a forward continuation of the pars plana and consists of veins and wide capillaries, mainly of veins, but in addition a capillary system is applied close to, and often in contact with, the basement membrane of the pigmented epithelium. The capillaries are almost venular in width and resemble those of the choriocapillaris. They are 15–30 μm in diameter, fenestrated (30–100 nm) (Taniguchi, 1962) and permeable to plasma proteins and blood-borne tracer materials. The fenestrations are found on all surfaces of the endothelial lining. Specialized junctions are identical to those found in the choriocapillaris (Raviola, 1977).

The capillaries which supply the muscle are sparse and less fenestrated. They have a smaller diameter and thicker endothelium. The capillaries merge into venules which consist of an endothelium and a basement membrane. Venous return from the ciliary processes is to the choroidal veins, and from the muscle, in part via these veins and in part via the anterior ciliary veins.

The endothelial cells of the iris vessels lack fenestrae and are joined by tight junctions (Vold, 1969; Hogan, Alvarado and Weddell, 1971; Vegge, 1971; Saari, 1972). Thus the major arterial circle of the iris root supplies the ciliary body with fenestrated capillaries of two types and the iris with unfenestrated endothelium. A similar situation obtains in the posterior segment of the eye, where ciliary arteries supply the fenestrated capillaries of the choriocapillaris and the unfenestrated capillaries at the optic nerve head.

The permeability of the ciliary body capillaries allows plasma proteins to diffuse into the ciliary body

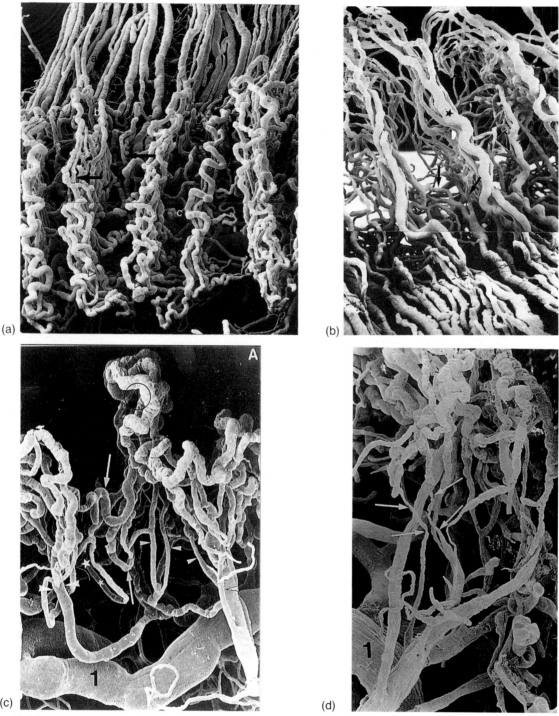

Fig. 10.29 (a) Scanning electron micrograph of a vascular resin cast of the human ciliary body. View from inside the first (a); second (b) and third (c) vascular territories. Arrows show marginal venules at the inner edge of the ciliary processes; the branching pattern of the vasculature in the anterior part of the pars plana is shown by arrowheads; (b) scanning electron micrograph of a vascular resin cast of the ciliary body in the human eye, oblique posterior aspect. Marginal venule at the inner edge of the ciliary processes; arrows show venule of the third vascular territory leading into zonules. The dotted line demonstrates the border between the pars plana and the ciliary body; (c) scanning electron micrograph of vascular resin casts of the human ciliary body, anterior aspect. The circled area shows the major ciliary process; 1 = major arterial circle of the iris; arrows, first vascular territory; *, venule of this territory. The casts are taken from a pair of eyes 4 h after death. Before plastic injection the eye on the left was immersed in Ringer's solution (control eye). The eye on the right was immersed in 50 ml Ringer's solution plus 1 mg adrenaline. In the anterior ciliary process arterioles of the treated eye marked constrictions were present in a segment of 60–100 μm (right-hand figure, arrows), but in a comparable segment of the anterior arterioles of the control eye (arrowheads) no, or only weak, reductions were found. (From Funk, R. and Rohen, J. W. (1990). *Exp Eye Res*, **51**, 651–661, with permission.)

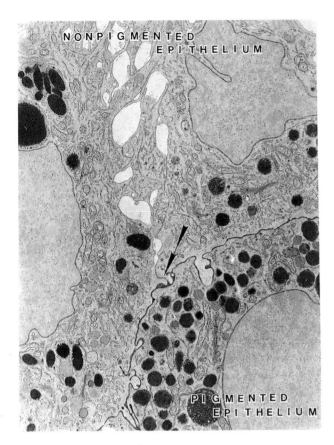

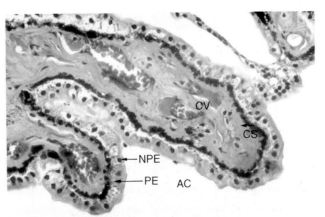

Fig. 10.31 High-power light micrograph of the ciliary processes. PC = Posterior chamber; CS = ciliary stroma; CV = ciliary vein; NPE = non-pigmented epithelium; PE = pigmented epithelium. Masson trichrome stain, original magnification ×420. (Courtesy of Dr D. Lucas.)

Fig. 10.30 Anterior part of the pars plicata of the ciliary body of the monkey (*Macaca mulatta*) following intravenous injection of horseradish peroxidase. Tracer, which has escaped from fenestrated vessels of the ciliary body stroma, has permeated the intercellular spaces between pigmented cells and between pigmented and non-pigmented cells. Diffusion is obstructed by the zonulae occludentes of the non-pigmented cell (arrow), which are the morphological counterpart of the blood–retina barrier. No reaction product is found in the intercellular spaces between the non-pigmented cells. Note the presence of melanosomes in the non-pigmented epithelium, a feature characteristic of the most anterior part of the pars plicata of the ciliary epithelium. Original magnification × 9800. (Courtesy of G. Raviola.)

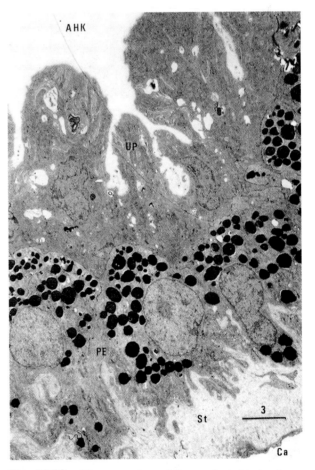

stroma. The continuity of the ciliary body and iris stroma at the iris root allows such macromolecules to diffuse forward into iris (Fig. 10.30). As the ciliary stroma adjoins the anterior chamber at the chamber angle this is a possible route of entry for plasma constituents which are found in normal aqueous, albeit in low concentrations (Raviola, 1977).

Epithelium

The epithelial layers of the ciliary body are the source of the aqueous humour. They are derived embryologically from the apposed layers of the optic cup. Occasionally a space may persist, or a cyst may form between the layers. There is an outer pigmented

Fig. 10.32 Ciliary processes of the monkey showing its two-layered structure. AHK = Posterior chamber; PE = pigmented epithelium; St = stroma; UP = unpigmented epithelium. Original magnification ×2000. (From van der Zypen, E. (1971) *Aging and Development*, published by F. K. Schattauer.)

and an inner non-pigmented epithelium; the apical surfaces of the epithelia are contiguous, while their free, basal surfaces are related to the basement membranes which they secrete (Figs 10.31 and 10.32). Specialized connections exist both within and be-tween the cell layers which are important to their secretory function.

External limiting membrane or anterior basement membrane

The external limiting membrane or anterior base-ment membrane is the product of the pigmented ciliary epithelium. It is continuous posteriorly with the basement membrane of the retinal pigment epithelium, which represents the inner 'cuticular' layer of Bruch's membrane (Figs 10.33, 10.34) and anteriorly with the basement membrane of the dilator of the iris. The basement membrane is of uniform thickness, is thin in the young, but thickens with age to form a multilamellar network (Figs 10.35, 10.36, 10.37), partly due to the accumulation of an amor-phous deposit in the deep stroma to which it is firmly bonded. It does not follow into the basal in-foldings of the pigment cell membranes. The outer, elastic and collagenous portions of Bruch's membrane are separate from this membrane and are prolonged forwards within the ciliary stroma to the level of the posterior border of the pars plicata (Hogan, Alvarado and Weddell, 1971). Over the pars plicata it is separated by a narrow space from the capillaries. Over the pars plana it is related to stromal collagen and veins (Fig. 10.22 and see p. 360).

Pigmented epithelium

The pigmented epithelium represents the outer layer of the optic cup, and as such is continuous with the retinal pigment epithelium posteriorly and with the dilator epithelium of the iris anteriorly. Where the photoreceptors cease at the ora serrata, the pig-

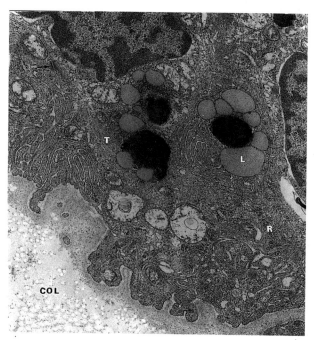

Fig. 10.33 The pigmented ciliary epithelial cells in mid pars plana of a young adult. The cytoplasm is electron dense with many tonofilaments (T). Lipid droplets (L) are present around dark lysosomal residual bodies. Desmosomes connect the cells (arrow). The basal surface and junctional areas are markedly infolded, and the basement membrane is moderately thick. Negative images of collagen fibres (COL) are seen in the dense stroma typical of this region. Original magnification ×26 000. (From Streeten, B. W. in Duane, T. D. and Jaeger, E. A. (eds) (1992) *Biomedical Foundations of Ophthalmology*, published by Harper and Row, with permission.)

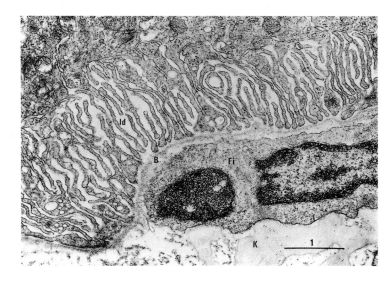

Fig. 10.34 Ciliary process of the monkey. Basal region of the pigment epithelium. Interdigitations increase the surface area of the plasmalemma. B = Basal lamina; Id = interdigitation; Fi = fibroblast; K = connective tissue. Original magnification ×8000. (From van der Zypen, E. (1971) *Aging and Development*, published by F. K. Schattauer.)

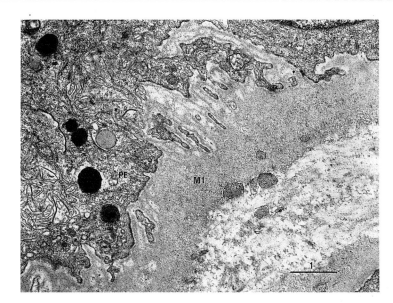

Fig. 10.35 Ciliary process. Basal region of the pigmented epithelium in a 75-year-old man. The membrana limitans externa becomes thickened with age, to form a layer about 2–3 μm wide. PE = Pigmented epithelium; MI = membrana limitans externa. Original magnification ×9000. (From van der Zypen, E. (1971) *Aging and Development*, published by F. K. Schattauer.)

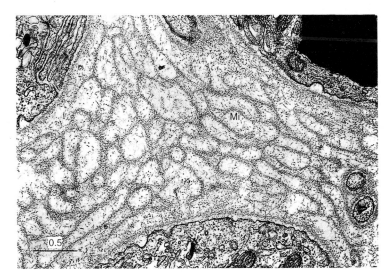

Fig. 10.36 Ciliary process of the monkey. Basal region of the pigment epithelium. The membrana limitans externa often extends deeply into the neighbouring stroma. MI = Membrana limitans externa. Original magnification ×18 000. (From van der Zypen, E. (1971) *Aging and Development*, published by F. K. Schattauer.)

ment cells are diminished in height and lose their processes. The cells are 8–10 μm wide, and taller over the pars plana (10–15 μm) than the pars plicata (8–12 μm). The rounded, or sometimes elliptical, pigment granules of the epithelium are about 3–4 times larger than those in the cells of the choroid and retina. Pigment obscures the oval nuclei of the cells, and is responsible for the darker colour (except over the ciliary processes). Foci of nodular hyperplasia, protruding into the stroma, regularly affect the pars plana, and less so the pars plicata.

Ultrastructural studies show the cells to be rich in organelles, although less so than the non-pigmented epithelium. Fibrillar structures resembling tonofilaments have been found (Misotten, 1964). The basal membranes of the cells are in-folded, and related to the anterior basal lamina which, however, does not follow the finest undulations. The lateral membranes interdigitate moderately, while the apical membranes are apposed to those of the non-pigmented cells, and undulate gently.

Non-pigmented epithelium

This is homologous with the inner layer of the optic cup and there is a relatively abrupt transition between the neuroretina and the epithelium at the ora serrata. The epithelium is continuous anteriorly with the posterior epithelium of the iris at the iris root. Some cells may be pigmented in this transition zone.

In youth, the cells are regular; cuboidal over the pars plicata (12–15 μm wide and 10–15 μm high over the crests of the ciliary processes) and columnar over the pars plana (6–9 μm wide and 30 μm high). Cell

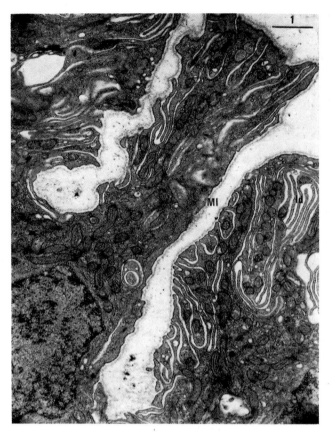

Fig. 10.37 Ciliary process of the monkey. Within the folds of the ciliary processes, in the non-pigmented epithelium, crypts and interdigitations (Id) extend in continuity with the superficial extensions of the plasmalemma. MI = Membrana limitans externa. Original magnification ×7000. (From van der Zypen, E. (1971) *Aging and Development*, published by F. K. Schattauer.)

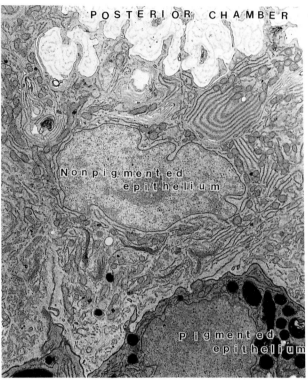

Fig. 10.38 Pars plicata of the ciliary body of *Macaca mulatta*; details of the interface between the two layers of the ciliary epithelium. The apices of the pigmented and non-pigmented epithelia face one another and are separated by an intercellular space of normal width. Original magnification ×11 000. (Courtesy of G. Raviola.)

height is greatest next to the ora serrata, possibly in response to vitreous traction, and increases with age.

Ultrastructural studies show abundant organelles, in keeping with the secretory functions of these cells (Fig. 10.38). Mitochondria, near the base of the cell, are very numerous and increase with age (Hara *et al.*, 1977) (Fig. 10.39a). There is a well-developed rough endoplasmic reticulum, often stacked in parallel perinuclear arrays, and the cisternae of the smooth endoplasmic reticulum are well distributed in the cell (Holmberg, 1959a; Fine and Zimmerman, 1963; Hogan, Alvarado and Weddell, 1971) (Fig. 10.39b). The apical surfaces of the cells are smooth and applied to those of the pigmented epithelium although, here and there, the space between them may be expanded to form a ciliary channel (Fig. 10.40). The lateral surfaces interdigitate along their basal third. With age, lateral intercellular spaces develop in which a glycosaminoglycan-like material may be

identified. It has been suggested that these cells, rich in Golgi complexes, secrete hyaluronic acid into the vitreous (Fine and Zimmerman, 1963). The basal surfaces are deeply in-folded at the perimeter of each cell in the pars plicata (34–62 folds per cell; Holmberg, 1955). With age, the epithelial cells become less regular. The basal in-foldings of the cells of the ciliary valleys and lateral walls of the ciliary processes become irregular while those of the pars plana become grossly elongated, as if stretched. The basal infoldings and lateral interdigitations of the plasma membrane increase the surface area of the cells. This is greatly exaggerated over the anterior half of the ciliary processes, supporting the notion that this region is the site of aqueous secretion (Baraiti and Orzalesi, 1966; Raviola, 1971, 1974; Rentsch and van der Zypen, 1971; van der Zypen and Rentsch, 1971; Smith and Rudt, 1973; Hara *et al.*, 1977; Raviola and Raviola, 1978; Ober and Rohen, 1979; Ohnishi and Kuwabara, 1979). The enzyme carbonic anhydrase is also located here in all species studied (Muther and Friedland, 1980).

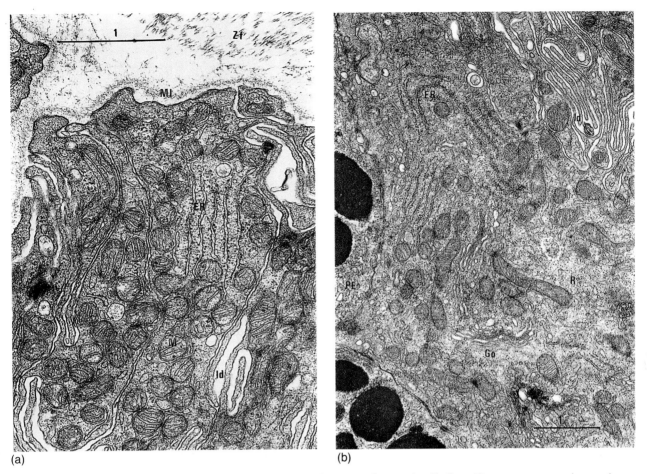

(a)   (b)

Fig. 10.39   (a) Ciliary process of the monkey; basal region of the non-pigmented epithelium. The numerous round or oval mitochondria show no relationship to the interdigitations (Id). ER = Endoplasmic reticulum; M = mitochondria; Ml = membrana limitans; Zf = zonular fibres. Original magnification ×18 000; (b) ciliary process of the monkey. Non-pigmented epithelial cell. The Golgi complex consists of lamellar and vesicular elements. The cell is well supplied with granular endoplasmic reticulum and free ribosomes. Original magnification ×10 000. (From van der Zypen, E. (1971) *Aging and Development*, published by F. K. Schattauer.)

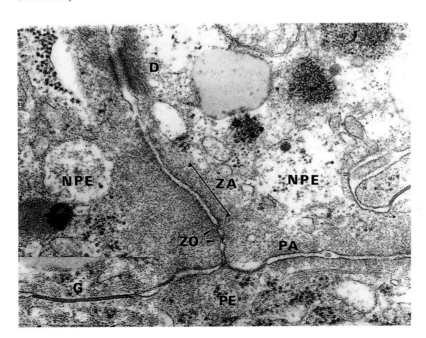

Fig. 10.40   Apical junction of two non-pigmented epithelial cells (NPE) showing focal zonula occludens (ZO), junctions (arrowheads), an adjacent zonula adherens (ZA), desmosome (D), puncta adhaerentes (PA) and gap junctions (G). PE = Pigmented epithelium. Original magnification ×58 700. (From Streeten, B. W. in Duane, T. D. and Jaeger, E. A. (eds) (1992) *Biomedical Foundations of Ophthalmology*, published by Harper and Row, with permission.)

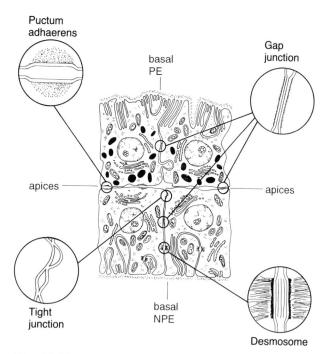

Fig. 10.41 Diagrammatic representation of the junctions between the ciliary epithelial cells. Redrawn from Raviola *et al.*, 1977.

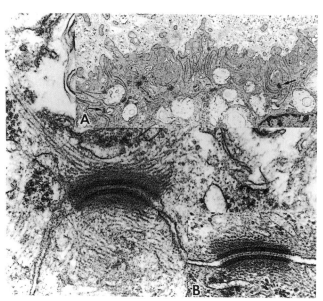

Fig. 10.42 A desmosome cut slightly obliquely showing tonofilaments inserting into the dense plaque material. Original magnification ×104 000. Inset A: Anterior pars plicata. The basement membrane does not enter the extensive surface infoldings and lateral interdigitations of the non-pigmented epithelium. Note large numbers of desmosomal intercellular junctions (arrows). Original magnification ×10 800. Inset B: Central dense core and plasmalemmal unit membranes of desmosomes cut perpendicularly. Original magnification ×104 000. (From Streeten, B. W. in Duane, T. D. and Jaeger, E. A. (eds) (1992) *Biomedical Foundations of Ophthalmology*, published by Harper and Row, with permission.)

Cellular junctions

The cellular junctions within and between the pigmented and non-pigmented epithelia are important to the secretory role of the ciliary processes (Cole, 1977) and have been summarized by Raviola (Raviola, 1971, 1974, 1977; Raviola and Raviola, 1975) (Fig. 10.41). **Zonulae occludentae** occlude the lateral surfaces of the non-pigmented cells close to their apices. They are morphologically more complex in the anterior pars plicata than the posterior, but complexity increases towards the pars plana. **Gap junctions** connect the lateral surfaces of the pigmented and (less frequently) the non-pigmented cells. A continuous row of **gap junctions** alternating with **puncta adhaerentia** is found at the interface between pigmented and non-pigmented cells. The puncta adhaerentes are thought to give strength to intercellular junctions and may provide attachment for actin-like cytoplasmic filaments (Raviola and Raviola, 1978). Their density is greatest in the ciliary valleys, where they may serve to counteract the pull of the ciliary zonules. Finally, **desmosomes** are commonly found between the lateral surfaces of the non-pigmented cells, less often between pigmented cells and at the apical interfaces (Fig. 10.42).

The zonulae occludentes are impermeable to the diffusion of macromolecular tracers from either side (Revel and Karnovsky, 1967). Freeze fracture

demonstrates the presence of anastomosing strands at the interfaces, and their varying complexity between different cells and at different regions probably explains why the ciliary epithelium is not totally impermeable to water and small ions (Raviola, 1977; Noske *et al.*, 1994). However, such diffusion is restricted, and the barrier is sufficiently tight for osmotic work to be performed across the epithelium. Thus, there is a selective transport of certain ions and molecules which are found in the aqueous humour in higher concentration than a plasma filtrate (e.g. bicarbonate and ascorbate) while others (e.g. calcium and urea) are transported at a lower concentration (Cole, 1977, 1984; Davson, 1980).

The presence of gap junctions in the epithelia suggests that the ciliary epithelial cells are electrically coupled and act as a functional syncytium. This coupling probably ensures co-ordination of the secretory activity of the ciliary epithelium. Most junctions occur at a smooth interface, but 'invaginating' gap junctions, occurring at sites of complementary interdigitation, are found between contiguous pigment cells, and between pigment cells and the non-pigmented cells. A few gap junctions are

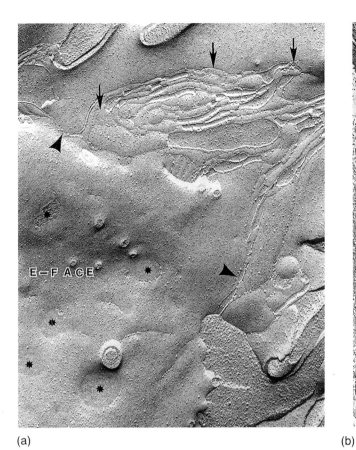

(a)

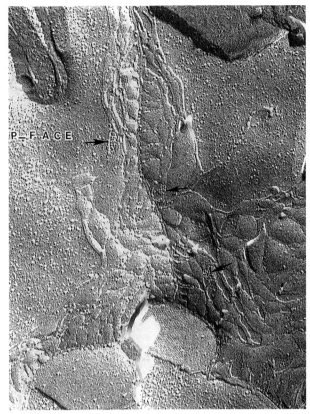

(b)

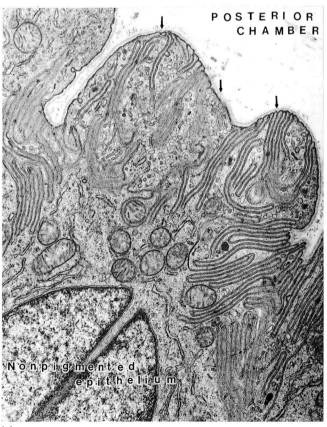

(c)

Fig. 10.43 (a) Freeze-fracture of rabbit ciliary epithelium. The fracture has exposed the E-face of the lateroapical surface of the non-pigmented cell. The zonula occludens is characterized by branching and anastomosing strands. Numerous small gap junctions between non-pigmented cells (arrows) are inserted into the tight junction. Note that the complexity of the zonula occludens varies in different regions of the cell surface; in places it consists of two or three strands only (arrowheads). This feature is typical of epithelia with high hydraulic conductivity. The asterisks at the lower left corner indicate gap junctions that connect a non-pigmented cell to a neighbouring pigmented cell. Original magnification ×75 000; (b) freeze-fracture of ciliary epithelium at the site where three or more cells abut. The zonula occludens is characterized by long strands that run parallel to the cell edge; these are interconnected in a ladder-like pattern by short strands oriented at right-angles. Gap junctions (arrows) are inserted into the zonula occludens. Original magnification ×125 000; (c) TEM of rabbit ciliary process, showing a part of the base of a non-pigmented cell. The basal plasma membrane rests on a basal lamina (arrows) and is deeply and repeatedly invaginated. Such a feature is typical of actively transporting epithelia. Original magnification ×15 000. (Courtesy of G. Raviola.)

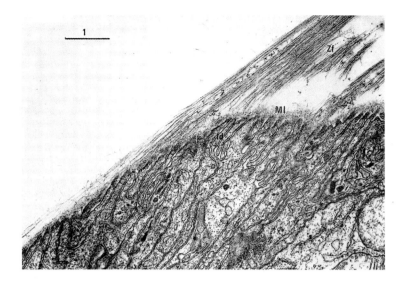

Fig. 10.44 Human ciliary process. Basal region of the non-pigmented epithelium to show the zonular fibres arising from the membrana limitans externa. Ml = Membrana limitans; Zf = zonular fibres; Id = interdigitations. Original magnification ×9000. (From van der Zypen, E. (1971) *Aging and Development*, published by F. K. Schattauer.)

associated with the zonulae occludentae between non-pigmented cells. Freeze-fracture studies show great variation in the intramembrane particles of the gap junctions, from discrete aggregates to hexagonal arrays (Fig. 10.43) (Raviola, 1977).

The internal limiting membrane (membrana limitans interna ciliaris)

The basal lamina of the non-pigmented epithelium lies on its basal (vitreal) surface, is thin and uniform, and is continuous with the internal limiting membranes of the retina posteriorly and the iris anteriorly. It gives origin to parts of the suspensory ligament of the lens (Fig. 10.44). In the infant this is a typical, thin basal lamina with granular layer (30 nm) separated from the plasma membrane by a lamina lucida (50 nm). From the age of 3 years the basal lamina remarkably thickened, and has the appearance of a multilaminar reticular layer. The thickening starts in the valleys of the posterior half of the pars plicata, extends posteriorly and onto the lateral walls of the ciliary processes, and affects most of the ciliary epithelium by the age of 50 years (Rentsch and van der Zypen, 1971; Streeten, 1982) (Fig. 10.45). The basal laminae of the pigmented and non-pigmented epithelia contains I, III and IV and also laminin.

THE NERVE SUPPLY OF THE CILIARY BODY AND IRIS

The short posterior ciliary nerves lie in the outer choroid and branch near the ora serrata to form a rich plexus of myelinated and unmyelinated nerves which supply the iris and ciliary body (Fig. 10.46). At each nerve bifurcation is a triangular thickening from which innumerable fibres emerge.

Parasympathetic fibres

The general features of the ciliary body innervation are as follows: parasympathetic fibres run from the Edinger–Westphal nucleus via the inferior division of the oculomotor nerve. These are mixed myelinated and unmyelinated fibres, the majority of which have their cell bodies (third neurone) in the ciliary ganglion. They form an extensive plexus within the ciliary muscle. They supply the iris sphincter and ciliary muscles. Ectopic ganglion cells, said to be parasympathetic in nature, have been demonstrated in the ciliary body plexus (Bryson, Wolter and O'Keefe, 1966) along the long posterior ciliary nerves, within the eye, and also between the ciliary ganglion and the globe. Ruskell (1982), in primate studies, could not demonstrate a significant contribution of such fibres to the iris and ciliary body musculature (Ruskell and Griffiths, 1979).

Sympathetic fibres

These run from the cervical sympathetic trunk. These fibres synapse (third neurone) in the superior cervical ganglion, not in the ciliary ganglion, and are distributed to the ciliary and iris muscles via the long ciliary nerve (Ruskell, 1973). In the monkey, about 1–2% of ciliary muscle terminals are of sympathetic origin. Sympathetic fibres which accompany the ciliary arteries are distributed extensively within the ciliary plexuses.

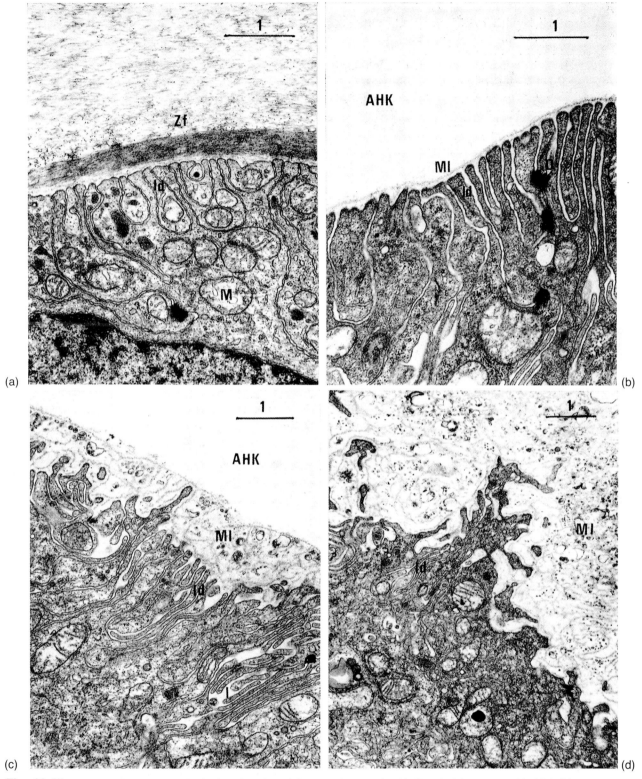

(a)

(b)

(c)

(d)

Fig. 10.45   Human ciliary process in the basal region of the non-pigmented epithelium in (a) a 4-year-old child; (b) an 8-year-old child; (c) a 17-year-old man; (d) an 85-year-old woman. The membrana limitans externa thickens with age and becomes increasingly netlike in structure. Osmiophilic granules are found in the meshes of the network. The basal interdigitations are fully developed by the age of 8 years. Later they become more complicated and are enveloped by cellular protrusions. AHK = Posterior chamber; D = desmosome; I = intercellular space; Id = interdigitation; M = mitochondria; Ml = membrana limitans; Zf = zonular fibres. Original magnifications: (a) ×11 000; (b) ×11 000; (c) ×10 000; (d) ×8000. (From van der Zypen, E. (1971) *Aging and Development*, published by F. K. Schattauer.)

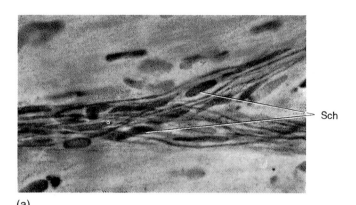

(a)

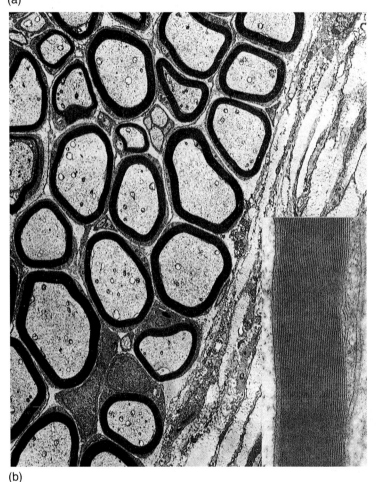

(b)

Fig. 10.46 (a) Basal nerve plexus between the sclera and ciliary body in the human. Frequent Schwann cell nuclei can be seen (Richardson stain; original magnification ×512). (From van der Zypen, E. *Aging and Development*, published by F. K. Schattauer, 1971); (b) Myelinated nerve fibres in the ciliary body (rhesus monkey, electron micrograph, ×75 000). Note the nuclei of satellite cells in the lower part of the filla. The inset shows myelin lamination in longitudinal section at higher magnification. (Courtesy of Dr John Marshall and Mr P. L. Ansell, Institute of Ophthalmology, London.)

Sensory fibres

These run from the nasociliary branch of the ophthalmic division of the trigeminal nerve, running in the long ciliary nerves. These fibres enter the ciliary body and terminate in iris, cornea and ciliary muscle. They are recognized by their club-shaped endings.

In 12% of human eyes, a loop of ciliary nerve (the intrascleral nerve loop of Axenfeld), 1–2 mm in size, may be found within the scleral channel of an anterior ciliary artery perforator, usually associated with pigment. The loops are most common inferiorly.

Nerve fibres pass from a plexus between the sclera and the ciliary body stroma to form an extensive plexus within the ciliary muscle. Fibres pass from here to form an additional plexus in relation to the ciliary epithelium. Nerve terminals containing synaptic vesicles can be found in relation to the pigmented epithelium (Fig. 10.47) and to capillaries (Fig. 10.48) within the ciliary body. Some terminals are characteristic of parasympathetic nerve endings

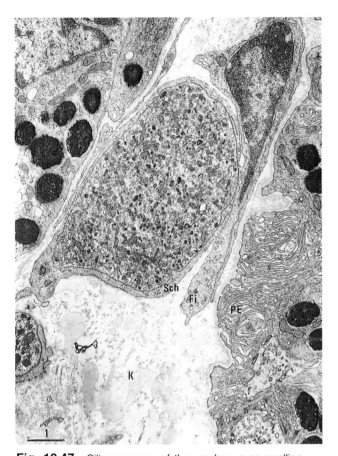

Fig. 10.47 Ciliary process of the monkey: axon swelling. Within the ciliary fold is an axon swelling 15 μm wide, which is stuffed with granular and agranular vesicles and full of small mitochondria and lamellar bodies. Fi = Fibroblast; K = collagenous connective tissue; PE = pigmented epithelium; Sch = Schwann cell. Original magnification ×6000. (From van der Zypen, E. (1971) *Aging and Development*, published by F. K. Schattauer.)

(Fig. 10.49), and some of adrenergic endings (but see below) (Fig. 10.50). Van der Zypen (1967) has demonstrated interaxonal synapses (Fig. 10.51) and occasional ganglionic synapses within the ciliary body (Fig. 10.52).

Ciliary smooth muscle

The ciliary muscle is a fast, multi-unit smooth muscle innervated by oculomotor, parasympathetic axons (Bozler, 1948). Each individual smooth muscle cell is surrounded by about 10–15 visceroefferent nerve endings, 0.5–1.0 μm wide, which stain intensely for synaptophysin. Extrinsic fibres arise in the Edinger–Westphal nucleus and synapse in the ciliary ganglion (Warwick, 1954; Ruskell, 1979). Degeneration studies in the monkey eye indicate that 97% of ciliary neurons supply the ciliary muscle and 3% supply the iris sphincter.

Ciliary muscle innervation

Individual ciliary muscle cells in monkeys (van der Zypen, 1967; Tamm *et al.*, 1990) and humans (Ishikawa, 1962) are richly innervated; the density of muscarinic and cholinergic nerve endings greater than in other tissues (Bárány *et al.*, 1982; Erickson-Lamy *et al.*, 1987). Sympathetic innervation is of minor physiological significance. Varicose nerve terminals are present which are positive for NPY, CGRP, VIP and SP.

In addition to its **extrinsic nerve supply**, there is also an **intrinsic ganglionic network** within the ciliary muscle (the plexus gangliosus ciliaris (Müller, 1859;

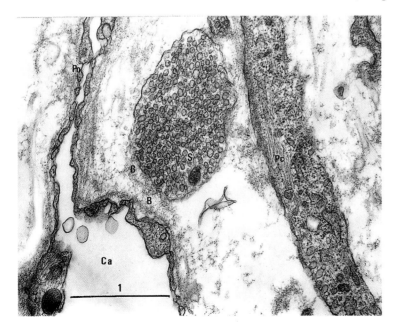

Fig. 10.48 Ciliary process in the monkey: nerve bundles. Free nerve endings, full of synaptic vesicles, are found close to a fenestrated capillary. B = Basal lamina; Ca = capillary lumen; Pc = pinocytotic vesicle; Po = pore; S = synaptic vesicles. Original magnification ×18 000. (From van der Zypen, E. (1971) *Aging and Development*, published by F. K. Schattauer.)

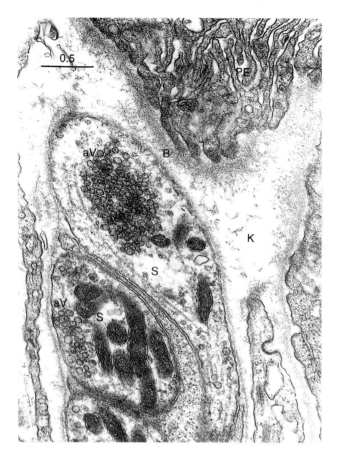

Fig. 10.49 Ciliary process of the monkey: innervation of the ciliary epithelium. A synaptic terminal supplied with neurotubules is shown, containing numerous agranular vesicles.
ac = Agranular vesicles; B = basal lamina; K = connective tissue; S = synaptic terminal; PE = pigmented epithelium. Original magnification × 18 000. (From van der Zypen, E. (1971) *Aging and Development*, published by F. K. Schattauer.)

Krause, 1861; Iwanoff, 1874; Lauber, 1936; Krummel, 1938; Kurus, 1955; Bryson, Walter and O'Keefe, 1966; Castro-Correira, 1967) whose features have recently been characterized by Tamm *et al.* (1995a). The plexus is located between the muscle bundles of the reticular and circular parts of the ciliary muscle, in the connective tissue spaces or close to the fibroblastic sheaths. **Ganglion cells** are not found within muscle bundles and are lacking entirely in the anterior longitudinal muscle. This presumably has a functional significance. Several ganglion cells may be found along the inner border of the ciliary muscle. The ganglion cells are usually solitary and only occasionally grouped in twos (Fig. 10.53).

Ganglia are oval in shape with large euchromatic nuclei, prominent nucleoli and clear cytoplasm. They are either small (70%), ranging from 10–14 μm in length, or large (30%), about 20–30 μm in length. On the whole, they are smaller than the ganglion cells associated with other viscera, which may explain the failure to identify them in some studies (Boeke, 1933; Hirano, 1941; van der Zypen, 1967). The ganglia are enclosed by a thin mantle of densely staining glial cells, and are closely related to numerous preterminal, unmyelinated axons and several terminal boutons (Figs 10.54 and 10.55). The boutons make axosomatic contact with perikarya and contain mitochondria, numerous small agranular vesicles (20–60 nm), and some large granular vesicles (60–120 nm). Some axodendritic synapses are also found, in which large granular vesicles are more frequent.

The ganglia and their axons, which are sometimes varicose, are nitrergic, staining positively for both NADPH-diaphorase and nitric oxide synthase (NO) (Fig. 10.56). In one donor eye studied by Tamm *et al.*

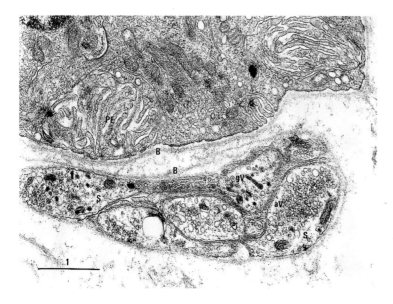

Fig. 10.50 Ciliary process of the monkey: innervation of the ciliary epithelium. In the neuroeffector region there are many synaptic terminals (S), containing both granular (gV) and agranular vesicles (aV). B = Basal lamina; PE = pigment epithelial cell. Original magnification ×12 000. (From van der Zypen, E. (1971) *Aging and Development*, published by F. K. Schattauer.)

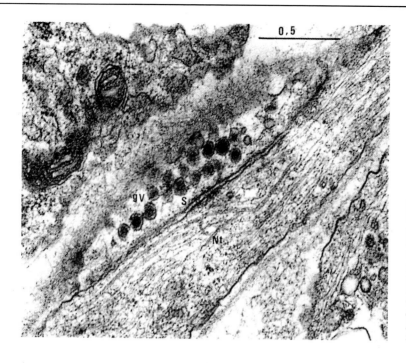

Fig. 10.51 Ciliary process of the monkey: innervation of the ciliary epithelium. Pre- and postsynaptic membrane thickenings are shown in the region of the interaxonal synapses. The region containing the granular vesicles (gV) is regarded as the presynaptic part of the axon.
Nt = Neurotubules; S = synaptic terminal. Original magnification ×20 000. (From van der Zypen, E. (1971) *Aging and Development*, published by F. K. Schattauer.)

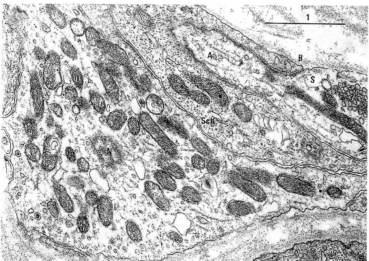

Fig. 10.52 Ciliary process of the monkey: ganglion cell. Occasionally, small ganglion cells, with light staining cytoplasm, may be found in stroma of the ciliary processes.
A = Axon; B = basal lamina; N = nucleus; S = synaptic terminal; Sch = Schwann cell. Original magnification ×12 500. (From van der Zypen, E. (1971) *Aging and Development*, published by F. K. Schattauer.)

(1995) there were 923 axons in the entire ciliary muscle (this compares with the total number of nerve cells in the ciliary ganglion of 1088 to 6835, mean 2394 (Perez and Keyser, 1986)). The perikarya receive arborizing or encircling terminal boutons which coexpress SP or CGRP.

There is faint staining of the endothelia of the ciliary muscle capillaries, in the absence of a perivascular neural network. By contrast, there is a rich nitrergic perivascular network in the major circle of the iris (lying within the circular part of the ciliary muscle), apparently connected with the ganglionic plexus.

The function of the ganglia in the ciliary body is not yet known. The nitrergic fibres of the ciliary muscle plexus may serve to relax it. Nitrergic stimulation will, for instance, relax isolated bovine ciliary muscle (Wiederholt *et al.*, 1994). Relaxation of the inner part of the ciliary muscle, where the ganglionic plexus is found, would facilitate disaccommodation. Tamm *et al.* (1995) have suggested that active relaxation might contribute to the accommodative microfluctuations said to be necessary for precise focusing (Campbell, Robson and Westheimer, 1959).

It is likely that the SP- and CGRP-positive neurons which synapse with the nitrergic ganglion cells have an extrinsic origin, perhaps in the Edinger–Westphal

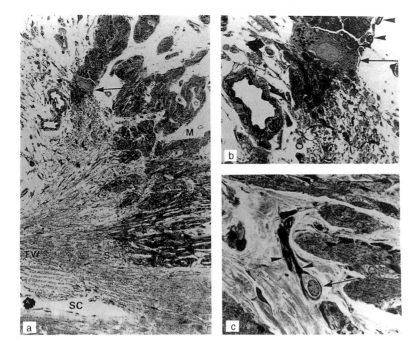

Fig. 10.53 Nerve cells in the human ciliary muscle (semi-thin sections, Richardson's stain); (a) an oval-shaped neuron (arrow) and a longitudinal diameter of 30 μm is situated between the muscle bundles of the circular portion. M = ciliary muscle; S = scleral spur; SC = Schlemm's canal; TW = trabecular meshwork; MA = major arterial circle of the iris. Donor age, 56 years (original magnification ×330); (b) higher magnification of (a) (original magnification ×1000). The nerve cell (arrow) is characterized by a large euchromatic nucleus, lipofuscin particles, and a clear cytoplasm. Myelinated axons (arrowheads) are seen close to the nerve cell; (c) small (longitudinal diameter 11 μm) ciliary muscle neuron (arrow) between the muscle bundles of the reticular portion. Similar to large neurons, small neurons are commonly associated with myelinated axons (arrowheads). Donor age, 71 years. (Original magnification ×1000). (Tamm, E. R., Flügel-Kock, C., Mayer, B. and Lütjen-Drecoll, E. (1995a) *Invest. Ophthalmol. Vis. Sci.*, **36**, 414–426, with permission.)

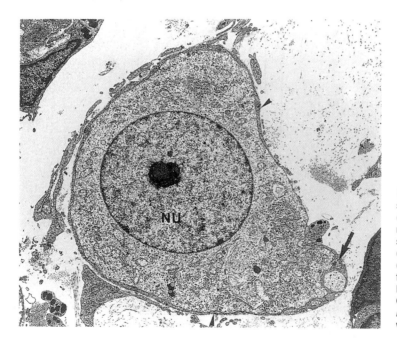

Fig. 10.54 Electron micrograph of a small ganglion cell in the ciliary muscle (consecutive section of Fig. 10.53; original magnification ×12 700). The neuron is surrounded by processes of glia cells (arrowheads). Contacts with nerve terminals (arrow) and preterminal axons are less frequent than in large neurons. NU = nucleus. (Tamm, E. R., Flügel-Kock, C., Mayer, B. and Lütjen-Drecoll, E. (1995a) *Invest. Ophthalmol. Vis. Sci.*, **36**, 414–426, with permission.)

nucleus as is found for SP-immunoreactive neurons in the cat (Maciewicz *et al.*, 1983), or in the ciliary ganglion, as is found for SP- and/or CGRP-positive neurons in the rat, cat and monkey (Stone *et al.*, 1988; Hardebo, 1992; Zhang *et al.*, 1994). These peptidergic neurons are also found in the trigeminal ganglion, and it is thought that their peptides could be released locally from collaterals (for instance through NO release) during an ocular irritative response (Unger, 1989; Bill, 1991). Thus ciliary muscle relaxation could be brought about by an axon reflex. An increase in uveoscleral outflow occurs in experimental iridocyclitis in cynomolgous monkeys (Toris and Pederson, 1987), and could be brought about by relaxation and widening of the ciliary muscle intermuscular spaces (Cuello, 1970).

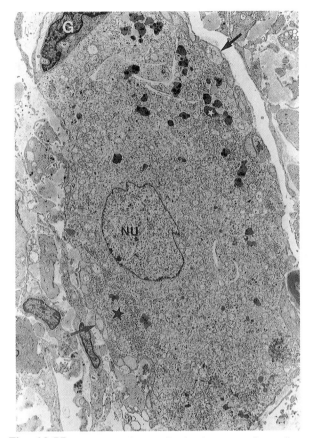

Fig. 10.55 Electron micrograph of a large ganglion cell (same neuron as in Figs. 10.53 and 10.54; original magnification ×7600). The perikaryon of the neuron contains numerous mitochondria and profiles of short, rough endoplasmic reticulum cisterns and free polysomes (black asterisk). Scattered throughout the cytoplasm are large granular vesicles and irregularly shaped lipofuscin granules (white asterisk). The neuron is surrounded by flat processes of glia cells (G), which also surround numerous preterminal, unmyelinated axons (arrows). NU = nucleus. (Tamm, E. R., Flügel-Kock, C., Mayer, B. and Lütjen-Drecoll, E. (1995a) *Invest. Ophthalmol. Vis. Sci.,* **36**, 414–426, with permission.)

10.3 ACCOMMODATION

Accommodation is the act of focussing from distance to near. Dysaccommodation is the reverse of this process. Accommodation is accompanied by pupil constriction, anterior movement of the iris, increase in the anterior and posterior curvatures of the lens, forward translation, and an increase in sagittal thickness (Brown, 1973; Koretz *et al.*, 1989; Brown and Bron, 1996). In the primate, the act of accommodation depends on the inward movement of the anterior part of the ciliary muscle (Rohen, 1979). Ciliary muscle contracts in a dose-related fashion in response to alpha muscarinic drugs such as carbachol, and this action is antagonized by atropine. Morphometric studies with pilocarpine and atropine show that contraction is associated with an increase in area of the circular and reticular part of the muscle, and a decrease in its meridional part. This shortens causing the posterior attachment to move forward and the ciliary muscle mass moves anteriorly and inward, reducing the internal diameter. The anterior end of the muscle is firmly attached to the scleral spur by tendons which are mainly collagenous, but which contain some elastic tissue. In this way, they gain insertion, via the trabecular meshwork into the peripheral cornea (Rohen, 1956; Kupfer, 1962b; Rohen, Lütjen and Bárány, 1967; Rohen *et al.,* 1989).

In contrast, in the young primate, the posterior end of the muscle is attached to the pars plana by a series of elastic tendons, which permit the muscle to move forward during accommodation and rapidly restore the muscle to its relaxed state in dysaccommodation (Iwanoff and Arnold, 1874; Salzmann, 1912a; Lauber, 1936b; Rohen, 1952, 1979). The tendons

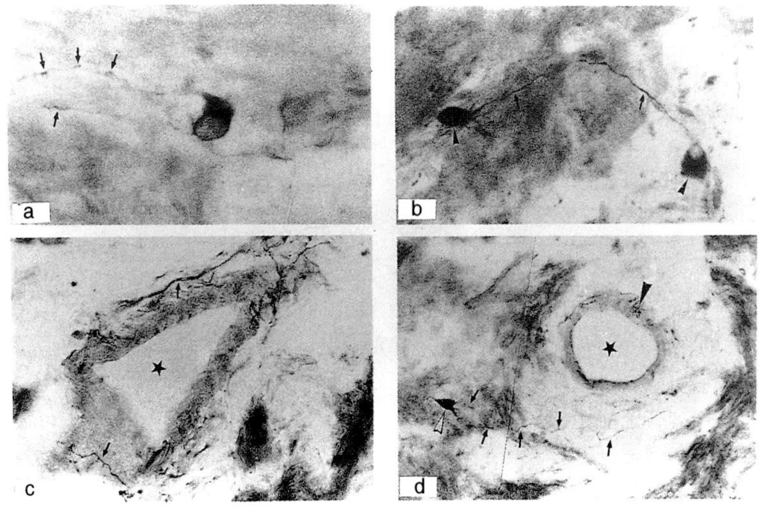

Fig. 10.56 NADPH-diaphorase (NADPH-d)-positive nerve cells in the ciliary muscle (tangential sections); (a) during their course along the muscle bundles, filamentous processes of ciliary muscle neurons express periodic swellings, suggesting varicosities (arrows; original magnification ×1000); (b) two neighbouring nerve cells are in contact with each other by axonal processes (arrows; original magnification ×250); (c) numerous NADPH-d-positive nerve fibres (arrows) are stained in the wall of the major arterial circle of the iris (asterisk; original magnification ×300); (d) the axon of an adjacent nerve cell runs close to and seems to contribute to the perivascular nervous network of the major arterial circle (asterisk; original magnification ×150). (Tamm, E. R., Flügel-Kock, C., Mayer, B. and Lütjen-Drecoll, E. (1995a) *Invest. Ophthalmol. Vis. Sci.,* **36**, 414–426, with permission.)

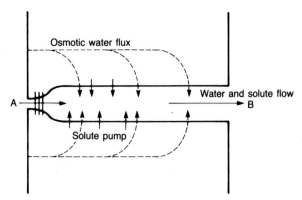

Fig. 10.57 Representation of standing gradient osmotic flow system. The system consists of a long narrow channel, the entry to which is restricted at the left-hand end (A). The density of dots indicates the solute concentration. Solute is actively transported from the cells into the intercellular channel by a solute pump, thus making the channel fluid hypertonic. As the solute diffuses towards the open end of the channel at the right-hand side (B), water enters across the walls because of the osmotic differential. In the steady state a standing gradient will be maintained, with osmolarity decreasing from the restricted to the open end and with volume flow directed towards the open end. In the limiting case, the emergent fluid approaches iso-osmolarity with the intracellular compartments. The arrow on the left-hand side (across the restriction) represents an element of hydraulic flow. (From Davson, 1993, with permission.)

are continuous with the elastic lamina of Bruch's membrane and are also connected to an elastic network in the stroma of the pars plana, between the ciliary muscle and the pigment epithelium. This network surrounds the efferent vessels of the ciliary body. In some places the tendons are in close contact with endothelial cells of pars plana capillaries. This relationship may explain the dilatation of such vessels after prolonged treatment with phospholine iodide in monkeys (Lütjen-Drecoll and Kaufman, 1979). The elastic tendons arise from sarcolemmal invaginations of the muscle cells or from their tips, which are completely embedded in elastic tissue. At sites of cell contact, the cell membranes form electron-dense bands with adhering myofilaments.

On accommodation, a similar process to that described in the monkey is thought to occur in human ciliary muscle. The action of all parts of the ciliary muscle is to slacken the suspensory ligaments of the lens. This results in decreased tension on the capsule of the lens, which therefore becomes more convex (Fincham, 1937). The circular fibres act directly as a sphincter diminishing the circumference of the ring formed by the ciliary body. This probably also applies to the radial portions of the muscle. The posterior attachments of the ciliary muscle, consisting largely of delicate elastic tissue, seem to be admirably

adapted to allow the posterior ends of the muscle to pass forwards during contraction and to guide them back to their original positions on relaxation. All fibres of the muscle, no matter what part, will thicken during contraction. The effect of this will be to increase the cross-sectional diameter of the whole muscle so that the inner border of the muscle moves inwards towards the outer edge of the lens. Thus the whole muscle (including the longitudinal fibres) will in effect act as a sphincter to the ciliary ring. In this connection it should be noted that the ciliary muscle is thickest approximately opposite the equator of the lens. It will therefore bulge most just where one would expect it to have the greatest effect on the zonular fibres.

Opinions have differed as to the mechanism of accommodation and of presbyopia, the loss of accommodative power with age. This has been clarified by the studies of Fisher (1973, 1977, 1982; Fisher and Hayes, 1979) and is admirably reviewed by Weale (1982). The unaccommodated lens has a flattened shape due to the transmission of zonular forces to the lens capsule. In the emmetrope the flattened anterior and posterior curvatures of the lens surfaces achieve a dioptric state giving a clear focus for distance. With age, the anterior and posterior surfaces become more curved, but because there is a reduction in the net refractive index of the lens, the emmetropic state is retained (Chapter 12). According to Rohen, the tension on the zonular fibres is directed radially from the ciliary body at the 'zonular fork' in the plane of the lens equator (Rohen, 1952, 1964b, 1979; Rohen and Rentsch, 1969). Farnsworth and Burke (1977) have described an alternative arrangement of the zonular fibres. Both authors have suggested that the differential change in anterior and posterior capsular curvature which occurs on accommodation is due to the zonular topography. In the dysaccommodated state the anterior lens surface is flatter than the posterior.

During accommodation the shape of the lens changes in such a way as to increase its refractive power, by an increase in the curvature of both the anterior and posterior surfaces; the anterior curvature increases more than the posterior. The anterior pole of the lens moves forwards and the posterior pole is essentially stationary or moves backwards slightly. The cortical thickness is unchanged during accommodation but the sagittal thickness of the nucleus increases and accounts for the thickening of the lens as a whole during accommodation.

In the adult lens, the posterior capsule is about 10% of the thickness of the anterior capsule centrally, and the anterior capsule is further thickened peripherally. Fincham (1937) argued that the change in lens shape during accommodation was generated by the differences in thickness of differing portions of the capsule. It has, however, been suggested that the peripheral thick zone of the anterior capsule is an artefact, and that the role of the capsule is not to mould the underlying lens, but to act as a force distributor (Handelman and Koretz, 1982; Koretz and Handelman, 1982, 1983, 1986). Coleman (1970, 1986) developed a hydraulic suspension theory of accommodation in which he proposed, on the basis of ultrasound studies, that the change in shape of the lens was caused by a rise in vitreous pressure during accommodation and the exertion of a peripheral force on the posterior lens.

It has been shown using ultrasound (Coleman, 1973), that the posterior pole moves back 40% less than the forward movement of the anterior pole. Fisher (1982), however, has shown that this difference in movement of the two poles of the lens in accommodation is independent of the presence of the vitreous body behind the lens, and that its elastic recovery depends solely on the intrinsic physical properties of the lens (its elastic anisotropy) which are thought to differ in the sagittal and equatorial planes.

Accommodation is mediated via the parasympathetic stimulation of the ciliary muscle. A small degree of parasympathetic tone may be abolished by atropine, to produce a hypermetropia of one dioptre in the emmetrope. A weak sympathetic inhibitory effect on accommodation has been suggested but the sympathetic contribution to ciliary muscular innervation is probably small. Thus cocaine, a sympathetic agonist, weakens accommodation slightly (Fuchs) and **tightens** the capsule after post-traumatic absorption of the lens substance to a greater extent in distance viewing (Graves), and in Horner's syndrome the near point of accommodation is said to be closer to the eye on the affected side.

10.4 PRESBYOPIA

Presbyopia is the reduction in the range of accommodation or accommodative power which occurs with ageing. It implies a recession of the near point, while the far point is unaffected. It also implies a reduction in the rate of both accommodation and dysaccommodation.

Various events occur within the ciliary body of the aged primate eye, which reflect a muscular component to presbyopia. A significant event which has been established in both the monkey (Nieder et al., 1990) and the human eye (Hollins, 1974; Enoch, 1976), is the reduced or absent forward movement of

the ciliary body, on accommodation, which occurs with age. The reduction in ciliary muscle area in meridional section, which occurs in the monkey, might indicate a loss of contractile cells, but although degenerative changes have been observed both in the ciliary muscle cells and nerves, these are not of marked degree, and have been discounted by some as the major factor in primate presbyopia. Of possibly greater relevance, at least for the loss of accommodative ability in the aged monkey, is the thickening and altered morphology which occurs in the posterior elastic tendons, consisting of a pronounced increase in the collagenous and microfibrillar content of the tendons. The tendons become almost completely ensheathed by collagenous fibrils, and the homogeneous part of the elastic tissue takes on an electronlucent fibrillogranular appearance under electron microscopy, and contains abnormal scattered microfibrils (Tamm et al., 1990). Lütjen-Drecoll and Rohen have postulated that this structural change causes a loss in compliance of the posterior insertion of the ciliary muscle in the monkey and limits the critical anterior-inward movement of the muscle during contraction, which is essential to achieve zonular relaxation.

These age-related ciliary muscle changes not only parallel a progressive decline in accommodative amplitude (Bito et al., 1982; Kaufmann et al., 1983), but in the primate are associated with a decreased responsiveness to pilocarpine (Lütjen-Drecoll et al., 1988) and to electrical stimulation of the Edinger–Westphal nucleus (Bito et al., 1987). These events are unassociated with any change in muscarinic receptor affinity or density, or in the muscle content of choline acetyl transferase or acetylcholinesterase (True-Gabelt et al., 1987).

Certain differences exist between the structure of normal human and monkey ciliary muscle, and differences have also been reported between the age-related changes in humans (Stieve, 1949; Rohen, 1989) and monkeys (Lütjen-Drecoll et al., 1988b). In the aged human muscle there is certainly a **marked** increase in extracellular material and a pronounced sclerosis and hyalinization of connective tissue lying between the muscle bundles. In the monkey, however, there is only a **limited** increase in intermuscular connective tissue and hyalinization is uncommon, except in monkeys of extreme age.

Accommodative power is at a maximum in youth (10–12 dioptres or more (Brückner, 1959)) and decreases in humans with age (Duane, 1912; Hamasaki et al., 1956). By 50 years of age, the accommodative amplitude is about 2 dioptres, and much of this is accounted for by the pinhole effect of the pupil, and the intrinsic depth of focus of the lens itself (Koretz, 1994).

Helmholtz (1855) supposed that presbyopia was due to a failure of the lens to change its shape with age, despite increasing power of the ciliary muscle. To some extent this view has been borne out by Fisher (1977), who has shown that the amount of ciliary force required to produce a given change in dioptric power of the human lens increases with age. This relates to such factors as increasing lens volume, lens mass and increasing stiffness of the lens. After the age of 30 years the force required to produce maximum accommodation rises steadily to about 50 years of age. Thereafter it probably falls slightly. It has been estimated that by the age of 50 years the ciliary muscle is probably 50% more powerful than in youth. Notwithstanding this, the rate of accommodation is said to be slower, for example at the age of 40 years, than at 10 years (Allen, 1956). As Koretz (1994) has pointed out, such a finding would be influenced by the topography of zonular attachment, as well as by factors confined to the lens itself.

Structural changes occur in the ciliary muscle with age (Stieve, 1949; van der Zypen, 1970). There is a marked increase in numbers of muscle fibres in the first few months of life and continuing through the first decade. From 10–60 years of age there is an increase in interstitial connective tissue with progressive replacement of muscle fibres posteriorly by connective tissue anteriorly, so that the muscle becomes expanded anteriorly. There is a continuous decrease in meridional area and length with age so that, after the age of 60 years, the longitudinal and radial (reticular) portions of the muscle atrophy while the area at the circular part increases. Tamm *et al.* (1992) have reported that the inner, apical region of the ciliary body moves forwards and inwards with age. This would be expected to cause a reduction in tension in the zonule and a reduced range of accommodation. It would also lead to an increase in curvature of the lens surfaces, simulating accommodative events in youth and causing a sagittal thickening normally attributed in part to lens growth. Such an increased sagittal width of the lens would be partly masked by nuclear compaction in the first two decades of life.

10.5 AMETROPIA

Morphological differences in ciliary muscle development have long been noted in ammetropia. The circular fibres are better developed in the hypermetrope than the myope, for instance (Iwanoff, 1874). This has been attributed to consistent differences in the need for accommodative effort in these two refractive states, but may also reflect differences in the length of the eye, the long myopic eye exhibiting a long ciliary muscle.

10.6 AQUEOUS SECRETION

Aqueous humour is secreted into the posterior chamber predominantly by a process of active transport in which ions are transported across the ciliary epithelium, creating an osmotic gradient leading to a flow of water (Fig. 10.57). Cole (1977) has suggested that the non-pigmented cells of the ciliary epithelium selectively absorb sodium ions from the ciliary stroma and transport them into the intercellular clefts. These are open at the aqueous humour side. The hyperosmolarity in the clefts leads to an osmotic flow of water from the stroma into the clefts and a continuous flow of fluid into the posterior chamber as aqueous humour. Shiose (1971) has localized ATPase in the membranes of the non-pigmented cells of the ciliary epithelium, and various workers have demonstrated a reduced transport of Na^+ into the aqueous humour by cardiac glycosides such as ouabain, which inhibit Na^+, K^+-activated ATPase and reduce aqueous secretion. The passage of other ions such as chloride, bicarbonate and potassium may also be controlled by independent active processes, whilst others may diffuse passively down concentration gradients established by the primary process; the same may apply to sugars and certain amino acids (Davson, 1980). Inhibition of bicarbonate secretion with the carbonic anhydrase inhibitor acetazolamide is used clinically to reduce aqueous secretion in patients with glaucoma. Beta-adrenergic and serotonergic receptors have been localized to the ciliary epithelium, and beta receptor antagonists are used clinically in glaucoma to reduce aqueous secretion (Coakes and Brubaker 1978).

CHAPTER ELEVEN

The choroid and uveal vessels

The uveal tract or **vascular tunic** of the eye consists of the iris, ciliary body and choroid which extend in continuity from before backwards. It is easily demarcated from sclera and cornea as a dark brown sphere attached to the optic nerve behind and exhibiting in front a central aperture, the pupil. Its name (*tunica uvea* or *uveal tract*) derives from its resemblance to a grape (*uva*), when exposed after scleral removal (Figs 6.4 and 6.5).

11.1   ARTERIES OF THE UVEAL TRACT

The arterial supply is divided into two more or less distinct parts: the **anterior** and **long posterior ciliary arteries** supply the iris and ciliary body and the anterior choroid is supplied by recurrent branches of the anterior ciliary arteries, perforating branches of the anterior ciliary arteries, and branches of the ciliary intramuscular artery; the **short posterior ciliary arteries** supply most of the choroid.

The ciliary arteries supply the whole of the uveal tract, the sclera, limbus and its adjacent conjunctiva, and comprise:

1.   the medial and lateral posterior ciliary arteries;
2.   the short posterior ciliary arteries;
3.   the long posterior ciliary arteries;
4.   the anterior ciliary arteries.

The posterior ciliary arteries and their branches have been extensively studied by Hayreh (1962, 1974a,b,c, 1975).

MEDIAL AND LATERAL POSTERIOR CILIARY ARTERIES

One medial and one lateral posterior ciliary artery arise from the ophthalmic artery while it crosses the optic nerve in the orbit (Fig. 11.1). There is an occasional superior posterior ciliary artery. These arteries divide into 10–20 branches which run forward, surround the nerve, and pierce the eyeball around it. Most constitute the short ciliary arteries, while one medial and one lateral branch become the long posterior ciliary arteries.

SHORT POSTERIOR CILIARY ARTERIES

The majority, and the largest of the short posterior ciliaries, after giving branches to the sclera, pierce it in the region temporal to the optic nerve and overlying the macula (Fig. 11.2). A small number, of smaller size, pierce the sclera around but closer to the optic nerve. The **scleral canals** are short and almost directly anteroposterior. The space around the vessels contains loose tissue which is a prolongation of the suprachoroid (Fig. 11.3). The short posterior ciliary arteries are formed by the second- and third-order divisions of the posterior ciliary arteries, close to the optic nerve head. As noted, there are more numerous, distal branches, and a smaller number of paraoptic branches, closer to the optic nerve head (Olver, Spalton and McCartney, 1990). The distal short posterior ciliary arteries arise more proximally on the temporal side (Ducournou, 1982). Olver, Spalton and McCartney (1990) have described the arrangement in further detail, based on the study of vascular casts (see Chapter 10).

The smaller, paraoptic arteries supply the peripapillary choroid and a vertical trapezoid strip of choroid above and below the optic nerve head either directly, or indirectly through branches of the anastomotic circle of Zinn (1755) and Haller (1754), which they form. The circle also supplies the

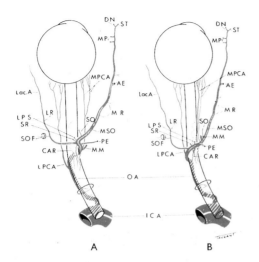

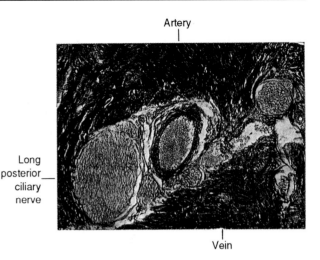

Fig. 11.1 The pattern of branching of the ophthalmic artery when it crosses (a) under and (b) over the optic nerve.
AE = anterior ethmoidal artery; DN = dorsal nasal artery;
CAR = central retinal artery; ICA = internal carotid artery;
LacA = lacrimal artery; LPS = artery to levator; LPCA = long posterior ciliary artery; LR = artery to lateral rectus;
MM = middle meningeal; MP = medial palpebral;
MPCCA = medial posterior ciliary artery; MR = artery to medial rectus; MSO = artery to superior oblique; OA = ophthalmic artery; PE = posterior ethmoidal artery; SO = artery to superior oblique; SR = artery to superior rectus; ST = supratrochlear.
(From Hayreh, S. S. in Cant, S. (ed.) (1976) *Vision and Circulation*, published by Henry Kimpton, with permission.)

Fig. 11.3 Transverse section of the canal showing a long posterior ciliary artery and nerve. Note the accompanying nerves and vessels. The veins are scleral veins and do not correspond to the long ciliary artery.

retrolaminar part of the optic nerve. There is disagreement as to the frequency of this vascular circle: Olver, Spalton and McCartney (1990) report that it is frequently present, while Hayreh (1964) found it only in a small proportion of normal eyes.

Most authors agree that the vascular circle is often incomplete and it may be this fact that has led to controversy. In the absence of this circular anastomosis, its place is taken by small branches of the paraoptic short ciliary arteries, which lie within the sclera and supply portions of the optic nerve head and sometimes the adjacent retina. It is absent in non-human primates (Hayreh, 1964).

In its complete form the circle (usually a horizontal ellipse) of Haller and Zinn is an intrascleral anastomosis between branches of the medial and lateral paraoptic short posterior ciliary arteries (Olver,

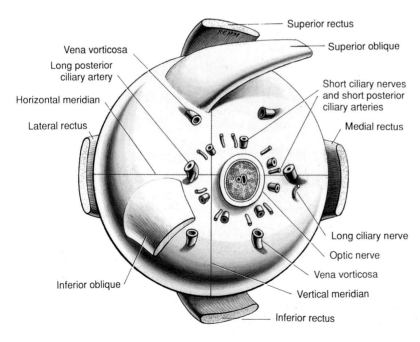

Fig. 11.2 The globe of the left eye seen from behind to reveal the attachment of the oblique muscles and the optic nerve, also the points of entry of the ciliary arteries and nerves and the exits of the venae vorticosae. Note that the inferior oblique is fleshy almost up to its insertion and that the venae vorticosae appear to converge towards a common trunk.

Spalton and McCartney, 1990). (This anastomosis must be distinguished from a more proximal extra-scleral anastomosis formed by separate short posterior ciliary arteries lying superiorly to the optic nerve in some eyes.) Incomplete, upper or lower arcuate anastomoses are also seen, or sometimes overlapping non-anastomosing upper and lower segments. The circle may be anteriorly placed, in which case it lies closer to the choroid within the sclera, or it may lie more posteriorly, when the superior and inferior parts are partially or completely extrascleral. Similarly, according to the radius of the circle, it may be situated close to or further away from the scleral opening.

The branches of the circle of Haller and Zinn are as follows:

1. Recurrent pial branches: four to seven of these arise from each segment, or may arise from two or three larger trunks. Small branches are given off to the retrolaminar nerve.
2. Recurrent choroidal branches supply the immediate peripapillary choroid, and extend toward the equator as straight vessels superiorly and inferiorly. Small centripetal branches of these arteries, and others from the choroid itself, also supply the laminar and retrolaminar regions of the optic nerve head.
3. Arteriolo-arteriolar anastomoses occur between the components of the circle and the pial and recurrent choroidal arteries.

The distal short posterior ciliary arteries supply large triangular areas of choroid whose apices are located approximately at the site of entry of each distal bundle of vessels (Figs 11.1 and 11.10). One of these vessels on the nasal and temporal side becomes the **long posterior ciliary artery** and the temporal of these only gives origin to a recurrent branch directed towards the posterior pole.

The supply of the anterior choroid from the short posterior ciliary arteries is supplemented by branches from the long posterior ciliary, the ciliary muscular arteries and perforating branches of the anterior ciliary arteries in the vertical meridian.

The short posterior ciliary arteries lie in the outermost layer of the choroid (Haller's layer) and give rise on their deep surface to the choroidal arterioles, which are in the intermediate layer (of Sattler) (Fig. 11.6b). At the peripapillary border a few sub-branches of the choroidal arterioles cross the disc margin to supply its prelaminar part (Fig. 11.12). Recurrent branches also contribute to the pial supply (Fryczkowski, 1992).

LONG POSTERIOR CILIARY ARTERIES

The nasal and temporal long posterior ciliary arteries pierce the sclera on each side of the optic nerve somewhat further anteriorly than the short ciliary arteries. Each passes forwards through the sclera in a very oblique canal about 4 mm long and then bends inwards at 45° to reach the interior of the eye. Each artery is accompanied by a ciliary nerve. The mouth of the canal is wide and may contain in addition a few short ciliary arteries, and nerves, arteries and veins of the sclera (Figs 11.2b,c, 11.3 and 11.4). Free space in the canal is filled with loose connective tissue. The canal narrows anteriorly but widens again slightly where it terminates in a sharp border. The arteries reach the suprachoroidal space and run forwards in the horizontal meridian (Fig. 11.4). Their course can be followed from the outside as a translucent blue line. Owing to the translucency of the sclera they appear as dark lines which form a useful landmark for the horizontal meridia after surgical disinsertion of the lateral and medial rectus muscles. Also, because of the accentuation of pigment in the fundus, near to the long ciliary vessel and nerve, they delineate the horizontal meridian ophthalmoscopically (Fig. 11.5).

The long posterior ciliary arteries bifurcate in the anterior choroid (or sometimes within the ciliary muscle), and after further divisions form the **major arterial circle of the iris**, for which they are the predominant supply. Funk and Rohen (1990) emphasize that the deep branches of the anterior ciliary arteries (mostly located in the superior and inferior quadrants) do not make a significant

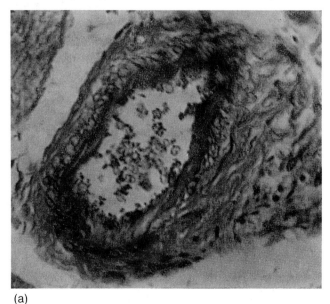

(a)

Fig. 11.4   (a) Posterior ciliary artery in the suprachoroid.

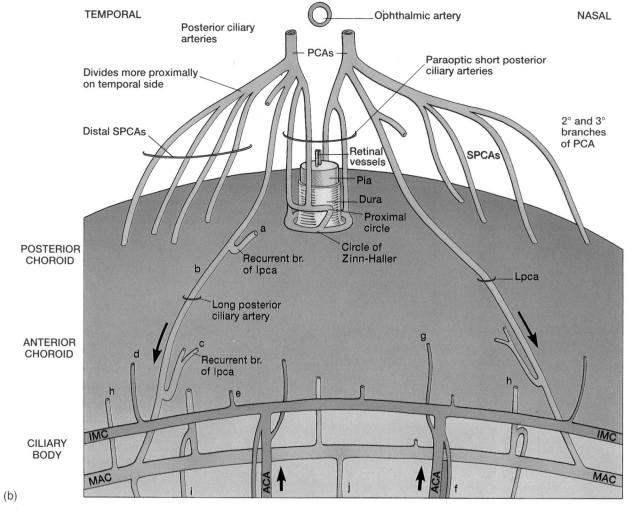

Fig. 11.4 (contd) (b) Schematic representation of the arterial supply of the uveal tract. The anterior ciliary arteries (ACAs) and posterior ciliary arteries (PCAs) arise from the ophthalmic artery. The PCAs divide into paraoptic and distal short posterior ciliary arteries (SPCAs). The short posterior ciliary arteries give rise to proximal and distal (Haller and Zinn) arterial circles in the region of the optic nerve head, and branches to the pia and directly to the nerve head itself (the scleral short posterior ciliary arteries). The distal SPCAs give rise to the long PCAs which are the chief supply to the major arterial circle of the iris (MAC) and also supply recurrent arteries to the anterior choroid. The temporal long posterior ciliary artery (lpca) also gives off a recurrent branch to the posterior choroid. The major arterial circle lies in the ciliary body, anterior to the circular part of the ciliary muscle. It supplies the iris and the ciliary processes, often by vessels with the same origin, and some recurrent vessels to the anterior choroid. The intramuscular arterial circle of the ciliary muscle (IMC) is formed chiefly by the penetrating branches of the ACAs, which also give off some branches to the anterior choroid and branches to the iris. The IMC supplies the outer and more posterior part of the ciliary muscle. There are scattered anastomoses between the branches of the ACAs and long PCAs.

contribution to the major circle of the iris but give rise to an **intramuscular arterial circle** (Leber, 1903) within the middle of the ciliary muscle. In all sectors (although they are often very thin) anastomoses occur between the branches of the anterior ciliary and long posterior ciliary arteries. Twigs from the anterior ciliary arteries supply the peripheral choroid as **recurrent choroidal arteries**, the canal of Schlemm and limbal sclera. Both the major arterial circle of the iris and the intramuscular circle of the ciliary muscle may be incomplete in some regions.

ANTERIOR CILIARY ARTERIES

The anterior ciliary arteries are derived from the arteries to the four recti which pass within their substance. Usually two arteries emerge from each tendon, except that of the lateral rectus which carries only one. These arteries, about 1.5 mm from the limbus, divide into deep (scleral) and superficial (anterior episcleral) branches (Fig. 11.6a). The former dip almost directly inwards through short scleral canals, to enter the ciliary muscle, where they join

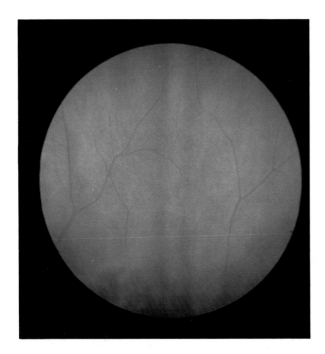

Fig. 11.5 Long posterior ciliary arteries visible in the fundus in the horizontal meridian.

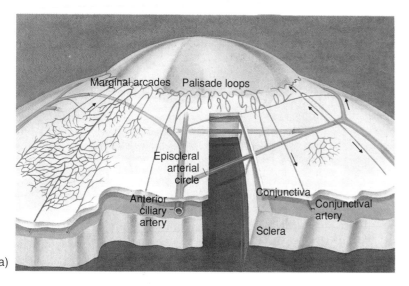

(a)

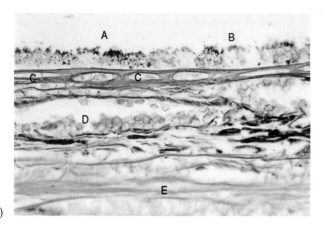

(b)

Fig. 11.6 (a) Distribution of the episcleral arteries and their branches. (b) Longitudinal section through the juxtapapillary choroid. A = Subretinal space; B = retinal pigment epithelium; C = choriocapillaris; D = large vessel layer of the choroid (Haller); E = suprachoroid. Original magnification × 840. (Courtesy of D. Lucas.)

the intramuscular circle and give off some direct branches to the iris and recurrent choroidal arteries to the peripheral choroid.

The point of scleral entry is often marked by pigment. The anterior episcleral arteries run forward and form an irregular, episcleral arterial circle whose anastomotic channels may be superficial or deep (Meyer and Watson, 1987; Meyer, 1989).

The episcleral arterial circle gives rise to branches supplying the sclera, limbus, perilimbal conjunctiva and iris via deep branches to its major circle. Some episcleral arteries emerge on the surface of the sclera at some distance anterior to, but in the meridia of, the rectus tendons or in the oblique meridia, and pursue a variable course in the episclera. Their origin has not been established.

It should also be noted that the anterior ciliary arteries supply the ciliary muscle, the iris, and the episclera. It is therefore easy to understand why inflammation of the iris or ciliary body is associated with dilatation of episcleral vessels at the limbus (ciliary flush), a classic sign of anterior uveitis. Multiple disinsertions of the rectus muscle during squint surgery deprive the ciliary muscle (and iris) of its anterior ciliary arterial supply and may give rise to anterior segment ischaemia (Stucci and Bianchi, 1957; von Noorden, 1976; Fells and Marsh, 1978; Hayreh and Scott, 1978; France and Simon, 1986; Olver and Lee, 1989). In the same way, during retinal detachment surgery, a tight encircling band placed around the globe may impair the blood supply to the ciliary body and iris by interfering with the long posterior ciliary supply to the major arterial circle. Vortex vein compression may also contribute to anterior ischaemic syndrome (Wilson and Irvine, 1955; Hayreh and Baines, 1973; Robertson, 1975; Hayreh and Scott, 1979; Chignell and Easty, 1971) (Fig. 10.23).

11.2 GROSS ANATOMY OF THE CHOROID

The choroid, the most posterior part of the uveal tract, is considered to be the homologue of the pia arachnoid, which vascularizes the brain. The choroid maintains but does not vascularize the outer retinal layers. It extends from the optic nerve to the ora serrata, the scalloped peripheral margin of the retina. It consists largely of vessels, and has been compared with cavernous tissue. The thickness of the choroid is difficult to determine because it diminishes after enucleation or fixation: it has been estimated at about 100 μm anteriorly and about 220 μm posteriorly, with greatest thickness over the macula. Central thickness in life has been estimated by ultrasound to be 500–1000 μm (Coleman and Lizzi, 1979) (Fig. 11.6). The choroid may be thinner in high myopia and congenital and chronic glaucoma.

The choroid is firmly attached to the margin of the optic nerve and loosely at points where vessels and nerves enter it. Its attachment to the sclera is strongest behind the equator.

The inner surface of the choroid is formed by Bruch's membrane. If the retina, including the pigment epithelium, is stripped away, this presents a smooth, brown, glistening and transparent aspect. On separating choroid from sclera, which is performed without difficulty, the outer surface appears roughened. This is partly because the deep layer of the suprachoroidal lamina remains with the choroid, and partly because the outer surface contains many interwoven vessels. The **lamina suprachoroidea** is interposed between choroid and sclera.

11.3 THE LAMINA SUPRACHOROIDEA (LAMINA FUSCA)

The lamina suprachoroidea is 10–34 μm in thickness. Anteriorly it is continuous with the supraciliary space. Its closely packed lamellae adjoin potential spaces, which become evident when the suprachoroid is pathologically distended by serous fluid or blood and they are seen to interlace at acute angles. The lamellae consist of a delicate mesh of collagen fibres and run from the sclera anteriorly to the choroid. They are shorter posteriorly, where they are more adherent to each other and to the sclera – hence, detachments of the choroid take place anteriorly and rarely pass behind the equator. However, ultrasound examination can reveal suprachoroidal effusions posteriorly in the absence of ballooning. The suprachoroidal space is traversed by the long and short ciliary arteries and nerves which supply the ureal tract.

MELANOCYTES

These occur spread out in the suprachoroid in the plane of the choroidal surface, interweave between lamellae and form an interlacing network with fibrocytes (Fig. 11.7). They are more stunted than those of the choroid, with shorter processes, and anteriorly their pigment may be deficient. Deeper cells are smaller, with longer processes. Their nuclei are flat and oval with long axes parallel to the choroidal curve. They are best seen in flat section. Non-striated muscle fibres also occur more frequently in front of the equator. Melanocytes are also described around the optic nerve (Fuchs). When

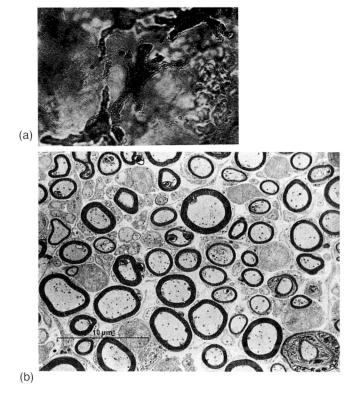

(a)

(b)

Fig. 11.7 (a) Human choroidal melanocytes (original magnification × 675). (Courtesy of J. Marshall and P. Ansell.) (b) Part of a myelinated ciliary nerve of the suprachoroid. The nerve also contains numerous unmyelinated nerve fibre bundles. (From Ruskell, G. L. (1971b) *Exp. Eye Res.*, **12**, 166, with permission.)

choroid and sclera are separated, part of the suprachoroid adheres to sclera and part to choroid, which accounts for the shaggy appearance of the external choroidal surface.

THE MUSCULO-ELASTIC SYSTEM

The whole vascular system of the choroid, excluding the choriocapillaris, is surrounded by an elastic network which extends from Bruch's membrane to the adventitia of the suprachoroid and partly into the elastica of the overlying sclera. This elastic network is best recognized in tangential sections of the uvea and can be demonstrated with special stains. It is recognized that fine elastic fibres, which surround the vessels, are distributed in a net-like manner throughout the whole thickness of the choroid. Anteriorly, this fine elastic net extends into the connective tissue stroma of the ciliary body, including Bruch's membrane of the pars plana. Into this net there inserts the posterior elastic tendon of the ciliary muscle. With contraction of the ciliary muscle during accommodation, the elastic tendon of the muscle, like the elastic net of the choroid, is stretched. The recoil of the elastica provides the energy required for disaccommodation (Rohen, 1952, 1964b; Tamm *et al.*, 1991). How the pull of the muscle tendon is transmitted to the elastic net of the choroid is unknown, and it is not known to what extent disaccommodation may influence choroidal blood flow (Lütjen-Drecoll, 1995).

Preparations of the suprachoroid have also shown that, close to the sclera, there is a network of smooth muscle cells (myofibroblasts or nonstriated muscle spindle of Salzmann) which stain positively with antibodies to alpha actinin. Electron microscopic studies of this network show very close contact with nerve endings, and partial attachment to the elastic network of the choroid and to the adventitia of the larger vessels. In the region of the equator, the quantity of contractile cells decreases distinctly. Only in the region of the vortex vein exits are more positively staining cells found. These cells are not present in the region of the ciliary muscle.

The function of this newly described musculoelastic system of the choroid is still not known. It may be that these smooth muscle cells transmit the forces of accommodation to the elastic network of the choroid. Thereby, the musculo-elastic system could play an important role for the retina itself. The vessels, together with the musculo-elastic system, could provide a compliant pillow for the neighbouring retina which could protect the retinal ganglion cells, and, above all, the photoreceptor outer segments, from deformation and damage during eye movement or eye rubbing, and also maintain the choroidal blood flow (Lütjen-Drecoll, 1995).

VESSELS AND NERVES

The suprachoroid contains the long and short posterior ciliary arteries and nerves, both myelinated (Fig. 11.7b) and non-myelinated, the latter showing nodes of Ranvier (Hogan, Alvarado and Weddell, 1971). They divide into progressively smaller branches which supply the choroid.

11.4 THE CHOROID

The choroid is composed almost entirely of vessels. Classically three superimposed strata are described: an outer layer of large vessels (Haller's layer); a middle layer of medium-sized vessels occupying the **choroidal stroma** (Sattler's layer); and an internal layer of capillary vessels (**choriocapillaris**). The choriocapillaris is fed by arterioles derived from the short posterior ciliary arteries. These arterioles do not pass directly into the choriocapillaris, but create a second capillary layer which shows few fenestrations and is covered by pericytes on its scleral side. These capillaries form, together with the first component of the draining venules, the two distinct layers of Haller and Sattler. Internal to this is a non-cellular connective tissue possessing two basal laminae, two layers of collagen and a single layer of elastin, termed the **membrane of Bruch**. This is intimately bound to the choriocapillaris and to the retinal pigment epithelium so this latter layer remains attached to the choroid in artefactual or clinical retinal detachment.

The outer and middle layers of stromal vessels separate in places but their interlacing and irregular distribution generally prevents this.

Three major choroidal layers may thus be described (Fig. 11.8):

1. the stromal layer (layer of large and medium vessels);
2. the choriocapillaris (layer of capillaries);
3. Bruch's membrane (non-cellular layer).

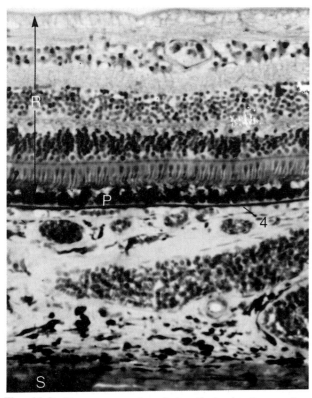

Fig. 11.8 Transverse section of choroid showing its overall architecture. 1, suprachoroidae; 2, stroma containing large and medium vessels, loose connective tissue, fibroblasts, and melanocytes; 3, choriocapillaris; 4, Bruch's membrane; S, sclera; PE, pigment epithelium; R, sensory retina (original magnification ×200). (From Tripathi, R. C. and Tripathi, B., in Davson, H. (ed.) (1974) *The Eye*, published by Academic Press, with permission.)

STROMAL LAYER

The stromal layer (substantia propria) contains vessels, nerves, cells and connective tissue. The stromal cells include melanocytes, fibrocytes, macrophages, mast cells and plasma cells. The vessels will be described last to provide a continuous account of their connections with the choriocapillaris.

Melanocytes

Melanocytes characterize the stroma and impart its brown colour (Figs 11.7 and 11.9). They form an almost continuous layer in the outer choroid spreading in the plane of the choroid and forming a thin three-dimensional network by their connections with adjoining layers, which is thinner in the suprachoroid. Even so, a whole cell is rarely seen in vertical section. Cell numbers vary regionally with age, race and general pigmentation: they are most numerous around the optic disc, less so in the periphery and in the inner choroid. They outline vessels, including the veins and ampullae of the venae vorticosae. Melanocyte nuclei are round, oval (or, rarely, reniform), and show an even chromatin dispersal and no nucleolus.

Melanosomes

Pigment granules (melanosomes) are fine, 0.3–0.4 (occasionally <0.2) μm wide, oval in shape, yellowish to dark brown in colour, and always smaller than those of the retinal pigment epithelium (which are up to 1 μm in diameter and 2–3 μm in length; Hogan, Alvarado and Weddell, 1971). Size is constant in any individual or cell but varies from race to race. They are evenly distributed within the cell body and processes, occupying about 70% of the cytoplasm. Only in the perinuclear region of the embryo is pigment lacking or absent. The more pigmented cells are also generally larger (Fig. 11.10a,b).

Fibrocytes

Fibrocytic processes intermingle with those of the melanocytes. They are most dense in the outer choroid, and are more numerous in males. The collagen framework of the stroma is loose and randomly oriented. The collagen encircles vessels to provide an adventitia. Reticulin and elastin fibres also occur, the elastin in flat ribbons up to 13 μm in length (Salzmann, 1912; Feeney and Hogan, 1961). There is a mucinous ground substance (Yanoff and Fine, 1972).

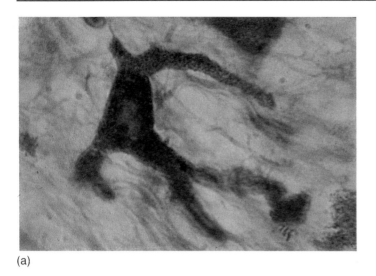

(a)

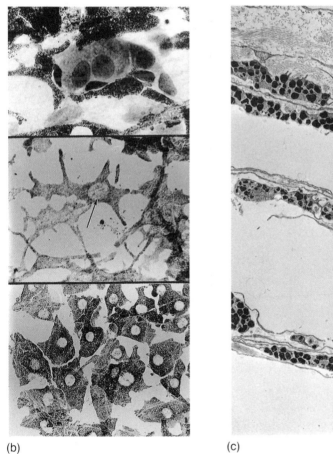

(b)

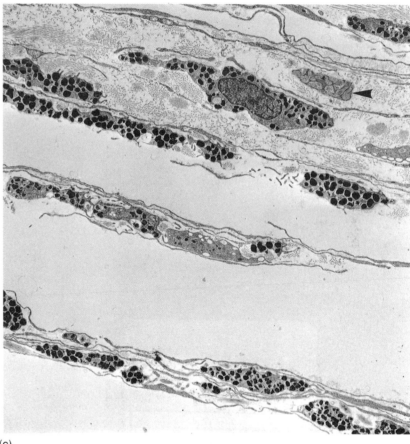

(c)

Fig. 11.9 (a) Choroidal melanocyte (flat section). Nucleus visible (Mallory's trichrome). (b) (Top) Unstained preparation of polygonal melanocytes in outer choroid. Faint, crisscrossing lines are imprints of collagen bundles. Connective tissue cells filling white spaces are not seen without appropriate staining (original magnification ×500). (Middle) Starlike clusters, with long thin processes from middle choroid. Nucleus is indicated by arrow (original magnification ×500). (Bottom) Ganglion cells in outer choroid surrounded by branching melanocytes. (Flat preparation, haematoxylin, original magnification ×1250.) (c) Melanocytes of the outer choroid and suprachoroid are filled with melanosomes and surrounded by collagen fibres. The nucleus (N) contains granular chromatin and the nucleolus. Suprachoroidal lamellae (below) are artificially separated by spaces. Thin cellular processes of melanocytes interdigitate. Unmyelinated nerve (arrowhead), suprachoroid, SC (×5510). ((b) and (c) from Torczynski, E. in Duane, T. D. and Jaeger, E. A. (eds) (1987) *Biomedical Foundations of Ophthalmology*, (published by Lippincott, with permission.)

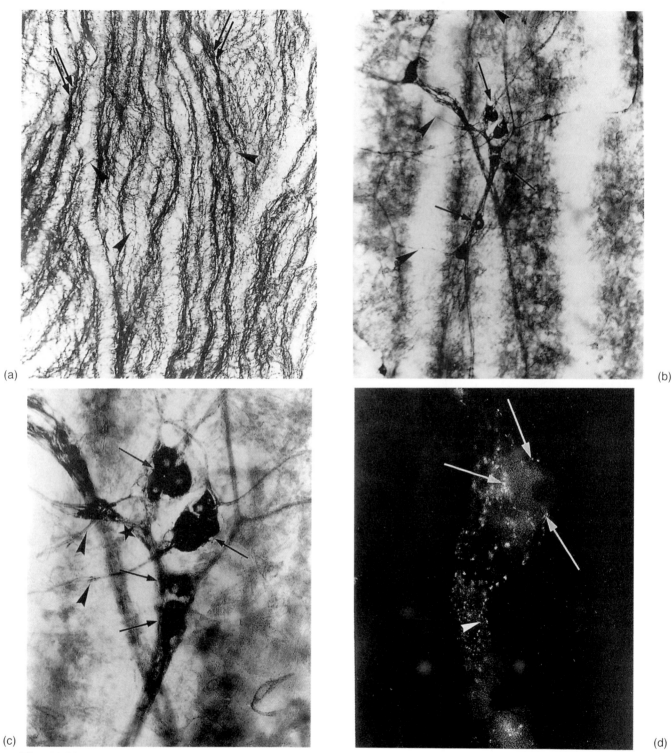

Fig. 11.10 (a) Whole mount of a rat choroid stained for NADPH–diaphorase. The temporal region in the vicinity of the optic nerve head is shown. Bundles of positively stained nerve fibres follow the course of arterial vessels (double arrows). Small axons originate from these bundles forming a delicate network around the vascular wall (arrowhead) (original magnification ×80). (b) Whole mount of a human choroid (temporal region) stained for NADPH-diaphorase (original magnification ×51). (c) Positively stained ganglion cells are shown (arrows). These cells are connected to each other by stained axons (asterisk). Additional nerve fibres lead to the perivascular fibre network (arrowheads) (original magnification ×160). (d) Frozen tangential section through the temporal quadrant of a human choroid after incubation for anti-synaptophysin. Two ganglion cells are surrounded by positively labelled varicosities (arrows). In addition, positive staining is also present in small vesicles lying in the cytoplasm of axons (arrowhead) (original magnification ×270). (From Flügel et al., (1994) Invest Opththalmol. Vis. Sci., **35**, 592 with permission.)

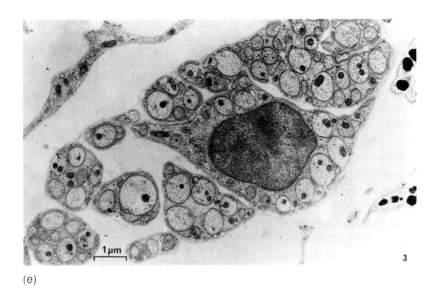

(e)

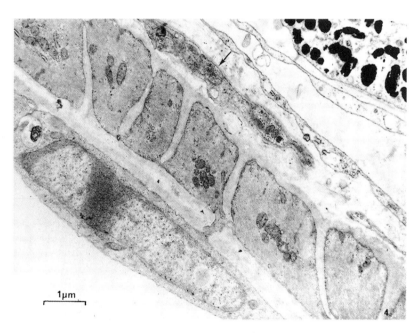

(f)

Fig. 11.10 (contd)   (e) Grouped unmyelinated nerve fibre bundles of the choroid. The section appears to be taken where a nerve has begun to break up into separate nerve fibre bundles. Rhesus. (f) Longitudinal section through the wall of a choroidal arteriole. The seven circularly orientated smooth muscle fibres are cut transversely. The flattening of their apposed faces is typical. Note the penetration of the internal elastic lamina by an endothelial cell (with nucleus) process that terminates adjacent to two muscle cells: this was a regular feature in arteriole walls. A terminal nerve fibre bundle (arrow) lies external to the muscle layer. Rhesus.

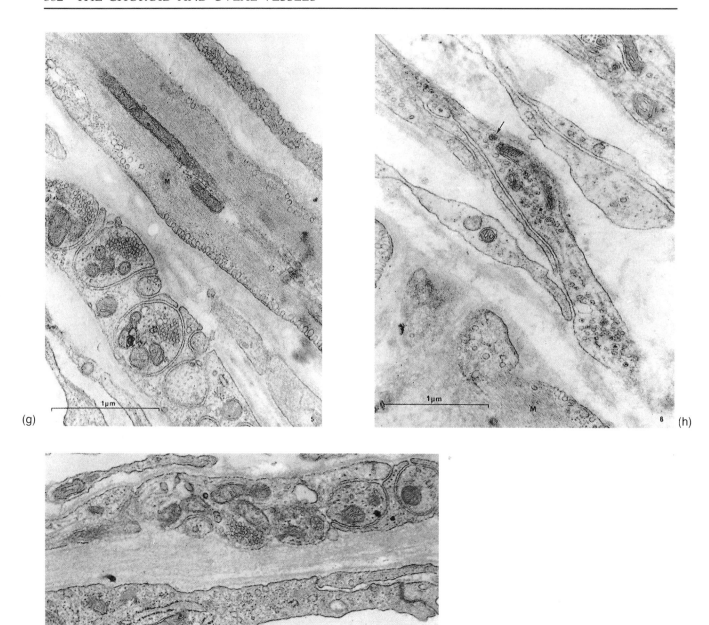

(g)

(h)

(i)

Fig. 11.10 (contd) (g) Three nerve fibre varicosities (lower left) with aggregated small agranular vesicles disposed towards the muscle wall (M) of an arteriole. Mitochondria occupy most of the remaining space of each varicosity. Note that a single Schwann cell process envelops the axons. Cynomolgous. (h) Consecutive varicosities of an arteriolar nerve fibre terminal. A large granular vesicle is present in one of them (arrow): small granular and small agranular vesicles are also present. The small granular vesicles reveal the sympathetic identity of the fibre. M, muscle cell. Rhesus. (i) A terminal nerve fibre bundle adjacent to the wall of a venule which consists only of an endothelial cell in this region. Cynomologous.

Innervation of the choroid (and see Chapter 16)

In the choroidal stroma each nerve bundle contains 50–100 axons which may lose their myelin sheaths as they enter the choroid but retain their neurolemmal (Schwann) cells. Postganglionic fibres arising from the ciliary ganglion remain myelinated. Ganglion cells, 40 μm in diameter, appear in this layer and are larger than other cells present. Their nuclei have prominent nucleoli and the usual organelles. Axons make contact with and indent the ganglion cells, and exhibit synaptic vesicles (Torczynski, 1987).

The vessels of the suprachoroid and stroma show a strikingly dense parasympathetic and sympathetic innervation. Sympathetic adrenergic fibres, which arise from the cervical sympathetic chain, have a vasoconstrictor action. The parasympathetic innervation of the choroid is from the facial nerve and pterygopalatine ganglion, and from the oculomotor nerve via the ciliary ganglion and short ciliary nerves. This contrasts with the innervation to the anterior segment (ciliary muscle and sphincter pupillae), which is from the latter supply alone.

Recent studies have increased our knowledge of the choroidal innervation (Lütjen-Drecoll, 1995). In various species (rat, rabbit and human), the arteries and arterioles of the choroidal stroma show a dense nitrergic and VIPergic **perivascular network** whose axons have varicose terminals and whose extrinsic origin, as noted, is the facial nerve via the pterygopalatine ganglion and the unmyelinated parasympathetic rami oculares of the retro-orbital plexus (Yamamoto *et al.*, 1993; Flügel *et al.*, 1994) (Fig. 11.10d–l).

In the human eye there is, in addition, an intrinsic network of nitrergic ganglion cells (NADPH-diaphorase and nitric oxide synthase positive) in the choroidal stroma whose neurons are connected to each other and to the perivascular network. Early studies by Müller (1859) and by Iwanoff (1874) described an elaborate system of intrinsic ganglion cells in the human choroid, and there have been more recent reports by Lauber (1936), Kurus (1955), Wolter (1960) and Castro-Correira (1967) (Fig. 11.10e,f). This intrinsic plexus appears to be confined to the choroid of foveate animals, and ganglia are found only sparsely in non-foveate species. It is not found in all primate eyes. For instance it is found in the foveate, cynomolgous monkey (which has ganglion cells which are smaller and more evenly distributed than in the human eye), but is absent from the choroid of the nocturnal owl monkey, which has no fovea centralis, and from the afoveate eyes of the tree shrew, cat and pig. The presence of an accommodative capacity does not influence this relationship; thus the owl monkey can accommodate but, as noted, shows no intrinsic plexus (Flügel-Koch, Kaufman and Lütjen-Drecoll, 1994).

In the human, the ganglion cells are concentrated chiefly in the temporal and central regions of the choroid, the latter, therefore, subjacent to the macula. The varicose terminals innervating the ganglion cell perikarya stain for synaptophysin (a marker for synaptic vesicles) (Fig. 11.10g). It is assumed that the perivascular and ganglionic networks receive extrinsic NOS fibres, for instance from the pterygopalatine ganglion as in the rat (Yamamoto, 1993).

The majority of the ganglion cells are solitary, polygonal cells, with diameters ranging from 10 to 40 μm. Occasionally, they lie in clusters of 2–10 cells (Fig. 11.10e,f). Most are located close to the walls of large arteries, but none is observed in the choriocapillaris. The total number in the human choroid is about 2000, asymmetrically distributed, with the largest cells and greatest number lying in the temporo-central region, and the remainder, smaller-diameter (<10 μm) cells distributed peripherally (Table 11.1) (Flügel *et al.*, 1994). The diameter of the ganglion cells increases with age, possibly due to an accumulation of lipofuscin granules. The increase occurs earlier in the central choroid where, it is suggested, light exposure may promote premature ageing in the neurons (Iwanoff, 1874; Lauber, 1936; Flügel *et al.*, 1994).

Neurons staining for nitric oxide synthase (NOS) use nitric oxide (NO) as a neurotransmitter. Nitric oxide (NO) is a mediator of endothelium-derived vascular relaxation, and the release of NO from perivascular nerves in various organs, including the cat choroid, causes vasodilatation (Sternschantz and Bill., 1980; Nilsson, Linder and Bill, 1985; Bill, 1991; Mann, 1993; Morris, 1993; Toda, 1993). Nitric oxide release also causes smooth muscle relaxation in other parts of the body, such as the intestine (Grozdanovic, Baumgarten and Bruning, 1992), gallbladder (Talmadge and Mawe, 1993) and trachea (Fischer *et al.*, 1993).

Table 11.1 Nitrergic ganglion cells of human choroid

Region	Left eye (48 year old)	Left eye (82 year old)
Temporo-central	1165 (45%)	1116 (70%)
Nasal	287 (27%)	89
Superior	146 (6%)	31
Inferior	986 (38%)	375
Total	**2579**	**1661**

NADPH-diaphorase positive cells of the intrinsic ganglionic plexus of the human choroid (data from Flügel *et al.*, 1994).

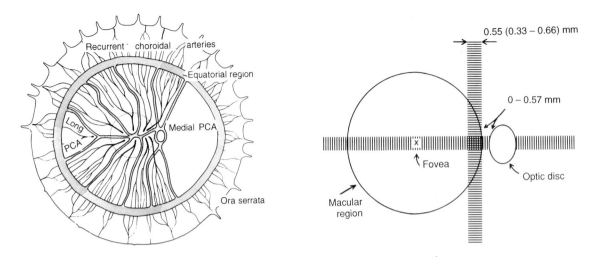

Fig. 11.11 (a) Diagrammatic representation of distribution of various temporal short posterior ciliary arteries (SPCAs) and their watershed zones in the posterior part of the fundus. Dotted circle in region of temporal SPCAs represents the macular region. Areas of supply by medial PCA and temporal long PCA are also shown. (b) Diagrammatic representation of the watershed zones of the vortex veins. (From Hayreh, S. S. (1974b) *A. von Graefes Arch. Klin. Exp. Ophthalmol.*, **192**, 197, with permission.)

In several organs, such as the choroid, NO is colocalized with VIP, which also has a vasodilator action (Miller *et al.*, 1983; Kummer *et al.*, 1992; Furness *et al.*, 1992; Talmadge and Mawe, 1993). The choroidal vessels are supplied by numerous VIPergic neurons (Uddman *et al.*, 1980; Miller *et al.*, 1983; Stone *et al.*, 1986) which probably arise from the pterygopalatine ganglion and run in the facial and greater petrosal nerve (Uddman *et al.*, 1980; Butler, 1984) (and see Chapter 16). In the rat, NOS-positive neurons arising in the pterygopalatine ganglion are probably also VIP-ergic (Yamamoto, 1993). It is likely that both NO and VIP contribute to the vasodilatation that accompanies facial nerve stimulation.

The perivascular and ganglionic neural plexuses appear to serve a vasodilator role in the choroid, perhaps adjusting blood flow in response to reduction in arterial blood pressure or protecting the retina from thermal damage associated with light exposure. Flügel *et al.* (1994) have suggested that the submacular location of the intrinsic choroidal ganglionic plexus in foveate animals may afford additional protection from light damage at a site where light is focused and the photoreceptors and RPE are most susceptible. Certainly Parva demonstrated a rise in blood flow in the choroid in response to light of high intensity falling on the retina.

The choroidal arterial supply

The short ciliary arteries, after piercing the sclera, are at first in the suprachoroid surrounded by pigmented tissue. They proceed forwards in a sinuous manner and gradually penetrate the choroid. They bifur-cate dichotomously and eventually divide into the choriocapillaris, the capillary bed of the choroid extending from optic disc margin to ora serrata. The larger arterial branches are less sinuous than the veins, which are hence cut more often in sections and appear more numerous than they are. Branches from the deep surface of the short posterior ciliary arteries, lying in the outer (Haller's) layer, give rise to the choroidal arterioles of the intermediate layer (of Sattler).

The **short posterior ciliary arteries** supply the posterior choroid up to the equator and a variable area anterior to it. The **temporal long posterior ciliary artery** supplies a wedge-shaped sector of choroid, starting from the point where it enters the choroid posterior to the equator and extending forwards (Fig. 11.11) (Hayreh, 1974b; Weiter and Ernest, 1974). The anterior part of the choroid is otherwise supplied by the recurrent ciliary arteries (Fig. 11.4, 11.11a and 11.13c) which arise in the ciliary body from the circulus iridis major and from the long posterior and anterior ciliary arteries before they join the muscular circle. Of varying size and number (10–20), they run back between numerous parallel veins in the pars plana, dividing dichotomously to supply the anterior choriocapillaris.

Classic descriptions of choroidal arteries based on post-mortem studies have suggested anastomoses between adjacent short posterior ciliary arteries and between these and recurrent ciliary arteries (Wybar, 1954; Ring and Fujino, 1967; Yoneyo and Tso, 1987). However, this is denied by Hayreh (Hayreh and Baines, 1972; Hayreh, 1975a), who considers that there are no functional anastomoses between individual short ciliary arteries or between arteries of supply to the anterior and posterior choroid. As will be seen, although the choroidal arterioles appear anatomically to be end arterioles, they are not completely so in the functional sense, because choroidovascular occlusions frequently recover over a matter of days.

ANATOMICAL AND FUNCTIONAL VASCULAR UNITS OF THE CHOROID (Figs 11.12 and 11.13)

Earlier observers of the choriocapillaris described it as a continuous intercommunicating sheet of wide-lumen capillaries disposed in a single plane. However, later experimental studies in pigs (Dollery *et al.*, 1968) demonstrated a fine segmental filling pattern, and Hayreh (1974b, 1974d, 1975, 1990) and Torczynski and Tso (1976) showed in human studies that each terminal arteriole appeared to supply an independent segment, or lobule of choriocapillaris comprising a central feeding arteriole, the capillary bed, and a series of peripheral draining venules (Fig. 11.12). Such lobules may be termed 'arteriocentric'. A lobular organization of the human choroid is now accepted (see Shimizu and Kaziyoshi, 1978; Yoneya and Tso, 1984, 1987), but further studies using methyl methacrylate vascular casting techniques have suggested that the arrangement of the lobules is not uniform over the whole of the choriocapillaris.

Peripheral to the disc (beyond 3 mm) and to the macula (beyond 2 mm), and excluding the region between the disc and macula, the choroid has a regular, lobulated pattern. A lobular pattern is absent, or difficult to recognize in the peripapillary or submacular regions, where the wide-bore capillaries are interconnected in a rich honeycomb pattern (Fryczkowski, 1992). The lobular organization is well developed at the posterior pole, where the lobules are round or polygonal, and exhibit triangular, pentagonal, or octagonal shapes. More anteriorly, the lobules increase in size and become less regular, and towards the ora serrata they are radially elongated.

In the posterior choroid, the arterioles and venules enter and leave the lobules at right angles to the plane of the choriocapillaris; more peripherally, and even within the posterior pole itself, arterioles and veins may be found to lie in the plane of the choriocapillaris. The diameter of the arterioles entering the choroid at right angles ranges from 1 to 70 μm, while the veins are 22–90 μm. Arterioles lying in the plane of the choriocapillaris are somewhat wider, 30–85 μm, while the venules are 35–95 μm wide. Dilated interlobular vascular structures are found in the equatorial region, whose function is unknown (Fryczkowski, 1992, 1993). Some of the larger veins of the equatorial choroid may show dilations where they overlie arteries, the so-called 'bulbiculi' described by Ashton (1952a,b).

The submacular choroid is fed by 8–16 precapillary arterioles, which show frequent interarteriolar anastomoses. These are uncommon elsewhere. The precapillary arteriole-to-venule ratio here is 3:1 (Fryczkowski *et al.*, 1988a–f). The average diameter of a lobule at the posterior pole is 515 × 450 μm, and the ratio of precapillary arteriole-to-venule is reversed compared to the submacular region, 1:2 to 1:5. At the equator the average size of a lobule is 645 × 550 μm, while the arteriole-to-venule ratio is about 1:2. Finally, at the choroidal periphery, the lobules are radially elongated and their size is in the region of 955–670 μm. The ratio of arterioles to venules here lies between 1:2 and 1:4 (Fryczkowski, Sherman and Walker, 1991).

Although the lobules described on the basis of fluorescein angiography and early vascular cast studies were arteriocentric, with a central feeding arteriole, Fryczkowski has suggested that the

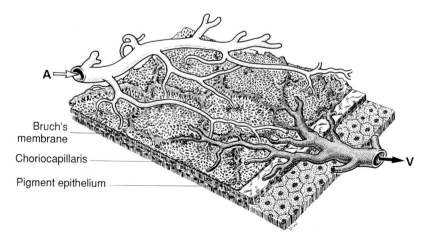

Bruch's membrane

Choriocapillaris

Pigment epithelium

Fig. 11.12 A three-dimensional representation of the choriocapillaris pattern. A = Choroidal arteriole; V = choroidal vein. Note that in this representation the choriocapillary unit is conceived as being fed by a centrilobular arteriole. (Redrawn from Hayreh, S. S. (1974a) *A. von Graefes Arch. Klin. Exp. Ophthalmol.*, **192**, 165, with permission.)

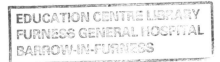

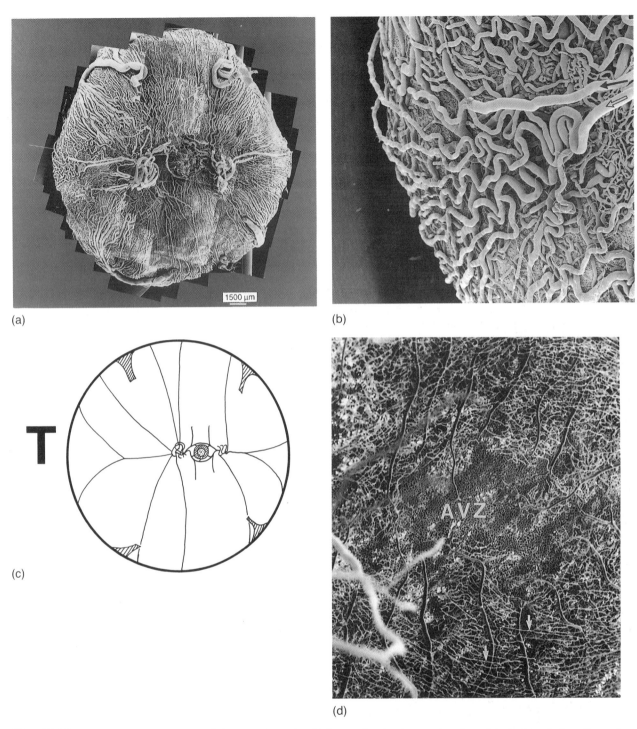

(a)

(b)

(c)

(d)

Fig. 11.13 (a) Photomontage of cast of the posterior pole of left eye showing temporal and medial short posterior ciliary artery (SPCA) bundles supplying choroidal vasculature and retrolaminar optic nerve vasculature. The paraoptic branches have divided on each side to form the 'circle' of Zinn and Haller which provides pial branches to the retrolaminar optic nerve, and recurrent choroidal branches to the peripapillary choroid and peripheral, vertical, meridional choroid. The lateral and medial long posterior ciliary arteries (LPCA) have been truncated at the equator. Vortex veins are clearly seen. (From Olver, J. (1990) *Eye*, **4**, 262, with permission.) (b) Higher power view of the lateral LPCA distribution shown in (a). (c) Diagrammatic representation of the montage in (b) to show the gross division of the choroid into triangular and trapezoid areas supplied by the SPCAs. T = Temporal. (d) Monkey macular area, anterior view. Retinal avascular zone (AVZ) with submacular choriocapillaris. Radial capillaries are arrowed. Vascular cast of SEM, original magnification ×25. (Courtesy of A. W. Fryczkowski.)

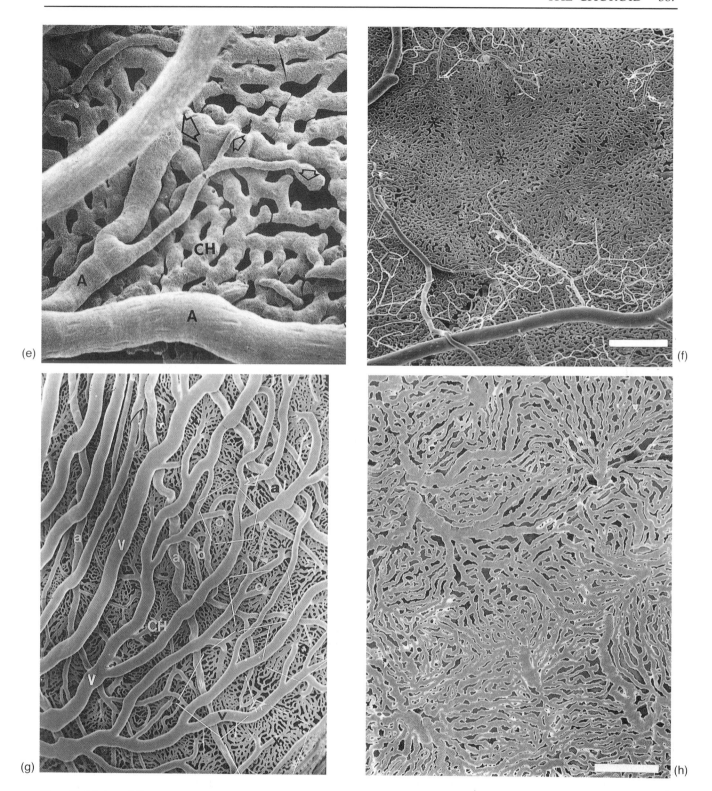

Fig. 11.13 (contd) (e) Human choroid. Submacular arteriolar openings (open arrows), posterior view. Arteriole (A), choriocapillaris (CH). Vascular cast, SEM original magnification ×500. Note linear nuclear impressions typical of arterioles. (Courtesy of A. W. Fryczkowski.) (f) Human choroid. Posterior pole choriocapillaris viewed from the retinal aspect. Remnants of the inferior retinal vessel arcade and retinal capillaries are visible. Lobular appearance is difficult to distinguish but can be identified. * = Choroidal arteriolar opening. Bar = 250 μm. (From Olver, J. (1990) *Eye*, **4**, 262, with permission.) (g) Monkey choroid. Posterior pole, posterior view. Venular openings 'in plane' (x) and at 90° (o) to the choriocapillaris (CH). a = Artery, v = vein. Arteriolar openings (open arrow) and centrifugal arterial capillaries distribution. Additional arteriolar openings are shown by arrowheads. Anatomical lobuli with centripetal course of the venular capillaries are outlined by boxes. Vascular cast, SEM original magnification ×39. (Courtesy of A. W. Fryczkowski.) (h) Human choroid: equatorial choriocapillaris viewed from the retinal aspect. The lobular pattern is more apparent. Terminal parts of arterioles and venules are visible. Bar = 250 μm. (From Olver, J. (1990) *Eye*, **4**, 262, with permission.)

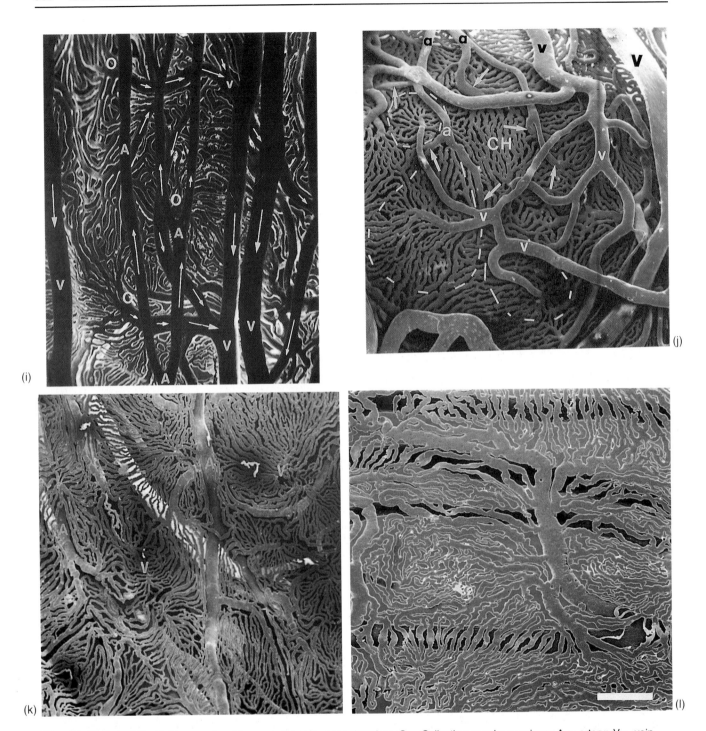

Fig. 11.13 (contd) (i) Human choroid: equatorial area, posterior view. O = Collecting venule openings; A = artery; V = vein. Directions of blood flow shown by arrows. Vascular cast, SEM original magnification ×60. (Courtesy of A. W. Fryczkowski.) (j) Human choroid: equatorial area, posterior view. Feeding arteriole (a) and collecting venule (v) connections with the choriocapillaris (CH) are 'in plane' – tangential (arrows) or at 90° to choriocapillaris (open arrows). Different sizes of the anatomical lobules are outlined. Vascular cast, SEM original magnification ×60. (Courtesy of A. W. Fryczkowski.) (k) Human choroid, midperiphery, anterior view. Feeding arteriole (A) and collecting venule (V) localized in the plane of the choriocapillaris. Vascular cast, SEM original magnification ×280. (Courtesy of A. W. Fryczkowski.) (l) Human choroid: peripheral choriocapillaris viewed from retinal aspect showing evident large fan-shaped lobules. Arterioles and venules lie in the same plane as the capillaries. Bar = 250 μm. (From Olver, J. (1990) *Eye*, **4**, 262, with permission.)

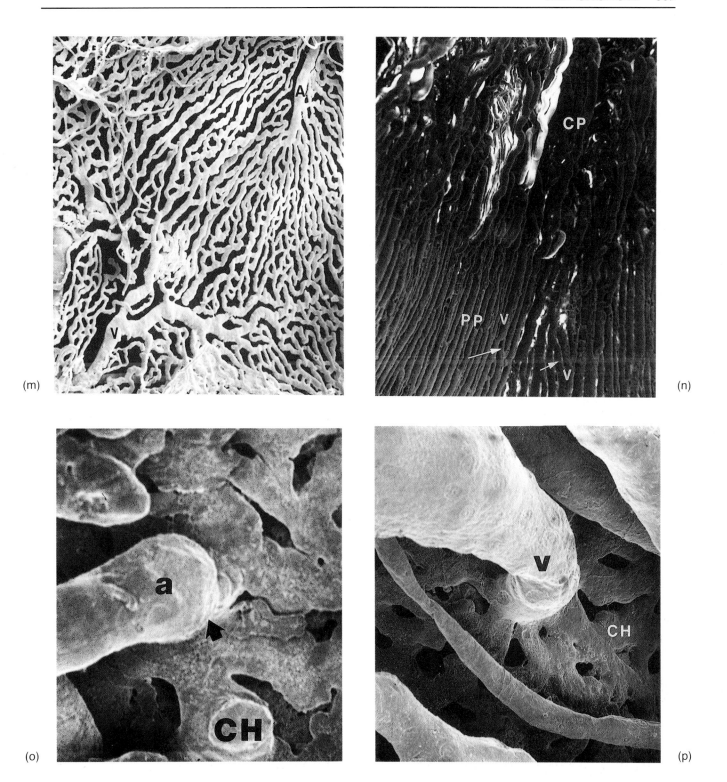

(m)

(n)

(o)

(p)

Fig. 11.13 (contd) (m) Human choroid: peripheral choriocapillaris, anterior view. A = Artery; V = vein. Vascular cast, SEM original magnification ×60. (Courtesy of A. W. Fryczkowski.) (n) Human choroid: pars plana (PP) and ciliary processes (CP), posterior view. Most of the vessels are veins (V). Multiple venous–venous anastomoses are visible (arrows). Vascular cast, SEM original magnification ×380. (Courtesy of A. W. Fryczkowski.) (o) Human choroid: arteriolar opening (a), posterior view. CH = Choriocapillaris. Vascular cast, SEM original magnification ×1400. (From Fryczkowski, A. W. (1989) *Int. Ophthalmol.*, **13**, 269.) (p) Human choroid: venular openings (V) forming 90° angles with the choriocapillaris (CH). Vascular cast, SEM original magnification ×1400. (From Fryczkowski, A. W. (1989) *Int. Ophthalmol.*, **13**, 269.)

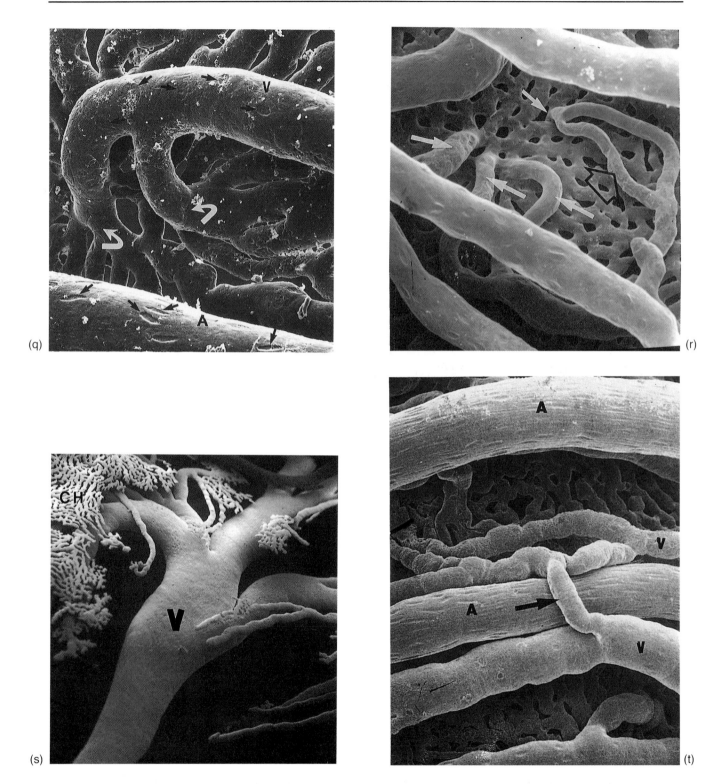

Fig. 11.13 (contd) (q) Human choroid: collecting venules, equatorial area, posterior view, 90° angle or tangential origination of venules from choriocapillaris (bent arrows). A = Artery; V = vein. Small arrows indicate the endothelial cell indentations (oval or round in veins and spindle-shape in arteries). Vascular cast, SEM original magnification ×670. (From Fryczkowski, A. W. (1989) *Int. Ophthalmol.*, **15**, 109.) (r) Human choroid: multiple collecting venules (arrows), posterior pole, posterior view. Venular collateral channel shown by open arrow. Vascular cast, SEM original magnification ×580. (From Fryczkowski, A. W. (1989) *Int. Ophthalmol.*, **15**, 109.) (s) Human choroid: vortex vein (V) and its tributaries from the choriocapillaris (CH). Vascular cast, SEM original magnification ×180. (Courtesy of A. W. Fryczkowski.) (t) Human choroid: venulo–venular anastomoses (arrow). A = Artery; V = vein. Vascular cast, SEM original magnification ×380. (Courtesy of A. W. Fryczkowski.)

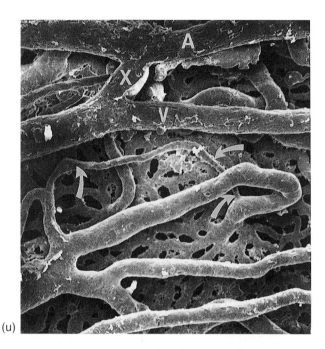

(u)

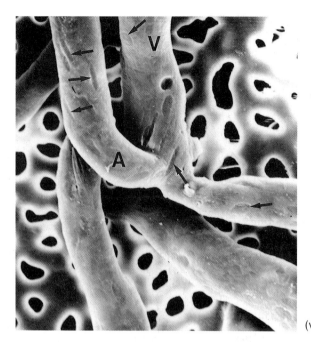

(v)

(w)

Fig. 11.13 (contd) (u) Human choroid: arteriovenous shunt (X), posterior pole, posterior view. A = Artery; V = vein. Venular collateral channel shown by arrows. Vascular cast, SEM original magnification ×580. (Courtesy of A. W. Fryczkowski.) (v) Human choroid: arteriovenous shunt. A = Artery; v = vein. Endothelial cells (arrows) are spindle-shaped in the artery and oval in the vein. Vascular cast, SEM original magnification ×500. (w) Scanning electron micrograph of the demarcating vascular loop at the peripapillary choroid (original magnification ×360). Courtesy of M. Araki.)

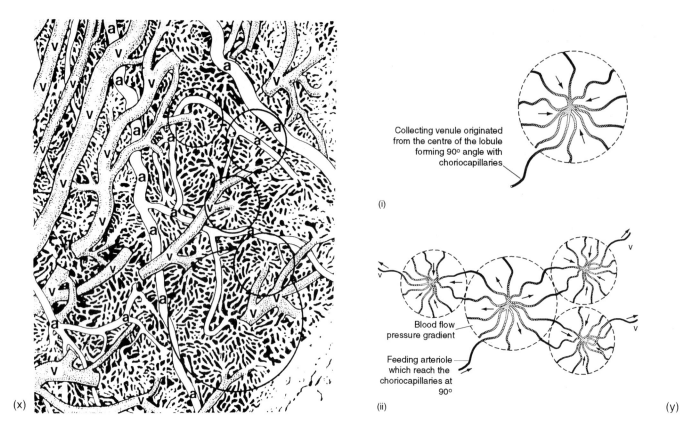

Fig. 11.13 (contd) (x) Anatomical lobuli, based on an SEM. Veins were partially removed to better visualize arteries and their feeding arterioles, and their course and connections with the choriocapillaries. a = Artery; v = vein. Anatomical lobuli are encircled (small circles) and an area slightly larger than the functional choroidal vascular unit is also outlined (large circle). (Courtesy of A. W. Fryczkowski.) (y) Drawings of the choroidal angioarchitecture based on Fryczkowski's concept. (i) The anatomical lobule with a centripetal arrangement of the capillaries and with the vein in the centre. (ii) The choroidal vascular functional unit – with artery (a) in the centre, with a centrifugal arrangement of the arterial capillaries and with venules (v) collecting from centripetally organized venous capillaries. The pressure gradient creates a functional barrier between the arterial and venous part of the capillaries (circular outline). This choroidal vascular unit is seen on fluorescein angiography and indocyanine green angiography as 'lobuli'.

predominant lobular anatomy at the posterior pole is with the feeding arteriole located peripherally and one or more draining venules located centrally (Fryczkowski *et al.*, 1989, 1991; Fryczkowski, 1992, 1993). The 'venocentric' lobular organization is also found in the equatorial choriocapillaris. Fryczkowski (1993) has suggested that the arteriocentric organization suggested by earlier fluorescein and histological studies may simply reflect the dynamic events occurring during fluorescein angiography that describe the 'functional vascular unit' (Fig. 11.13y,z), as opposed to the 'anatomical unit' suggested by vascular cast studies. The interpretation of later cast studies has been greatly aided by the establishment of specific criteria to differentiate arterial from venous vessels. Arterial endothelial nuclei form spindle-shaped impressions which run along the axis of the vessel cast, while venous nuclei produce round impressions which are randomly disposed along the vessel (Risco, Grimson and Johnson, 1981; Berger

et al., 1987; Fryczkowski and Sherman, 1988; Fryczkowski, Sherman and Walker, 1991; Olver, Spalton and McCartney, 1990). The lobules are conceived as a functional unit arranged in a mosaic, with little anastomosis between them; similarly each short posterior ciliary artery has its separate territory of supply, with limited functional anastomosis between adjacent territories. Experimental evidence has come from the injection of microspheres (Stern and Ernest, 1974; Uyama *et al.*, 1980) or from studies involving the division of posterior or short posterior ciliary arteries (Hayreh, 1974a,b,c, 1975a; Hayreh and Baines, 1972). These territories vary widely in size and shape, but temporal to the disc, where they have been most studied, they spread radially from the submacular region towards the periphery, reflecting the entry of the short posterior ciliary arteries at this location (Hayreh, 1974c).

The deficient anastomosis between each zone creates vascular watersheds, which are regarded as important determinants of the shape and location of occlusive events in the choroid and at the optic nerve head (Fig. 11.11). Occlusion of the posterior ciliary or short posterior ciliary arteries gives rise to triangular zones of ischaemia, or vertically disposed zones, lying above or below the disc (Amalric, 1963, 1973). Occlusion of choroidal arterioles produces small foci of ischaemia which give rise to pale lesions seen ophthalmoscopically as 'Elschnig spots'. Whatever recovery occurs after such ischaemic injury has been attributed to the presence of limited intervenular or interarteriolar anastomoses, for instance at the posterior pole (Ring and Fujino, 1967; Weiter and Ernest, 1974; Yoneya and Tso, 1984, 1987; Lee and Olver, 1990; Olver, 1990; Fryczkowski, 1992). Interarteriolar anastomoses are found particular in the submacular choroid (Fryczkowski, 1992), while rare intercapillary and interarteriolar anastomoses have been demonstrated between the anterior and posterior uvea (Olver, Spalton and McCartney, 1990: see also Ashton, 1961; Wybar, 1954; Hayreh, 1974a, 1975; Risco, Grimson and Johnson, 1981; Woodlief and Eifrig, 1982; Krey, 1975).

The medial and lateral ciliary arteries each supply, by their short posterior ciliary branches, the nasal and temporal halves of the choroid. The **lateral posterior ciliary artery** may supply up to two-thirds of the choroid (Hayreh, 1976). The watershed between nasal and temporal territories is vertical and usually centred on the optic disc; occasionally the watershed is obliquely disposed.

The vessel density in the macular region is much greater than elsewhere. The almost inextricable mass of vessels of various size resembles cavernous tissue. The veins anastomose freely (Fig. 11.14) but a venous watershed along the horizontal meridian has been proposed. A special submacular arterial supply was proposed by Weiter and Ernest (1974) but has not been generally confirmed.

The choriocapillaris subjacent to the macula and posterior pole forms a close meshwork fed by precapillary arterioles (lumen 20–40 μm) entering its posterior surface or sometimes in the plane of the capillaries. These arterioles may be short and perpendicular to the surface, or, particularly near the equator and periphery, may run a course parallel to the capillary bed before supplying it. The capillaries are of wide bore (20–50 μm) and the meshes of the capillary net are of variable width, 3–18 μm in the posterior eye, where the lobules are densely packed and less easily distinguished from one another or even absent. They are wider and longer at the equator (6–36 × 36–400 μm; Hogan, Alvarado and Weddell, 1971), thus forming a remarkable intercon-

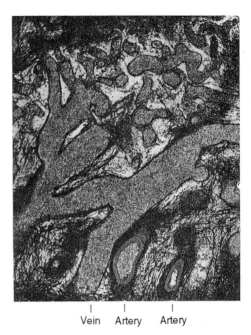

I   I   I
Vein   Artery   Artery

Fig. 11.14 Flat section of the choroid at the macula to show anastomosing choroidal veins (Zenker, Mallory's trichrome). The arteries have a well-developed tunica media and generally thicker walls than the veins.

necting capillary channel. The postcapillary venules have lumens of 10–40 μm width. In the periphery the capillary lobules are larger and are more radially disposed. The capillaries are wider, with flattened elliptical cross-sections, and are more widely separated. The arterioles and venules here lie in the same plane as the choriocapillaris.

A different arrangement exists at the optic nerve head and in the peripheral choroid. The **peripapillary choriocapillaris** has a smooth margin as it abuts the nerve but some arterial twigs may enter the nerve head (Fig. 11.13t,u). The capillaries show an approximately radial elongation for about 100 μm around the nerve. The meshes of the **peripheral choriocapillaris** are wider than those at the posterior pole, and no longer form a flat capillary sheet because the terminal arterioles and postcapillary venules occur in the same plane. A single terminal arteriole serves a larger zone of capillaries (Shimizu and Kazuyoshi, 1978). The choriocapillaris stops at the ora serrata.

Intercapillary septa

Between the capillary meshes are bundles of collagen fibres which form so-called intercapillary septa (Wybar, 1954; Klein, 1966; Ring and Fujino, 1967; Torczynski and Tso, 1976; Araki, 1977). Because these occupy spaces between capillaries, they are round, oval or square in tangential section posteriorly and

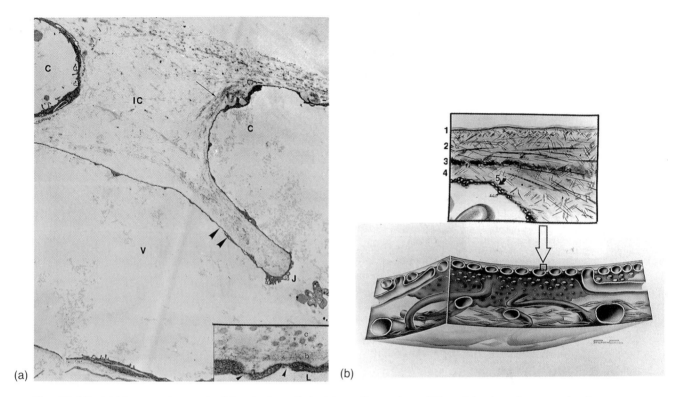

(a)

(b)

Fig. 11.15 (a) Electron micrograph of the choriocapillaris. Intercapillary column (IC) contains loosely arranged collagen; longitudinal section of collagen (arrow) near lateral wall of capillary (C) gives shape to the vessel. The capillary floor (arrowheads) slants outward at junction (J) of capillary and venule (V). Platelet is in lumen (original magnification ×5510). Inset: endothelium of inner wall of choriocapillaris with fenestrations (arrowheads). Layers of Bruch's membrane (b) of capillaris. L = Lumen of capillary (original magnification ×98 600). (b) Schematic view of the choroid. Arteriole shown in cross-section on the right as it joins the choriocapillaris perpendicularly, venule in cross-section on the left. Capillaries are separated by intercapillary pillars of connective tissue continuous with Bruch's membrane. Detail of Bruch's membrane above, showing (1) basement membrane of retinal pigment epithelium; (2) collagen; (3) elastic tissue; (4) collagen; (5) basement membrane of the choriocapillaris, which is discontinuous at the intercapillary columns. (From Torczynski, E., in Duane, T. D. and Jaeger, E. A. (eds) (1987) *Biomedical Foundations of Ophthalmology* published by Lippincott, with permission.)

form elongated fillets at the equator and anteriorly. Occasional gaps permit intercapillary anastomoses. The septa are reinforced by fibres from the collagenous zones of Bruch's membrane and their fibres intermingle with collagen in the supraciliary layer (stromal aspect of the choriocapillaris). The capillaries are thus held in a relatively rigid collagen framework which prevents their collapse (Hogan, Alvarado and Weddell, 1971) (Fig. 11.15). As in the retina (Friedman, Kopald and Smith, 1964), there appears to be a continuous flow in the choroidal capillaries (Friedman and Oak, 1965). In the iris, a great number of capillaries seem not to be perfused at any one time (Bill, Tornqvist and Alm, 1980).

Structure of choroidal vessels

The **arteries** have a muscular tunica media and an adventitia of fibrillar collagenous tissue containing thick elastic fibres. According to Wolfrum (1908) the **arterioles** possess muscular fibrils with long

processes which surround the vessels like the tentacles of an octopus. The vascular **adventitia** is more or less continuous with the choroidal adventitia. The

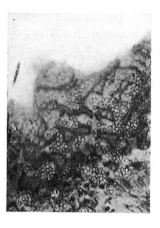

Fig. 11.16 Flat section of the choriocapillaris. Note the areas of connective tissue (staining denser at the periphery than the centre) between streams of corpuscles in the capillaries.

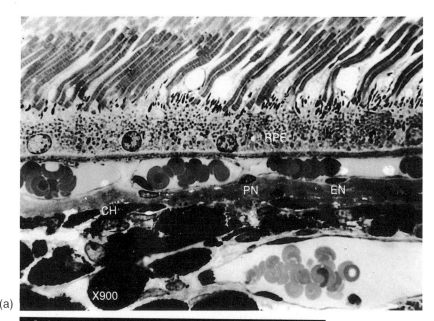

(a)

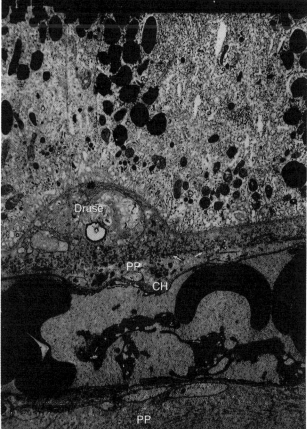

(b)

Fig. 11.17 (a) Low-power TEM to show the relationship between Bruch's membrane and the choriocapillaris. (b) Low-power TEM showing the presence of a druse of Bruch's membrane. CH = Choriocapillaris; PP = pericyte processes; RPE = retinal pigment epithelium (Courtesy of J. Duvall.)

veins have a perivascular sheath, outside which there is an adventitia of connective tissue.

Capillaries

Capillaries of the choriocapillaris are large in calibre, allowing several erythrocytes to pass along together (Figs 11.16, 11.17 and 11.18). They are tubes of endothelial cells, with pericytes disposed only on the scleral face of the capillaries, and incompletely investing them. Whereas the ratio of pericytes to endothelial cells is about 1:2 in the retinal capillaries, the ratio is 1:6 in the choriocapillaris. **Pericytes** are

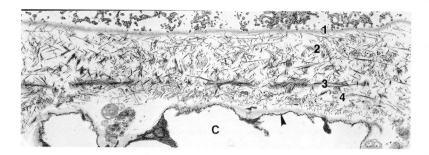

Fig. 11.18 The five layers of Bruch's membrane include (1) the basement membrane of the retinal pigment epithelium; (2) the inner collagenous layer; (3) the elastic layer; (4) the outer collagenous layer; (5) the basal lamina of the choriocapillaris (arrowhead). C = Lumen of capillary (original magnification ×5510). (From Torczynski, E., in Duane, T. D. and Jaeger, E. A. (eds) (1987) *Biomedical Foundations of Ophthalmology* published by Lippincott, with permission.)

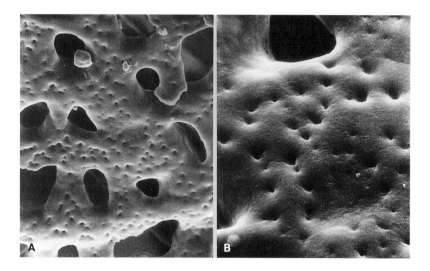

Fig. 11.19 (A) SEM of corrosion cast of choriocapillaris of cynomolgus monkey injected with plastic monomer; posterior pole. Large, dark oval areas are intercapillary columns. Inner surface of the capillaries shows many indentations, the fenestrations or pores (original magnification ×1200). (B) Fenestrations at high magnification (original magnification ×3600). (From Araki, M. (1977) *Acta Soc. Ophthalmol. Jpn*, **80**, 315, with permission.)

contractile cells, which in other tissues regulate blood supply or serve a nutritive function. Their disposition in choroidal capillaries would suggest that contraction is unlikely to bring about regulation of flow; this is in keeping with the constant high flow in the choroid. Pericytes are more numerous at the fovea.

The capillaries are fenestrated like those of the viscera and account for the permeability of the choroid to small molecules, including sodium fluorescein and even proteins (Bill, 1968; Shiose, 1970). Fenestrations are 60–80 nm in diameter, and are covered by a thin diaphragm of attenuated cytoplasm which is thickened centrally (30 nm) (Fig. 11.19). The circular fenestrations are evenly and abundantly disposed on the interior face of the capillaries which adjoin Bruch's membrane, except for a narrow rim at the periphery of each endothelial cell. There are fewer fenestrations on the lateral and external aspects of the cells. The endothelium is enveloped by a thin basal lamina which also surrounds the pericytes (Feeney and Hogan, 1961; Matsusaka, 1975). The lateral interfaces of the endothelial cells are sloping.

The endothelial lining of the choroidal arterioles shows typical occluding zonules between cells, but the junctions between the endothelial cells of the choriocapillaris, and also of the venules, are of a special type, similar to those in hepatic sinusoids (Yee and Revel, 1975) and venules of the mesentery (Simionescu, Simionescu and Palade, 1975). Freeze-fracture techniques show that the reciprocal folds and grooves on the P and E faces of junctions lack the typical interconnecting strands of the tight junction (Fig. 11.20). Instead, there are discontinuous zonulae occludentae (maculae or fasciae occludente) which might be expected to perform as leaky junctions (Raviola, 1977; Spitznas and Reale, 1975). Gap junctions are present at the scleral end of the lateral interfaces between endothelial cells and pericytes (Spitznas and Reale, 1975). The capillary bed is supported by a collagenous framework, with some fibrocytes, within meshes of the choriocapillaris and in the overlying supracapillary layer (Fig. 11.15).

BRUCH'S MEMBRANE

Bruch's membrane (lamina vitrea) is a thin non-cellular lamina between the choriocapillaris and retinal pigment epithelium, derived from each of them. It is described in this chapter partly for convenience. Its fused elements cannot be separated in the normal eye and adhere to the choriocapillaris

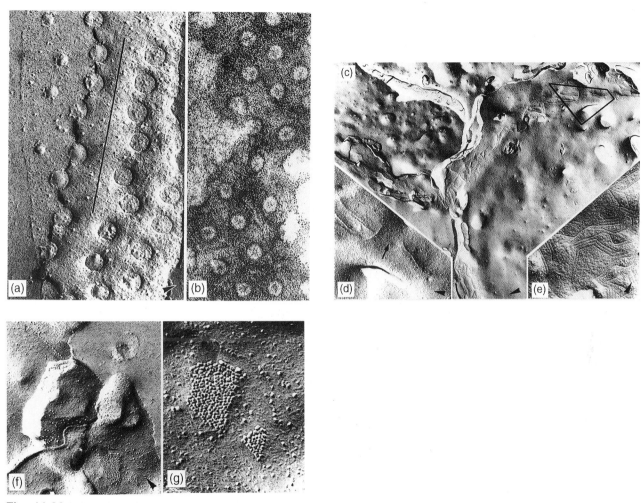

Fig. 11.20 Composite of fracture faces of zonulae occludentes between endothelial cells of a choroidal venule. (a) and (b) Fenestrated endothelium of a choroidal capillary. (a) On the left of the dark line the smooth central prominence bridging the fenestrae is clearly seen; on the right small particles are seen; (b) grazing section: central thickenings are seen in most of the sections. (c) Extensive zonula occludentes centrally. In most places the strands are branching and interconnected; in limited areas they are missing. (d) Higher magnification of area delineated in (c) with interruption (arrow) of the zonula occludens (original magnification ×46 000). (e) Typically angulated strands of a zonula occludens, seen as imprinted grooves on cell surface (original magnification ×42 000). (f) and (g) Gap junction on the plasma membrane of a choroidal capillary endothelial cell. The junction lies close to an intercellular suture (original magnification ×62 000 and ×160 000). (From Spitznas, M. and Reale, E. (1975) *Invest. Ophthalmol. Vis. Sci.*, **14**, 98, with permission.)

when the pigment epithelium is scraped from the choroid in dissection.

Bruch's membrane extends from the margin of the optic disc to the ora serrata. It is smooth and regular and averages 2 μm in thickness in early adult life but increases in thickness with age. It is thickest near the disc (2–4 μm) and tapers in the periphery to 1–2 μm. Earlier light microscopy studies showed a featureless glassy membrane, while more selective stains later showed an inner 'cuticular' zone and an outer connective tissue zone. However, ultrastructural studies (Feeney and Hogan, 1961; Hogan, 1961; Hollenberg and Burt, 1969; Hogan, Alvarado and Weddell, 1971) have shown it to be a complex structure with the following layers (Figs 11.21 and 11.22):

1. inner basal lamina (of retinal pigment epithelium) (0.3 μm);
2. inner collagenous zone (1 μm);
3. elastic zone;
4. outer collagenous zone;
5. outer basal lamina (of choriocapillaris) (0.14 μm).

Inner basal lamina

The inner basal lamina is a continuous layer in continuity with the basal lamina of the ciliary epithelium. It is synthesized by the retinal pigment

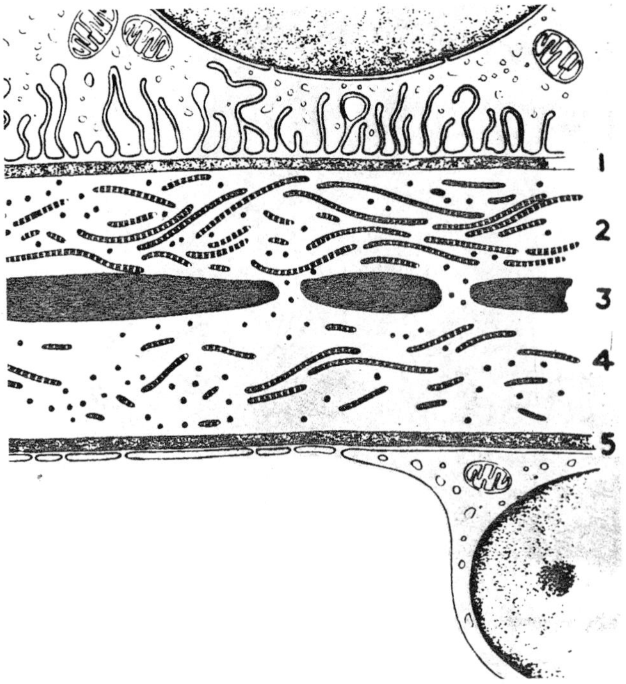

Fig. 11.21 Diagram of the layers of Bruch's membrane. (1) Basement membrane of the retinal pigment epithelium; (2) anterior collagenous zone; (3) elastic layer; (4) narrow, outer collagenous layer; (5) basement membrane of the choriocapillaris. (From Hogan, M. J., Alvarado, J. A. and Weddell, J. E. (1971) *Histology of the Human Eye*, published by W. B. Saunders.)

epithelium and separated from it by a radiolucent zone 100 nm wide. It does not follow the many infoldings of the retinal pigment epithelium, but may project towards them. Its fine filaments blend with fibres of the adjacent collagenous zone (Fig. 11.23).

Inner collagenous zone

This is composed of interweaving collagen fibres, some in the plane of the layer and others traversing the elastic layer to reach the outer collagenous zone. It is 1 μm thick, but thicker towards the ora.

Elastic zone

The elastic layer is composed of rod-like fibres with a dense cortex and homogeneous core. These form a narrow strip which in cross-section is interrupted irregularly by collagen fibres passing between the collagenous zones. In flat section there are interwoven bands of elastic fibres of varying thickness.

Outer collagenous zone

This is similar to the inner zone. It is traversed by collagen fibres from the inner zone which then pass

through the interruptions in the outer basal lamina to join collagen fibres of the intercapillary septa and the supracapillary region, thus contributing to the collagenous investment of the capillaries. Vesicles, linear structures and dense bodies occur in the collagenous and elastic zones but predominantly in the inner collagenous layer.

Outer basal lamina

The outer basal lamina is the deep stratum of the lamina which invests capillaries in the choriocapillaris and is therefore not a continuous sheet across the outer aspect of Bruch's membrane. At the ora serrata the inner basal lamina continues forwards into the ciliary body, but the outer lamina becomes separated from it by a well-marked connective tissue layer between them.

Drüsen

Over the age of 40 years focal aggregations of debris are observed immediately external to the retinal pigment epithelium; these excrescences are called **drüsen** (or colloid bodies) (Farkas, Krill and Sylvester, 1971; Sarks, 1976; Foos and Trese, 1982) (Fig. 11.17b). These should not be confused with the congenital glial inclusions found rarely within the papilla, and termed drüsen of the optic nerve head (Spencer, 1978).

11.5 ARTERIAL SUPPLY OF THE CILIARY BODY AND IRIS

As noted earlier, the major circle of the iris is formed predominantly by the long posterior ciliary arteries, while the intramuscular circle of the ciliary muscle is formed by the penetrating branches of the anterior ciliary arteries.

CIRCULUS IRIDIS MAJOR

The circulus iridis major is really located in the ciliary body, anterior to the circular part of the ciliary muscle (Figs 6.18, 11.24 and 11.25) and anterior to the muscular circle. The arteries of the ciliary muscle are numerous and dichotomize to form a dense capillary plexus markedly different from that of the ciliary processes. The latter arteries spring from the major arterial circle, often with those of the iris. Each process usually receives a separate artery, but a larger branch may supply two, or even three, adjacent processes (Fig. 11.25b). These arteries, like those in the iris, pierce the ciliary muscle to enter the ciliary

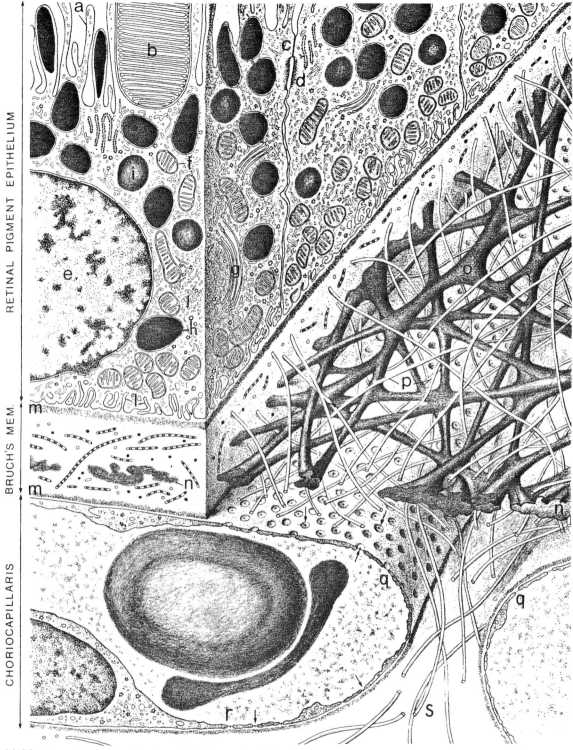

RETINAL PIGMENT EPITHELIUM

BRUCH'S MEM.

CHORIOCAPILLARIS

Fig. 11.22   Three-dimensional drawing of the inner choroid and retinal pigment epithelium. The villi of the pigment epithelium (a) extend internally to enclose the outer segments of the rods and cones (b). The intercellular junctions are characterized by a zonula occludens (c) and a desmosome (d); otherwise the cell relations are of the usual type. The cytoplasm of the pigment cells contains a nucleus (e), mitochondria (f), a Golgi apparatus (g), pigment granules (h), phagosomes (i) and is characterized by a large amount of smooth-surfaced endoplasmic reticulum (j). The external cell membrane shows complex infoldings (l) and a basement membrane (m). Bruch's membrane shows an apparently interrupted elastic zone (n) in meridional section, but the elastica is layered and continuous in flat section (o). Collagen fibrils (p) which form the inner and outer collagenous zones have a random orientation around the elastic zone. The choriocapillaris (q) shows a fenestrated endothelium internally, laterally and to a lesser extent externally (r). The intercapillary zone shows considerable collagen (s). The lumen of the capillary contains two red cells. (From Hogan, M. J., Alvarado, J. A. and Weddell, J. E. (1971) *Histology of the Human Eye*, published by W. B. Saunders.)

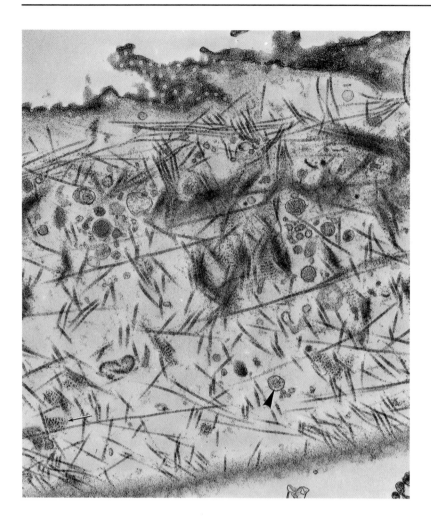

Fig. 11.23 TEM of Bruch's membrane in a 13-year-old girl. This slightly oblique section shows membrane-bound vacuoles (arrowhead) and bundles of long-spacing collagen (arrow) scattered throughout the middle layers. Endothelial fenestrations with central densities are shown below (original magnification ×31 900). (From Torczynski, E., in Duane, T. D. and Jaeger, E. A. (eds) (1987) *Biomedical Foundations of Ophthalmology*, published by Lippincott, with permission.)

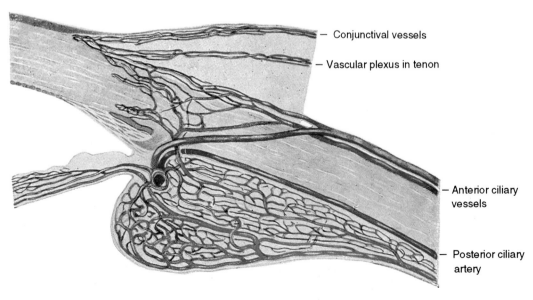

— Conjunctival vessels

— Vascular plexus in tenon

— Anterior ciliary vessels

— Posterior ciliary artery

Fig. 11.24 The vessels of the anterior segment (from Lauber, after Maggiori).

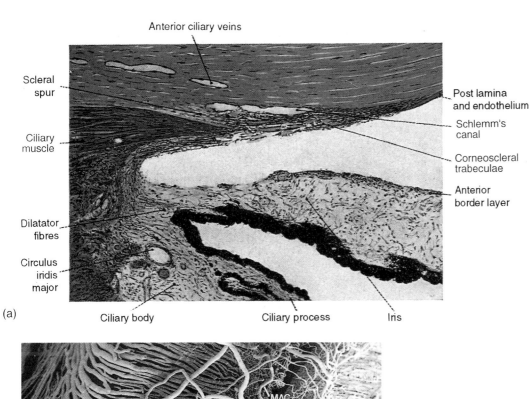

(a)

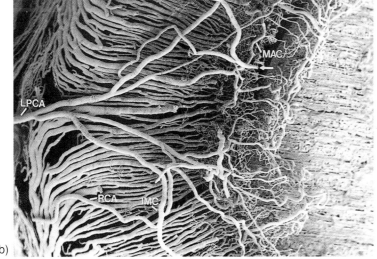

(b)

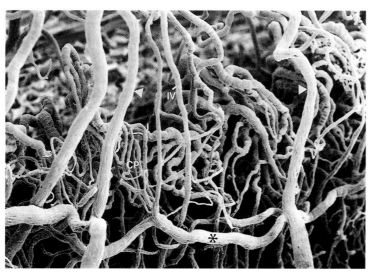

(c)

Fig. 11.25 (a) Section of the angle of the anterior chamber. (b) Anterior view of cynomolgous monkey lumenal castings after removal of ciliary muscle capillaries. The long posterior ciliary artery (LPCA) and the perforating branches (arrows) of the anterior ciliary arteries join within the ciliary muscle to form the intramuscular circle (IMC). Branches from the intramuscular circle contribute to the segmental, discontinuous, major artery circle (MAC). RCA = Recurrent ciliary artery (original magnification ×30). (From Morrison, J. C. and van Buskirk, E. M. (1986) *Trans. Ophthalmol. Soc.*, **105**, 13, with permission.) (c) Anterior view of the 'major' arterial circle (*) composed of circumferentially oriented vessels derived from the intramuscular circle. Note frequent iris arterial (arrowheads) and ciliary process arterials (CP). IV = Iris vein, passing posterior to the major arterial circle to enter the choroidal veins (original magnification ×150). (From Morrison, J. C. and van Buskirk, E. M. (1986) *Trans. Ophthalmol. Soc.*, **105**, 13, with permission.)

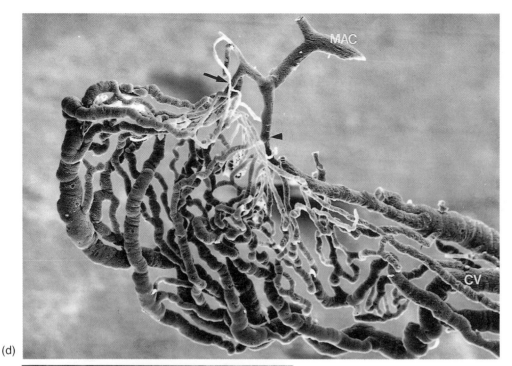

(d)

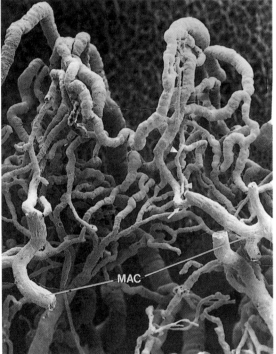

(e)

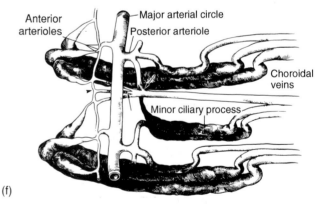

(f)

Fig. 11.25 (contd)   (d) Microvascular cast of a major ciliary process in the monkey. Constricted arterioles (arrow) from the major arterial circle (MAC) supply irregularly dilated capillaries in the anterior region and crest of the ciliary process. Large artery (arrowhead) supplies capillaries in the central portion of the process. All capillaries empty posteriorly into the choroidal veins (CV) (original magnification ×75). (From Morrison, J. C. and van Buskirk, E. M. (1986) *Trans. Ophthalmol. Soc.*, **105**, 13, with permission.) (e) Posterior view of two contiguous ciliary processes. An arterial and arteriole (arrow) from the major arterial circle (MAC) directly enters a ciliary process and overlies one of its own branches (arrowheads), obscuring its destination (original magnification ×205). (From Morrison, J. C. and van Buskirk, E. M. (1986) *Trans. Ophthalmol. Soc.*, **105**, 13, with permission.) (f) External view of the interconnections of two contiguous major ciliary processes. Lateral anterior arteriole branches join to form interprocess intracapillary networks (arrowhead) that provide communication between major processes. Laterally directed posterior arterioles form posterior interprocess networks through which the minor ciliary processes receive blood; additionally both anterior and posterior interprocess networks drain directly into the choroidal veins (arrows). (From Morrison, J. C. and van Buskirk, E. M. (1986) *Trans. Ophthalmol. Soc.*, **105**, 13, with permission.)

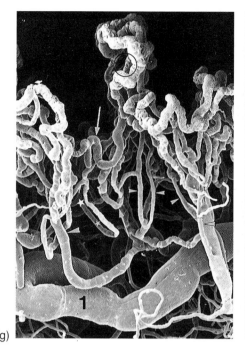

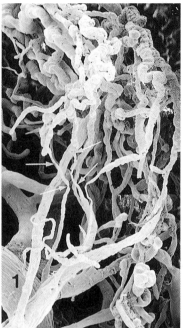

Eye A   Eye B

Fig. 11.25 contd (g) Scanning electron micrographs of vascular resin casts of the ciliary body in the human eye: anterior aspect. Circle = Major ciliary process; 1 = MACI; arrows = first vascular territory; ** = venules of this territory. This cast is from a pair of autopsy eyes (4 hours post mortem). Before plastic injection, eye A was immersed in Ringer's solution (control eye) and eye B was immersed in 50 ml Ringer's solution plus 1 mg adrenaline. In the anterior ciliary process arterioles of the treated eye, marked constrictions were present in a segment of 60–100 μm (arrows in B), whereas in a comparable segment of the anterior arterioles of the control eye (arrowheads in A) no, or only weak calibre reductions were found. (From Funk, R. and Rohen, J. W. (1990) *Exp. Eye Res.*, **51**, 651, with permission.)

process anteriorly, where they branch and anastomose into a dense plexus of wide capillaries forming the main mass of the processes. The veins anastomose extensively and drain into the venae vorticosae. They are internal to the ciliary muscle.

11.6   VASCULATURE OF CILIARY MUSCLE AND PARS PLANA

The inner and anterior part of the ciliary muscle is mainly fed by arterioles derived from the **major arterial circle** of the iris, whereas the outer and more superficial part is supplied by the **intramuscular circle**, formed by the anterior ciliary arteries. This arrangement is consistent with the demonstration that the muscle consists of two histochemically and probably functionally different parts (Flügel, Bárány and Lütjen-Drecoll, 1990). Venules drain into the ciliary valleys, or directly back into the pars plana. The pars plana receives tributaries from the iris, from the (basal) venules of the first and third territories of the ciliary processes, and from the marginal venules of the second vascular territory (see below).

The anterior zone exhibits capillary interconnections with the third vascular territory of the ciliary processes (see below), especially those in the ciliary valleys, and some small arterioles and capillaries from the ciliary muscle pass into this layer. The mid zone has more large, flat venules lying in parallel with sparse interconnections or bifurcations and the

posterior zone increasingly takes up the pattern typical of the choriocapillaris.

11.7   VASCULATURE OF THE CILIARY PROCESS

The arterioles of the ciliary processes derive from the major arterial circle of the iris (i.e. anterior to the intramuscular circle) (Fig. 11.24b,e). They often show luminal constrictions once they have reached the processes.

Three vascular territories may be recognized (see Chapter 10 and Funk and Rohen, 1990).

FIRST VASCULAR TERRITORY

The first vascular territory lies anteriorly, in the crest of each major ciliary process. This is fed by a fan of short arterioles. The capillary network has separate venules which turn towards the bases of neighbouring ciliary processes and then run posteriorly.

SECOND VASCULAR TERRITORY

Also in the anterior part of the major processes is the second vascular territory. This has two components.

Main capillary network

The main capillary network lies centrally in the depth of the ciliary process and drains into the marginal venules formed by the superficial capillary network.

Superficial capillary network

This is sparse and forms an almost direct connection between the feeding arteriole and the large marginal venule (sometimes two) situated sagittally at the inner edge of the ciliary process and forming the efferent venous segment. This continues as a **pars plana venule**.

THIRD VASCULAR TERRITORY

This consists of the capillary networks within the minor ciliary processes and the posterior third of the major ciliary processes. Those within the major processes drain partly into the marginal venule and partly into the basally arranged venules. Those of the minor ciliary processes also drain into a marginal venule leading to pars plana vessels. There are also fine anastomosing capillaries in the valleys between the major and minor ciliary processes here. Interconnections exist between these vascular beds and those in the ciliary muscle.

FUNCTIONAL ASPECTS

Studies in monkeys and rabbits show that the terminal arterioles supplying the first and second vascular territories are constricted by adrenergic drugs (Fig. 11.27i). The first territory in these species may also be functionally different from the others and more susceptible to breakdown of the blood–aqueous barrier, for instance after paracentesis (Funk and Rohen, 1989; Funk, 1991; Ohnishi and Tanaka, 1981). The venular drainage of this territory is relatively discrete from the other two territories, in the human as well as in monkeys and rabbits (Morrison, 1987a; Funk and Rohen, 1987). In human ciliary processes there is a *marginal route* (as in the rabbit), which is thought to offer a rapid flow system with a high venous pO_2 and a high venous pressure which may favour filtration rather than aqueous absorption.

11.8   NERVES OF THE CILIARY BODY

These are branches of the long and short ciliary nerves (Fig. 11.25h). They form a plexus in the ciliary muscle. Their fibres, at first medullated, are among the muscle fibres. At each bifurcation is a triangular thickening from which innumerable fibrils emerge. **Sensory fibres** are recognized by their club-shaped endings. **Vasomotor nerves** also occur, surrounding the vessels in the ciliary processes, and are not medullated.

11.9   ARTERIES OF THE IRIS

The arteries of the iris arise from the circulus major, often with those to the ciliary processes. There is also a supply from the perforating branches of the anterior ciliary arteries. They enter the iris at the attachments of the ciliary processes, usually several to each process (Leber) and in intervals between the peripheral crypts. Anastomosing occasionally, they converge radially from ciliary to pupillary margin. In pupillary miosis their course is straight, but they become sinuous as the pupil dilates. Like the veins, their walls are thick in comparison with their calibre (Fig. 9.15).

The vessels are visible as radial streaks united with each other here and there. They are more visible in blue irides than brown and are apparent only in the ciliary part. Dense iridial pigment obscures them in coloured races, and blood is only slightly visible in albinotic eyes. At the collarette, a few anastomoses occur, which, with corresponding venous anastomoses, make an incomplete vascular circle, the so-called **circulus arteriosus iridis minor**. Most vessels reach the pupillary margin where, after breaking up into capillaries, they bend round into the veins.

CAPILLARY PLEXUS

A dense capillary plexus surrounds the sphincter muscle and another, less dense plexus is anterior to the dilator. In the ciliary region the capillary plexus is less dense and is sparse or absent in the anterior limiting layer.

STRUCTURE OF IRIDIAL VESSELS

These vessels are usually said to have a markedly thick and hyaline adventitious coat: this is only partly true and is the appearance given by stains such as haematoxylin and eosin, etc. The adventitia is certainly thick, but if Mallory's connective tissue stain is used a much more accurate idea of the real structure is obtained. The adventitia may be more or less uniform or may be thinner in its inner region. Mostly typically, however, the vessel appears to consist of two tubes, one within the other. The outer is the adventitia proper which stains deep blue, and is made up of very fine connective tissue fibres, while the inner consists of the essential blood channel, that is, the endothelial lining to which are added, in the case of the arteries, muscle cells and elastic fibres.

Between these is a relatively wide zone filled with a loose collagenous **tunica media** peculiar to these vessels (Fig. 9.15). The zone is no doubt associated with the constant concertina-like movement of the iris in pupillary dilatation and constriction of the pupil, and thus with the repeated straightening and wrinkling of the vessels.

The arteries and veins are distinguished not by the thickness of the adventitia, which is proportional to the size of the vessels, but by the structure of the inner tube, which is much thicker in the arteries. These have a media of circular non-striated muscle cells, which can be followed to the capillaries, and elastic fibres in the intima which reach almost as far. The arterial wall shows four layers of cells: (1) endothelial cells, with nuclei elongated in the axis of the vessel; (2) muscle cells, with nuclei at right-angles to this axis; (3) loosely packed media with pale-staining fibrocytes and collagen; and (4) fibrous adventitia (Fig. 9.15b).

The iris capillary endothelium has a thick (0.5–3 μm), often multilayered basal lamina, outside which are numerous round or oval bodies. Pericytes also exist outside the basal lamina. The endothelial cell borders are not fenestrated and are joined together by tight junctions, impermeable to protein tracers (Vegge, 1971; Raviola, 1974). Although they resemble retinal capillaries in this respect, they differ in some species in that exposure to histamine renders them permeable to macromolecules (Ashton and Cunha-Vaz, 1965), while the retinal capillaries are insensitive to this. However, whereas paracentesis increases the permeability of iridial vessels in cats, rabbits and rats, it does not influence their permeability in monkeys (Raviola, 1974). The endothelial cells are unusual in the possession of rod-shaped electron-dense structures within a unit membrane lying close to the Golgi apparatus. They are similar to Weibel–Palade bodies found in retinal capillaries.

11.10 INNERVATION OF THE IRIS

Nerves arise as numerous branches of the ciliary plexus, composed largely of non-myelinated fibres. They form plexuses in the anterior border layer (possibly sensory), around vessels, and anterior to the dilator pupillae. From the last, many non-myelinated fibres innervate muscle cells by endings which may contain synaptic vesicles and form close contacts (20 nm). Sympathetic and parasympathetic fibres occur. Adrenergic and cholinergic activity has been demonstrated in both the sphincter and dilator (Lowenstein and Loewenfeld, 1969).

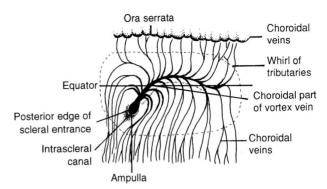

Fig. 11.26 Ampulliform dilatation at the confluence of vortex vein tributaries. (After Rutin, U. (1967) *Am. J. Ophthalmol.*, **64**, 281.)

11.11 VEINS OF THE UVEAL TRACT

The venae vorticosae drain blood from all parts of the choroid and practically the whole uveal tract. The anterior ciliary veins drain part of the ciliary muscle. These two sets communicate, which may explain compensatory changes in circulation in certain circumstances; thus in acute glaucoma, where outflow of venous blood through venae vorticosae is impeded, the anterior ciliary veins carry larger quantities of blood than usual (Fig. 11.26).

VENAE VORTICOSAE (POSTERIOR CILIARY VEINS)

There are usually four veins (two superior and two inferior), which pierce the sclera obliquely on each side of the superior and inferior rectus muscles about 6 mm behind the equator of the globe (Fig. 11.2). No veins leave the eye in the region where the posterior ciliary arteries enter (except, very rarely, in myopic eyes). The superior veins leave the eye further back than the inferior, while the lateral veins tend to be nearer the mid-vertical plane than the medial. The superior lateral vein is the most posterior (8 mm behind the equator), and is close to the insertion of the superior oblique (Fig. 11.2). The inferior lateral vein is the most anterior (5.5 mm behind the equator). Often there are more than four veins. At times, especially in myopic eyes, they may leave the globe much further back, even close to the optic nerve.

The passage of the vortex veins through the sclera is as oblique as that of the long posterior ciliary arteries. The canals, about 4 mm long, point posteriorly towards the mid-vertical plane of the eye so that the four veins appear to converge towards a common parent trunk (Leber). Their course in the canals is visible externally, as, because of the translucency of the sclera, they appear as dark lines. The veins may divide in the canals so that six or more vessels may emerge. The stems of the venae vorticosae undergo ampulliform dilatation just before they enter the sclera (Fig. 11.26). They are joined by radial and curved tributaries which give the whole a whorl-like appearance, apparent on the outer surface of the choroid, and visible during ophthalmoscopy in blonde, myopic or albinoid fundi (Figs 11.28 and 11.29). It is this appearance which is responsible for the name venae vorticosae.

Choroidal veins

The choroidal veins form the venae vorticosae. The posterior tributaries arise from posterior choroid, optic nerve head, and sometimes peripapillary retina. The branches from around the optic disc run more or less directly to the venae vorticosae, and are longest draining the posterior choroid (Fig. 11.27). The more they enter the vein from the sides, the shorter and more curved they are. It is obvious that here the veins do not follow the course of the corresponding arteries.

Anterior tributaries

The anterior tributaries of the vorticose veins come from the iris, the ciliary processes, the ciliary muscle

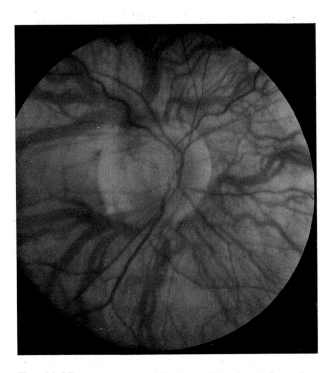

Fig. 11.27 Arrangement of the choroidal veins at the optic disc of a myope.

and anterior region of the choroid. The veins are parallel with each other in the pars plana but at the ora serrata turn obliquely towards the corresponding vena vorticosa, receiving branches from the choroid as they do so.

Veins of the ciliary processes

These pass backwards as a series of parallel anastomosing vessels in the pars plana to the inner side of the ciliary muscle to reach the choroid and join the venae vorticosae.

Veins of the ciliary muscle

These mostly pass back to join the parallel veins from the ciliary processes. A few, however, pass forwards and pierce the sclera to join the anterior ciliary veins.

Iris veins

The veins of the iris run like the arteries, anastomose with each other, and at the ciliary border enter the ciliary body to join the veins of the ciliary processes and so to the venae vorticosae.

Hayreh and Baines (1973) have suggested that, in primates, the vortex veins drain a well-defined segmental territory extending the full sagittal length of the uveal tract, from the iris through the ciliary body to the choroid. Experimental occlusion of a single vortex vein produces congestion of this elongated drainage territory. It is supposed that in humans there is little communication between adjacent territories and that the watershed between the four drainage areas roughly forms a Maltese cross centred on the disc (Fig. 11.11b). This will be modified according to the number of vortex veins present.

The two superior vorticose veins open into the superior ophthalmic either directly or via its muscular or lacrimal tributaries. The two inferior veins open into the inferior ophthalmic, or into its anastomotic connection with the superior ophthalmic vein.

SMALL BRANCHES FROM THE SCLERA

These correspond to the scleral branches of the short ciliary arteries. They carry only blood from the sclera, none from the choroid, and are therefore smaller than the corresponding arteries.

ANTERIOR CILIARY VEINS

The anterior ciliary veins are, like the arteries, tributaries of the muscular veins. Because they drain

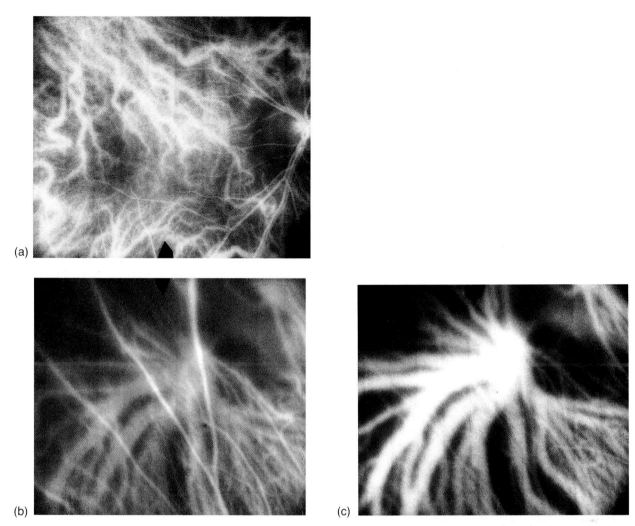

Fig. 11.28 (a) Choroidal veins at the posterior pole (II): watershed zone in the submacular choroid of a 39-year-old patient with myopia, right eye. The watershed zone of the four vortex veins is located in the submacular choroid. (b) Angiography of choroidal arteries and the vortex vein in the early filling phase in a 30-year-old patient with diabetic retinopathy. In the early filling phase of this angiogram, taken in the region of the temporal superior vortex vein, the radial choroidal arteries are filled and the vortex vein also begins to show up. (c) Vortex vein, same patient, 4 s later. The vortex vein is maximally filled. Note the huge calibre of this vessel compared to the normal central retinal vein. The choroidal circulation carries much more blood than the retinal circulation. (Courtesy of P. Bischoff.)

only the ciliary muscle, they are smaller than the corresponding arteries. Thus the arteries and veins of the uveal system of vessels do not correspond either in number, course or mode of branching. Moreover, the arteries are often larger than the veins, which is unusual elsewhere. The veins, like those of the retina, have no valves.

11.12 CHOROIDAL CIRCULATION

The ocular circulation has been studied extensively in experimental animals, including primates, and this work has been fully reviewed by Bill (1975a) who has made a major contribution in this field.

In monkeys the choroidal flow is extremely high,

about 20 times that of the retinal blood flow (iris 8 ($\pm$1) mg/ml; ciliary body 81 ($\pm$6) mg/ml; choroid 677 ($\pm$67) mg/ml; retina 34 ($\pm$2) mg/ml). Because of the high flow, choroidal venous blood oxygen saturation is only 3% lower than arterial blood saturation (Alm and Bill, 1970, 1987), although the choroid supplies oxygen to the outer part of the central retina (arteriolovenous anastomoses make a small contribution to this high oxygen saturation). The extraction rate of the retinal vessels is much higher than that of the choroidal vessels, and the oxygen saturation of retinal venous blood is about 60% (65% in the pig; Tornquist and Alm, 1979) and 60% in human retinal veins by reflective densitometry (Hickam, Fraser and Ross, 1963; Fraser and Hickam, 1965).

On this basis, it appears that the choroid, and also the anterior uvea, is perfused at a rate which exceeds its nutritive needs. It has been suggested that the high uveal blood flow performs a thermoregulatory function, for instance offsetting heat loss from the anterior surface of the eye, and preventing overheating of the outer retina during exposure to bright light. It may also buffer the ocular pressure rise induced by external pressure, as when rubbing the eyes, because blood is expressed from the venous side of the system.

REGULATION OF BLOOD FLOW

Metabolic regulation of blood flow differs in retina and choroid. Retinal blood flow increases slightly in response to raised pCO_2 (Alm and Bill, 1972; Friedman and Chandra, 1972; Wilson, Strang and Mackenzie, 1977), while hyperoxia causes slight vasoconstriction and reduced flow (Epron et al., 1973). Retinal flow is autoregulated, and is not influenced by wide changes in perfusion pressures induced for instance by altering ocular pressure.

Choroidal blood flow is also increased by a raised pCO_2, but is not influenced by a raised pO_2 (Bill, 1962a,b; Wilson, Strong and Mackenzie, 1977). The net effect of raising both inspired oxygen and carbon dioxide is to cause a major rise in oxygen tension in the retina: breathing a 94% O_2, 6% CO_2 mixture increases retinal oxygen tension by 300% (Alm and Bill, 1972).

Choroidal blood flow is not autoregulated (Alm and Bill, 1973). Changes in perfusion pressure cause a proportional change in blood flow, but because choroidal blood flow is normally greatly in excess of nutritional need, quite large changes in blood flow cause only minor changes in choroidal tissue fluid composition (Bill, Tornqvist and Alm, 1980). There is some autoregulation of iris and ciliary body blood flow. Parva demonstrated a rise in blood flow in the choroid in response to bright light falling on the retina.

Neuroregulation of uveal flow is governed by a number of mechanisms. Sympathetic stimulation causes marked choroidal vasoconstriction and a fall in ocular pressure due to a fall in ocular blood volume (Alm and Bill, 1973; Alm, 1977). This is an alpha-adrenergic response (Bill, 1962a,b). The choroid is normally under a vasoconstrictor tone and it has been suggested that this may protect the retina and nerve head from overperfusion in certain circumstances such as arterial hypertension (Bill, Linder and Linder, 1977b). Vasomotor terminals end chiefly on arterioles

and less on arteries. There is some innervation of veins and venules but none of the choriocapillaris (Ruskell, 1971b).

The choroid responds to cholinergic stimulation by vasodilatation (Stjernschantz and Bill, 1979) and it appears that parasympathetic cholinergic fibres synapsing in the ciliary ganglion supply the choroid via the short ciliary nerves.

As noted earlier, Ruskell (1971b), in addition, has demonstrated nitrergic and VIPergic choroidal vasodilator fibres of facial nerve origin which synapse in the pterygopalatine ganglion (Uddman et al., 1980; Nilsson, Linder and Bill, 1980; Nilsson and Bill, 1984; Stjernschantz and Bill, 1980; Flügel et al., 1994).

The fenestrated capillaries of the choroid and ciliary processes are like those of the intestinal mucosa or kidney. Tracer studies with horseradish peroxidase demonstrate leakage of large molecules into the extravascular compartment. The movement of proteins such as albumin or IgG, or even smaller molecules, from the choroid across the retina is prevented by the tight junctions between retinal pigment epithelial cells (Cunha-Vaz, Shakib and Ashton, 1966; Grayson and Laties, 1971; Smith and Rudt, 1975). The protein leakage across the capillaries of the choroid or ciliary processes exceeds that across the fenestrated capillaries of the kidney by fivefold, and that across the non-fenestrated capillaries of cardiac or skeletal muscle tenfold (Bill, Tornqvist and Alm, 1980). The extravascular albumin and IgG concentrations in the ciliary processes and choroid is in the region of 60–70% of that in the plasma (Bill, 1968), which creates a high osmotic pressure in the tissue fluid of (say) the choroid, which exceeds that in the retina by about 15 mmHg. This causes a net filtration of fluid from retina to choroid and is thought to be a force which 'sucks' the neuroretina onto the retinal pigment epithelium and balances forces tending to separate these layers and cause retinal detachment.

The choroidal capillary fenestrations may also be important in allowing the entry of vitamin A into the extravascular compartment for uptake by the retinal pigment epithelium. Vitamin A is carried in a macromolecular complex combining retinol-binding protein with prealbumin. The availability of this large molecule in the choroidal extracellular space must depend on the presence of fenestrated capillaries.

The permeability to low molecular weight substances such as glucose is also high, i.e. more than twenty times greater than that in heart muscle and up to eighty times that in skeletal muscle. This contrasts with the situation in the retinal vessels, which are non-fenestrated. Here, glucose requires a

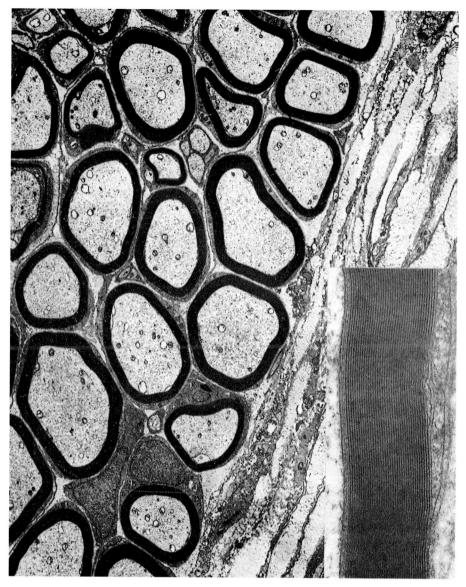

Fig. 11.29 Myelinated nerve fibres in the ciliary body (rhesus monkey, electron micrograph original magnification ×75 000). Note nuclei of satellite cells in lower part of filla. The insert shows myelin lamination in longitudinal section at higher magnification. (Courtesy of Dr John Marshall and Mr P. L. Ansell, Institute of Ophthalmology, London.)

transporter for delivery to the retinal tissues (Törnqvist and Alm, 1979).

CHOROIDAL CHANGES WITH AGEING OR GLAUCOMA

In the aged, the elastic tissue of the uvea degenerates and presumably leads to a reduction in the elasticity of the tissues (Streeten, 1995). One such situation in which elasticity is lost with old age is the ciliary muscle. As Tamm, Tamm and Rohen (1992) were able to show in a large study in the aged, the ciliary

muscle moves progressively forwards with age and gradually takes on the form of the accommodated muscle. This change in shape may explain why, although the ciliary muscle fibres are still able to contract, the muscle is no longer able to return to its disaccommodative state because of the ageing elastica.

In the eyes of healthy animals, the oxygen tension of the retina remains largely constant despite rises in intraocular pressure of over 50–70 mmHg, but it seems conceivable that the implication of the reduction in choroidal elastica might be a functional disturbance of blood flow in response to blood pressure changes.

A recent study of the human choroid shows, also, that there is a distinct reduction in thickness with age (Ramrattan *et al.*, 1994). Histologically, sagittal sections show compression of the choroid. In many eyes, a sheath develops around the larger vessels which resembles the sheath of the iris vessels. Possibly this investment could hinder vessel movement, for instance during variations of blood pressure. In addition to sclerosis, there may be a reduction in the number and calibre of the vessels which would contribute to decreased thickness of the choroid (Tripathi and Tripathi, 1974). It is not known whether these changes with age have a functional effect.

In human donor eyes with primary open-angle glaucoma, and also in secondary glaucoma (Kubota, 1993), choroidal thickness is reduced. There is also a parallel reduction in the number of ganglion cells in the choroid, while the choriocapillaris remains unchanged despite the reduction of choroidal innervation. Only in patients with long-standing glaucoma were changes in the choriocapillaris, and a reduction in capillary surface, found.

CHAPTER TWELVE
The lens and zonules

12.1   THE LENS

The lens of the eye is a transparent, biconvex, elliptical, semisolid, avascular body of crystalline appearance located between the iris and the vitreous (Fig. 12.1a). Laterally, the equatorial zone of the lens projects into the posterior chamber and is attached by the zonules to the ciliary opithellum. It enables the eye to focus images on the retina of objects lying at distances from near to infinity. In order to perform this role the lens must be both transparent and elastic, the former to allow the passage of incident light and the latter to facilitate the repeated changes in shape accompanying accommodation. The lens is unique among organs in that it contains cells solely of a single type, in various stages of cytodifferentiation, and retains within it all the cells formed during its lifetime. The oldest cells are contained within the core or nucleus of the lens, and throughout life new cells are added superficially to the cortex, in a series of concentric layers. A proper understanding of these relationships can be obtained by referring to the embryonic development of the lens. As cells become older and more embedded within the lens they undergo several changes, losing organelles, and to some extent their structural integrity, and becoming progressively more inert metabolically. As no cells are shed, the lens demonstrates cells at varying states of senescence and is remarkable for its ability to preserve its specialized function of transparency, throughout the human life span.

The equatorial **diameter** of the adult lens is 9–10 mm. By direct measurement, its **axial sagittal width** is about 3.5–4.0 mm at birth, about 4 mm at 40 years, and increases slowly to 4.75–5.0 mm in extreme old age. It varies markedly with accommodation. In contrast its **equatorial diameter** is 6.5 mm at birth, 9–10 mm in the second decade and changes little thereafter (Fig. 12.1b–d).

Like all lenses, that of the eye presents for examination two surfaces, anterior and posterior, and a border where these surfaces meet, known as the equator (equator lentis) (Fig. 12.2).

The anterior surface, less convex than the posterior, is the segment of a sphere whose radius averages 10 mm (8.0–14.0 mm). This surface is in relation in front with the anterior chamber of the eye through the pupillary aperture, and with the posterior surface of the iris, the pupillary part of which rests on it. The lateral surface is related to the posterior chamber of the eye and through the zonules to the ciliary processes.

The centre of the anterior surface is known as the **anterior pole**, and is about 3 mm from the back of the cornea.

The posterior surface, more curved than the anterior, presents a radius of about 6 mm (4.5–7.5 mm). It is usually described as lying in a fossa lined by the hyaloid membrane on the front of the vitreous, but it is separated from the vitreous by a slit-like space filled with aqueous. This retrolenticular space was described by Berger (1882) and is confirmed by slit-lamp examination (see Fig. 13.2).

The **equator** of the lens forms a circle lying 0.5 mm within the ciliary processes. The equator is not smooth, but shows a number of dentations corresponding to the attachment of the zonular fibres (Figs 12.2 and 12.3). These tend to disappear during accommodation when the tension of the zonular fibres is relaxed. The refractive index of the lens (1.39) is slightly more than that of the aqueous and vitreous humours (1.33) and hence, despite its smaller radii of curvature, it exerts much less dioptric effect than the cornea. The dioptric contribution of the lens is about 15 out of a total of about 40 dioptres for the normal eye. At birth the accommodative power is 15–16 dioptres, diminishing to half of this at about 25 years of age and to 2 dioptres or less at age 50 years.

With the pupil dilated, many features of the lens may be seen with the slit-lamp microscope. In the slit-beam a stratification of the lens into concentric

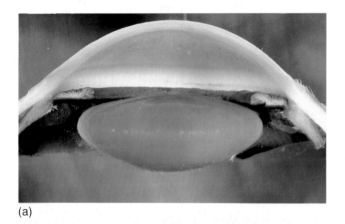

(a)

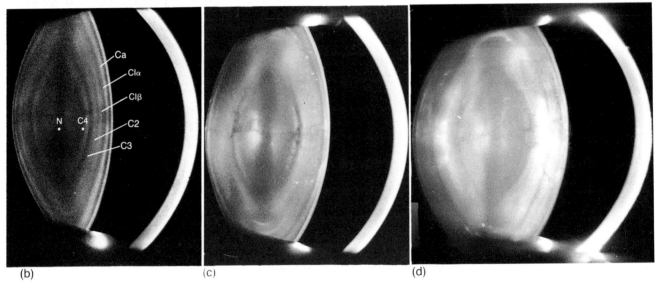

(b)   (c)   (d)

Fig. 12.1   (a) Parasagittal section of the globe to show an intact lens suspended by the ciliary zonule. (Courtesy of J. Marshall.) The normal human lens viewed by slit-image (Schleimpflug) photography at different ages: (b) 20 years; (c) 50 years; (d) 80 years. Note the increasing size and light scatter from the lens with increasing age. Ca = capsule; C1α = first cortical clear zone; C1β = first zone of disjunction; C2 = second cortical clear zone; C3 = light-scattering zone of the deep cortex; C4 = clear zone of the deep cortex; N = lens nucleus. Note the lack of scattering by the central part of the nucleus in the younger lenses. (Courtesy of N. A. P. Brown.)

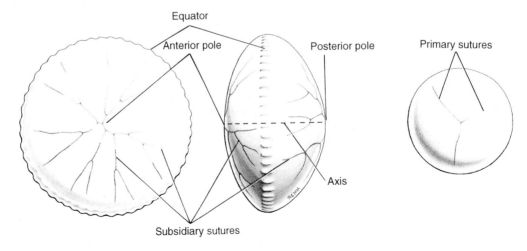

Fig. 12.2   The lens. Adult lens left, fetal lens right.

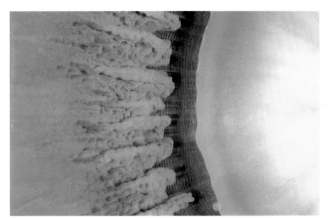

Fig. 12.3 Microphotograph of the posterior aspect of part of the ciliary body and lens. Note the major and minor ciliary processes and the slightly crenated equator of the lens. The zonular fibres are faintly seen. (Courtesy of J. Marshall.)

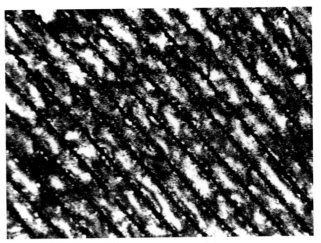

Fig. 12.5 Confocal reflected image of the *in situ* crystalline lens. The spacing between the lenticular fibres is 7µm. The image is back-scattered light in the confocal mode. Reflected light confocal microscope image of the enucleated *in situ* rabbit eye. BioRad MRC 600 confocal microscope. Light wavelength 488 µm, objective Leitz 25×, 0.8NA water objective. (Courtesy of B. R. Masters.)

layers may be made out (Fig. 12.1). From the front backwards are: capsule; subcapsular clear zone (cortical zone C1α); a bright narrow, scattering zone of discontinuity (C1β); the subclear zone of the cortex (C2). These make up the superficial cortex. Then there are two deep cortical or perinuclear zones which autofluoresce a brilliant green under blue exciting light. The first of these zones (C3) is a bright, scattering zone and the second is relatively clear (C4). The nucleus which follows represents the *prenatal* part of the lens. It shows further stratification, with a central clear interval which has been termed the 'embryonic' nucleus. However, its sagittal width suggests that it also includes some early fetal lens fibres (Bron and Brown, 1994). The sutures of the lens (see below) can also be made out with the slit-beam.

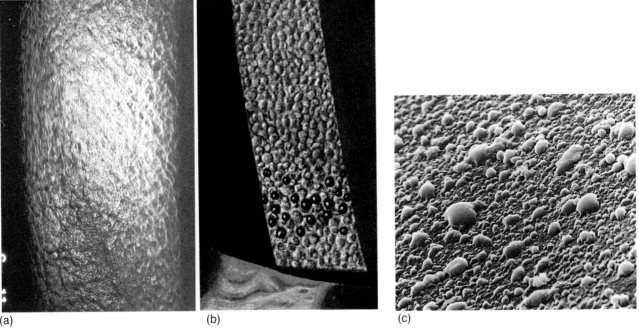

(a) (b) (c)

Fig. 12.4 (a) Capsular shagreen, shown by specular photography. A few scattered blebs are seen, which are occasional features of the capsule. (b) Capsular blebs as depicted by Vogt, 1921. (c) Surface blebs on the anterior surface of the lens capsule seen by scanning electron microscopy. (From Tripatni R. C. and Tripathi, B. J. (1984) in Davson, H. (ed.) *The Eye*, third edition, published by Academic Press.)

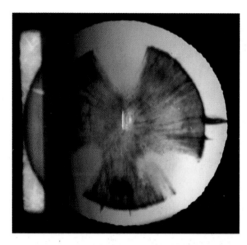

Fig. 12.6 Lamellar cataract, to show wedge-shaped opacities corresponding to opacified fibres at the periphery of the lens nucleus. (Courtesy of N. A. P. Brown.)

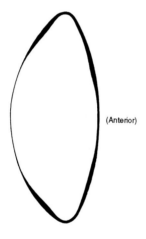

(Anterior)

Fig. 12.7 Very schematic anteroposterior section of the lens capsule to show the relative thickness of its different zones. (From Fincham.)

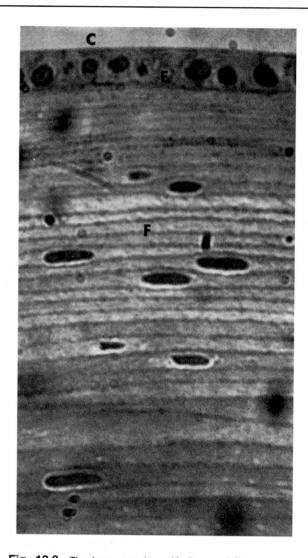

Fig. 12.8 The lens capsule, epithelium and fibres (photomicrograph, original magnification ×500).

With specular microscopy a beaten metal appearance is visible at the interface between aqueous and anterior capsule, termed the **lens shagreen** (Fig. 12.4). Although its structural basis is not known, scanning electron microscopy reveals a pebble-like appearance of the lens capsule which seems to correspond to the shagreen (Fig. 12.4c) (Tripathi and Tripathi, 1984). Specular microscopy at high magnification will also demonstrate the lens epithelial cells and the sub-epithelial lens fibre system (Fig. 12.5). By retro-illumination the lens appears entirely clear, but any opacification (cataract) is visible as a shadow, which may sometimes mirror the architecture of the lens (Bron and Brown, 1986) (Fig. 12.6).

STRUCTURE

The lens consists of (Fig. 12.7):

1. the lens capsule;
2. the lens epithelium;
3. the lens cells or fibres.

The lens capsule

The capsule completely envelops the lens and is unique in that its cells of origin are completely contained by it. The capsule is the basement membrane of the lens epithelium and is the thickest basement membrane in the body. It is much thicker in front than behind and the anterior and posterior portions are thicker towards the periphery (equator)

THE LENS 415

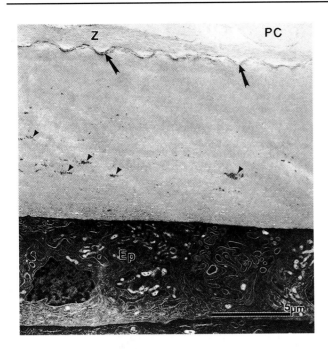

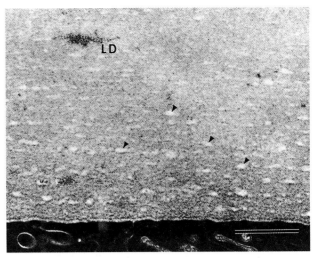

Fig. 12.10 Higher power view of lens capsule. The linear density (LD) exhibits a periodicity of about 60 μm due to axial banding of its constituent fibrils. Electronlucent 'bubbles' (arrowheads) occur between adjacent lamellae. Bar indicates 1 μm. (Courtesy of G. E. Marshall and S. Cameron.)

Fig. 12.9 Transmission electron micrograph of anterior equatorial lens capsule in a 13-year-old girl. Linear densities (arrowheads) are scattered throughout the substance of the capsule. The interface of the capsule with the posterior chamber (PC) is bounded by a pericapsular membrane (zonal lamella) (arrows), above which lies a zonular process (Z). Note the smooth interface between the single layer of lens epithelial cells (Ep) and the lens capsule. (Courtesy of G. E. Marshall and S. Cameron.)

just within the attachment of the suspensory ligament, than at the poles. Fincham (1925, 1937) recorded figures of 2.8 μm at the posterior pole and 15.5 μm at the anterior (Figs 12.7 and 12.8).

Capsule thickness increases anteriorly with age but there is little change at the posterior pole (Salzmann, 1912; Fisher, 1969). This reflects that the epithelium, which is the secretory source of the basement membrane, is itself situated anteriorly and is involved in the remodelling of the capsule which occurs with lens growth. In the rat, some postnatal growth of the posterior capsule does occur, which suggests that the posterior portion of the elongating fibre has some ability to secrete basal laminar material (Parmigiani and McAvoy, 1989). The capsule receives the insertion of the zonular fibres anteriorly and posteriorly at the lens periphery as well as at the lens equator.

Under the light microscope (Fig. 12.8) the capsule appears transparent, homogeneous, and under polarized light, birefringent with an indication of a lamellar structure with fibres arranged parallel to its surface (Grignolo, 1954). Its basement membrane origins are displayed by a positive reaction to Periodic acid–Schiff reagent which stains the glycoprotein matrix.

Even under the electron microscope, the capsule appears to have a relatively amorphous appearance in which a lamellar structure is suggested by coarse scattered filamentous elements. There are up to 40 lamellae, each of which is about 40 nm thick (Wulle and Lerche, 1969). At higher resolution fine fibrils may be identified which are in the region of 2.5 nm in diameter (Fisher and Hayes, 1979, rat). The lamellae run parallel to the capsular surface (Figs 12.9 and 12.10).

There is some suggestion that the lamellar structure becomes modified with age since it disappears from the posterior pole during the first decade and from the anterior aspect four or five decades later (Seland, 1974). Fisher (1971) has shown that 90% of the age-related losses in accommodation result from changes in capsular elasticity, although this is questioned and Weale (1982) has proposed that the loss of lamellae may be a morphological manifestation of this process.

In the anterior and equatorial capsule there is an occurrence of electron dense inclusions which consist of collagen fibrils 15 nm in diameter and with periodicity of 50–60 nm. These are attributed to epithelial activity and increase with age (Seland, 1974) as does the occurrence of long-spacing collagen (periodicity 110 nm).

The layer of inserting zonular fibres and the related capsular layer were termed the zonular lamella by

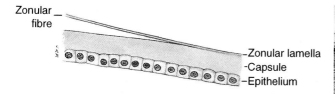

Fig. 12.11 The lens capsule and zonular lamella.

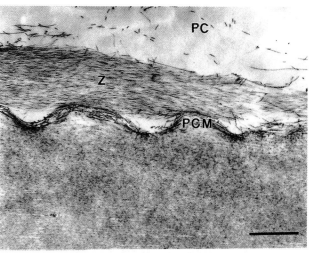

Fig. 12.12 Superficial portion of human lens capsule. The pericapsular membrane (PCM), also referred to as the zonular lamella, is composed of fibrils morphologically indistinguishable from those of zonules (Z). Note the faint fibrillar nature of the capsule. PC = posterior chamber of eye. Bar indicates 1 μm. (Courtesy of G. E. Marshall and S. Cameron.)

Berger (1882) (Figs 12.11 and 12.12). (It is also termed the pericapsular membrane.) This superficial layer of the capsule, 0.6 to 0.9 μm thick, is less compact, and richer in glycosaminoglycans than the rest of the capsule. The zonular lamella may contribute to zonular adhesive mechanisms, due to the presence of fibronectin (Goldfischer, Coltoff-Schiller and Goldfischer, 1985; Inoue *et al.*, 1989), vitronectin (Li Z-Y, Streeten and Wallace, 1991) and other matrix proteins. The fibrils of this fibrogranular layer are only 1 to 3 nm wide (compared to the 10 nm width of the zonular fibrils).

Earlier histochemical studies (McCulloch, 1954) had suggested that the zonular lamella was a distinct superficial zone involving the whole extent of the capsule. However, electron microscopy has shown that such a structure is confined to a narrow zone around the equator, related to the insertion of the zonule (Fig. 12.12). Like other basal laminae, the capsule is rich in type IV collagen. It also contains types I and III collagens, in addition to a number of extracellular matrix components, which include laminin, fibronectin, heparin sulphate proteoglycan and entactin. Among the fibrillar features seen on electron microscopy in the more superficial layers (Seland, 1974), linear densities are also found. These may be granular, or contain coarse filaments parallel to the surface. They have been identified to contain laminin and are not found in the posterior capsule (Marshall *et al.*, 1991).

Human capsular permeability has been investigated by Hess (1911), Friedenwald (1930), Francois and Rabaey (1958), Fisher (1969, 1973a) and Hockwin *et al.* (1973). The capsule is freely permeable to water, ions and other small molecules, and offers a barrier to protein molecules the size of albumin (Mr 70 kDa; molecular diameter 74 Å) and haemoglobin (Mr 66.7 kDa; molecular radius 64 Å). Neither Freidenwald (1930) nor Fisher (1974b) noted a difference in permeability of capsules between normal and cataractous lenses, but Fisher noted a correlation between permeability and cortical water content.

The lens epithelium

The epithelium consists of a single sheet of cuboidal cells spread over the front of the lens, deep to the capsule and extending outwards to the equator. Its cells are cuboidal in sagittal section, but polygonal in surface view (Fig. 12.13). There are about 500 000 cells in the mature lens (Young, 1991) with a central density of about 5009/mm² in men, and 5781/mm² in women (Gugenmoos-Holzmann *et al.*, 1989) and an increased density towards the periphery (Hogan *et al.*, 1971) (Fig. 12.14). Cell density is higher in women than in men, and declines with age. There is no corresponding posterior layer because the posterior epithelium of the embryonic lens is involved in the formation of the primary lens fibres which come to occupy the centre of the lens nucleus (Chapter 17).

Central zone

The central zone represents a stable population of cells whose numbers, like those of the corneal endothelium, slowly reduce with age. They are polygonal in flat section, 11–17 μm wide, 5–8 μm high and present a smooth apical surface to the most superficial lens fibres, which they adjoin. Their nuclei are round and located slightly apically.

The nuclei are large and indented, have numerous nuclear pores, and have two nucleoli. The cells have nominal numbers of ribosomes, polysomes, smooth and rough endoplasmic reticulum and Golgi bodies and their small mitochondria have irregular cristae.

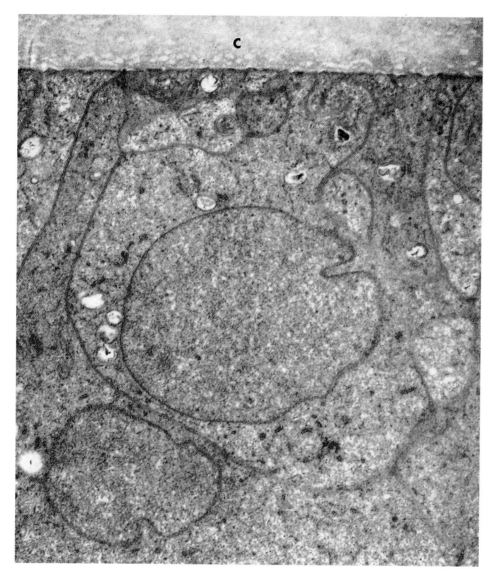

Fig. 12.13 The lens capsule (C) and epithelium (Rhesus monkey, electron micrograph, original magnification ×20 000). (Courtesy of Dr C. Pedler, Institute of Ophthalmology, London. Preparation by Mrs R. Tilly.)

Lysosomes, dense bodies and glycogen particles are also present. Cytoskeletal proteins include actin, intermediate filaments (vimentin), microtubules and the proteins spectrin, alpha-actinin and myosin. These provide a well-defined cytoskeleton which compartmentalizes the cell interior (Ramaekers and Bloemendahl, 1981; Benedetti *et al.*, 1981; Alcala and Maisel, 1985; Aster, Brewer and Maisel, 1986 and Allen *et al.*, 1987). In many vertebrates, and notably the primate, actin filaments have been found in the form of polygonal arrays or 'geodomes', immediately subjacent to the apico-lateral and baso-lateral membranes (Rafferty and Scholz, 1984, 1989; Yeh *et al.*, 1986) (Fig. 12.15). Alpha crystallin is present in the epithelium, but not beta or gamma.

Hemidesmosomes attach the basal aspects of the cell to the lens capsule (Porte *et al.*, 1975).

The central cells do not normally mitose, but they can do so in response to damage, including a wide variety of injuries (Harding *et al.*, 1959; Rafferty, 1963; Rothstein *et al.*, 1964; Rothstein *et al.*, 1965; Rafferty, 1967; Rothstein, 1968; Harding *et al.*, 1971; Rafferty, 1972a, 1972b; Weinsieder *et al.*, 1973; including uveitis; Wiensieder *et al.*, 1975; Reddan *et al.*, 1979; Worgul and Merriam, 1979).

Intermediate zone

The intermediate zone is peripheral to the central zone and its cells are smaller, more cylindrical

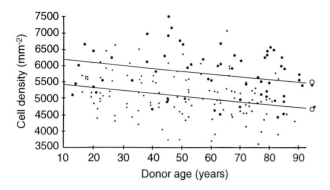

Fig. 12.14 Lens epithelial cell density: ● males; * females. Note that the density is higher in females than males and that the density falls with age in both sexes. (From Googenmoos-Holzmann, I. *et al.* (1989) *Invest. Ophthalmol. Vis. Sci.* **30**, 330–332, with permission.)

and with a central nucleus. These cells show complex basal interdigitations and the basal surface is irregular. Mitoses are occasionally seen.

Germinative zone

The germinative zone is the most peripheral and is located just pre-equatorially. It is the major site of cell division although, even here, mitotic figures are rare in adults. The cell nuclei are flattened and lie in the plane of the cell axis. From this region new cells migrate posteriorly to become lens fibres, though some may migrate forwards into the intermediate zone.

Electron microscopy (Cohen, 1965) of the epithelial cells shows few organelles lying in a coarse granular cytoplasm. There are short segments of rough-surfaced endoplasmic reticulum, ribosomes, small mitochondria and a Golgi complex. The number of organelles increases in the equatorial region where elements of the cytoskeleton assume a particular prominence together with other organelles (Rafferty and Goossens, 1978).

Cytoskeletal proteins include actin, vimentin (intermediate filaments), **microtubular protein**, spectrin, alpha-actinin and myosin. There are prominent actin networks subjacent to the apico- and baso-lateral membranes ('geodomes') which are thought to perform a structural function (Fig. 12.16) (Rafferty and Scholz, 1984, 1989; Yeh *et al.*, 1986). Alpha crystallin is present, but not beta and gamma crystallin.

Fibre elongation

Following terminal cell division, one or both daughter cells pass into the adjacent transitional

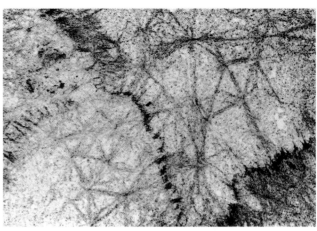

(a)

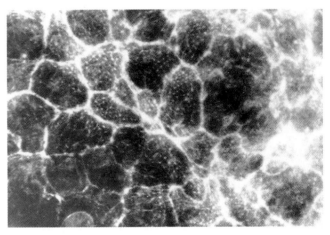

(b)

Fig. 12.15 Polygonal arrays of geodomes, demonstrated at the apical ends of lens epithelial cells. (a) Rabbit TEM (original magnification ×6600; bar = 0.5 μm). (b) Human, rhodamine–phalloidin fluorescence microscopy (original magnification ×750; bar = 10 μm). (From Rafferty, N. S. and Scholz, D. L. (1989) *Curr. Eye Res.*, **8**, 569–579, with permission.)

zone, in which the cells are organized into meridional rows (Figs 12.16 and 12.17). They differentiate into secondary lens fibres, rotating through 180° and elongating anteriorly and posteriorly. The new lens fibres retain their polarity, so that the posterior (basal) part of the fibre remains in contact with the capsule (basal lamina) while the anterior (apical) part is separated from it by the epithelium. These transitional cells are rich in ribosomes (polysomes) and multivesicular bodies, and also have pronounced microtubules. With increasing differentiation, they become columnar and then pyramidal, with their bases towards the capsule. Worgul (1992) has hypothesized that the parallel organization of the meridional rows is achieved in part by the staggered

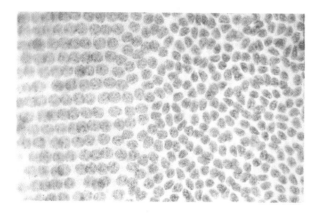

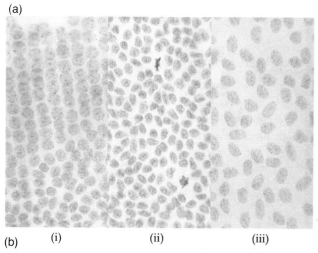

Fig. 12.16 Whole mount of normal rat lens epithelium. (a) The meridional rows of epithelial cells lie in perfect register in the pre-equatorial, germinative zone of the lens. (b) i. Bermunative zone; ii. Cells in the peripheral lens, relatively densely packed and with occasional mitoses; iii. Cells in the central zone are larger and rarely divide.

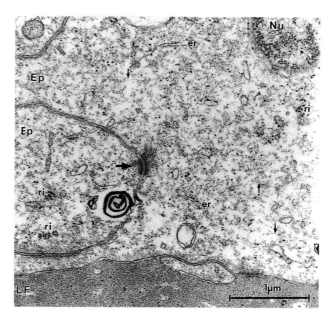

Fig. 12.17 Lens epithelium, showing two epithelial cells (Ep) and adjacent lens fibre (LF). A desmosome (arrow) is present between the two epithelial cells. The cells contain a nucleus (Nu), fibrils (small arrows), ribosomes (ri) and endoplasmic reticulum (er). (Courtesy of G. Vrensen.)

arrangement of the central cells, which permits new cells to dock into furrows between alternating cells. Their continued alignment is then thought to be achieved by intralenticular tension and the cell pressure of contiguous fibres (Worgul and Rothstein, 1977; Worgul, 1992). Loss of meridional row arrangement is associated experimentally (Worgul and Merriam, 1979; Worgul and Rothstein, 1977; Eguchi, 1964) and in human disease, with cataract (Streeten and Eschagian, 1978).

Epithelial mitosis is accompanied by DNA synthesis, while fibre elongation involves increased transcriptional activity and RNA synthesis, as specific structural, membrane and other proteins are formed (Yamada, 1972). The fibres undergo a process of terminal differentiation, in which the nuclei become pyknotic and finally disappear, and the cell organelles are lost (Jurand and Yamada, 1967; Papaconstantinou, 1967; Modak, Morris and

Yamada, 1968; Modak and Bollum, 1972; Kuwabara and Imaizumi, 1974). Basnett (1992a,b) and Basnett and Beck (1992) have noted in the rabbit lens that the loss of fibre nuclei, mitochondria and other cells occurs abruptly, across a single generation of fibres. Loss of nuclear DNA is preceded by increasing evidence of DNA strand scission (Fig. 12.18) (Modak, 1972). Little information about epithelial mitosis in the human is available, but in the rat, mitosis falls with age. In the young rat about five new fibres are formed a day, while in the old rat it drops to about one a day (Brolin, Diderholm and Hammar, 1961; Mikulicich and Young, 1963; Hammar, 1965; Worgul et al., 1976).

The nucleoli of the elongating fibres enlarge (Hertl, 1955; Srinavasan and Iwamoto, 1973; Kuwabara, 1975) and the cells become more basophilic due to their increased ribosomal content (Eguchi, 1964; Karasaki, 1964). The latter is related to the synthesis of cell components necessary for the process of cell elongation and differentiation, such as plasma membrane (Benedetti et al., 1976), cytoskeleton (Ramaekers and Bloemendahl, 1981) and the lens crystallins (Wistow and Piatagorsky, 1988).

The germinative zone, unlike the central zone which lies in the pupillary aperture, is protected from the potentially harmful effects of radiant energy in UV range, 300–400 nm (e.g. sunlight) by its location behind the iris.

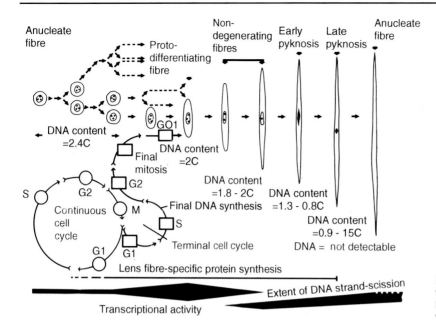

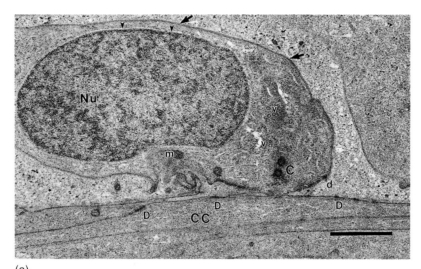

Fig. 12.18 A schematic representation of terminal lens fibre differentiation. (From Modak, S. P. (1972) *Ophthalmic Res.*, **3**, 23, with permission.)

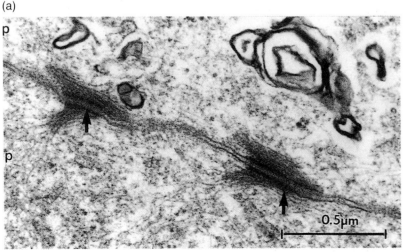

Fig. 12.19 (a) Lens epithelial cells in the anterior equatorial region of a 73-year-old female. Transmission electron micrograph illustrating lateral membranes of adjacent cells (arrows) with desmosomal attachments (d). Desmosomes (D) also secure the apical epithelial membrane to underlying cortical fibre cells (CC). Part of the nuclear envelope is evident (arrowheads) as are the pair of centrioles (C). Coated vesicles are present in the cytoplasm and mitochondria (m) and lie close to the basal membrane. (Bar = 2 μm.) (b) The desmosomes (arrows) have filaments extending into the cytoplasm TEM.

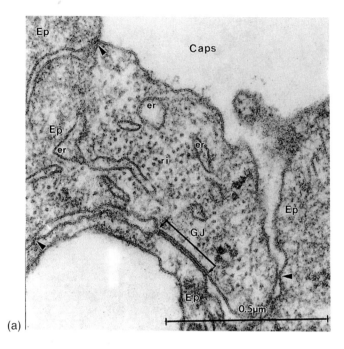

(a)

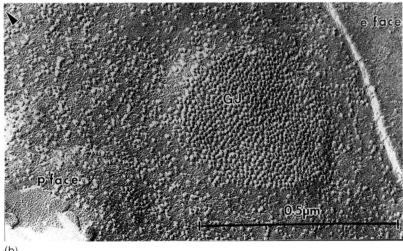

(b)

Fig. 12.20 (a) Junctions between epithelial cells (Ep). A gap junction (GJ) is present. In addition the membranes are confluent at three sites suggesting the presence of tight junctions. Within the cells are ribosomes (ri) and endoplasmic reticulum (er) (TEM). (b) In the freeze fracture the gap junction (GJ) is marked by 90-μm particles. The cytoplasmic face (p face) surface has many isolated intramembranous particles. These are scarce on the extracellular surface (e face). Arrow indicates direction of platinum shadowing (SEM). (Courtesy of G. Vrensen and B. Willekens.)

Membrane specialization in the epithelium

With the exception of the basal membrane, which interfaces with the lens capsule, the cell membranes of the epithelial cells are relatively complex. The lateral margins of the cells show gentle undulations, whilst the apical membranes enter into extensive interdigitation with underlying fibres. The basal aspects of the cells are attached to the anterior capsule by hemidesmosomes. The lateral aspects of the cells are attached to one another by desmosomes (Fig. 12.19).

Gap junctions are found within the lateral membranes of contiguous cells, which permit the free movement of small molecules between them (Kuwabara, 1975) (Fig. 12.20). These have the classic morphology of intercellular communicating junctions of liver type, i.e. the presence of tightly packed, complementary aggregates of hexameric transmembrane proteins conjoined with those from adjacent cells, across a narrowed (2–4 nm) extracellular space (Kreutziger, 1968; McNutt and Weinstein, 1970; and Chalcroft and Bullivant, 1970). Gap junctions of this type are found only infrequently between the lens fibres.

The apical membranes of the epithelial cells interface with the apical membranes of the youngest fibres, as they advance towards their sutural destinations (Kuszak and Rae, 1982). There are infrequent gap junctions across this interface, and these are similar to those between the fibres themselves. Although earlier studies had suggested that the movement of substances between these cells occurred via gap junctions (Goodenough, 1979; Goodenough, Dick and Lyons, 1980), freeze etch analysis of the complete apical membranes shows that gap junctions are extremely rare at the epithelial–fibre interface. This is not unexpected, since gap junctions are typically lateral membrane specializations, and apico–apical junctions are uncommon (Simons and Fuller, 1985; Rodriguez-Boulan and Nelson, 1989; Kuszak, Novak and Brown, 1995). Although epithelial cells are coupled ionically to underlying elongating fibre cells, they are not coupled using tracer dyes (Rae and Kuszak, 1983). Both sets of apical membranes display abundant evidence of receptor-mediated endocytotic processes of importance to the transfer of metabolites between these cells (Brown et al., 1990). This may reflect the presence of a number of defined receptors in the epithelium, e.g. to insulin, growth hormone, and beta-adrenergic agonists, and their likely involvement in epithelial metabolism and the traffic between the fibres and the epithelial cells. The apical membranes of lens epithelial cells are characterized by orthogonally arranged particles (OAPs) measuring 6–7 nm in diameter (Kreutziger, 1968; Stahelin, 1972; Dermietzel, 1973; Landis and Reese, 1974 and Hatton and Ellisman, 1981) which form patches of square array membrane. Immediately subjacent to the epithelial cell apical membrane, frequent examples of clathyrin-coated pits can be found. These are thought to provide a route by micropinocytosis for the transfer of nutrients and metabolites between these cells (Brown et al., 1990; Kuszak et al., 1993). This morphology is also encountered along the basal epithelial cell membrane, and the basal lens fibre membrane, at their junction with the lens capsule.

Although tight junctions were reported to be present between epithelial cells in the lens (Lo and Harding, 1983, 1984) they are now thought to be virtually absent (Kuszak, Petersen and Brown, 1991). Only a few simple strands of IMPs are found between the apico-lateral borders of adjacent cells. The resistance presented across the epithelium is therefore not high (Gonzalez-Mariscal et al., 1989; Cereijido et al., 1978, 1983; Claude, 1978; and Claude and Goodenough, 1973), and there does not appear to be a significant barrier to extracellular flow between the lens cells (Rae and Stacey, 1979; Goodenough, Dick and Lyons, 1980).

The lens fibres

The transition between epithelial cells in the germina-tive zone to the elongated nucleated lens fibre cell is accompanied by a reduction of lateral interdigitations and the onset of a pronounced elongation of the basal and apical portions of the cell, which extend backwards along the inner surface of the capsule, and forwards under the epithelium, respectively. The deposition of successive generations of lens fibres is associated with the formation of the nuclear bow, in which the now-flattened nuclei of successive generations of lens fibres form an arch forwards when traced into the deeper portions of the lens. This forms an S- or C-shaped curve in meridional section (Fig. 12.21).

The means by which the lens bow is formed is not known, but its formation is unlikely to involve differential fibre elongation alone, since fibre elongation will have ceased in the deeper regions of the cortex where the deeper parts of the bow are present. A significant participation of cytoskeletal proteins may be assumed. The deeper, older lens fibres, about 150 μm into the cortex, lose their nuclei and this represents the termination of the nuclear bow (Fig. 12.21). At the equator, the nucleated zone in the adult lens averages 300–500 μm thick (Kuwabara, 1975).

The fibres are laid down in concentric layers, the outermost of which lie in the **cortex** of the lens and the innermost in the core or **nucleus**. The division between the cortex and the nucleus of the lens is arbitrary and for convenience may be taken to be the junction between fetal and postnatal lens fibres. Because the lens is about 6.5 mm wide at birth, this represents the width of the postnatal nucleus.

The lens fibres are strap-like or spindle-shaped cells which arch over the lens in concentric layers from front to back. They are hexagonal in equatorial cross-section and in the cortex can be seen to form radial rows (Figs 12.22, 12.23 and 12.24) (Rabl, 1903) which lose their regularity with increasing depth within the lens. Their average width is 10–12 μm and average thickness 1.5–2 μm at the adult equator. The primary fibres of the embryonic bovine nucleus are less than 250 μm in length, while those of the adult lens may be over 7 mm long. The fibres are thinner posteriorly, which explains the asymmetrical shape of the lens in sagittal section and the greater thickness of the anterior cortex (Kuszak et al., 1984, 1989). The tips of the fibres meet those of other fibres to form **sutures**. These lines of junction are accompanied by an expansion, flattening and curving of the tips as they insert into the suture, with overlapping and interlocking below the tenth layer of cortical cells. The area of overlap is about 70 μm wide. Flattening is greater in the cortex (2 μm) than in the nucleus (5 μm).

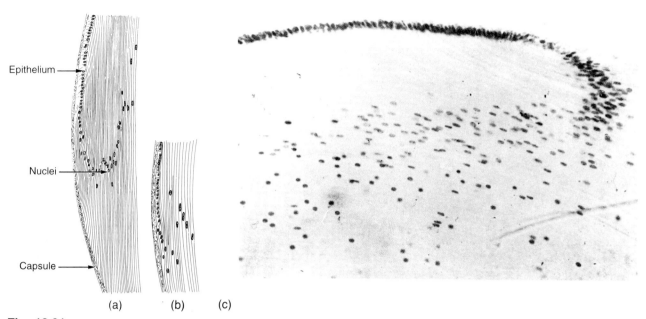

Epithelium ——

Nuclei ——

Capsule ——

(a) (b) (c)

Fig. 12.21 The human lens fibre nuclear bow: (a) in new-born, (b) in old man. As cortical fibres age, and recede from the surface of the lens, their nuclei pass forwards in a C- or S-shaped fashion and spread out before fragmenting and disappearing. (c) Equatorial region of the lens in meridional section in a 6-month-old fetus showing a large nuclear bow and many nucleated fibres (original magnification ×260).

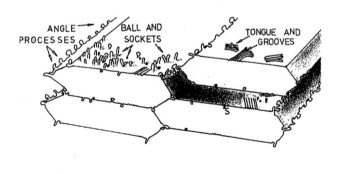

Fig. 12.22 The form and junctions of the primate cortical fibres. (Courtesy of M. Travers.)

Lens sutures

The suture arrangements of the lens become increasingly complex with the growth of the lens. In the fetal nucleus there is an anterior erect Y and a posterior inverted Y suture (Fig. 12.25). After birth more branch points are added to succeeding suture lines, so that in the adult nucleus the sutures have a stellate structure. The suture system may be envisaged as a means of accommodating the growth and packing of the lens fibres while retaining the cross-sectional configuration of the lens. The sutural arrangement

may be reflected in certain forms of cataract (Brown and Bron, 1994).

Earlier textbooks depicted the fibre tips as tapering towards the suture. This does occur in lower vertebrates (Kuszak, Bertram and Rae, 1984), but not in animals with star-shaped sutures, including primates. It has been shown *in vivo* by specular microscopy (Figs 12.26 and 12.27) and scanning electron microscopy (Fig. 12.28) that the fibres flare in width, and also curve, as the suture is approached (Brown *et al.*, 1987; Kuszak, Peterson and Brown, 1996; Kuszak, 1995).

Kuszak *et al.* (1984) and Kuszak, Bertram and Rae (1986) have studied the geometry and construction of the lens sutures in great detail. As noted, in the fetal human lens there is an anterior Y-suture and an inverted, posterior Y. With further growth, there is additional symmetrical branching of the suture ultimately to form the 9-point star of the mature cortex. Later, in senescent lenses, there is further, irregular sub-branching (Fig. 12.29).

It has been suggested that, collectively, these growth shells are responsible for the zones of optical discontinuity seen in adult and senescent lenses (Kuszak, Brown and Deutsch, 1993b). This is a reasonable proposition for most of the cortical zones but seems less likely for the first zone of discontinuity (Koretz *et al.*, 1984; Koretz and Handelman, 1988; Koretz *et al.*, 1988), since the suture architecture is a

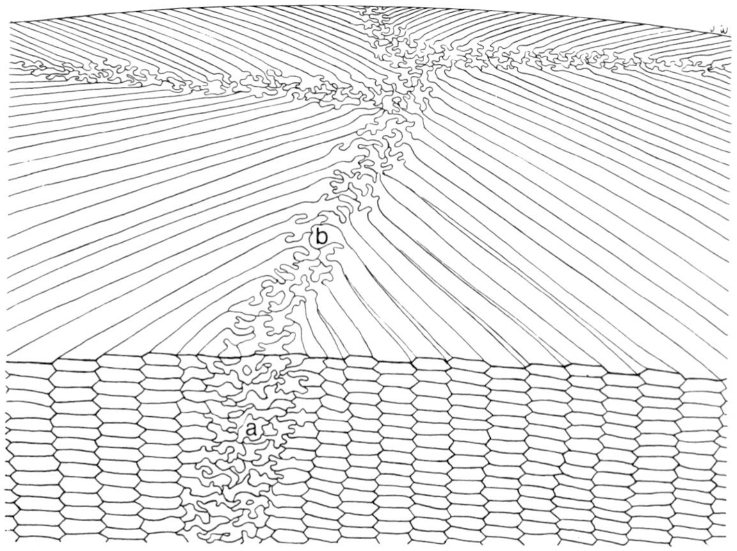

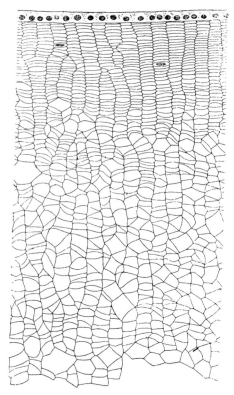

Fig. 12.23 Schematic drawing of the sutures of the adult lens showing the continuity of the suture throughout its thickness. In cross-section (a) lens fibres have complex interdigitations. They become broader and thinner as the fibres approach the suture. In flat section (b) the cells become wider and form branches that interdigitate in a complex manner at the suture. (From Hogan, M. J., Alvarado, J. A. and Weddell, J. E. (1971) *History of the Human Eye*, published by W. B. Saunders.)

stable feature of the lens, and this zone of discontinuity moves outwards as the lens grows, like the ripple of a wave, while maintaining a constant distance from the lens surface.

The manner in which the lens fibres are arranged with respect to the adult 9-point suture is as follows: eighteen fibres are found to run precisely in the meridia at 20° apart. Half of these originate at the anterior pole and end slightly posteriorly (at 10° latitude) while the other half start at the posterior pole and end slightly anteriorly (at 10° latitude). On either side of these straight fibres the fibre tips curve away from the polar axis as they insert into their respective sutures. This end curve is in an opposite sense, anteriorly compared to posteriorly. Because the equatorial circumference of the fibres is shorter than the length of the sutures into which they insert, the fibre tips are expanded as well as curved. (Thus in a 9-star suture, the group of fibres occupying 20 longitudinal degrees of the equator inserts over greater than 75 degrees at the suture.)

This situation is different at the Y-sutures of the lens nucleus, since fibres arising over a span of 60 longitudinal degrees insert into suture branches measuring 30 latitudinal degrees. These fibres are thus wider at the equator than at the sutures (Kuszak, Bertram and Rae, 1986). Because there are only six branches associated with the Y-sutures, the end curves are more pronounced.

Also in relation to the Y-suture, since fibre length varies only slightly with meridian, the overlap of fibre cells within successive growth shells produces ordered meridional columns (of Rabl, 1903). In the fetal nucleus, there is also a superimposition of the suture zones, which is visible on biomicroscopy as

Fig. 12.24 Peripheral portion of an equatorial section of the human lens to show the radial lamellae.

a suture plane because of the light-scattering behaviour of the overlapping membranes within the sutures. Each successive star position is generated over a period of about 15 years. In the post-natal lens, where fibre length is not a function of radial location, the sutures do not lie in register but are offset, so that

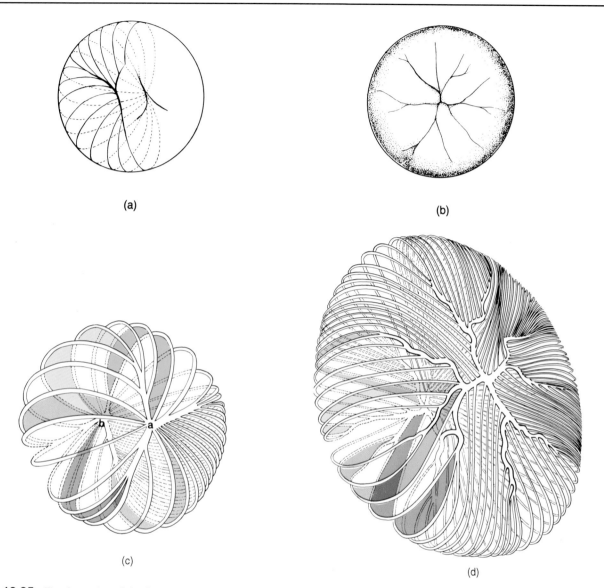

(a)

(b)

(c)

(d)

Fig. 12.25 The formation of the lens sutures. (a) Fetal pattern; (b) later adult pattern, in superficial view. (c) Drawing of the embryonal nucleus. The anterior Y suture is at (a) and posterior at (b). At the lens cells lens fibres are depicted as wide bands. Those fibres that attach the tips of the Y sutures to one pole of the lens are attached to the fork of the Y at the opposite pole. (d) The adult lens cortex. The organization of anterior and posterior sutures is more complex. Those fibres that arise from the tip of a branch of the suture insert further anteriorly or posteriorly into a fork at the posterior pole. This arrangement conserves the shape of the lens. The fibre termination is normally flared. (From Hogan, M. J., Alvarado, J. A. and Weddell, J. E. (1971) *History of the Human Eye*, published by W. B. Saunders.)

continuity of the suture plane is more difficult to see with the slit-lamp. It has been shown that the suture is a site of increased spherical aberration in the lens (Kuszak, Sivak and Weeheim, 1991a).

It has been pointed out that, as the lens grows, an increase in equatorial circumference can be achieved in two ways, either by an increase in fibre width, or by an increase in number of rows. Although the former has been demonstrated in lower vertebrates (Bron *et al.*, unpublished) it appears that in the primate lens this is achieved chiefly by an increase

in the number of rows. It has been noted that the increase in row number is associated with sites of fibre cell fusion. These fused cells are pentagonal in cross-section instead of hexagonal, and are thought to possess positional information which directs the formation of the additional radial columns (Kuszak *et al.*, 1989) (Fig. 12.30). Fibre cell fusions are found throughout the superficial and deep cortex and also in the nucleus, but rarely between elongating fibres (Kuszak *et al.*, 1985). They may also have a role related to cell–cell communication.

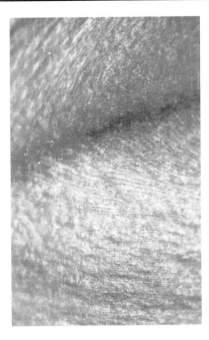

Fig. 12.26 Lens fibres joining at a suture, shown by specular reflex photography in the living eye. (Courtesy of N. A. P. Brown.)

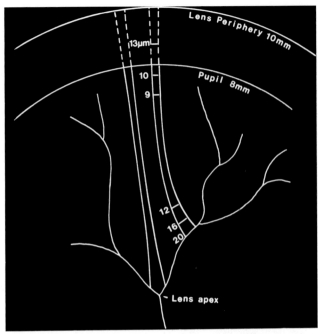

Fig. 12.27 The shape of the human lens fibre, showing flaring as the suture is reached. As it is not possible to draw a single fibre, the figure shows a group of 20 fibres. (From Brown *et al.*, with permission.)

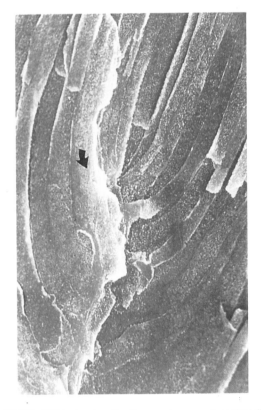

Fig. 12.28 TEM showing the flare and curve of cortical fibres joining a lens suture. (Courtesy of M. Travers.)

The fine structure of the youngest lens fibres compared to their parent epithelium shows fewer organelles and a denser, amorphous granular cytoplasm. This cytoplasmic appearance is due to high concentration of protein in the lens fibres, the fibres containing both beta and gamma crystallins in addition to the alpha crystallin present in the lens epithelium. Lens fibres contain the highest protein content of any cell in the body, with about 35% of its wet weight as protein. The fibres of the nucleus and deeper cortex are free of organelles and fibre membrane definition is poor. It has not been established whether this loss of definition is artefactual, due to the problems of fixation which exist for this tissue.

Membrane specialization

Ball-and-socket and tongue-and-groove interdigitations

The cell membranes of the lens fibres enter into a variety of associations with those of their neighbours and to some extent these vary with the degree of displacement from the lens surface. In the superficial 8–10 layers of the anterior cortex the short, or lateral, sides of the hexagon undulate and interlock into adjacent fibres a series of 'ball and socket'-like joints arranged regularly along the length of the fibre (Figs

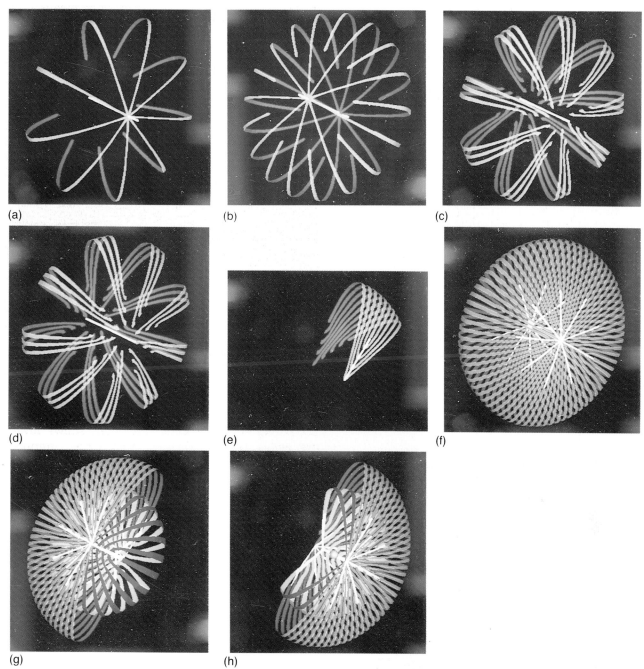

Fig. 12.29 Scale (approximately 6:1) computer-assisted drawings depicting the essential suture parameters in young adult primate lenses. (a) The positions of the nine straight fibre cells that extend to confluence at the anterior pole and define the position of the nine posterior sutures. (b) The positions of the 18 straight fibre cells that extend to confluence at the anterior and posterior poles to define the positions of both the anterior and posterior sutures. (c) The nine groups of fibres with clockwise anterior end curvature and counterclockwise posterior end curvature positioned within a single growth shell. (d) The nine groups of fibres with counterclockwise anterior end curvature and clockwise posterior end curvature positioned in a single growth shell. (e) Two groups of fibres with overlapped anterior ends forming one of the nine symmetrically positioned anterior suture branches. Note that as a result of opposite end curvature the groups of fibre cells that overlap to form an anterior suture will not overlap with the same fibre cells to form a posterior suture. (f) The symmetrical crystalline latticework formed by exactly offsetting anterior and posterior star sutures. (g) The position of Y suture characteristic of primate lenses at birth exposed by removing several sutural branches of the star suture. (h) The position of the embryonic nucleus, a portion of the fetal nucleus and a portion of the adult nucleus shown schematically. (Courtesy of J. Kuszak.)

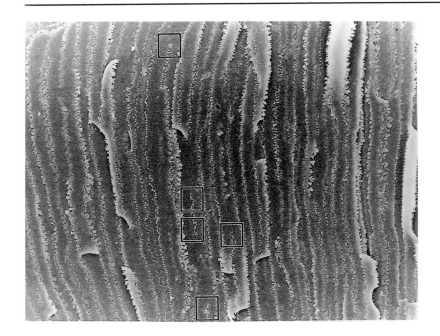

Fig. 12.30 Scanning microscopy of cortical lens fibres in the Macaque monkey to show points of fusion of fibres (outlined). (Courtesy of J. Kuszak.)

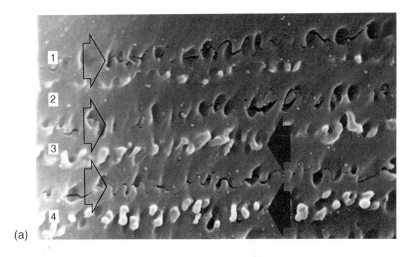

(a)

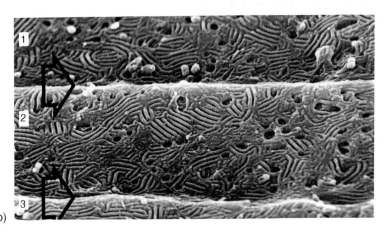

(b)

Fig. 12.31 SEM of superficial lens cortex from the posterior aspect of a 43-year-old adult lens. (a) The superficial lens fibres are roughly hexagonal in cross-section, with the hexagon having two long sides and four short ones. This view shows the short sides and points of four fibres (1, 2, 3, 4). Where adjacent fibres meet (open arrows) they enter into a series of interlocking 'ball and socket' joints. Balls can be best seen on the apex of fibres 3 and 4 (closed arrows). (b) SEM of deep cortical perinuclear fibres from the posterior cortex. Surface undulations become more complex as the fibres are displaced deeper into the cortex as shown on three fibres (1, 2, 3) and their inter-fibre junctions (open arrows). The ball and socket joints still occur, but at a reduced frequency. (From Marshall, J., Beaconsfield, M. and Rottery, S. (1982) *Trans. Ophthalmol. Soc. UK*, **102**, 423–440, with permission.)

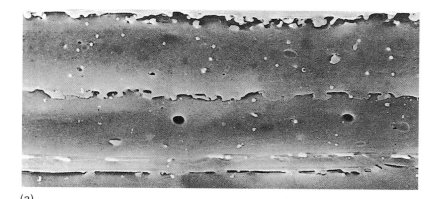

(a)

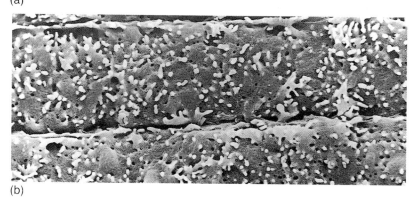

(b)

Fig. 12.32 SEMs showing the dramatic transition from the surface membrane morphology of the fibre cells as a function of development, maturation and growth. (a) The surface morphology of newly formed fibres is relatively smooth with developing lateral interdigitations (original magnification ×12 000). (b) As fibres mature their smooth surfaces are altered by the development of numerous microplicae (original magnification ×10 000). The changes in mature primate fibres are seen in Fig. 12.33. (Courtesy of J. Kuszak.)

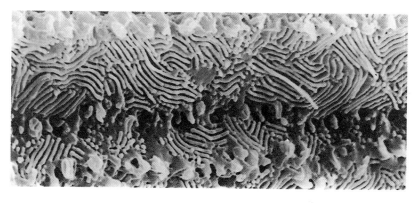

Fig. 12.33 SEM of mature primate fibres featuring polygonal domains of furrowed membrane, many with overlying microvilli (original magnification ×10 000). (Courtesy of J. Kuszak.)

12.31 and 12.32). In this way, cells within a given layer are firmly attached to each other while having only loose connections with preceding and succeeding layers. This arrangement may be important for the movement of fibres during accommodation. In the primate lens the ball-and-socket interdigitations are more prevalent in the mid periphery of the cortex, which is the appropriate position to resist zonular stresses. In the deeper fibres miniature 'ball and socket' joints spread on to the broad sides of the hexagons in a random fashion, thus interlocking fibres of different generations and depths. In the deepest layers of the cortex and in the nucleus, the 'ball and socket' systems are further supplemented by a complex series of ridges and troughs or tongue

and groove joints. These surface corrugations are found regularly along the narrow, lateral faces of the fibres (Kuwabara, 1975) and also at the angles of the narrow fibre interfaces (Willekens and Vrensen, 1982). Deeper in the nucleus of the primate lens, Kuszak and others have demonstrated polygonal domains of 'furrowed membrane' borne by the primary lens fibres, the oldest fibre cells of the lens (Fig. 12.33). These zones exhibit numerous, elongated microvilli (Lo and Harding, 1983; Kuszak *et al.*, 1988). All of these interlocking devices are thought to be specializations for the maintenance of fibre order, which is deemed to be essential for the continuing transparency of the lens, whilst allowing a limited degree of fibre sliding and a certain amount

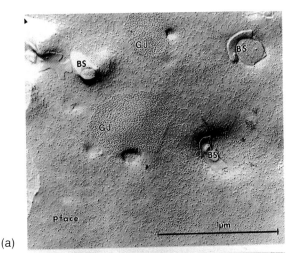

(a)

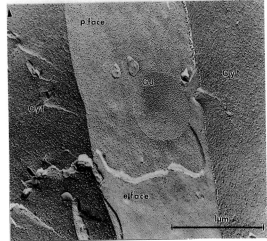

(b)

Fig. 12.34 (a) Cytoplasmic surface (p face) of superficial cortical fibre showing gap junctions (GJ) and fractured ball-and-socket joints (BS). (b) Intramembranous particles are common on the cytoplasmic surface (p face) and scarce on the extracellular surface (e face). Fibre cytoplasm (Cyt). Arrow indicates direction of platinum shadowing (SEM). (Courtesy of G. Vrensen and B. Willekens.)

of flexing of the whole lens structure which is a requirement of accommodation.

Desmosomes are reported between elongating fibre cells (Lo, 1987), but not between mature fibre cells. It may be that they perform a coordinating role during the growth of new fibres which is no longer required once elongation has ceased. However, since each adjacent fibre within a generation of elongating fibres has a slightly different sutural destination than its neighbour, some topographic fluidity must be necessary even in these cells.

Gap junctions

A second order of junctional complexes is found in human lens fibres: these are the gap junctions (Phillipson, Hanninen and Balazs, 1975) which are thought to fulfil two roles. First by conjoining large areas of membrane they further contribute to fibre order and therefore transparency (Kuszak, Maisel and Harding, 1978). Secondly, they are considered to contribute to lens function by providing pathways between terminally differentiated lens fibres which lack the cellular organelles for metabolic co-operation. Gap junctions are of two types, crystalline (or high-resistance) junctions and non-crystalline (or low-resistance) systems, and in some cells, such as the liver, they may change from one form to the other in response to changes in ionic composition (e.g. calcium concentration). In the lens fibre they are incapable of carrying out such a transformation (Goodenough, 1979) and in the lens the former are found in association with lens epithelial cells, whilst only the latter are found between fibres. The gap junctions of the developing fibres are intermediate between those of the epithelium and the mature fibre (Benedetti et al., 1976; Kuszak et al., 1982). These low-resistance junctions have intramembranous particles which are less densely packed and an inter-membranous gap of less than 2 nm. This determines that the interiors of all the lens fibres exist in a state of relatively open communication with each other, and that the levels of concentration of ions and small molecules in individual fibres rapidly equilibrate (Fig. 12.34).

Gap junctions are present between the lateral face of contiguous fibre membranes as in other epithelia (Fig. 12.20). Less numerous gap junctions are found within the interdigitating processes (ball and socket, tongue and groove) and more sparsely along the broad faces of the fibres. In the human lens only 5% of the lateral fibre membrane is specialized in this way while in the frog this is 15%, in the rat lens 30% and in the chick lens 60% (Kuszak et al., 1978, 1985; Lo and Harding, 1986). Gap junctions are not found at the anterior and posterior tips of the fibres, and therefore not within the sutural zone. Their density increases towards the lens equator and therefore their location along the fibre will vary according to the meridional position of the fibre and the anteroposterior disposition of the fibre with respect to the equator. In other words, the highest density of gap-junctions is not located in the same region along every fibre.

The apico-lateral border of the superficial fibre cell is comparable to the apico-lateral border of the lens epithelial cell. Both share endocytotic processes and pits, square array membrane, and an absence of gap or tight junctions. The square array membrane is more prominent in the fibre. Endocytotic events and

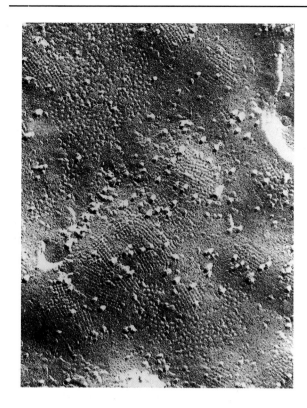

Fig. 12.35 Transmission electron micrograph of an E-face freeze-etch replica showing the ultrastructure of superficial cortical fibre cell apico- or basolateral membrane. Note the numerous sites of orthogonal arrays of proteins (OAPs) of 'square array membrane' and the less frequent gap junctions (original magnification ×150 000). (Courtesy of J. Kuszak.)

undulating membranes of the tongue-and-groove interdigitations characteristic of the inner cortex and nucleus of the lens (Lo and Harding, 1984; Costello, MacIntosh and Robertson, 1984, 1985; Dickson and Crock, 1972, 1975). Intervening areas of smooth senescent membrane express gap junctions. The relationship between gap junctions and square-array membrane is not entirely clear. Both gap junctions and square array membrane contain the main intrinsic polypeptide MP 26, which in the past has been considered to be the channel protein of the gap junction. However, it appears that MP 70 is located exclusively in gap junctions, found predominantly in the cortex, while MP 26 is associated with square-array membrane, found predominantly in the lens nucleus (Zampighi *et al.*, 1989). These findings are in accord with the observation that MP 26 is the most abundant membrane protein in both cortex and nucleus, whilst MP 70, another lens-specific protein, is more abundant in the cortex (Kistler and Bullivant, 1987; Costello *et al.*, 1984).

Electron microscopy and freeze fracture analysis show these junctions to be morphologically different. Gap junctions are thick symmetrical pentalaminar structures (16–18 nm) with intramembranous particles distributed symmetrically on either side of the junctional membranes. They are generally held to be communicating junctions. Square arrays are thin asymmetrical junctions (11–13 nm) in which one side of the membrane contains the square crystalline array of protein particles, while the membrane facing it is nearly devoid of them (Lo and Harding, 1984; Costello *et al.*, 1985). This protein distribution is mirrored by the distribution of MP 26 in the junction demonstrated by Zampighi *et al.* (1989). Costello *et al.* (1989) have suggested that the asymmetrical arrangement of protein particles in square arrays would be unlikely to afford an intercellular communication between conjoined cells, and have suggested that they participate in forming the curved shape to the tongue-and-groove folds of the deeper lens fibres and maintain a narrow extracellular space between these cells. Zampighi *et al.* (1989), however, suggest that the arrays, formed by MP 26, provide single-membrane, unidirectional channels which regulate the volume of the extracellular space.

Kuszak *et al.* (1993) speculate further that the square arrays, which occupy polygonal domains of furrowed membrane and are oriented at acute angles to the fibre axis, serve to enhance the drainage of expelled substances along the extracellular space and towards the suture planes. Here it is postulated that substances would be expelled by transcytosis anteriorly, and diffusion posteriorly.

square array membrane are also typical of the basal membranes of lens epithelial and superficial fibre cells. With ageing, the lens fibre membranes show remarkable senescent changes (Lo and Harding, 1984; Kuszak *et al.*, 1988). These are most extensive in the primary embryonic fibres, for instance in the primate lens, where virtually the entire surface of the fibres features polygonal areas of 'furrowed membrane', varying in size from 2.0 to 9.0 $(\mu m)^2$ and arranged at acute angles to the length of the cell. The ridges within these domains display microvilli, about 0.14 μm in diameter and from 1.25 to 4.75 μm in length. Each microvillus appears to possess a cytoskeleton. These features are also seen in younger primate nuclear fibres and in the nuclei of lenses from other, less long-lived primates.

The zones can be shown, by freeze-etch analysis, to exhibit patches of square-array membrane. Square arrays are more common than gap junctions in membranes isolated from whole lens (Zampighi *et al.*, 1989), and have been found extensively in membranes from the lens nucleus (Dunia *et al.*, 1985). These membranes are found frequently on the

PHYSIOLOGY AND BIOCHEMISTRY OF LENS GROWTH

The human lens grows continuously throughout life, adding about 29 μm to its sagittal thickness each year (Niesel, 1982; Brown, 1973). The events associated with lens growth are as follows (see chapter 17, and also Brown and Bron, 1994, 1996; Bron and Brown, 1994):

From the 6th–7th week of intrauterine life (18 mm embryo) the lens is elongated in the anteroposterior plane, in the direction of the primary lens fibres. During the 18–24 mm stage the lens is approximately spherical. With the appearance of the secondary lens fibres, at the 26 mm stage, the lens becomes wider in its equatorial diameter. The zonule, which appears later, at the 65 mm stage of fetal life, plays no role in this initial widening of the lens. There is no information as to whether compaction occurs in the intra-uterine lens (but see later). Intrauterine growth is rapid. The lens increases in mass and volume and expands in both the sagittal and equatorial planes. At birth it is almost spherical, but is wider in the equatorial plane. In the first two decades after birth, expansion ceases in the sagittal plane and continues in the equatorial plane alone (Fig. 12.36). Zonular tension, increasing with the continued growth of the globe in the transverse plane, could account in part for the preferential enlargement of the lens in the equatorial plane; this enlargement is more than just a simple redistribution of lens volume towards the equator. A vigorous compaction of the nucleus, which occurs at this time, is probably the most potent factor determining the plateau of sagittal growth, while zonular tension acting in the earliest period probably assists in the change in shape of the lens (for a fuller account see Brown, 1976; Brown et al., 1988; Brown and Bron, 1996) (Fig. 12.37 illustrates schematically the sagittal growth of the lens). The specific gravity of the lens remains more or less constant throughout life and there is no evidence in the normal lens that nuclear density is significantly increased in the ageing eye. (Bours and Fodisch (1986), and Bours et al. (1987) by direct measurement, demonstrated a small dehydration of the nucleus with age based on a study of lens slices, but Siebinga et al. (1991) using Raman spectroscopy found hydration to increase with age.) Although the increase in thickness in the lens is due to the addition of fibres to the superficial cortex, there is evidence of a compaction of the central lens fibres with time, so that a traumatic lens opacity formed at the lens recedes from the surface at approximately twice the speed at which the lens is growing (Brown et al., 1988).

The surfaces of the lens are bathed by aqueous humour which is replenished by its bulk flow anteriorly. Posteriorly, movement of aqueous is restricted by the presence of the zonular apparatus. The biochemistry of the lens is discussed by Berman (1991). The glucose content of the aqueous is similar to that of plasma (100 mg) and is slightly lower in the vitreous (90 mg). Aqueous oxygen is 60 mmHg (Cole, 1974). The metabolism of the lens is chiefly anaerobic through the glycolytic pathway. Only 3% of the glucose utilization is aerobic, via the Krebs cycle, and this activity is confined to the epithelium and most superficial cortical fibres. Nonetheless this may supply up to 20% of the energy requirements of the lens (van Heyningen, 1969). Energy is required for active transport and synthetic processes involved in the growth, synthesis and turnover of membrane constituents, crystallins, cytoskeletal proteins and nucleoproteins. A pentose shunt pathway exists in the lens and is involved in ribonucleoprotein synthesis, and a sorbitol pathway is present which may, among other things, provide coenzyme for the pentose shunt. However, the significance of the sorbitol pathway in lens metabolism has been questioned by Harding (1991, 1993).

The lens capsule is a modified basement membrane, and as such consists mainly of collagen (Kefalides, 1978) embedded in a glycoprotein matrix (Dische, 1970). About 10% of the capsule is carbohydrate. The capsule forms a barrier to particulate matter such as bacteria and inflammatory cells, but will allow the diffusion of molecules smaller than the size of haemoglobin (Fisher, 1969; 1973). Although the capsule contains no elastin, it is thought by many (but not all) to be highly elastic in behaviour. The configuration of the collagen is thought to be in the form of superhelices which uncoil under tension (Fisher and Wakely, 1964; Fisher and Hayes, 1969). The capsule is normally under tension, so when cut or ruptured its edges roll out and then curl up. This property of **elastic recoil** is used during extracapsular lens extraction when the capsule is incised to release the lens contents, or in the operation of YAG-capsulotomy when a gap is cut in the posterior capsular sheet.

The high refractive index of the lens is achieved by the high protein content of the fibres and its transparency results from the organization and regularity of fibre packing, the homogeneous structure of fibres within each generation, and the small size of the extracellular space (under 1% of lens volume). In addition to this, the fibres and epithelial cells themselves are not rich in organelles. The cell nuclei of the epithelium are present in a monolayer, and the nuclei

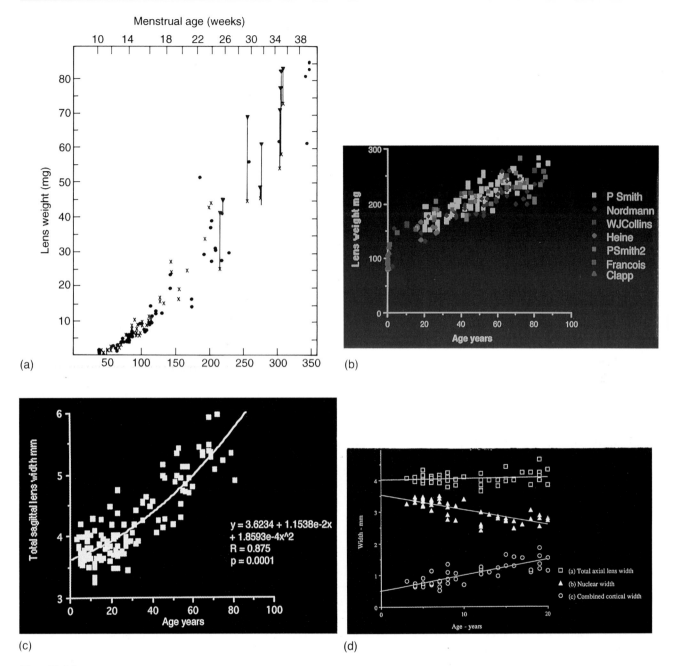

Fig. 12.36 (a) The growth in mass of the fetal lens in utero (Ehlers, N., Mathiessen, M. E. and Anderson, H. (1968) *Acta Ophthalmol.*, **46**, 329–349); (b) Growth in mass of the postnatal lens, from various authors. (c) The change in postnatal sagittal width of the lens with age. Note that the sagittal width is relatively stationary in the first two decades after birth, while over that same period, (d), nuclear width is decreasing. This phenomenon is explained by nuclear compaction (see text for a fuller explanation) (b), (c), (d) from Forbes *et al.*, 1992.

of the multilayered lens fibre system are either displaced to the periphery in the nuclear bow of the cortex or absent from the deeper fibres. All these factors combine to minimize fluctuations in backscattering over small domains between fibres. There are, however, graded changes of refractive index in the lens passing inwards from cortex to nucleus which correlate with changes in protein content and account for the overall refractive power of the lens and its relative freedom from chromatic aberration (Phillipson, 1969). Regulation of ionic and water content of the lens fibres is essential to their structural integrity, and hence to the maintenance of the optical homogeneity and transparency of the lens. The lens

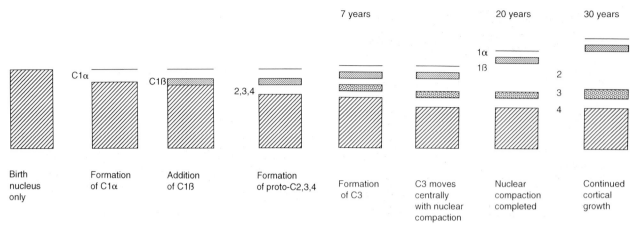

| | 7 years | 20 years | 30 years |

Birth nucleus only

Formation of C1α

Addition of C1β

Formation of proto-C2,3,4

Formation of C3

C3 moves centrally with nuclear compaction

Nuclear compaction completed

Continued cortical growth

Fig. 12.37 Schematic drawing of the sagittal growth of the lens. Only the half width of the lens is shown. At birth only the lens nucleus is present. It is not known whether a cortical clear zone (C1α) exists in utero. It is depicted here that C1α develops postnatally over a small number of generations. The fibres in the older generations then increase their scattering properties and in that way creat C1β. As the lens grows, the fibres which were in C1β, age, and scatter light less. They thus generate a zone which may be called proto-C2,3,4. At some point, very roughly around the age of 7 years, a zone of increased scattering appears in this region, which is C3. The scattering properties of this zone increase throughout life. It separates a deeper perinuclear C4 from a more superficial C2. In the first approximately 20 years of life there is negligible sagittal growth of the lens, because growth is concentrated equatorially. This period is associated with central compaction of the lens. From about the age of 20 years, while nuclear compaction has been completed, sagittal growth resumes and there is now negligible equatorial growth of the lens.

epithelium and possibly some superficial cortical fibres serve as the major pump system of the lens, transporting sodium forwards and outwards by the activity of Na^+K^+ activated ATPase. There is also a calcium-activated pump. Potassium moves into the lens anteriorly. At the posterior aspect of the lens there is passive diffusion of sodium inwards and potassium outwards. This pump–leak system (Kinsey and Reddy, 1965), in addition to others, controls the ionic environment of the lens, and equilibration between individual fibres and the epithelium is facilitated by the provision of gap junctions (Fig. 12.38).

The lens at birth is perfectly transparent. With growth of the lens there is an increasing yellowing of its nucleus due probably to the effect of absorbed u.v. (mainly 315–400 nm) of sunlight by certain **chromophores**, which leads to the production of visible and fluorescent pigments. It has been suggested that these pigments may serve to screen the retina from the damaging effects of short-wave 'blue light' radiation (Sliney and Wolbarsht, 1980). Cortical pigments render the perinuclear cortex autofluorescent in blue exciting light while others may accumulate in the nucleus with age and in some individuals produce the brunescent colour of senile nuclear cataract (Fig. 12.39). In the ageing lens nucleus, and particularly the nuclear cataractous lens, an increasing quantity of insoluble protein is found which is due to the presence of cross-linked and macromolecular aggregates of crystallins. Metabolic activity

at the centre of the lens is negligible and the proteins do not turn over significantly (Harding and Dilley, 1976). They are therefore extremely long-lived and vulnerable to oxidative and other influences which may unfold the protein structure and expose sulphydryl groups. These groups may then engage in disulphide bonding, which results in further crosslinking and conformational changes. The opacity of cataract is due to zones of increased scattering within its substance. This may be caused by a breakdown of fibre regularity, the products of membrane degradation, and by the scattering produced by macromolecular protein aggregates. Swelling and fibre disorganization are produced by disturbances of ion and water regulation. (For further details, see Harding, 1991; Brown and Bron, 1996.)

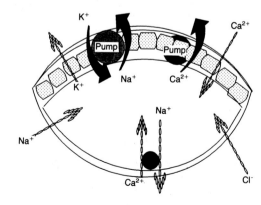

Fig. 12.38 Schematic diagram of ion movement in the lens. (Courtesy of K. Hightower.)

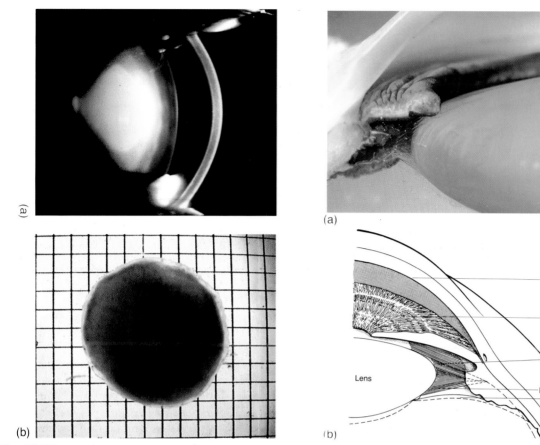

Fig. 12.39 (a) Slit image of a brunescent cataract. (b) Highly brunescent lens in vitro.

Fig. 12.40 (a) Micrograph of the chamber angle to show the relationship between the lens iris and ciliary body. (b) Schematic view of the lens zonule.

Accommodative changes in shape of the lens are best understood in relation to the attachments of the suspensory ligament.

12.2 THE CILIARY ZONULE (zonule of Zinn, suspensory ligament of the lens)

The ciliary zonule consists essentially of a series of fibres passing from the ciliary body to the lens. It holds the lens in position and enables the ciliary muscle to act on it during accommodation. The lens and zonule form a diaphragm which divides the eye into a smaller anterior portion and a larger posterior portion. The zonule forms a ring which is roughly triangular in meridional section. The base of the triangle is concave and faces the equatorial edge of the lens. The apex is elongated and curved, and follows the valleys of the ciliary processes to be prolonged over the pars plana ciliaris to the ora serrata (Figs 12.1a; 12.30 and 12.40).

The fibrils are composed of a noncollagenous glycoprotein containing O- and N-linked oligosac- charides, which explains their positive histochemical reaction to PAS stain. Fibril size, tubular ultrastruc- ture (Raviola, 1971; Fischer and Hayes, 1969), cross- reactivity (Streeten et al., 1981) and amino acid and peptide profiles (Ross and Bornstein, 1969; Streeten et al., 1983; Streeten and Gibson, 1988) all resemble elastin, as do their resistance to collagenase and susceptibility to digestion by trypsin. This property is utilized in intracapsular lens extraction in which alphachymotrypsin dissolves the zonules but has no effect on the collagenous capsule (Ley, Holmberg and Yamashita, 1960). Recently it has been shown that the zonular fibril is a cysteine-rich microfibrillar com- ponent of the elastic system, fibrillin, which in other tissues provides a template for elastin deposition during elastogenesis (Ross and Bornstein, 1969). Fibrillin, however, like oxytalan, another microfibril- lar component of the elastic system, never becomes elasticized. Fibrillin maps to chromosome 15 q21.1 (Lee et al., 1991; Magenis et al., 1991). The zonular fibres are strongly immunoreactive for fibrillin (Saiki, Keene and Engvall, 1986, 1991; Streeten, 1992). The

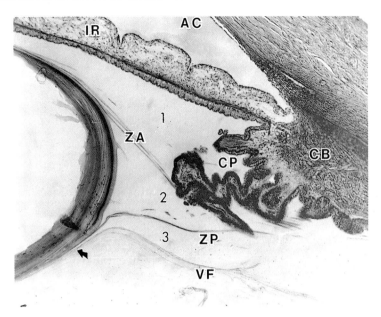

Fig. 12.41 Light micrograph of a meridional section of the anterior segment to show the drainage angle, iris, lens and ciliary body. AC = anterior chamber; CB = ciliary body; CP = ciliary processes; VF = vitreous face; ZA = anterior zonule; ZP = posterior zonule; 1 = posterior chamber; 2 = canal of Hanover; 3 = canal of Petit.

Marfan syndrome, which is associated with lens dislocation, cardiovascular and joint disease, has been shown to be due to mutations in the fibrillin gene, and some Marfan phenotypes may be linked to defects in fibrillin genes on other chromosomes.

Each zonular fibre is composed of fibrils averaging 10 nm in cross-section (8 to 12 nm), and tubular in profile. They show a microperiodicity of 12–14 nm, or occasionally 40–55 μm when the fibrils are densely aggregated. Granular and finely fibrillar material can be demonstrated in and between the fibrils (using cationic dyes which stain for polysaccharides) (Raviola, 1971; Streeten, 1992). Rotary shadowing shows that individual fibres consist of beads (29 nm wide) held together by about four filaments 3–6 nm in diameter. The beads have a periodicity which varies from 30 to 57 nm from fibril to fibril, which may be an expression of the elastic properties of the fibrils (Wallace *et al.*, 1991). Similar features have been observed in other tissues (Wallace *et al.*, 1991; Ren *et al.*, 1991; Keene *et al.*, 1991).

Although it can be seen that the main components of the suspensory apparatus run a more or less complex but continuous course from the ora serrata to the edge of the lens, it is useful to keep in mind four main topographic zones: the **pars orbicularis** (lying on the pars plana), the **zonular plexus** (between the ciliary processes), the **zonular fork** (the point of angulation of the zonule at the mid zone of the ciliary valleys), and the anterior, equatorial and posterior limbs of the zonule (Figs 12.41 and 12.42).

Structurally the **anterior zonule** runs mainly from the pars plana to the pre-equatorial lens, but is supplemented from the pars plicata, while the **posterior zonule** runs chiefly from the pars plicata to the post-equatorial lens and is supplemented from the pars plana. The **equatorial zonule** passes from pars plicata to lens equator. The **hyaloid zonule** is a flimsier structure and can be imagined as being plastered as a thin layer deep to the main suspensory apparatus to run a course from pars plana to the lens at the edge of the patellar fossa where it attaches

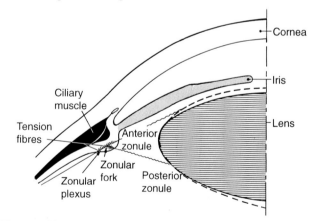

Fig. 12.42 Schema for the accommodative mechanism according to Rohen. Accommodating eye ciliary muscle contracted, forming an edge; the tension fibre system is stretched, taking up the traction from the posterior zonular fibres and choroid. Thus the anterior zonular fibres become relaxed and the lens more spherical (dotted line). The arrow indicates the direction of ciliary muscle movement during accommodation. In the non-accommodating state the ciliary muscle is relaxed and the anterior zonular fibres are stretched by the traction from the posterior (pars plana) zonular fibres. The lens is therefore flattened. (Modified from Rohen, 1979, with permission.)

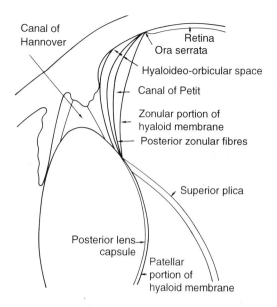

Fig. 12.43 Relationship of anterior vitreous to posterior chamber. Canal of Hanover (HAN); pars plana (PP); retina (R); ora serrata (OS); hyaloideo-orbicular space (HOS) (Garnier); canal of Petit (CP); zonular portion of hyaloid membrane (ZAHM); posterior zonular fibres (PZF); posterior lens capsule (PLC); superior plica (SP); patellar portion of hyaloid membrane (PAHM).

to the hyalocapsular zonule (corresponding to the annular fibres of Wieger's ligament) (Farnsworth and Burke, 1977; Rohen, 1979; Nishida, 1982).

Scanning electron microscopy has contributed greatly to our understanding of the anatomy of the zonule. The vast majority of the zonules arise from the posterior end of the pars plana up to 1.5 mm from the ora serrata, where they either run into its inner limiting membrane without entering the cytoplasm of the underlying cells (Rohen, 1979) or become continuous with fibres of the anterior vitreous (Nishida, 1982). Most fibres arise as bundles of 2–5 fibrils which blend with the basement membrane of the non-pigmented epithelium of the pars plana (Figs 12.43, 12.44 and and 12.45). Some fibrils occasionally penetrate between these cells in the absence of basement membrane. Fibrils have also been reported between the ciliary pigmented epithelium, its basement membrane, and extending into the elastic lamina of Bruch's membrane (McCulloch, 1954; Roll *et al.*, 1975). However, Streeten (1992) suggests that these are more likely to be a mixture of fibrils found in ageing basement membrane, and microfibrils related to the elastic tissue of ciliary body stroma.

The fibres pass forward over the pars plana as a feltwork until they reach the posterior margin of the pars plicata. Here they segment into the zonular plexuses, which pass through the valleys between

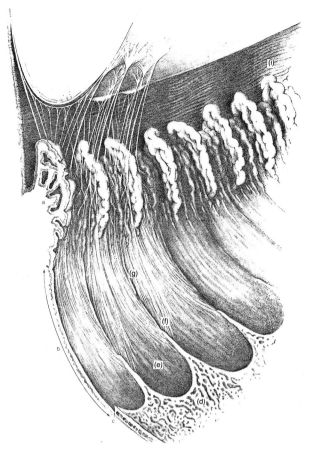

Fig. 12.44 Drawing of the inner aspect of the ciliary body to show the pars plicata (a) and pars plana (b). The ora serrata is at (c). Posterior to it the retina shows cystoid degeneration (d); the base (e) and dentate processes (f) of the ora are shown: linear ridges or striae (g) project forward from the dentate processes across the pars plana to enter the valleys between the ciliary processes. The zonular fibres arise from the pars plana beginning 1.5 mm from the ora serrata. They curve forward from the sides of the dentate ridges into the ciliary valleys, then from the valleys to the lens capsule. Zonules coming from the valleys on either side of a ciliary process have a common point of attachment on the lens. The zonules attach up to 1 mm from the equator posteriorly and up to 1.5 mm from the equator anteriorly. At the equatorial border the attaching zonules give a crenated appearance to the lens. The ciliary processes vary in size and shape and often are separated from each other by lesser processes. The radial (h) and circular furrows (i) of the peripheral iris are shown. (From Hogan, M. J., Alvarado, J. A. and Weddell, J. E. (1971) *History of the Human Eye*, published by W. B. Saunders.)

the ciliary processes to whose lateral walls they are closely attached (Figs 12.42 and 12.46). Each zonular plexus consists of broad flattened fibre strands which cross and join each other in a regular pattern. The zonular plexuses are firmly attached to the bases of the ciliary valleys by fine and coarse fibrils which leave the main strands and run anteriorly at an acute angle. These **tension fibres** find anchorage to the basement membrane within the depths of the valleys

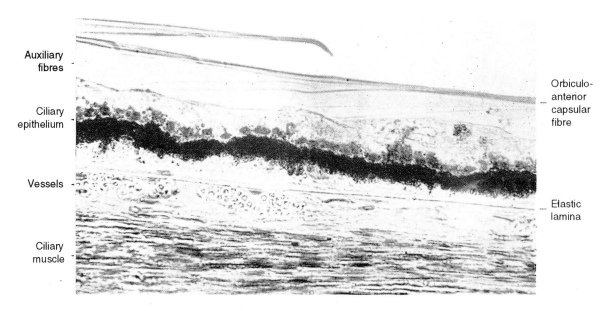

Auxiliary fibres

Ciliary epithelium

Vessels

Ciliary muscle

Orbiculo-anterior capsular fibre

Elastic lamina

Fig. 12.45 Zonular fibres emerging from the pars plana.

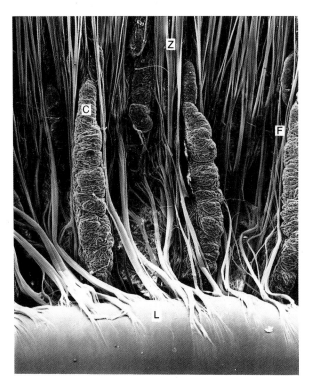

Fig. 12.46 Scanning electron micrograph of zonules passing through the valleys in the pars plicata. The zonules (Z) pass between the ciliary processes (C) and then divide into three main systems at the zonular fork (F) before reaching the surface of the lens (L). At the posterior margin of the ciliary processes the zonular fibres rearrange themselves to form a series of zonular plexuses (P). (From Marshall, J., Beaconsfield, M. and Rottery, S. (1982) *Trans. Ophthalmol. Soc. UK*, **102**, 423–440, with permission.)

and are thought to play an important role in the accommodation process by stabilizing the zonules. Towards the anterior margin of the pars plicata each plexus divides into a zonular fork consisting of three fibre groups running to the anterior, equatorial and posterior lens capsule, respectively (Fig. 12.42) (Rohen, 1979). In scanning preparations the entire zonular apparatus is always bent at the zonular fork, showing the strength of the anchorage of the zonular plexuses to the ciliary processes. This secondary anchorage is thought to be extremely important in relation to accommodation as it explains how an equatorial force is exerted upon the lens by fibres that originate partly in the pars plana (Rohen, 1979) without involving the older and unacceptable theories of a fulcrum of resistance being provided by the hyaloid face of the vitreous (Wolff, 1976).

The pre-equatorial, equatorial and post-equatorial insertions of the zonules into the lens capsule are macroscopically different. The pre-equatorial insertions are relatively dense, as they all insert at approximately the same distance from the equator (1.5 mm), as an irregular double row of bundles, 5–10 μm wide (Fig. 12.47). Bundles decrease in width to insert over a zone of 0.3 to 0.4 mm in meridional width (Fig. 12.47). Their zonular insertions flatten in the plane of the capsule, and then split up into ever smaller finger-like processes which fan out and finally run into the lens capsule to form the zonular lamella. They join a surface of loosely arranged microfibrils which blend into the fibrogranular matrix of the capsule. These fibrils are lost, 1 mm central to the

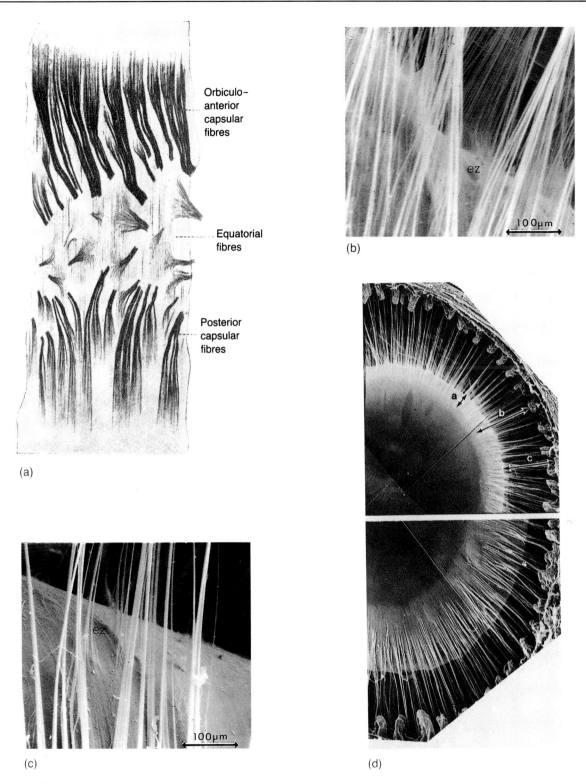

Fig. 12.47 (a) Equatorial zone of the lens capsule, with the insertion of the zonular fibres. (b) The equatorial region of a 46-year-old lens showing numerous fine equatorial zonules (ez) (original magnification ×200). (c) The equatorial region of a 73-year-old lens showing a shift anteriorly of all zonules and the presence of equatorial-like zonules (ez) on the anterior lens face (original magnification ×200). (d) The anterior surface of two suspended human lenses (ages 46 and 85) showing an increase in insertion-equatorial distance, a, with age, a consistent insertion-ciliary body distance, b, and a decrease in the circumlental space, c, (original magnification ×20). Any apparent size difference in the ciliary processes in the two sections is related to observed changes due to age and to the varying amounts of the ciliary processes exposed by dissection.

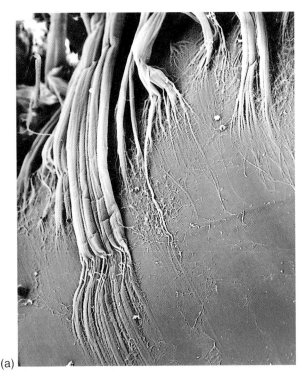

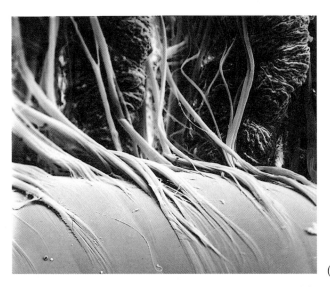

(a)   (b)

Fig. 12.48   (a) Zonular insertions into the pre-equatorial lens capsule. (b) Scanning electron micrographs of the post-equatorial surface of a human lens to show the sparsity of the zonules and the variety of levels at which they insert. This discontinuity in fibre insertions gives rise to the dentations of the lens. (From Marshall, J., Beaconsfield, M. and Rottery, S. (1982) *Trans. Ophthalmol. Soc. UK*, **102**, 423–440, with permission.)

zonular insertion, where the capsule resumes its normal patina. At the point of insertion, the anterior zonule sends fibres and smaller fibrils (0.07 to 0.5 μm) to a depth of 0.6 to 1.6 μm into the capsular surface. The zonular lamella thickens from 1.0 to 1.7 μm, lateral to the anterior zonular insertions. The insertion of the meridional zonular fibres, 0.5 to 1.0 μm wide, creates an anteroposterior ribbing. It has been suggested that anterior zonules decrease in number with age and that the site of the anterior insertion becomes displaced more centrally (Weale, 1982). The origin of the zonule from the pars plana is also thought to move anteriorly with age (Farnsworth and Shyne, 1979).

The equatorial fibres are sparse and poorly developed but again fan out in a brush-like manner to insert into the capsule almost perpendicularly to the surface. They rarely insert into the equator and are usually either just anterior or posterior to it. Fibres are usually 10 to 15 μm wide but may be up to 60 μm wide. They merge with the meridional fibres, which arch over the equatorial capsule (Fig. 12.48).

The posterior fibres insert in two or three layers, over a zone of 0.4 to 0.5 mm wide. They fan out more and show less interconnections than the anterior zonule. Anteriorly they insert at the posterior edge

of the lens equator, close to the margin of the lens epithelium; posteriorly they extend about 1.25 mm from the equatorial margin. The fibres of the zonule insert into the capsule to a depth of about 2 μm. Both the posterior and meridional fibres are partly obscured by a thick layer of loosely arranged fibrils, which are of zonular type (Streeten, 1992).

The post-equatorial fibres appear relatively less well developed than the anterior ones but this is probably illusory and results from the fact that they insert into the capsule at a variety of levels, with the hyaloid zonules being most central. The hyaloid zonule is a single layer connecting the anterior hyaloid at the border of the patellar fossa with the pars plana and pars plicata. It is undistinguished in the untouched eye because its fibres are closely apposed to those of the posterior zonule (Eisner, 1973).

The space between the anterior and posterior zonules is known as the canal of Hannover. Actually, it is subdivided into larger and smaller spaces by the equatorial fibres. Streeten (1992) has speculated that the mucoid character of the zonular fibres might offer a diffusion barrier between the posterior chamber and the vitreous. The space between the hyaloid zonule and the posterior zonule is the canal of Petit.

The arrangement of the zonular fibres is shown in Fig. 12.43. These fibres with their relatively large interspaces give rise to the dentations of the lens equator with the crests corresponding to insertions and the valleys between.

A narrow band of fibres extends forwards on the lens capsule from the point of attachment of the hyaloid zonule to the point of insertion of the posterior zonule. This hyalocapsular zonule probably corresponds to the ligament of Wieger (Wieger, 1883) and its fibres are mainly radial (Albrecht and Eisner, 1982). Where it joins with the anterior hyaloid membrane at the rim of the patellar fossa, there is a circular band of fibres. There is a similar attachment of the anterior hyaloid to circular zonular girdles (the anterior and posterior orbicular bands of Daicker, 1972) over the posterior third of the ciliary processes, and the middle of the pars plana.

CIRCUMFERENTIAL ZONULAR GIRDLES

A few, flimsy circumferential structures lying in relation to the ciliary body have been noted by Eisner (1975). The anterior ciliary girdle lies over the ciliary crests and arises from branches of the posterior zonular bundles. It lies in and on the surface of the anterior hyaloid membrane, binding it to the ciliary processes and resisting the pull of the coronary vitreous tract, which inserts here (Eisner, 1975). Neighbouring vitreous collagen fibrils may have a circumferential orientation. It readily pulls away with the vitreous when it becomes detached.

A posterior girdle of circularly disposed zonular fibres has been demonstrated *in vitro* over the ciliary processes, pars plana and posterior insertion of the zonule, by several authors (Garnier, 1892; Graf Spee, 1892; Salzmann, 1912; McCulloch, 1954; Kaczurowski, 1967; Garzino, 1953; Davanger, 1975a,b; Farnsworth and Burke, 1977; Streeten and Pulaski, 1978; Rohen, 1979). It has also been shown by biomicroscopy on postmortem eyes (Eisner, 1975).

The posterior zonular bundle lies on the pars plana at the internal surface of the main zonule, 1 to 2 mm anterior to the ora serrata, at a site into which the median vitreous tract inserts (Eisner, 1975). Its fibrils have the same circumferential direction as those of the adjacent vitreous, perhaps reflecting the influence of similar tractional forces on both structures. They are more aggregated and easier to observe in older eyes (Streeten, 1992).

Aberrant zonular fibres, which are separate from the main zonular streams, are commonly found, close to the ora serrata, in relation to retinal abnormalities such as zonular traction tufts, meridional folds,

enclosed ciliary bays, and peripheral rosettes or granulations. Some zonular bundles may also pass back across the ora into the vitreous at all ages without attachment to the ciliary body (Foos, 1969).

After the second decade, occasional bundles of fibrils may be found in the equatorial capsule. These are believed by some to represent deep zonular insertions. However, no connection with the zonules has been demonstrated (Dark *et al.*, 1969; Seland, 1974). Some material shows a banding at 45 to 55 nm, and resembles fibrillar material found in ageing basement membranes. Other fibrillogranular material with the characteristics of zonular fibrils is found superficially, but has no connection with the surface zonules. It has been suggested that this may represent a secretory product of the lens epithelium.

AGEING OF THE ZONULE

The fetal and infantile zonular fibres are finer and less aggregated than in the adult, and richer in proteoglycans. In the elderly, the fibres are finer and more sparse, especially the meridional ones, and they rupture more readily (Buschmann *et al.*, 1978; Weale, 1982). In the first two decades of life the zonular attachments are narrow. With time they broaden and move more centrally, both anteriorly and posteriorly. Anteriorly, the zonule-free area of the capsule reduces from 8 mm at age 20 years, to 6.5 mm in the eighth decade or as low as 5.5 mm, so that the insertion may intrude into the region selected for capsulotomy during extracapsular cataract surgery (Farnsworth and Shine, 1979; Stark and Streeten, 1984) (Fig. 12.48).

In childhood, the anterior hyaloid membrane is closely attached to the whole posterior zonular insertion and the lens. In the adult, the anterior hyaloid membrane may be peeled back to the zonular insertion, its strongest point of attachment at all ages. During intracapsular extraction a superficial flap, or even the full thickness of lens capsule, may be separated by this attachment, the posterior zonular complex and the circumferential complex (see below).

During intracapsular cataract extraction most of the zonular complex is torn from the capsule, with only the tips of the anterior zonular insertions and a few meridional fibres remaining. The zonule may also tear partially, during extracapsular cataract surgery, with rupture, or a preferential separation of the posterior and meridional fibres from the capsule. About 5% of these dehiscences may be detected at the time of surgery, occurring during the removal of lens material as traction is applied to the zonule

(Guzek *et al.*, 1987). More are identified at postmortem (Wilson *et al.*, 1987).

The zonule is weak in the disorder pseudoexfoliation of the lens capsule, and is four times more likely to rupture during cataract surgery than normally (Skuta, 1987). Each zonular bundle associated with a major ciliary process forms a unit which emerges as a flat ribbon of bundles 30–60 μm wide: 6–10 per ciliary unit. It has been suggested that rubbing of the posterior iris across the zonule is responsible for iris pigment loss in pigmentary glaucoma (Campbell, 1979).

CHAPTER THIRTEEN
The vitreous

13.1   GROSS APPEARANCES

The vitreous humour is a transparent colourless gel of a consistency somewhat firmer than egg white (Fig. 13.1). It fills the posterior four-fifths of the globe and is in contact with the retina behind, and the ciliary body, zonule and lens, in front (Fig. 6.7). The vitreous body is roughly spherical, but is flattened anteriorly. It exhibits a cup-shaped anterior depression, the **patellar fossa**, which accommodates the lens and is separated from it by the capillary space of Berger (Figs 13.2 and 13.3). At the margin of the patellar fossa the vitreous is adherent to the lens capsule over a ring-shaped zone (the ligamentum hyaloideo capsulare of Wieger) 8–9 mm in diameter.

Although anatomic fusion of these tissues has not been demonstrated, the union is strong in youth. By the sixth decade, however, it becomes sufficiently weak to permit intracapsular extraction of the lens without pulling on the anterior face of the vitreous. This site also receives the insertion of the hyaloid portion of the zonule.

Outside the ring of attachment, the vitreous is intimately apposed to the ciliary processes, which indent its anterior face, or to the fibres of the ciliary zonule.

The hyaloid canal (of Cloquet) runs from the post-lenticular space of Berger, from a point slightly nasal to the posterior of the lens, to the funnel-shaped space (the area of Martegiani) in front of the optic disc (Fig. 13.2). The canal is 1–2 mm wide and

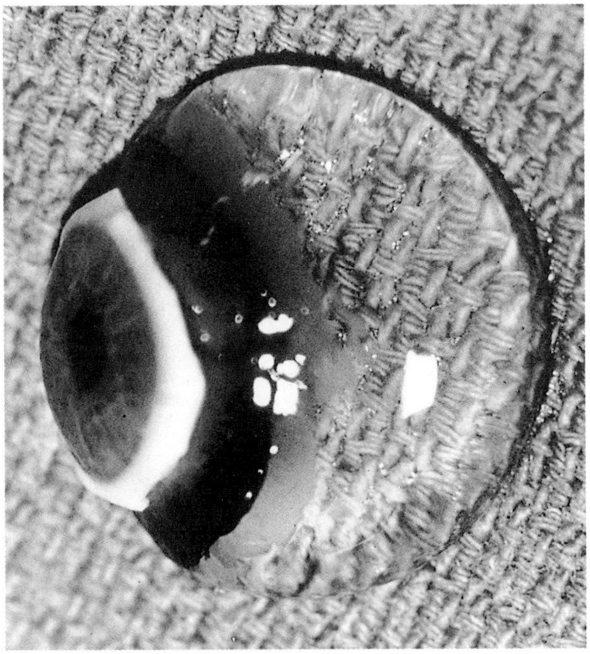

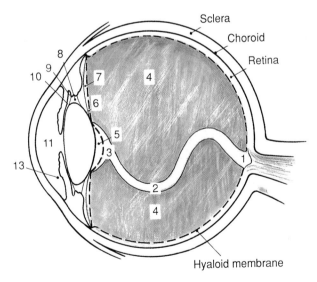

Fig. 13.2   Intraocular spaces 1 = posterior part of Cloquet's canal (space of Martegiani); 2 = mid portion; 3 = anterior portion; 4 = secondary vitreous; 5 = Berger's space (exaggerated); 6 = canal of Petit; 7 = hyaloideo-orbicular space (Garnier); 8 = canal of Hannover; 9 = iridozonular; 10 = iridocapsular; 11 = anterior chamber. (After Cibis, P. A., (1965) *Vitreoretinal, Pathology and Surgery in Retinal Detachment*, published by C. V. Mosby Co.)

Fig. 13.1   Eye of a 9-month-old human from which the sclera, choroid and retina have been dissected. The posterior extent of the vitreous base is seen as a grey band at the ora serrata. (Courtesy of J. Sebag.)

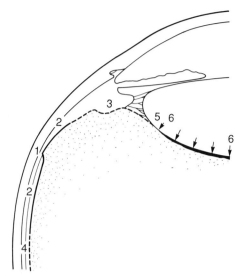

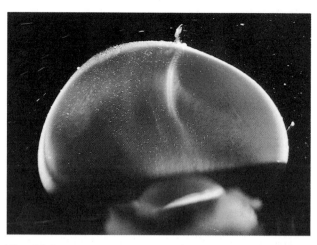

Fig. 13.3 The relations of the vitreous in the anterior eye. The ora serrata (1) is the termination of the retina, The vitreous base (2) extends forwards for about 2 mm over the ciliary body and posteriorly about 4 mm over the peripheral retina. Collagen in this region is oriented at a right-angle to the surface of the retina and ciliary body. Anteriorly over the pars plana it has a more parallel orientation to the inner surface of the ciliary body. The posterior hyaloid (4) is continuous with the retina and anterior hyaloid (3) and with the zonules and lens. Ligamentum hyaloideocapsulare is at (5) and the space of Berger at (6). (From Hogan, M. J., Alvarado, J. A. and Weddell, J. E., (1971) *Histology of the Human Eye: An Atlas and Textbook*, published by W. B. Saunders.)

Fig. 13.4 Dark-field horizontal optical section of vitreous in a 33-week gestational age human. Anterior segment is below and posterior pole is above. Hyaloid artery remnant is seen coursing towards the prepapillary vitreous cortex. (Courtesy of J. Sebag.)

runs a sinuous course from lens to disc. It represents the sites of the primary vitreous and the fetal hyaloid artery. Its walls are formed by condensation of vitreous (Mann, 1927; Goldmann, 1954; Busacca, Goldmann and Schiff-Wertheimer, 1957). Multilayered fenestrated structures have been found in Cloquet's canal in adult human and primate eyes and have been thought to represent the sheaths of the media of the embryonic hyaloid artery and its branches. The multilaminar structure of the sheath may contribute to its visibility during slit-lamp examination. Occasional cells are found within the canal and a network of fine collagen outside it (Balazs, 1973). Eisner believes that the hyaloid canal of prenatal life disappears completely after birth and is replaced by a retrolental tract that develops anteriorly in the first four years of life and extends posteriorly in adolescence.

Histological studies of vitreous structure in the eighteenth and nineteenth centuries provided four different hypotheses: The **alveolar** theory (Demours, 1741); the **lamellar** theory (Zinn, 1780); the **radial sector** theory (Hannover, 1845); and the **fibrillar theory** (Szent-Gyorgi, 1917). In 1849 Bowman claimed that these descriptions were incorrect, due to fixative artefacts. Although introduction of the slit-lamp biomicroscope enabled *in situ* observation of the vitreous, an equal variety of descriptions followed: Gullstrand (1912) described membranes, Koeppe (1917) saw fibres and Friedenwald and Stiehler (1935) observed concentric sheets.

Eisner, using slit-lamp microscopy in both living and dead eyes with special conditions of illumination, has proposed the following account (Eisner, 1971, 1973a,b, 1975, 1982).

At birth, vitreous structure is homogeneous, and shows a finely striated pattern (Figs 13.4 and 13.5). At this stage a denser outer cortex and an inner central vitreous are not established. Here and there, narrow **transvitreal 'channels'** of lower density

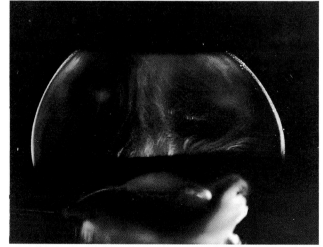

Fig. 13.5 Dark-field horizontal optical section of vitreous in a 4-year-old human. Dissolution of the walls of the hyaloid Artery is noted. Light scattering in the central vitreous arises from Cloquet's canal. (Courtesy of J. Sebag.)

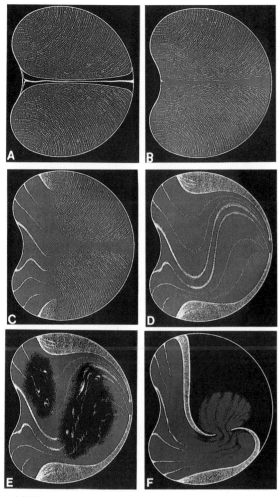

Fig. 13.6 Growth and ageing of the vitreous. (a) Late stage of fetal life. The hyaloid artery extends from disc to lens, surrounded by a transparent material within a channel to delineate it from the definitive vitreous by a membrane-like condensation (intravitreal limiting membrane of Dejeane); (b) infant. The hyaloid artery and intravitreal limiting membrane have disappeared. The definitive vitreous shows a regular finely striated pattern (infantile striation radiation); (c) adolescent. Vitreous tracts begin to develop in the anterior vitreous. The posterior vitreous still shows the infantile striation; (d) adult. Vitreous tracts extend into the posterior vitreous; (e) senile destruction of the framework; development of liquified cavities interspersed with irregular strands; (f) senile posterior vitreous detachment. Destroyed vitreous empties through a gap into the retrovitreal space; the vitreous collapses. (From Eisner, G. in Duane, T. D. and Jaeger, E. D. (eds) (1987) *Biomedical Foundations of Ophthalmology*, published by Harper and Row.)

traverse its substance from the periphery. These overlie the optic disc, fovea and retinal vessels, and presumably reflect variations in vitreous synthesis during the growth of the eye. The shape of these channels is altered accordingly at different vitreous depths. Such channels are also found in relation to congenital (or experimentally induced) retinal anomalies (Eisner, 1973a,b, 1975, 1978; Eisner and van den Zypen, 1981).

From infancy into adult life, the homogeneous structure of the vitreous changes, with a decrease in density of the central vitreous, while the cortex retains its relatively higher density (Eisner, 1971, 1973a,b; Eisner and Bachmann, 1974a–d). Formation of the cortical vitreous starts anteriorly and proceeds posteriorly, and the posterior vitreous is the last to lose its infantile striations. It is of interest that there is a marked interspecies variation in vitreous density; in dogs and cats the central vitreous has the highest density (Eisner and Bachmann, 1974a,b), in cattle and sheep the vitreous is homogeneous (Eisner and Bachmann, 1974c) while in the horse, the entire vitreous is of low density (Eisner and Bachmann, 1974d).

The second post-natal development, also beginning anteriorly, is the formation of the so-called **vitreous tracts**: fine, sheet-like condensations of vitreous structure which radiate backwards into the vitreous space from defined points on the circumference of the ciliary body and anterior retina (Figs 13.6–13.9). It is these tracts which give rise to the concentric 'onion skin' arrangement of the adult vitreous. The vitreous tracts arise as follows.

RETROLENTAL TRACT

The retrolental tract is inserted into a circular zone on the lens capsule, near to the hyaloideocapsular ligament, and extends posteriorly into the central vitreous. It is conspicuous as a highly reflecting boundary, the membrana plicata of Vogt (Vogt, 1941).

CORONARY TRACT

The coronary tract passes backwards into the central vitreous from a circular zone overlying the posterior third of the ciliary processes (the **coronary ligament**). It is of variable density and fairly indistinct optically.

MEDIAN TRACT

The median tract is inserted into a circular zone at the anterior margin of the vitreous base, about the middle of the pars plana, which is termed the **median ligament**. The tract extends backwards as a faint veil into the central vitreous.

PRERETINAL TRACT

The preretinal tract is inserted at the ora serrata and is more strongly reflecting than the preceding two.

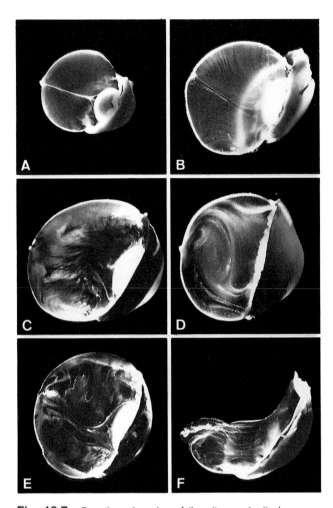

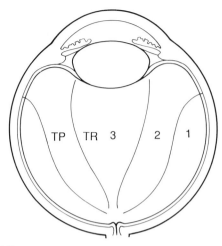

Fig. 13.8 Topographic subdivisions of the vitreous space. 1 = preretinal zone, bounded on the outer side by the retina; 2 = intermediate zone, bounded anteriorly by the epiciliary portion of the anterior hyaloid membrane and by the ciliary epithelium of the posterior pars plana (ciliary vitreous base); 3 = retrolental zone, bounded anteriorly by the patellar fossa of the lens. The intermediate zone is delineated from the retrolental zone by the retrolental (or hyaloid) tract (TR), from the preretinal zone by the preretinal tract (TP). (From Eisner, G. in Duane, T. D. and Jaeger, E. D. (eds) (1987) *Biomedical Foundations of Ophthalmology*, Vol. 1, published by Harper and Row.)

Fig. 13.7 Growth and ageing of the vitreous (optical dissection of autopsy eyes in the hyaloidean plane). (a) Premature infant at the 32nd week of pregnancy. The hyaloid artery and its retrolental ramifications as well as the remnants of Bergermeister's papilla are still present. The structure of the remaining vitreous is homogeneous; (b) child aged 7 months. Only tiny remnants of the hyaloid artery remain. There is a prepapillary channel of even width traversing the vitreous. The other vitreous structures show a homogeneous finely striated pattern. There are no vitreous tracts; (c) adolescent, aged 14 years. In the anterior vitreous the cortex is delineated from the more transparent vitreous centre; vitreous tracts appear. The posterior vitreous still shows the infantile radial striation; (d) adult 70 years of age. The vitreous tracts nearly reach the posterior pole. They now follow a typical S-shaped course descending first behind the lens, ascending then in the centre of the cavity, descending finally towards the disc; (e) early vitreous destruction in an adult, 31 years of age. At several points cavities develop, some of them in the anterior zone of the adult pattern, some in the posterior vitreous of the infantile striation; (f) posterior vitreous detachment in an adult of about 75 years of age. The vitreous has collapsed. Coarse strands pass from the intravitreal into the retrovitreal space. (From Eisner, G. in Duane, T. D. and Jaeger, E. D. (eds) (1987) *Biomedical Foundations of Ophthalmology*, Vol. 1, published by Harper and Row.)

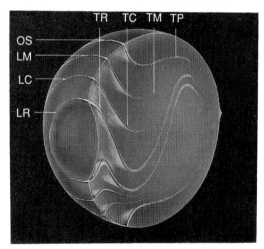

Fig. 13.9 Schema of the vitreous tracts in human eyes: TR = tractus retrolentalis ('hyaloideus'), inserting at the retrolental ligament (LR); TC = tractus coronarius, inserting at the ligamentum coronarium (LC); TM = tractus medianus inserting at the ligmanetum medianum (LM); TP = tractus preretinalis inserting at the ora serrata (OS). (From Eisner, G. in Duane, T. D. and Jaeger, E. D. (eds) (1987) *Biomedical Foundations of Ophthalmology*, Vol. 1, published by Harper and Row.)

These tracts show a gentle curvature in younger eyes, which gradually becomes more sinuous and extensive with ageing, the precise configuration depending on the effects of gravity (Nordmann & Roth, 1967; Eisner, 1971).

Also, starting in adolescence, a process of liquefaction and fibrillar degeneration of the vitreous occurs, which also breaks up the basic pattern of the tracts.

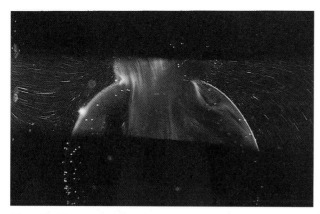

Fig. 13.10 Dark-field horizontal optical section of an 8-year-old human, showing the absence of fibrous structures even though vitreous is seen extruding out of the 'hole' in the premacular vitreous cortex (above). (Courtesy of J. Sebag.)

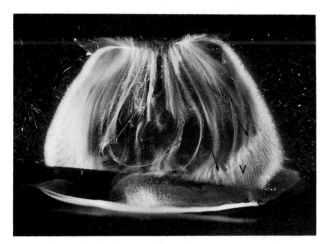

Fig. 13.11 Dark-field sagittal optical section of vitreous structure year demonstrating prominent vitreous fibres coursing in an anterior–posterior direction, and orientated towards the premacular hole. Fibres inserting into the vitreous base are also seen (lower right-hand aspect of photo). (Courtesy of J. Sebag.)

The tractus preretinalis is least affected by these changes (Fig. 13.7).

Using dark-field slit microscopy in fresh unfixed human vitreous, Sebag and Balazs have shown that the homogeneous appearance persists in childhood apart from the visibility of Cloquet's canal (Figs 13.14 and 13.8). By middle age, macroscopic 'fibres' appear which traverse the vitreous in an anteroposterior direction and insert into the vitreous base both anterior and posterior to the ora serrata (Figs 13.10 and 13.11) (Sebag, Balazs and Flood, 1984). At the posterior pole the fibres appear oriented towards the macula (Sebag and Balazs, 1984).

13.2 MICROSCOPIC STRUCTURE

The vitreous has the following components:

1. cortex:
   anterior hyaloid;
   vitreous base;
   posterior hyaloid;
   peripapillary and perimacular attachments;
2. central vitreous;
3. vitreous cells.

CORTEX (Fig. 13.12)

Clinically, the term cortex is applied to the dense broad zone, up to 0.2 or 0.3 mm in width, adjoining the retina. Eisner has also used the term **posterior cortex** for this zone, while adopting the term **anterior cortex** for the very thin zone corresponding to the anterior hyaloid of the clinician and lying external to the preretinal tract. Eisner (1982) regards the central vitreous as lying internal to this tract and further subdivides it into intermediate vitreous (between the preretinal and retrolenticular tracts) and retrolenticular vitreous (lying internal to the retrolenticular

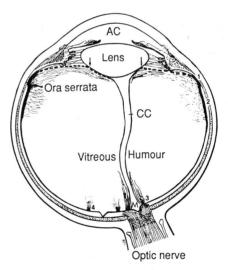

Fig. 13.12 Schematic view of vitreous attachments. In young eyes, the vitreous face is adherent to the posterior lens capsule in the region of the hyaloideocapsular ligament (arrows). The vitreous body is firmly attached (solid line) to about a 2 mm zone of the pars plana (1) and continues posteriorly to about a 4 mm width of the peripheral retina (2). The dotted line anteriorly represents the anterior vitreous face, which in places is in contact with the posterior zonular fibres. Posteriorly the vitreous face is attached at the edge of the optic disc (3), although not as firmly as at the vitreous base. A similar anular attachment 3–4 mm in diameter is seen in young eyes at the macular region (4). AC = anterior chamber; CC = Cloquet's canal; M = space of Martegiani. (From Tripathi, R. C. and Tripathi, B. J. in Davson, H. (ed.) (1984) *The Eye*, 3rd edition, published by Academic Press, 1984.)

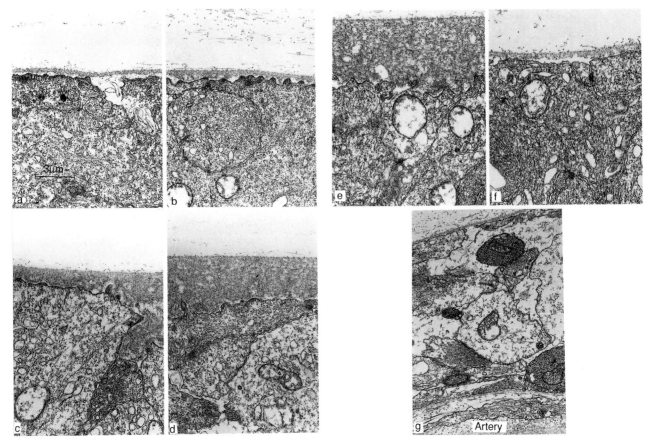

Fig. 13.13 Vitreoretinal junction in various zones of the retina (eye nucleated from a woman aged 45 years with orbital tumour and optic atrophy). (a) Region of the ora serrata; (b) equatorial region; (c) intermediate region; (d) posterior region; (e) fovea: margin of the pit; (f) fovea: centre of the pit; (g) overlying a retinal vessel at the posterior pole. The inner limiting lamina progressively increases in thickness from the periphery towards the posterior pole. Extreme thinning is found at the centre of the fovea and overlying the vessels. The inner limiting membrane is separated from the cell membrane of Müller by an electronlucent zone. This sublaminar space is crossed by fibrils that increase in number at the site of densifications in the surface cytoplasm of Müller cells ('attachment plaques'). Original magnification a–e × 23 000, f × 20 000, g × 19 800. (From Duane, T. D. and Jaeger, E. D. (eds) (1987) *Biomedical Foundations of Ophthalmology*, Vol. 1, published by Harper and Row; originals courtesy of E. van der Zypen, Institute of Anatomy, University of Berne.)

tract). Many authors, however, use the term cortex, for the outer vitreous zone at any site. Microscopically, the cortex is regarded as the outer 100–200 μm of the vitreous and is formed by a condensation of its constituent fibrils, cells and glycosaminoglycan (Balazs, 1961). Its fibrils are in the region of 12 nm wide and insert into the internal limiting membrane of the retina posteriorly, blending with the basal lamina of the Müller's cells, or with the basal lamina of the ciliary body epithelium anteriorly. In places, such as the **vitreous base** and margin of the **disc and macula**, and overlying the retinal vessels, a firm bond is achieved, which is strong in youth and weakens with age; elsewhere the attachment is loose (Fig. 13.12).

In healthy young eyes the attachments between the Müller's cell membranes, basal lamina and cortical collagen fibrils are so strong that if vitreous is pulled away from the retina the cell membrane of the

Müller's cell breaks, while the basement membrane remains attached to the vitreous fibrils and the cell membrane (Sebag, 1989).

The thickness of the basal lamina varies between 20 and 100 nm, and is thicker over the posterior part of the retina, except at the fovea and optic nerve head. This thickness increases with age and may reach 3 μm in width (Foos, 1972). The basal lamina serves partially as a barrier to large molecules, and may in part prevent macromolecules of 7 nm or over from entering the vitreous across the retina. The continuity of the basal lamina is interrupted at the pars plana and at the ciliary processes. At these points, vitreous fibrils are in direct contact with the cell membranes of the epithelial cells. It appears that these breaks in basal lamina increase with age, and basal laminar fragments may be found in the cortical vitreous in adult eyes (Rentsch and van der Zypen, 1971) (Fig. 13.13).

The condensation at the vitreous surface does not constitute a distinct hyaloid membrane but does constitute a fragile envelope which is present everywhere except just anterior to the vitreous base (the zonular cleft of Salzmann) and at the area of Martegiani. Salzmann recognized anterior and posterior limiting layers which are now termed the anterior and posterior hyaloid. They extend to the margins of the anatomical vitreous base (Fig. 13.12).

The anterior hyaloid

The anterior hyaloid is the portion of the vitreous surface that stretches forwards typically from the anterior margin of the vitreous base at the ora serrata. Its epiciliary portion passes anteriorly to reach the ligamentum hyaloideocapsulare. Central to this, its retrolental portion is thinned and less distinct. Clinically, the epiciliary portion may be seen with the slit-lamp microscope to be floating freely to a variable extent in some adult eyes (Eisner, 1973a,b). Thus it may run from the edge of the hyalocapsular ligament to the coronary ligament, to the mid pars plana region, to the ora serrata or to some intermediate point. Alternatively, it may be in contact with and adherent to the most posterior fibres of the zonule. The retrolental portion is less distinct, but may be seen more clearly after the extracapsular lens extraction when the posterior capsule flattens and loses its posterior curvature.

Using specific staining techniques and a certain amount of traction, fibres may be detected *in vitro*, running from the anterior hyaloid to other structures such as the valleys between the ciliary processes (the **hyalociliary zonule**) (Fig. 13.14). There are also three circular sets of zonules which are attached to or traverse the anterior hyaloid (Graf Spee, 1902). These are the **retrolental ligament**, corresponding to the ligamentum hyaloideocapsulare, the **coronary ligament** whose fibres run circumferentially across the inner face of the posterior third of the ciliary processes, and the **median ligament** whose fibres are also circumferential, at the level of the mid zone of the pars plana. The fibres of these so-called 'ligaments' are interwoven into the anterior vitreous cortex and give off radial fibres to the ciliary body or lens (Daicker, 1972). Their relationship to the vitreous tracts has already been mentioned.

The collagen fibrils of the anterior cortex are arranged in compacted lamellae, parallel with the plane of the pars plana ciliaris and woven into a mesh-like structure (Fine and Tousimis, 1961; Faulborn and Bowald, 1982) (Figs 13.2 and 13.8).

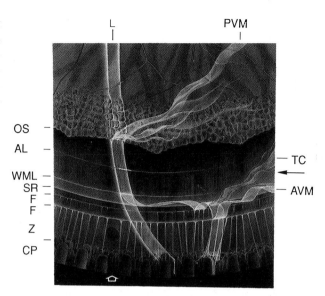

Fig. 13.14 The biomicroscopic appearance of the hyalociliary zonular fibres and retrolental ligament in a patient of 62 years. After intracapsular cataract extraction the ciliocapsular and hyalocapsular zonular fibres were disrupted. The hyalociliary zonular leaf then became visible at the anterior hyaloid membrane (AVM), connecting the circular zonular fibres of the retrolental ligament (LR) to the ciliary body. More posteriorly the ligamentum coronarium (LC) with the tractus medianus (TM) are seen. At the ora serrata (OS), the preretinal tract (TP) is inserted. The posterior hyaloid membrane (PVM) is detached and – an exception at this age – is inserted just behind the ora serrata. AL, accessory ligament; SL, slit light. (From Eisner, G. in Duane, T. D. and Jaeger, E. D. (eds) (1987) *Biomedical Foundations of Ophthalmology*, Vol. 1, published by Harper and Row.)

Vitreous base

The vitreous base is a broad band of vitreous condensation and attachment which runs circumferentially from a point 2.0 mm anterior to the ora serrata to a point 2–4 mm behind it. Collagen fibrils are most densely packed at the vitreous base and in the adult insert throughout its width (Sebag, Balazs and Flood, 1984). Anterior to the ora, the vitreous fibrils blend with the basal lamina of the nonpigmented epithelium of the pars plana ciliaris, while behind it they blend with the internal limiting membrane of the retina (Fig. 13.13); this provides a firm bond of attachment. Over the retinal surface they are organized as groups of tapering bundles which pass out into the vitreous substance approximately at right-angles to the retinal surface. More anteriorly the fibres are finer and fan out towards the lens. Collagen fibrils at the vitreous base are wider than elsewhere in the cortex, in the region of 45 nm.

At the vitreous base in the aging eye small crypts may be found between the Müller's cell foot plates at the level of the internal limiting membrane. Here vitreal fibres may perforate the inner limiting membrane and in many cases fill the crypt (see p. 458 and Fig. 14.7). Traction on the vitreous base may create a retinal tear, the forerunner of a retinal detachment (Chaine, Jebay and Coscas, 1983).

The most established portion of the vitreous base is a narrow band overlying the ora serrata. In infancy it is said to lie just posterior to the ora. With age, the vitreous base broadens anteriorly and posteriorly (Hogan, 1963; Daicker, 1972), having a relatively straight course temporally where the oral bays are flattened and a more wandering course nasally where the bays are most marked. There are also racial differences, with the vitreous base lying more posteriorly in the African and Chinese.

The posterior hyaloid

Just posterior to the vitreous base the fibrils of the vitreous cortex curve backwards along the inner retina as thin layers which pass towards the central vitreous. Posterior to the equator the fibrils blend with the inner limiting membrane of the retina (Fig. 13.13). These fibrils are more readily identified in fetal eyes.

The peripapillary and perimacular cortex

The peripapillary cortex is firmly united to a narrow zone of marginal retina 10 μm wide at the edge of the disc. This is where the Müller's fibres and associated inner limiting membrane end. A similar but less dense attachment to perimacular retina occurs. Both attachments are more developed in young eyes (Fig. 13.15).

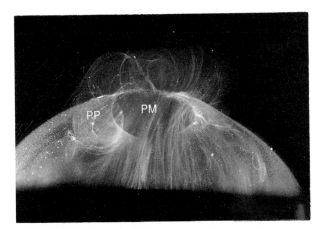

Fig. 13.15 Dark-field horizontal optical section of posterior vitreous in a 56-year-old human demonstrating the premacular (large and to the right, PM) and prepapillary 'holes' (PP) in the posterior vitreous cortex. (Courtesy of J. Sebag.)

CENTRAL VITREOUS

The general structure of the central vitreous is like that of the vitreous cortex. However, cells are infrequent and collagen fibrils are sparse and do not insert into peripheral structures. Throughout the vitreous substance collagen is probably loosely bonded to the hyaluronic acid ground substance. Balazs proposed that the large molecules of hyaluronic acid maintain a physical separation of collagen filaments and hence maintain a high degree of optical transparency. With age this framework breaks down so that in the adult central vitreous the collagen fibrils become aggregated in parallel bundles that coalesce to form macroscopic 'fibres' (Sebag, Balazs and Flood, 1984) (Fig. 13.16).

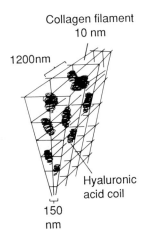

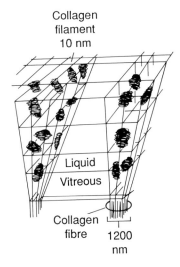

Fig. 13.16 Schematic representation of collageo fibrils and sodium hyaluronate molecules in gel vitreous. (Courtesy of E. Balazs.)

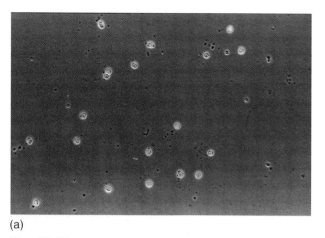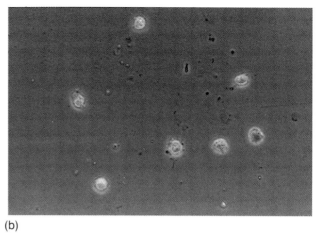

(a)   (b)

Fig. 13.17 (a) Phase contrast microscopy of flat mount preparation of hyalocytes in the vitreous cortex from the eye of an 11-year-old girl obtained *post mortem*. Mononuclear cells are distributed in a single layer within the vitreous cortex; (b) higher magnification demonstrates the mononuclear round appearance of these cells. Pseudopodia are present in some cells. (From Sebag, J., *The Vitreous: Structure, Function and Biology*, published by Springer Verlag, 1989.)

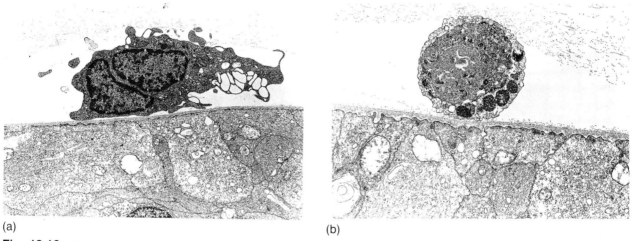

(a)   (b)

Fig. 13.18 Cells in the cortical vitreous at the surface of the posterior retina. (a) Migratory cell with pseudopodia and vacuoles; (b) round cell rich in intracytoplasmic filaments. (From Duane, T. D. and Jaeger, E. D. (eds), *Biomedical Foundations of Ophthalmology*, Vol. 1, published by Harper and Row, 1987; originals courtesy of E. van der Zypen, Institute of Anatomy, University of Berne.)

VITREOUS CELLS (OR HYALOCYTES)

Cells are present only in the cortex adjacent to the retina and ciliary body. The central vitreous and cortex adjacent to the lens and posterior chamber are completely cell-free in normal adult eyes. Cells are most prominent at the vitreous base, over the optic nerve head or in relation to retinal vessels. The vast majority of cells are mononuclear phagocytes (macrophages) called hyalocytes. Some fibrocytes and various glial cells may also be found (Figs 13.17 and 13.18).

Hyalocytes

The hyalocytes are phagocytic cells which contain many lysosomes, some phagosomes and a prominent Golgi complex. They have an affinity for neutral red, show an intense red autofluorescence and possess large, electron-dense inclusions. They have been demonstrated to have phagocytic properties *in vivo* and *in vitro* and hydrolytic enzymes have been found in their lysosomes. They are capable of synthesizing hyaluronic acid. In the normal vitreous, the hyalocytes form a resting population in the cortex, usually not in contact with the basal lamina. However, with inflammation of the vitreous, their numbers increase and they may be found in the central vitreous and also penetrating the basal lamina in their passage to and from the retina or ciliary body. In such situations the macrophage population is expanded by other cells of monocytic origin or, after retinal damage, by retinal pigment epithelial cells (Hogan, Alvarado and Weddell, 1971; Balazs, 1973).

13.3   COMPOSITION

The vitreous is 99% water and its volume is about 4.0 ml. The liquid phase of the vitreous gel contains hyaluronic acid and it is this high molecular weight proteoglycan (33–61 kDa) which is responsible for its characteristic high viscosity. The concentration in human vitreous is 0.03–0.1% (Balazs, 1973). The molecular diameter of the hyaluronic acid is in the region of 0.1–0.5 μm.

The vitreous contains a fine fibrillar collagen, relatively resistant to trypsin and α-chymotrypsin, but digested by pepsin and collagenase, which is different from that found in the ocular coats or lens capsule. Biochemically it is type II collagen, and has a moderate sugar content, though lower than that of the basement membrane collagens. Types IX and XI collagen are also present. Fibrillar diameter is in the region of 6–16 nm with a microperiodicity of 22 nm. A 64 nm periodicity can be shown using a phosphotungstic acid staining and shadow casting (Schwarz, 1956; Balazs, 1961; Fine and Tousimis, 1961; Hogan, 1963; Swan, 1980). The collagen fibrils are coated with glycosaminoglycan, stainable with ruthenium red and removed with hyaluronidase (Brini, Porte and Stoeckel, 1968).

The composition of vitreous is in other respects similar to that of aqueous, apart from quantitative and regional differences and there is a free diffusion of water between the vitreous and aqueous compartments (Davson, 1980). However, the movement of large solute molecules across the vitreous is restricted by its gel-like structure, and this may influence the distribution, delivery and removal of drugs and other materials into and from the vitreous body.

13.4   AGEING AND VITREOUS DETACHMENT

In the young eye the vitreous appears to be relatively empty optically on slit-lamp biomicroscopy. With increasing age a veil-like scattering of light may be seen which undulates with movements of the eye. This is presumably due to an alteration of the gel structure, but the fibrillar appearance is not caused by a visibility of collagen fibrils, which are of molecular dimensions. In old age or in the younger myopic eye a breakdown in structure occurs as indicated by increased scattering properties and the appearance of optically empty spaces (syneresis) (Figs 13.19 and 13.20); the altered gel may collapse, so that its outer surface pulls away from the internal coats of the eye (vitreous detachment). This detachment of vitreous is facilitated by the weakening of the adhesion between

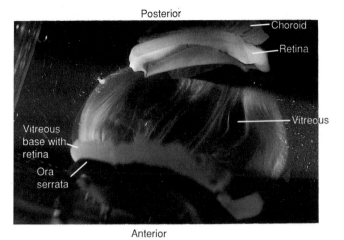

Fig. 13.19 Preparation of the human vitreous from a 79-year-old subject. The sclera, choroid and retina have been dissected from the mid zone of the globe but remain attached posteriorly (above). A fringe of retina is present overlying the vitreous base and the ora serrata is seen. The fibrillar structure of the vitreous is well seen by dark-field illumination. (Courtesy of J. Sebag.)

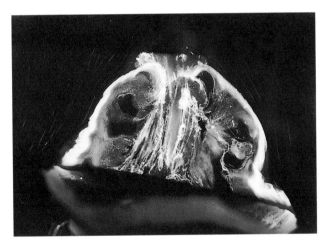

Fig. 13.20 Dark-field horizontal optical of vitreous in an 88-year-old human. The overall structure is collapsed (syneresis). Fibres are tortuous, aggregated and thickened. Large lacunae of liquid vitreous are seen peripherally. (Courtesy of J. Sebag.)

vitreous and structures external to it, which occurs with age. Detachment may merely split the internal limiting membrane of the retina at the points of attachment of the vitreous, may separate vitreous from the internal limiting membrane, may split the cortical vitreous or may at times tear the retina itself leading to a retinal hole. This event may be a precursor of a retinal detachment (Balazs, 1973; Foos, 1975; Daicker, Guggenheim and Guyat, 1977).

Vitreous detachment may be regarded as a normal consequence of ageing, and is frequently found in otherwise normal eyes in old age (Jokl, 1927). It is usually precipitated by the formation of a hole in the posterior vitreous face which may come about when the vitreous separates from its normally strong attachment around the macula or optic disc. In this situation, the fluid central vitreous can pass posteriorly through such a hole, while the posterior hyaloid itself moves forwards (Eisner, 1982; Sebag and Balazs, 1984).

CHAPTER FOURTEEN
The retina

The retina (Latin: *rete* = net), in the most comprehensive sense, includes all structures that are derived from the optic vesicle (namely, the sensory layers of the retina (pars optica retinae), the pigmented epithelium of the retina), as well as the epithelial linings of the ciliary body (pars retinae ciliaris) and of the iris (pars retinae iridis). In the vernacular sense, however, the retina has two main components: a sensory layer and a pigmented layer (Fig. 14.1), derived from the inner and outer layers of the optic vesicle, respectively. The two layers are attached loosely to each other by the extracellular matrix that fills the space between the apical villi of the pigment epithelium and the outer segments of the photoreceptors as well as the interphotoreceptor space (Fig. 14.1). The tenuous nature of this adhesion becomes apparent after death and in pathological conditions when the sensory retina detaches from the underlying pigmented layer, which usually remains firmly attached to Bruch's membrane of the choroid.

14.1 TOPOGRAPHY OF THE RETINA

The retina proper is a thin, delicate layer of nervous tissue that has a surface area of about 266 mm^2. The major landmarks of the retina are the **optic disc**, the **retinal blood vessels**, the **area centralis** with the **fovea** and **foveola**, the peripheral retina (which includes the equator) and the **ora serrata**. The retina is thickest near the optic disc, where it measures 0.56 mm. It becomes thinner towards the periphery, the thickness reducing to 0.18 mm at the equator and to 0.1 mm at the ora serrata (Sigelman and Ozanics, 1982; Tripathi and Tripathi, 1984; Ogden, 1989a,b).

THE OPTIC DISC

In the normal human eye, the optic disc is a circular to slightly oval structure that measures approximately 1.5 mm in diameter. Centrally, it contains a depression which is known as the physiological cup; however, the size and shape of this excavation depends on several factors such as the course of the optic nerve through its canal, the amounts of glial and connective tissues, the remnants of the hyaloid vessels and the anatomical arrangement of the retinal and choroidal vessels.

THE AREA CENTRALIS

The area centralis or central retina is divisible into the fovea and foveola, with a parafoveal and a perifoveal ring around the fovea (Fig. 14.2). This region of the retina, located in the posterior fundus temporal to the optic disc, is demarcated approximately by the upper and lower arcuate and temporal retinal vessels and has an elliptical shape horizontally (Fig. 14.3). With an average diameter of about 5.5 mm, the area centralis corresponds to approximately 15° of the visual field and it is adapted for accurate diurnal vision and colour discrimination (Tripathi and Tripathi, 1984).

The fovea

The fovea, which marks the approximate centre of the area centralis, is located at the posterior pole of the globe, 4 mm temporal to the centre of the optic disc and about 0.8 mm below the horizontal meridian

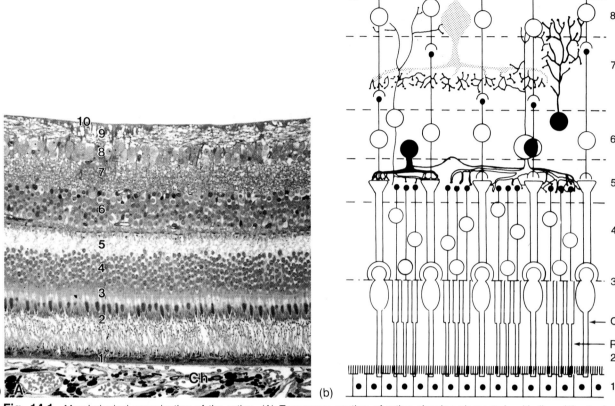

Fig. 14.1 Morphological organization of the retina. (A) Transverse section of retina showing pigmented epithelium (1) attached to the sensory retina that consists of photoreceptor layer (2); external limiting membrane (3); outer nuclear layer (4); outer plexiform layer (5); inner nuclear layer (6); inner plexiform layer (7); ganglion cell layer (8); nerve fibre layer (9); and internal limiting membrane (10). Ch = Choroid. Photomicrograph, original magnification × 245.
(B) Diagrammatic representation of the elements that comprise the retina. 1 = Pigment epithelium; 2 = photoreceptor layer consisting of rods (R) and cones (C); 3 = external limiting membrane; 4 = outer nuclear layer; 5 = outer plexiform layer; 6 = inner nuclear layer; 7 = inner plexiform layer; 8 = ganglion cell layer; 9 = nerve fibre layer; 10 = internal limiting membrane. (From Tripathi, R. C. and Tripathi, B. J. in Davson, H. (ed.) (1984) *The Eye*, published by Academic Press.)

(Fig. 14.2a). It has a diameter of 1.85 mm (which represents 5° of the visual field) and an average thickness of 0.25 mm. At the centre of the fovea, the layers of the retina are thinner so that a central concave indentation, the foveola, is produced. The downward-sloping border which meets the floor of the **foveal pit** is known as the **clivus** (Fig. 14.4).

The foveola

The foveola, which measures 0.35 mm in diameter and 0.13 mm in thickness, represents the area of the highest visual acuity in the retina, even though its span corresponds to only 1° of the visual field. This is due partly to the sole presence of cone photoreceptors (Fig. 14.5) and partly to its avascular nature. The foveola usually appears deeper red than does the adjacent retina because of the rich choroidal circula-

tion of the choriocapillaris which shines through it. The colour of the fovea persists and is even accentuated as the so-called 'cherry-red spot' when the surrounding retina becomes cloudy as occurs after obstruction in the central retinal vasculature and in certain metabolic storage diseases.

The macula lutea

The macula lutea is an oval zone of yellow colouration within the central retina. It is not easily discernible on ophthalmoscopic examination of the living eye, but in red-free light and in darkly pigmented individuals it is seen as a horizontally oval zone that includes the fovea. In freshly enucleated eyes, the macula lutea appears as a greenish-yellow elliptical region some 3 mm in diameter, with the centre being the foveola, which itself is colourless. With special

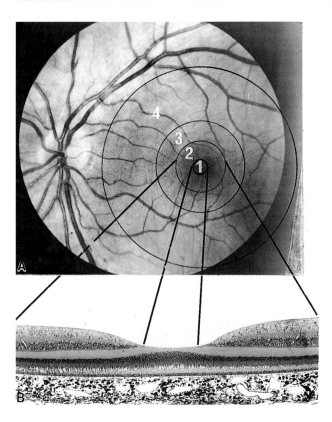

Fig. 14.2 (A) Fundus photograph of left human eye showing topographic demarcation of the area centralis that measures 5.5–6 mm in diameter (outermost circle) and its sub-divisions (inner circles). From an anatomic standpoint, the zones demarcated are in fact horizontally elliptical rather than circular as depicted here. The central area of the macular region is represented by the fovea centralis (2), approximately 1.85 mm in diameter, which has a central pit, the foveola (1), 0.35 mm in diameter. The anatomically distinguishable retinal belts that surround the fovea centralis are the parafovea (3), 0.5 mm wide, and the perifovea (4), 1.5 mm wide. (B) Transverse section of the foveal retina matched to the fundus photograph shown in (a). Photomicrograph, original magnification × 70. (From Tripathi, R. C. and Tripathi, B. J. in Davson, H. (ed.) (1984) *The Eye*, published by Academic Press.)

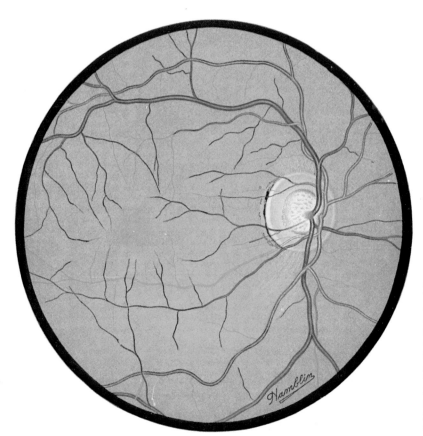

Fig. 14.3 Fundus of right human eye showing the upper and lower arcuate and temporal retinal vessels that demarcate the approximately elliptical shape of the central retina. The macula is seen as an area darker than the remainder of the fundus. Its centre, the fovea, is seen as a whitish reflex located below the centre of the optic disc. At the edge of the disc are the pigmented 'choroidal' crescent and a scleral ring. The normal striation, which is often seen above and below the disc, is due to the non-medullated nerve fibres and is over-exaggerated in this figure.

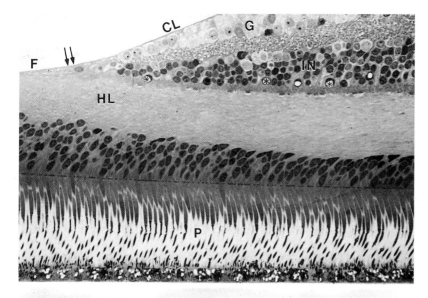

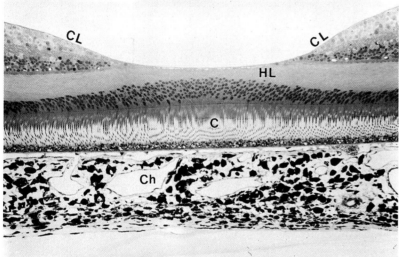

Fig. 14.4 Higher magnification of the retina in Fig. 14.2(B), showing the slope or clivus (CL) meeting the floor of the foveola (F). The junction (arrows) marks the termination of the inner nuclear layer (IN) and of the retinal capillaries (asterisks). The ganglion cells (G) terminate about 30 μm before the inner nuclear layer. The internal limiting membrane continues uninterrupted. HL = Henle's fibre layer; P = photoreceptors of retina. Photomicrograph, original magnification × 485. (From Tripathi, R. C. and Tripathi, B. J. in Davson, H. (ed.) (1984) *The Eye*, published by Academic Press.)

Fig. 14.5 Transverse section through the foveal retina showing the exclusive presence of cone photoreceptors (C) and the absence of capillaries from the foveola. CL = Clivus; HL = Henle's fibre layer; Ch = choroid. Photomicrograph, original magnification × 190.

optical devices, however, the faint yellow colour can be observed as a wider zone, approximately 5 mm in diameter, in the central retina. This finding may explain the apparent confusion in the use of the terms macula, macular area, and macula lutea clinically and histologically. The yellow colouration probably derives from the presence of the carotenoid pigment, xanthophyll, in the ganglion and bipolar cells. The yellow colour remains for several hours to a few days in enucleated eyes kept at 4°C and can be visualized in flat, unfixed preparations of the central retina. In specimens that have been fixed in aldehyde and stored appropriately, the yellow colour remains for several weeks or months. However, the pigment may be extracted from retinas treated with alcohol (Tripathi and Tripathi, 1984).

Within the area centralis two other regions are distinguished outside the fovea: the **parafovea** (0.5 mm in width) and the **perifovea** (1.5 mm in width) (Fig. 14.2).

THE PERIPHERAL RETINA

The peripheral retina increases the field of vision and is divided into four regions: the near periphery, the mid-periphery, the far periphery and the ora serrata. The near periphery occupies a circumscribed region of 1.5 mm around the area centralis, and the mid-periphery is a 3 mm-wide zone around the near periphery. The far periphery is a region that extends from the optic disc, 9–10 mm on the temporal side and 16 mm on the nasal side in the horizontal meridian. This asymmetry is accounted for by the location of the optic nerve on the nasal side of the globe (Sigelman and Ozanics, 1982; Tripathi and Tripathi, 1984).

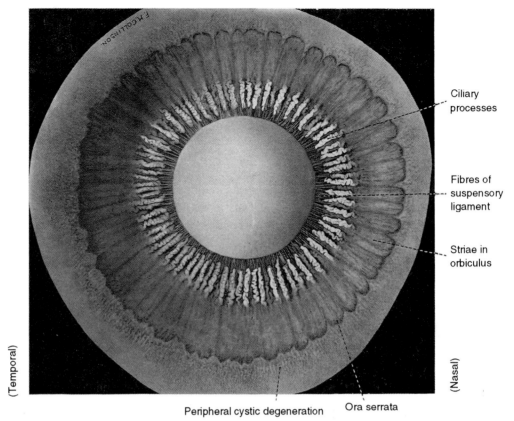

Ciliary processes

Fibres of suspensory ligament

Striae in orbiculus

(Temporal)

(Nasal)

Peripheral cystic degeneration   Ora serrata

Fig. 14.6   The ora serrata, showing its greater width temporally than on the nasal aspect. The serrations are also less developed temporally where cystic degeneration (depicted by the mottled appearance) is most evident.

The most anterior region of the retina is the ora serrata, which consists of a dentate fringe, and which denotes the termination of the retina (Straastma, Landers and Kreiger, 1968; Tripathi and Tripathi, 1984). It is 2.1 mm wide temporally, 0.7–0.8 mm wide nasally (Fig. 14.6) and is located 6.0 mm nasally and 7.0 mm temporally from the limbus, 6–8 mm from the equator and 25 mm from the optic nerve on the nasal side. The ora serrata marks the transition between the attenuated retina and the inner, columnar, non-pigmented cells of the pars ciliaris retinae; the retinal pigment epithelium continues anteriorly as the outer cuboidal cell layer of the ciliary body (Fig. 14.7). Beginning at a young age, cystoid degeneration occurs, usually in the outer plexiform layer of the sensory retina at the ora serrata (Fig. 14.7). The cystic spaces that form are pronounced in the elderly and are more marked on the nasal than on the temporal aspect (Sigelman and Ozanics, 1982; Tripathi and Tripathi, 1984). They extend between the inner and outer limiting membranes and may communicate with the vitreous and give rise to retinal detachment.

14.2   GENERAL ARCHITECTURE OF THE RETINA

As seen in cross-section by light microscopy, the retina is represented by 10 layers (Fig. 14.1; see table 14.1). Sclerad to vitread they are:

1. retinal pigment epithelium;
2. photoreceptor layer of rods and cones;
3. external limiting membrane;
4. outer nuclear layer;
5. outer plexiform layer;
6. inner nuclear layer;
7. inner plexiform layer;
8. ganglion cell layer;
9. nerve fibre layer;
10. internal limiting membrane.

At the fovea the only layers that are present are the retinal pigment epithelium, the photoreceptors (cones only), the external limiting membrane, the outer nuclear layer (which contains the nuclei of the cone cells), the inner fibres of the photoreceptors (the so-called 'Henle's fibre' layer), and the internal limiting membrane.

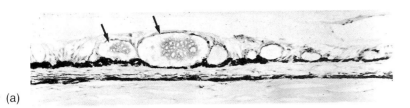

(a)

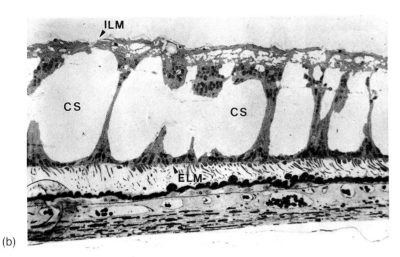

(b)

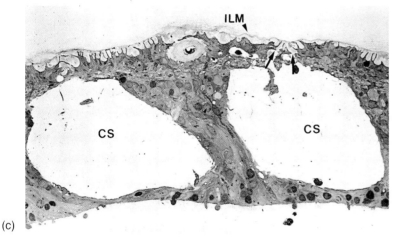

(c)

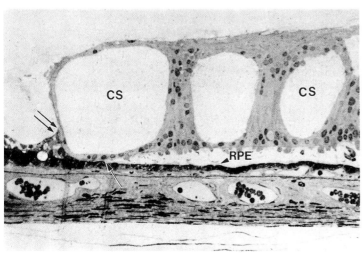

(d)

Fig. 14.7 The far peripheral retina and ora serrata showing the transition of the attenuated retina and the inner, non-pigmented cells of the pars ciliaris retinae, as well as various profiles of cystic spaces. (a) This paraffin-embedded section stained with alcian blue demonstrates the presence of glycosaminoglycans within the cystic spaces (arrows). Photomicrograph, original magnification × 145.
(b) The cystic spaces (CS) extend from the internal limiting membrane (ILM) and the external limiting membrane (ELM). Photomicrograph, original magnification × 250.
(c) The cystic space (CS) is in communication (arrows) with the thickened internal limiting membrane (ILM). Photomicrograph, original magnification × 490.
(d) Section of ora serrata showing termination of sensory retina and its abrupt transition (double arrows) into non-pigmented neuroepithelium of the ciliary pars plana. The retinal pigmented epithelium (RPE) continues as the pigmented epithelial layer of the ciliary pars plana. Note the union of the external limiting membrane with the retinal pigment epithelium (single arrow). CS = Cystic space in sensory retina. Photomicrograph, original magnification × 390. (From Tripathi, R. C. and Tripathi, B. J. in Davson, H. (ed.) (1984) *The Eye*, published by Academic Press.)

Table 14.1 Layers of the retina

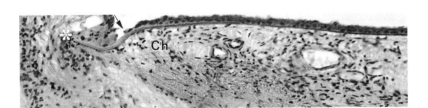

1. Pigment epithelium		
2. Photoreceptor layer		
3. External limiting membrane	Neuron I (percipient elements)	Neuroepithelial layer (rod cell, cone cell)
4. Outer nuclear layer		
5. Outer plexiform layer		
6. Inner nuclear layer	Neuron II (conductive and associative elements)	Cerebral layer (bipolar, ganglion, horizontal, and amacrine cells, centrifugal bipolars Müller fibres, astrocytes)
7. Inner plexiform layer		
8. Ganglion cell layer		
9. Nerve fibre layer	Neuron III (conductive elements)	
10. Internal limiting membrane		

Fig. 14.8 Termination of Bruch's membrane at the edge of the optic disc (asterisk). Note that the pigment epithelium falls short of the termination (arrow), but the choroid (Ch) continues further medially. Photomicrograph, original magnification × 195. (From Tripathi, R. C. and Tripathi, B. J. in Davson, H. (ed.) (1984) *The Eye*, published by Academic Press.)

The primary neurons in the visual pathway are the photoreceptors, which (with their end organs, perikarya, axonal processes and synapses) constitute the layer of rods and cones, the outer nuclear layer and the outer plexiform layer. The external limiting membrane is a histologically identifiable attachment site between the photoreceptors and the Müller cells. Bipolar, horizontal, amacrine and interplexiform cells constitute the second-order neurons. The ganglion cell layer and the nerve fibre layer form the conductive network internal to the inner plexiform layer and external to the internal limiting membrane. This network of third-order neurons and their respective axonal processes send the information gathered by the photoreceptors for further processing by the visual cortex. The internal limiting membrane makes intimate contact with the vitreous body, which also contributes in part to the architecture of the former (Fig. 14.1). The Müller cells extend between the two limiting membranes and, together with other glial cells, constitute the neuronal connective tissue cells of the retina.

14.3 THE RETINAL PIGMENT EPITHELIUM

Removal of the vitreous and sensory retina from a bisected globe reveals the retinal pigment epithelium (RPE) to be a continuous brown sheet that extends from the optic nerve to the ora serrata, from which it continues forward as the pigmented layer of the ciliary epithelium (Tripathi and Tripathi, 1984). At the

optic nerve Bruch's membrane stops abruptly; the pigment epithelium, however, falls short of the basal lamina of the choroid and the terminal, somewhat depigmented, cells may heap up to form the choroidal ring at the edge of the optic disc (Fig. 14.8). Grossly, the RPE is more pigmented in the macular region than it is at the ora serrata. Microscopically, individual pigmented epithelial cells also display variation in their pigmentation. The fine mottling is due to the unequal distribution of pigmentation within individual cells, and this gives the fundus a granular appearance when it is viewed with an ophthalmoscope (Figs 14.9 and 14.10).

STRUCTURE OF THE RPE

The RPE consists of a single layer of approximately five million cells firmly attached to its basal lamina, the lamina vitrea of Bruch's membrane. The

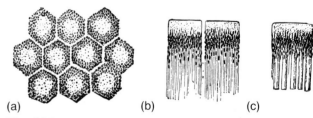

(a) (b) (c)

Fig. 14.9 Pigment epithelium of the human retina. (a) Surface appearance; (b) two cells with cytoplasmic extensions seen in profile; (c) a cell showing interconnection with outer segments of rod photoreceptors.

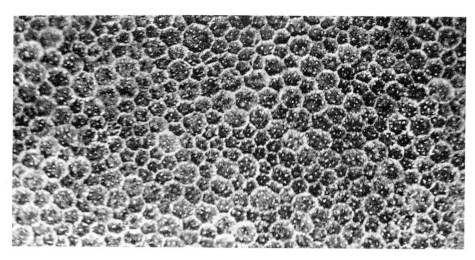

Fig. 14.10 Flat section of human retinal pigment epithelium showing approximately hexagonal shape of the cells and their variable size. (Courtesy of Dr John Marshall and Mr P. L. Ansell, Institute of Ophthalmology, London.)

microfibrils that originate from this lamina extend into the lamina elastica of Bruch's membrane. The apical region of the RPE is only loosely adherent to the sensory retina. The absence of specialized adhesion molecules, such as laminin and fibronectin in the interphotoreceptor matrix, and the lack of junctional complexes between apical microvilli of pigmented epithelial cells and the outer segments of the photoreceptors leave the sensory retina prone to detachment in pathological conditions.

Size and shape of cells

Viewed from above, RPE cells have 4–8 sides and give the appearance of cobblestones (Figs 14.10 and 14.11). The total number of pigmented epithelial cells ranges from 4.2 to 6.1 million. In the area centralis, each pigment cell measures 12–18 μm in width and 10–14 μm in height. As the RPE layer approaches the ora serrata, the cells become flatter and may measure

up to about 60 μm in width. With increasing age, the pigmented cells in the macular region increase in height and decrease in width; the inverse occurs in cells at the periphery (Watzke, Soldevilla and Trune, 1993). The pattern of pigmentation also changes with increasing age: the cells in the area centralis become less pigmented and those at the ora serrata acquire more pigmentation.

Paracellular space

By light microscopy, the RPE cells frequently appear to be separated by an optically empty space that is probably caused by an artefact created by fixation and processing of the specimen. However, suitably fixed specimens, and especially those prepared and examined by transmission electron microscopy, demonstrate close cellular approximation, and adjacent cells are joined at their lateral apical margins by **terminal bars** (Figs 14.12 and 14.13). From top to

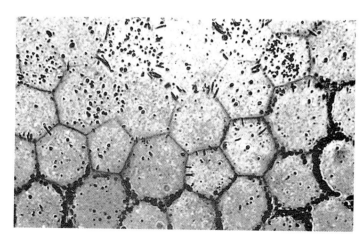

Fig. 14.11 Tangential section of retinal pigment epithelium showing the predominantly hexagonal pattern of the cells. The mottled appearance is due to variation in the pigmentation in each cell. Photomicrograph, original magnification × 3375. (Courtesy of Dr John Marshall and Mr P. L. Ansell, Institute of Ophthalmology, London.)

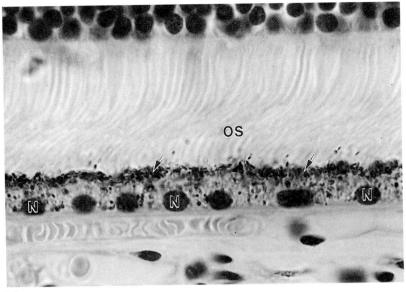

(a)

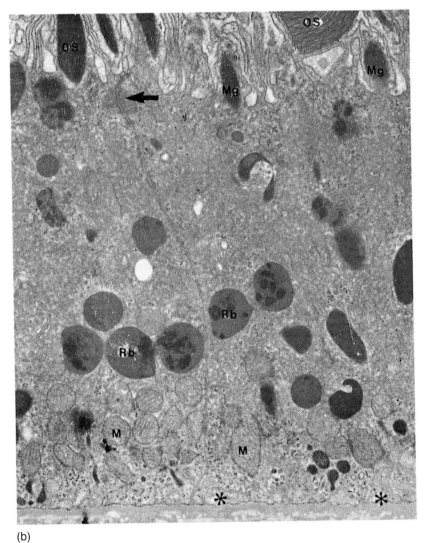

(b)

Fig. 14.12 (a) Photomicrograph of retinal pigment epithelium showing the close approximation between adjacent cells and the interdigitation of their apical processes with the outer segments of the photoreceptors (OS). Note also the basal location of the cell nuclei (N) and the mainly apical location of the melanin pigment granules (arrows). Original magnification × 1400. (b) Transmission electron micrograph of two adjacent retinal pigment epithelial cells showing the location of the terminal bars (arrow) at their lateral apical margins. The plasma membrane of the basal cell surfaces has numerous complex infoldings (asterisks), whereas the apical surface has microvilli that surround the outer segments (OS) of the photoreceptors. Melanin granules (Mg) are located towards the apex of the cell and residual bodies (Rb) that result after phagocytosis and digestion of the outer segments accumulate towards the basal region. M = Mitochondria. Original magnification × 22 000. (Courtesy of Dr John Marshall and Mr P. L. Ansell, Institute of Ophthalmology, London.)

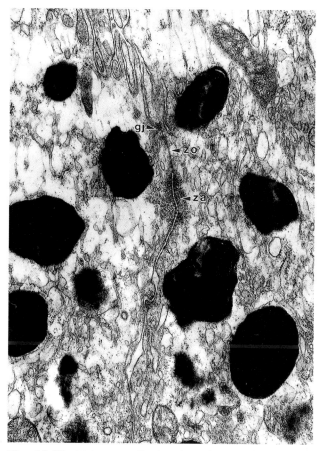

Fig. 14.13 Higher magnification view of the terminal bar at the lateral apical margin of two adjacent retinal pigment epithelial cells. This junctional complex (from cell apex to base) consists of a gap junction (gj), zonula occludens (zo), and zonula adherens (za). Transmission electron micrograph, original magnification × 40 000.

bottom these bars consist of a **gap junction**, a **zonula occludens** and a **zonula adherens** (Hudspeth and Yee, 1973). Nutrients from the choriocapillaris diffuse through the basal lamina and between the paracellular space up to the terminal bars, where the zonulae occludentes form the external component of the blood–retinal barrier. The residual space that is not occupied by the terminal bars is filled with extracellular matrix. Verhoeff's membrane, as seen by light microscopy, encompasses both the extracellular matrix and the terminal bars.

ULTRASTRUCTURE OF RETINAL PIGMENT EPITHELIUM

The basal aspect of RPE cells is characterized by myriad complex infoldings of the plasma membrane that may extend for up to 1 μm into the basal surface (Figs 14.12a and 14.14). This region of the cells is populated by numerous mitochondria and annulate lamellae, which are active in protein synthesis. The central portion houses a large, round to oval nucleus (5–12 μm in diameter) that contains one or two nucleoli and diffuse chromatin. This area is often obscured by round to spindle-shaped **melanin** granules that measure 2–3 μm in the longest axis. **Lipofuscin** granules, when present, also occupy this mid-portion of the cell. The apex of the cell makes contact with the sensory retina through microvillus-like processes of two types: processes of 5–7 μm that extend between the outer segments of the photoreceptors and 3 μm processes that form a

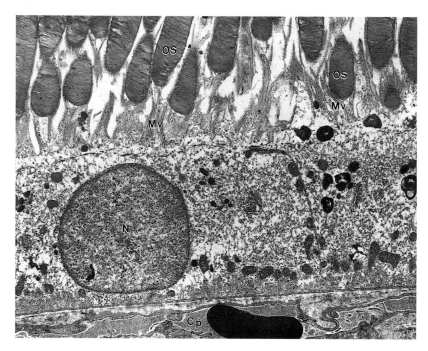

Fig. 14.14 Transmission electron micrograph of retinal pigment epithelium, showing the microvillus-like projections (Mv) that extend from the apical surface of the cells and ensheath the outer segments (OS) of the photoreceptors. N = Nucleus; Cp = capillary of choriocapillaris. Original magnification × 9000.

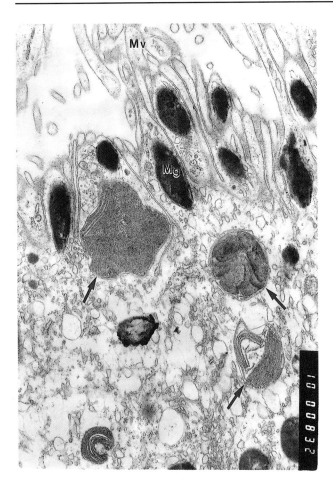

Fig. 14.15 Higher magnification of the apical region of a pigment epithelial cell showing the phagocytosed outer-segment discs of the photoreceptors (arrows) undergoing various stages of digestion. Mg = Melanin granules; Mv = microvillous projections. Transmission electron micrograph, original magnification ×25 000.

sheath around the outer third of the outer segments (Fig. 14.14). However, no specialized junctional complexes exist between these processes and the photoreceptors. Despite the lack of any adherent function, the 3 μm apical villi of the RPE are involved in phagocytosis of outer segment discs, and thus they promote the renewal of photoreceptor cells (Spitznas and Hogan, 1970; Steinberg, Wood and Hogan, 1977; Zinn and Benjamin-Henkind, 1982). The engulfed 30–40 photoreceptor discs are recognizable as phagosomes or lamellated bodies which, after further digestion, accumulate as residual bodies at the base of the cell (Figs 14.12a and 14.15).

Melanin granules

Spindle-shaped melanin granules, 1 μm in diameter and 2–3 μm long, are abundant at the apex of the RPE cell; they assume a spherical shape in the para-apical cytoplasm and an ovoid or fusiform structure in the villi (Figs 14.13 and 14.15). Dark-staining granules have an intense concentration of melanin because of the conversion of dihydroxyphenylalanine into melanin by tyrosinase. Light-staining granules have scant melanin or tyrosinase activity. Throughout the three regions of the RPE cell (basal, mid-portion, apical) there is a well-developed network of smooth endoplasmic reticulum that assumes a tubular, vesicular or lamellar appearance.

FUNCTIONS OF THE RPE

In addition to photoreceptor renewal and recycling of vitamin A, the RPE is involved in the absorption of scattered light by the melanin granules, transport of nutrients and metabolites through this extraretinal–blood barrier and elaboration of the extracellular matrix (Zinn and Benjamin-Henkind, 1982). Nutrients from the choriocapillaris must pass selectively through the RPE cells to reach the sensory retina. Uptake and transport of retinol (vitamin A) are mediated by receptors (serum retinol binding protein) on the basolateral sides of the RPE and by cytosolic retinol binding proteins that carry retinol to the interphotoreceptor matrix to be distributed to the photoreceptors. Once in the interphotoreceptor matrix, the retinol is carried by the interstitial retinol binding protein to the photoreceptors. This retinol-binding protein is the most abundant glycoprotein in the interphotoreceptor matrix elaborated by the RPE cells (Hewitt and Adler, 1989). The interphotoreceptor matrix, which is also elaborated by the RPE, is devoid of collagen, laminin and fibronectin, but is rich in sialic acid (25%) and the proteoglycans, hyaluronic acid (15%) and chondroitin sulphate (60%) (Varner *et al.*, 1987; Tien, Rayborn and Hollyfield, 1992). The chondroitin-6-sulphate in particular forms a sheath around cone photoreceptors (Iwasaki *et al.*, 1992). It has been postulated that the interphotoreceptor matrix participates in the retinal attachment of the retina to the RPE and facilitates phagocytosis of the shed discs of the outer cone segments. The absence of such a sheath around rod photoreceptors, however, implies involvement in other physiological processes, such as mechanical and electrical isolation of cone photoreceptors from the surrounding environment. On their basal surfaces, RPE cells produce type IV collagen, heparin sulphate and laminin, which become incorporated in the lamina vitrea of Bruch's membrane.

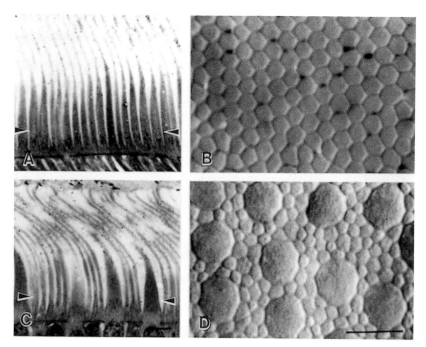

Fig. 14.16 Comparison of vertical histological (A, C) and *en face* optical (B, D) sections through photoreceptors in the fovea (A, B) and near the periphery (C, D) of the human retina. Arrowheads in (A) and (C) indicate the approximate level through the ellipsoid portion of the photoreceptor inner segments where the photographs (B) and (D) are taken. All profiles in (B) and the large profiles in (D) are cones. Scale bar = 10 μm. (From Curcio, C. A. *et al.* (1990), *J. Comp. Neurol.*, **292**, 497.)

14.4 THE SENSORY (NEURAL) RETINA

In the living eye the retina is a diaphanous tissue that is purplish-red because of the **visual pigment** (visual purple or rhodopsin) incorporated in the rod photoreceptors. However, this colour disappears rapidly on exposure to light and 5–10 minutes after death, so that the retina becomes white and semi-transparent (Tripathi and Tripathi, 1984). In freshly excised eyes, opened transversely and with the vitreous removed, the pigmented choroid and pigment epithelium are visible through the sensory retina.

14.5 THE LAYER OF RODS AND CONES

There are between 77.9 and 107.3 million (average 92 million) **rods** and 4.08 to 5.29 million (average 4.6 million) **cones** in the human eye. Flat preparations of the retina viewed by optical or scanning electron microscopy reveal that the photoreceptors are arranged as a mosaic. However, individual variations in the density of both rods and cones occur in different regions of the retina, so that the composition of the mosaic varies (Curcio *et al.*, 1990). The greatest variability occurs near the fovea and at the ora serrata; it is minimal at the mid-periphery (Figs 14.16–14.18). The numbers of rods and cones are similar (within 8%) in eyes from the same individual, but their topography is only similar, not identical (Fig. 14.19).

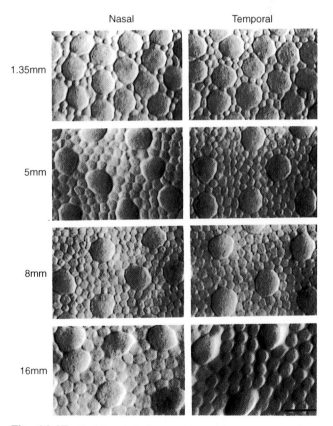

Fig. 14.17 Peripheral photoreceptor mosaic at corresponding eccentricities in nasal (left) and temporal (right) retina showing eccentricity-dependent changes in photoreceptor density and inner segment diameter. The eccentricity is given at the left. Cones are large profiles and rods are small profiles. Scale bar = 10 μm. (From Curcio, C. A. *et al.* (1990), *J. Comp. Neurol.*, **292**, 497.)

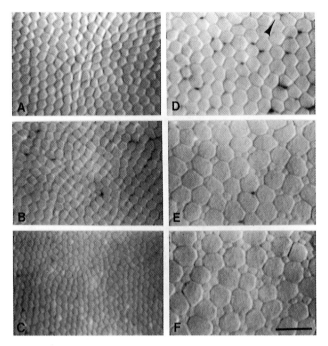

Fig 14.18 Optical sections of the foveal cone mosaic showing variability in cell size and density in three individuals in the fourth decade of life. (A–C) Foveal centres; (D) edge of rod-free zone, 0.125 mm temporal to the foveal centre (arrowhead denotes a rod); (E) point of equal rod and cone density, 0.42 mm nasal to foveal centre; (F) foveal slope, 0.66 mm temporal to foveal centre where the small rods outnumber the cones by approximately 4:1 and encircle them incompletely. Scale bar = 10 μm. (From Curcio, C. A. *et al.* (1990), *J. Comp. Neurol.*, **292**, 497.)

CONE DENSITY AND DISTRIBUTION

The density of cones is maximal at the fovea, with an average of 199 000 cones/mm^2, but their number is highly variable and ranges from 100 000 to 324 000 cones/mm^2 with the highest density in an area as large as 0.032 degree^2 (Curcio *et al.*, 1990). The number of cones at the fovea is similar even among eyes with widely different total counts, which suggests that differences in the lateral migration of the photoreceptors occur during development (Curcio *et al.*, 1990). With increasing eccentricity from the fovea, the density of cones decreases rapidly. Nevertheless, this density is 40–45% greater on the nasal than on the temporal aspect of the human retina, and slightly lower in the superior than in the inferior retina at the mid-periphery. The number of cones increases some threefold again in 1 mm wide band at the periphery of the retina and this cone-enriched rim is most highly developed along the nasal margin (Williams, 1991).

The spatial disposition of the foveal cones is generally assumed to be the limiting factor for the resolving power of the eye. However, the mean centre-to-centre cone spacing increases from 2.53 ($\pm$0.29) μm to 6.16 ($\pm$1.04) μm as a function of retinal eccentricity, which is approximately 9% to 17% of the mean (Hirsch and Curcio, 1989). Furthermore, the variation in the centre-to-centre cone angular position deviates from 60° by as much as 14–25%. Based on the variability of the peak densities of cones at the human foveola, the Nyquist limits (the highest anatomical resolving power) ranges from 48 to 86 cycles/degree with a mean of 66 cycles/degree (Curcio *et al.*, 1990). Because psychophysical measurements yield a range of 53–60 cycles/degree which are consistent with visual acuity (Williams, 1988), the data suggest that factors other than cone spacing are involved in producing the functional variation. Some potential spacing resolution may be lost, either by the foveal optics or by the neural processing beyond the sampling stage (Hirsch and Curcio, 1989; Curcio *et al.*, 1990). The only region in the retina where acuity overlaps the anatomical resolving power is between approximately 0.2 and 2.0° of retinal eccentricity (Hirsch and Curcio, 1989).

VISUAL ACUITY

Visual acuity in human (and monkey) neonates is two orders of magnitude lower than that in adults (Boothe, Dobson and Teller, 1985). During fetal and postnatal development, the cones, rods and pigment epithelial cells are displaced progressively toward the foveal centre and during this process differentiation of the photoreceptors is slower in the central than in the peripheral retina (Hendrickson, 1994). Based on studies in monkeys, in which the adult packing density of cones at the fovea is not attained until 15–18 months of age (Packer, Hendrickson and Curcio, 1990), it has been estimated that human cone density increases until 5–8 years of age (Hendrickson, 1994). However, the foveal immaturity is probably not the major factor in the lower visual acuity of neonates because the calculated cone acuity is significantly higher than visual performance (Curcio and Hendrickson, 1991). In monkeys up to 12 months of age, visual acuity deficits also occur because of changes in neural connectivity peripheral to neurons of the lateral geniculate nucleus, at the geniculocortical synapses and at the level of the striate cortex (Jacobs and Blakemore, 1988). However, virtually all of the increase in visual acuity after 12 months (equivalent to 4.3 years in humans) occurs due to maturation of the fovea (Jacobs and Blakemore, 1988). Defects in foveal development may account, at least in part, for the reduced visual acuity in individuals

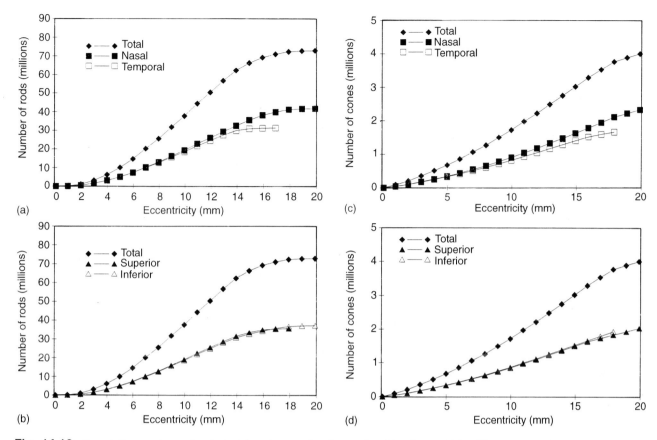

Fig. 14.19 Cumulative numbers of rods (a, b) and cones (c, d) as a function of eccentricity. The top curve in each graph represents the entire average retina. (a, c) Nasal and temporal hemiretinas; (b, d) superior and inferior hemiretinas. (From Curcio, C. A. *et al.* (1990), *J. Comp. Neurol.*, **292**, 497.)

with ocular albinism; in this condition the adult fovea is reported to be comparable to that of a neonate, both morphologically and psychophysically (Guillery *et al.*, 1984; Wilson *et al.*, 1988a,b).

ROD DENSITY AND DISTRIBUTION

The average horizontal diameter of the rod-free area at the fovea is 0.35 mm, which corresponds to 1.25° of the visual field. The highest concentration of rods occurs along a contour that describes a broad, horizontally oriented ellipse with the same eccentricity as the centre of the optic disc and extending towards the nasal and superior retina. The density of rods slowly decreases from this area to the far periphery. The entire nasal retina has 20–25% more rods than does the temporal retina, and the superior region has 2% more than the inferior region. A one-to-one ratio of rods to cones is seen 0.5 mm nasal and temporal, and 0.4 mm superior and inferior, to the centre of the fovea (Curcio *et al.*, 1990).

THE INNER AND OUTER SEGMENTS

Extending from their cell bodies, the photoreceptors have two morphologically distinct regions: the inner and outer segments (Fig. 14.20). The outer segment lies embedded in the interphotoreceptor matrix just internal to the retinal pigment epithelium. Its major function is the conversion of light energy into electrical impulses that are propagated through the neural retina and along the optic nerve to reach the visual cortex in the brain. Phototransduction is accomplished by a sequence of events that begins with the photochemical stereoisomerization of the visual pigment which is arranged as a single molecular layer of the membranous discs and constitutes the outer segments of the photoreceptors.

Visual pigments

Different visual pigments in the rods and cones reflect their functional specializations: the visual purple in the rods allows for scotopic vision whereas photopic vision originates in the cones by the

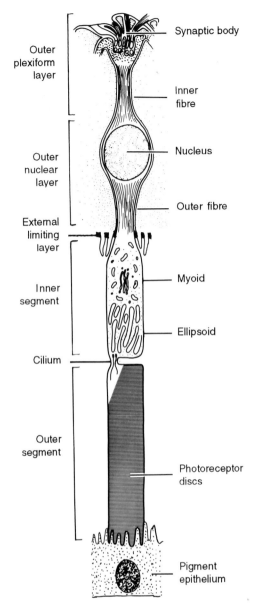

Outer plexiform layer

Outer nuclear layer

External limiting layer

Inner segment

Cilium

Outer segment

Synaptic body

Inner fibre

Nucleus

Outer fibre

Myoid

Ellipsoid

Photoreceptor discs

Pigment epithelium

Fig. 14.20 Diagrammatic representation of a generalized photoreceptor in the human retina, showing its various components and their location relative to the retinal layers. (Modified from Newell, F. W., (1982) *Ophthalmology, Principles and Concepts*, 5th edn, published by C. V. Mosby Co., St Louis.)

respectively (Dacey and Lee, 1994). Except for the putative 'blue' or S-cone, the types of cones are not distinct morphologically. The 'blue' cone has been identified by its longer inner segment that projects into the subretinal space, large diameter inner segment, and increased staining intensity (Ahnelt, Kolb and Pflug, 1987). Cones with this morphology constitute 3–5% of the total photoreceptors at the centre of the fovea and increase to a maximum of 15% on the foveolar slope; at the periphery of the retina they account for 7–10% of the total cone population. By using antibodies to visual pigments it has been possible to distinguish the three types of cones in a variety of mammalian species, as well as the additional ultraviolet-sensitive cone in the avian retina (Cserhati, Szel and Rohlich, 1989; Szel, Diamantstein and Rohlich, 1988). Immunocytochemistry using an affinity purified antibody to a 19-amino acid peptide sequence at the N-terminus of blue opsin has revealed that foveal blue cones are sparse, irregularly spaced, and absent in a zone about 100 μm (0.35°) in diameter near the site of peak cone density (Curcio *et al.*, 1991). The highest density of blue cones (more than 2000 cells/mm^2) is present in a ring at 0.1–0.3 mm eccentricity.

Segment size

The outer segment is attached to an inner segment through a cytoplasmic isthmus with its specialized cilium (Fig. 14.21). The combined length of both segments varies with topography and with the type of photoreceptor. In rods the inner and outer segments are 40–60 μm long throughout the retina; in cones the length is maximal at the fovea (80 μm) and gradually reduces to 40 μm at the periphery. At the ora serrata the end organs of cones are short and stout, measuring approximately 4 μm in length. The slender outer segment (25–28 μm long and 1–1.5 μm in diameter) and the slightly thicker inner segment of rods do not show much variation in morphology from the fovea to the periphery. However, the cones appear rod-like at the fovea, and the inner region of the outer segment becomes wider towards the periphery (Fig. 14.22). The outer segments of the cones away from the fovea have a diameter of 6 μm at the base and 1.5 μm at the tip (Sigelman and Ozanics, 1982; Tripathi and Tripathi, 1984).

Rod outer segments

The outer segments of the rods are cylindrical in shape and contain stacks of flattened double lamellae

presence of trichromatic pigments. The visual pigments are formed from the attachment of the protein opsin to retinal, which is an aldehyde of vitamin A. Rhodopsin, the visual pigment in rods, has the greatest sensitivity for blue-green light (λ_{max} 493 nm). Each cone, however, contains one of three different iodopsin molecules that absorb light at three distinct peaks at 440 nm (blue), 540 nm (green) and 577 nm (orange) referred to as S- (short), M- (medium), and L- (long) wavelength cones,

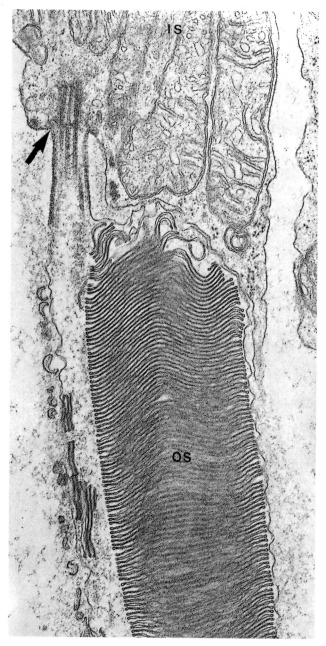

Fig. 14.21 Transmission electron micrograph, showing the attachment of the photoreceptor outer segment (OS) to its inner segment (IS) through a cytoplasmic isthmus that contains a specialized cilium (arrow). Original magnification × 9200. (Courtesy of Dr John Marshall and Mr P. L. Ansell, Institute of Ophthalmology, London.)

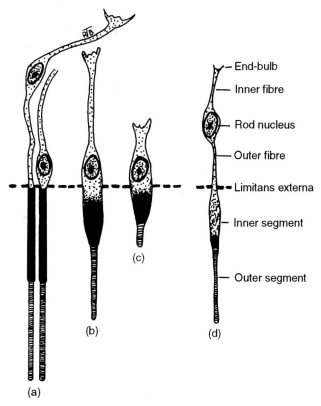

Fig. 14.22 Schematic representation of photoreceptors of human retina. (a) Cones from the foveola; (b) cones from midway between the ora serrata and the optic disc; (c) cone from near the ora serrata; (d) rod. (From Tripathi, R. C. and Tripathi, B. J. in Davson, H. (ed.) (1984) *The Eye*, published by Academic Press.)

in the form of discs (Fig. 14.23). The number of discs varies between 600 and 1000 per rod, depending on the species, and each disc has a thickness of 22.5–24.5 nm, with an average interdisc space of 21 nm (Sigelman and Ozanics, 1982). There are no specialized attachments between discs or between discs and the ensheathing plasma membrane. In longitudinal sections, clefts at the periphery of discs appear as furrows along the surface of the outer segments. The external aspect of each outer segment is surrounded by a layer of neurokeratin. The discs contain 90% of the visual pigment, whereas the remaining pigment is scattered on the surface of the plasmalemma.

A modified cilium (or basal body) connects the outer segment to the inner segment (Sigelman and Ozanics, 1982). This region shows a marked constriction, measuring only 0.3 μm in width and 1 μm in length. The basal body arises from one of a pair of centrioles located in the cytoplasm of the outer region of the ellipsoid (see below) of the inner segment, slightly to one side of the central axis. In this region, the cilium consists of nine doublets of microtubules that are arranged in a ring-like configuration but, towards the outer segment, the microtubules form nine singlets that gradually become attenuated and merge imperceptibly with the electron-lucent material of the basal third of the outer segment. Bundles of filaments arise from the basal body and extend across the ellipsoid to terminate in the cytoplasm of the myoid region (Fig. 14.21). Where

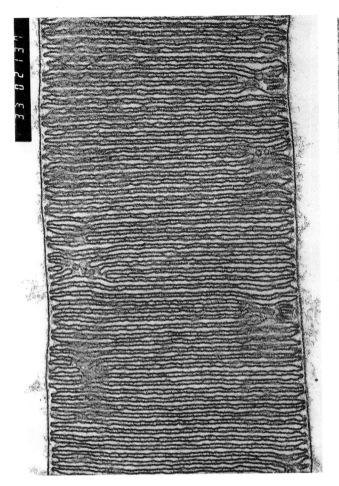

Fig. 14.23 Ultrastructure of rod outer segment that contains stacks of flattened double lamellae in the form of discs. Transmission electron micrograph, original magnification × 82 500.

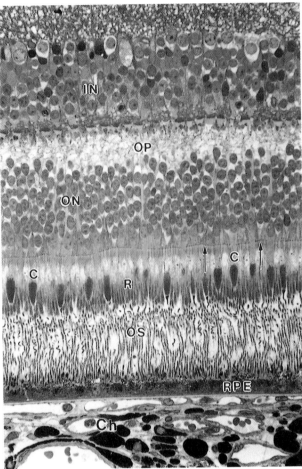

Fig. 14.24 Transverse section of posterior retina, showing the morphology of the inner segments of the rods (R) and cones (C). Ch = Choroid; RPE = pigment epithelium; OS = outer segments of photoreceptors; ON = outer nuclear layer; OP = outer plexiform layer; IN = inner nuclear layer; arrows = external limiting membrane. Photomicrograph, original magnification × 475. (From Tripathi, R. C. and Tripathi, B. J. in Davson, H. (ed.) (1984) *The Eye*, published by Academic Press.)

the cilium emerges from the inner segment in rods, the cytoplasm forms 9–12 microvilli that extend over the surface of the outer segment for approximately 12.5 µm. They constitute the calyx, but no function has been ascribed to these calyceal processes. Similarly, the exact function of the cilium is unknown, but it may represent an evolutionary vestige of photoreceptors.

Rod inner segments

The rod inner segment is cylindrical and is composed of a finely granular cytoplasm (Fig. 14.24). Histologically, two regions are discernible: an outer eosinophilic ellipsoid and an inner basophilic myoid, although the staining characteristics vary with the metabolic activity of the photoreceptor. The ellipsoid derives its staining characteristic from the large number of long and slender mitochondria (usually

20–30 per cross-section). The cytoplasm also contains smooth endoplasmic reticulum, neurotubules, free ribosomes and glycogen granules. The basophilia of the myoid is accounted for by the high concentration of free ribosomes. The myoid, which is the site of major protein synthesis, houses rough endoplasmic reticulum, glycogen granules and a Golgi apparatus that is located close to its innermost portion. The cytoplasm also contains microtubules and microfilaments that are arranged parallel to the long axis of the cell and extend to the level of the external limiting membrane and of the synapse, respectively. A thin cytoplasmic process (the outer fibre) extends from the basal portion of the inner segment, through the

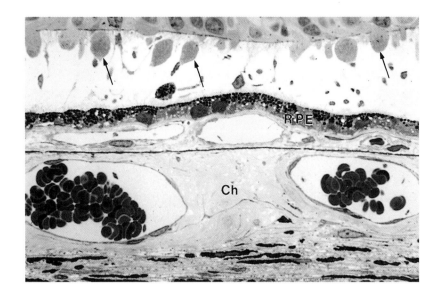

Fig. 14.25 Transverse section of peripheral retina, showing the morphology of the cone photoreceptors (arrows). RPE = Pigment epithelium; Ch = choroid. Photomicrograph, original magnification × 1025.

external limiting membrane, to the perikaryon of the rods located in the outer nuclear layer.

Cone outer segments

The outer segments of the cones assume a morphology that differs depending on their location in the retina (Sigelman and Ozanics, 1982; Tripathi and Tripathi, 1984). At the ora serrata and at the near periphery the cone outer segments are short and conical (Fig. 14.25); at the fovea centralis, however, they have long outer segments and resemble those of the rods. Ultrastructurally, the cone outer segments have more discs (1000–1200 per cone) than do rod outer segments. The intradisc and interdisc spaces are also wider in cones (3.5 nm and 16.5 nm, respectively). Unlike the rod discs, cone discs are attached to each other as well as to the surface plasma membrane over short segments of their circumference and thus, they are not detached easily. However, cone outer segments are relatively more fragile than those of rods.

Cone inner segments

As in the rods, the outer and inner segments of the cones are connected to each other through a thin cytoplasmic isthmus containing a short modified cilium. The inner segments of the cones display variations that depend on the topography. At the fovea centralis inner segments are long and tapered, but in the periphery they are distinctly conical in shape. The ellipsoid assumes a more engorged conical shape than does its counterpart in the rods because it has many more mitochondria (200–300 per

cross-section). Even so, the cytoplasmic contents that are common to both the ellipsoid and myoid are equivalent in both rod and cone inner segments. The outer fibre that connects the innermost inner segment to its soma is both short and wide in the cones because the nuclei of the cones in the outer nuclear layer are apposed closely to the external limiting membrane.

Myoids

Along the surface of the myoids of both the rods and cones, villus-like extensions of the Müller cells form the 'fibre baskets of Schultze', so that no communications between adjacent myoids are seen by electron microscopy (Sigelman and Ozanics, 1982). The villi of the Müller cells are long and numerous, and their probable function is to regulate the composition of the extracellular milieu of the photoreceptors. These cytoplasmic processes also serve to maintain precise alignment of the rods and cones.

Cell body histology

The cell bodies of the rods and cones stain differently with selective dyes (Fig. 14.26). With Unna's orcein–polychrome methylene blue–tannin stain, the outer segments of the rods are colourless and the cones appear deep blue. By using Mallory's trichrome stain after fixation with Zenker's fluid, the foveola can be demonstrated to be devoid of rod inner segments. Ordinarily in this preparation rod inner segments stain blue, whereas cone inner segments stain red. In the foveola, however, all photoreceptors stain red, which indicates the absence of rods in this region.

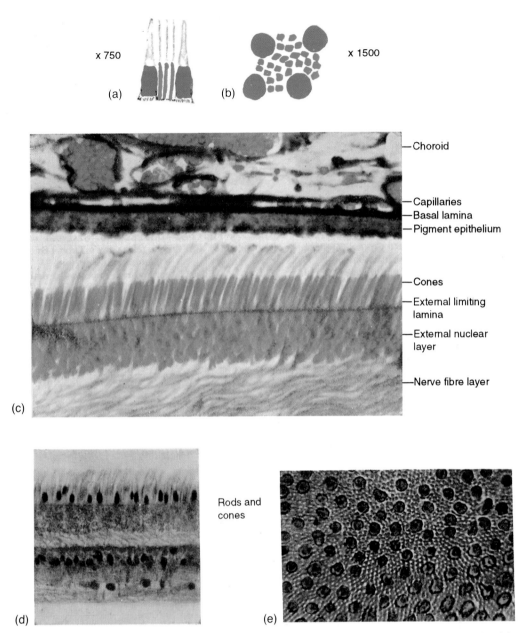

Fig. 14.26 Differential staining of rods and cones after fixation with Zenker's fluid and staining with Mallory's triple stain. (a, b) Photoreceptors in longitudinal and cross-section, respectively. The cones are red and the rods blue. Original magnification (a) × 750; (b) × 1500. (c) Vertical section through the macula. Although the cones appear rod-like in morphology, they stain red with Mallory's triple stain. The space between the retinal pigment epithelium and the cone outer segments is an artefact. (d) Vertical section of peripheral retina showing rods which stain blue and cones which stain red. (e) Tangential section of photoreceptors, showing large red-stained cones and small blue-stained rods.

14.6   THE EXTERNAL LIMITING MEMBRANE

Under the light microscope the external limiting membrane appears to separate the layer of rods and cones from the overlying outer nuclear layer (Figs 14.24 and 14.27). It extends from the optic disc to the ora serrata, where it becomes continuous with the basal lamina between the pigmented and non-pigmented portions of the ciliary epithelium. The external limiting membrane is revealed by electron microscopy to be composed of the terminal bars (zonulae adherentes) between Müller cells and photoreceptors, between adjacent Müller cells and, rarely, between adjacent photoreceptor cells (Figs 14.27 and 14.28). The external limiting membrane is not a true membrane, because small molecules pass freely through the junctional complexes. The main

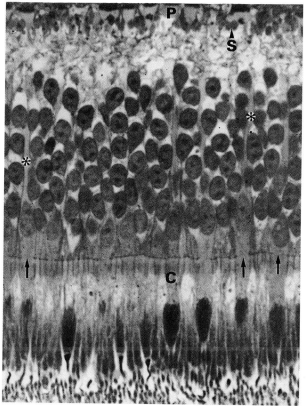

Fig. 14.27 Section of retina, showing photoreceptor cell bodies passing through the external limiting membrane (arrows), which is formed by dense junctional complexes (zonulae adherens) around the circumference of the cells. The nuclei of the cones (C) lie close to the external limiting membrane and have extremely short (or no) intervening fibre. Their long inner fibres (asterisk) synapse through cone pedicles (P). The rod synaptic bodies or spherules (S) are smaller. Photomicrograph, original magnification × 1175. (From Tripathi, R. C. and Tripathi, B. J. in Davson, H. (ed.) (1984) *The Eye*, published by Academic Press.)

functional implications of the external limiting membrane include providing a selective barrier for nutrients that pass between the adjacent Müller cells as well as stabilization of the position of the transducing portion of the photoreceptors.

14.7   THE OUTER NUCLEAR LAYER

The outer nuclear layer lies internal to the external limiting membrane and contains the soma and nuclei of the photoreceptor cells (Figs 14.24 and 14.27). Topographically the width of this layer varies, primarily because of the number of rows of nuclei. Nasal to the disc the outer nuclear layer is 45 μm thick and has 8–9 rows of nuclei, at the temporal disc only four rows of nuclei are present and the thickness is reduced to 22 μm and in the fovea the 10 rows of cone nuclei increase the width of the outer nuclear layer to 50 μm. Except at the ora serrata, the outer nuclear layer in the remainder of the retina has a single row of cone nuclei that are apposed closely to the external limiting membrane and four rows of rod nuclei internal to them; the thickness is about 27 μm. The different nuclei of the two types of photoreceptors may be distinguished because the nuclei of the rods stain orange and those of the cones red with Mallory's (and often with Heidenhain's azan) stains.

PHOTORECEPTOR NUCLEI

The cone nuclei measure 5–7 μm in diameter, appear oval, and are located 3–4 μm internal to the external limiting membrane (Fig. 14.27). Rod nuclei are also oval and measure 5.5 μm in width, but contain

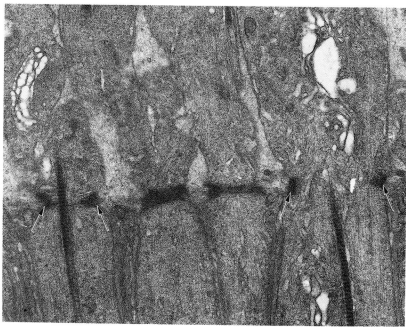

Fig. 14.28 Transmission electron micrograph of a transverse section through the region of the external limiting membrane, which is formed by zonulae adherens (arrows) that attach photoreceptors to adjacent Müller cells and, in places, Müller cells to Müller cells. Original magnification × 24 900.

dispersed chromatin and a visible nucleolus. The cytoplasm that surrounds the nuclei of both cells is scant; externally it is continuous with the photoreceptor outer fibres and internally with the inner fibres or axonal processes that pass into the outer plexiform layer. The outer fibres of cones are short because of the close proximity of their nuclei to the external limiting membrane and to their inner segments but the outer fibres of the rods are long, thin and varicose (Fig. 14.27). The outer fibres of both rods and cones contain mitochondria, smooth endoplasmic reticulum, free ribosomes and perinuclear neurotubules. The cytoplasmic content of the inner fibres of the cones includes endoplasmic reticulum, mitochondria and abundant microtubules. Because the rod nuclei are positioned more external to the external limiting membrane than are the cone nuclei the inner fibres of the rods traverse a shorter distance to reach their connecting second-order neurons in the outer nuclear layer than do the cone inner fibres (Sigelman and Ozanics, 1982; Tripathi and Tripathi, 1984).

14.8   THE OUTER PLEXIFORM LAYER

The outer plexiform layer marks the junction of the first- and second-order neurons in the retina (Tripathi and Tripathi, 1984). The outer two-thirds of this layer is composed of the **inner fibres of photoreceptors** surrounded by processes of the Müller cells and the remaining one-third consists of the **dendrites of the bipolar and horizontal cells** as well as Müller cell processes. The outer plexiform layer is thickest at the macula, measuring approximately 51 μm, and consists predominantly of oblique fibres that have deviated from the fovea. This layer is also known as Henle's fibre layer (Figs 14.4 and 14.5).

The inner fibres in the outer layer represent the axons of the rods and cones. The diameter of a rod axon is some four times greater than that of a cone axon. However, both contain similar organelles, mainly occasional mitochondria, a few free ribosomes, smooth endoplasmic reticulum, glycogen granules and uniformly packed microtubules interspersed in a fairly dense cytoplasm. The rods synapse with second-order neurons through round or oval cytoplasmic expansions 1 μm in diameter that are known as spherules (Fig. 14.29). Cone synapses have cytoplasmic expansions known as pedicles that are larger (7–8 μm in diameter at the parafovea and 5 μm at the fovea) than the rod spherules (Fig. 14.27). Immunocytochemical studies have demonstrated a conspicuous reaction product for glutamate in all photoreceptors (rods more strongly than cones) and

an enrichment of immunoreactivity at the spherules and pedicles (Davanger, Ottersen and Storm-Mathisen, 1991; Crooks and Kolb, 1992).

ROD SYNAPSES

The synaptic complex of a rod consists of a **presynaptic spherule**, a **ribbon synapse** and **postsynaptic processes** that belong either to a horizontal or a bipolar cell. The spherule contains numerous presynaptic vesicles filled with acetylcholine, mitochondria and neurotubules. The density of the pre- and postsynaptic membranes increases at the site of their close apposition (the synaptic cleft, which measures 15 nm). Perpendicular to the presynaptic membrane is the ribbon synapse (Fig. 14.29a) consisting of three dense layers, each measuring 12 nm thick and separated by a clear zone of 40 nm and surrounded by a halo of vesicles (Sigelman and Ozanics, 1982). Only one ribbon is present at each synaptic complex. The synaptic ribbon is found exclusively in the photoreceptor cells of the visual system.

Both horizontal and bipolar cells make contact with the rod spherule (Fig. 14.29). The axons of horizontal cells invaginate the spherule deeply, whereas the invagination made by the bipolar cell is more shallow (Linberg and Fisher, 1988). A horizontal cell contacts each spherule only once, but each spherule may be contacted by several different horizontal cells. One to four bipolar cells contact an individual spherule at separate points. Each bipolar cell contacts up to 50 rods at the perifovea and hundreds at the periphery of the retina. The total number of synaptic complexes varies from two to seven per rod spherule, with four being most common. The spherules also form lateral connections with adjacent telondendria of pedicles. These associations lack synaptic vesicles and ribbons and probably couple the two photoreceptor terminals chemically and electrically.

CONE SYNAPSES

The **cone pedicle** has a pyramidal shape, with the axon forming its apex and the synaptic surface delineating the base (Fig. 14.30). The synaptic indentations on the pedicles receive three neurons, which also contact each other; this arrangement has been designated as the 'triad' (Sigelman and Ozanics, 1982). The central axon of the triad belongs to a midget bipolar cell that may contact the same cone at 10–25 different points. The two dendrites on either side of the triad originate from different horizontal cells. Although only one bipolar cell contacts one

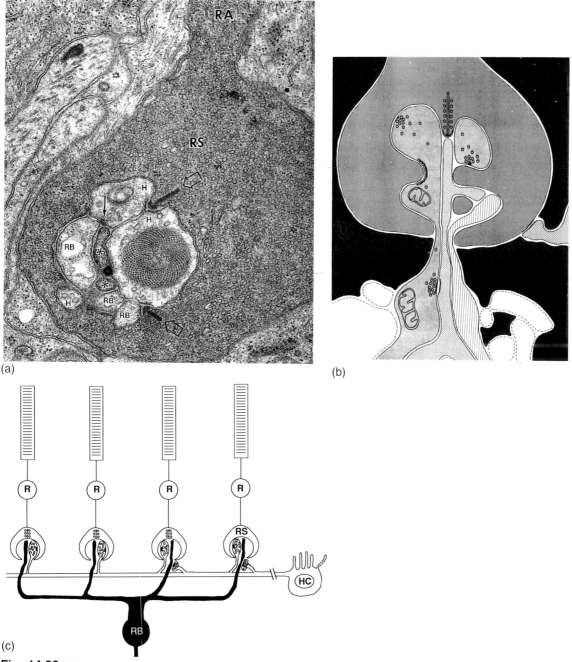

(a)

(b)

(c)

Fig. 14.29 (a) Transmission electron micrograph of a single rod spherule (RS), with its synaptic invagination. The large crystalloid structure in one of the horizontal cell processes is a 'cylinder organelle' and is found only in horizontal cells. All of the horizontal cell axon terminal processes contain small vesicles and one of them shows an accumulation of vesicles adjacent to a region of membrane densification (solid arrow). Open arrows = Synaptic ribbons; asterisks = projections of rod spherule cytoplasm; RA = axon of rod photoreceptor; RB = rod bipolar cell; H = processes of type I horizontal cell axon terminal. (b) Diagrammatic representation of the structure and organization of rod spherule and horizontal cell axon terminals within the spherule. The horizontal cell axon terminals contain synaptic vesicles which are clustered at certain sites and have densification of the membrane associated with them. In some cases, the postsynaptic element is the cytoplasm of the rod spherule, while in others (within the outer plexiform layer) it is a rod bipolar dendrite. In some instances, rod bipolar dendrites could assume the 'lateral position' among the postsynaptic elements, although they do not invaginate as deeply as do the horizontal cell axon terminals. (c) Diagrammatic representation of the synaptic connections and circuitry between the rod photoreceptors (R), horizontal cells (HC) and rod bipolar cells (RB). One of the type I horizontal cell axon terminals makes contact within each synaptic invagination of the rod terminal. Beneath almost every rod spherule (RS), horizontal cell axon terminals also make presynaptic contact with the invaginating rod bipolar dendrites. Because these axon terminals are isolated electrically from their cell body, they may provide a circuit for altering the receptive field of the rod bipolar cell. (Modified from Linberg, K. A. and Fisher, S. K. (1988), *J. Comp. Neurol.*, **268**, 281.)

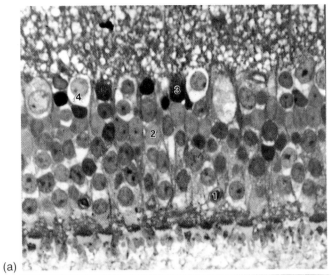

(a)

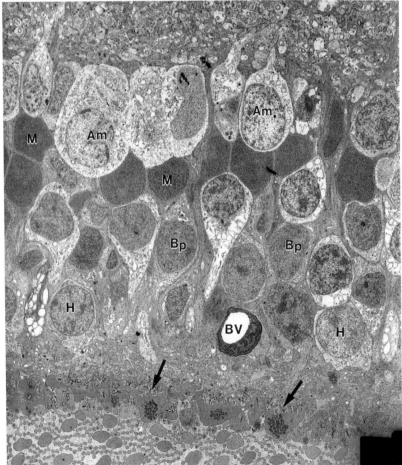

(b)

Fig. 14.30 (a) Transverse section of posterior retina showing cone pedicles abutting against the inner nuclear layer which is made up of 8–12 rows of closely packed nuclei. 1 = Horizontal cells; 2 = bipolar cells; 3 = Müller cells; 4 = amacrine cells. The inner plexiform layer (top) contains the synaptic connections between these cells and the ganglion cell dendrites. Photomicrograph, original magnification × 1175. (From Tripathi, R. C. and Tripathi, B. J. in Davson, H. (ed.) (1984) *The Eye*, published by Academic Press.)
(b) Survey transmission electron micrograph of posterior retina, showing cone pedicles (arrows) and the nuclei of the horizontal (H), bipolar (Bp), Müller (M) and amacrine (Am) cells that constitute the inner nuclear layer. BV = Capillary within inner nuclear layer. Original magnification × 3100.

cone pedicle, contact is made by all horizontal cells in that field, usually 6–8 in number.

Each pedicle also has many small superficial indentations (the so-called 'basal junction'), which are the sites of contact with the flat, diffuse bipolar cells. This type of bipolar cell synapses with as many as six cones. At the site of contact the membranes of the pedicle and of the bipolar cells thicken slightly; however, no synaptic vesicles or ribbons are present (Linberg and Fisher, 1986). The basal junctions represent classic excitatory synapses, and they function similarly to gap junctions.

Except for their greater number in the pedicles (up to 25), the synaptic ribbon and the arciform density in the pedicles share the same ultrastructure and position as those in the spherules. Cone pedicles, like rod spherules, communicate laterally with adjacent photoreceptor cells through some 6–12 neurotubule-rich expansions of cytoplasm.

The presence of numerous junctions, some of which are of the occluding zonule type, between the intertwining processes of the outer plexiform layer impedes free passage of metabolites, fluids and exudates. This arrangement probably aids in the homeostasis of this region of the retina.

14.9   THE INNER NUCLEAR LAYER

The inner nuclear layer consists of 8–12 rows of closely packed nuclei of the bipolar cells, horizontal cells, amacrine cells, interplexiform cells and supportive Müller cells (Tripathi and Tripathi, 1984). Four layers can be distinguished by light microscopy (Fig. 14.30):

- the outermost layer with horizontal cell nuclei;
- the outer intermediate layer with bipolar cell nuclei;
- the inner intermediate layer with Müller cell nuclei;
- the innermost layer with amacrine and interplexiform cell nuclei.

HORIZONTAL CELLS

The flat horizontal cells serve to modulate and transform visual information received from the photoreceptors. Unlike bipolar cells, information from which is relayed radially through the retina, horizontal cells form a network of fibres that integrate the activity of the photoreceptor cells horizontally. The concentration of horizontal cells is highest at the fovea and their number decreases towards the periphery, but their processes branch extensively as one proceeds from the central retina towards the ora serrata.

Horizontal cells are seen by light microscopy to have short processes that radiate symmetrically from the perikaryon and long processes that stem from the base of a short process or directly from the perikaryon. The **long neurite** does not branch within 200–300 µm of the parent horizontal cell, and may reach up to 1 mm in length.

Depending on the size of the cell, as well as the extent and type of the synapses made by the dendrites and axons, three types of horizontal cells,

designated HI, HII, and HIII, are identified (Fig. 14.31). The HI cell has long, stout dendrites that contact only cones at the triad, as well as a single axon up to 2 mm long terminating in elaborate arborizations that make one or two small punctate synapses within the invagination of the rod spherule (Kolb, 1991; Kolb, Linberg and Fisher, 1992; Kolb *et al.*, 1994). Before these processes enter the invagination the axon also makes distinct synapses onto the dendrites of rod bipolar cells. This arrangement constitutes a form of feed-forward which expands the receptive field of the rod bipolar cells beyond their dendritic field. The HIII cells are 30% larger than the HI cells and contact more cones, but are otherwise similar. The HII cells have slim overlapping dendrites and a short (100–300 µm) curved axon, both of which contact cones only. The HI cells contact all spectral types of cones but their communication with the short-wavelength or blue cones is minor; the HII cells have a relatively large input from blue cones and the HIII cells have no contact with these cones (Kolb *et al.*, 1994). Thus, HI cells are presumed to function as luminosity cells, and the HII and HIII types as chromaticity cells (Fig. 14.32).

Morphology

Except for the extent of their dendrites and axons, all horizontal cells have a similar morphology. The cell body is usually flattened and has a diameter of 6–8 µm. The nucleus is round and is surrounded by a Golgi apparatus that is frequently electron-optically empty. The cytoplasm also contains smooth and rough endoplasmic reticulum, slender mitochondria and many free ribosomes, a unique finding in retinal neurons (Sigelman and Ozanics, 1982). A characteristic feature of horizontal cells is the presence of an intracytoplasmic inclusion, the **Kolmer crystalloid** or body (Fig. 14.29a). This body consists of stacks of 5–30 parallel dense tubules, which are separated from one another by a space of 2–6 nm. Each tubule is composed of 2–3 membranes arranged concentrically and decorated on the inner and outer surfaces with ribosome-like particles (Sigelman and Ozanics, 1982). Although the function of Kolmer's crystalloid is unknown, it may represent a structured rough endoplasmic reticulum.

BIPOLAR CELLS

The bipolar cells are the second-order neurons in the visual circuitry. Each retina contains some 35 676 000 bipolar cells (Sigelman and Ozanics, 1982). Oriented radially in the retina, the perikarya of these cells are

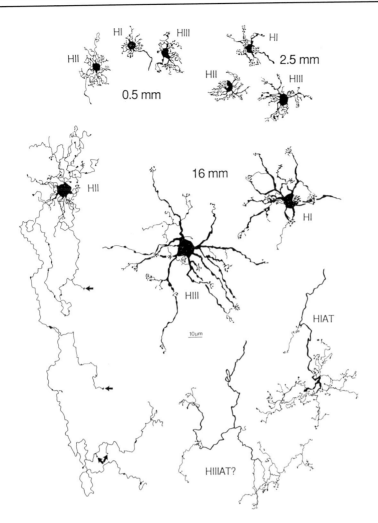

Fig. 14.31 Whole mount views of horizontal cells in a Golgi-impregnated preparation of the human retina. The cells at the fovea (0.5 mm, top) are small and difficult to distinguish into the three types. By 2.5 mm eccentricity, HI, HII and HIII types are more discernible. In the peripheral retina (16 mm) the HIII cell is clearly larger than HI and has an asymmetric dendritic field. HII cells have a woolly appearance, which distinguishes them from the HI and HIII types. The short curled axon of the HII cell gives rise to occasional terminals (arrow). The HI axon terminal ends as a fan-shaped structure with many 'lollipop' terminals (HIAT), while a finer, more loosely clustered terminal (HIIIAT?) is assigned putatively to the HIII horizontal cell. Scale bar = 10 μm. (From Kolb, H. *et al.* (1992), *J. Comp. Neurol.*, **318**, 147.)

located in the inner nuclear layer and their processes extend to the outer and inner plexiform layers. The cell bodies are approximately 9 μm in diameter at the fovea and 5 μm at the periphery of the retina (Sigelman and Ozanics, 1982). On the basis of morphology and synaptic relationships, nine main types of bipolar cells have been distinguished (Kolb, Linberg and Fisher, 1992):

1. rod or mop (Fig 14.33);
2. invaginating midget;
3. flat midget;
4. flat diffuse or brush;
5. invaginating diffuse;
6. ON-centre blue cone;
7. OFF-centre blue cone;
8. giant bistratified;
9. giant diffuse invaginating.

Rod bipolar cells

The rod bipolar cells constitute 20% of the total population and are present 1 mm from the fovea. The diameter of their dendritic tree increases from the central to the peripheral retina (Kolb, Linberg and Fisher, 1992). In the outer plexiform layers the main dendrite divides into 2–3 secondary branches, which, after passing between the cone pedicles, arborize further into a brush-like array of processes that penetrate the invaginations of the rod spherule. The axons of the rod bipolar cells pass into the inner plexiform layer to synapse with processes of the amacrine cells and with the dendrites and cell bodies of the diffuse ganglion cells.

Midget cells

The invaginating midget cells are the smallest of the bipolar cells. Their dendrites penetrate as the central tuft in the triad of the cone pedicles. The apical dendrite of the extrafoveal midget bipolar cells divides into two parts so that it may synapse with two different cones. The axons proceed through the inner plexiform layer and form synapses with processes of amacrine cells and dendrites of the midget ganglion

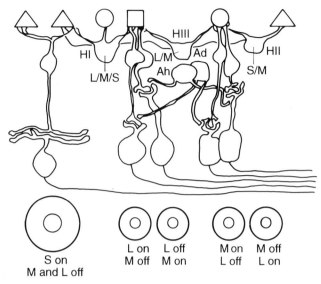

Fig. 14.32 Summary diagram showing the possible synaptic circuits responsible for the construction of the M- and L-wavelength colour-opponent midget ganglion cell or P-cell receptive fields, and the S-wavelength M- and L-opponent receptive fields of the blue-cone system. On- and off-centre pathways for the midget system are provided by the dual parallel midget bipolar to midget ganglion cell connectivity. The colour-opponent surrounds could be formed at the outer plexiform layer by the horizontal cell types (HI, HII and HIII), and the spatially and colour-opponent surrounds could be fortified at the inner plexiform layer by the small-field amacrine cell types (centre hyperpolarizing, Ah, and centre depolarizing, Ad). L-, M-, and S-wavelength input is indicated by colour. (From Kolb, H. (1991), *Vis. Neurosci.*, **7**, 61.)

cells. The flat midget bipolar cells resemble the invaginating type, except that their dendrites do not deeply invaginate the cone pedicles. Instead, they only indent them slightly and make a superficial contact. At the fovea there is a one-to-one ratio of midget bipolar cells and the cones (Kolb, Linberg and Fisher, 1992).

Flat diffuse and invaginating bipolar cells

The small-field, flat diffuse and invaginating bipolar cells have many dendritic processes, which have a broad expanse and terminate in the pedicles of many cones. The apical dendrite of these bipolar cells arborizes in the outer plexiform layer, and their branches extend horizontally. The branches divide further into very fine tufts that terminate as aggregates in shallow depressions on the pedicles. In addition, the small-field, diffuse bipolar cells, which are present across the entire retina, form an extensive overlay in the perifovea (Kolb, Linberg and Fisher, 1992).

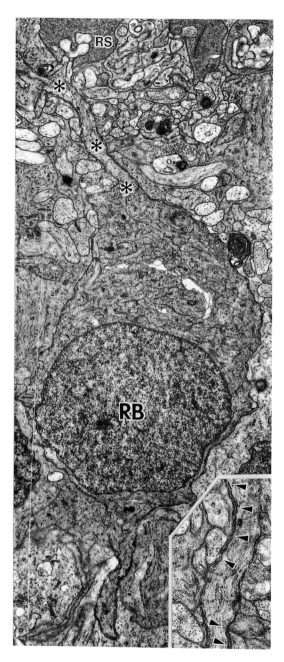

Fig. 14.33 Transmission electron micrograph of a rod bipolar cell (RB), with one of its dendrites (asterisks) extending from the synaptic invagination of a rod spherule (RS). Inset is a higher magnification of the dendrite just above the cell body, showing that it contains cisternae of smooth endoplasmic reticulum (arrowheads) lining its membrane in a configuration known as the helical organelle. Original magnification × 8600; inset × 17 000. (From Linberg, K. A. and Fisher, S. K. (1989), *J. Comp. Neurol.*, **268**, 281.)

Blue-cone bipolar cells

Like the diffuse bipolar cells, blue-cone bipolars innervate more than one cone pedicle (Kolb, Linberg and Fisher, 1992). The ON-centre or BBb variety is characterized by its axon terminal arborizing in stratum 5 of the inner plexiform layer; the OFF-centre or BBa type has its axon terminal ending in stratum 1 immediately under the amacrine cell bodies. The BBb bipolar occurs at 4 mm eccentricity from the foveola and its axon terminal, with its widely ramifying varicose structure, extends over an area of 30 μm. This cell also has two sturdy dendrites that converge on the same cone as well as fine branches that end either on another cone or in the neuropil of the outer plexiform layer. The BBa bipolar is present more towards the periphery of the retina (10 mm eccentricity).

Giant bipolar cells

The two types of giant bipolar cells are distinguished by the extent of their dendritic spread, which exceeds 50 μm in the central retina and 100 μm at the periphery (Kolb, Linberg and Fisher, 1992). The giant diffuse bipolar cell has a thick major dendrite that divides into three long sinuous branches and a bistratified axon which terminates in strata 1 and 4 of the inner plexiform layer. Except for the size of its dendritic field, the giant diffuse bipolar cell has a morphology similar to that of the flat diffuse cells (Kolb, Linberg and Fisher, 1992).

Ultrastructure

All types of bipolar cells have a similar ultrastructure (Fig. 14.33). The nucleus is round or oval with one or two nucleoli. The Golgi apparatus is prominent and is located with the centrioles at the site of origin of the main dendrite. Ribosomes, rough endoplasmic reticulum and mitochondria fill the cytoplasm, and microtubules are present in the dendrites. These processes are 0.1–0.2 μm thick at the fovea and contain a few vesicles, 20 nm diameter filaments and many long, thin mitochondria. The axon hillock is situated opposite the origin of the dendrite. Adjacent to the cell membrane of both the dendrite and the axon are small, regularly arranged, helical tubules. These structures are usually found more frequently in rod bipolar cells than in other types of bipolar cells, which also contain numerous mitochondria and neurofibrils that are located centrally within the cell (Sigelman and Ozanics, 1982). The axons of bipolar cells contain 12.5 nm diameter neurotubules, vesicles that resemble dilated neurotubules and sparse mitochondria (Fig. 14.33). Up to the inner plexiform layer, the axon is surrounded by processes of the Müller cells. After shedding this glial coat, the axon makes a sudden transition into the telodendrion.

The telodendrion of bipolar cells has characteristic boutons, which contain numerous large and complex mitochondria (Sigelman and Ozanics, 1982). Synaptic vesicles are present throughout the cytoplasm in this region, but they are also concentrated around the synaptic ribbon. The afferent or postsynaptic telodendrion has conventional synapses, whereas the efferent processes which are presynaptic to amacrine or ganglion cells have typical ribbon synapses.

Most of the midget and diffuse bipolar cells (but not the rod bipolar cells) are glutamatergic. In addition, a subpopulation of bipolar perikarya (18%) and terminals (32%) exhibit strong immunolabelling for glycine (Crooks and Kolb, 1992; Davanger, Storm-Mathisen and Ottersen, 1994). The glutamate/glycine-positive terminals establish contact with amacrine cell processes and ganglion cell dendrites and are located to between 44% and 88% of the depth of the inner plexiform layer. These cells are believed to correspond to the ON-cone/bipolar system (Davanger, Storm-Mathisen and Ottersen, 1994).

MÜLLER CELLS

Most of the inner intermediate layer of the inner nuclear layer is occupied by the cell bodies of Müller cells, although their perikarya can be present in any sublayer (Fig. 14.34). The mean density of Müller cells is 8–13 000 cells/mm^2 (Dreher, Robinson and Distler, 1992). Embryonically, Müller cells are derived from the inner layer of the optic vesicle. During development of the retina these cells have an important role in the orientation, displacement and positioning of the developing neurons. As the principal glial cells of the retina, they conserve the structural alignment of its neuronal elements. Müller cells are the largest of all cells in the retina, and extend from the external to the internal limiting membranes. Their shape is similar to that of columnar epithelial cells. Müller cells are characterized by their cytoplasmic expansions, which fill all intercellular spaces and envelop the cell bodies of the neurons.

Four types of Müller cell processes are distinguishable (Sigelman and Ozanics, 1982):

1. radial processes that extend from both sides of the Müller cell body in the inner plexiform layer;
2. fine horizontal processes that extend laterally in both of the plexiform layers as well as in the nerve fibre layer;
3. thin, villus-like projections that form fibre baskets around the inner segment of the photoreceptors (see p. 471);

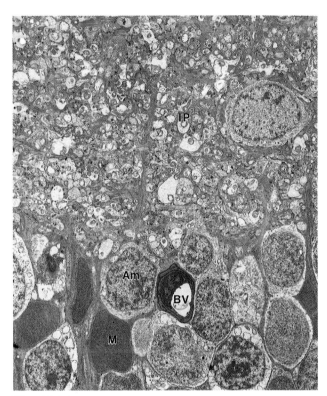

Fig. 14.34 Transmission electron micrograph of transverse section of the posterior retina. The inner plexiform layer (IP) contains the synaptic connections between the bipolar cells, amacrine cells and the ganglion cell dendrites. Am = Nucleus of amacrine cell; M = nucleus of Müller cell; BV = small arteriole within the inner nuclear layer. Original magnification × 4300.

4. processes that form a honeycomb meshwork which envelops the perikarya of the ganglion cells and the cells of the inner plexiform layer.

Except at the external limiting membrane where zonulae adherentes are found, tight junctions exist between Müller cells and other neuronal cells.

Morphology

The cytoplasm of the Müller cells shows regional morphological differences that reflect variations in the metabolic activity of these cells (Sigelman and Ozanics, 1982). The inner half of the cell contains rough and smooth endoplasmic reticulum, Golgi apparatus, slender mitochondria, free ribosomes and filaments 10–20 nm in diameter that are oriented radially. The cytoplasm is moderately electron-dense, and the organelles suggest the function of protein synthesis. The cytoplasm around the nucleus contains ribosomes and an extensive smooth endoplasmic reticulum. The outer or scleral half of the cell appears to be adapted to absorption and intracellular

transport. Numerous microtubules are present, and mitochondria are concentrated in the cytoplasm close to the external limiting membrane; presumably these organelles provide the energy required for active transport across the outer plasma membrane. The outer region of the cell also contains a large amount of glycogen, although this varies with the degree of oxygenation of the retina.

Retinal metabolism

Müller cells have an important role in the metabolism of the retina. Immunohistochemical studies have revealed the presence of cellular retinaldehyde-binding proteins, glutamine, taurine and glutamine synthetase in their cytoplasm (Lewis *et al.*, 1988; Milam *et al.*, 1990; Pow, Crook and Wong, 1994). Hybridization *in situ* has revealed the mRNA for carbonic anhydrase II (Rogers and Hunt, 1987; Herbert, Cavallaro and Martone, 1991), which is suggested to help buffer variations in extracellular CO_2 in the retina (Newman, 1994). Furthermore, as revealed by hybridization *in situ*, Müller cells cultured from the rat retina contain the mRNA for insulin, which may function in the control of glucose metabolism (Das, Pansky and Bud, 1987). Müller cells are also known to degrade neurotransmitter substances (e.g. γ-aminobutyric acid: GABA). The membrane potential across the Müller cell indicates that it has a role as a K^+ electrode. The available evidence suggests that K^+ ions liberated through the activity of the retinal neurons (mostly bipolar cells) are taken up and discharged at the endfoot surface of the Müller cells into the vitreous and, in at least some species with vascularized retinas, into the retinal capillaries; in this way they contribute to the b-wave of the electroretinogram (Newman and Odette, 1984; Newman, 1987; Wen and Oakley, 1990). Experimental studies in the salamander retina have shown that activation of glutamate uptake leads to accumulation of K^+ outside the Müller cells. Suppression of glutamate release from the photoreceptors by light is suggested to reduce the efflux of K^+ from the Müller cells, which contributes to the light-evoked fall of K^+ in the outer retina (Amato *et al.*, 1994).

AMACRINE CELLS

The somas of the amacrine cells lie internal to the nuclei of the Müller cells (Figs 14.30 and 14.34). Each amacrine cell has a single process that branches extensively and has characteristics in common with both axons and dendrites. The amacrine processes extend over a wide area in the inner plexiform layer.

The cell body of the amacrine cells has a flask or urn shape with a diameter of 12 μm and, except in the fovea (where they are absent), is located in the inner nuclear layer. The nucleus is round and has prominent infoldings in the membrane which give it a lobulated appearance. The abundant cytoplasm is located on the inner side of the nucleus and contains numerous mitochondria, granular endoplasmic reticulum (Nissl substance) and many electron-dense, round bodies that are probably lipoidal. A cilium is present on the inner side of the cell close to the nucleus (Sigelman and Ozanics, 1982).

Morphology

Amacrine cells have a diverse morphology; up to 24 varieties have been described in the human retina (Kolb, Linberg and Fisher, 1992). On the basis of the Golgi impregnation technique, two major types of amacrine cells are distinguishable: (1) diffuse and (2) stratified. The main process of the **diffuse** cell type extends through the inner plexiform layer and, on the inner side of this region, arborizes to give a dense horizontal plexus. Depending on the extent of these processes, the diffuse amacrine cells are further sub-divided into **narrow-field cells**, which cover an area 10–50 μm wide (average 25 μm) and **wide-field cells**, which spread 30–50 μm in the inner plexiform layer and up to 600 μm in the ganglion cell layer. The wide-field diffuse amacrines make contact with rod bipolar terminals and ganglion cells. Depending on the layer in which the processes lie, the stratified amacrine cells are also further classified as unistratified, multistratified and diffuse or polystratified. The **unistratified amacrine cells** are located in the outer half of the inner plexiform layer, where their processes radiate horizontally for up to 500 μm. The main process of **multistratified cells** extends from the cell body and divides into branches that spread horizontally for 400–600 μm at two or more levels, usually in the central region of the inner plexiform layer and near the ganglion cell layer. The **stratified diffuse cells** have smaller nuclei than the other amacrine cells and their processes cover a field of only 50 μm width.

Neurotransmitters

Amacrine cells are also classified according to the neurotransmitter that they produce; however, no correspondence exists between this physiological

classification and the morphological description. The transmitter substances associated with amacrine cell function include both neuroactive substances (acetylcholine, GABA, glycine, dopamine, serotonin) and neuropeptides (cholecystokinin, enkephalin, glucagon, neurotensin, somatostatin, substance P, neuropeptide Y and vasoactive intestinal peptide). Two or more of these neuromodulating chemicals may be present in one cell. Most amacrine cells contain γ-aminobutyric acid and glycine, which have an inhibitory action on the ganglion cells (Crooks and Kolb, 1992; Davanger, Ottersen and Storm-Mathisen, 1991).

INTERPLEXIFORM CELLS

The nuclei of the interplexiform cells occupy the innermost part of the inner nuclear layer. Because the perikarya of these cells are located among those of amacrine cells, some authors do not regard them as a separate class of cells. However, their processes extend to both plexiform layers (Kolb, Linberg and Fisher, 1992). The processes to the outer plexiform layer may arise directly from the cell body or from an interplexiform cell process in the inner plexiform layer (Fig. 14.35).

Sensory input to the interplexiform cell occurs in the inner plexiform layer, and most synapses are in the outer plexiform layer. Thus, information is carried between the two plexiform layers and the neurons appear to be centrifugal in nature. In the human retina interplexiform cells synapse onto cone horizontal cells and receive input mainly from amacrine cell processes (Linberg and Fisher, 1986). Some interplexiform cells are dopaminergic.

14.10 THE INNER PLEXIFORM LAYER

The inner plexiform layer marks the junction of the second-order neurons, the bipolar cells, with the third-order neurons, the ganglion cells (Figs 14.1 and 14.36). However, although the bipolar cell terminals provide input to this layer and the ganglion cells carry the output, the amacrine cells also mediate interactions within the layer and the interplexiform cells receive input from the amacrine cells. In addition to the synaptic connections among bipolar, ganglion, amacrine and interplexiform cells, the inner plexiform layer contains processes of the Müller cells, an abundant microvasculature and an occasional displaced nucleus of a ganglion or an amacrine cell. The inner plexiform layer is thicker (18–36 μm), has more synapses per unit area (more than 2 million per mm^2) and contains a greater variety of synapses than the

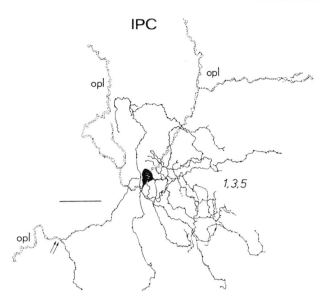

IPC

opl

opl

1,3,5

opl

Fig. 14.35 An interplexiform cell (IPC) of the human retina. This cell has its major dendritic tree in the inner plexiform layer, with dendrites obvious at strata 1, 3 and 5. Two ascending processes from the cell body and one from a dendrite in stratum 1 (arrows) pass to the outer plexiform layer (opl) and course therein over approximately the same distance as the dendritic span in the inner plexiform layer. The ascending processes and those in the outer plexiform layer are indicated by dashed lines. Scale bar = 25 µm. (From Kolb, H. *et al.* (1992), *J. Comp. Neurol.*, **318**, 147.)

outer plexiform layer. The inner plexiform layer is absent from the foveola.

ULTRASTRUCTURE

The axons of the bipolar cells in this layer have an abundance of neurotubules and neurofilaments,

as well as occasional mitochondria (Sigelman and Ozanics, 1982). Bipolar cells make contact with the processes of amacrine cells and the dendrites of ganglion cells. Two elements are present at synapse in an arrangement that is known as a 'dyad'. Most often, in the human retina, one of these elements is a dendrite of a ganglion cell and the other is a process of an amacrine cell; this seems to correlate with the presence of many contrast-sensitive ganglion cells. Occasionally, two amacrine cell processes or, more rarely, two dendrites of ganglion cells, are present. A ribbon synapse, similar to those in the photoreceptor spherules and pedicles, is a characteristic that is unique to bipolar cells in the inner plexiform layer.

The dendritic tips of all bipolar cells have receptors for GABA-A (Vardi and Sterling, 1994). Immunoreactivity for this receptor is strongest on membrane apposed to horizontal cells, but is also concentrated on the tips of flat and invaginating bipolar and rod bipolar cells as well as at the base of the cone pedicles. The presence of the GABA-A receptor on bipolar dendritic tips suggests that horizontal cells can affect bipolar cells directly, and their presence on the bipolar axon terminals suggests that inhibition feedback from amacrine cells is mediated by GABA-A (Vardi and Sterling, 1994).

SYNAPTIC CONTACTS

The processes of amacrine cells interface with bipolar cell axons, with somas and dendrites of ganglion cells and with processes of other amacrine cells through conventional synapses. The interplexiform cells also have conventional synapses, mainly with

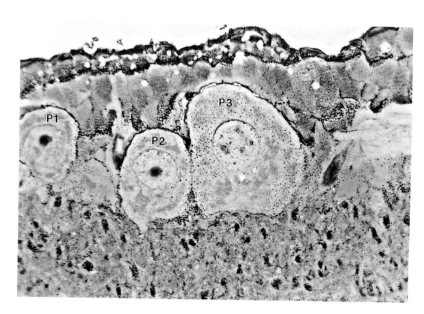

Fig. 14.36 Ganglion cells in the peripheral retina showing, from left to right, P1 (midget), P2 (small bistratified) and P3 (parasol) cell types. Nissl granules are seen as dense intracytoplasmic patches. Silver stained photomicrograph, original magnification × 1350. (From Tripathi, R. C. and Tripathi, B. J. in Davson, H. (ed.) (1984) *The Eye*, published by Academic Press.)

the processes of amacrine cells. Two distinct synapses are unique to the amacrine cells: the reciprocal and the serial synapse. In the **reciprocal synapse**, the process of an amacrine cell in a dyad causes a nearby synapse to back onto the bipolar terminal, thus allowing for feedback between amacrine and bipolar cells near the ribbon synapse. The **serial synapse** consists of two consecutive synapses between two amacrine processes and a third synapse with a ganglion cell dendrite, a bipolar axon or another amacrine process. This network fosters local inter-action between neighbouring amacrine cells. The synapses of amacrine cells have a stratified distribu-tion; at the foveal slope two main layers are recog-nized, whereas in the peripheral retina this increases to five strata (Koontz and Hendrickson, 1987).

14.11   THE GANGLION CELL LAYER

The ganglion cell layer is composed mainly of the cell bodies of the third-order ganglion cells, although other elements such as processes of Müller cells, other neuroglia and branches of retinal vessels are also present. The ganglion cells form a single layer in the peripheral retina (Figs 14.36 and 14.37), but two layers are formed at the temporal side of the optic disc and 6–8 layers at the edge of the foveola (Figs 14.4 and 14.5). At the foveola and optic nerve head the ganglion cell layer is absent. The depth of the layer ranges from 10 μm to 20 μm in the nasal retina and from 60 μm to 80 μm in the macular region.

Adjacent cells are packed closely together, except at the periphery, where they are separated by a distance of 400 μm. Some 1.2 million ganglion cells are present in the retina; each of these produces a single axon. These converge and exit from the eye as the **optic nerve** (Sigelman and Ozanics, 1982; Tripathi and Tripathi, 1984). Within the central area of the retina, the density of ganglion cells is 32–38 000 cells/mm^2 in a horizontally oriented elliptical ring 0.4–2.00 mm from the foveola (Curcio and Allen, 1990). In the peripheral retina the densities in the nasal quadrant exceed those at corresponding eccentricities in the temporal quadrant by more than 300% and the superior exceeds the inferior by 60%. Overall, the ratio of cones to ganglion cells ranges from 2.9:1 to 7.5:1 in different individuals. Displaced amacrine cells account for 3% of the total cells in the ganglion cell layer in the central retina and nearly 80% in the far periphery (Curcio and Allen, 1990).

MORPHOLOGY

Ganglion cells are large, with diameters that range from 10 μm to 30 μm, and are round, piriform or oval in shape. The smaller cells are especially prominent in the macular region. They have a large nucleus and abundant cytoplasm that contain rough endoplas-mic reticulum (**Nissl substance**) and a prominent Golgi apparatus near the nucleus (Fig. 14.37). Dis-integration of the Nissl substance represents an early sign of physiological or pathological distur-

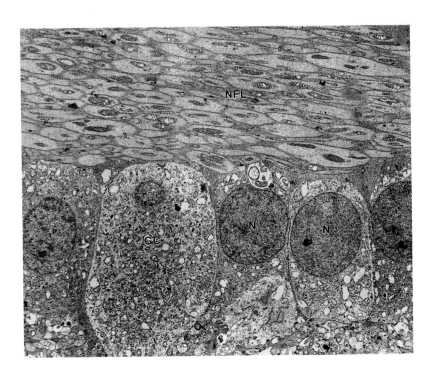

Fig. 14.37 Transmission electron micrograph of peripheral retina, showing ganglion cell bodies (GC) and the nerve fibre layer (NFL). N = Nucleus. Original magnification × 19 800.

bance in the retina. Smooth endoplasmic reticulum, mitochondria, lipoidal and pigment granules are dispersed throughout the cytoplasm. The increase in the number of lipofuscin bodies that occurs with age is thought to account in part for the increase in the yellow colouration of the macula lutea. Ganglion cells have numerous neurofilaments; these make the cytoplasm dense and easily distinguishable from that of Müller cells (Sigelman and Ozanics, 1982).

CLASSIFICATION

In general the ganglion cells are multipolar, with dendrites that extend horizontally in the retina and radially into the inner plexiform layer. Their non-branching axons are directed towards the nerve fibre layer, where they become aligned parallel to the surface of the inner retina (Fig. 14.37). Ganglion cells are classified according to their size, degree of arborization and spread of their dendrites, and the pattern of synaptic connection with amacrine and bipolar cells.

Some 18 different types of ganglion cells have been described recently, but it is not yet clear whether these merely represent variations of major categories, or how their morphology relates to their physiology (Kolb, Linberg and Fisher, 1992). Two major types of cells, which are designated M (or parasol) and P, with P cells further subdivided into two subclasses, P1 or midget and P2 or small bistratified, have been identified in the human eye (Fig. 14.36). The M cells project to the magnocellular layers of the lateral geniculate body and exhibit non-opponent responses. Physiologically, the M cells resemble the α-ganglion cells of the cat retina, whereas the P cells seem to be specialized cells in primates for colour vision and have no correlation with any of the feline ganglion cells.

P ganglion cells

The P ganglion cells project to the parvocellular layers. The P1 cells correspond to the midget cell and have the smallest dendritic trees. These cells exhibit opponent responses to M- and L-wavelength stimuli and receive input from a single cone. The P1 ganglion cells occur as pairs with a high-branching (a-type, which show OFF-centre responses) and low-branching (b-type, which show ON-centre responses) member across the entire retina (Kolb and DeKorver, 1991; Kolb, Linberg and Fisher, 1992). At the fovea, P1 cells constitute 90% of the total ganglion cell population. In this region of the retina their elongated cell bodies measure $8\,\mu m \times 12\,\mu m$, but the size enlarges and

reaches a maximum of $14\,\mu m \times 16\,\mu m$ at a distance of 8 mm from the fovea, where they account for 40–45% of the ganglion cells (Dacey, 1994). The single apical dendrite has few terminals, covers an area 5–7 μm in diameter and shows limited branching in the outer (a-type) or inner (b-type) one-third of the inner plexiform layer (Kolb and DeKorver, 1991; Dacey, 1993a,b). The a-type cells synapse with the axon terminals of the flat midget bipolar cells and the b-type cells with the invaginating bipolar cells. Between 55 and 81 ribbons are present at the dyad or monad terminals. The number of amacrine cell processes that synapse onto the dendritic tree of these ganglion cells is approximately equal to the number of bipolar ribbon inputs (Kolb and DeKorver, 1991). The spread of the P1 dendrites is 5–10 μm in the central retina, but increases tenfold between 2 mm and 6 mm eccentricity, and reaches a maximum of 225 μm at the periphery (Kolb, 1991; Dacey and Petersen, 1992; Dacey, 1993a,b).

At the fovea it is difficult to distinguish P1 cells from P2 cells; however, 1.5 mm from the foveola, the P2 cells are noticeably larger (Fig. 14.38a), with a dendritic field that measures 30–50 μm across, up to 60 μm at 8 mm from the centre of the fovea, and 400 μm at the far periphery (Dacey, 1993a,b). P2 cells exhibit a strong blue-ON response to stimulation of the S-cones (Dacey and Lee, 1994). They represent 1% of the total ganglion cells at the fovea and 10% at the periphery of the retina (Dacey, 1994).

M ganglion cells

Overall, M cells have larger cell bodies than do P cells, and their dendritic trees cover an area 25–30 μm in diameter, which increases to 160 μm at 8 mm from the foveola, and to 270 μm at 14 mm (Dacey and Petersen, 1992). At the periphery of the retina the M cell body is 25–30 μm and gives rise to two or more thick dendrites (Fig. 14.38b). M cells constitute 5% of the total ganglion cell population at the fovea and 20% at the periphery of the retina (Dacey, 1994).

14.12 THE NERVE FIBRE LAYER

The nerve fibre layer contains the axons of the ganglion cells (the so-called 'centripetal' or 'afferent' fibres), glial cells, a rich capillary bed and centrifugal (or efferent) fibres. The axons are arranged in arcades delineated by the processes of Müller and other glial cells. Individual afferent fibres measure from 0.6 μm to 2.0 μm in diameter. They contain prominent microtubules, mitochondria and smooth endoplasmic reticulum (Fig. 14.37). They have a bidirectional

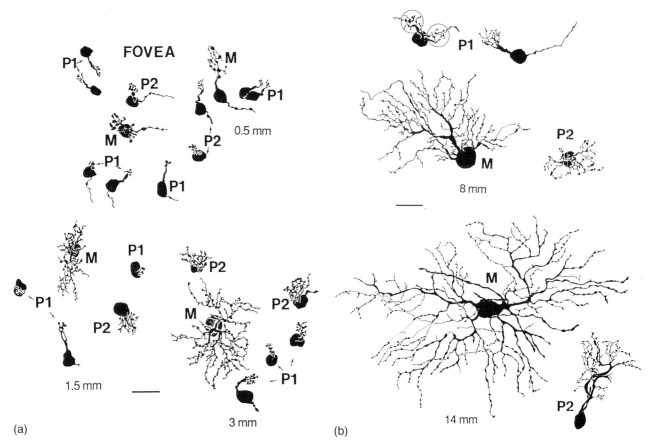

Fig. 14.38   Whole mount views of ganglion cells in a Golgi-impregnated preparation of the human retina. (a) P1, P2 and M cells of the fovea and central retina. The three types can be distinguished by the size of their dendritic trees when they occur adjacent to each other: P1 ganglion cells have minute dendritic trees at the fovea, which expand to be no more than a small bouquet of varicosities that measure 9–12 μm in diameter at 3 mm eccentricity; P2 cells have dendritic trees that are about the size of P1 cells; M cells are, on average, three times the size of P2 cells in the extent of their dendritic trees. All three types occur as a and b subtypes depending on the level of their dendritic trees in sublamina a or b of the inner plexiform layer. (b) Ganglion cells of the mid- and far periphery of the retina. All three cell types show a continuation from (a) of increasing size of their dendritic trees at greater eccentricities. P1 cells are rarely encountered past the mid-periphery (10 mm); many in this region have two dendritic heads (circled), others have the normal single head. P1 cells reach a maximum dendritic tree size of 25 μm; P2 and M cells occur at the far periphery and are clearly distinguishable on the size of their bodies and dendritic trees. Scale bar = 25 μm. (From Kolb, H. *et al.* (1992), *J. Comp. Neurol.*, **318**, 147.)

axoplasmic flow that occurs at two rates: at the slow rate (0.5–5 mm/day) the flow carries high-molecular-weight proteins that are utilized for axonal growth, maintenance and repair; the fast rate (10–2000 mm/day) caters to molecules that are involved in synaptic function (Sigelman and Ozanics, 1982). The axons remain unmyelinated until they reach the lamina cribrosa of the optic nerve.

The afferent fibres take a radial course parallel to the inner limiting membrane and converge on the optic nerve, except for those axons that arise from ganglion cells immediately temporal to the optic disc, which are the first to develop and form the centre of the optic nerve (Fig. 14.39). These fibres are distinguished as the papillomacular bundle. The axons originating from ganglion cells temporal to the fovea

take an increasingly arcuate course to bypass this region (Siegelman and Ozanics, 1982; Tripathi and Tripathi, 1984). The superior and inferior fibres are separated at their origin by a horizontal raphe that extends from the fovea to the extreme temporal periphery of the retina (Fig. 14.39).

The nerve fibre layer is thickest at the nasal edge of the disc, where it measures 20–30 μm. The thickness decreases from the optic disc to the ora serrata, where the ganglion cell layer and the nerve fibre layer blend to form a single layer. The **papillomacular bundle** represents the thinnest portion of the nerve fibre layer around the optic disc; it is the last portion of the optic disc to be affected in papilloedema. Because axons are so numerous close to the optic nerve head they become heaped up, especially on the

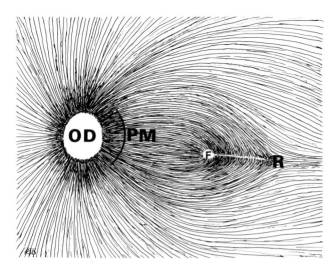

Fig. 14.39 Schematic representation of the course of the nerve fibres to the optic nerve. OD = Optic disc; PM = papillomacular bundle; F = foveola; R = raphe. (From Tripathi, R. C. and Tripathi, B. J. in Davson, H. (ed.) (1984) *The Eye*, published by Academic Press.)

nasal side, which causes an elevation (the papilla) to be formed towards the vitreal surface. Thus, the nasal aspect of the optic disc is the most susceptible to changes of papilloedema because of its greater collection of nerve bundles and blood vessels.

Centrifugal fibres that originate from the central nervous system terminate in the inner plexiform layer or in the innermost part of the inner nuclear layer. Usually they associate with amacrine cells or capillary walls, where they exert vasomotor effects.

NEUROGLIA

The neuroglial cells that are present in the nerve fibre layer are categorized as **macroglia** and **microglia** (Sigelman and Ozanics, 1982; Ogden, 1989a,b).

Macroglia

Macroglia are derived embryonically from the cells of the neural crest and are distinguished as fibrous and protoplasmic astrocytes. The two types of astrocytes display certain similarities in morphology, such as the presence of prominent cytoplasmic filaments 10 nm in diameter, endoplasmic reticulum, glycogen granules, elongated mitochondria and an occasional centriole and a cilium (Sigelman and Ozanics, 1982). Fibrous astrocytes have many cytoplasmic processes and a dense round or oval nucleus that is located in the nerve fibre layer. These cells have fewer mitochondria and a greater filamentous content than found in protoplasmic astrocytes. The processes of the protoplasmic

astrocytes are short and blunt, and they often extend into the inner plexiform layer. Their nuclei are irregular in shape and have coarse chromatin granules. Although astrocytes make contact with the abluminal aspect of blood vessels through gap junctions on their pedicles or footplates, they seem to have no role in dispersing nutrients to the neural elements; rather, they function to segregate the receptive surface of neurons from extraneous influences. In response to injury, astrocytes hypertrophy, increasing in number and size. Their proliferation results in the formation of scars in the retinal tissue (Ogden, 1989a,b).

Microglia

Microglia are small cells that are derived from mesodermal invasion of the retina at the time of vascularization (Sigelman and Ozanics, 1982). The cytoplasm of these cells is similar to that of astrocytes, but it lacks glycogen granules and has fewer filaments. The nucleus has prominent clumps of chromatin and is surrounded by scant cytoplasm. A distinctive feature of microglial cells is the long and winding configuration of the cisternae of the rough endoplasmic reticulum. These cells populate the retina from the nerve fibre layer to the outer plexiform layer and are the only glial cells present in Henle's fibre layer of the fovea. Unlike macroglia, microglial cells do not have a structural role in the retina; they take the role of wandering tissue histiocytes in response to tissue injury and phagocytose debris which is carried to the vasculature for removal from the retina.

14.13 THE INTERNAL LIMITING MEMBRANE

The internal limiting membrane forms the innermost layer of the retina and the outer boundary of the vitreous. Both the retina and the vitreous contribute to the formation of this membrane, which consists of four elements: (1) collagen fibrils and (2) proteoglycans (mostly hyaluronic acid) of the vitreous; (3) the basement membrane; (4) the plasma membrane of the Müller cells and possibly other glial cells of the retina (Fig. 14.40). The basement membrane stains positively with periodic acid–Schiff and red with Mallory trichrome stains. However, the vitreal contribution to the internal limiting membrane stains blue with Mallory trichrome, which is indicative of its collagenous nature. By electron microscopy, the collagen fibrils of the vitreous are seen enmeshed in the vitreal proteoglycans and finally

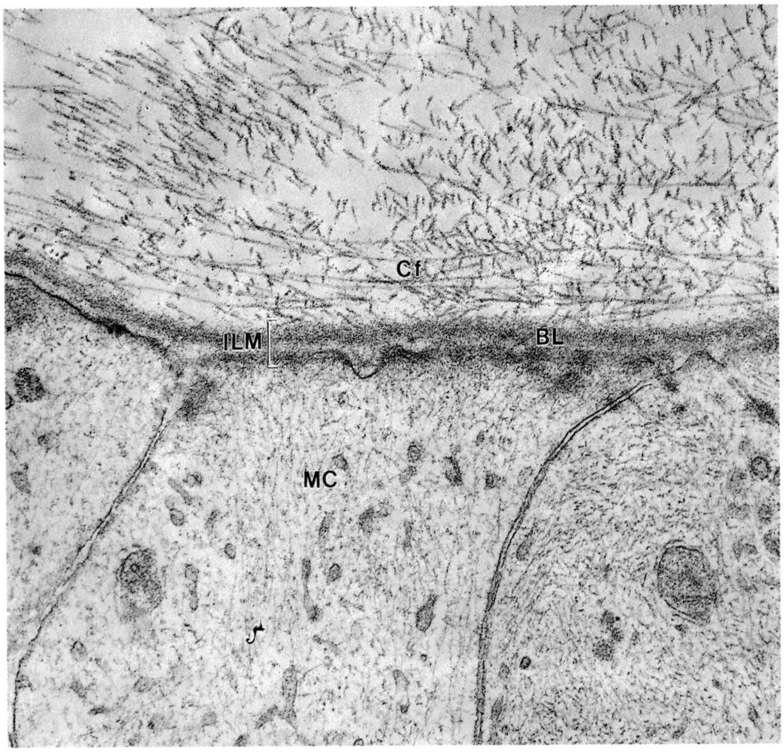

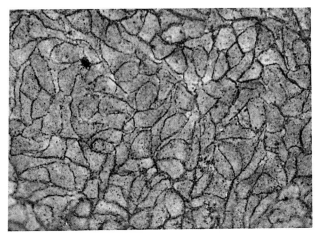

Fig. 14.40 Transverse section of the surface of the retina, showing the insertion of collagen fibrils (Cf) of the vitreous into the basal lamina (BL) of the Müller cells (MC), which, together with the plasma membrane of their foot processes, constitutes the internal limiting membrane (ILM) of the retina. Transmission electron micrograph, original magnification × 50 000.

insert into the basement membrane of the glial cells.

In flat preparations of the retina (Fig. 14.41) the external portion of the internal limiting membrane exhibits a mosaic pattern that depicts the irregularities of the foot processes of the Müller cells (Ashton and Tripathi, 1972). The irregularities form

Fig. 14.41 The mosaic pattern of the internal limiting membrane of the retina is revealed by a flat preparation stained with silver, which outlines the footplates of the Müller cells and accessory glial cells that attach to the internal limiting membrane. Photomicrograph, original magnification × 1500. (From Tripathi, R. C. and Tripathi, B. J. in Davson, H. (ed.) (1984) *The Eye*, published by Academic Press.)

pockets which are filled by the overlying basement membrane. These pockets are called basement membrane facets. The vitreous portion of the membrane appears smooth in flat sections of the retina, except at the retinal periphery where it may be irregular.

In the posterior retina the internal limiting membrane attains a thickness of 0.5–2.0 μm. It continues uninterrupted at the fovea where it is thickest (Heegaard, 1994), but is absent at the edge of the optic disc. At the periphery of the retina, the membrane is continuous with the basal lamina of the ciliary epithelium. With ageing, the internal limiting membrane becomes generally thicker and interrupted at the ora serrata (Fig. 14.7c).

The inner portion of the internal limiting membrane is also known as the hyaloid membrane of the vitreous. It gives the posterior retina a characteristic sheen when observed with the ophthalmoscope. When the vitreous detaches from the retinal surface, as in ageing, artefact or pathological conditions, the posterior surface condenses and produces the 'membrana hyaloidea posterior'. Normally, the vitreous has a firm attachment to the retina at the optic disc, the fovea and at the ora serrata. The site at the fovea is more tenuous and the vitreous can detach and produce an annular ring in ageing and myopic eyes (see also p. 452).

CHAPTER FIFTEEN
The visual pathway

The visual pathway from the retina may be divided into seven levels (Fig. 15.1):

1. optic nerve;
2. optic chiasma;
3. optic tract;
4. lateral geniculate body;
5. optic radiation;
6. striate cortex;
7. prestriate cortex.

15.1 OPTIC NERVE

The optic nerve has the following parts:

1. intraocular nerve head;
2. intraorbital;
3. intracanalicular;
4. intracranial.

It is in essence a tract of the brain, an outgrowth of the cerebral vesicle, whose fibres possess no neurolemma and which is surrounded by meninges, unlike any peripheral nerve. Most cogently, the 'primary' and 'secondary' sensory neurons of the pathway are in the retina, the ganglion cells corresponding, for example, to those in the gracile or cuneate nuclei in the medulla oblongata.

Ensheathed in pia the optic nerve extends posteromedially from the globe at the optic nerve head (papilla) to the chiasma in the cranial cavity. Where it leaves the eye, the centre of the optic nerve is just above and 3 mm medial to the posterior pole of the globe (Fig. 4.32e). Within the orbit its cross-section is rounded. As it passes to the optic foramen, the optic nerve takes a sinuous course which allows for ocular movements. In the canal it is oval in section. The dura mater lines the canal as periosteum, and the nerve is covered by arachnoid mater within the canal, so that both here and in the orbit the nerve is covered by all meninges and is bathed with cerebrospinal fluid (Fig. 5.3). As the nerve leaves the canal it is piriform in cross-section with a rounded end medially; it becomes a flat band as it inclines posteromedially and slightly upwards to the chiasma (Fig. 5.2). The total length of the nerve is about 5 cm (intraocular 0.7 mm, intraorbital 3 cm, canalicular 6 mm and intracranial 1 cm).

INTRAOCULAR NERVE HEAD (OPTIC PAPILLA, OPTIC DISC)

The intraocular portion of the optic nerve (Figs 15.2–15.5) extends from its anterior surface in contact with the vitreous to a plane which is level with that of the posterior scleral surface (about 1 mm). The choroid ends abruptly here, as do all elements of the retina except its axons. These bend at a right-angle into the nerve head and pass posteriorly through the scleral canal. The nerve head exhibits three zones but

Superficial nerve fibre layer

This is covered by the inner limiting membrane of Elschnig (1901), which is composed of astrocytes and is in continuity with the inner limiting membrane of the retina. Glial cells and interaxonal processes are relatively sparse here but increase progressively towards the retrolaminar nerve (Minckler, McLean and Tso, 1976). Astrocytes make up approximately 10% of the volume of the nerve head (Quigley, 1986).

Topographic organization of nerve fibres

In the retina   The nerve fibres converge towards the disc. On the temporal side is the papillomacular bundle. There is no overlap between the upper and lower halves of the fibres of the peripheral parts of the retina. In the retina the line dividing nasal from temporal fibres (in the sense of those that will cross in the chiasma and those that will not) passes through the centre of the fovea. Hence the temporal macular fibres remain on the same side, while the nasal ones cross.

The upper temporal retinal fibres (and some of the nasal portion as well) are separated from the lower by the macular fibres, an arrangement which holds throughout the central visual pathway.

The retinotopic organization of the nerve axons is rigidly preserved at the nerve fibre layer, just anterior to the ganglion cell layer, as they reach the periphery of the nerve head (Fig. 15.6). The process observed in the retina, by which newly arising axons pass through the nerve fibre layer to reach its (internal) surface, includes the peripapillary retina. Axons arising here cross those of peripheral origin and pass at the vitreal surface of the nerve fibre layer to the centre of the nerve head. Axonal bundles from ganglion cells near the fovea along the horizontal raphe occupy an intermediate location in the nerve fibre layer near the disc and remain between fibres of peripheral or peripapillary origin (van der Hoeve, 1920; Minckler, 1980) (Fig. 15.7). Those fibres subserving vision in areas of the visual field which are characteristically lost in glaucoma (the Bjerrum areas) are confined primarily to a wedge-shaped area (approximately the central 30°) of the superior and inferior temporal quadrants of the disc (Radius and Anderson, 1979a,b; Minckler, 1980).

In the optic nerve   Behind the eye (Fig. 15.78a) the peripheral fibres are distributed exactly as in the retina; those from the temporal side are lateral in the nerve, those from the nasal side medial. The macular

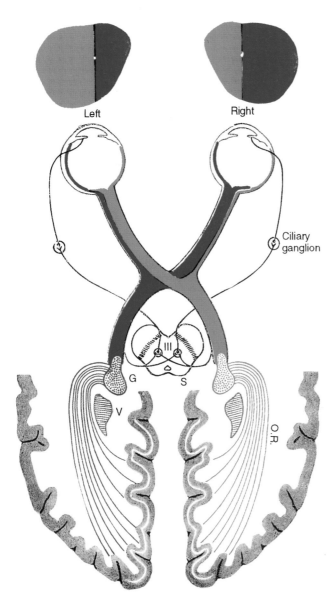

Fig. 15.1 The course of the visual and pupillary fibres and the corresponding fields of vision. The cell station in the pretectal nucleus is not shown. G = lateral geniculate nucleus; S = superior colliculus; III = oculomotor nucleus; V = posterior horn of lateral ventricle; O.R. = optic radiations.

the immediately retrolaminar nerve is usually described with it as follows:

1. the superficial nerve fibre layer, a prelaminar zone anterior to the level of Bruch's membrane (pars retinalis) (Figs 15.2 and 15.4);
2. the prelaminar zone level with the choroid (pars choroidalis);
3. the lamina cribrosa (pars scleralis);
4. the retrolaminar portion immediately behind the lamina.

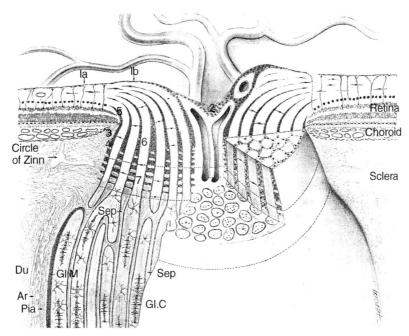

Fig. 15.2 Drawing of the intraocular and part of the orbital optic nerve. The Müller cells (1a) are in continuity with the astrocytes where the retina terminates at the optic disc edge. The Müller cells form the internal limiting membrane of Elschnig (1b). In some specimens, Elschnig's membrane is thickened in the central part of the disc to form the central meniscus of Kuhnt (2). At the posterior termination of the choroid on the temporal side, the border tissue of Elschnig (3) lies between the astrocytes surrounding the optic nerve canal (4) and the stroma of the choroid. On the nasal side choroidal stroma is directly adjacent to the astrocytes surrounding the nerve. This collection of astrocytes (4) surrounding the canal is known as the border tissue of Jacoby. This is continuous with a similar glial lining called the intermediary tissue of Kuhnt (5) at the termination of the retina. Astrocytes (6) segregate the nerve fibres of optic nerve into approximately 1,000 fascicles. Upon reaching the lamina cribrosa (upper dotted line), the nerve fascicles (7) and their surrounding astrocytes are separated by connective tissue. This connective tissue is a cribriform plate which is an extension of scleral collagen and elastic fibres through the nerve. The external choroid also sends some connective tissue to the anterior part of the lamina. At the external part of the lamina cribrosa (lower dotted line) the nerve fibres become myelinated and columns of oligodendrocytes (black and white cells) and a few astrocytes are present within the fascicles. The astrocytes surrounding the fascicles form a thinner layer here than in the laminar and prelaminar portion. Bundles continue to be separated by connective tissue all the way to the chiasm. This connective tissue is derived from the pia mater and is known as the septal tissue (Sep). A mantle of astrocytes (Gl.M) is continuous anteriorly with the border tissue of Jacobi, and surrounds the nerve along its course. The dura (Du), and arachnoid (Ar) and pia mater (Pia) are shown. The central retinal vessels are surrounded by a perivascular connective tissue throughout its course in the nerve; this connective tissue blends with that of the cribriform plate in the lamina cribrosa. Here, it is called the central supporting connective tissue strand. (From Anderson, D. and Hoyt, W. (1969) *Arch. Ophthalmol.* **82**, 506, with permission.)

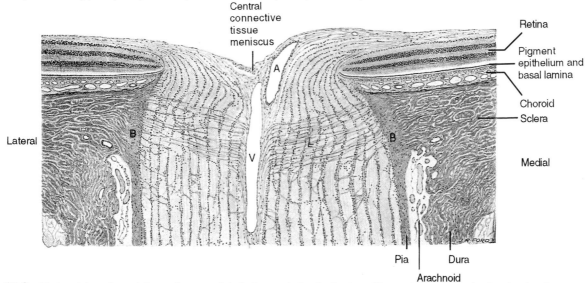

Fig. 15.3 Horizontal section of the optic nerve head. A = central retinal artery; V = central retinal vein; B = border tissue; L = lamina cribrosa.

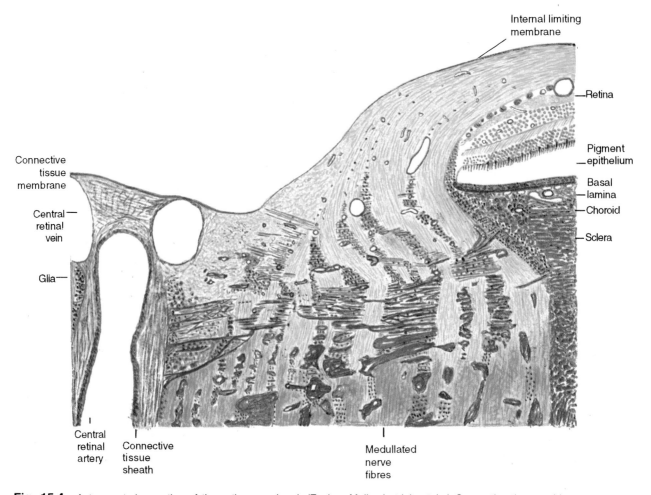

Fig. 15.4 Anteroposterior section of the optic nerve head. (Zenker, Mallory's triple stain.) Connective tissue – blue; non-medullated nerve fibres – light red; medullated nerve fibres – darker red; neuroglia – darkest red. Note that the anterior portion of the lamina cribrosa is glial; the posterior consists of alternating layers of glia and connective tissue, but mainly the latter. Glia separates the anterior portion of the sclera and the whole thickness of choroid from the nerve fibres and is continued anteriorly behind the basal lamina (hyaloid membrane) and pigment epithelium to form the 'intermediary tissue' of Kuhnt. This lies in the concavity of the nerve fibres as they sweep into the nerve.

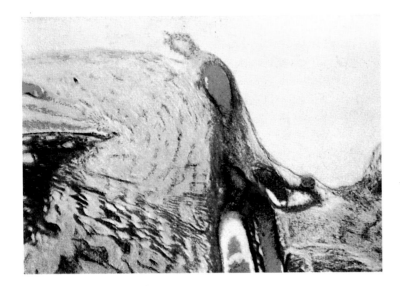

Fig. 15.5 Section across the optic nerve head. (Mallory's triple stain.) Red-staining glia covers the physiological cup. Note remains of the hyaloid artery.

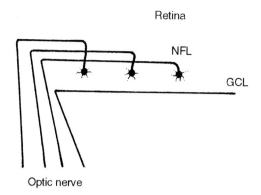

Retina

NFL

GCL

Optic nerve

Fig. 15.6 Anterior–posterior organization of ganglion cell axons projecting from peripheral middle and peripapillary retina to the optic nerve. NFL = nerve fibre layer; GCL = ganglion cell layer. The representation of axon lamination in the retina is speculative. (From Minckler, D. S. (1980) *Arch. Ophthalmol.*, **98**, 1630, with permission.)

fibres, which constitute almost one-third of the whole nerve (whereas the macular area is only one-twentieth of that of the retina), are placed laterally in the nerve, occupying a wedge-shaped area; but as the chiasma is approached they insinuate themselves so that near the chiasma they are centrally placed (Fig. 347,B). Retinotopic organization tends to become less precise, towards the chiasm.

Prelaminar zone

The prelaminar region contains bundles of axons lying within astrocytic channels (Fig. 15.8). The astrocytic processes are largely circumferential. Although Wolter (1957) described glial processes around axonal bundles and between individual axons here, Anderson (1969) found only occasional processes passing through at right-angles to the

fibres. This loose glial tissue does not bind the axon bundles together as do the Müller cells of the retina and therefore fibres here are more easily separated. This may explain why the disc swells so easily in papilloedema while the adjacent retina does not.

The trabeculae between the axon bundles carry capillaries, most of which are surrounded by a narrow perivascular connective tissue space (Anderson, 1969). A limiting membrane formed from glial footplates surrounds this region (Hayreh and Vrabec, 1966).

The presence of glial cells in this (as in other parts of the optic nerve) accords with its development. The optic peduncle is predominantly neuroglial before optic nerve fibres grow into it. Moreover, when the hyaloid artery (which arises from the arteria centralis) degenerates, the neuroglial cells surrounding its origin persist anteriorly as an astrocytic lamella, the **central tissue meniscus of Kuhnt**. This is in continuity with the inner limiting membrane at the surface of the disc and with glial tissue surrounding the adventitia of the central vessels (**the intercalary tissue of Elschnig** (Elschnig, 1901)).

The only connective tissue located on the disc is that sparse amount associated with the central vessels and the capillaries running between the axon bundles. Astrocytes are the only glial cells found in the prelaminar part of the nerve head. Oligodendrocytes, which in the central nervous system are responsible for formation of the myelin sheaths, are found only in the myelinated part of the nerve, behind the lamina cribrosa. The astrocytes form a shallow, cap-like 'wicker basket' which supports the axon bundles and performs a protective and nutritive function. The basket is closely connected to the lamina cribrosa and forms a rounded convexity towards the vitreal surface of the nerve head (Wolter,

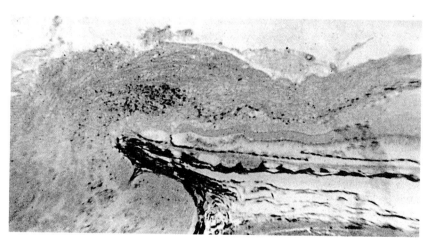

Fig. 15.7 Margin of the optic disc and adjacent retina of a rabbit with a peripheral retina lesion inflicted one month previously. (Marchi.) Degenerating fibres as shown by the Marchi technique are deep in the nerve-fibre layer and peripheral at the nerve-head. (From Wolff E. and Penman, C. G. (1950) *Proc. Int. Cong. Ophthalmol. Lond.*, **2**, 625, with permission.)

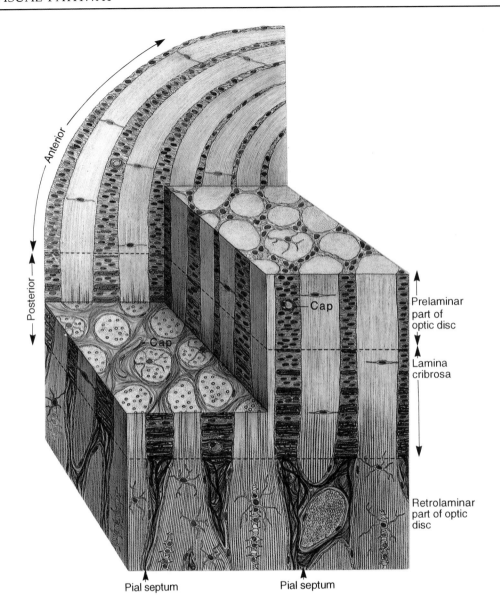

Fig. 15.8 Detailed view of the prelaminar, laminar and postlaminar optic nerve. In the prelaminar region the nerves coming from the retina become segregated into bundles that are invested with a tube-like layer of astrocytes. The astrocytes and their processes are oriented perpendicular to the nerve bundles. Capillaries course within the astrocytic tubes in the prelaminar region. As the lamina cribrosa is reached (upper dotted line), the nerve fascicles are separated from each other by a layer of astrocytes, which in turn is covered by a mantle of connective tissue containing collagen, elastic fibres, fibroblasts and capillaries. In the posterior lamina cribrosa (lower dotted line), the nerves become myelinated, and columns of oligodendrocytes and a few astrocytes are found within the fascicles. The astrocytes separating the nerve fascicles in the laminar and postlaminar regions form a thinner layer than in the prelaminar portion. The connective tissue of the lamina cribrosa is continuous posteriorly with the pial septae. (From Anderson, D., *Arch. Ophthal.* (1969) **82**, 506, with permission.)

1957). Hayreh and Vrabec (1966) did not observe an anterior limit to this basket.

As in other parts of the optic nerve, neuroectodermal derivatives are at all times separated from connective tissue elements by glial cells (Anderson, Hoyt and Hogan, 1967). The only exception appears to be the unmyelinated fibres which are found enclosed within the adventitia of the central retinal artery within the intraorbital portion of the optic nerve (Ikui, Tominaga and Mimura, 1964). Thus, at the periphery of the prelaminar part of the optic nerve, the axons are separated from the connective tissue of the scleral canal and/or choroid by a cuff of astrocytes of varying thickness, termed the **border**

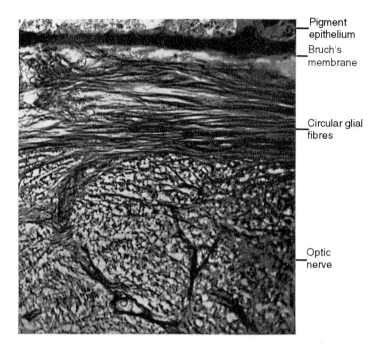

Pigment epithelium
Bruch's membrane
Circular glial fibres
Optic nerve

Fig. 15.9   Transverse section of edge of optic nerve at level of Bruch's membrane. (Zenker, Mallory's triple stain.)

tissue of Jacoby. It then extends forwards to intervene between prelaminar axons and the termination of the posterior retinal layers, as the intermediary tissue of Kuhnt. Here it appears as a mass of nuclei and circular fibres in the concavity of the stratum opticum as it curves round the edge of the disc to enter the optic nerve (Figs 15.15 and 15.20). This glial cuff may in turn be traced backwards across the periphery of the lamina cribrosa in continuity with the **glial mantle** of the intraorbital part of the nerve where it lies immediately deep to the pia mater (Figs 15.4, 15.8 and 15.9).

The rim of sclera at the scleral foramen is termed the **border tissue of Elschnig**. It is sometimes prolonged forwards, especially on the temporal side, to intervene between the peripapillary choroid and the glial, border tissue of Jacoby. It is composed of dense collagenous tissue with many glial and elastic fibres and some pigment (Salzmann, 1912).

Some further comment can be made here about the glial cells of the central nervous system.

Astrocytes are of two types, varying in size, morphology and location. These are:

Protoplasmic astrocytes which range in size from 10 to 40 μm. They are found frequently in grey matter in relation to capillaries and have clearer cytoplasm than fibrous astrocytes. They contain 9 nm glial filaments, microtubules 24 nm in diameter, glycogen, and organelles such as lysosomes and lipofuscin-like bodies. Various morphological sub-types exist.

Fibrous astrocytes contain glial filaments (9 nm in diameter) which are distinguished from neurofilaments by their close packing and by an absence of side arms. Desmosomal and gap junctions exist between neighbouring astrocytes, particularly among the subpial astrocytes which exhibit specialized membrane thickenings in relation to the blood vessels.

Functions of astrocytes

Astrocytes have six main functions:

1. They provide physical support for neurons.
2. They isolate the synaptic regions and the neuronal perikarya.
3. They have an important role in repair. Both types of astrocyte proliferate and swell, and accumulate glycogen, in response to injury. They express greater amounts of glial fibrillary protein (GFAP) and proceed to produce a state of diffuse or focal gliosis leading to the formation of a glial scar. Fibrous astrocytosis may occur in both grey and white matter.
4. The astrocytic glia are the most resistant cells of the CNS, although they are damaged in alcoholism.
5. They may have an important functional role in the blood–brain barrier.
6. They provide a protective function to the CNS by the active transport of selected molecules, such

as potassium, from the extracellular space into the neuronal capillary.

Oligodendrocyte somata are about 10–20 μm wide. These cells are more globular and have a denser cytoplasm than that of the astrocytes. The cellular characteristics of oligodendrocytes include few cytoplasmic processes, abundant organelles, lack of GFAP and 24 nm microtubules which frequently marginate the cell and extend into the cytoplasmic loops of the myelin sheaths. Desmosomes and gap junctions occur between interfascicular oligodendrocytes.

Three classes of oligodendrocyte are described: Satellite cells are small (10 nm wide), restricted to grey matter and closely applied to neurons. Potentially myelinating cells are interfascicular in location, larger during myelination (20 μm wide), and smaller (10–15 μm wide) in the mature nervous sytem. Intermediate cells also exist.

The role of the oligodendrocyte is in myelinogenesis, during which process there are connections between the glial cell body and the nerve sheath. However, unlike its Schwann cell counterpart in the peripheral nervous system, this connection is lost in the adult. A single myelinated oligodendrocyte may produce multiple myelinated internodes, for instance, 30–50 such internodes in the optic nerve.

Oligodendrocytes have a low mitotic rate and a poor regenerative capacity. The cell soma supports many times its own volume of membrane and cytoplasm, so that the ratio between the surface area of the soma and the myelin it sustains may be in the region of 1:3000.

Lamina cribrosa

The lamina cribrosa forms a band of dense compact connective tissue across the scleral foramen (Fig. 15.10). Its sieve-like arrangement (the cribriform plate) transmits the axon bundles of the nerve and the central retinal vessels, through a series of round or oval apertures embraced by strong trabeculae (Figs 15.4, 15.8, 15.10–15.14). Its trabecular structure derives from the disposition of collagen bundles connecting the sclera across this foramen.

The structure of the lamina cribrosa is illuminated by its development, which posteriorly is like that of the optic nerve septa. Each trabecula results from the ingrowth of a branch of the short ciliary arteries or circle of Zinn, accompanied by glia and scleral connective tissue. Each trabecula, therefore, has a vessel in it surrounded by collagen bundles and elastic fibres. External to this are glial cells, which line the trabecular beams and separate the axon bundles

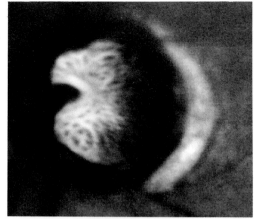

(a)

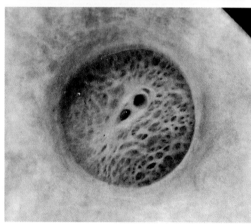

(b)

Fig. 15.10 (a) Imaging of the human lamina cribrosa in vivo. The figure shows the pores of the lamina cribrosa imaged with the Zeiss confocal scanning laser ophthalmoscope in a patient with primary open angle glaucoma. A series of 64 images was digitized by computer, aligned to compensate for eye movements, averaged and the contrast stretched to improve image quality. In normal imaging these structures are difficult to discern because the neural substance diffuses the light and reduces the contrast. By taking narrow optical sections with confocal imaging, the deeper layers of the optic nerve head can be imaged at higher contrast. (Courtesy of F. W. Fitzke and A. Bhandari.) (b) Digested right optic nerve head viewed from the vitreous side by light microscopy. Superior nerve head above. Largest laminar pores are found at upper and lower poles. Original magnification ×50. (From Quigley, H. A. and Addicks, E. M. (1980) *Arch. Ophthalmol.*, **99**, 137, with permission.)

from direct contact with scleral connective tissue (Anderson, Hoyt and Hogan, 1967). Interaxonal glial processes constitute about 40% of the total tissue mass within individual axonal bundles (Minckler, McLean and Tso, 1976).

The anterior part of the lamina cribrosa has been said to consist of astrocytes but these are merely accumulated between nerve fibre fascicles in the prelaminar part of the nerve, suggesting such an interpretation in stained sections (Fig. 15.13). Posteriorly, it attaches to the connective tissue septa of

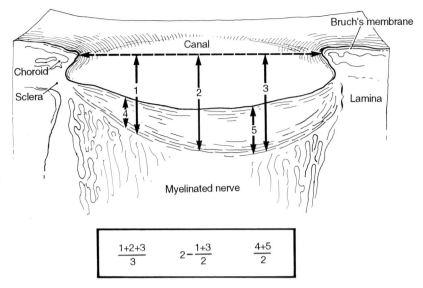

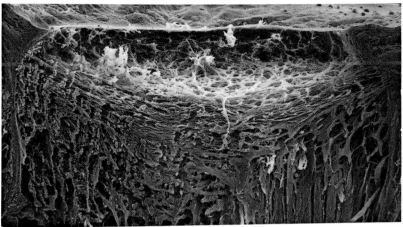

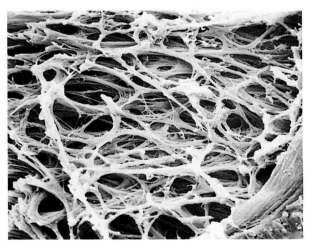

Fig. 15.11 Sectional view of optic nerve head in glaucoma. (From Quigley, H. A. (1983) *et al.*, *Am. J. Ophthalmol.*, **95**, 673, with permission.)

Fig. 15.12 Partial view of a digested optic nerve head with the nasal part at the upper right and the inferior below (SEM). Laminar sheets at lower pole are thinner and sparser, leading to larger pores here compared to the nasal periphery or central zone. Original magnification ×250. (From Quigley, M. A. and Addicks, E. M. (1981) *Arch. Ophthalmol.*, **99**, 137, with permission.)

the retrolaminar nerve and has been regarded simply as a continuation of this framework. The histological transition between the lamina and prelaminar zones is gradual: the striking, angular, collagen-rich septa give way to a fine reticulin structure dominated increasingly by glial cells (Lieberman, Maumenee and Green, 1976).

The bulk of the lamina cribrosa is made up of a series of 3–10 dense connective tissue sheets, the cribriform plates, which blend peripherally with the sclera and alternate with a series of glial sheets in a lamellar fashion. Posteriorly the sheets are more prominent. The most posterior are directed posterointernally to the central connective tissue, level with the surface of the globe to form a V, concave forwards (Fig. 15.4). More anterior sheets extend more directly inwards but are still concave anteriorly. At the posterior boundary of the lamina a thick trabecula often emerges from the sclera, containing a large artery with much muscle and elastic tissue, a strong muscularis and well-marked elastica.

Border tissue

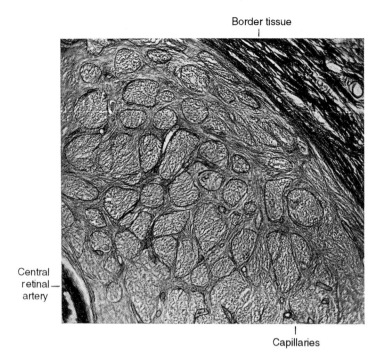

Central
retinal —
artery

Capillaries

Fig. 15.13 Transverse section through the anterior prelaminar part of the optic nerve. (Zenker, Mallory's triple stain.)

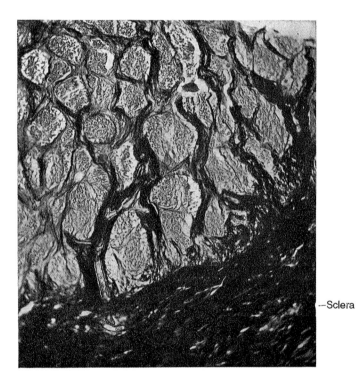

—Sclera

Fig. 15.14 Transverse section through the lamina cribrosa. (Zenker, Mallory's triple stain.) The elasto-collagenous trabeculae correspond in pattern to the neuroglial arrangement in the prelaminar region (Wolff's preparation.)

The pores which admit the axon bundles are not of uniform size across the lamina. Scanning microscopy has demonstrated that the largest pores are found above and below, implying that there is less structural support for the nerve bundles in this region (Quigley and Addicks, 1981) (Fig. 15.10). Radius and Gonzales (1981) have confirmed a regional variation in the distribution of supportive glial and connective tissue between nerves of different individuals. In general, there was a greater tissue density circumferentially than axially, though in some nerves tissue density was distributed fairly uniformly. Where an increased density was found it was in the horizontal meridian and often denser nasally than temporally.

In some nerves there was a deficiency of support tissue superiorly and inferiorly. Both groups of authors suggest that the regional variation in density of support determines the location of the early backward bowing and collapse of sheets of the lamina in chronic simple glaucoma (Quigley *et al.*, 1981, 1983, 1986; Vrabec, 1976).

Immunohistochemical investigations have revealed that the cribriform plates consist of a core of elastin fibres together with sparsely distributed type III collagen fibrils, and are coated by type IV collagen and laminin (Hernandez *et al.*, 1987). The mRNA for type IV collagen is expressed by astroglial cells as well as by cells within the plates, in the glial columns, pial septae, and vascular walls (Hernandez *et al.*, 1991). However, the mRNAs for collagen types I and III are expressed only by cells of the cribriform plates in the adult human lamina cribrosa (Hernandez *et al.*, 1991, 1994). The elastin fibres are oriented longitudinally in the plates and with age, become thicker and tubular in appearance and surrounded by densely packed collagen fibres (Hernandez, 1992). Age-dependent increases in collagen types I, III, and IV also occur (Hernandez *et al.*, 1989).

Retrolaminar portion

The retrolaminar nerve axons are myelinated, unlike those of the retina and nerve head proper. The change is not abrupt, for some fibres lose their myelin sheath proximal to and some distal to the posterior face of the lamina cribrosa (Figs 15.4 and 15.15). Developmentally, myelination proceeds anteriorly in the optic nerve and ceases postnatally at the nerve head. Occasional patches of myelination are found in the prelaminar part of the optic nerve or even within the retina at a distance from the nerve head. Myelination accounts almost entirely for the doubling of nerve diameter from 1.5 to 3.0 mm after traversing the lamina cribrosa; however, glial cell numbers also increase in a centripetal direction (Minckler, McLean and Tso, 1976).

The retrolaminar nerve is part of the intraorbital optic nerve, and as such is invested in a thick sheath of dura, arachnoid and pia mater. The nerve bundles lie in polygonal spaces formed by connective tissue septa (Figs 15.16 and 15.17). These septa are attached to pia peripherally, the lamina anteriorly and the connective tissue adventitia of the central retinal vessels centrally; they carry blood vessels to the optic nerve. The axons are separated from the vessels and other connective tissue by an astroglial layer at all times.

Within the axon bundles are rows of supporting astrocytes, oligodendrocytes (responsible for formation of myelin sheaths) and scattered microglial (reticuloendothelial) cells as seen elsewhere in the optic nerve (Figs 15.18 and 15.19).

The nerve axons show an increase in average diameter at the level of the lamina cribrosa and there are focal constrictions and expansions as they pass through the cribriform plate (Minckler, 1980).

The nerve head has important relations to neighbouring structures.

Relation to neighbouring retina

The layers of the retina, except the stratum opticum, are separated from the optic nerve by the **inter-**

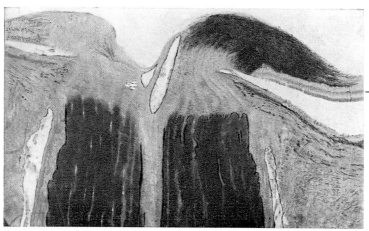

Retina with medullated nerve fibres

Fig. 15.15 Section of the optic nerve to show congenitally-medullated nerve fibres in the retina. (Weigert's stain.) Note that the normal medullation stops behind the lamina cribrosa, in which region the fibres are non-medullated. (From a section kindly supplied by Mr Percy Fleming.)

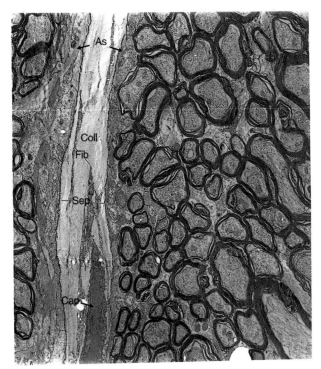

Fig. 15.16 Monkey optic nerve with myelinated fibres of various sizes. Astroglial tissue (As) forms a complete lining for septum (Sep) composed of collagen (Coll), fibroblasts (Fib) and capillaries (Cap). Original magnification ×8,300. (From Anderson, D. and Hoyt, W. (1969) *Arch. Ophthalmol.*, **82**, 506, with permission.)

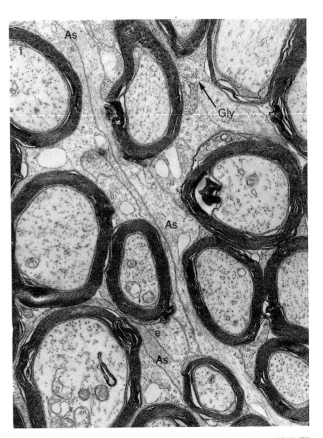

Fig. 15.17 Human optic nerve astrocyte processes (As) fill spaces between myelinated axons cut in cross-section; some contain glycogen (Gly). Note labelled internal (i) and external (e) mesaxons of myelin sheaths. Original magnification ×25,000. (From Anderson, D. and Hoyt, W. (1969) *Arch. Ophthalmol.*, **82**, 506, with permission.)

mediary tissue of Kuhnt (Figs 15.2, 15.4 and 15.20). These glial cells lack tight junctions and therefore no blood–brain barrier exists between the peripapillary choriocapillaris and the optic nerve head at this level, as indicated in primates by tracer studies (Tso, Shih and McLean, 1975) (Fig. 15.21). This probably explains the late fluorescence of the nerve head which occurs with fundus fluorescein angiography. It is said that this tissue can be seen with the ophthalmoscope, but neuroglia is transparent and the tissue is covered by the stratum opticum as it curves into the optic nerve (however, its bulk can be appreciated in stereoscopic viewing). In this region optic nerve fibres are in fasciculi, separated by columns of neuroglial nuclei, processes and vessels. Rarely, individual fibres have extremely fine glial processes around them.

The discal boundary of the retina is usually oblique, and more so nasally, where it may be vertical. The inner layers end before the outer. Rods and cones diminish to half the normal size, and cease before the pigment epithelium which reaches almost to the intermediary tissue. The basal lamina may be separated from the nerve fibres merely by glia. The retina may fall short enough of the disc to expose the choroid which is visible ophthalmoscopically as a pigmented **choroidal crescent**. A localized accumulation of retinal pigment epithelium may cause a similar crescent. Where both choroid and retina fall short of the nerve, a pale **scleral crescent** may be seen ringed by pigment; this is a common feature of the myopic eye (Fig. 15.22).

Relation to neighbouring choroid

The posterior termination of the choroid correlates with variations in the profiles of the scleral canal; it may be oblique, pointed, or almost rectangular in section. The two layers of the basal lamina of Bruch's membrane end almost together, at the entry of the nerve. The pigment epithelium continues almost as far, but rods and cones disappear earlier (Fig. 15.4). The vascular choroidal stroma ends further from the disc than the basal laminae of Bruch's membrane, the capillaries reaching nearer than the layer of smaller vessels (Figs 15.4 and 15.20). The non-vascular stroma is dense and contains

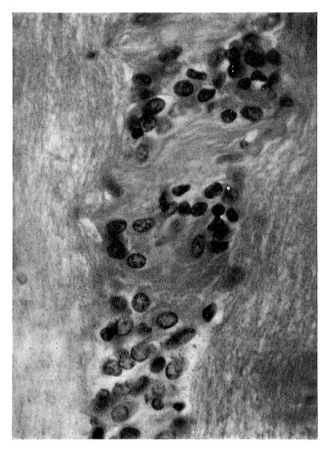

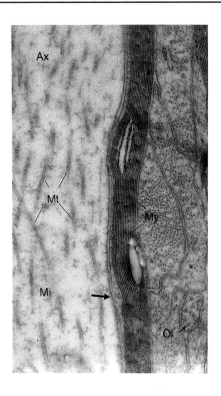

Fig. 15.18 Normal optic nerve (original magnification ×220). (Masson's stain.) Longitudinal section. Columns of glial nuclei. Note pale and dark types.

Fig. 15.19 Human optic nerve in longitudinal section at high magnification. Axoplasm (Ax) contains microtubules (Mt) and a mitochrondrion (Mi). Note small amount of oligodendroglial cytoplasm (arrows) just within myelin (My). Oligodendrocyte processes (Ol) identifiable by presence of microtubules. Remaining processes are astrocytes and contain many tonofilaments. Original magnification ×51,000. (From Anderson, D. and Hoyt, W. (1969) *Arch. Ophthalmol.*, **82**, 506, with permission.)

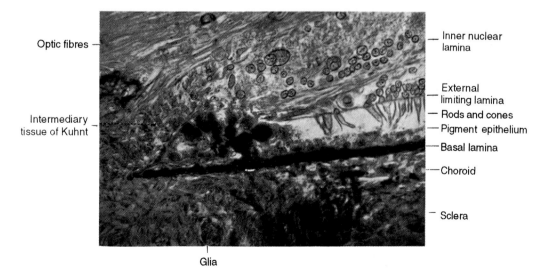

Fig. 15.20 Edge of optic nerve (anteroposterior section). Drüsen have formed on the basal lamina.

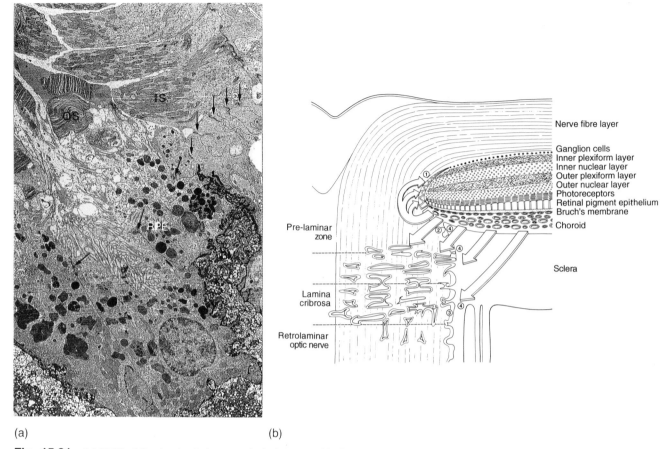

(a)   (b)

Fig. 15.21 (a) TEM of the border between retinal pigment epithelium and glia (intermediary tissue of Kuhnt) at the border of the optic nerve head, five minutes after the intravenous injection of horseradish peroxidase in the rhesus monkey. A series of tight junctions are seen (thin arrows) between adjoining glial cells and also a pigment epithelial cell. Tracer material (heavy arrows) permeates between glial cells but is prevented by the tight junctions from entering the subretinal space. RPE, retinal pigment epithelium; BM, Bruch's membrane; IS, inner segment of photoreceptor cells; OS, outer segment (original magnification ×17.92). (Courtesy of AFIP.) (b) Schematic diagram of the blood–brain barrier at the optic nerve head. Plasma proteins may leak readily from the choroid via the highly fenestrated choriocapillaris and into the nerve head across the sclera, through the glial mantle, and directly, at the level of the choroid. Entry of proteins into the retina is blocked by the presence of a series of tight junctions between the lining glial cells and the adjacent pigment epithelium. (From Tso, M. O. M., Shih, C.-Y. and McLean, I. W. (1975) *Arch. Ophthalmol.*, **93**, 815, with permission.)

many pigment cells. Pigment cells from different sources may thus adjoin on opposite sides of the basal membrane. Stromal lamellae of the choroid do not reach the nerve, being separated by border tissue. The suprachoroidal laminae between sclera and choroid proper, but near the optic nerve, become meridional and parallel with sclera. Pigmentation is also dense nearer the nerve.

Relation to neighbouring sclera

Near the optic nerve most internal scleral fibres are meridional; intermediate fibres are meridional and circular and the most superficial are circular. The last, approaching the optic nerve, interlace with the outer longitudinal fibres of the dura as they do at the limbus with the cornea. Pigment cells increase towards the optic nerve. The marginal tissue (of Elschnig) (Figs 15.4, 15.9, 15.23 and 15.24) is an annular region of neuroglia between choroid, sclera and optic nerve fibres. Basically collagenous, with some glia, it is a scleral derivative, unlike the intermediary tissue (of Kuhnt) and the border tissue (of Jacoby), its backward continuation. Both regions are part of a sleeve of astrocytes around the optic nerve, interrupted only by scleral tissue of the lamina cribrosa. In longitudinal section the marginal tissue is a denser strip around the optic nerve, continued forwards between choroid and nerve fibres: thus nothing other than glia in the eyeball, except the stratum opticum, is in direct contact with the optic nerve itself. Even the basal lamina of the choroid is separated from it by neuroglia (Fig. 15.4).

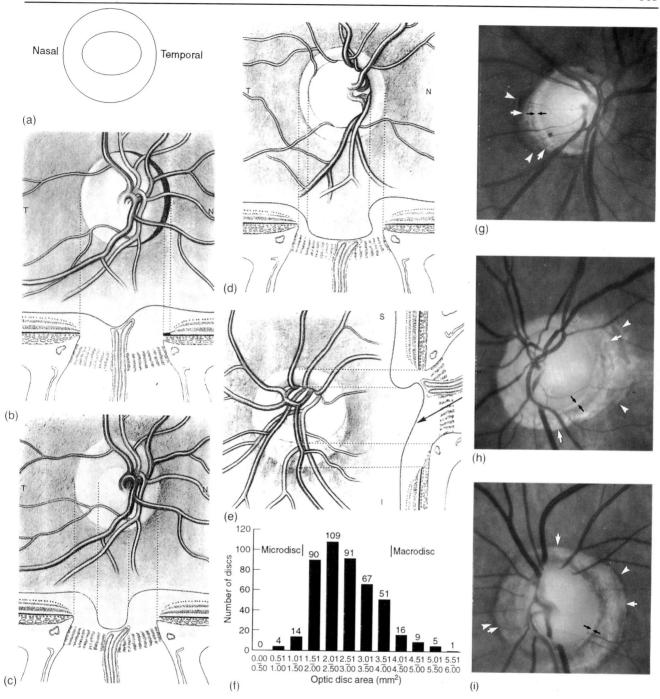

Fig. 15.22 (a) Diagram of the left optic disc. Note that since the cup is horizontally oval, the neuroretinal rim is widest below then above and then nasally. (Modified from Jonas, J. B., Gusek, G. C. and Naumann, G. O. H. (1988) *Invest. Ophthalmol. Vis. Sci.*, **29**, 1151, with permission.) (b) Normal disc with small shallow cup. A hyperpigmented alpha zone is present on the nasal side. (c) Normal right disc with a small cup with steep margins. (d) Primary right macrodisc with large cup. (e) Disc from a myopic eye showing oblique entry of the vessels, which are directed inferiorly. This is associated with a large inferior parapapillary crescent (Fuchs). ((b)–(d) from Hogan, M. J., Alvarado, J. A. and Weddell, J. E. (1971) *Histology of the Human Eye*, published by W. B. Saunders, with permission.) (f) Histogram to show the frequency distribution of disc areas in a group of 450 normal human nerve heads. Macrodiscs are defined as lying two standard deviations above the mean, and microdiscs, two standard deviations below the mean, see text for detail. (From Jonas, J. B., Gusek, G. C. and Naumann, G. O. H. (1988) *Invest. Ophthalmol. Vis. Sci.*, **29**, 1156. (g) Right optic nerve head to show the scleral ring (black arrows), zone alpha (arrowheads) and zone beta (short white arrows). There is a small haemorrhage on the neuroretinal rim. (Courtesy of J. Jonas.) (h) Left disc showing glaucomatous enlargement of the cup, a circular circumferential beta zone (white arrows) and a faint irregular alpha zone (arrowheads). The scleral ring lies between black arrows. (Courtesy of J. Jonas.) (i) Left disc showing a large glaucomatous cup, a broad circular beta zone (white arrows), faint alpha zones present as fringes (arrowheads) and the scleral ring (black arrows). (Courtesy of J. Jonas.)

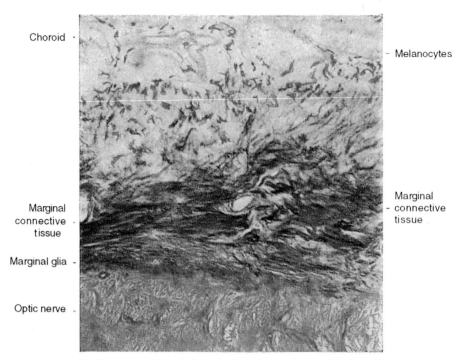

Choroid

Melanocytes

Marginal connective tissue

Marginal connective tissue

Marginal glia

Optic nerve

Fig. 15.23   Transverse section of optic nerve a little posterior to Bruch's membrane. (Zenker, Mallory's triple stain.)

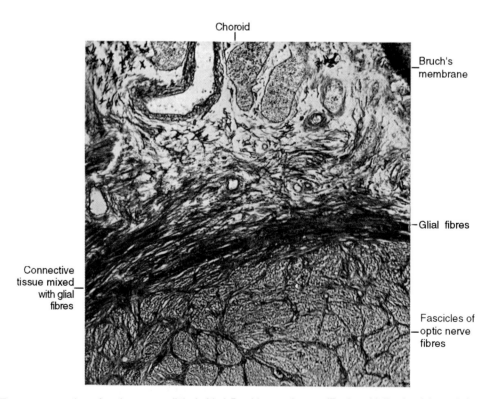

Choroid

Bruch's membrane

Glial fibres

Connective tissue mixed with glial fibres

Fascicles of optic nerve fibres

Fig. 15.24   Transverse section of optic nerve a little behind Bruch's membrane. (Zenker, Mallory's triple stain.)

Scleral canal

The scleral canal is bounded by the border tissue, which separates nerve fibres from choroid and sclera. About 0.5 mm in length, it may be straight or directed slightly nasally, temporally, or downwards.

Three shapes of scleral canal are recognizable: a cone narrowest at the basal lamina; narrowing to the inner third of the sclera, and uniform beyond this; hourglass-shaped, with a 'waist' in the intermediate third of the sclera. In the first two shapes a scleral ring is present, visible by ophthalmoscopy.

Ophthalmoscopic features of the optic nerve head (Fig. 15.22)

That part of the nerve head visible with the ophthalmoscope is termed the **optic disc**. Its intrapapillary parts are the **optic cup** and the **neuroretinal rim**, which are separated, by the **scleral ring** of Elschnig, from a zone of parapapillary atrophy variably present on the temporal side. The scleral ring represents the border tissue of the nerve. The definition of intra- and parapapillary structures is discussed by Jonas, Gusek and Naumann (1988). Features such as disc, cup and rim areas or diameters and vessel width do not correlate with age after the age of 10 to 15 years, or with sex, or side in eyes with refractive errors within the range ±5 dioptres.

Optic disc colour

The pink colour of the disc is due to the rich capillary supply to its rim, which can be demonstrated by fluorescein angiography. This is most noticeable inferotemporally where the rim is widest. The white appearance of the cup is due to scattering of light by the lamina cribrosa and the sparse vascularity of this region. There is little light-scattering by the nerve axons themselves, which are unmedullated and relatively transparent. Nerve fibre loss in chronic glaucoma leads to increasing exposure of the lamina as axons are lost so that its pores become more visible as the cup enlarges.

Disc shape

The optic disc may be round, but is usually oval in shape, its vertical diameter being on average 9% longer than its horizontal. The cup is 8% wider in the horizontal, so that the rim is wider above and below (Fig. 15.22; Table 15.1).

Disc size

Normal disc area ranges widely, from 0.86 mm^2 to 5.54 mm^2 with a mean of 2.69 ± 0.7 mm^2 (Jonas, Gusek and Naumann, 1988). Ophthalmoscopically, the disc corresponds in size to the internal opening of the scleral canal. The distribution of areas is nearly gaussian in eyes with refractive errors lying between ±5 dioptres (Fig. 15.22) but at each end of this range Jonas and Naumann (1991) have identified primary **macrodiscs**, whose areas lie greater than two standard deviations above the mean (>4.09 mm^2), and **microdiscs** whose areas are less than two standard deviations below (<1.29 mm^2). Primary macrodiscs may be associated with conditions such as pits of the optic nerve 'Morning Glory' syndrome. Secondary macrodiscs are associated with the acquired globe enlargement which accompanies high myopia and buphthalmos and may reach up to 20 mm^2 in area. A difference in area of 0.1 mm^2 or less between the two sides occurs in 28% of normal subjects, of 0.2 mm^2 or less in 46% and of 0.5 mm^2 or less in 84% of normal subjects.

Certain morphological features of the disc may predispose to optic nerve head disease. Small optic discs have a smaller number of optic nerve fibres than large discs and a smaller scleral canal

Table 15.1

Optic disc	Mean	+/−	Range
Disc area (mm^2)	2.69	0.7	0.86–5.54
Disc width (mm)			
horizontal	1.76	0.31	0.91–2.61
vertical	1.92	0.29	0.96–2.91
Cup area (mm^2)	0.72	0.70	0.0–3.41
Cup diameter (mm)			
horizontal	0.92	0.48	0.0–2.08
vertical	0.84	0.47	0.0–2.13
Cup volume' (mm^3)			
median	0.279	0.012	
average	0.342	0.013	0.126–0.675
Cup depth' (mm)			
median	0.214	0.027	
average	0.236	0.007	0.123–0.391
Rim area (mm^2)	1.97	0.50	0.80–4.66
Cup/disc ratio			
horizontal	0.51	0.23	0.0–0.87
vertical	0.43	0.21	0.0–0.85
Parapapillary zones			
alpha: frequency	84.4%		
beta: frequency	15.2%		
alpha (mm^2)	0.41	0.37	0.0–2.21
beta (mm^2)	0.13	0.42	0.0–3.65

'From Rohrschneider et al., 1994.
All other data from Jonas, Guesk and Naumann, 1988.

(Quigley, Coleman and Dorman-Pease, 1991; Jonas et al., 1992a). Hence, there is a smaller anatomical reserve. Non-arteritic ischaemic optic neuropathy (Beck et al., 1984) is commoner in smaller optic nerve heads due to problems of vascular perfusion and of limited space. The same is true for optic nerve head drüsen when it is assumed that blockade of orthograde axoplasmic flow is an important factor (Jonas et al., 1987). Pseudopapilloedema is also encountered with smaller optic nerve heads, particularly in highly hypermetropic eyes whose discs are usually of small size.

Various morphological factors may be relevant to axon loss in glaucoma. Rim loss occurs, for instance, in regions furthest from the central retinal trunk (Jonas and Fernandez, 1994). The susceptibility of the superior and inferior disc regions to damage (Quigley et al., 1981a) may be associated with the higher pore-to-disc area in these regions (Quigley and Addicks, 1981; Radius, 1981). The ratio decreases with decreasing optic disc size (Jonas, 1994) which might be thought to be a protective influence in smaller discs. Although large nerve heads have a greater neuronal reserve than small ones, the pressure gradient across the lamina cribrosa is believed to produce more displacement in such discs (Chi et al., 1989). Jonas, Fernández and Naumann (1991) indicated, however, that where there is asymmetry of disc size in patients with chronic glaucoma, there is no difference in susceptibility and it may be that opposing factors also relating to disc size cancel out in effect.

In a histological study by Jonas, Fernández and Naumann (1991) the area of the lamina was 2.88 (± 0.84) mm^2 and ranged from 1.62 to 5.62 mm^2 (ratio 1:3.5). Laminar area was independent of age in those over 15 years, sex, and side. The form was slightly oval, with the vertical slightly longer than the horizontal. Maximal diameter was on average 14% larger than minimal. Histologically, the pore count on the inner surface of the laminar averaged 227 ± 36.00 (168–292) with no age, sex or side differences. The count increases with lamina area. The mean single pore area (0.00387 ± 0.00091 mm^2) and the total pore area was larger in the inferior and superior regions than in the temporal regions. The mean single pore area and total pore areas are greater in the peripheral part of the lamina.

The optic cup

The optic disc is excavated by a funnel-shaped depression, the optic cup, which varies in form and size and is usually off-centre towards the temporal side. Cup area correlates with disc area and, hence, is large in large discs and small in small discs. It is common for the cup to be absent from a small disc.

The cup is usually defined on the basis of contour change in relation to the plane of the rim and this criterion has been used by Jonas and colleagues in photographic studies of the disc. Other workers have chosen to use the pallor of the cup as a basis of definition (Tuulonen et al., 1992; Brigatti and Caprioli, 1995). The cup was absent in one-third of the discs in the study of Jonas, Gusek and Naumann (1988), and such discs were smaller than average. Witusek (1966) found cups to be shallow in 23% of subjects, of medium depth in 31% and deep in 25%. In other studies using the direct ophthalmoscope, the optic cup was present in about 75% of subjects (72%, Ford and Sarwar (1963), 78%, Witusek (1966)) and more commonly present in emmetropes (86%) than in hypermetropes (34%) or myopes (5%) (Bednarski, 1925). The cup tends to be larger in discs with steep, punched out cups (1.37 ± 0.62 mm^2) than in those whose cups have flat temporal slopes (0.59 ± 0.39 mm^2). Mean optic cup area is 0.72 ± 0.7 (0.0–3.41) mm^2.

Recently it has been possible to make three-dimensional measurements of cup shape using stereoscopic techniques or confocal microscopy. Rohrschneider et al. (1994), using the scanning laser ophthalmoscope, found median cup volume to be 0.28 mm^3 and median cup depth 0.63 mm in a group of normal subjects and similar data is reported by Gierek-Lapinska et al. (1995). A comparison of photographic and confocal measurements is reported by Dichtl, Jonas and Mardin (1996). Further data are given in Table 15.1.

The neuroretinal rim

The tissue outside the cup is termed the neuroretinal rim and contains the retinal nerve axons as they enter the nerve head. Rim area ranges from 0.8–4.66 mm^2 (1.97 ± 0.5 mm^2) and correlates with disc area (Jonas, Gusek and Naumann, 1988). It is broadest in the lower segment of the disc, then above, then nasally and then temporally. It is narrowest in the temporal horizontal disc region in 99.2% of all discs. This typical rim configuration correlates with the diameter of the retinal artery and vein, which is larger below and temporal than above and temporal, with the nerve fibre visibility more detectable in the inferior temporal arcade than the superior and with the location of the foveola inferior to the optic disc centre (0.53 ± 0.34 mm below). This implies that there is a greater retinal axonal mass and vascularity in the

the inferotemporal sector. A difference of rim area between the two eyes of 0.1 mm² or less is encountered in 31% of normals, of 0.2 mm² or less in 52% and of 0.5 mm² or less in 84%. Rim area is not correlated with ametropia (±5 dioptres) or with sex or side.

In primary open angle and other forms of chronic glaucoma a progressive loss of retinal ganglion cells occurs. This leads to a characteristic pattern of axonal loss at the neuroretinal rim, with enlargement of the cup, particularly at the upper and lower poles of the disc. The vertically-oval cup of chronic glaucoma contrasts with the horizontally-oval cup of the normal disc. Another characteristic feature of glaucomatous optic nerve damage is the occurrence of flame-shaped haemorrhages on the rim, usually at the inferior or superior temporal margin, an early sign of glaucoma, rarely seen in normal eyes.

Cup/disc ratio

The cup/disc ratio is the ratio of cup and disc width, measured in the same meridian, usually the vertical or horizontal. Because the disc is vertically oval and the cup horizontally oval (Fig. 15.22), the cup/disc ratio is normally lower in the vertical meridan in the majority of individuals (i.e. 93.2% or normals). It increases in chronic glaucoma.

The ratio has a median value of 0.3. It does not differ by more than 0.1 between the two eyes in 92% of subjects, or more than 0.2 in 99% of subjects. Thus as a rule of thumb, an asymmetry of greater than 0.2 has been taken to signify enlargement and to be of diagnostic importance in glaucoma.

In the same way, the vertical ratio is used as a simple index of rim integrity in chronic glaucoma, since earliest tissue losses affect the infero- and supero-temporal parts of the rim. A vertical cup/disc ratio of 0.4 or less is often taken to imply the absence of glaucoma. However, it is important to remember that since the cup/disc ratio correlates with disc area in normals, the size of the disc must be taken into account when assessing the possibility of glaucomatous nerve damage. Since small discs commonly have no cup, the presence of a cup/disc ratio of 0.2–0.3 in a small disc may in fact indicate early glaucomatous nerve damage, whereas in a primary macrodisc, a cup/disc ratio of 0.8 may be entirely normal.

Parapapillary chorioretinal atrophy

A crescentic region of chorioretinal atrophy is a common finding at the temporal margin of normal discs and may be exaggerated in chronic glaucoma

or in high myopia. Two zones of parapapillary chorioretinal atrophy are described, both usually found, if present, at the temporal margin of the disc (Jonas et al., 1989a, 1989b; Jonas, Fernández and Naumann, 1992b). They correspond to the older terms of choroidal and scleral crescent (Hogan, Alvarado and Weddell, 1971) (Fig. 15.22).

Zone alpha is the more peripheral zone and is an irregular hypo- or hyperpigmented region associated histologically with irregularities of the retinal pigment epithelium and parapapillary choiroid. Peripherally, it is adjacent to the retina and centrally, to zone beta if present, or directly to the scleral ring if not. This zone corresponds to the **choroidal crescent**, in which it was envisaged that the pigment epithelium failed to extend to the disc margin. Sometimes a narrow, deeply pigmented crescent is seen, often on the nasal side of the disc, which has been called a **pigment crescent** in the past.

Zone beta is related to the disc centrally and to the retina or zone alpha peripherally. It consists of a marked atrophy of the pigment epithelium and choriocapillaris, with good visibility of the larger choroidal vessels. It corresponds to the **scleral crescent** (Hogan, Alvarado and Wedell, 1971) and is always closer to the optic disc than zone alpha. In the normal nerve head, zone alpha is significantly larger and found more frequently (83.9%) than zone beta (16.3%). Both zones are significantly larger in the temporal horizontal meridian, then inferotemporally, then superotemporally and then in the nasal region. The area of the optic nerve head, scleral ring and parapapillary atrophic zones correlates with the size of the blind spot, zone alpha contributing a relative scotoma and zone beta to an absolute scotoma (Jonas, Fernández and Naumann, 1991).

The zones are larger in total area and individually in the presence of chronic glaucoma, when parapapillary atrophy may surround the disc. In primary open angle glaucoma the area of zone alpha averages 0.65 (±0.49) mm² compared to 0.4 (±0.32) mm² in normal subjects and zone beta averages 0.79 (±1.17) mm² compared to 0.13 (±0.42) mm². Zone beta is found significantly more frequently than in normal subjects. However, there are patients with advanced glaucomatous atrophy who show no abnormal parapapillary atrophy and atrophy may surround the disc in the absence of glaucoma.

Retinal vessels

The retinal vessels emerge on the medial side of the cup, slightly decentred superonasally, the temporal arteries taking an arcuate course as they leave the disc, while the nasal ones take a more direct, though curved course. The course of the veins and arteries is similar but not identical and this avoids excessive shadowing of the rods and cones. The arteries (which are actually of arteriolar size) are narrower and brighter red than the veins and the image of the ophthalmoscope light produces a well-marked light streak along their axes. The light streak on the veins is broader and dimmer. The light reflex is lost in papilloedema as the vessels bend over the elevated disc margin, since the image of the light source is thrown beyond the pupil.

When the scleral canal is straight, the end of the **arteria centralis** is seen in optical section and branches appear to come off at a right angle. If the intraneural part of the optic nerve is directed anterolaterally, the nasal wall of the cup may be steep or overhanging and the arteria centralis may be obscured so that only its first divisions are seen, directed temporally. If the canal is directed anteromedially, the artery is seen for some distance and the vessels are displaced towards the temporal side. In so-called situs inversus of the disc, the scleral canal is directed nasally and the vessel divisions sweep nasally for a considerable distance before assuming their usual course. The condition is frequently associated with a high degree of corneal astigmatism.

In normal eyes, the diameter of the inferior temporal parapapillary vessels is larger than the superior, corresponding to the broader inferior disc, the greater visibility of the retinal nerve fibres below and the location of the foveola inferior to the optic disc centre (0.53 ± 0.34 mm below). Vessel diameter is independent of age (Jonas and Naumann, 1989).

Venous pulsation is observed at the disc in 15–90% of normal subjects (Hedges *et al.*, 1994) and is due to the pulsatile collapse of the veins as ocular pressure rises with arterial inflow into the uvea. Visible retinal arterial pulsation is rare and usually pathological, implying, for example, aortic incompetence or high ocular pressure.

The **retinal nerve fibre layer** is most visible inferotemporally, then superotemporally, then supero- and inferonasally (Jonas *et al.*, 1989d). This correlates with the configuration of the neuroretinal rim, which is broadest inferiorly and then superiorly, and with the juxtapapillary calibres of the retinal vessels, which are widest inferotemporally, then superotemporally and then supero- and inferonasally (Jonas and Schiro, 1993). It also relates to the location of the fovea, below the horizontal. Retinal nerve fibre layer thickness and visibility decreases with age, in keeping with the age-related loss of optic nerve axons (at a rate of about 4–5000 axons per year (Jonas and Naumann, 1991). Axonal loss in experimental glaucoma has been shown to involve apoptosis (at least in part) (Quigley, 1995), and this is likely to be true for age-related loss. Nerve fibre layer thickness is not correlated with sex or side.

Retinal photoreceptor count, surface area and optic disc size were correlated in normal eyes shorter than 26 mm in axial diameter (Panda-Jonas *et al.*, 1994). Eyes with large optic nerveheads have higher rod and cone counts and retinal surface area (Panda-Jonas *et al.*, 1994). This is in keeping with other studies showing a correlation between optic nerve fibre count and disc size.

RELATIONS OF THE OPTIC NERVE IN THE ORBIT (Figs 1.15, 5.18, 5.23)

As the nerve traverses the annular tendon at the optic foramen, the attachments of the superior and medial recti are adherent to its dural sheath: this may explain the pain (in extreme movement) so characteristic of retrobulbar neuritis. Between the nerve and lateral rectus are the oculomotor, nasociliary, sympathetic and abducent nerves and sometimes the ophthalmic vein or veins (Fig. 5.6). Further forwards, orbital fat separates the muscles from the nerve. The nasociliary nerve, ophthalmic artery and superior ophthalmic vein cross the nerve superiorly to its medial side.

The **ciliary ganglion** lies between the nerve and lateral rectus (Figs 5.18, 5.22). The long and short ciliary nerves and arteries gradually surround the nerve as it approaches the back of the eyeball. The **arteria centralis retinae**, a branch of the ophthalmic artery near the optic foramen, runs forwards within or outside the dural sheath and with its vein crosses the subarachnoid space to enter the nerve inferomedially about 12 mm behind the eye. The nerve is oval or crescentic in section where the vessels enter; in two places if they enter separately (Kuhnt, 1890).

RELATIONS OF THE OPTIC NERVE IN THE OPTIC CANAL

The pial sheath is adherent to the nerve. The dura, lining the canal as periosteum, splits at its orbital end to become the periorbita and the dural sheath of the optic nerve. According to Hovelacque (1927) a short sleeve of arachnoid penetrates the cranial end of the canal for 1–2 mm, but is absent beyond this. With slight variations, the intracranial subarachnoid space is continuous with that around the nerve and there-

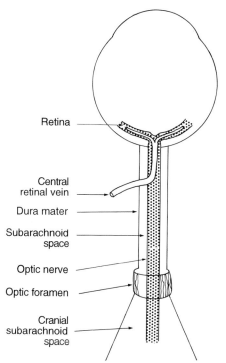

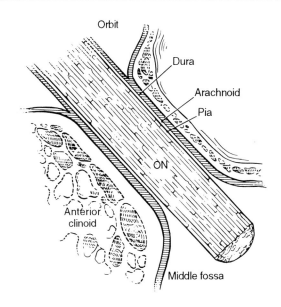

Fig. 15.25 Diagram to show the continuation of the cranial subarachnoid space around the optic nerve. Note how the central vessels cross the space and may be compressed if the intracranial pressure be raised.

Fig. 15.26 Schematic drawing of the optic nerve sheaths showing their relationship to the optic nerve (ON) and to the surrounding sphenoid bone. The dura is tightly adherent to the bone within the optic canal. Within the orbit it divides into two layers, one of which remains as the outer sheath of the optic nerve, the other becoming orbital periosteum (periorbita). Intracranially the dura leaves the optic nerve to become the periosteum of the sphenoid bone. (From Miller, N. R. (1985) *Clinical Neuro-Ophthalmology*, 4th edition, Vol. 1, published by Williams and Wilkins, with permission.)

fore exposes the central retinal vein and artery as they cross the space around the nerve to the cerebrospinal fluid pressure (Figs 15.25 and 15.26). The dura mater, being in part periosteum, is attached to bone. It is variably adherent at some points in the canal to pia mater, thus to some degree fixing the nerve in the canal. This adhesion varies in position and density. If it is superior to the nerve (Schwalbe) the subarachnoid space exists inferior to it, but Hovelacque (1927) stated that adhesion might be anywhere in the circumference of the nerve and that it is usually adjacent to the ophthalmic artery (Fig. 15.27). Weaker trabeculae cross from the dura to pia.

The ophthalmic artery crosses inferolateral to the nerve in the dural sheath and leaves the dura near the anterior end of the canal. Thus the internal carotid artery is to some extent tethered by its ophthalmic branch (Fig. 15.28) and is attached indirectly to the optic nerve by the dural adhesion and branches to it from the ophthalmic artery.

Medial to the nerve is the sphenoidal air sinus (Fig. 15.27) or a posterior ethmoidal sinus, separated by a thin plate of bone, which may explain retrobulbar neuritis as a complication of sinusitis. Occasionally either sinus may invade the roots of the lesser wing of the sphenoid, and even the wing itself, surrounding the nerve.

INTRACRANIAL RELATIONS OF THE OPTIC NERVE

The nerve is superior to, first, the **diaphragma sellae**, then the anterior part of the **cavernous sinus**. Between the nerves and anterior to the chiasma is a triangular space covered by the diaphragma, overlying part of the **hypophysis cerebri**. Above is the **anterior perforated substance, medial root of the olfactory tract**, and **anterior cerebral artery**, which cross superiorly to reach the medial side of the nerve (Figs 15.29 and 15.30). The **internal carotid artery** is then lateral. The **ophthalmic artery** usually leaves the internal carotid under the optic nerve (Fig. 5.18) but, because it is inferoposterior and passes anterolaterally to leave the nerve, it may at first be medial before passing laterally. The nearer the origin of the artery to the optic foramen, the nearer it is to the **medial** side of the nerve (Fig. 15.31).

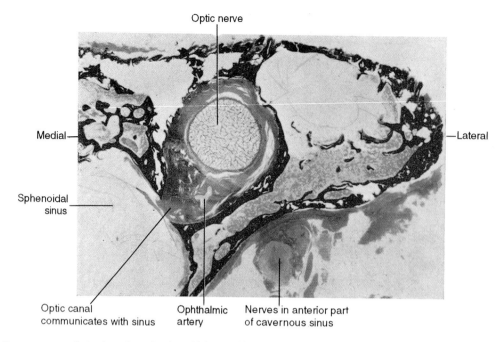

Optic nerve

Medial

Lateral

Sphenoidal
sinus

Optic canal
communicates with sinus

Ophthalmic
artery

Nerves in anterior part
of cavernous sinus

Fig. 15.27 Transverse section of portion of sphenoid bone with optic canal (bone decalcified). Note dense connective tissue around artery.

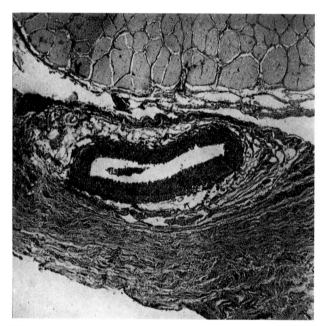

Fig. 15.28 Transverse section of the sheaths of the optic nerve in its canal. The ophthalmic artery is here in the dura mater.

SHEATHS OF THE OPTIC NERVE (Fig. 15.32)

In the cranial cavity the optic nerve is surrounded only by pia, but in the optic canal arachnoid and dura are present. At the optic foramen the cranial dura splits into periosteum (periorbita) and the dural covering of the optic nerve, as already noted. Thus in the canal and in the orbit the nerve is surrounded by sheaths of all three meninges. Between the dura and arachnoid is the so-called **subdural space** and between arachnoid and pia the **subarachnoid space**, both of which communicate with corresponding intracranial spaces. Fluid injected into the cranial subarachnoid space spreads into its perioptic prolongation; accidental injection into the subarachnoid space of the orbital optic nerve may occur during retrobulbar injection of local anaesthetic and give rise to CNS complications. The subdural space, though often seen in microscopic preparations, is an artefact: it is only **potential** and appears chiefly in pathological states.

Dura mater

The dura mater is tough compacted collagen tissue, whose fibres are larger than those of sclera. Among them are numerous elastic fibres. The dura is 0.35–0.5 mm thick, and is thickest where it becomes continuous with the sclera. Its internal fibres are mostly circular, the peripheral (nearest the supravaginal space) are longitudinal and oblique (Fig. 15.33a,b). Most are collagenous, but elastic fibres are interspersed in small numbers. The collagen fibres have a diameter of 600–700 μm, but finer ones occur. The longitudinal outer layer often divides into two to five lamellae, between which are fusiform nuclei, more numerous in childhood, that

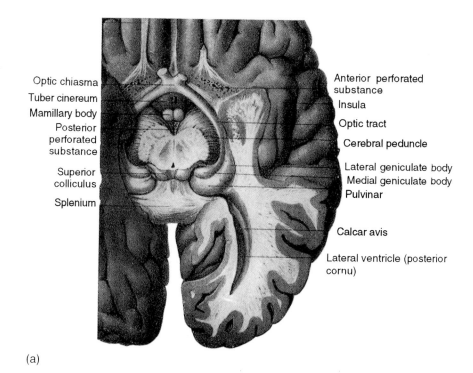

Optic chiasma
Tuber cinereum
Mamillary body
Posterior perforated substance
Superior colliculus
Splenium

Anterior perforated substance
Insula
Optic tract
Cerebral peduncle
Lateral geniculate body
Medial geniculate body
Pulvinar
Calcar avis
Lateral ventricle (posterior cornu)

(a)

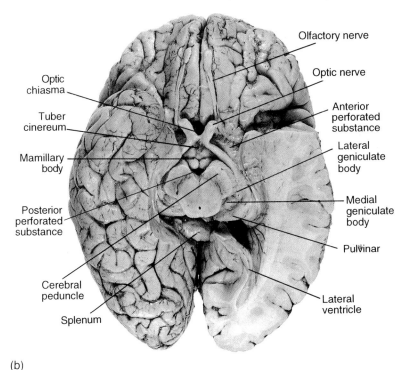

Optic chiasma
Tuber cinereum
Mamillary body
Posterior perforated substance
Cerebral peduncle
Splenum

Olfactory nerve
Optic nerve
Anterior perforated substance
Lateral geniculate body
Medial geniculate body
Pulvinar
Lateral ventricle

(b)

Fig. 15.29 (a) Inferior aspect of the brain. (From Hirschfeld and Leveillé) (b) Inferior aspect of the brain. Similar view to that in (a), with lower part of the temporal lobe and parieto-occipital lobe on the left removed.

belong to flat star-shaped cells in close relation with numerous elastic fibres.

The internal aspect of the dura has a mesothelial lining one (or sometimes two) cells thick. The dura is very easily detached from the underlying arachnoid (Fig. 5.33b). Around the dural sheath of the optic nerve is the so-called **supravaginal space**, described by Schwalbe (1887) as a 'lymph space'. It has, however, the structure of loose connective tissue easily distensible with fluid. There are no orbital lymphatics.

The dura blends imperceptibly with the outer two-thirds of the sclera (Fig. 15.20). Its external fibres enter the sclera and bend acutely at about 110° away

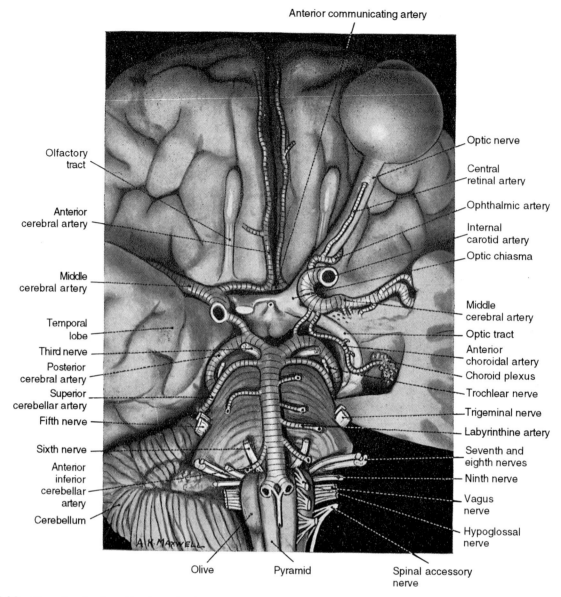

Fig. 15.30 Dissection to show blood supply of optic pathway and relations of vessels to ocular nerves. Basal aspect. (Wolff's preparation.)

from the optic nerve; internal fibres pass in more obliquely.

Arachnoid mater

The arachnoid mater, a very thin layer some 10 μm thick, consists basically of an interrupted core of collagenous tissue covered by several layers of flattened mesothelial (or meningothelial) cells (Fig. 15.34) held together by desmosomes and (rarely) tight junctions, forming a multilaminar membrane in contact with cerebrospinal fluid. Nowhere is the collagen in direct contact with the subarachnoid

space. A faint, discontinuous basal lamina may be present at the external surface of some collagen bundles where they abut the layered mesothelial cells. The external cells tend to proliferate, even forming mesothelial pearls (corpora amylacea) (Fig. 15.35a).

Numerous trabeculae pass to the **pia**, forming a network in the subarachnoid space. Each trabecula consists of collagenous tissue surrounded by mesothelial cells which are in continuity with those of the arachnoid and pia (Fig. 15.35b–d). The mesothelial layer is one or two cells thick, but may be several layers over the larger trabeculae such as

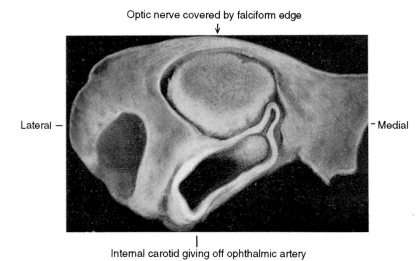

Optic nerve covered by falciform edge

Lateral —   — Medial

Internal carotid giving off ophthalmic artery

Fig. 15.31   Transverse section of portion of the sphenoid bone with the optic canal at the level of the falciform edge. Note the ophthalmic artery is medial here.

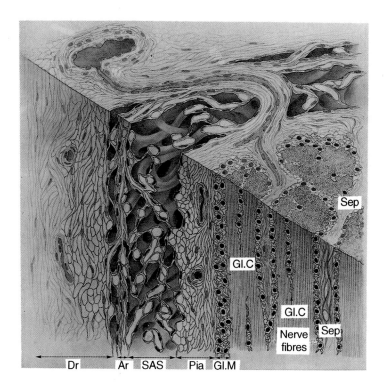

Sep

Gl.C

Gl.C

Nerve
fibres

Sep

Dr   Ar   SAS   Pia   Gl.M

Fig. 15.32   Schematic drawing of vaginal sheaths of human optic nerve, showing relationships of dura mater (Dr), arachnoid mater (Ar), subarachnoid space (SAS), pia mater (Pia), peripheral glial mantle of Fuch's (Gl.M), pial septa (Sep), and glial columns (Gl.C). Meningothelial cells are shown in colour, illustrating how they are the main component of arachnoid mater and form linings for dura mater, arachnoid trabeculae and pia mater. (From Anderson, D. R. (1969b) *Arch. Ophthalmol.*, **82**, 800, with permission.)

those which contain blood vessels; elastin and reticulin fibres also occur. This continuity has led to the concept of a compound pia arachnoid meninx, containing the cerebrospinal fluid. The arachnoid ends at the lamina cribrosa by becoming continuous with the sclera (Fig. 15.3).

Pia mater

The pia mater is composed of loose connective tissue of fibroblasts, collagen, elastin, and reticulin fibres.

Its surface presents mesothelial cells like those of the arachnoid (Fig. 15.36). Its deeper layers, next to the optic nerve, may be of neuroectodermal origin and unite with glial elements, leading to the term 'pia–glia', an astrocytic condensation or glial mantle (Fuchs, 1885; Greeff, 1899).

Numerous pial septa enter the optic nerve, dividing fibres into fascicles (Figs 5.3, 15.37a,b), and it is hence separated from the nerve with difficulty. Numerous vessels in the pia are mostly between its longitudinal and circular fibres: pia is thus much

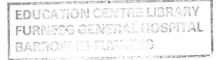

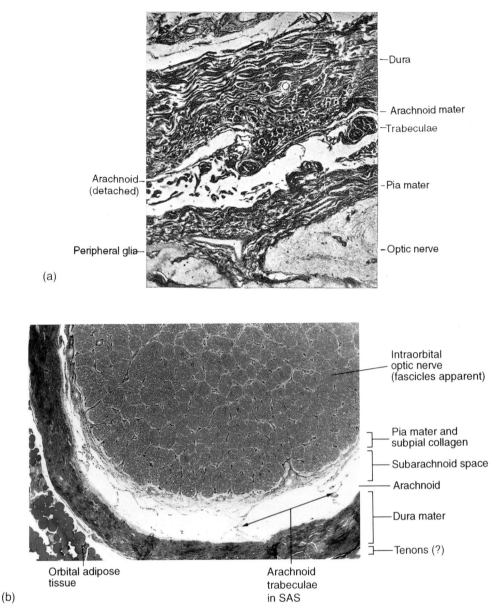

Dura

Arachnoid mater

Trabeculae

Pia mater

Optic nerve

Arachnoid (detached)

Peripheral glia

(a)

Intraorbital optic nerve (fascicles apparent)

Pia mater and subpial collagen

Subarachnoid space

Arachnoid

Dura mater

Tenons (?)

Orbital adipose tissue

Arachnoid trabeculae in SAS

(b)

Fig. 15.33 (a) Longitudinal section of optic nerve sheaths. (b) Low-power micrograph of the intraorbital part of the optic nerve in transverse section. (Courtesy of M. Greaney.)

more vascular than dura. As in the optic nerve itself, the pial vessels have a non-fenestrated endothelium and adjacent endothelial cells are connected by tight junctions. According to Anderson (1969) the mesothelial cells are ultrastructurally indistinguishable from fibroblasts found embedded within the collagen bundles of the meninges, except that the mesothelial cells are more likely to be connected by desmosomes. The pia mater does not form a complete barrier to diffusion (Waggener, 1964; Brightman, 1965), although tight junctions may be observed where mesothelial cells overlap (Fig. 15.38).

The pia, turning outwards, also becomes continuous mostly with sclera, but some fibres merge with the choroid and some with the border tissue round the optic nerve. The pia thickens as it nears the eye, by addition of circular fibres. External pial fibres extend into the dense meridional fibres of the inner scleral layers. This union of pia with the meridional fibres of sclera and of dura with its outer circular fibres gives this transition zone an extremely dense structure. The innermost layers of pia pass to the basal lamina between the choroid and nerve, becoming continuous with the choroid. Some circular

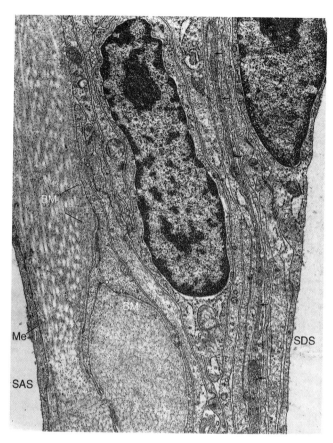

Fig. 15.34 Human arachnoid mater separating the subdural space (SDS) and subarachnoid space (SAS). Several layers of meningothelial cells make up the surface facing the dura. One cell (arrows) is darker than the rest. Discontinuous basement membrane (BM) is present on the under surface of the innermost cell abutting the collagenous bundle at the subarachnoid surface. Complete mesothelium (Me) separates the arachnoid from the subarachnoid space. Original magnification ×25,000. (From Anderson, D. R. (1969b) *Arch. Ophthalmol.*, **82**, 800, with permission.)

pial fibres intervene between fused lamellae of the suprachoroid lamina, and some extend into its border tissue.

Subarachnoid space

The subarachnoid space ends in a scleral cul-de-sac reaching the back of the lamina cribrosa (Fig. 15.3). It is widest anteriorly, where the optic nerve is thinnest, and in a temporally directed scleral canal is wider on the nasal side.

The dura is largely connected through arachnoid to the pia by trabeculae, which mostly tear easily, so that the dura can be made to slide backwards and forwards on the pia. (Normally, with movements of the eye a slight amount of this sliding probably also takes place.) Near the globe the linkage is stronger, and the dura is firmly attached to bone in the optic canal.

STRUCTURE OF THE OPTIC NERVE

The optic nerve is concerned with **vision**; but although most of its axons, derived from retinal ganglion cells, terminate in the lateral geniculate nucleus *en route* to the visual cortex, a minority establish mesencephalic connections for visual reflexes in eye movements and pupillary responses. Some optic fibres are therefore **pupillomotor**, and exercise no direct effect on vision. Pupillomotor fibres are still sometimes described as collateral branches of **visual** fibres, but the evidence is equivocal. The optic nerve also carries some centrifugal fibres, probably vasomotor. The evidence for supposed 'trophic' and 'retinoretinal' nerve fibres is negligible.

In section the pial sheath of the nerve is seen to pass in as many septa, dividing it into 800–1200 fascicles (Deyl, 1895). There are about one million fibres in the optic nerve, amounting to almost 40% of all afferent fibres in the cranial nerves (Bruesch and Arey, 1942). Polyak (1941) estimated the number of human optic fibres to be 800 000–1 000 000, with more recent estimates being 1 190 000 (Oppel, 1963) and 1 060 000–1 130 000 (Kupfer, Chumbley and de Downer, 1967).

Each axon is bounded by its own plasma membrane with a membrane of glial origin in close apposition. A thin lining of glial cytoplasm may be trapped between this and the enclosing myelin sheath. The axons vary focally in diameter along their length and exhibit nodes of Ranvier resembling those in other parts of the central nervous system (Fig. 15.39). The unmyelinated gap is bounded by myelin terminations exhibiting cytoplasm-filled loops. The gaps are occupied by astrocytes. Where myelination terminates at the lamina cribrosa, half of the nodes of Ranvier are formed. The axons contain microtubules 20–25 nm in diameter and oriented lengthwise, in addition to fine (6–7 nm) filaments, mitochondria and occasional smooth endoplasmic reticulum (Anderson and Hoyt, 1969).

The connective tissue is more obvious in the more vascular region of the nerve, distal to the entrance of the central vessels and in the optic canal. Near the chiasma a distinct glial septum passes obliquely down and medially to the centre of the nerve. This and all trabeculae disappear in the chiasma and optic tracts.

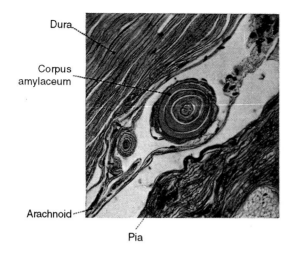

Dura

Corpus amylaceum

Arachnoid

Pia

(a)

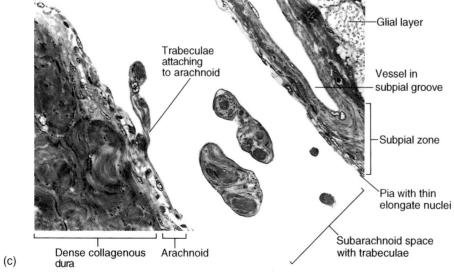

Nerve

Glial layer

Subpial collagen

Pial cell nucleus

Pia - single cell layer

Cross-section of trabeculae

(b)

Glial layer

Trabeculae attaching to arachnoid

Vessel in subpial groove

Subpial zone

Pia with thin elongate nuclei

Dense collagenous dura

Arachnoid

Subarachnoid space with trabeculae

(c)

Fig. 15.35 (a) Corpus amylaceum in arachnoid. (b) Detail of the subarachnoid space to show the monolayer of pial cells overlying the sub-pial collagenous zone and lining the collagenous, subarachnoid trabeculae. (Courtesy of M. Greaney.) (c) Light micrograph of the subarachnoid space. Each trabecula has a collagen core and is invested by pial cells. (Courtesy of M. Greaney.)

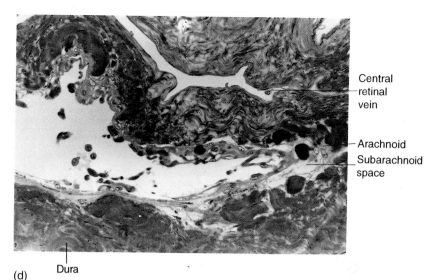

(d)

Dura

Central retinal vein

Arachnoid

Subarachnoid space

Fig. 15.35 (contd) (d) Point of reflexion of the arachnoid over the dura mater at the site of exit of the central retinal vein of the retina. (Courtesy of M. Greaney.)

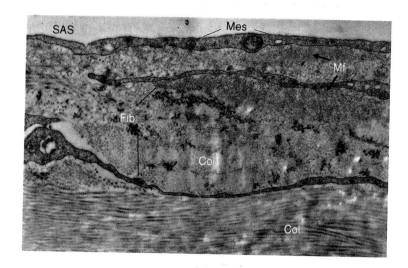

SAS

Mes

Mf

Fib

Col

Col

Fig. 15.36 Surface of the pia mater of human optic nerve. Most of the surface layer is a thin covering of meningothelial cytoplasm (Mes), similar in appearance to the cytoplasmic strands of fibroblastic cells (Fib). Microfibrils (Mf) are close to some cells. Original magnification ×48,000. (From Anderson, D. R. (1969b) *Arch. Ophthalmol.*, **82**, 800, with permission.)

The septa

The developing optic nerve is surrounded by glia, which is carried into it by invading septal vessels at about the fourth month. In each septum, a single artery enters surrounded by collagen tissue and neuroglia (Fig. 15.37) enters the nerve (radially), divides dichotomously and, anastomosing with others, forms a vascular plexus which reaches the centre of the nerve or central vessels. Anterior and posterior branches, also extend between nerve fascicles. There are between six and nine thick primary septa dividing the nerve into sectors, and between these many thinner secondary septa which, like the blood vessels, divide repeatedly and dichotomously and rejoin each other to divide the nerve into fascicles. The interseptal spaces are rounded in the human optic nerve but usually polygonal in other mammals.

The anteroposterior septal branches anastomose together and with transverse branches to form a longitudinal vascular plexus around each fascicle. The septa surround the fascicles like tubes, which are fenestrated for communication between fascicles. Thus in longitudinal section the longitudinal septa are not continuous. Hiatuses, occupied by glial cells, represent the fenestrations (Fig. 15.40). In transverse section also, gaps appear in septa, completed by glia (Fig. 15.41).

Each trabecula shows a central vessel which in larger septa has muscular and elastic layers. Externally is a variable amount of loose connective tissue surrounded by dense connective tissue and then a layer of glial cells (Fig. 15.37). Most of these are

Glial membrane

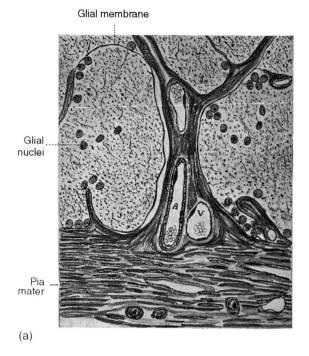

Glial
nuclei

Pia
mater

(a)

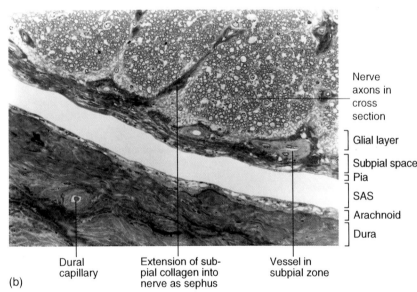

Nerve
axons in
cross
section

] Glial layer

] Subpial space
] Pia
] SAS
] Arachnoid
] Dura

Dural
capillary

Extension of sub-
pial collagen into
nerve as sephus

Vessel in
subpial zone

(b)

Fig. 15.37   (a) Transverse section of a septum of the optic nerve (Zenker, Mallory's triple stain) to show that each septum contains a vessel (or vessels); around this is connective tissue and then a glial membrane. (Wolff's preparation.) (b) High-power micrograph of the optic nerve in transverse section. (Courtesy of M. Greaney.)

astrocytes, but oligodendrocytes and microglial cells occur in small numbers.

The pia is continuous with the septa which tether it to the nerve and allow separation with difficulty. Lining the pia is the 'glial mantle' of Fuchs, a layer of glial tissue (Fig. 15.42) which is prolonged into the nerve to line the septa, penetrating also into the nerve bundles. Glial cells are scattered in these prolongations. The glial mantle varies but is usually thin, although it is much thicker in the floor of the third ventricle and just behind the optic canal, in the superolateral quadrant of the nerve.

A prominent, somewhat triangular, glial septum extends downwards and posteromedially to a point anterior to the chiasma. Thin extensions of it radiate to trabeculae. It separates the nerve into ventromedial and dorsolateral parts, the former fibres crossing in the chiasma. This septum marks the end of septation in the nerve, which is absent from its most proximal part. This accords with the unhindered course of anterior decussating fibres (see Fig. 15.62). The end of the septum also marks the actual beginning of decussation where crossed fibres first separate from uncrossed fibres, anterior to the macroscopic chiasma.

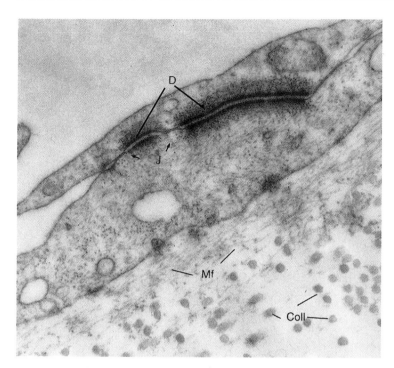

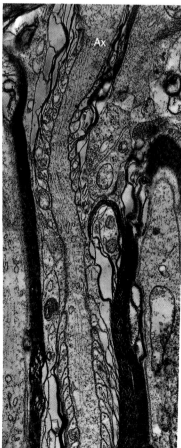

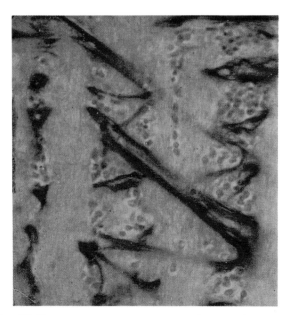

Fig. 15.38 Surface of the pia mater over the human optic nerve. Where two mesothelial cells overlap, they are held together by tight junctions (J) and desmosomes (D). Subjacent tissue includes microfibrils (Mf) and collagen fibres (Coll). Original magnification ×64,000. (From Anderson, D. R. (1969b) *Arch. Ophthalmol.*, **82**, 800, with permission.)

Fig. 15.39 Human optic nerve axon (Ax) in longitudinal section through a node of Ranvier. Original magnification ×28,000. (From Anderson, D. R. and Hoyt, W. (1969) *Arch. Ophthalmol.*, **82**, 506, with permission.)

Fig. 15.40 Longitudinal section of the optic nerve. (Mallory's triple stain.) Note columns of glial nuclei and parts of connective tissue septa (stained blue).

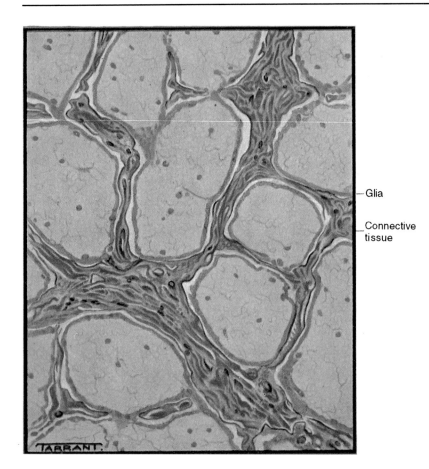

—Glia

—Connective tissue

Fig. 15.41 Section of the optic nerve. (Mallory's triple stain.) To show nerve fascicles. Connective tissue is blue, glia is red.

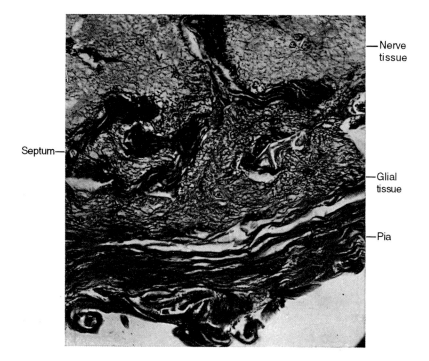

—Nerve tissue

Septum—

—Glial tissue

—Pia

Fig. 15.42 Transverse section of the optic nerve (Zenker, Mallory's triple stain) to show the glial mantle.

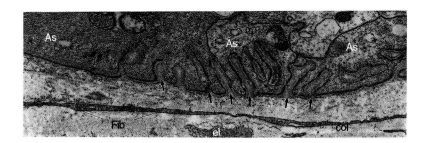

Fig. 15.43 Astrocyte foot processes (As) abutting upon septum of human optic nerve. Strand of fibroblast cytoplasm (Fib) and elastic fibre (el) lie within collagen (col) of septum. Basement membrane material extends into the invaginated spaces within and between astroglial feet. Original magnification ×23,000. (From Anderson, D. and Hoyt, W. (1969) *Arch. Ophthalmol.*, **82**, 506, with permission.)

Within the septa, astrocyte feet (or less often cell bodies) are apposed to the connective tissue stroma and a dense layer is formed by the insertion of cytoplasmic filaments into their processes. The glial membrane is separated from connective tissue by a basal lamina and is indented in places by invaginations 120–150 μm wide both between and within simple footplates (Fig. 15.43). This achieves a firm attachment of the glia to the septa. In the chiasma, where there are no connective tissue septa, the astrocytes abut capillaries directly with only basal lamina intervening (Anderson and Hoyt, 1969).

Fibres of the optic nerve vary in diameter from 0.7 to 10 μm; class A sensory fibres (up to 20 μm) are absent. Of these myelinated axons about 92% are less than 1 μm (Oppel, 1963; Kupfer, Chumbley and de Downer, 1967). Of larger fibres most are less than 2 μm (Chacko, 1948). Smaller fibres appear to be derived from midget ganglion cells, the largest from the peripheral retinal area.

Ultrastructural studies demonstrate few peculiarities (Yamamoto, 1966; Cohen, 1967; Anderson and Hoyt, 1969). Neuroglial processes are distinguishable from non-myelinated nerve fibres; the latter are concentrated peripherally in nerve fascicles. Branching of fibres is described by some, denied by others.

BLOOD SUPPLY OF THE OPTIC NERVE

The optic nerve, an outgrowth from the brain, has a vascular supply modelled on that organ. The resemblance is great, but not absolute, for in the optic nerve there is no grey matter and there are no nerve cells. The optic nerve, chiasma, and tracts are covered with pia mater identical with that of the brain: only those portions of the chiasma and tracts adherent to the base of the brain are bare of pia.

All the arteries which will eventually supply the nerve tissue do so through the pial network of vessels (Fig. 15.44). This network is rich and fine and extends to the back of the globe. In the intracranial portion of the nerve it is situated on the surface of the pia: in the orbital portion, between the longitudinal and circular fibres.

As in the case of the cerebral convolutions there are actually two networks, one inside the other. The outer is the larger and formed of arterioles of fair size; the other, lying within the first, consists of vessels of microscopic size. The network is supplied by arteries which probably anastomose slightly in the network, but not before they reach it.

When the vessels pass into the nerve they take with them a coat of pia and also a covering of glia, which constitute the septa. In fact, the distribution of the septa is exactly that of the blood vessels. Also, the thickness of each septum is proportional to the size of the contained vessel. While this is obvious in the orbital portion of the nerve, it is more difficult to discern in the tract and chiasma. In the most posterior portion of the optic nerve (where the septa gradually disappear), in the chiasma, and in the optic tract even the larger vessels are surrounded by only a slight covering of connective tissue which gets less with the smaller vessels and seems to disappear entirely in the capillaries. They are, however, always separated from the nerve tissue by the perivascular gliae.

There is a striking contrast between the great vascularity of the pia mater and the relatively few vessels in the dura mater. The pial network acts as a distributing centre which provides for a regular supply of blood to the nerve. As the vessels pass into the nerve in the septa, they divide dichotomously and send branches anteriorly and posteriorly.

The vessels which join the optic nerve ultimately come from the internal carotid artery and, because the eye has grown out from the brain, its vessels have followed it. This explains why the vessels to the chiasma are short and those to the globe relatively long.

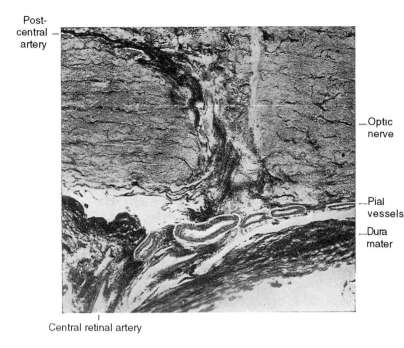

Post-central artery

Optic nerve

Pial vessels

Dura mater

Central retinal artery

Fig. 15.44 Longitudinal section of the optic nerve, showing a large branch from the central artery passing forwards in the subarachnoid space to the pial plexus; also a post-central artery passing backwards. (Wolff's preparation.)

Intracranial part (Fig. 15.45)

This region has been considered as a 'no-man's-land' between the territories of the ophthalmologist and neurologist, and as a result has not received detailed study.

Perichiasmal artery

A perichiasmal artery running back along the medial side of the optic nerve joins its fellow of the opposite side along the anterior border of the chiasm and supplies both. It is probably the largest supply to the intracranial optic nerve. Hayreh (1963) and Steele and Blunt (1956) regard the origin to be the superior hypophyseal branch of the internal carotid, although Dawson (1958) believed the ophthalmic artery to be its source.

Ophthalmic artery

The ophthalmic artery gives rise to a variable number of small collateral arteries which run backwards along the inferior surface of the nerve, winding round its margins to its superior aspect (Hayreh, 1963). Magitot (1947) and Steele and Blunt (1956) also demonstrated ophthalmic artery branches supplying its upper surface.

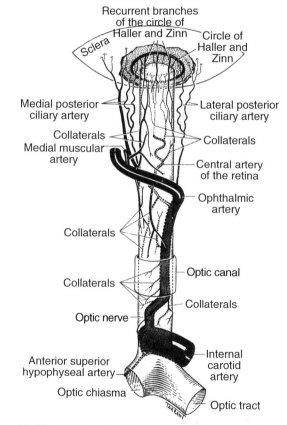

Recurrent branches of the circle of Haller and Zinn

Sclera

Circle of Haller and Zinn

Medial posterior ciliary artery

Lateral posterior ciliary artery

Collaterals

Medial muscular artery

Collaterals

Central artery of the retina

Ophthalmic artery

Collaterals

Optic canal

Collaterals

Collaterals

Optic nerve

Internal carotid artery

Anterior superior hypophyseal artery

Optic chiasma

Optic tract

Fig. 15.45 Relationship between the optic nerve and chiasm, the internal carotid artery, the ophthalmic artery and its branches. Right eye seen from above. (From Hayreh, S. S., In Cant, J. S. (ed.) (1972) *The Optic Nerve*, published by Kimpton, with permission.)

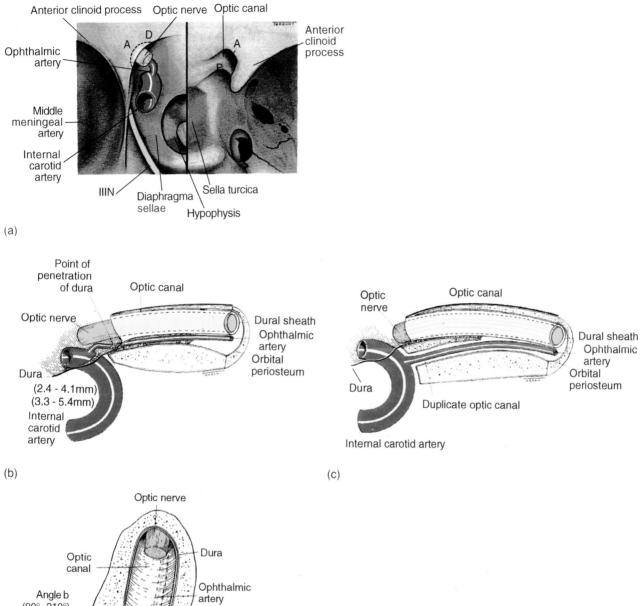

(a)

(b)

(c)

(d)

Fig. 15.46 (a) Right half shows cranial opening of the optic canal and surrounding bony landmarks, as seen at the base of the skull. Left half shows cranial opening of the optic canal with dural margin intact, optic nerve, ophthalmic artery, internal carotid artery, hypophysis and diaphragma sellae, as seen after removal of the brain. (b) Lateral view of the optic canal and intracranial part of the internal carotid artery, showing details of origin and intracranial and intracanicular course of the ophthalmic artery. The diameters of the lumen of the internal carotid artery before and after the origin of the ophthalmic artery are shown. (c) Same as in (b), but the figure shows an extradural origin of the ophthalmic artery and its course through duplicate optic canal. (d) Origin and intracanicular course of the ophthalmic artery and its subdivisions as seen on opening the canal. (From Hayreh, S. S. (1963) *J. Surg.*, **227**, 938, with permission.)

Additional branches

Additional branches from the anterior cerebral artery and anterior communicating artery, described by Behr (1935), Wolff (1939) and Francois and Neetens (1954), were not demonstrated by Hayreh (1963).

Various arterial sources feed a pial plexus of vessels which supplies centripetal end arteries to the whole substance of the nerve.

Intracanalicular nerve (Figs 15.45 and 15.46)

The ophthalmic artery has several branches: intra-canalicular; intraorbital; and the central retinal artery.

For more details on the branches of the ophthalmic artery see Chapter 3. Hayreh (1963) found the ophthalmic artery to be the sole supply to this portion of the nerve, except for an occasional branch from the central retinal artery on its inferior aspect. Branches of the ophthalmic artery arise within the canal or in the orbit (Steele and Blunt, 1956) and also from its other intraorbital branches. A supply from the internal carotid, anterior cerebral and anterior communicating arteries (Magitot, 1947; Francois and Neetens, 1954) was not confirmed by Hayreh.

The nerve substance is supplied by a pial network, which in this region is relatively poor. Because the arteries reach the pia along connective tissue bands binding the nerve to the surrounding dural sheath, this supply is vulnerable to shearing injury in skull fracture.

Intraorbital part (Fig. 15.45)

The optic nerve in the orbit is 3 cm long and the central retinal artery enters at 5–15.5 mm behind the eyeball. The arterial supplies proximal and distal to this point of entry are different; the proximal part being supplied by centripetal branches of the pial network, while the distal part, carrying the central retinal vessels, exhibits an axial supply in addition. The embryonic origin of arteries supplying these two segments of the intraorbital nerve is also different (Mann, 1927a).

Posterior to the entry of the central retinal artery

The proximal part of the nerve, like the intra-canalicular and intracranial portions, is supplied throughout its substance by centripetal vessels from the pial network of arteries (Fig. 15.47). This network is supplied by collaterals from the ophthalmic artery or its branches, of smaller size than those branches themselves. They arise near to the nerve as the ophthalmic artery lies close to it. Their origin and location depend on whether the ophthalmic artery crosses over the nerve (in 82–85% of cases) or under it (Fig. 15.48). As they arise, they are more often directed posteriorly.

The supply is thus:

1. direct branches of the ophthalmic artery;
2. extraneural part of the central retinal artery;
3. other branches of the ophthalmic artery.

When the ophthalmic artery crosses above the optic nerve direct branches reach the pia in 75% of cases,

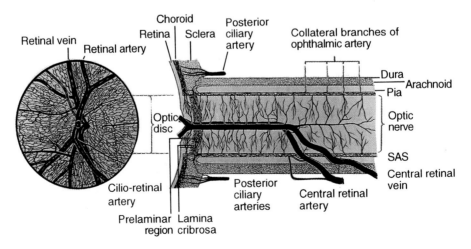

Fig. 15.47 Diagrammatic representation of blood supply of optic nerve head. (SAS), Subarachnoid space. (From Hayreh, S. S., In Cant, J. S. (ed.) (1972) *The Optic Nerve*, published by Kimpton, with permission.)

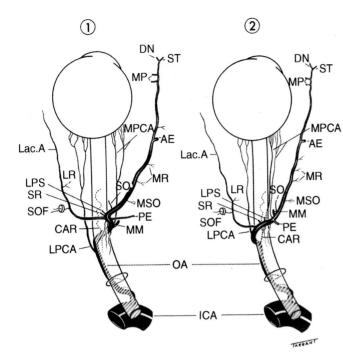

Fig. 15.48 The pattern of branches of the ophthalmic artery when it crosses (1) under and (2) over the optic nerve. AE = anterior ethmoid artery; CAR = central artery of retina; DN = dorsal nasal artery; ICA = internal carotid artery; Lac. A = lacrimal artery; LPCA = lateral posterior ciliary artery; LPS = muscular artery to levator palpebrae superioris; LR = muscular artery to lateral rectus; MM = medial muscular artery; MP = medial palpebral artery; MPCA = medial posterior ciliary artery; MR = muscular artery to medial rectus; MSO = muscular artery to superior oblique; OA = ophthalmic artery; PE = posterior ethmoid artery; SO = supraorbital artery; SOF = superior orbital fissure; SR = muscular artery to superior rectus; ST = supratrochlear artery. (From Hayreh, S. S. (1963) with permission.)

while branches from medial muscular, posterior ciliary or central retinal arteries are found in 25% of cases for each group. (Posterior ethmoidal, supraorbital or muscular branches to the medial and superior rectus or superior oblique muscle are rare sources.) When the ophthalmic artery passes below the nerve direct branches arise in 50% of cases, with 25% of each of the medial posterior ciliary, central retinal and lacrimal arteries. (Posterior ethmoidal and, very rarely, the lateral posterior ciliary artery or branch to medial rectus muscle supply occasionally.)

Not unexpectedly, collaterals lie mostly superior when the ophthalmic artery is above and inferior when it crosses below, with vessels arising less frequently at the obverse side of the nerve, or medially. Hayreh (1963) rarely found collaterals located at the lateral side of the nerve although they were reported by Hughes (1954).

Anterior to the entry of the central retinal artery

The peripheral part of the nerve is supplied by the pial plexus of arteries while its axial part is supplied in a complementary, but variable manner by the intraneural portion of the central retinal artery. These sets of arteries supply interconnected transverse and longitudinal capillary systems lying within the septal framework of the nerve, anastomosing posteriorly with capillaries in the proximal nerve and anteriorly with those at the nerve head. The supply is thus via the pial plexus and the central artery of the retina (Fig. 15.45).

Pial plexus   The pial plexus of arteries anastomose in a tortuous manner throughout the length of the orbital portion of the optic nerve. The pial plexus receives branches from along its length, and at the junction of optic nerve and globe it is reinforced by branches from the scleral short posterior ciliary arteries or arterial circle of Zinn.

Multiple branches from the pial plexus enter the nerve substance centripetally to supply its axons, each lying within a central core of connective tissue lined externally with a glial coat of astrocytes.

Central artery   The central retinal artery is a branch of the ophthalmic artery (or, rarely, of the middle meningeal artery). Its origin varies with the course of the ophthalmic artery:

1. When the ophthalmic artery crosses above the nerve it arises independently or in conjunction with the medial posterior ciliary artery at the angle between the first and second parts of the ophthalmic artery.
2. When the artery crosses below the nerve it arises independently as its second branch.

The central retinal artery runs forwards tortuously to pierce the dura 5–15.5 mm behind the globe inferomedially. Its intravaginal course (0.9–2.5 mm) is mainly within the subarachnoid space. It enters the nerve vertically, and makes a right-angled bend on reaching its central axis to pass forward to the nerve head. Its branches are: intraorbital (about 5); intravaginal (about 3); intraneural (about 8); and terminal retinal branches.

Hayreh (1963) found branches arise in orbit, sheath or nerve in all but 3.1% of nerves he examined. No branches were ever demonstrated to the lamina cribrosa and in this Hayreh agreed with Francois and Neetens (1954). Branches were lacking from the intraorbital part of the artery in 47.8% of nerves examined, from the intravaginal part in 5.3% and from the intraneural part in 25%. The intraorbital branches supply the pia from globe to canal in about half the nerves. Intravaginal branches to the pia arise close to the entry of the artery, usually passing forwards, and sometimes posteriorly in addition. In keeping with its origin, the territory of supply of the artery to the pia always includes the inferior surface of the nerve, and the lateral and medial surfaces in about half the cases; the superior surface is least often supplied. The remaining pial territories are supplied in a complementary manner by other branches of the ophthalmic artery.

The pial branches of the central retinal artery anastomose with one another, with other pial vessels derived from branches of the ophthalmic artery and with recurrent pial branches from the choroid, scleral short ciliary arteries or circle of Zinn, in the retrolaminar region. Some anastomoses occur within the substance of the nerve.

Structure of the central retinal artery   The **intima** of the central retinal artery (Fig. 15.49) is lined by a continuous endothelium lying on basement membrane and this layer is expanded by a zone of basement membrane-like material which thickens

with age (Ikui, Tominaga and Mimura, 1964) and may contain smooth muscle cells and collagen in the later decades of life, as in the intracranial arteries (Flora, Dahl and Nelson, 1967; Anderson and Hoyt, 1969). Outside the intima is the **internal elastic lamina** similar to that of the intracranial arteries, whose surface, particularly on the luminal side, is irregular. It disappears at the lamina cribrosa (Anderson, 1969) and is absent from the retinal arteries (Hogan and Feeney, 1963). In giant cell arteritis only those vessels possessing an internal elastic lamina are affected. Thus the posterior ciliary, choroidal and central retinal arteries are affected while the retinal arteries themselves show no direct involvement (Cogan, 1974).

The **media** consists of about six layers of smooth muscle intermingled with collagen, elastin and basement membrane material. In the monkey, the number of smooth muscle cells increases to 7–12 at the lamina and in proximal retinal arteries. There is no discrete external elastic lamina. The **adventitia** consists of dense connective tissue, with occasional elastic fibres, continuous with that of the optic nerve septa. It is of interest that both myelinated and unmyelinated nerve fibres enclosed by Schwann cell

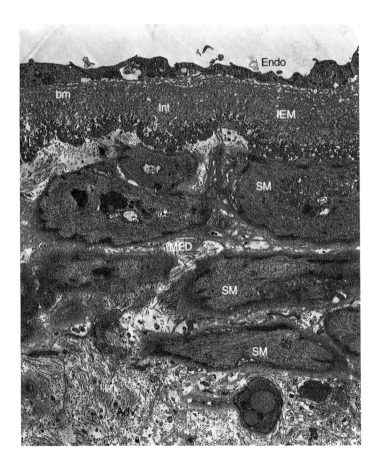

Fig. 15.49 Central retinal artery in the intraorbital portion of the human optic nerve. Intima (Int) consisting of endothelium (Endo) and reduplicated basement membrane (bm) bounded by internal elastic membrane (IEM). Media (MED) consist of several layers of smooth muscle (SM) and surrounded by collagenous adventitia (Adv). Original magnification ×12,000. (From Anderson, D. and Hoyt, W. (1969) *Arch. Ophthalmol.*, **82**, 506, with permission.)

cytoplasm are observed in the connective tissue adventitia of the central retinal artery (Ikui, Tominaga and Mimura, 1964; Anderson and Hoyt, 1969). These fibres, therefore, differ from the axons of the retinal ganglion cells, which are at all times insulated from contact with mesodermal derivatives within the optic nerve (Anderson and Hoyt, 1969).

The nerve fibres within the adventitia of the central retinal artery, a few of which may be found in association with the central retinal vein, include sympathetic and parasympathetic fibres and exhibit terminals along the artery up to the level of the lamina cribrosa, where they are rare. Unmyelinated nerve bundles, with or without a perineurium, are most frequent immediately outside the media. Occasional neurons accompany the proximal 2 mm of the retinal arteries, and terminals have not been identified.

Adrenergic, sympathetic nerve fibres have been demonstrated in the central artery of the retina as far forward as the optic disc in a variety of animals (Ehinger, 1964, 1966; Malmfors, 1965; Laties and Jacobowitz, 1966). It is likely that their cell bodies are located mainly in the superior cervical ganglion with some additional in ectopic ganglia *en route* to the artery (Ruskell, 1972).

Ruskell (1972) has demonstrated in monkeys and humans a parasympathetic innervation of orbital vessels, including lacrimal, ciliary and choroidal arteries, and it appears that the central artery of the retina is no exception. Cell bodies are located in the pterygopalatine ganglion and distributed to the **orbital plexus** of autonomic nerves, via the rami orbitales of that ganglion. (Although the ganglion receives sympathetic fibres from the nerve of the pterygoid canal, few if any are distributed to the orbit via this route (Ruskell, 1970).) The orbital plexus receives its sympathetic fibres from the internal carotid nerve. Tiedeman (1824) traced a fine nerve branch from the ciliary ganglion which entered the optic nerve with the central artery of the retina in humans: in contrast, Ruskell (1970) found a fine nerve of similar distribution arising from the retro-orbital plexus in the monkey.

A number of authors described a separate arterial supply to the axial part of the intraorbital optic nerve termed the central artery of the optic nerve. This was said to arise from the ophthalmic artery just proximal to the central retinal artery and to divide into anterior and posterior divisions centrally in the nerve at this level, to supply the papillomacular bundle and vasa vasorum of the central retinal artery (Kuhnt, 1879; Vossius, 1883; Behr, 1935; Wolff, 1939, 1954; Francois and Neetens, 1954; Francois, Neetens and Collette,

1955, 1956). Despite the number of reports, this supply appears to be extremely infrequent, if it exists at all (Steele and Blunt, 1956; Beauvieux and Ristich, 1924; Hayreh, 1963).

Venous drainage of optic nerve

The venous drainage of the optic nerve is chiefly by the central retinal vein and to a lesser extent via the pial venous system. Both systems drain into the ophthalmic venous system in the orbit and less commonly directly into the cavernous sinus:

1. pial veins;
2. central retinal vein(s);
3. posterior central vein.

Pial veins

The pial veins in the orbit and optic canal drain into the ophthalmic system. The intracranial pial veins drain into the adjacent venous sinuses.

Central retinal vein(s)

The central retinal vein is formed on the optic nerve head by the union of the retinal venous tributaries. The vein runs on the lateral side of the central artery in the axial part of the nerve, in a fibrous envelope in common with the artery or separated from it by axon bundles. At times two veins enter the nerve head and unite within the substance of the nerve. This reflects the embryonic origins of the vein as two venous channels at the third month of intrauterine life lying on either side of the hyaloid artery, which fuse prenatally. Failure to do so results in a doubled vein. Sometimes two separate channels persist.

The site of exit of the vein from the optic nerve varies. The vein exits from the same aspect of the nerve as the point of entry of the central retinal artery in 42% of nerves, in which case the vein is anterior to the artery in 81% of cases (Fry, 1930). Sometimes the vein exits laterally and curves inferiorly to leave the dura with the artery. The intravaginal course (3.8–8 mm) is longer than that of the artery and a greater fraction resides in the dura.

The vein receives tributaries from the retina, the optic nerve head at all levels (including choroidal tributaries and those from the peripapillary sclera), the pia and from the posterior central vein.

The central retinal vein joins the orbital plexus of veins, to drain into the superior and/or inferior ophthalmic vein, and/or cavernous sinus directly.

Because of these multiple connections blockage of the blood flow in the cavernous sinus will not block blood flow in the central retinal veins, though it may impede it.

Posterior central vein

Hayreh (1963) describes a vein draining the proximal part of the intraorbital optic nerve, posterior to the exit of the central retinal vein and running forward to empty into the latter at its bend. This is often present and is usefully termed the posterior central vein. Cone and MacMillan (1932) also gave this name to a vein described by Kuhnt which exits from the nerve inferiorly where the ophthalmic artery lies in its dural sheath and runs backward on the lateral side of the nerve to the cavernous sinus (Greeff, 1932).

Structure of the central retinal vein

The structure of the central retinal vein is simpler than that of the central retinal artery. The continuous endothelium lies on a basement membrane. Outside this is a cell which may be smooth muscle or pericyte and media is represented by a separation of occasional smooth muscle cells from basement membrane. A connective tissue adventitia is present.

OPTIC NERVE HEAD

The optic nerve head is a watershed zone between the retina and the optic nerve whose vessels are exposed to significantly different hydrostatic pressures. The disc and retina are exposed to the intra-ocular pressure, and the retrolaminar and proximal nerve to the cerebrospinal fluid pressure. This special arrangement, and the importance of diseases affecting the nerve head, has directed considerable attention of researchers to the vasculature of the zone, with a substantial contribution to the literature from Hayreh. The reader should consult articles by Singh and Dass (1960), Hayreh (1963, 1974), Beauvieux and Ristich (1924), Steele and Blunt (1956), Anderson (1969), Francois and Neetens (1954), Levitzky and Hendkind (1969), Hendkind and Levitzky (1969) and Lieberman, Maumenee and Green (1976).

It is generally agreed that, excluding the superficial nerve fibre layer, the disc and retrolaminar nerve receive their blood supply mainly, if not entirely, from the short posterior ciliary artery system. It is also accepted that there is a major variation in the vascular architecture between individual nerve heads so that any schematic representation is bound to differ in some particular, from case to case. Nevertheless, there is sufficient agreement to provide a coherent account of the blood supply and indicate where major differences have been reported.

Arterial supply (Figs 15.50 and 15.51)

Retrolaminar optic nerve

Pial arteries   The retrolaminar nerve receives its supply mainly from the arteries and arterioles of the pial sheath of the neighbouring leptomeninges.

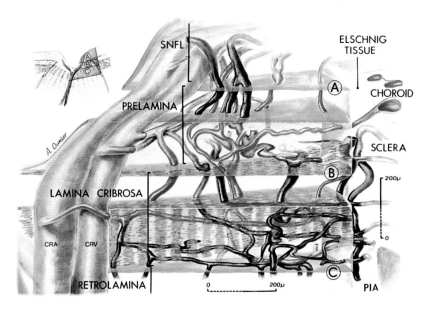

Fig. 15.50 Vascular supply of the optic nerve head. (From Lieberman, M. F., Maumenee, A. E. and Green, W. R. (1976) *Am. J. Ophthalmol.*, **82**, 405, with permission.)

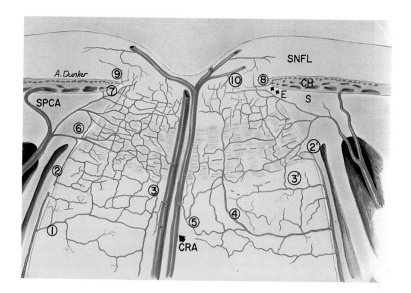

Fig. 15.51 Vascular supply of the optic nerve head. Retrolamina: ① = Pia mater as source of vessels; ②, ② = recurrent short posterior ciliary artery and pial vessels; ③, ③ = pial-derived longitudinal arterioles; ④ = large pial arteriole; ⑤ = intraneural branching of central retinal artery. Lamina cribrosa: ⑥ = scleral short posterior arteries. Prelamina: ⑦ = branch of short posterior ciliary artery enters nerve; ⑧ = occasional choroidal vessel to prelamina, S indicates sclera. Superficial nerve fibre layer (SNFL): ⑨ = Choriocapillaris capillary anastomosis; ⑩ = both epipapillary and peripapillary branches of central retinal artery. (From Lieberman, M. F., Maumenee, A. E. and Green, W. R. (1976) *Am. J. Ophthalmol.*, **82**, 405, with permission.)

Hayreh (1974) is of the opinion that these arise chiefly as recurrent branches from the peripapillary choroid, but these were not noted by Lieberman (1974).

Occasional longitudinal vessels of pial origin   The pial system occasionally gives rise to curved longitudinal arterioles and precapillaries which pass forwards and often may be traced through to the vascular networks of the lamina and prelaminar regions (Fig. 15.51) (Leiberman, Maumenee and Green, 1976).

Recurrent scleral short posterior ciliary arteries   Lieberman, Maumenee and Green (1976) give the name scleral short posterior ciliary arteries to those direct branches of the short posterior ciliary arteries supplying the optic nerve, pial sheath, episclera and choroid. These vessels supply the interconnecting system of the arterioles at the meningoscleral interface and pass through the pia to the retrolaminar nerve. The circles of Zinn and Haller have been found infrequently by some authors who thus regard them as an uncommon source of supply to the retrolaminar nerve (Hayreh, 1974). However, more recent studies have suggested that it is commonly present and that it provides an important supply to both the retrolaminar and laminar parts of the nerve head (Olver *et al.*, 1990).

Direct choroidal arteries   Some choroidal arteries supply the retrolaminar region (Hayreh, 1975; Anderson and Braverman, 1976).

Intraneural branch   The central retinal artery gives off a small number of branches in the retrolaminar

2 mm of the optic nerve which are short, narrow rapidly, and run anteriorly or posteriorly to anastomose with the septal system of arterioles and capillaries within the substance of the nerve. Their contribution is small relative to the pial supply, and in many instances there may be no branches to the region immediately behind the lamina cribrosa (Hayreh, 1974).

The intraseptal vessels of the retrolaminar region are primarily large precapillaries and capillaries confined to the connective tissue septae and arranged as both transverse and longitudinal polygonal units surrounding axon bundles. There is extensive anastomosis and no uniformity of size of these intraseptal vessels. Their numbers increase near the posterior bowing of the lamina. Anteriorly the system anastomoses with vessels of the lamina itself and posteriorly with the septal system of the intraorbital nerve (Fig. 15.52).

Laminar region (Figs 15.50 and 15.51)
There is controversy concerning the vascular supply of this region. Lieberman, Maumenee and Green (1976) use the term scleral short posterior ciliary arteries to describe direct branches of the short posterior ciliary arteries which are a major supply to both the retrolaminar region and the lamina cribrosa itself. However, there is increasing support for the view that both regions commonly receive a substantial arterial supply from a complete, or incomplete, intrascleral anastomosis around the optic nerve head. The anastomotic 'circles' of Zinn (1755) and Haller (1754) are formed by the paraoptic branches of the

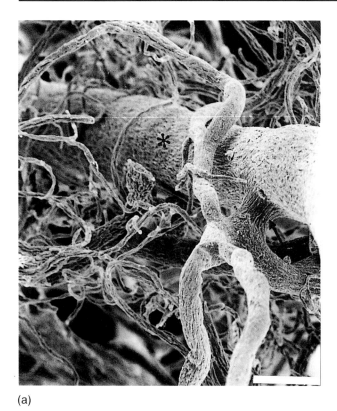

(a)

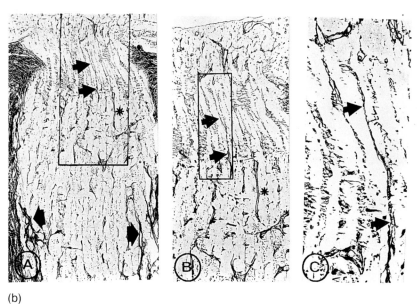

(b)

Fig. 15.52 (a) A branch (arrow) from the intraneural central retinal artery (star) arising approximately 1.5 mm posterior to the lamina cribrosa, to anastomose with optic nerve capillaries. Bar = 125 μm. (From Olver, J. M., Spalton, D. J. and McCartney, A. C. E. (1990) *Eye*, **4**, 7, with permission.) (b) Longitudinal microcirculatory pattern of anterior optic nerve. A, pial-arterioles (large arrows) in retrolaminar nerve, one of which (asterisk) traces on serial sections into the laminar portion. Precapillaries (thin arrows) extend through the lamina cribrosa anteriorly to the prelaminar region. B, Enlargement of insert in A; C, Enlargement of inset in B. (Modified silver reticulin stain.) Original magnifications: A ×40; B ×60; C ×145. (From Lieberman, M. F., Maumenee, A. E. and Green W. R. (1976) *Am. J. Ophthalmol.*, **82**, 506, with permission.)

short posterior ciliary arteries (Fig. 15.53) (Olver and McCartney, 1989; Olver, Spalton and McCartney, 1990). There is disagreement as to the frequency of this vascular circle; Olver, Spalton and McCartney (1990) report that it is frequently present, while Hayreh found it only in a small proportion of normal eyes. Most authors agree that it is often incomplete (Levitzky and Henkind, 1969) and it may be this fact that has led to controversy. In the absence of this

circular anastomosis, its place is taken by small branches of the paraoptic short ciliary arteries, which lie within the sclera and supply portions of the optic nerve head and sometimes the adjacent retina. It is absent in sub-human primates (Hayreh, 1964).

In its complete form the 'circle' (usually a horizontal ellipse) is an intrascleral anastomosis between branches of the medial and lateral paraoptic short posterior ciliary arteries (Fig. 15.54) (Olver,

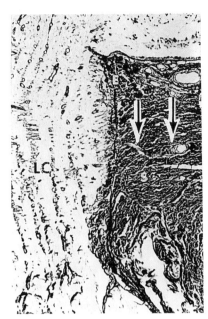
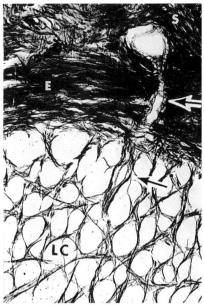

Fig. 15.53 Short posterior ciliary arteries in sclera (S) give rise to branches to the lamina cribrosa (LC). (a) Longitudinal section; scleral short posterior ciliary artery contributes branch (arrows) to the lamina as traced in serial sections; (E) Elschnig's tissue. (b) Transverse section through a different nerve showing scleral short posterior cililiary artery (arrows) coursing through Elschnig's border tissue (E) to the septal system of the lamina. (Modified silver reticulin stain.) Original magnification (a) ×40; (b) ×205. (From Lieberman, M. F., Maumenee, A. E. and Green, W. R. (1976) *Am. J. Ophthalmol.*, **82**, 506, with permission.)

Maumanee and Green, 1990). (This anastomosis must be distinguished from a more proximal, extrascleral anastomosis formed by separate short posterior ciliary arteries lying superiorly to the optic nerve in some eyes). Incomplete, upper or lower arcuate anastomoses are also seen, or sometimes overlapping non-anastomosing upper and lower segments. The circle may be anteriorly placed, in which case it lies closer to the choroid within the sclera, or it may lie more posteriorly, when the superior and inferior parts are partially or completely extrascleral (Fig. 15.54f). Similarly, according to the radius of the circle, it may be situated close to, or further away from, the scleral opening.

The branches of the anastomosis of Zinn and Haller are as follows:

1. Recurrent pial branches: four to seven of these arise from each segment, or they may arise from two or three larger trunks. Small branches are given off to the retrolaminar nerve.
2. Recurrent choroidal branches supply the immediate peripapillary choroid and extend towards the equator as straight vessels superiorly and inferiorly. Small centripetal branches of these arteries and others from the choroid itself, supply the laminar and retrolaminar regions of the optic nerve head.
3. Direct branches to the retrolaminar and laminar parts of the nerve head are relatively infrequent.
4. Arteriolo–arteriolar anastomoses occur between

the circle, and pial and recurrent choroidal arterioles at the optic nerve head.

Ruskell (1984) has noted that as some of the centripetal vessels enter the lamina at the margin of the scleral canal, they turn abruptly in a circumferential direction at the level of the glial cuff in continuity with the border tissue of Jacoby anteriorly and glial mantle of the optic nerve posteriorly (Fig. 15.54). These **interfacial precapillaries** then run a short distance within the glial border tissue and then turn abruptly inwards again to enter the septal system of anastomoses. This arrangement is more developed in the monkey eye. Ruskell (1984) suggests that these thin-walled vessels would be vulnerable to closure with raised intraocular pressure and could be related to the disc haemorrhages which occur in chronic glaucoma.

The transverse system of anastomoses established within the septa of the connective tissue plates of the lamina cribrosa dominate the vascular architecture. Those of the posterior lamina tend to be larger (arterial and arteriolar) than the anterior (arteriolar to capillary). The transverse capillary beds anastomose with longitudinal precapillary and capillary beds along paths which are tortuous rather than geometrically axial.

Prelaminar optic nerve (Figs 15.50 and 15.51)

The prelaminar nerve receives its supply mainly from the scleral short posterior ciliary system and the

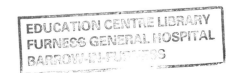

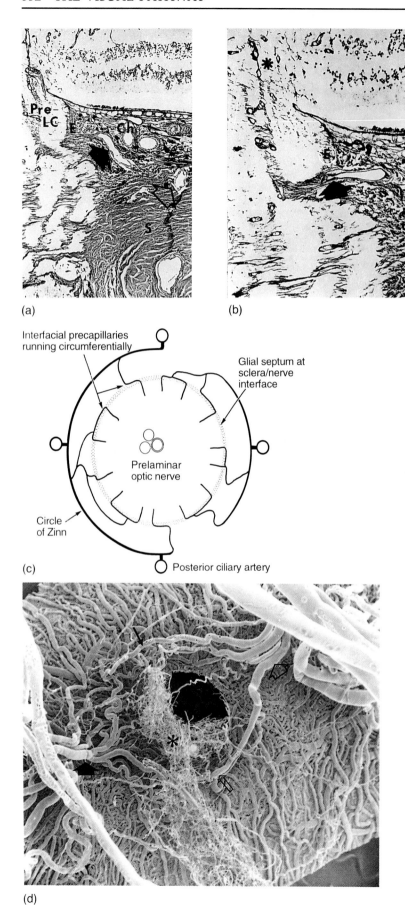

(a)

(b)

Interfacial precapillaries
running circumferentially

Glial septum at
sclera/nerve
interface

Prelaminar
optic nerve

Circle
of Zinn

Posterior ciliary artery

(c)

(d)

Fig. 15.54 (a) Branch of short posterior ciliary artery courses through Elschnig's border tissue (E) at level of choroid (Ch) to prelaminate (Pre-LC). Arterial branch (solid arrow) traces in serial sections to originate in short posterior ciliary artery (open arrow) in sclera (S). (b) Several sections later, the branch vessel seen in (a) penetrates Elschnig tissue and on further serial sections can be traced continuously with capillary lumens (*) in prelamina. (Modified silver reticulum strain.) Original magnification: (a) ×35; (b) ×175. (c) Diagram to show interfacial precapillaries arising from the short ciliary system, lying within the glial cuff at the level of the lamina cribrosa. (Courtesy of G. Ruskell.) (d) SEM of the 'circle' of Zinn and Haller formed by branches of the lateral short posterior ciliary arteries (short empty arrow) and a medial short posterior ciliary artery (short solid arrow) forming a superior (straight solid arrow) and inferior anastomosis (straight empty arrow). *, optic nerve capillaries. (From a right eye.) (From Olver, J. M., Spalton, D. J. and McCartney, A. C. E. (1990) *Eye*, **4**, 7, with permission.)

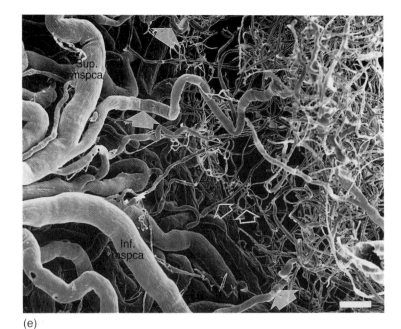

(e)

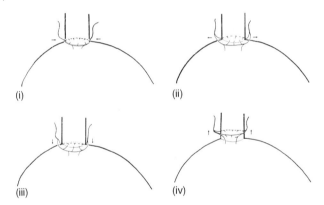

(i)   (ii)

(iii)   (iv)

(f)

Fig. 15.54 (contd) (e) Higher magnification of the branches of the medial short posterior ciliary arteries (mspca) from the specimen (d), as they diverge, enter the sclera, and form the superior (sup) and inferior (inf) parts of the anastomotic circle. Pial branches (solid arrows) and small centripetal branches from both the choroid and recurrent choroidal branches (empty arrows) enter the laminar and retrolaminar nerve. Bar = 200 µm. (f) Diagram showing the position of the 'circle' of Zinn and Haller in relation to the optic nerve. (i), tightly apposed to the optic nerve; (ii), at some distance from the nerve; (iii), anterior (intrascleral); (iv), posterior (extrascleral). (g) SEM showing axial position of the anterior (intrascleral) 'circle', with inferior anastomosis (empty arrow), recurrent choroidal branches (short solid arrows) and pial branches (long arrows). The central retinal artery (*) is surrounded by residual optic nerve capillaries. (Right eye. Bar = 400 µm). (e, f and g, from Olver, J. M., Spalton, D. J. and McCartney, A. C. E. (1990) *Eye*, **4**, 7, with permission.) (h) SEM of the vessels at the optic nerve head. The central retinal artery (A) and vein (V) are seen, together with the epipapillary (e) and peripapillary (p) capillaries of the nerve head and retina. Capillary free zones (arrows) are seen in relation to the retinal arterioles. (Courtesy of J. M. Olver.)

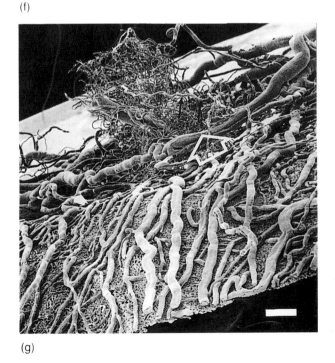

(g)

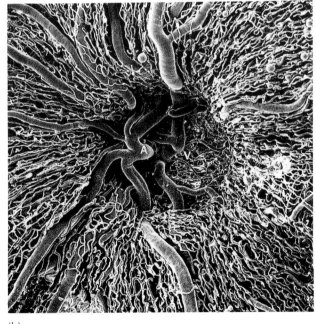

(h)

recurrent choroidal arteries but there is no full agreement as to their relative contribution.

Scleral short posterior ciliary artery Lieberman, Maumenee and Green (1976) emphasize the role of branches of the scleral short posterior ciliary arteries, which course through the sclera and the border tissue of Elschnig to reach the prelaminar space without traversing the choroid (Fig. 15.54). They supply transverse precapillaries and capillaries in this region. Hayreh (1974) gives such vessels a negligible role.

Recurrent choroidal arteries Hayreh (1974) attributes the major supply to the centripetal branches of the peripapillary choroid, a view supported by Levitzky and Henkind (1969), Anderson (1969) and Theodossiadis (1971). Lieberman, Maumanee and Green (1976) in their careful study, found that only 10% of vessels entering the prelaminar region originate from choroidal arteries although about 30% of the prelaminar depth is in contact with peripapillary choroid.

Although the capillary networks of the choroid (choriocapillaris) and disc are quite distinct and separate (Hayreh, 1975; Anderson and Braverman, 1976), a microvascular cuff is present between disc and choroid immediately external to the peripheral bundle of optic nerve axons. This may be regarded as the anterior extension of the pial vascular bed, and exhibits in addition to its capillary-sized circumferential vessels, some longitudinally disposed arteries of choroidal origin, passing posteriorly to supply the retrolaminar pia mater.

Cilioretinal arteries Cilioretinal arteries passing from sclera or choroid are infrequent sources of prelaminar precapillaries.

Laminar vessels There is a longitudinal continuity of precapillaries and capillaries between the laminar, prelaminar and superficial nerve layer systems which anastomose with the transverse networks supplied by the scleral short posterior ciliary arteries. The temporal part of the region is much more vascular than the remainder.

Superficial nerve fibre layer

This layer is supplied by:

1. peripapillary arterioles of central retinal artery origin;
2. epipapillary arterioles of central retinal artery origin;
3. rich anastomoses with the prelaminar region;
4. occasional anastomoses with the chorocapillaris;
5. precapillary branches from cilioretinal arteries when present.

The central retinal artery is the major supply to the superficial nerve fibre layer, with those peripapillary arterioles arising around the disc being more important than epipapillary arterioles arising on the disc (Anderson and Hoyt, 1969; Hayreh, 1974). There are rich anastomoses between the prelaminar and nerve fibre layer vessels and between the latter and the radial peripapillary network described by Michaelson and Campbell (1940), Toussaint, Kuwabara and Cogan (1961) and Henkind (1967). Those vessels of central retinal artery origin are generally arteriolar or precapillary while those of the prelaminar region are of precapillary and capillary size.

Venous drainage

The venous drainage of the optic nerve head is much simpler than its arterial supply. In each zone, venules drain into the central retinal vein, or when present into a duplicated vein (probably an embryological persistence of hyaloid veins (Hayreh, 1963)). Occasional septal veins in the retrolaminar region drain into pial veins. Some small venules from the prelaminar region or from the nerve fibre layer (opticociliary veins) drain into the choroid (Lieberman, Maumenee and Green, 1976). They may enlarge in association with optic nerve sheath meningiomas.

BLOOD–BRAIN BARRIER AT THE OPTIC NERVE

The capillaries of the optic nerve head, as in the remainder of the optic nerve (Anderson, 1969; Anderson and Hoyt, 1969), the retina (Ishikawa, 1963; Cunha-Vaz, Shakib and Ashton, 1966; Shakib and Cunha-Vaz, 1966) and the central nervous system generally (Reese and Karnovsky, 1967), have non-fenestrated endothelial linings with tight junctions between adjacent endothelial cells. These junctions are responsible for the blood–tissue barrier to the diffusion of small molecules (such as proteins and tracer materials) across these capillaries. However, the blood–brain barrier at the optic nerve head is incomplete as a result of the continuity between the extracellular spaces of the choroid and the optic nerve head at the level of the choroid (in the prelaminar region, or the pars choroidalis).

There is no barrier to diffusion across the highly fenestrated capillaries of the choroid. Cohen (1973) noted that there was a potential route from the choriocapillaris, along Bruchs' membrane to the glial sheath of cells which invests the axons of the optic nerve in the prelaminar zone (border tissue of Jacoby). Tso, Shih and McLean (1975), using horseradish peroxidase as a tracer molecule in monkeys, demonstrated a deficiency of the blood–brain barrier in this region allowing the diffusion of tracer. This entered the extracellular space of the choroid into the extracellular space of the peripheral optic nerve at the prelaminar level. Peroxidase could be traced into the nerve head, across the glial sheath of astrocytes (at prelaminar level), along the septa of the lamina cribrosa and into the retrolaminar portion of the nerve head. Tracer also diffused around the axon bundles of the nerve head itself. These results confirm the earlier fluorescein studies of Grayson and Laties (1971) in the monkey and are in keeping with supportive studies in the human eye by McMahon *et al.* (1975) and Ben Sira and Riva (1975).

An important observation by Tso, Shih and McLean (1975) is the presence of tight junctions between those astrocytes which make up the marginal tissue of Kuhnt (Fig. 15.21b). This arrangement forms a glial 'gasket' which seals off the extracellular space of the optic nerve head from the peripapillary termination of the outer retina. Diffusion across the choriocapillaris and Bruch's membrane is impeded by the tight junctions between the retinal pigment epithelial cells themselves. This arrangement may have important implications for the behaviour of eyes with optic pits and papilloedema.

15.2 OPTIC CHIASMA

The crossing of neural tracts in the central nervous system is common, and the chiasma is no exception. Complete crossing of the retinal axons from right to left and vice versa is a characteristic of the bony fishes, most reptiles, amphibians and birds. In all mammals, except monotremes (Lund, 1978), a variable fraction of the fibres fail to cross, the proportion decreasing as the eyes become more forward placed. A partial crossing at the chiasma is associated with the development of overlapping visual fields and binocular function. In the equidae with laterally placed eyes and panoramic vision, only 15% of fibres are uncrossed while in the carnivora with more forward-directed eyes 25–30% of fibres are uncrossed (see Walls, 1963).

Partial decussation of human retinal axons was first

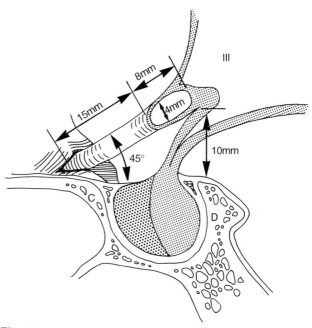

Fig. 15.55 Relation between the optic nerve and chiasm, the sellar structures and the third ventricle (III). C = anterior clinoid; D = Dorsum sellae. (From Olver, J. M., Spalton, D. J. and McCartney, A. C. E. (1990) *Eye*, **4**, 7, with permission.)

suspected by Isaac Newton who postulated the value of such an arrangement for binocular vision, providing for the representation of the homonymous retinal halves together in the same cerebral hemisphere. The idea was confirmed anatomically by Gudden (1874–9) and Cajal (1909) many years later (see Duke-Elder, 1961).

The optic chiasma is a flattened band, embedded in the anterior wall of the third ventricle between the two thalami and projecting into the chiasmatic cistern. This point may be overlooked by the student, because the chiasma is often separated from the third ventricle in dissection, but it is well demonstrated in Fig. 15.55. It overlies the sphenoid body but is separated from it by a variable distance of 0–10 mm (Traquair, 1916; Cope, 1916; Schweinitz, 1923). The chiasma lies obliquely, continuing the inclination of the optic nerves of 45° to the horizontal (Figs 15.55 and 15.56). Its anterior concavity is therefore directed downwards and forwards towards the anterior clinoid processes (Figs 15.57 and 15.58).

The chiasma is about 13 mm transversely (range 10–20 mm), 8 mm in sagittal diameter (range 4–13 mm) and 3–5 mm thick (Whitnall, 1932; Hoyt, 1969). It lies at the junction of anterior wall and floor of the third ventricle, forming the floor of a ventricular (supraoptic) recess reaching almost to its anterior border (Fig. 15.57). Covered by pia it lies obliquely, with its posterior border above the anterior

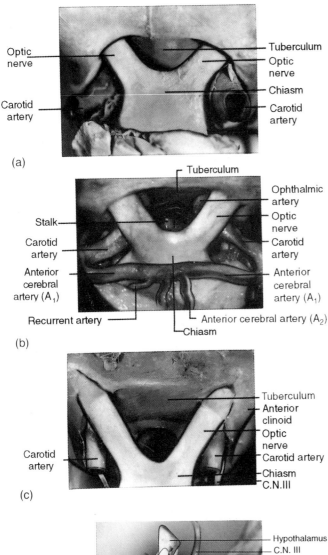

(a)

(b)

(c)

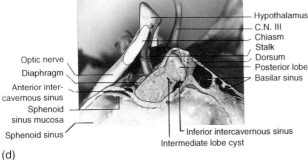

(d)

Fig. 15.56 Dorsal view of the sellar region. A, prefixed chiasm; B, normal chiasm. The anterior cerebral arteries pass dorsal to the chiasm. The left recurrent artery arises from the A-1 segment of the left anterior cerebral artery. The pituitary stalk is between the optic nerves. C, post-fixed chiasm. Diaphragma sellae and pituitary gland removed. The IIIrd cranial nerves lie ventral to the carotid arteries. D, midsagittal section of the sellar region showing the optic nerve and chiasm, IIIrd cranial nerve, inferior part of the hypothalamus and the pituitary stalk and gland. The anterior and inferior intercavernous sinuses are small. Note the 45° obliquity of the optic nerves as they emerge from the optic canals. (From Renn, W. H. and Rhoton, A. L. (1975) *J. Neurosurg.*, **43**, 288, with permission.)

in the interpeduncular cistern above the diaphragma sellae, posterosuperior to the chiasmal groove.

In its most common location (79% of cases) it overlies the dorsum sellae, with the pituitary fossa below and anterior. In 12% it is more anterior (prefixed) and overlies the diaphragma, in which case the tuberculum sellae may project about 2 mm behind the anterior border of the chiasma: in only 5% (also prefixed) does the chiasma lie in the sulcus chiasmaticus (Rhoton, Harris and Renn, 1977), while in a further 4% the chiasma lies over and behind the dorsum sellae (post-fixed) about 7 mm behind the tuberculum sellae (Schweinitz, 1923; Schaeffer, 1924; Bergland, Ray and Torack, 1968; Rhoton, Harris and Renn, 1977). The chiasma is not in contact with the diaphragma, but is separated from it by 5–10 mm. Hence part of the cisterna interpeduncularis is inferior to the chiasma (Fig. 15.57).

The optic chiasma is in contact with the cerebrospinal fluid of the chiasmatic cistern anteriorly and below and with that of the third ventricle posteriorly, except where it is continuous with the cerebrum (Fig. 15.59). The chiasmatic cistern is an expanded region of the subarachnoid space which extends from the pituitary stalk forwards around the optic nerves into the olfactory sulci and above into the cisterna lamina terminalis. Its caudal part may be narrowed to a slit-like zone filled with a trabecular membrane, which extends across the lateral margins of the infundibulum to fuse with the arachnoid around the carotid arteries and up over the inferior surface of the chiasm (Lindgren, 1957).

RELATIONS (Figs 15.57 and 15.58)

Anterior

Anteriorly are the anterior cerebral and anterior communicating arteries. These may lie above or on the surface of the optic nerve and chiasm. In a study by Rhoton, Harris and Renn (1977) the anterior communicating artery was usually above the chiasma rather than the optic nerves. Aneurysms arising from it or from the proximal (A1) segment of the anterior cerebral artery may compress either the chiasma or one or both optic nerves. The anterior cerebral arteries at their origins from the carotid arteries pass forwards and medially above the chiasma to the interhemispheric fissure where they turn backwards over the corpus callosum. When the proximal segment is short it is smoothly apposed to the chiasma, but otherwise passes anteriorly over the optic nerves (Figs 15.60 and 5.2).

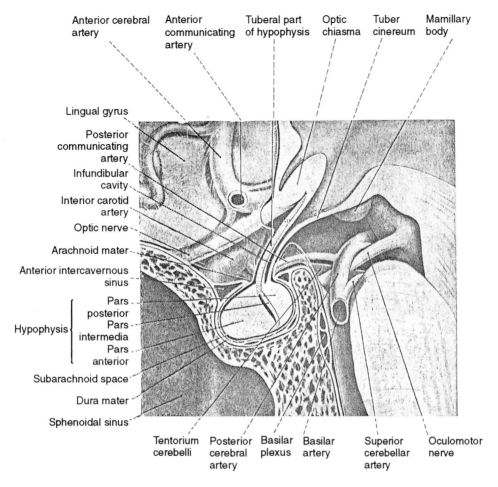

Fig. 15.57 Diagrammatic median section of hypophysis (*in situ*). (The existence of a subarachnoid space around the gland in the pituitary fossa is doubtful.) (From Cunningham's 'Anatomy'.)

Lateral

Laterally the chiasma is in continuity with the anterior perforated substance. The internal carotid artery as it ascends from the roof of the cavernous sinus is in contact with the chiasma between optic nerve and tract (Figs 5.2, 15.58 and 15.30). Also lateral is the anterior perforated substance. Posteriorly is the quadrilateral, interpeduncular space, with the chiasm and anterior tract forming anterior boundaries and cerebral peduncles the posterior. Within this is the tuber cinereum and then the mammillary body behind (Fig. 15.27). From the apex of the chiasma depends the infundibulum (hypophyseal stalk), a hollow conical process descending forwards through a hole in the posterior part of the diaphragma sellae to the posterior lobe of the gland. The infundibulum is thus very close to the posteroinferior part of the chiasma, which it joins at an acute angle.

Superior

Above is the third ventricle, into the floor of which the chiasma projects. It is continuous anteriorly with the lamina terminalis which closes the anterior end of the diencephalon and extends up to the anterior commissure (Fig. 15.61). This location explains its vulnerability to compression or stretching by tumours of the third ventricle, or the raised ventricular pressure of internal hydrocephalus. The medial root of the olfactory tract is superolateral to the anterior part of the chiasma (Fig. 15.29a).

Inferior

Inferior is the hypophysis, and laterally the cavernous sinus (with its contents), with the oculomotor nerve the closest on the diaphragma before entering the sinus.

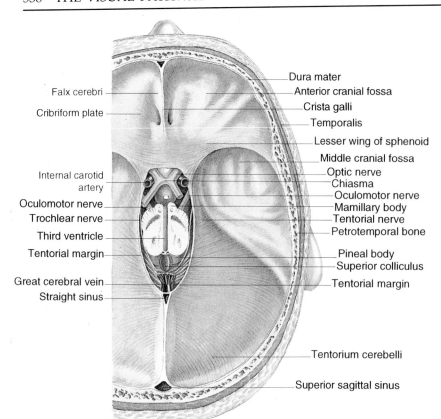

Falx cerebri

Cribriform plate

Internal carotid artery

Oculomotor nerve

Trochlear nerve

Third ventricle

Tentorial margin

Great cerebral vein

Straight sinus

Dura mater

Anterior cranial fossa

Crista galli

Temporalis

Lesser wing of sphenoid

Middle cranial fossa

Optic nerve

Chiasma

Oculomotor nerve

Mamillary body

Tentorial nerve

Petrotemporal bone

Pineal body

Superior colliculus

Tentorial margin

Tentorium cerebelli

Superior sagittal sinus

Fig. 15.58 Section of cranium just above tentorium cerebelli. (From Hirschfield and Leveillé.)

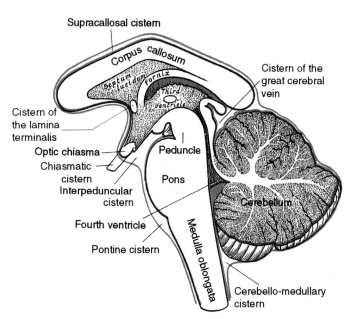

Supracallosal cistern

Corpus callosum

Septum lucidum

Fornix

Third ventricle

Cistern of the great cerebral vein

Cistern of the lamina terminalis

Optic chiasma

Chiasmatic cistern

Interpeduncular cistern

Peduncle

Pons

Cerebellum

Fourth ventricle

Pontine cistern

Medulla oblongata

Cerebello-medullary cistern

Fig. 15.59 Diagram to show the positions of the principal subarachnoid cisterns. Red: pia mater. Blue: arachnoid mater. (From *Gray's Anatomy* (1995) 38th Edition, ed. P. L. Williams, Churchill Livingstone, with permission.)

The arachnoid spreads between the optic nerves, and is attached to the pole of the temporal lobe and internal carotid artery laterally and anteriorly to the frontal lobes (Fig. 5.3).

NEURAL ORGANIZATION WITHIN THE CHIASMA

It is agreed on the basis of human and primate studies that the retinotopic distribution of retinal axons continues within the chiasma though here, because of the complication of the chiasmal decussation and perhaps also because of the oblique placement of the chiasma, the detailed organization in the human is not precisely established. The degree of retinotopy is less than previously thought. Human information has been derived from clinical studies relating field defect to chiasmal compression and from studies of autopsy material in patients with optic neuropathies and other anterior visual pathway disease (e.g. Henschen, 1893; Wilbrand and Saenger, 1906; Ronne, 1914). Degeneration studies in monkeys gave some support to such human data (Brouwer and Zeeman, 1925, 1926) and culminated in the studies

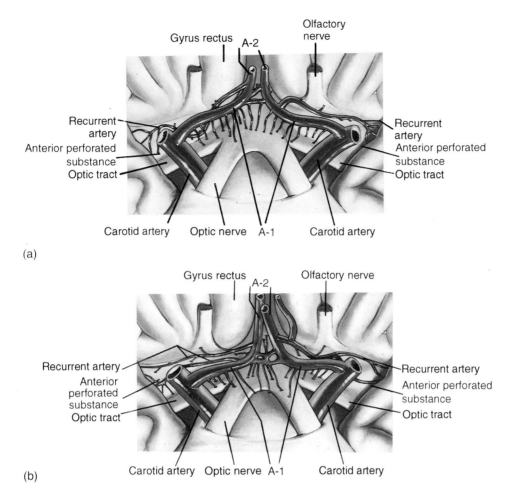

Fig. 15.60 Anterior views of the A-1 and proximal A-2 segments of the anterior cerebral arteries, anterior communicating arteries, and recurrent arteries showing variations in blood supply to the intracranial optic nerves and chiasm. Gyrus recti and olfactory nerves are located superiorly. (From Perlmutter, D. and Rhoton, A. L. Jr (1976) *J. Neurosurg.*, **45**, 259, with permission.)

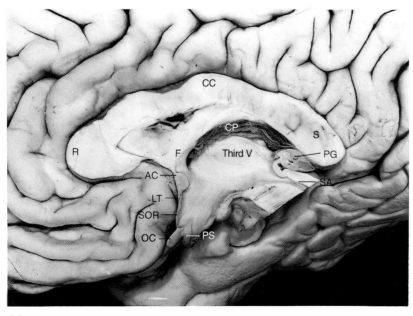

(a)

Fig. 15.61 (a) Medial surface of the brain following sagittal section passing through the corpus callosum and third ventricle. AC, anterior commissure; CC, corpus callosum; CP, choroid plexus; F, fornix; LT, lamina terminalis; OC, optic chiasm; PG, pineal gland; PS, pituitary stalk; R, rostrum; S, splenium; SA, sylvian aquaduct; SOR, supraoptic recess; Third V, median part of the thalamus seen in the third ventricle. (Courtesy of A. Duvernoy.)

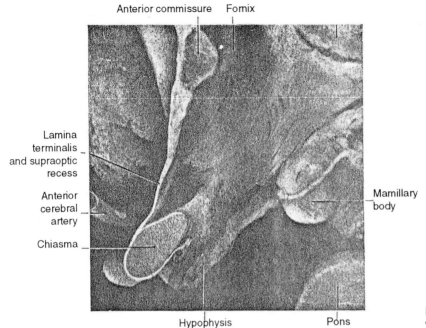

Anterior commissure   Fornix

Lamina
terminalis
and supraoptic
recess

Anterior
cerebral
artery

Chiasma

Mamillary
body

Hypophysis
(pituitary)

Pons

Fig. 15.61 (contd) (b) Higher power view of the relationship between the optic chiasm and third ventricle.

(b)

of Hoyt and Louis (1963) tracing axons in human nerves instead of myelin degeneration in monkeys.

The concept of semidecussation of the optic nerve fibres at the chiasma was well reviewed by Rucker (1958). The uncrossed, temporal and crossed, nasal retinal axons begin to separate in the most proximal nerve and anterior chiasm, the crossing fibres lying medial to the end of the pial septum in the nerve. The macular representation is high in both neural streams.

Uncrossed fibres

Uncrossed fibres maintain the relationship in the chiasma that they held in the optic nerve, travelling backwards as a flattened compact bundle in the lateral part of the chiasma, carrying axons from the ipsilateral, temporal hemiretina. Fibres from the upper retina come to lie in the dorsal and slightly medial part of the tract (eventually coming to lie medially as they reach the lateral geniculate body). Those from the lower retina occupy a ventral and slightly lateral position as they enter the tract (and will be lateral as the tract enters the lateral geniculate body). In the chiasma they mingle not only with the nasal fibres from the same side, but also with those of the opposite side looping forward into the proximal nerve. In cases of unilateral optic atrophy, this is not demonstrated in horizontal sections, but

only in coronal, where the uncrossed bundle of the fellow eye survives laterally in the chiasma as a reniform area with its hilum medially.

Crossed fibres

Crossed fibres arising from the nasal hemiretinae (53% of the total; Kupfer, Chumbley and de Downer (1967)) decussate to join the contralateral optic tract, but not all by the shortest route. As the nasal fibres approach the chiasma they spread out horizontally across almost the whole width of the optic nerve to form a roughly quadrilateral sheet of fibres, some of which loop posteriorly into the ipsilateral optic tract and others which loop anteriorly into the contralateral optic nerve, before joining the contralateral tract (Fig. 15.62). Fibres from the inferior nasal retinal quadrants decussate anteriorly in the chiasma; the most anterior of these loop forward in the proximal part of the contralateral optic nerve for a distance of up to 3 mm and then pass backwards to the inferomedial part of the optic tract. These anterior loop fibres mingle with optic nerve fibres still parallel to the nerve axis to form a characteristic interlacing basketwork (the knee of Wilbrand).

It is because of these anterior loop fibres that compression of the proximal optic nerve may affect both the field of that eye and that of the opposite side. These fibres probably cross low in the chiasma

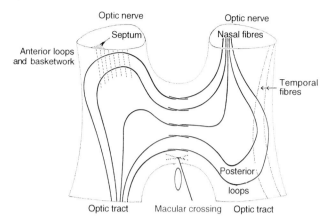

Fig. 15.62 The decussation of nerve fibres in the optic chiasma. To avoid confusion, only the fibres from one side are shown (except at the actual decussation).

because chiasmal involvement by pituitary tumours is often heralded by an upper bitemporal quadrantanopsia.

Fibres from the superonasal retinal quadrant pass at first backwards in the chiasma somewhat to the lateral side (Fig. 15.62) and mix with the uncrossed temporal fibres. The most lateral, loop backwards into the ipsilateral optic tract before crossing the chiasma to the superomedial part of the contralateral tract. These posterior loops are less prominent than the anterior.

Actual decussation is central in the chiasma, anterior fibres crossing at more acute angles than posterior. Fibres decussate not only from side to side, but also in ascending and descending directions (see Traquair, 1957; Polyak, 1957; Duke-Elder and Cook, 1963).

Macular fibres

In the posterior part of the optic nerve the macular fibres are central and maintain this position as they enter the chiasma. The crossing fibres separate from the non-crossing fibres and pass as a bundle obliquely and upwards to decussate with those fibres of the opposite side, somewhat posteriorly in the chiasma (what Traquair referred to as 'a little chiasma within the chiasma and within its posterior part'). Macular axons and those from the central retina occupy most of the central part of the chiasma to the exclusion of peripheral decussating fibres. Lesions here, therefore, cause a central bitemporal hemianopic scotoma.

Non-visual commissural fibres

Supraoptic commissural fibres have been noted in some species but not confirmed in humans or monkeys. Polyak (1957) found interretinal fibres in primate optic nerves. Magoun and Ransom (1942) identified a **dorsal commissure** of Ganser and **ventral commissures** of Gudden and Meynert. Gitlin and Lowenthal (1969) were not convinced of their existence (see also Crosby, Humphrey and Laver, 1962; Williams and Warwick, 1975).

VASCULAR SUPPLY

The chiasma is supplied by a rich collateral anastomosis of chiasmatic arteries; blockage of any single vessel is unlikely to have a marked effect on visual fibres.

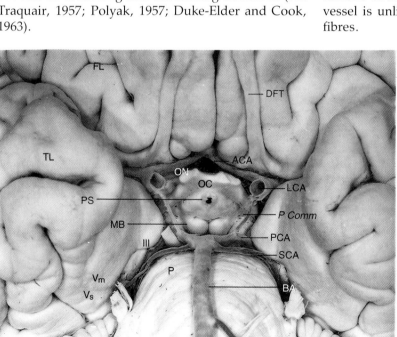

Fig. 15.63 Ventral aspect of the brain to show the relation of the circle of Willis to the cerebral hemispheres and brain stem. aca, anterior cerebral artery; b/a, basilar artery; FL, frontal lobe; ica, internal carotid artery; MB, mamillary body; OC, optic chiasm; OLFT, olfactory tract; ON, optic nerve; PCA, posterior cerebral artery; P, pons; PCOMMA, posterior communicating artery; SCA, superior cerebellar artery; TL, temporal lobe. III, third cranial nerve; IV$_m$; V$_s$; motor and sensory branches of the fifth cranial nerve.

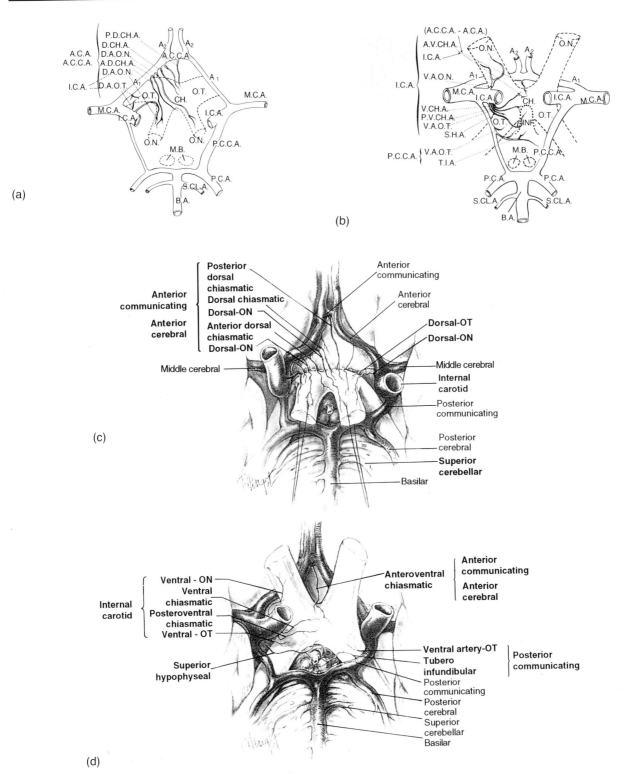

Fig. 15.64 Schematic representation of the blood supply to (a) the ventral optic chiasma and optic nerves, (b) the dorsal optic chiasma and optic nerves. A₁ = anterior cerebral artery, horizontal part; A₂ = anterior cerebral artery, distal to the anterior communicating artery; A.C.C.A. = anterior communicating artery; A.D.CH.A. = antero (dorsal) (rostrodorsal) chiasmatic artery; B.A. = basilar artery; CH. = chiasm; D.A.O.N. = dorsal artery of the optic nerve; D.A.O.T. = dorsal artery of the optic tract; D.CH.A. = dorsal chiasmatic artery; I.C.A. = internal carotid artery; M.B. = mamillary bodies; M.C.A. = middle cerebral artery; O.N. = optic nerve; O.T. = optic tract; D.C.A. = posterior cerebral artery; P.C.C.A. = posterior communicating artery; P.D.CH.A. = posterodorsal (caudodorsal) chiasmatic artery; S.CL.A. = superior cerebellar artery. (c) the dorsal optic chiasm and optic nerves; (d) the ventral optic chiasm and nerves. (From Wollschlaeger *et al.* (1971) *Ann. Ophthalmol.*, **3**, 862.)

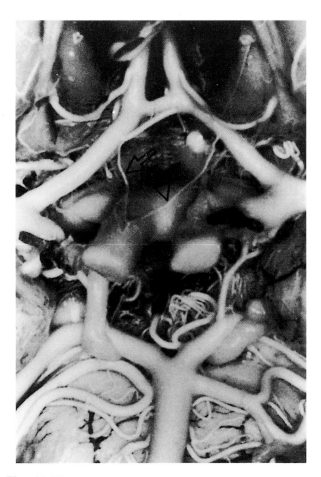

Fig. 15.65 Two arteries supplying the right optic nerve (arrows). (The optic nerves are retracted into a ventral position.) (From Wollschlaeger, *et al.*, (1972) *Ann. Ophthalmol.*, **3**, 862, with permission.)

Injection studies by Wollschlaeger *et al.* (1971) in 630 autopsy specimens demonstrated the following supplies (Figs 15.64 and 15.65).

1. A **dorsal supply** mainly from the proximal (A1) segments of the anterior cerebral arteries and a lesser supply from the internal carotid and anterior communicating arteries. Perlmutter and Rhoton (1976) always found a contribution from central branches of the distal (A2) segment of the anterior cerebral arteries.
2. A **ventral supply** mainly from the internal carotid and anterior communicating arteries. Unlike Bergland and Ray (1969) Wollschlaeger *et al.* did not identify contributions from posterior communicating, posterior cerebral and basilar arteries.

Small additional 'feeders' may be supplied by the superior hypophyseal and middle cerebral arteries.

Wollschlaeger *et al.* (1971) have classified two groups of chiasmatic arteries: **dorsal**, with antero- and posterodorsal branches, and **ventral**, with antero- and posteroventral branches. There are anastomoses between corresponding members of each group.

The optic tracts and remainder of the retrochiasmal pathway are dealt with on p. 544.

HYPOPHYSIS CEREBRI (PITUITARY GLAND)

The hypophysis consists of an **anterior lobe**, derived from the stomatodeum, glandular in structure; a **posterior lobe**, the pars nervosa, an outgrowth from the cerebral vesicle, composed largely of neuroglia and fine non-myelinated nerve fibres. A vestigial cleft of the oral cavity, Rathke's pouch, separates the major part of the anterior pituitary from a thin zone of tissue, the pars intermedia, which lies adjacent to the posterior pituitary (Fig. 15.66).

The pituitary gland is small and ovoid, with maximum and minimum diameters of about 12 and 8 mm. It is situated in the hypophyseal fossa of the sella turcica on the superior (cranial) surface of the sphenoid, about midway between the cribriform plate and the foramen magnum. In front are the tuberculum sellae and groove behind the dorsum sellae. The roof of the fossa is formed by the dural diaphragma sellae (Fig. 15.57), perforated centrally for the infundibulum, which connects the hypophysis to the floor of the fourth ventricle. On each side the hypophysis is flanked by dura mater, which separates it from the cavernous sinus and structures within it. In the lateral wall of the sinus are the oculomotor, trochlear, ophthalmic and maxillary nerves in descending order. Within the sinus are the internal carotid artery and lateral to it the abducent separated from it by the internal carotid artery. Joining the cavernous sinuses in the hypophyseal fossa are anterior and posterior inter-cavernous sinuses, forming a 'circular sinus', which is usually plexiform.

In the body of the sphenoid, below the hypophysis, are two sphenoidal sinuses separated by a median septum, and each presenting in its lateral wall the carotid buttress, a ledge of bone, often discernible in radiographs and an important landmark in approaching the gland by the nasal route. The circulus arteriosus (of Willis) is superior to the level of the hypophyseal fossa and may encircle an enlarging tumour. The trigeminal ganglion, on the apex of the petrous bone, is lateral to the cavernous sinus, and above this is the uncus, pressure on which by a tumour may evoke olfactory hallucinations.

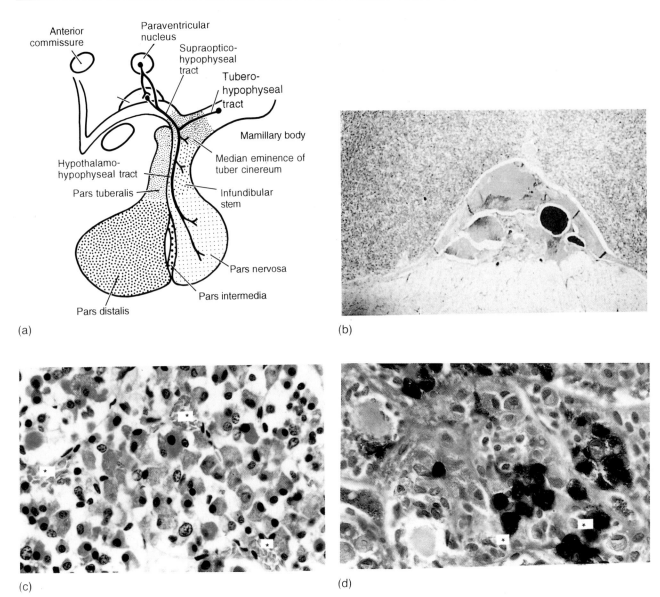

Fig. 15.66 (a) Diagram of the pituitary gland with the origin and distribution of the hypothalamo-hypophyseal tract. (From Miller (1985), redrawn from Crosby, E. C., Humphrey, T. and Laver, E. W. (1962) *Correlative Anatomy of the Nervous System*, published by Macmillan.) (b) Normal pituitary gland. Junction between the anterior (above) and posterior (below) lobes. A small cyst is present in the posterior lobe. (c) Cells of the anterior pituitary stained with PAS and orange G. *, blood vessels. (d) Anterior pituitary gland immunostained for growth hormone secreting cells. *, dark. The typical microacinar architecture of the gland is well shown. ((b), (c) and (d) courtesy of M. Esiri.)

The meninges blend with the capsule of the hypophysis, obliterating the subarachnoid space, and cannot be identified as such (Warwick and Williams, 1973). The hypophysis is supplied from the internal carotid artery by upper and lower hypophyseal branches, which supply the stalk and posterior lobe, from the capillaries of which a portal system of vessels provides the major supply to the anterior lobe (Xuerer, Prichard and Daniel, 1954). The hypophyseal veins drain to the intercavernous plexus and cavernous sinuses (Stanfield, 1960).

15.3 OPTIC TRACTS

The optic tracts, often described as if extracerebral, are completely integral with the inferior aspect of the cerebrum. Moreover, the fibres of the optic nerve, chiasma and tract are axons of 'secondary' neurons, which are confined to the central nervous system.

Each optic tract is a slightly flattened cylindrical band, travelling posterolaterally from the angle of the chiasma, between the tuber cinereum and anterior perforated substance (Fig. 15.29). It is the antero-

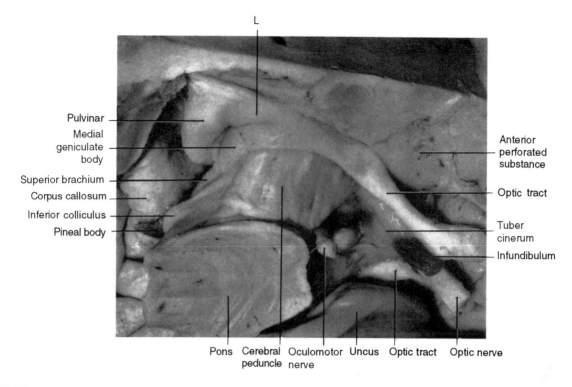

L

Pulvinar

Medial
geniculate
body

Superior brachium

Corpus callosum

Inferior colliculus

Pineal body

Anterior
perforated
substance

Optic tract

Tuber
cinerum

Infundibulum

Pons   Cerebral   Oculomotor   Uncus   Optic tract   Optic nerve
peduncle   nerve

Fig. 15.67 Relations of the optic tract. A further stage in the dissection of Fig. 15.71. The uncus and hippocampus have been removed.

lateral boundary of the interpeduncular space. Becoming flatter the tract skirts the anterolateral aspect of the cerebral peduncle, united to it and close to the entry of the peduncle into its hemisphere (Fig. 15.67). Below and parallel to the tract is the **posterior cerebral artery**, and even closer the **anterior choroidal**, which arises from the internal carotid lateral to the posterior communicating artery, lateral to the commencement of the optic tract (Figs 15.30, 15.68–15.70). Turning posteromedially the anterior choroidal artery crosses below the optic tract to become medial, maintaining this relation to the anterior part of the lateral geniculate body. It is frequently a branch of the middle cerebral.

Anteriorly the optic tract is continuous with the wall of the third ventricle only along a narrow medial zone. It passes posterolaterally, ascends slightly round the cerebral peduncle, and rotates slightly so that the zone of continuity with the cerebrum is first dorsomedial and finally dorsolateral, its lateral border becoming ventral. The dorsal fasciculi are said to be partially surrounded by the supraoptic 'commissures' (of Meynert and Gudden), which are really decussations, while the ventral bundles are free and covered by thin pia mater.

Anteriorly, the optic tract is superficial to the

inferior cerebral surface (Fig. 15.29), above the dorsum sellae, and the tract crosses with the oculomotor nerve to its lateral side (Fig. 15.58). Above is the posterior part of the anterior perforated substance and floor of the third ventricle, medially the tuber cinereum.

In the middle part of its course, the tract is overlapped by the uncus and cerebral peduncle. Its flattening here begins to conform with the upper surface of the uncus (Figs 15.71 and 15.72). Here the optic tract crosses the corticospinal tract in the middle segment of the cerebral peduncle, and dorsal to the substantia nigra are main sensory tracts (lemnisci). A single lesion at this site may affect vision and the large motor and sensory tracts. The optic radiations also cross and come close to the motor and sensory tracts in the posterior part of the internal capsule, so that here a single lesion may affect all three pathways.

Posteriorly the optic tract is deep in the hippocampal sulcus near the inferior horn of the lateral ventricle. It has the globus pallidus above, the internal capsule medially, and the hippocampus below (Figs 15.72 and 15.73). The tract here develops a superficial sulcus which is more apparent as it approaches the lateral (geniculate) and medial (collicular) parts, or so-called 'roots'.

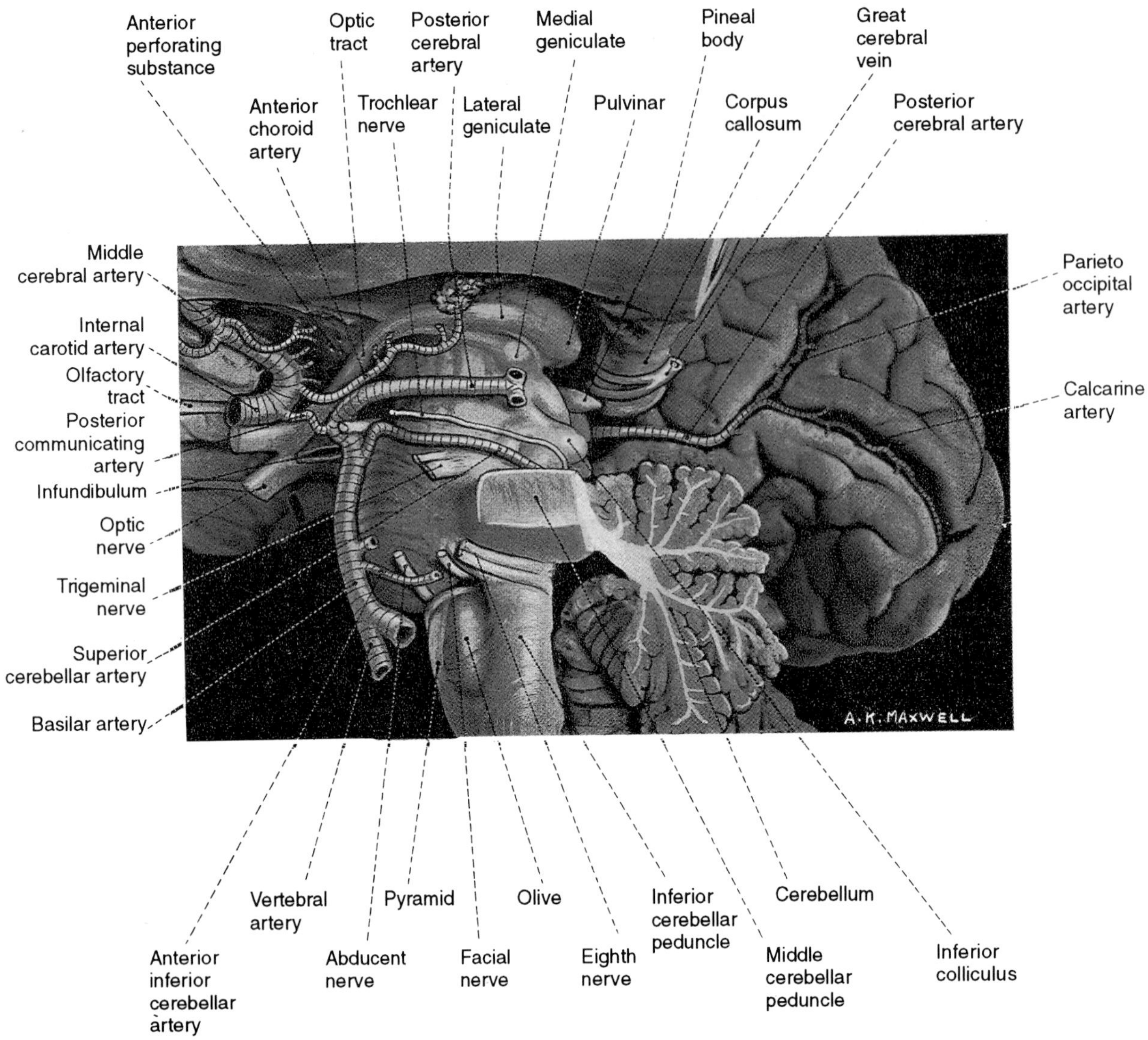

Fig. 15.68 Dissection to show the blood supply of the visual pathway and the relations of the vessels to the ocular nerves. (Wolff's preparation.)

MEDIAL ROOT

The medial root, the 'commissure' of Gudden, is sometimes still described as a supraoptic pathway connecting the two medial geniculate bodies by passing to the medial side of each optic tract and behind the chiasma, and even to be an auditory commissure. These concepts are no longer tenable. The elevation ascribed to the medial 'root' is partly due to the lateral geniculate nucleus, whose medial part is immediately superior (Figs 15.74 and 15.75) and may thus augment the elevation (Figs 15.76 and 15.77). Nerve fibres in the medial part of the tract are therefore very close to the lateral geniculate nucleus, but any participation of them in vision is completely obscure in humans.

LATERAL ROOT

The lateral root spreads over the lateral geniculate body, and mostly ends in it. The groove between the roots runs into the hilum of the body, which is usually a definite cleft (Figs 15.76 and 15.77).

The fibres of the optic tract, axons from retinal ganglion cells, reach four major destinations: (1) lateral geniculate nucleus for relay to the visual cortex; (2) each pretectal nucleus as part of the pupilloconstrictor path; (3) superior colliculus for reflex responses to light; (4) the nucleus of the optic tract (NOT) and nuclei of the supraoptic pathway, concerned with the optokinetic reflex (see Chapter 4).

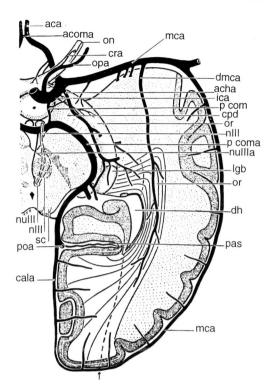

Fig. 15.69 Total blood supply to the visual pathways, viewed from the ventral aspect: semi-schematic. (Abbie.) Note the different sources of supply to the optic radiation. The arrow at the bottom of the figure marks the point of anastomosis between the calcarine and middle cerebral arteries.
ac = anterior commissure; aca = anterior cerebral artery; a ch a = anterior choroidal artery; acoma = anterior communicating artery; bol = olfactory bulb; cala = calcarine artery; cals = calcarine sulcus; cc = corpus callosum; cpd = cerebral peduncle; cplx = choroidal plexus; cra = central artery of the retina; do mca = deep optic branch of the middle cerebral artery; f = fornix; h = hilum of lateral geniculate body; ha = hilar anastomosis; ica = internal carotid artery; lgb = lateral geniculate body; luns = lunate sulcus; mca = middle cerebral artery; mgb = medial geniculate body; nIII = oculomotor nerve, nuIII = oculomotor nucleus; nu III a = artery to the oculomotor nucleus; nur = red nucleus; och = optic chiasma; on = optic nerve; or = optic radiation; ot = optic tract; opa = ophthalmic artery; pca = posterior cerebral artery; p com a = posterior communicating artery; poa = parieto-occipital artery; po = pons; pcals = posterior calcarine sulcus; pos = parieto-occipital sulcus; pth = pulvinar thalami; sc = superior colliculus; sn = substantia nigra; tp = temporal pole.

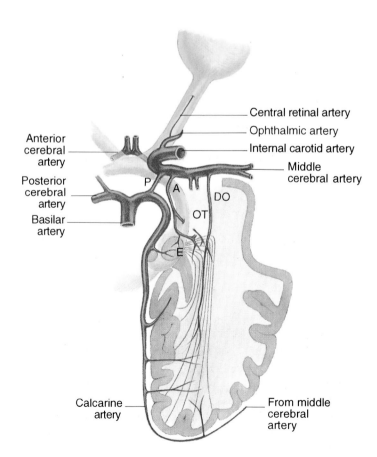

Fig. 15.70 The arteries of the visual tract, inferior view. (Modified after Abbie.)

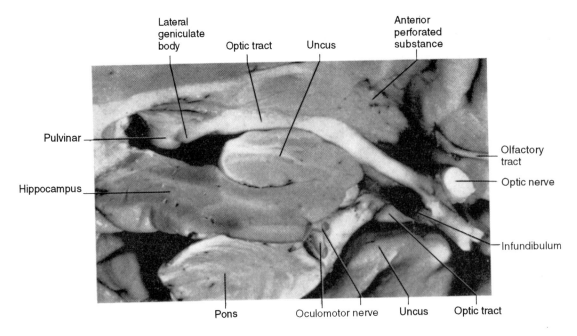

Fig. 15.71   Relations of the optic tract. The uncus and hippocampus have been divided vertically.

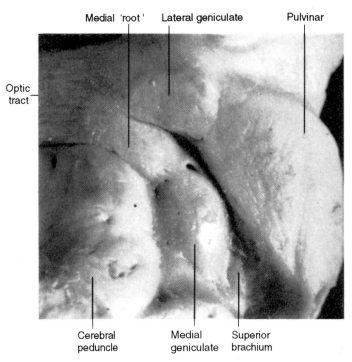

Fig. 15.72   Section of the brain in the plane of the brain stem from in front. On the left the section through the hemisphere is somewhat dorsal to that on the right. I, II and III indicate the anterior, medial and lateral nuclei of the thalamus. (From Sabotta.)

LOCALIZATION IN THE OPTIC TRACT

In the chiasma, crossed and uncrossed fibres are intermingled and when they reach the optic tract they are rearranged to correspond with their position in the lateral geniculate body, i.e. the macular fibres (crossed and uncrossed) occupy an area of the cross-section dorsolaterally; the lower retinal quadrants are lateral, those from the upper are medial. The fibres from the peripheral portions of the retina lie more anteriorly.

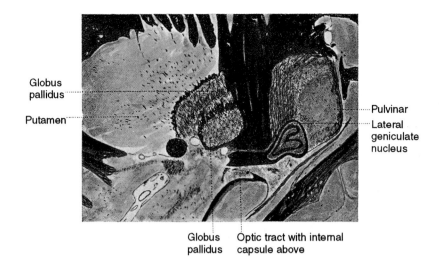

Globus pallidus

Putamen

Pulvinar

Lateral geniculate nucleus

Globus pallidus

Optic tract with internal capsule above

Fig. 15.73 Para-sagittal section of the brain (Weigert). Showing optic tract dividing to form capsule to lateral geniculate body; also its relation to the internal capsule.

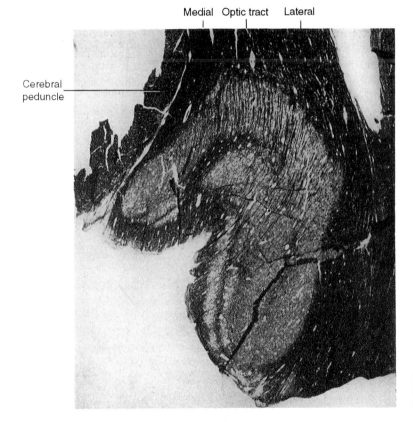

Medial Optic tract Lateral

Cerebral peduncle

Fig. 15.74 Horizontal section of human lateral geniculate body with termination of optic tract. (Stained Wiegert-Pal.)

TOPOGRAPHIC ORGANIZATION IN THE OPTIC NERVE, CHIASMA AND TRACT

It is no longer possible to sustain the view that the chiasma simply represents the site at which a retinotopic organization of the optic nerves is rearranged into hemiretinotopic organization in the tracts (Guillery, 1991). It has become clear from studies in non-primate species such as the ferret, cat and mouse that, despite the retinotopic maps which may be demonstrated within the layers of the lateral geniculate nucleus, the level of spatial organization changes from the optic nerve head to the nucleus itself. This also applies, although information is more scarce, to the human visual pathway. The basic retinotopic map is modified in three important ways along the retinogeniculate pathway.

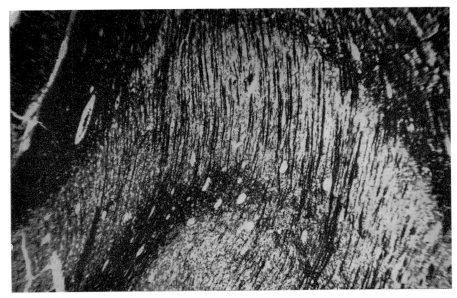

Fig. 15.75 As Fig. 15.74, but at higher magnification. Note medullated fibres entering lateral geniculate nucleus from the tract. No line of demarcation is visible between medial and lateral portion of the tract.

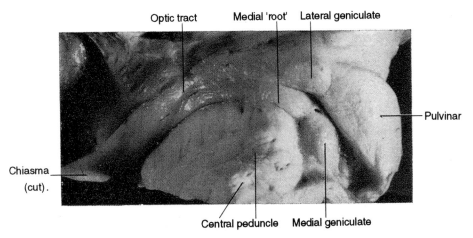

Fig. 15.76 The optic tract, etc, from below. Note two portions of the lateral geniculate body with hilum between them. See caption to Fig. 15.67.

1. There is a loss of retinotopic organization in the optic nerve as the chiasma is approached. Horton *et al.* (1979) found no precise retinotopic map in the normal cat optic nerve or tract, near-neighbour axons in the retina became widely separated in the proximal pathway.
2. Fibres destined to cross or to remain uncrossed at the chiasma are not strictly segregated in the optic nerve, and within the tract, the crossed fibres from the contralateral nasal hemiretina do not lie in perfect register with the uncrossed fibres from ipsilateral temporal hemiretina. This partial segregation of crossed and uncrossed fibres within the tract has been used to explain incongruous homonymous hemianopic field defects in patients with partial optic tract lesions (Bender and Bodis Wollner, 1978; Savino *et al.*, 1978; Newman and Miller, 1983).
3. The retinal axons also become segregated according to fibre size in both the optic nerve and tract. Because retinal ganglion cell size and axon diameter correlate with the input into the magno- and parvocellular layers of the lateral geniculate nucleus, this probably has important functional implications. As noted elsewhere, the largest fibres in the cat (Y – over 4 μm wide) are destined

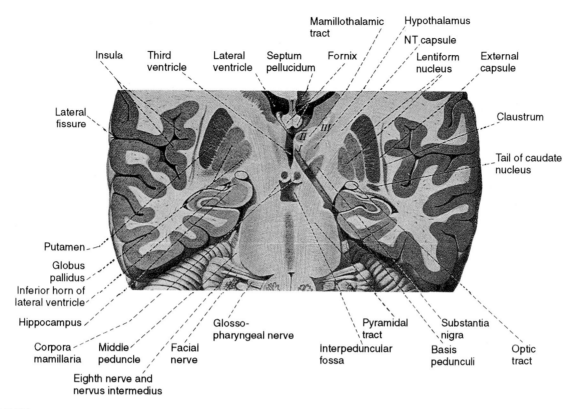

Fig. 15.77 Enlarged view of a portion of Fig. 15.71. The elevation marked as 'medial root' is in part due to the medial rim or spur of the lateral geniculate nucleus. The cleft between this and the main lateral geniculate elevation or 'body' corresponds approximately to the hilum of the nucleus. See also Fig. 15.71.

for the magnocellular layers of the nucleus, and are equivalent to the M fibres of the monkey. Medium-sized fibres (X fibres, 2–4 μm) are equivalent to P fibres in the monkey, and are distributed to the parvocellular layers. The smallest fibres of the cat optic nerve (W fibres, <1.5 μm) may also be represented in the primate.

It has been known since the 1970s that, although fibres of different diameter are mingled in the optic nerve, they become segregated in the optic tract (van Crevel and Verhaart, 1963; Donovan, 1967). Guillery, Polley and Torrealba, (1982) have shown that in the cat X axons lie deepest in the tract, the Y are superficial, and the W axons are found throughout the nerve's cross-section but are concentrated superficially just deep to the pia. It has been further shown in both cat and ferret that it is the time of arrival of the retinal axons at the chiasma during development which determines their location in the optic tract. Thus, fibres that are the latest to arrive lie most superficially, nearest to the pia (Guillery, Polley and Torrealba, 1982; Torrealba *et al.*, 1982). In the cat the order of appearance of retinal axons is first the X axons, and then the Y axons. The appearance of the W axons is more distributed in time, but is concentrated in late development (Walsh *et al.*, 1983; Walsh and Guillery, 1985; Walsh and Polley, 1985). It can therefore be seen that the spatial organization of the fibre classes (X deepest, Y more superficial, and W the most superficial) is determined by developmental timing (i.e. there is a series of chronotopic maps). It follows that the spatial maps for each fibre class are not in register in the tract, just as the retinal axons from the contralateral hemiretinae are not in register.

In developing fish and amphibia, ganglion cell axons arise in a perfect central-to-peripheral sequence, so that the chronotopic order maintains the retinopic relationships throughout the retinofugal pathway. In mammals such as the cat, retinofugal axons appear in waves which show only a rough central-to-peripheral order (Walsh and Polley, 1985).

A group of pure crossed fibres, arising from the most peripheral contralateral nasal retina and corresponding to the monocular crescent of the visual field, can be demonstrated in the optic tract. In the cat, for instance, this lies ventrally in the tract. However, another pure crossed group of fibres is present in the dorsal part of the tract. This is made up of fibres arising from the ventral contralateral nasal retina, which originate earlier than their counterparts in the ipsilateral temporal retina and are therefore segregated from them in the tract. As noted, birth order of the retinal ganglion cells corresponds to the deep-to-superficial order in the tract. Examination of the growth cones of retinofugal axons in the developing ferret shows that, although they are distributed throughout the section of the optic nerve, they are heavily concentrated near the subpial surface of the optic tract, next to the subpial end feet of the glia (Guillery and Walsh, 1987; Colello and Guillery, 1987; Colello, 1990). At some point in their course they are deviated towards the pial surface. This changeover point moves proximally during development and coincides with a change in organization of the glial cells. In the optic nerve the glia have an interfascicular distribution, with their nuclei scattered and their processes enveloping fibre bundles as they extend towards the pial surface. More proximally, nearer to the brain, the glial nuclei are periventricular (adjacent to the ventricular cavity of the eye stalk), and they extend radial processes away from the axon bundles towards the ventral pia. Guillery suggests that the advancing growth cones, on reaching these processes, are guided down them towards the ventral pial surface (Guillery and Walsh, 1987). The time of arrival of axons in the chiasmal region during development, and glial factors such as those mentioned above, are important determinants of the nasotemporal segregation of fibres at the chiasma although selective fibre loss also plays a role (Lund, 1978; Lund and Hankin, 1995; Cowan et al., 1984; Leventhal et al., 1988).

The segregation of axons according to class has also been recorded in primates. Hoyt and Luis (1963) described this in the monkey chiasma, and noted larger fibres in the lower, more superficial parts of the tract. Reese and Guillery (1987) found a non-homogeneous distribution of fibre diameters in the optic nerve and tract, with the wider fibres, destined for the magnocellular layers (nearest to the pia), lying nearer to the surface. Bender and Bodis-Wollner (1978) noted that tract lesions in patients can produce

a dissociation of perceptual loss, with colour and form losses appearing earlier than losses to movement. This is in keeping with the possibility that fibre classes, and the functions that they subserve, are segregated in the tract.

SUPRAOPTIC COMMISSURES (OF GUDDEN, MEYNERT, GANSER, etc.)

It is clear that in many vertebrates, including mammals (and humans), there are fibres other than retinogeniculate and retinocollicular connections, which traverse the optic tracts and chiasma in such a way as to appear commissural, though they are almost certainly mere decussations. The supraoptic commissures are fibre pathways which lie in the chiasma and connect diencephalic to mesencephalic structures across the midline, including the ventral lateral geniculate nucleus, pretectal and tectal areas. They are probably nonvisual in nature, and persist in the chiasma after binocular enucleation. They lie in the dorsal and posterior part of the chiasma itself and postero-lateral to it in the hypothalamus. In dorsoventral order they are the commissures of Gudden, Ganser and Meynert.

TRANSVERSE PEDUNCULAR TRACT (ACCESSORY OPTIC TRACT)

This arises from the optic tract, at entry into the mid brain, skirts the ventral aspect of the cerebral peduncle, and enters the brain close to the exit of the oculomotor nerve (Gillilan, 1941) to supply the three terminal nuclei: the dorsal, medial and lateral terminal nuclei. The dorsal is essentially part of the pretectum, joining with the nucleus of the optic tract. These three nuclei have a role in the control of eye movement, signalling retinal slip in three planes corresponding to the planes of the three semicircular canals.

TRACT OF DARKSCHEWITSCH

This is an uncertain connection, said to link the optic tract to the habenular nucleus (in the wall of

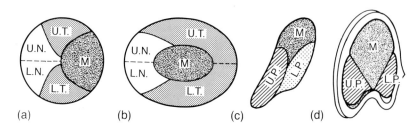

(a)   (b)   (c)   (d)

Fig. 15.78 Distribution of the visual fibres. (Note that in (d), LeGros Clark and Penman (1934) have shown that only the macular area occupies the posterior two-thirds of the geniculate body.)

the third ventricle, near the pineal stalk and posterior commissure), and ultimately to the oculomotor nucleus. Such connections in the human brain are largely unknown. (For discussion consult Crosby, Humphrey and Lauer, 1962.) There is, however, considerable experimental evidence for a pathway from the retina, leaving the optic tract to pass by relay through the suprachiasmatic nucleus and thence to the pineal gland (see Mason and Lincoln, 1976; Sawaki, 1977), a connection almost certainly concerned with circadian rhythms but not yet elucidated in humans.

BLOOD SUPPLY OF THE OPTIC TRACT

The optic tract also has its **pial plexus**, continuous anteriorly with that of the chiasma, and fed partly from the posterior communicating but mainly from the **anterior choroidal artery** (Figs 15.60, 15.68–15.70, 15.79). The latter supplies several branches to the tract, but its largest traverse it to enter the base of the brain and supply, among other structures, part of the optic radiation.

According to Shellshear (1927) these perforating arteries traverse the tract between the crossed and uncrossed fibres. Sometimes they circle round the tract before entering it. (In this case pressure on the tract might obstruct the arteries rather than act directly on the nerve fibres.) There is considerable reciprocity in size between the anterior choroidal and posterior communicating arteries, and occasionally one predominates to the complete exclusion of its fellow (Abbie, 1938).

Injection studies (Francois, 1959) show that the optic tract is supplied not only by the anterior choroidal artery but also by branches of the middle cerebral, overlapping and intermingling, but without anastomosis. Overlap of such end arteries may explain absence of hemianopia after occlusion of the anterior choroidal.

15.4 THE LATERAL GENICULATE NUCLEUS

The lateral geniculate body is an elevation produced by the lateral geniculate nucleus, in which most optic tract fibres end. At the simplest level, the lateral geniculate nucleus provides a relay station for retinal axons synapsing with neurons of the geniculocalcarine pathway, transferring information from the optic tract to optic radiation and thence to visual cortex (Fig. 15.80). Certainly, there is a roughly 1:1 relationship between retinal axons entering the lateral geniculate nucleus and geniculocalcarine neurons leaving it. Eighty per cent of the synaptic connections of the lateral geniculate nucleus are with retinofugal axons.

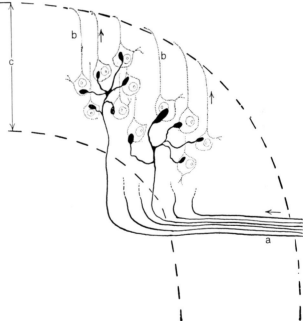

Fig. 15.80 Diagram showing the termination of optic fibres in relation to the cells of the lateral geniculate body in a monkey. A fasciculus of optic fibres (a) is shown entering the geniculate body from the right. From this fasciculus individual fibres turn out at right-angles to enter their appropriate cell lamina (c). Each fibre ends in a spray of 5–6 branches, and each of these terminates in an end-bulb which lies in contact with the body of one geniculate cell. The axons of the geniculate cells (b) pass into the fibre laminae of the nucleus and run through these to reach the optic radiations. (From Glees, P. and Le Gros Clark, W. E. (1941) *J. Anat.*, **75**, 295.)

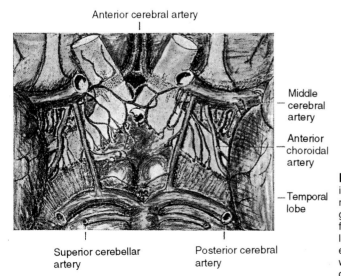

Anterior cerebral artery

Middle cerebral artery

Anterior choroidal artery

Temporal lobe

Superior cerebellar artery

Posterior cerebral artery

Fig. 15.79 The arterial Circle of Willis showing the arteries supplying the optic nerve, chiasma and tract.

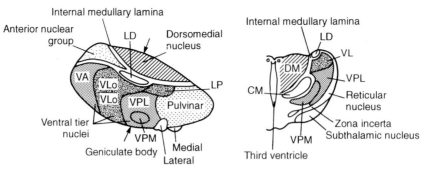

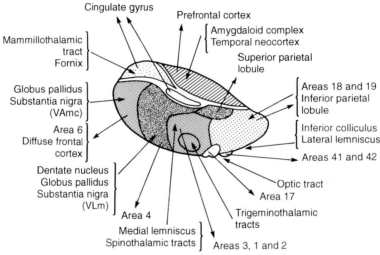

Fig. 15.81 Schematic diagrams of the major thalamic nuclei. (a) Left, an oblique dorsolateral view of the thalamus and its major subdivisions; right, a transverse section of the thalamus at level of arrows. This indicates: (1) the relationships between VPM and VPL, and (2) the location of CM with respect to the internal medullary lamina of the thalamus; (b) the principal afferent and efferent projections of particular thalamic subdivisions. While most cortical areas project fibres back to the thalamic nuclei from which fibres are received, not all of these are shown. (Redrawn from Carpenter, M. B. (1976) *Human Neuroanatomy*, published by Williams and Wilkins.)

The nucleus is one of the nuclei of the thalamus (making, with the medial geniculate nucleus, the **metathalamus**). It lies anterolateral to the medial geniculate nucleus and is in effect applied to the outer surface of the junction between the ventroposterolateral nucleus of the thalamus and the pulvinar, which overhangs it (Fig. 15.81).

The lateral geniculate nucleus consists of a **dorsal** nucleus, and a phylogenetically older **ventral** nucleus. The ventral nucleus is rudimentary in humans, consisting of a few interspersed neurons (pregeniculate nucleus) lying rostral to the dorsal nucleus (Polyak, 1957). In lower mammals it is concerned with primitive photostatic responses, and does not receive input from the optic tract (Hines, 1942) or project to the visual cortex (Ingvar, 1923; Woollard, 1926).

The dorsal, or principal, nucleus makes up the major portion of the lateral geniculate nucleus and

is a laminated saddle-shaped mass whose hilum is directed ventromedially. Its shape was well demonstrated by the model of Pfeifer (1925) and reconstructions of Chacko (1948, 1955) (Figs 15.82 and 15.83).

The lateral geniculate body is an asymmetrical cone with a rounded apex. An inferior, incomplete rim extends laterally as a 'peak' and is largely responsible for the surface elevation of the lateral geniculate body. Part of the rim is superior to the 'medial root' of the optic nerve and contributes variably to this surface elevation, which appears to lead dorsally to the medial geniculate body (Figs 15.76 and 15.77) (Wolff, 1953; Polyak, 1957). The anterior part of the rim is obscured by optic fibres. Inferiorly the nucleus is hollowed as a kind of hilum, which also extends to the dorsal aspect of the nucleus. Here this has no rim. The hilum may be indicated by a superficial cleft or depression.

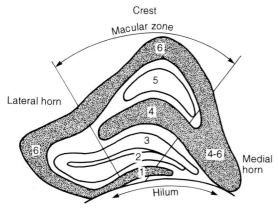

Fig. 15.82 Schematic representation of a coronal section through the lateral geniculate body viewed from its posterior aspect. (From Miller, N. R. (1985) *Clinical Neuro-ophthalmology*, 4th Edition, published by Williams and Wilkins, with permission.)

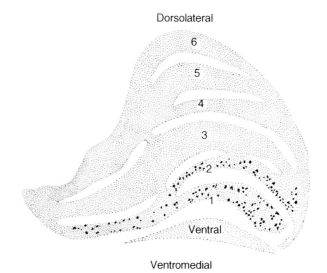

Fig. 15.83 Drawing of the cellular lamination of the lateral geniculate body. Laminae 1 and 2 constitute the magnocellular layers; the ventral nucleus is shown below. Crossed fibres of the optic tract terminate in laminae 1, 4 and 6, and uncrossed fibres terminate in laminae 2, 3 and 5. (From Carpenter, M. B. (1976) *Human Neuroanatomy*, published by Williams and Wilkins, with permission.)

Much of the lateral geniculate nucleus is hidden, being overlapped by the pulvinar and visible only in sections. In coronal section it is like a peaked cap, the peak projecting laterally (Fig. 15.73). In horizontal section, it is related anteriorly to the optic tract which ends in it, laterally with the retrolenticular part of the internal capsule, medially with the medial geniculate body, posteriorly with the hippocampal gyrus and posterolaterally with the inferior cornu of the lateral ventricle.

At a higher level, the lateral geniculate nucleus projects into the pulvinar (Fig. 15.73). Anteriorly is the pregeniculate grey matter, anterolaterally the temporopontine fibres and posterior part of the internal capsule, laterally the zone of Wernicke and medially the medial geniculate nucleus (Fig. 15.84).

The zone of Wernicke is the innermost portion of the internal capsule, a triangular zone containing the origin of the optic radiation. It contains transverse and longitudinal fibres including fibres from the medial geniculate body and pulvinar. The fibres of the optic radiation are dorsal and lateral to the lateral

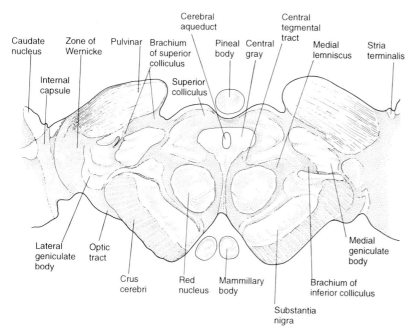

Fig. 15.84 Transverse section through rostral midbrain demonstrating the relationship of midbrain and caudal portions of the thalamus. (Original: Weigert's stain: redrawn from Carpenter, M. B. (1976) *Human Neuroanatomy*, published by Williams and Wilkins, with permission.)

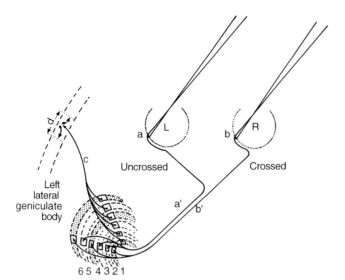

Fig. 15.85 Diagram illustrating certain points in the central representation of the retina. Impulses from equivalent spots (a, b) in the two retinae pass back in the optic tract to the same region of the lateral geniculate body. Crossed impulses (b) terminate in laminae 1, 4 and 6 and uncrossed impulses (a) in laminae 2, 3 and 5. Thus the receptive unit in the lateral geniculate body with respect to each retina is a band of cells radiating from the hilum of the nucleus, and involving three laminae. On the other hand, the projection unit of the lateral geniculate body on to the visual cortex is a band of cells involving all six laminae. (Clark (1941), *J. Anat.*, **75**.) It is important to note that while 'a' and 'b' in this diagram may represent single retinal ganglion cells, the geniculostriate connection, 'c', must represent a minimum of six neurons, each with a soma in one lamina alone.

geniculate nucleus while the white matter tracts of the acoustic radiation lie dorsal and medial. The auditory radiation connects the medial geniculate body with the primary projection area for hearing in the transverse convolution of Heschl in the temporal lobe. The white matter between the junction of the auditory cortex and insula, and the dorsal inferior ventricular horn is called the temporal isthmus. The optic and auditory radiations pass through this narrow bridge, as does the fibre tract connecting the auditory or sensory speech area (of the first temporal convolution) to the motor speech area (of the precentral gyrus of the third frontal convolution) (Miller, 1982).

In sagittal section the fibres of the optic tract divide into two layers (Fig. 15.73), the inferior forming the white layer of the hilum, the superior the dorsal part of the body, so that the nucleus is enveloped in a kind of capsule. Between these layers are the alternating laminae of myelinated fibres and cells which give the body its characteristic laminated appearance.

The lateral geniculate body is connected to the superior colliculus by a slender band called the superior brachium (Figs 15.13 and 15.68).

Even macroscopic sections of the lateral geniculate nucleus show its lamination (Fig. 15.85) indicative of a high level of organization (Figs 15.82 and 15.83). In primates, including humans, there are six laminae of 'grey matter' and intervening 'white' strata composed of axons and dendrites (but see below). The grey laminae are like six irregularly stacked cones, numbering from one ventrally, at the hilum, to six dorsally. The two inner layers consist of loosely arranged large cells (the magnocellular layers 1 and 2) and the four outer layers consist of polar staining small and medium-sized cells (the parvocellular

layers, 3–6). They contain the neurons which receive the retinal projection and project to the visual cortex, and also a large number of interneurons. The functional significance of the magnocellular and parvocellular layers is discussed on p. 583.

Crossed fibres of the optic tract end in laminae 1, 4 and 6, uncrossed in 2, 3 and 5 (Fig. 15.85) so that fibres from corresponding parts of the two hemiretinae (e.g. right temporal and left nasal retina) end in neighbouring laminae. It will be noted that fibres from each retina pass to both magnocellular (1 and 2) and parvocellular (3–6) laminae. This segregation is achieved within the nucleus itself, since the crossed and uncrossed fibres are still intermingled as they enter the lateral geniculate nucleus (see Minkowski, 1913; Brouwer and Zeeman, 1926; Le Gros Clark and Penman, 1934; Glees, 1941; Polyak, 1957; Meikle and Sprague, 1964; von Noorden and Middleditch, 1975).

Extensive studies by Hickey and Guillery (1979) have shown a topographic variation in the number of human laminae usually present. Anteriorly the number is more variable although it is always possible to identify small segments with six, four or two layers. (The latter is the 'monocular segment'.)

Kaas *et al.* (1978) have proposed that the basic anthropoid plan consists of two ventral magnocellular and two dorsal parvocellular laminae, each with a full representation of the visual hemifield. In Old World monkeys, certain apes and humans, in which four parvocellular layers are customarily described, they believe that two fundamental parvocellular laminae (one with ipsilateral and the other with contralateral input) split and interweave, especially in the region representing central vision, to give the appearance of four laminae.

Interlaminar cells between parvo- and magnocellular layers are found in several species of monkey (Kaas *et al.*, 1978; Hendrickson, Wilson and Ogren, 1978) and a further row of cells receiving ipsi- and contralateral inputs (sometimes called the S lamina) is often found in the optic tract, external to the magnocellular layer.

CONNECTIONS OF THE LATERAL GENICULATE NUCLEUS (Fig. 15.86)

Afferent connections

Retinogeniculate projection

There is a point-to-point retinoptic projection from corresponding points in each hemiretina to each lamina of the lateral geniculate nucleus. Each map contains a representation of the contralateral hemifield and the maps are conceived to be in vertical register across the laminae. A slight discontinuity identifies the 'blind spot'. Minute experimental retinal lesions produce transneuronal degeneration in small, well-defined clusters in three laminae on each side (Matthews, Cowan and Powell, 1960; Nobak and Laemle, 1970; Polyak, 1957). Similarly, a focal lesion or injection of tracer in part of the visual cortex leads to axonal or cellular labelling in a line extending across all laminae at the same level. Such units would have receptive fields in the same point in visual space. Sanderson (1971) refers to this as a projection column. That portion of the map in layers 2, 3 and 5 representing the **monocular crescent**, and corresponding to most peripheral, temporal, ipsilateral retina, is inevitably lacking in layers 1, 4 and 6. The apparent monocular crescent of vision is estimated by comparing the field of binocular single vision with that achieved by superimposing the two visual fields – the binocular field. This over-estimates the monocular crescent, because each field is obstructed nasally in the primary position of gaze by the presence of the nose, which prevents light from a target reaching the most temporal retina. However, this temporal retina is functional, and will project to the ipsilateral lateral geniculate nucleus. There is a **true monocular crescent**, which reflects that the nasal retina extends further from the fovea in the horizontal meridian than the temporal.

Information on the retinotopic organization of the retinofugal fibres in the optic nerve, chiasma tract and lateral geniculate nucleus in humans and monkeys is based on the studies of Brouewer and Zeeman (1926), Polyak (1957) and Hoyt and Luis (1963). Considering **non-macular** fibres: uncrossed

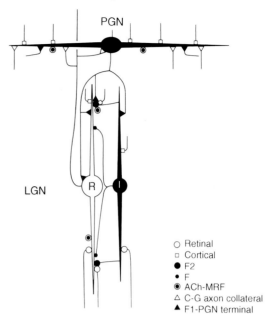

Fig. 15.86 Schematic diagram of excitatory and inhibitory neural circuits in LGN. The GABAergic inhibitory interneurons (I) support two different types of terminals: (1) The dendritic F2 boutons, which in microcircuits are postsynaptic to dendrites of relay (R) cells. The retinal terminals frequently form triadic synaptic arrangements with F2 boutons and with relay dendrites. ('Tails' of terminals indicate renotopy.) (2) The axonal F terminals, which are not postsynaptic to other terminals and are presynaptic to dendrites of relay cells. Contrary to the F2 terminals, the axonal F terminals would be under the influence of retinal, cortical, and perigeniculate terminals synapsing on the dendrites of the interneurons, especially with respect to those synapsing near the soma (Hamos *et al.*, 1985; Montero, 1986). Contrary to the orientation of the dendritic and axonal arborizations of interneurons along projection lines in LGN, the dendrites of the GABAergic perigeniculate (PGN) neurons are oriented perpendicular to the projection lines. PGN cells are synapsed by axon collaterals of geniculocortical relay cells and of other PGN cells, and by cortical and cholinergic terminals. The F1 axon terminals of PGN cells synapse on all regions of relay cells, especially on the soma, and on F2 terminals and dendrites of interneurons. (From Montero, V. M. (1987) *J. Comp. Neurol.*, **264**, 268, with permission.)

fibres from the superior temporal quadrant of the retina are dorsomedial in the chiasma while corresponding crossed fibres (superonasal retina) are medial. These project to the medial part of the lateral geniculate nucleus. Uncrossed fibres from the inferior temporal quadrant of the retina are inferolateral in the chiasma while crossed (inferonasal retina) are ventrolateral. These project to the lateral part of the geniculate nucleus. The **macular** region of the retina projects to a wedge-shaped sector in the posterior two-thirds to three-quarters (Kupfer, 1962; Malpeli and Baker, 1975).

It will be noted that the representation of the visual hemifields in the visual pathway 'twists' at the level of the lateral geniculate nucleus so that the vertical meridian becomes horizontal, with the upper retina medial, and the lower lateral. This twist is reversed in the optic radiations so that when the visual cortex is reached, the superior retinal quadrants lie in the upper part of the pathway and the inferior lie below.

Malpeli and Baker (1975), using microelectrode techniques in the monkey, demonstrated a distribution of macular and central retinal axons to all six layers of the lateral geniculate nucleus and of peripheral retinal axons to four layers (two parvocellular and two magnocellular). (Projection from the monocular crescent involved one parvo- and one magnocellular layer.) Bunt *et al.* (1975), using horseradish peroxidase to label retinogeniculate axons, found that all ganglion cells project to parvocellular laminae while only peripheral large ganglion cells, and some parafoveal ganglion cells (26%), project to the magnocellular laminae.

Enroth-Cugell and Robson (1966) established the presence of three morphologically and functionally distinct ganglion cell types in cat retina: the X, Y and W cells (see Chapter 14, The Retina). X cells represent 80% of the retinal ganglion cells and are particularly concentrated in the foveal region. They are of medium size, with smaller dendritic arborizations in the retina, narrow axons, and a circumscribed, vertically organized, terminal distribution across the laminae. They are distributed to both magno- and parvocellular laminae (Sur and Sherman, 1982a).

Y cells, about 10% of the ganglion cell population, are found increasingly in the peripheral retina. They have large dendritic trees, larger axons, terminate on more than one layer of the lateral geniculate nucleus and branch extensively within a layer, but little within the medullary laminae. Y cells also supply collaterals to the superior colliculus in the cat via the superior brachium.

W cells, about 10% of the ganglion cell population, project entirely to the superior colliculus. No W-type cell projections to the lateral geniculate nucleus were found (Leventhal, Rodieck and Dreher, 1981).

Shapley and Perry (1986) have summarized the comparative morphologic and functional features of cat and monkey ganglion cells as follows.

In the cat there are, as noted, the X and Y cells, which are highly sensitive to contrast. X cells are driven by a single receptor mechanism, Y cells receive centre and surround signals and a non-linear input from other units within their receptive fields. Both cells project to the A and A1 layers of the lateral geniculate nucleus while Y cells also project to layer C and to superior colliculus. W cells are of several classes, one of which is colour-coded.

The X and Y cells are of the greatest importance for pattern perception because of their high sensitivity to spatial patterns and their direct connection to the lateral geniculate nucleus. The X cells are most sensitive to fine detail and signal accurate location. Their response characteristics include linear summation to sinusoidal stimuli. At the peak or trough of the wave form there is a null response, which is not shown by Y cells. The X-cell response is more sustained than that of the Y cell, especially at high contrast. The X cell modulates its firing rate at the temporal frequency rate of the stimulus.

The Y cells show a linear response at the fundamental frequency of the stimulus, but not at the second harmonic. If the responses to the fundamental and second harmonic frequency are plotted against spatial frequency the curves intersect, and the point of intersection is called the Y cell 'signature'. The non-linear component of the response is dependent on the network of connections between the photoreceptors and ganglion cells.

The dendritic field size of X and Y cells increases with eccentricity from the fovea, and the receptive field size increases correspondingly. The larger receptive field size of Y cells probably explains their greater response to large targets and higher target velocities. The Y cells resolve patterns about as well as X cells but have about three times poorer spatial frequency resolution at the same eccentricity.

Monkey ganglion cells   Old World monkey (e.g. macaque) retinal ganglion cells can also be sorted into cell classes (Gouras, 1968; Schiller and Malpeli, 1978; De Monasterio, 1978). There are three clear subdivisions. The most numerous type is the P cell, which projects only to the four most dorsal parvocellular laminae of the lateral geniculate nucleus.

P ganglion cells   The P cells have the smallest dendritic fields and the smallest receptive field centres. The width of the dendritic tree is almost invariant with eccentricity, within the central 8° of the retina, especially for the midget ganglion cells (Polyak, 1941). The receptive field radius near the fovea averages 0.03°, with the smallest around 0.01°. (This compares with values in the cat of 0.1 for X cells and 0.3 for Y cells.) The radii of P-cell receptive fields does not vary greatly within the central 5° (Linsenmeier *et al.*, 1982; De Monasterio, 1978).

The P cells give sustained responses to light when the wavelength is at the peak of the cells' spectral sensitivity curve. They respond phasically to white light and to other broad-band illumination. They have concentric centre-surround organization, often with colour-opponent properties. Almost all P cells resemble cat X cells when tested for linear signal summation, and their target lateral geniculate nucleus cells share this X-cell-like property. For this reason, and because X and P cells have the smallest receptive fields and dendritic trees, some authors have equated parvocellular lateral geniculate nucleus cells (Dreher, Fukada and Rodiesk, 1976) and their P cell retinal inputs (De Monasterio, 1978; Schiller and Malpeli, 1978) with X cells and X-like behaviour. However, P cells are very unlike cat X cells in their contrast gain and other visual characteristics. The P cells show a much lower contrast gain than X cells (and indeed M cells – see below) with a lower response up to 64% contrast. P cells are wavelength selective, unlike X cells. Shapley and Perry (1986) suggest that the primate P cell has no exact functional equivalent in the cat, but represents the colour-coded class of W cell in the cat which projects to the C-laminae and responds like the blue-on, yellow-off cells of the monkey.

M ganglion cells.   The other major class of ganglion cell, less numerous than the P cell, is the M ganglion cell (Gouras, 1968), which projects chiefly to the magnocellular cells of the lateral geniculate nucleus, but also to the superior colliculus. They have larger dendritic trees and receptive fields than P cells. M cell tree width increases with retinal eccentricity. The M cells have concentric centre-surround receptive fields and respond in a transient manner to a step of broad-band illumination, like P cells. They show little wavelength selectivity but may receive antagonistic signals from different cones. Kaplan and Shapley (1982) have proposed that M cells can be subdivided into those with X cell and those with Y cell features (M–X and M–Y). This proposal is based on the following considerations (Shapley and Perry, 1986):

1. A large majority of magnocellular neurons and their M-cell inputs (80%) are X-like in their spatial filtering and summation properties.
2. A small fraction of magnocellular neurons and M cells have the Y-cell 'signature'.
3. All monkey ganglion cells have transient responses to white light and most have more or less sustained responses to monochromatic light.
4. The contrast gain of M cells is comparable to that of X and Y cells in the cat and about ten times greater than the contrast gain of parvocellular neurons and P cells.
5. Most M cells synapse only with magnocellular lateral geniculate nucleus neurons while most cat

Y cells branch three or four times to contact the A and C laminae and colliculus.
6. P cells and parvocellular lateral geniculate nucleus neurons are wavelength selective while cat X cells are not.

A third class of cell, the 'rarely encountered' cell is not wavelength selective and provides the bulk of cells projecting to the superior colliculus.

Functional role of monkey M and P cells   The high gain and high sensitivity of monkey M cells are probably responsible for pattern perception at low contrasts and at low and intermediate spatial frequencies. At high contrast, where the M responses saturate, the P cells may contribute to extend the dynamic range of vision but P cells, despite their small receptive fields, do not resolve well because their contrast gains are so low. Human colour perception is a low-gain, low-resolution system and it is possible that the small fields are needed for wavelength selectivity.

Shapley and Perry (1986) suggest that there is a one-to-one connection at the fovea, with red (560 nm) or green (530 nm) cones, and thence with midget P_1 ganglion cells. This is supported by the small increase in dendritic field size within the 0–14° for P cells compared with M cells. P cells within 1.6 mm of the fovea (8°) show invariant dendritic fields; fields increase outside this. The former are colour-opponent cells, and the latter are mainly hidden opponent cells dominated by red cones.

In the peripheral retina it is impossible to elicit perceptions of saturated colours, particularly green. Deterioration of colour perception begins about 10° out from the fovea, although the ratio of red to green cones does not change with eccentricity. It is suggested that in the periphery P cells become red cone-dominated hidden opponent cells.

Corticogeniculate projections

Corticogeniculate axons arising in layer VI of the visual cortex are distributed to all laminae and to the interlaminar zones. A small cortical lesion, therefore, causes atrophy in all six layers of the lateral geniculate nucleus (Garey, Jones and Powell, 1968; Giolli and Guthrie, 1969; Hollander and Martinex-Milan, 1975). Terminal boutons are small and end on fine dendrites of geniculocalcarine and interneurons in the absence of a glomerular organization (Guillery, 1971a,b; Famiglietti and Peters, 1972). They contain densely packed and rounded synaptic vesicles.

Tectogeniculate projections

Fibres arising in the stratum griseum superficiale of the colliculus terminate in the S layers and interlaminar regions of the more ventral layers (Kaas *et al.*, 1978; Harting *et al.*, 1980). Cells here project widely to layers I–III of the visual cortex.

Efferent connections

Geniculocalcarine projections

The optic radiation is dealt with in greater detail on p. 566. In monkeys P cell axons project only to the parvocellular laminae while the faster-conducting M cells project to the magnocellular laminae. The geniculocortical axons are of comparably different conduction velocities (Marrocco and Brown, 1975). The magno- and parvocellular layers project to different levels of the striate cortex. Parvocellular axons project to the deeper half of layer IV (IVc), with a smaller termination in the upper part (IVa) and with occasional fibres to layer I. Magnocellular axons terminate just above the deeper terminations of the parvocellular axons in layer IVc (see Jones, 1985). The independent relay of P- and M-like axons to the cortex is in keeping with the segregation of their functions to influence separate populations of cortical neurons.

Other connections

Other connections of the lateral geniculate nucleus are with the pulvinar and the ventral and lateral thalamic nuclei (Carpenter, 1976).

Interneurons of the lateral geniculate nucleus

The presence of short axon interneurons confined to the lateral geniculate nucleus was once controversial. Polyak (1934) found in the monkey and Rae (1961) found in humans that loss of the occipital cortex was associated with a total loss of neurons on the same side; however, Minkowski (1913) demonstrated the persistence of short axon cells in primate experiments, and it is now accepted that such cells exist. Some have invoked their presence to explain the extremely intricate synaptic structures found, for example, by Szentagothai (1963).

SYNAPTIC INTERACTIONS WITHIN THE LATERAL GENICULATE NUCLEUS

As mentioned earlier, retinofugal fibres may synapse with several lateral geniculate nucleus neurons and

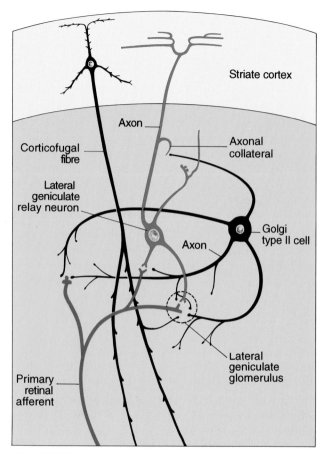

Fig. 15.87 Schematic diagram of the neuronal arrangements in a glomerulus of the lateral geniculate body. A primary retinal afferent is indicated in red, while the LGB relay neuron is in blue. A corticofugal fibre and Golgi type II are in black. The golmerulus contains a terminal of a primary retinal afferent, several club-shaped terminals of an LGB relay neuron and contributions from both Golgi type II neurons and corticofugal fibres. This synaptic complex is enclosed in a capsule of glial processes, indicated by the dashed line. (From Carpenter, M. B. (1976) *Human Neuroanatomy*, published by Williams and Wilkins, after Szentagothai, 1970.)

each geniculocalcarine neuron may receive inputs from several retinal axons, so that there is evidence of both divergence and convergence of pathways (Szentagothai, 1963). Various types of synaptic contact are established (Colonnier and Guillery, 1964; Campos-Ortega, Glees and Neuhoff, 1968; Lieberman, 1974). Fibres may terminate axosomatically, axodendritically on primary or secondary dendrites, in boutons en passage, or in complex 'glomerular' endings (Figs 15.86 and 15.87).

The **synaptic glomeruli** of the lateral geniculate nucleus constitute a complex of interlocking nerve processes of various origins, and are arranged in a specific manner. In the cat, the glomerulus is separated from the environment by a capsule of glial

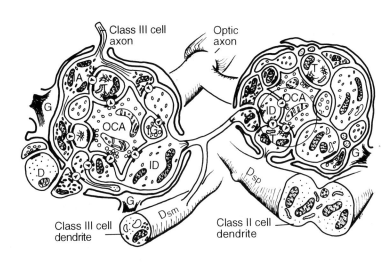

Fig. 15.88 Semidiagrammatic drawing of two synaptic glomeruli in the lateral geniculate nucleus of the cat. Optic tract axon is shown dividing and entering two adjacent glomeruli where it forms the central element (OCA). Dendrites of geniculocortical cells contribute thorns (T) that enter the glomeruli and receive direct input from the visual axons. Dendrites of interneurons (ID) have multilobed dendritic terminals that may enter adjacent glomeruli. These interneuronal dendrites form most of the profiles within the glomeruli. Interneuronal dendrites are frequently interposed between optic axons and geniculocortical dendrites in a triad (*circled region* on *right*). In addition, some interneuronal dendrites synapse with other interneuronal dendrites from adjacent glomeruli (IG) to form serial synapses. Interneuronal axons (IA) form clawlike terminations as the periphery of the glomeruli and end on interneuronal dendrites and geniculocortical dendrites. All glomeruli are surrounded by a sheath of astroglial processes (G). (From Famiglietti, E. V. and Peters, A. (1992) *J. Comp. Neurol.* **144**, 285–334.)

processes (Szentagothai, 1970; Famiglietti and Peters, 1972), but this is absent in the primate (Colonnier and Guillery, 1964). Synaptic glomeruli entail the synaptic apposition of terminal retinal axons, geniculocalcarine neurons and interneurons (Fig. 15.88). (Corticogeniculate neurons do not participate.) This triad of synapses should be compared with a similar arrangement in the retina, with the lateral geniculate nucleus interneurons being homologous with the retinal amacrine cells.

Each glomerulus consists of a region of closely packed neurons and terminals, within which a central retinogeniculate axon is presynaptic to a geniculocortical neuron and an interneuron (Fig. 15.88). Dendrites of the geniculocortical neurons enter the glomeruli as **thorns** which synapse with, and receive direct input from, retinal axons. Interneuronal dendrites have multilobed terminals interposed between retinal axons and geniculocortical dendrites to form the synaptic triad. The dendrites of interneurons may synapse with those of adjacent glomeruli to form serial synapses between them.

Lieberman (1974) has described pre- and postsynaptic inhibiting and exciting dendrodritic and glomerular synapses. These glomeruli, like those in the cerebellum and thalamus, are complex aggregations of synapses between axons and dendrites and may provide the anatomical basis for the inhibitory and excitatory receptive field phenomena identified by unit recording (Hubel and Wiesel, 1961). It is to be emphasized that these findings appear to indicate intralaminar coordination. Interlaminar integration

has been propounded by some observers (Guillery and Colonnier, 1970) and the point is important because such connections would provide a basis of interretinal coordination at the geniculate level. According to Hubel and Wiesel (1977) there is no adequate evidence for such geniculate integration: in electrophysiological terms at any rate, no geniculate cell responds to stimulation of both retinas and fusion of biretinal signals is to be sought at cortical levels. (However, see Jones (1985) for a fuller discussion.)

FUNCTIONAL BEHAVIOUR OF GENICULATE CELLS

Because each lateral geniculate nucleus neuron receives input from only a few retinal ganglion cells, the receptive fields resemble those of the retinal ganglion cells. However, the receptive fields of the geniculate neurons are wider but respond to small spots of light rather than to diffuse illumination.

Electrophysiological studies in the cat have demonstrated that cells in the lateral geniculate nucleus show a similar 'on' centre or 'off' centre organization to that of the ganglion cells which project to them, even retaining a segregation into X-cell (sustained) and Y-cell (transient) characteristics. The receptive fields show some evidence of increased lateral inhibition and hence of integration of incoming signals (Hubel and Wiesel, 1961). Suzuki and Kato (1966) were able to demonstrate postsynaptic inhibition of responses on stimulation of the optic nerve. This inhibitory relay is envisaged as involving a geniculocalcarine and corticogeniculate feedback pathway (Miller, 1982).

In the monkey lateral geniculate nucleus, three types of response are encountered (Hubel and Wiesel, 1962): type I cells are most common and exhibit three types of spectral response corresponding to the three cone types; type II cells give opponent colour responses in their receptive fields, suggesting inputs from opponent cones; type III cells show typical 'on' or 'off' centre receptive fields to stimuli of the same wavelength. (An 'on' centre cell responds preferentially to a bright central stimulus with dark surround, an 'off' centre to the reverse conditions.) These three cell types are thought to be associated with macular cone function concerned with colour vision and with processing of complex wavelength data in the visible range.

BLOOD SUPPLY OF THE LATERAL GENICULATE NUCLEUS

Posterior cerebral and posterior choroidal arteries

The main supply of the lateral geniculate nucleus, particularly the posteromedial aspect, is the posterior cerebral artery directly or via its posterior choroidal branches (Fig. 15.89). These vessels are therefore nutritive to the superior homonymous retinal quadrants.

Anterior choroidal artery

The anterior choroidal artery supplies almost the entire anterior and lateral aspects of the lateral geniculate nucleus and therefore fibres projecting from the inferior retinal quadrants (Beevor, 1908; Abbie, 1933, 1938). The artery arises from the internal carotid (or sometimes middle cerebral artery) just distal to the origin of the posterior communicating artery. These arteries pass posteriorly to cross the outer surface of the optic tract which they supply. The anterior choroidal artery turns laterally on reaching the anterior pole of the lateral geniculate nucleus giving off a variable number of branches, before entering the inferior horn of the lateral ventricle to supply the choroidal plexus.

The hilum and intervening region radiating dorsally from it and containing the macular projection are supplied by both vessels (see Francois, Neetens and Collette, 1956; Fujino, 1961, 1962; Fuju, Lenkey and Bhoton, 1980).

The well-developed arterial anastomosis in the overlying pia-arachnoid provides arterioles which penetrate the lateral geniculate nucleus perpendicularly and end in the rich capillary bed of the laminae. From this arises a sparse capillary network within the medullary zones (Francois, Neetens and Collette, 1956).

The description of the optic radiation and retrogeniculate pathway continues on p. 566.

15.5 THE SUPERIOR COLLICULI

The superior colliculi are small rounded elevations of the dorsal surface of the mid brain, separated by a vertical median groove in which depends the pineal body, while a transverse groove separates the superior from the inferior colliculi (Fig. 5.13). Above the superior colliculi is the thalamus and, in the mid line, the great cerebral vein passing into the straight sinus. Posterosuperior to the whole **tectum**, which comprises all four colliculi, is the cerebellum; both structures are covered by pia-arachnoid tissue, between layers of which is the cisterna of the great cerebral vein, a local dilatation of the subarachnoid space (Fig. 15.90a).

AFFERENT FIBRES

Afferent fibres pass from the optic tract via the superior brachium, which runs alongside the lateral geniculate body to the superior colliculus (Fig. 5.13).

From the occipital cortex via the optic radiations (corticofugal fibres) to the lateral geniculate body, and thence via the superior brachium.

From the spinotectal tract, connecting it with the sensory fibres of the cord and medulla.

EFFERENT FIBRES

Of the fibres which arise from collicular neurons, some cross to the opposite superior colliculus, but many decussate (**fountain decussation of Meynert**) to connect with the contralateral ocular nuclei and form the tectospinal tract. No fibres pass from the superior colliculus to the cortex.

For further details see Chapter 4.

15.6 THE THALAMUS

The thalami are two large ovoid ganglionic masses above the cerebral peduncles, flanking the third ventricle and extending posterior to its cavity. Each measures about 4 cm anteroposteriorly, and 2.5 cm in width and height. The **anterior extremity** is narrow, near the mid line, and is the posterior boundary of the interventricular foramen (Fig. 15.57). The

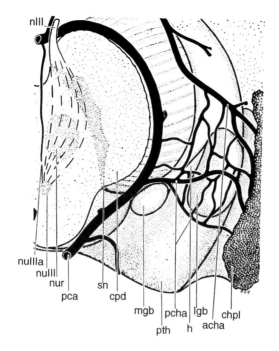

(a)

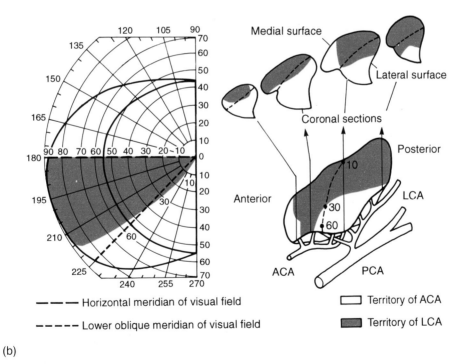

——— Horizontal meridian of visual field

----- Lower oblique meridian of visual field

□ Territory of ACA

■ Territory of LCA

(b)

Fig. 15.89   (a) The arterial network over the lateral geniculate body (simplified) (Abbie). Note its derivation from the anterior and posterior choroidal arteries. The specific end-artery from posterior cerebral to the oculomotor nucleus is indicated. acha = anterior choroidal artery; chpl = choroidal plexus; cpd = cerebral peduncle; h = hilum of lateral geniculate body; lgb = lateral geniculate body; mgb = medical geniculate body; nIII = oculomotor nerve; nuIII = oculomotor nucleus; pca = posterior cerebral artery; pcha = posterior choroidal artery; sn = substantia nigra. (b) Schematic representation of the right lateral geniculate body (LGB) seen from its medial side and in coronal section and the homonymous visual field defects that may result from ischemia within the territory of the lateral choroidal artery (LCA). ACA = anterior choroidal artery; PCA = posterior cerebral artery. (From Frisen *et al.*, 1978, with permission.)

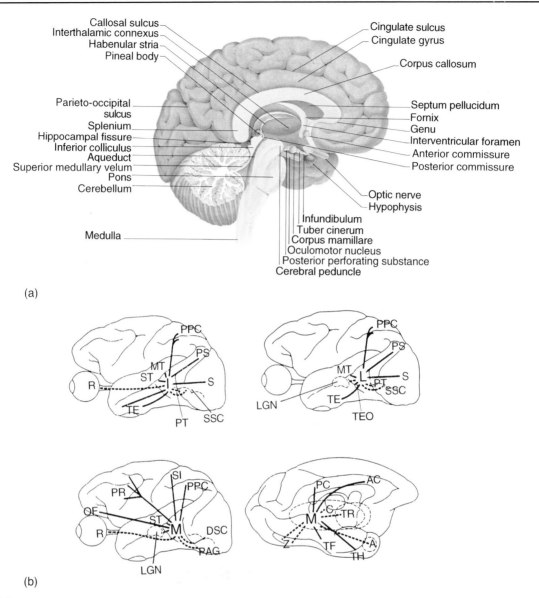

(a)

(b)

Fig. 15.90 (a) The medial surface of the left half of the brain. (From Hirschfield and Leveillé.) (b) Anatomical connections of subdivisions of the pulvinar. (i) The cortical and subcortical pathways of the cytoarchitectonically defined inferior pulvinar (I). (ii) The relationship of the cytoarchitectonic lateral pulvinar (L) with other parts of the brain. (iii) Lateral and (iv) medial surfaces of the brain showing pathways of the cytotechtonically defined medial subdivision of the pulvinar (M). Since most cortical connections are reciprocal, directions are not specified. Dashed lines indicate subcortical structures and pathways. A = amygdala; AC = anterior cingulate cortex; C = claustrum; DSC = deep layers of the superior colliculus; LGN = lateral geniculate nucleus; MT = middle temporal cortex; OF = occipitofrontal cortex; PAG = periaqueductal gray; PC = posterior cingulate cortex; PPC = posterior parietal cortex. PR = prefrontal cortex; PS = prestriate cortex; PT = pretectum; R = retina; S = striate cortex; SI = primary somatosensory cortex; SSC = superficial layers of superior colliculus; ST = superior temporal cortex; TE, TEO, TF and TH, von Bonin and Bailey subdivisions of temporal cortex; TR = thalamic reticular nucleus. 'Z' = brainstem sites including locus coeruleus, abducens, penduculo-pontine tegmental and dorsal raphe nuclei. (From Robinson, D. L. and Petersen, S. E. (1992) *TINS*, **15**, 127, with permission.)

expanded posterior pole or **pulvinar** overlaps the superior colliculus, and presents medially a prominent **posterior tubercle** which continues laterally into the lateral geniculate body. Inferomedial to the pulvinar, separated by the superior brachium, is the **medial geniculate body** (Fig. 15.68). Laterally the thalamus is separated from the **lenticular nucleus** of the **corpus striatum** by the posterior part of the **internal capsule** (Fig. 15.73).

Each thalamus is an immense collection of neurons of varying size, dendritic fields and interconnections. By such criteria it has been divided and subdivided into a series of topographical and, sometimes, functional entities. The basic division into anterior, **medial** and **lateral** parts is by laminae of myelinated nerve fibres accumulated between these major groups of nuclei. There are also **intra-laminar**, mid line (periventricular), and **reticular** groups. The pulvinar and geniculate nuclei belong to the lateral group, the pulvinar (phylogenetically late in development, reaching its zenith in higher mammals) forming almost one-quarter of the thalamus at its posterior or caudal pole. The lateral geniculate nucleus appears topographically as an elevation on part of the thalamus, and some intercommunication between the two seems likely; the existence of this is an old controversy. Although Minkowski (1913), Brouwer and Zeeman (1926) and others denied any visual connections to the pulvinar, it is now accepted that a geniculothalamic tract exists (Cajal, 1909; Elliot Smith, 1928; Le Gros Clark, 1932; Walker, 1938). The lateral group of thalamic nuclei, to which the pulvinar is ascribed, is, according to some experimenters (e.g. Mountcastle and Henneman, 1952), concerned with pain but it also has extensive reciprocal connexions with the whole of the occipital lobe of the cerebrum, including the visual cortex. Neurons are present within the pulvinar that respond to features of a visual target such as colour, direction and orientation (Allman *et al.*, 1972; Mathers and Rapisardik 1973; Gattas, Oswaldo-Cruz and Souza, 1979; Benevento and Miller, 1981; Bender, 1982). Early studies did not clarify whether this implied a functional role for these cells in the visual process. Recent studies suggest that the pulvinar is involved in determining the interest of visual stimuli, in several ways:

1. the selection of targets of interest;
2. the filtering out of irrelevant visual stimuli; and
3. utilizing information of visual interest ('visual salience') to initiate directed movements of the eyes or other parts of the body (Robinson and Petersen, 1992).

Retinotopic maps have been identified in the anterior pulvinar (Bender, 1981) in its inferior (PI) and lateral parts (PL). Area PL contains a complete map of the contralateral field. These two areas receive strong projections from the superior colliculus, the visual cortical and other areas, including the prefrontal cortex, striate and prestriate cortex and the posterior parietal and superior temporal cortex (Fig. 15.90). They also project back to these areas (Robinson and McLurkin, 1989). Adjacent to these maps, in the dorsomedial part of the lateral pulvinar (Pdm), is another, smaller area, which has connections with the middle temporal area (cortical area 7) and with the parieto-occipital area (Trojanowski and Jacobson, 1976; Baleydier and Maguiere, 1977; Ungeleider *et al.*, 1984; Colby *et al.*, 1989). The visual receptive fields are wider, and the latencies of response are longer in the Pdm than in the PI and PL areas.

Various studies suggest that the pulvinar is concerned with visual attention and is activated in relation to targets of visual interest, but is actively suppressed in relation to visual stimuli which must be disregarded. Neurons in the Pdm appear to be concerned with visual spatial attention, while the retinotopically mapped regions respond to saccadic eye movements. In the Pdm cells the response is enhanced before a saccade, or during attention to a peripheral stimulus in the absence of a saccade (Petersen, 1985). Enhancement occurs only when the stimulus is placed in the receptive field of the cell. This spatially selective, movement-independent enhancement is also found in cells of area 7 of the parietal cortex (Wurtz, Goldberg and Robinson, 1980), which is traditionally associated with spatial attention (Posner *et al.*, 1984; Petersen, Robinson and Currie, 1989). It has been shown in monkeys that visual spatial attention can be facilitated by the injection of a GABA agonist into the Pdm, and inhibited by injection of an antagonist. Rafal and Posner (1987) have described patients with lesions of the pulvinar who showed reduced visual attention in their contralateral visual field. Cells in PI and PL show such enhanced responses only when the stimuli are the targets for eye movements (Wurtz, Goldberg and Robinson, 1980). Such movement-related, spatially non-selective responses may signal relevance of targets for specific eye movements. About 30% of pulvinar cells, however, give a response after an eye movement has been completed. They appear to signal the act of refixation, or the beginning of a new visual scan.

Although many PI and PL neurons respond in relation to saccades, these same cells show no response to stimulation by visual targets which are not the object of regard during saccades or pursuit movements, for example, stimuli which are not fixated, but are part of the moving visual scene during an eye movement. This suggests that there is an active suppression of activity in these cells. The superficial layers of the superior colliculus project to PI and PL (Benevento and Fallon, 1975; Partlow, Colonnier and Szabo, 1977; Raczkowsky and Diamond, 1978; Harting *et al.*, 1980), and contain cells with the same properties (Robinson and Wurtz, 1976). Robinson and Petersen (1992) have suggested that the modulations induced in the pulvinar by eye movements are mediated by the superior colliculus.

Visual activation of pulvinar cells unrelated to movement is dependent on connections with the striate cortex and not the superior colliculus (Bender, 1983). Thus the visuomotor properties of the pulvinar cells may be the result of a convergence of collicular and geniculostriate streams. The visual excitation of yet another group of pulvinar neurons is gaze-locked; that is, excitation occurs only when the eye is directed at a particular location (Robinson, McClurkin and Kertzman, 1990). Here again it appears that a suppression mechanism exists which can determine the attention given to a visual target (Davidson and Bender, 1991). Other studies also support the view that a role of the pulvinar is to suppress unwanted, distracting visual information as well as signalling information about visual space. (For details and discussion of these and other thalamic problems consult Hassler, 1955; Crosby, Humphrey and Lauer, 1962; Purpura and Yahr, 1966; Dewulf, 1971; Williams and Warwick, 1980; Jones, 1985.)

15.7 OPTIC RADIATION

The optic radiation, or geniculocalcarine pathway, arises in the lateral geniculate nucleus and is the relay of fibres carrying visual impulses to the occipital lobe (Figs 15.92 and 15.93). The description of Meyer (1907) is accepted as representing the exact course of the radiation. The fibres ascend anterolaterally (through the so-called zone of Wernicke) as the **optic peduncle**, anterior to the lateral ventricle, traversing the retrolenticular part of the internal capsule behind the somaesthetic fibres and medial to the auditory tract. They diverge widely as the **medullary optic lamina**, which is at first vertical but becomes horizontal near the striate cortex. It consists of dorsal, lateral and ventral bundles which occupy the **external sagittal stratum**. The dorsal and lateral bundles pass directly backwards lateral to the temporal and **occipital cornua** of the lateral ventricle, separated from the ventricle by the **tapetum of the corpus callosum** (Figs 15.94 and 15.95).

The ventral bundle sweeps forwards and laterally into the temporal pole superior to and around the inferior horn of the lateral ventricle, before swerving posteriorly through the sublenticular portion of the internal capsule to reach the visual cortex (Figs 15.96 and 15.97) (Ranson, 1943). Interference with this temporal loop (of Meyer) may cause a superior homonymous quadrantanopsia. It reaches forward in the temporal lobe no further than 5 cm from its anterior pole. Its most anterior fibres lie 0.5–1 cm lateral to the tip of the temporal horn and amygdala (Probst, 1906).

The optic radiation, as it passes back in the white matter of the cerebral hemisphere, is internal to the

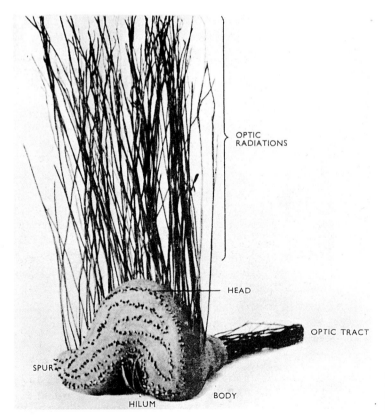

OPTIC RADIATIONS

HEAD

OPTIC TRACT

SPUR

HILUM

BODY

Fig. 15.91 Model of the left lateral geniculate nucleus from behind and medial side. (After Pfeifer, 1925.)

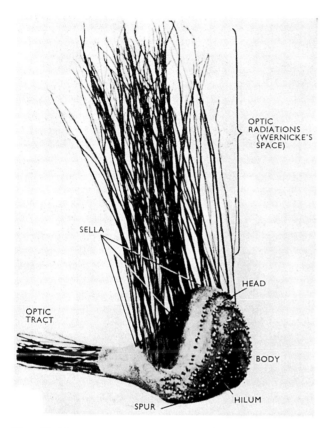

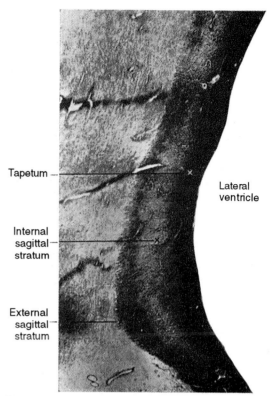

Fig. 15.93   Strata sagittalia. (From Brouwer.)

Fig. 15.92   Model of left geniculate nucleus from behind and lateral side. The origin of the optic radiations from the anterior portion of the saddle (Sella) is seen. This is the stalk of the lateral geniculate nucleus, or Wernicke's field, as it is also called. (From Pfiefer, 1925.)

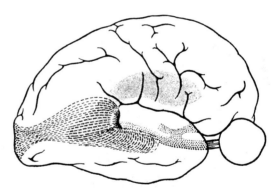

Fig. 15.94   Diagrammatic representation of the course of the fibres of the optic radiation. The geniculo-cortical fibres from the geniculate nucleus (not visible) curve around the concavity of the lateral ventricle to reach the striate area. (From Brodal, after Cushing, 1922.)

middle temporal gyrus, and tumours of this region may cause visual defects. The optic radiation ends in an extensive area of thin occipital cortex (the **striate cortex**, 1.4 mm or less in thickness), in which is the distinctive white stripe, the **stria of Gennari**.

Apart from corticofugal fibres, the optic radiations also contain corticogeniculate fibres and corticocollicular fibres in some animals, including primates, but these have not been substantiated in humans. The radiation may also contain fibres descending to the nuclei of the ocular motor nerves, but it is likely that this pathway is interrupted at such loci as the para-abducent interstitial nuclei, or the posterior commissural nuclear complex (Carpenter and Peter, 1970).

ORGANIZATION OF FIBRES IN THE OPTIC RADIATION

The retinoptic organization found in the lateral geniculate nucleus is continued in the geniculolcarine pathway. A **dorsal** bundle of fibres, representing superior peripheral retinal quadrants, arises from the medial aspect of the lateral geniculate nucleus and passes to the dorsal lip of the calcarine fissure (Fig. 15.97). The **ventral** bundle, representing peripheral inferior retinal quadrants, originates in the lateral aspect of the lateral geniculate nucleus and passes to the ventral lip of the calcarine fissure. This upper and lower peripheral projection is thought to lie medial to the macular projection in the radiation (Spalding,

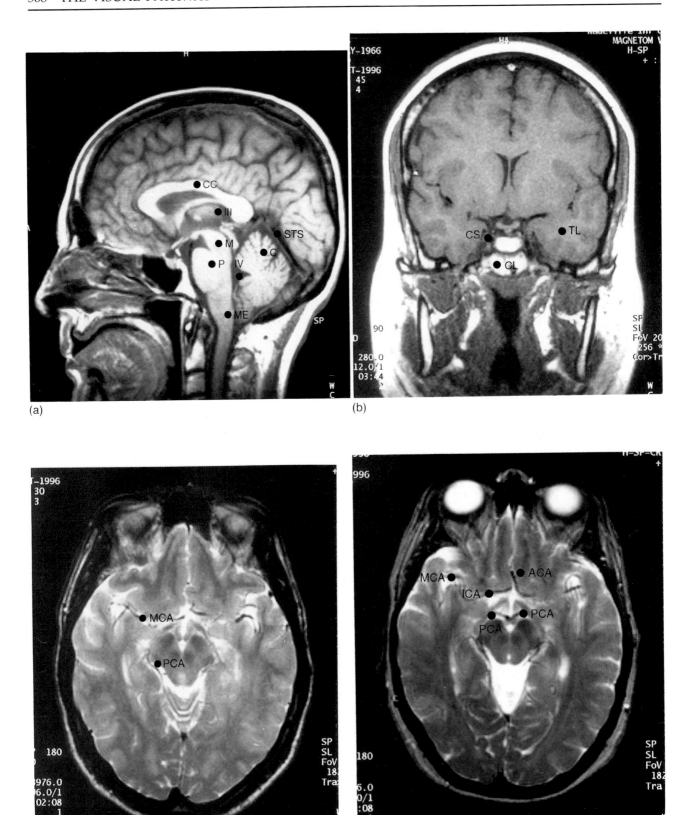

(a)

(b)

(c)

(d)

Fig. 15.95 Magnetic resonance images (MRI) of the brain: (a) sagittal view; (b) coronal slices passing through the pituitary fossa; (c, d) horizontal slices at the mid brain level;

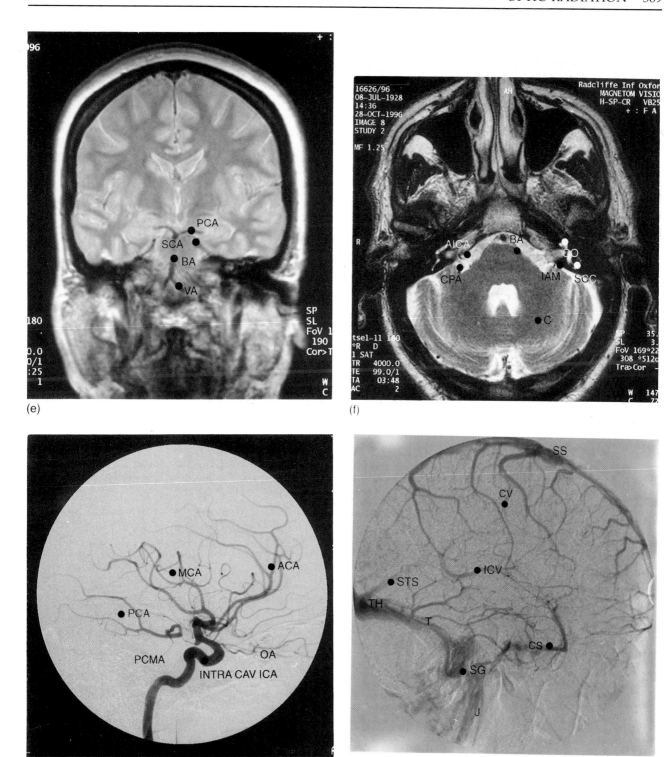

Fig. 15.95 (contd)   (e) coronal slices demonstrating the vertebro-basilar arteries; (f) horizontal slices showing the cerebello-pontine angle; (g) carotid angiogram demonstrating the main vascular territories of the cerebrum; (h) venous phase of the carotid angiogram demonstrating the disposition of the venous sinuses. AICA = anterior inferior cerebellar artery; ACA = anterior cerebral artery; BA = basilar artery; C = cerebellum; CL = clivus; CC = corpus callosum; CO = cochlea; CPA = cerebello-pontine angle; CS = cavenous sinus; CV = cortical veins; IAM = internal auditory meatus; ICA = internal carotid artery; ICV = internal cerebral vein; INTRACAV = intracavernous portion of internal carotid artery; J = jugular vein; L = lateral sinus; M = midbrain; MCA = middle cerebral artery; ME = medulla; P = pons; PCA = posterior cerebral artery; PCMA = posterior communicating artery; SCA = superior cerebellar artery; SCC = semicircular canals; SG = sigmoid sinus; SS = sagittal sinus; STS = straight sinus; T = torcular herophylli; TL = temporal lobe; VA = vertebral artery; III = third ventricle; IV = fourth ventricle.

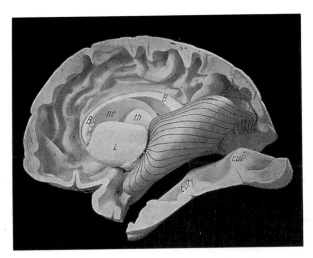

Fig. 15.96 The form and position of the geniculostriate pathway. K = temporal bend of optic nerves; B = corpus callosum; L = lentiform nucleus; nc. = nucleus caudatus; th. = thalamus; col. = grey matter of the collateral sulcus; cul. = highest level of grey matter of collateral sulcus.

1952; Harman and Teuber, 1959) (but see below). Macular fibres spread out anteriorly within the large central portion of the radiation as a base-out wedge, which converges posteriorly to its distribution into the upper and lower lips of the calcarine fissure at the occipital pole. Because of this separation of peripheral and central projections within the radia-

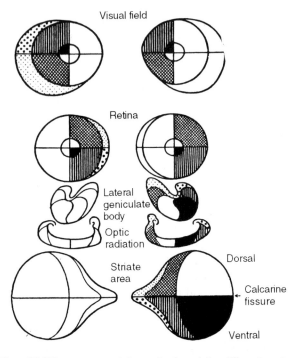

Fig. 15.97 Diagram of the projection of the different parts of the retina in the lateral geniculate nucleus, the optic radiation and the striate area.

tion a lesion may result in a quadrantic visual field defect with a sharp horizontal border.

Field defects caused by lesions of the anterior radiation were found to be congruous by a number of authors, who suggested that fibres representing corresponding points are in juxtaposition in the temporal loop (Spalding, 1952; Hughes, 1954; Falconer and Wilson, 1958; Wendland and Nerenberg, 1960). This view conflicts with that of other authorities who found incongruous field defects with damage to this region (Meyer, 1907; Archambault, 1906, 1909; Cushing, 1921). Van Buren and Baldwin (1958) and Marino and Rasmussen (1968) concluded from their studies that: (1) projections from ipsilateral points lie lateral to contralateral corresponding retinal points; (2) macular projections are not discretely separated from peripheral; and (3) macular projections are medial, not lateral, to peripheral fibres in the temporal loop.

The far peripheral nasal retinal projections, representing the monocular crescent, are thought to congregate at the upper and lower borders of the dorsal and ventral bundles of the radiation (Polyak, 1934; Bender and Strauss, 1937; Bender and Kanzer, 1939).

BLOOD SUPPLY OF THE OPTIC RADIATION

The blood supply can be described at three levels (Abbie, 1933).

1. Where the radiation passes laterally, superior to the inferior horn of the lateral ventricle, the supply is by perforating branches of the **anterior choroidal artery**.
2. Posteriorly, and lateral to the descending horn of the ventricle, the supply is from the **deep optic branch of the middle cerebral artery**, which enters through the anterior perforated substance with the lateral striate arteries (Figs 15.69 and 15.70).
3. As the radiation spreads towards the striate cortex, the supply is by perforating cortical vessels, mainly from the **calcarine branch of the posterior cerebral artery**, but also from the **middle cerebral artery**. It is said that perforating vessels which supply the radiation do not supply cortex.

Francois, Neetens and Collette (1959) added some details. Where optic fibres pass anteriorly from the lateral geniculate nucleus, the middle cerebral and the posterior cerebral arteries overlap the anterior without anastomosis. They confirmed that all perforating branches are end arteries. The optic radiation

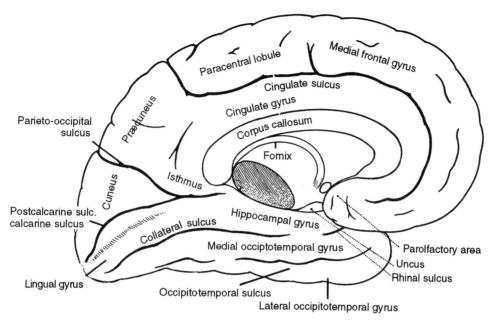

Fig. 15.98 The medial surface of the left cerebral hemisphere. (From *Gray's Anatomy* (1995) 38th edition, ed. by P. Williams, published by Churchill Livingstone.)

itself receives few arterioles; these branch superficially and enter it as non-anastomosing precapillaries. This plexus is completely separate from that of the cortex.

Duvernoy, Delon and Vannson (1981) have studied these vessels in great detail. They noted no capillaries in pia, but arterial and venous anastomoses were present. A stratified pattern of intracortical vessels was observed, and this could be correlated with cellular layers. Glomerular loops and coiled arteries were noted in the cortex; these and other peculiarities may have pathological significance.

15.8 CORTICAL GYRI AND SULCI

The location of the various cortical gyri and sulci is shown in Fig. 15.98. The primary visual area is found mainly in relation to the calcarine sulcus.

CALCARINE SULCUS

The calcarine sulcus is largely confined to the medial surface of the hemisphere, but its anterior end is inferior and posteriorly it may curve round the occipital pole to the lateral surface.

The sulcus is deep and extends from near the occipital pole, usually beginning in the centre of the lunate sulcus (Fig. 15.98). From here it curves anteriorly convex upwards, and ends below the splenium of the corpus callosum. The lunate is sometimes separated from the calcarine sulcus.

The calcarine sulcus is usually just above the inferomedial margin of the occipital lobe which adjoins the junction of falx cerebri and tentorium cerebelli, but may be above it. The **parieto-occipital sulcus** joins the calcarine at an angle a little anterior to its mid point, dividing it into anterior and posterior portions (Fig. 15.99).

If the parieto-occipital and calcarine sulci are opened they seem to be separated by a small vertical **cuneate gyrus**, which sometimes appears on the surface, then visibly separating the two sulci.

The posterior part of the calcarine sulcus develops independently of the stem, which is derived from a fissure of the fetal hemisphere, the posterior part being formed much later by two depressions which ultimately coalesce; the anterior part of the sulcus is hence often called the **calcarine fissure** to distinguish it from a postcalcarine sulcus. The anterior part crosses the inferomedial cerebral margin to reach the inferior surface, forming the inferolateral boundary of the isthmus (Fig. 15.100), which connects the cingulate and parahippocampal sulcus as it does in many other primates. The anterior end of the calcarine sulcus is sometimes close to the colliculi and even the pulvinar and lateral geniculate nucleus, but its termination varies (Figs 15.99 and 15.100).

SULCUS LUNATUS

The sulcus lunatus is not always easily identifiable, although it is constant and marked on the lateral

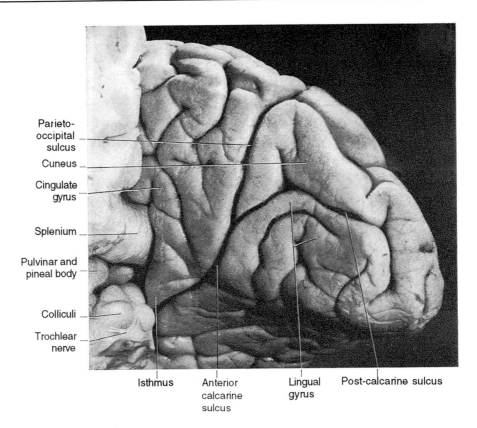

Parieto-occipital sulcus

Cuneus

Cingulate gyrus

Splenium

Pulvinar and pineal body

Colliculi

Trochlear nerve

Isthmus   Anterior calcarine sulcus   Lingual gyrus   Post-calcarine sulcus

Fig. 15.99 Medial and inferior aspects of right occipital lobe, etc.

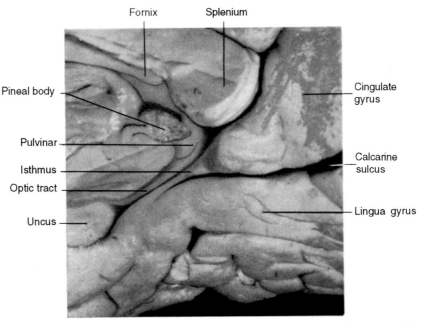

Fornix   Splenium

Pineal body

Pulvinar

Isthmus

Optic tract

Uncus

Cingulate gyrus

Calcarine sulcus

Lingua gyrus

Fig. 15.100 The relations of the anterior part of the calcarine sulcus. Further stage in the dissection of Fig. 15.99.

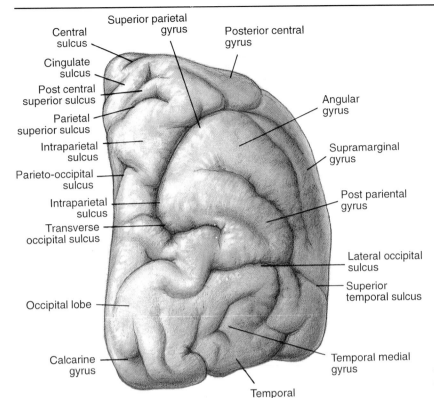

Central sulcus — Cingulate sulcus — Post central superior sulcus — Parietal superior sulcus — Intraparietal sulcus — Parieto-occipital sulcus — Intraparietal sulcus — Transverse occipital sulcus — Occipital lobe — Calcarine gyrus — Superior parietal gyrus — Posterior central gyrus — Angular gyrus — Supramarginal gyrus — Post pariental gyrus — Lateral occipital sulcus — Superior temporal sulcus — Temporal medial gyrus — Temporal inferior gyrus

Fig. 15.101 Right cerebral hemisphere from behind. G = gyrus, S = sulcus. (After Quain's Anatomy.)

aspect of the occipital lobe in apes and monkeys. The human sulcus is small, often continuous with the calcarine sulcus, which it crosses like a T. It is a limiting sulcus, separating the striate and peristriate areas of the cortex, but the parastriate area is hidden in the walls of the sulcus and intervenes between them. The lunate sulcus is the posterior boundary of the gyrus descendens, posterior to the occipital gyri. Two curved sulci, the superior and inferior polar, are often discernible near the ends of the lunate sulcus. The **superior polar sulcus** arches upwards to the medial aspect of the occipital lobe from the upper limit of the lunate sulcus; the **inferior polar sulcus** arches downwards and forwards to the inferior aspect from its lower limit. These polar sulci enclose crescentic extensions of the striate area and may result from expansion of the visual cortex associated with an enlarging macular area.

LINGUAL GYRUS

The lingual gyrus (containing area V4 in the monkey) separates the calcarine and collateral sulci. Posteriorly it reaches the occipital pole. Anteriorly it is continuous with the **hippocampal gyrus** which is lateral to the mid brain (Fig. 15.98) and continuous with the **uncus**, a recurved area forming the posterolateral boundary of the anterior perforated substance. The depression between uncus and hippocampal gyrus is near the tip of the inferior cornu of the lateral

ventricle, and here the anterior choroidal artery enters the choroid plexus of the lateral ventricle. The **lateral occipital sulcus** divides the lateral aspect of the occipital lobe into superior and inferior gyri (Fig. 15.101).

PARIETO-OCCIPITAL SULCUS

The parieto-occipital sulcus appears as a deep cleft on the medial surface of the hemisphere descending anteriorly from the superomedial cerebral border, about 5 cm from the occipital pole, to the posterior extremity of the corpus callosum to join the calcarine fissure at an angle which encloses a region, the cuneus. On the convex superolateral cerebral surface the sulcus is continued for a variable distance, usually a few millimetres, as the lateral part of the parieto-occipital sulcus, where it marks the boundary between parietal and occipital lobes. In other primates its lateral end is in a deep sulcus lunatus, intervening between the parietal and occipital lobes, the cleft extending obliquely backwards, with its occipital edge overlapping the parietal lobe (Fig. 15.102).

15.9 THE STRIATE CORTEX (PRIMARY VISUAL AREA)

The striate cortex (area 17 of Brodman, area V1 in the monkey) is largely on the medial aspect of the

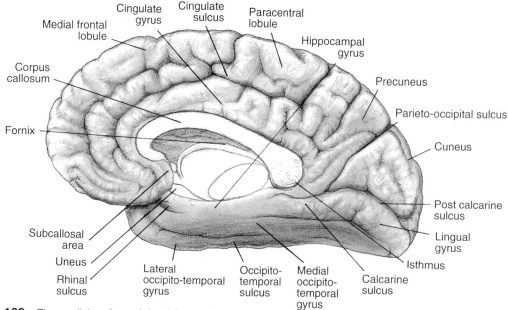

Fig. 15.102 The medial surface of the right cerebral hemisphere.

occipital lobe, around and in the calcarine sulcus, with extensions into the cuneus and lingual gyrus; it extends variably on the lateral aspect of the occipital pole, limited by the sulcus lunatus. It is characterized by the **white line** (or stria) **of Gennari**, visible to the naked eye: hence the term **area striata** (Fig. 15.103). The stria, in the fourth layer of the cortex (IVB), is partly formed by fibres of the optic radiation but mainly by intracortical connections. The fibres run vertically, transversely and obliquely (Fig. 15.104). In the posterior part of the calcarine sulcus the stria appears above and below it (Fig. 15.105), while in the anterior part it is only apparent in cortex below the sulcus (Fig. 15.106).

The approximate limit of the area striata, above, is the cuneate sulcus and below, the collateral sulcus.

The whole of the striate cortex is an elongated ovoid 3000 mm² in area; its narrow end is close to the splenium of the corpus callosum (Fig. 15.106), from which it expands backwards to the occipital pole and

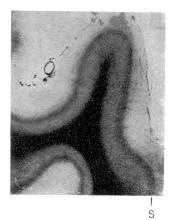

Fig. 15.103 Visual stria (S). (Weigert's stain.) Coronal section of posterior calcarine sulcus.

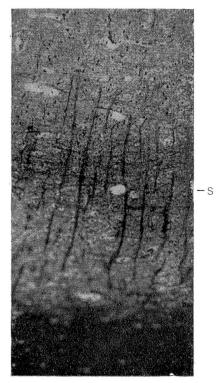

Fig. 15.104 Visual stria (S). (Part of Fig. 15.103 enlarged.)

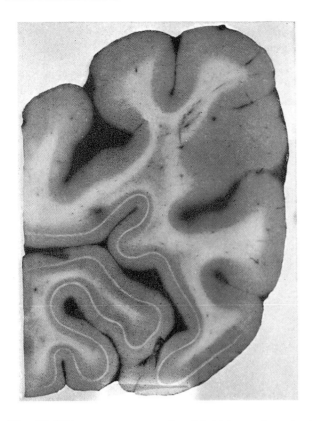

Fig. 15.105 Coronal section of occipital lobe to show visual stria of Gennari in both walls of posterior calcarine sulcus.

beyond it to the lunate sulcus. At about the sixth month of intrauterine life it becomes folded along its axis, the anterior part producing the prominence of the calcar avis in the posterior cornu of the lateral ventricle (hence Huxley's term 'calcarine fissure'). This anterior part is deeper, more constant in form and position, and appears earlier in development and phylogeny than the posterior.

The position of the sulcus lunatus is variable, depending perhaps on the development of parietal and temporal association areas, which may push the sulcus and visual area on to the medial aspect of the occipital lobe; but in some brains it may be lateral and like that found in apes (the *Affenspalte*) (Fig. 15.107). Hence, perhaps, the variable effect of localized injuries of the occipital lobe.

The cerebral cortex (except the allocortex of the hippocampal formation, or archipallium) has a laminar arrangement of neurons and their processes. This is apparent whether staining is aimed at cell bodies or neurites. Varying accounts of this pattern exist (Campbell, 1905; Brodmann, 1909; Cajal, 1909; Von Economo and Koskinas, 1925; Conel, 1939; Woolsey, 1964), but in basic details there is much agreement (Billings-Gagliardi, Chan-Palav and Palay, 1974). The generalized pattern is as follows (Figs 15.108–15.111).

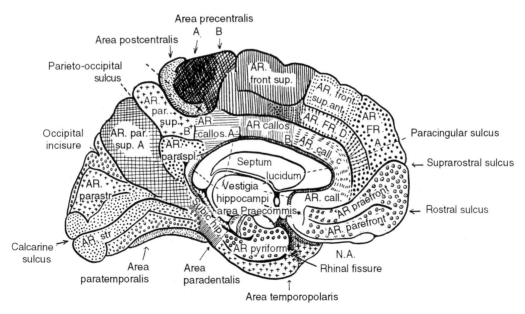

Fig. 15.106 Topography of cortical areas (medial surface). Note area striata on both sides of the posterior part of the calcarine sulcus, but only inferior to its anterior part. The nomenclature is partly superceded, but is preserved for its historical value. (AR = area; S = sulcus.) (Elliott Smith.)

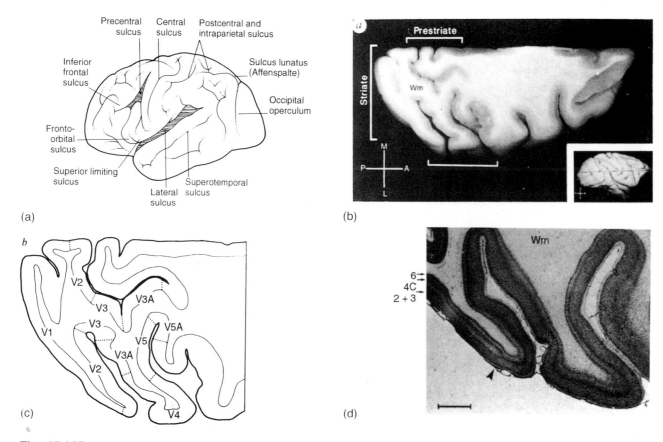

Fig. 15.107 Striate and extrastriate areas of the brain. (a) Left hemisphere of the monkey brain to show the disposition of the sulci. Both in man and macaque monkey, shown here, the cerebral cortex is a highly convoluted sheet, much of it buried inside the folds or sulci, seen in (b), a section through the brain at the level indicated in the inset. Visual cortex occupies the posterior third of the cortex and can be divided into many distinct visual areas, shown in (c) on a drawing of a section at the same level as in (b). A section through the posterior third of the macaque brain treated to stain the cell bodies (d) shows two distinctive regions, the primary visual striate cortex, area V1 (left) and the prestriate cortex lying in front of it. The border is indicated by an arrowhead. (From Zeki and Shipp, 1988.)

LAYER I: PLEXIFORM LAMINA

This is the most external layer, a dense interweaving of neurites (axons and dendrites), or neuropil, derived from intrinsic cortical neurons (mostly stellate cells; see below) and pyramidal cells (both situated in deeper layers), and the terminations of afferent fibres from other parts of the central nervous system, including other parts of the cortex (association fibres).

LAYER II: EXTERNAL GRANULAR LAMINA

Internal to the plexiform lamina is the external granular lamina, so called because of the large number of nuclei of cells visible in it. The layer contains the bodies of neurons, shaped by their array of dendrites and axons, some being pyramidal, some stellate (multipolar), and so optic nerve axons and dendrites from this layer make contacts within it and adjacent layers. Afferent fibres arriving here form

innumerable synapses with local neurons, especially with apical dendrites of pyramidal cells.

LAYER III: PYRAMIDAL LAMINA

The pyramidal lamina is dominated by the familiar 'pyramidal' nucleus, somewhat conical in shape, with apical and basal dendrites and an axon continuous with the base. There are also many stellate interneurons, including neurons with processes oriented both vertically (fusiform cells) and horizontally ('basket' cells). Their axons and dendrites extend far beyond their own lamina.

Layers I–III are sometimes referred to as the **supragranular layers**.

LAYER IV: INTERNAL GRANULAR LAMINA

This is thin and contains largely stellate interneurons and a few pyramidal cells. Many axons and dendrites

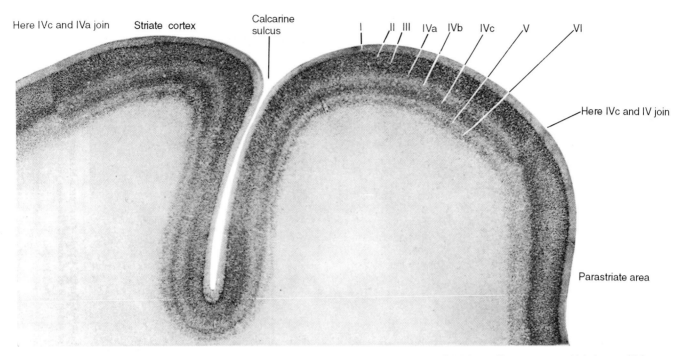

Here IVc and IVa join   Striate cortex   Calcarine sulcus   I   II III   IVa IVb   IVc   V   VI

Here IVc and IV join

Parastriate area

Fig. 15.108   Lamination of the visual cortex. I, the plexiform lamina is the clear superficial layer. Next comes a thick layer which really consists of three portions: layers II, III and IVa. II, the external granular layer is the outermost portion of the thick dark layer. III, the pyramidal lamina is the middle portion of this layer. IVa, the internal granular layer is the innermost layer of the thick dark layer. IVb, the internal granular layer (the stria of Gennari) is the clear layer that follows. IVc, the internal granular is the next dark layer. V, the ganglionic layer is the clear layer that follows. VI, the multiform lamina is the innermost dark layer. Note that the stria of Gennari corresponds to IVb and that it is cut off from the parastriate area by the blending of IVa and IVc. (After Vogt, *Journ. F. Psychologie*, 1902–1904.)

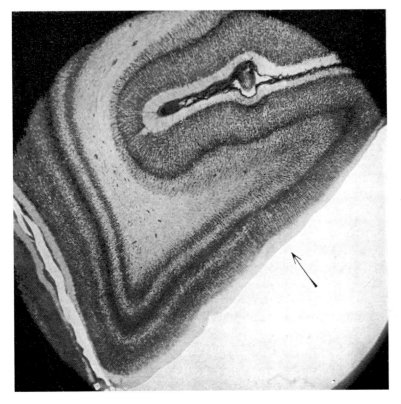

Fig. 15.109   Sagittal section of neonatal visual area—inferior margin of calcarine sulcus. Note the sudden termination of the stria of Gennari. The area parastriata is to the right. (From Pfeifer.)

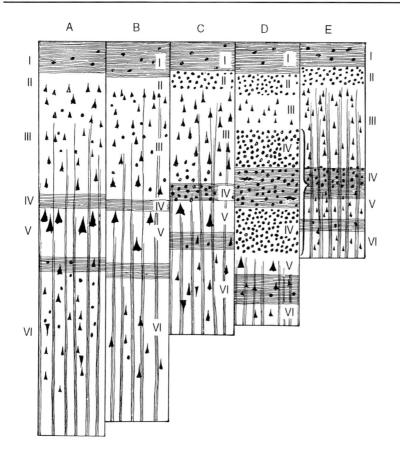

Fig. 15.110 Diagram to show five different types of cerebral cortex. A = motor cortex. Note the absence of granular layers and the presence of giant pyramidal (Betz) cells in small clumps. B = premotor cortex. Note absence of granular layers and giant pyramidal cells. Large discrete, pyramidal cells are present in layer V. C = sensory cortex, post central area. Granular layers are well developed. D = visuosensory cortex. Note reduction of layer III and enormous increase of layer IV, which is traversed by the visual stria. E = visuopsychic area. The granular layers are well developed, but large cells are absent from layer V. The relative depths of individual layers and the relative depths of the whole cortex are approximately accurate. (From P. Williams *et al.* (eds) (1995) *Gray's Anatomy* published by Churchill Livingstone, with permission.)

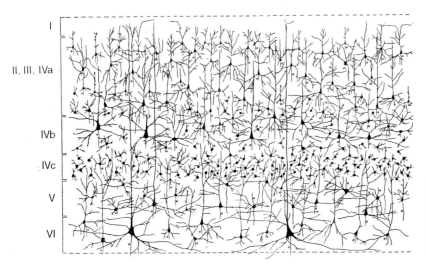

Fig. 15.111 Composite drawing of a section of the visual cortex of a macaque monkey, made from Golgi material. Two Meynert cells are represented in the multiform lamina. The approximate extents of the cell laminae are indicated on the left. The axonal processes of the cells are marked a. (From Le Gros Clark, 1942.)

extend vertically, but there is a special condensation of horizontal processes (Fig. 15.109), the so-called external band of Baillarger (Fig. 15.110), which is particularly prominent in the striate cortex. The layer is subdivided into IVA, IVB and IVC.

LAYER V: GANGLIONIC LAMINA

The ganglionic lamina also contains stellate and pyramidal cells, and here the pyramidal neurons are

largest of any cortical area. Like other laminae, it is permeated between the neuronal cell bodies, by a dense neuropil of dendrites and axons, both local, in passage (arriving at or departing from the cortex), and extending to other levels of the cortex.

LAYER VI: MULTIFORM LAMINA

Next to the central 'white matter' of the cerebrum, this layer consists of small neurons, mostly of 'granular' or stellate interneuron type with a few small pyramidal cells. Some of the latter (Martinotti neurons) send a long centrifugal axon into the plexiform layer and vertically arranged dendrites ramify into deeper layers of the cortex.

Layers V and VI are sometimes referred to as the **infragranular layers**.

Much is known of the processes of cortical interneurons and of pyramidal neurons whose axons leave the cortex for the basal ganglia, thalamus, hippocampus, brain stem nuclei and spinal cord. The types of synapses – axodendritic, axosomatic, axoaxonal, and so on, excitatory or inhibitory – have been studied extensively in recent decades, and certain repetitive arrangements of neurons interacting groups have been recognized, in terms of both structure and function (consult Eccles, Ito and Szentagothai, 1967; Szentagothai, 1975). In many parts of the cortex these congeries of interacting neurons are arranged in a columnar manner, although complex horizontal interconnections also exist. The methods of 'unit-recording' have been instrumental in revealing this vertical organization and the striate cortex has received particular attention (see below).

The cell types, actual numbers, and their intrinsic and extrinsic connections vary in different regions of the cerebral cortex. Certain patterns are recognized: one, in which pyramidal cells predominate, is typical of 'motor' areas, whereas another, in which 'granular' cells are preponderant, is associated with sensory areas. This granular type of cortex is at its most elaborate in the striate area. Even here, in lamina IV, a few pyramidal neurons (cells of Meynert) appear in a single row. Their axons descend through the optic radiations to the superior colliculus and possibly ocular motor nuclei. The profusion of granular cells is remarkable; although a mere 3% of the total cortex, they constitute 10% of the area of the total population of cortical neurons. Lamina IV is commonly further subdivided in this area (Figs 15.110 and 15.111). (For further details see Polyak, 1957; Crosby, Humphrey and Lauer, 1962; Colonnier, 1967, 1974; Billings-Gagliardi, Chan-Palav and Palay, 1974.)

DISTINGUISHING FEATURES OF THE STRIATE CORTEX

1. The visual **stria of Gennari** distinguishes the striate cortex from all other cortical areas.
2. Like other sensory areas, the inner granular lamina (IV) is augmented and here the cells are more densely arranged than in any other cortical area. The outer (and more especially the inner) granular layers consist of a great number of small cells packed closely together, but the whole granular layer (IV) is wider here than in any other cortical area.
3. The basic sexilaminar pattern is complicated by the stria in lamina IV, which divides it into sublamina IVA and IVC, with the stria (IVB) between.
4. The visual stria (IVB) contains a few large, horizontally placed stellate neurons (Fig. 15.110).
5. The ganglionic layer (V) contains the solitary neurons of Meynert, which are pyramidal in shape, measure about 3 μm across, and are widely spaced in a row. The cells project to the superior colliculus and possibly to ocular motor nuclei.
6. Their dendritic pattern suggests an integrative function in the cortex (Chan-Palay, Palay and Billings-Gagliardi, 1974).

While there is no doubt that the striate cortex (area 17 in Brodman's terminology) is the main receptor area for the optic radiation from the geniculate body, the surrounding peristriate and parastriate zones (areas 18 and 19 of Brodman), also receive such fibres directly as well as through connections with the striate cortex itself.

LOCALIZATION IN THE VISUAL CORTEX

It is in the primary visual areas that the impulses from corresponding parts of each retina meet. A lesion of the striate area affects all laminae of the lateral geniculate nucleus. There is a point-to-point localization of the retina in the cortex, each area in the retina being precisely represented in a corresponding area of the striate cortex, and in adjoining visual areas. All visual stimuli to corresponding halves of the retinas are transmitted to the one geniculate nucleus, and finally to the ipsilateral striate area of that side. Visual stimuli from the left field fall on the right halves of both retinas. The fibres from the right eye pass to the right optic tract, those from the left eye decussate in the chiasma to join the uncrossed fibres in that tract to reach the right lateral geniculate nucleus and relay to the striate area. This is the neural substrate for the perception of the left visual field and accords with the mediation in the right hemisphere of motor and sensory activities in the left half of the body.

The upper and lower quadrants of the retina are represented respectively above and below the

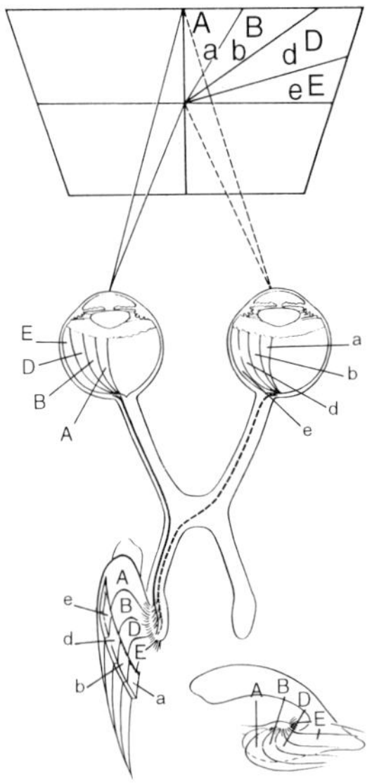

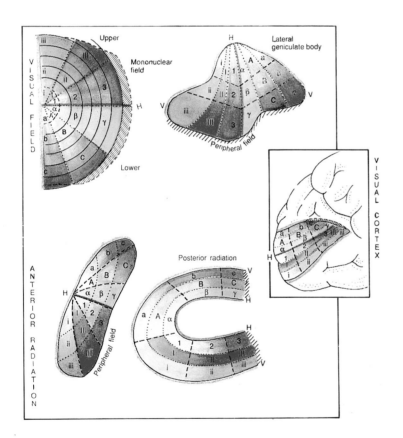

Fig. 15.112 Representation of the right upper quadrant of the visual field in the visual pathway. Objects are imaged on the inferior left retinal quadrants and information is transmitted via the optic nerves and left optic tract to the optic radiation, after synapse in the left lateral geniculate body. Information from the visual field close to the vertical meridian is carried by fibres looping forwards from the radiation. Note that the tip of the temporal horn of the lateral ventricle is not capped by the radiation. Information from the visual field close to the horizontal is transmitted by fibres passing more directly backwards. The distribution from each retina extends anteriorly to an equal degree. Representation of the *ipsilateral* retina lies lateral to that from the *contralateral* retina. The macular fibres at all levels are considered to lie medial to fibres representing the peripheral retina. The representation is based on the study of Van Buren and Baldwin concerning visual field defects following temporal lobectomy. (From Miller, N. R. (1985) *Clinical Neuro-Ophthalmology* 4th Edition, Vol. 1, published by Williams and Wilkins, with permission.)

Fig. 15.113 Representation of the visual field (a), projected onto (b) the lateral geniculate body, (c) the anterior radiation and (d) the posterior radiation. Note that in the lateral geniculate body central vision is represented superiorly and peripheral vision inferiorly. The upper quadrant of the field is lateral, the lower medial and the horizontal meridian roughly vertical. In the anterior radiation the fibres rotate through almost a right angle; central vision lies mainly over the lateral aspect of the radiation, but concentrated in its intermediate part, while peripheral vision is on the medial aspect, particularly above and below. The horizontal meridian is once again anatomically horizontal. In the posterior radiation, central field is represented by intermediate fibres, lying lateral to the posterior horn of the lateral ventricle as they pass back to the occipital pole. Peripheral field is represented by fibres in the margins of the radiation (at the end of the 'horseshoe'), in readiness to enter the calcarine cortex. (From Miller, D. N., redrawn from Spalding, J. M. K. (1952) *J. Neurol. Neurosurg. Psychiatr.* **15**, 101.)

calcarine sulcus. The periphery of the retina is represented anteriorly and the macula towards the occipital pole. The most anterior part of the striate area represents the extreme nasal periphery of the retina, corresponding to the monocular temporal crescent in the visual fields (Figs 15.112–15.114).

While there is some degree of macular representation around the posterior part of the calcarine fissure and extending onto the lateral surface of the occipital pole, it is possible that this overlaps that of more peripheral parts of the retina. The macular area of the cortex is relatively much larger in proportion to the

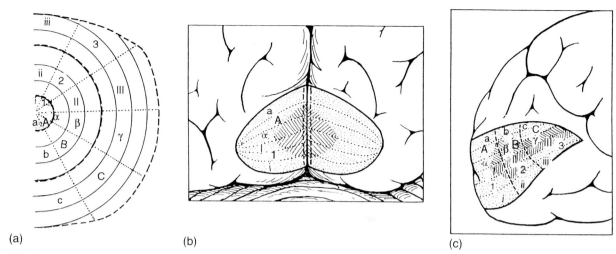

Fig. 15.114 Representation of the visual field and striate cortex according to Spalding. (a), right visual field; (b), the striate cortex viewed from the posterior aspect showing principally the macular representation; (c), the striate cortex viewed from the medial aspect. The hatched area of the cortex represents the walls of the calcarine fissure, illustrated as though it were pulled open; the stippled area represents the visual cortex that faces both posteriorly and medially. (From Miller, D. N., after J. M. K. Spalding (1952) *J. Neurol. Neurosurg. Psychiatr.*, **15**, 101.)

striate area than is the macular region of the retina relative to the whole retina. This contrast relationship resembles the ratios of representation of the hand, face, and larynx, in the pre- and post-central gyri, as conveyed so forcefully by Cushing's 'homonunculus' (see Warwick and Williams, 1976).

In a horizontal section the area striata undergoes a sudden change in appearance just posterior to its mid point. The stria diminishes and the dark band internal to it disappears. These changes mark the beginning of the macular area, which extends around the occipital pole onto the lateral surface of the hemisphere to the lunate sulcus. It is possible to identify the macular area in many human brains by simple features of the surface. Three semilunar sulci (lunatus, polaris superior, and polaris inferior) are often grouped around the calcarine sulcus in the axis of the area striata like a trefoil. The rapid phylogenetic expansion of the posterolateral part of the area striata for representation of the macula leads to formation of three opercula bounded by these three semilunar sulci (Elliot Smith, 1930).

An old view, that the macula has a double representation (i.e. that each point in the macula is represented in both occipital poles), was dispelled by the observations of Holmes and Lister (1915) on the effects of gunshot wounds. The same observers also explained the phenomenon of 'sparing of the macula' in cases of lesions of the posterior cerebral artery by anastomosis at the occipital pole between the middle and posterior cerebral arteries (Fig. 15.70). Polyak (1957) has reviewed this problem most exhaustively

and favours this vascular explanation, as did Brodal (1969). However, in one study (admittedly on cats; Stone and Hansen, 1966), the possibility of a bilateral macular representation at the geniculate level in this species was suggested.

THE UNIOCULAR VISUAL FIELDS

The fibres mediating uniocular and binocular fields run separately at some levels of the visual pathway. According to Brouwer and Zeeman (1926) the binocular field (in the rabbit, where it is only 20°) occupies a very small area in the lateral geniculate nucleus, the whole of the remainder being uniocular. But this animal, with lateral orbital axes, represents those with well-developed panoramic vision and little or no true binocular vision.

The human uniocular field, seen by one eye only, is the extreme temporal field. The retina involved is the most nasal. Its fibres form the nasal crescent medial to the crossed bundle and then a small ventral strip in the tract and lateral geniculate nucleus with the superior fibres medial and inferior fibres lateral (Bender and Kanzer, 1939) (Fig. 15.78).

In the radiation the superior fibres are in the upper quadrant and inferior in the lower quadrant. The uniocular field is localized anteriorly in the lower lip of the calcarine sulcus.

The clinical importance of this is that it is possible to have a lesion of the optic radiation, for instance, affecting one field only.

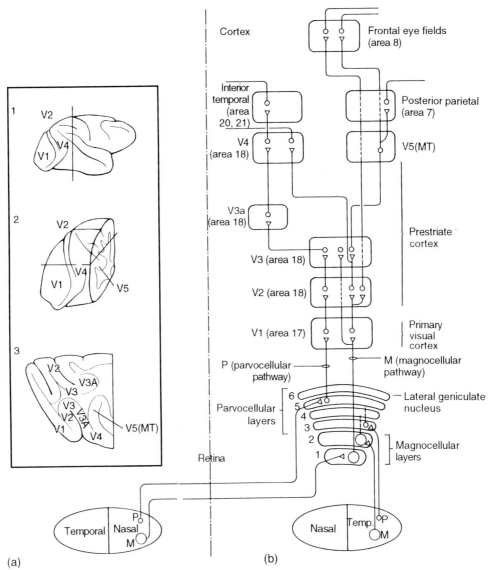

Fig. 15.115 (a) Schematic diagram of the visual projections from retina to various visual areas of the primate cerebral cortex. (a) Visual cortical areas in the Macaque monkey as seen in the intact hemisphere (1, 2), and in histological section (3). 1, lateral view of the right hemisphere; 2, an expanded view showing the location of the buried middle temporal area in the superior temporal sulcus at the rostral border of the occipital lobe. 3, horizontal section through the occipital lobe (as shown in 2) showing the approximate location of visual areas at this level. (b) Diagram of the visual pathways emphasizing two key aspects. First, there appears to be a hierarchy of processing. Second, there are major pathways by which aspects of visual information can be processed in parallel. The parvocellular pathway P (equivalent to the X pathway in the cat) is concerned with detail, form, and colour, while the magnocellular pathway (M—the Y pathway in the cat) is concerned with the gross features of the stimulus. (From Kandell and Schwartz (1985), adapted from van Essen, 1979, with permission.)

15.10   THE PRESTRIATE CORTEX (VISUAL ASSOCIATION AREAS)

The belt of cortex surrounding the striate cortex (area 18 of Brodmann – parastriate cortex – and area 19 – peristriate cortex) has long been regarded as the seat of higher visual functions. Kuypers *et al.* (1965) demonstrated a direct projection to it from the striate cortex, and a projection from it to the inferior temporal cortex, the seat of visual memory. Certainly

this accords with the knowledge that lesions of area 17 affect sight but not visual memory, while prestriate lesions induce visual disorientation including loss of topographical memory, visual agnosia and inability to judge distances.

The **parastriate cortex** (18) lies immediately adjacent to area 17 and is a six-layered granular cortex which lacks the stria of Gennari of the visual cortex (Fig. 15.115).

The **peristriate cortex** (19) completely surrounds

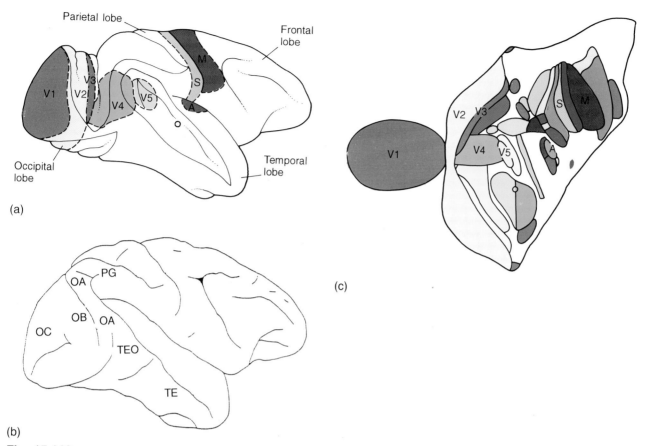

Fig. 15.116 (a) Right hemisphere of primate brain with sulci unfolded to display visual areas. (b) Representation of the right hemisphere opened out to show visual areas (V = red and yellow), auditory areas (A = green), somatic areas (S = blue) and areas controlling movement (M = grey). (c) Cortical visual areas in the rhesus monkey. Arrows signify two cortical visual pathways arising in the primary visual cortex (OC), which diverging in the prestriate cortex either ventrally, into the temporal cortex (TEO and TE) or dorsally into the parietal cortex (PG). The ventral pathway is crucial for object vision and the dorsal for spatial vision. (Modified from Mishkin, M., Ungerleider, L. G. and Macko, K. A. (1913) *TINS*, **6**, 414.)

the parastriate cortex on the lateral aspects of the hemisphere encroaching above and below its medial aspect. Most lies in the posterior parietal lobe, but inferiorly it forms part of the temporal lobe. It resembles parietal lobe histologically, lacking large pyramidal cells in layer V.

LOCALIZATION IN THE PRESTRIATE CORTEX

The prestriate cortex differs from striate cortex in a number of ways. Studies by Cragg and Ainsworth (1969) and Zeki (1969, 1970, 1971, 1975) showed that the prestriate cortex could be subdivided into multiple zones receiving projections from the striate cortex (V1 in the monkey). Callosal association fibres connect striate and prestriate cortex in one hemisphere to prestriate cortex in the fellow hemisphere. These fibres terminate in cells representing the sagittal meridian of the hemifield (Whitteridge, 1965).

Zeki found, in degeneration studies following callosal section, that this saggital meridian was represented in multiple regions of the prestriate cortex and has inferred from this structural segregation a functional segregation of these zones (Zeki, 1975; Zeki and Sandeman, 1976; Zeki, 1977, 1984a,b). Thus in the monkey the zones are V2, V3, V3a, V4, V4a, V5 and V6. The modalities represented preferentially, though not exclusively, are orientation (V2, 3, 3a), colour V4, and motion (V5) (Fig. 15.116).

These functionally distinct areas are located in cortex with distinct cytoarchitectonic features (Bailey and von Bonin, 1951) (Fig. 15.117c). Area V1 is the striate cortex OC; area V2 corresponds to prestriate area OB, and V3 and V4 are contained in prestriate area OA exclusive of its dorsal part. Prestriate area MT (corresponding to medial temporal cortex in the owl monkey) is located in the caudal portion of the superior temporal sulcus, mainly within dorsolateral OA. Of four further dorsal areas concerned with

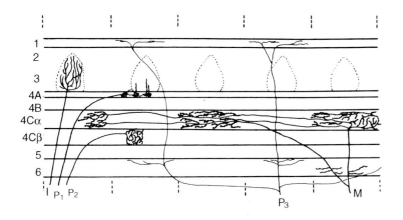

Fig. 15.117 Summary diagram of the pattern of lateral geniculate termination in the striate cortex. I, input from the intercalated layers; P$_1$, P$_2$, P$_3$, input from the parvocellular layers; M, input from the magnocellular layers; perhaps two components (Hubel and Wiesel, 1972; Hendriksen *et al.*, 1978; Blasdel and Lund, 1983; Fitzpatrick *et al.*, 1983). The ocular dominance bands are indicated by dashed lines 400–500 μm apart. (Courtesy of M. Hawken.)

visual processing, two are in the upper superior temporal sulcus and two are in the depths of the intraparietal sulci. The more anterior parietal one is in the cytoarchitectonic area PG in inferior parietal lobule. Additional extrastriate visual areas, which will be discussed later, are found in the inferior temporal cortex as far forward as the temporal pole (areas TEO and TE).

Cells in the prestriate cortex of the monkey have much larger receptive fields than corresponding ones of the striate cortex and there is not the precise retinotopic mapping in the prestriate cortex encountered in the anterior visual pathway. The topographic map on V2 is almost as precise as in V1; in V4 and V5 the representation is less well defined.

15.11 CONNECTIONS OF THE STRIATE AND PRESTRIATE CORTEX

STRIATE CORTEX

Afferents from the lateral geniculate nucleus are mapped retinotopically to layer IVC of the striate cortex (area 17). A few pass to layers I and VI. The distribution of fibres from parvocellular and magnocellular layers is not identical and the axons of the parvocellular cells show lower conduction velocities.

Histochemical staining of the striate cortex for the mitochondrial enzyme cytochrome oxidase provided fresh insights into the organization of this area (Wong-Riley, 1979; Hendrickson, 1982, 1985). The termination zones for lateral geniculate nucleus neurons in IVA and IVC stain dark (positive), while IVB remains light. Staining is heavy in layer III and less intense in II. Tangential sections at the level of II/III show positive staining to be arranged in a series of 'blobs' 150–200 μm in diameter in the monkey. The blobs are arranged in parallel rows, with lighter-

staining 'interblobs' between them (Fig. 15.118). Each row of blobs is centred on an ODC band. Blob spacing changes with cortical eccentricity. Topographically the blob density is five per mm^2 at the foveal representation and eight per mm^2 at the representation of far periphery (Horton, 1984; Livingstone and Hubel, 1984). Parvocellular neurons, conveying high spatial acuity and colour (wavelength)-coded information, terminate in layers IVA, IVCβ and VIA. Spiny stellate neurons in IVCβ provide a major input into the lower layer of III of the blob region. There is also a direct input from parvocellular lateral geniculate nucleus cells to layer III of the striate cortex. There is some input from magnocellular neurons into the blob region. The blobs contain cells highly selective for wavelength or brightness.

Input from the parvocellular neurons also reaches the interblob region, containing cells selective for orientation but not for wavelength or movement. Magnocellular input passes to layer IVB of the striate cortex. Cells in this layer are selective for orientation and movement.

Layer IVC connects with layers superficial and deep to it by cortical loops. It connects with layers II and III, which in turn connect with layer V. Layer V connects with VI and with IV (Fig. 15.117). Layer I of the visual cortex consists of bundles of parallel axons.

Projections from pyramidal cells of the striate cortex establish imperfect retinotopic maps in several extrastriate cortical areas as well as in the brain stem. Axons pass from layers II and III to area 18 and the medial temporal lobe. Layer V projects to the superior colliculus and integrates with the inputs from the lateral geniculate nucleus, while layer VI provides the rich reciprocal projection to all layers of the lateral geniculate nucleus including the interlaminar zones. Fibres to the magnocellular layers arise in the deepest part of layer VI, those to the parvocellular layers in its superficial parts.

Summary of the connections of the visual cortex (area 17)

1. With the opposite visual cortex by commissural fibres through the splenium of the corpus callosum. The striate cortex (area 17) is less profusely connected by such fibres, which are more numerous in the peristriate regions (areas 18 and 19).
2. With the frontal eye fields, especially from the peristriate area (19) to areas 6, 8 and 9 (frontal fields I and II).
3. With pyramidal 'association' areas.
4. With the superior colliculus (from area 19).
5. With the oculomotor nuclei and other nuclei by descending fibres which run in the optic radiations (especially from area 19).

The striate visual cortex is directly connected with other parts of the visual cortex and with the frontal, pyramidal and temporal lobes by abundant association fibres, to provide an anatomical basis for visuotactile, visuoauditory and other associative functions, including eye movements.

PRESTRIATE CORTEX

Area 18 connects with areas 17 and 19 of the same hemisphere and, via the corpus callosum, with areas 18 and 19 of the opposite hemisphere. It is connected by long association fibres with other ipsilateral association areas including the prefrontal, sensory motor and auditory association cortex, the insula, and, by polysynaptic pathways, the anterior temporal lobe.

The superior longitudinal and inferior fronto-occipital bundles to the frontal region are thought to provide visual feedback for the voluntary control of eye movements. Corticotectal projections are concerned with the initiation of slow vertical or oblique eye movements.

There are reciprocal connections with many of the cortical zones, and also the tectum and pulvinar. Recently, a small but definite projection from the lateral geniculate nucleus to the prestriate cortex was demonstrated (Fries, 1981; Yukie and Iwai, 1981), but no reciprocal corticogeniculate projection. The function of this connection, by-passing the striate cortex, is not known.

Area 19 also projects to the tectum (Mettler, 1935). An occipital projection probably arises from the medial surface of area 19, while an occipitopontine projection arises from its lateral surface (Hines, 1942).

Extensive studies by Zeki (1984a,b) in the monkey have demonstrated rich parallel and serial connections between striate and prestriate cortex. Almost all these connections are reciprocal. However, a hierarchical relationship can be recognized based on the laminar origin and termination of the neurons involved. In general, those areas which are higher in the hierarchy show greater complexity of structure and processing functions and have larger receptive fields. A retinotopic relationship is maintained, but mapping is less precise in the prestriate cortex than in the anterior visual pathway.

Forward projections to higher functional areas arise primarily in the **supragranular** layers (i.e. superficial to layer IV and especially to IVC, which is the only true granular layer). They terminate for the most part in layer IV (the **granular** layer) and also in the lower part of layer III. Feedback projections to lower functional areas originate partly in supragranular cortex, but chiefly in the **infragranular** layers; they terminate in supra- and infragranular layers, most densely in layers I and VI (Maunsell and Van Essen, 1983).

Striate cortex (V1) projects to V2–V6 of the prestriate cortex. As noted earlier, Wong-Riley (1979) demonstrated that certain repetitively occurring regions of the cat striate cortex showed up as dark bands or 'blobs' when stained for the respiratory enzyme cytochrome oxidase (Fig. 15.118). They also showed a regular periodicity in the monkey striate cortex (Hendrickson, 1982; Horton and Hubel, 1981). Similar cytochrome oxidase-positive stripes occur in V2 (Livingstone and Hubel, 1982; Zeki, 1984a,b). Most of the cells in the blob region of V1 and V2 are wavelength selective rather than orientation selective, suggesting a functional segregation here (Livingstone and Hubel, 1981; Zeki, 1984a).

Studies with horseradish peroxidase injection have demonstrated a projection from V1 blobs selectively to cytochrome oxidase stripes in V2 (Livingstone and Hubel, 1984) while (layers 2 and 3 of) these regions in turn project to V4 complex (Fries and Zeki, 1983; Shipp and Zeki, 1984), and are the predominant source of input from V2 to V4. V4 complex is rich in colour-coded cells. There are reciprocal connections between V4 complex and the inferotemporal cortex, projections from the latter region arising in layers 2, 3, 5 and 6, with projections from V4 complex ending in layer 4. The input from V1 to V4 complex arises from scattered cells in layer 2, while that from V3 complex may arise from superficial or deep layers.

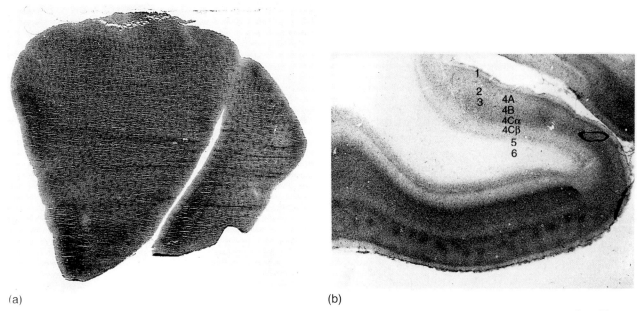

(a)   (b)

Fig. 15.118 (a) Tangential section through layer 3 of a flattened region of the occipital operculum of a rhesus monkey. The central area of the visual field is represented in this part of the striate cortex. The preparation is stained for cytochrome oxidase activity and shows the 'blob' (dark) and 'interblob' regions. (Courtesy of M. Hawken and I. D. Thompson.) (b) Vervet monkey. Border of area 17 (top) and area 18. Transverse section stained for cytochrome oxidase activity. Notice label in layers 4 and 6 and extending up into superficial layers as 'blobs'.

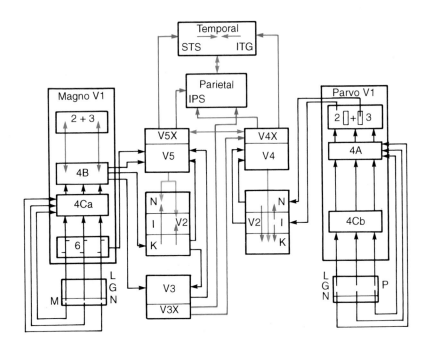

Fig. 15.119 Connectivity of the V areas in the macaque monkey. (Courtesy of S. Zeki.)

Connections with the 'motion' area, V5, also exist (Fries and Zeki, 1983) (Fig. 15.119).

V2 projects to V3 and V5, in addition to V4, and has reciprocal connections with V1. V5 projects to V2 and, independently, to layer IVb of V1. Projections from V1 to V5 arise in a different layer. The prestriate zone V5a projects to the pons, while V6 projects to tectum.

The **corpus callosum** is a massive slab of association fibres connecting the neopallium of the two

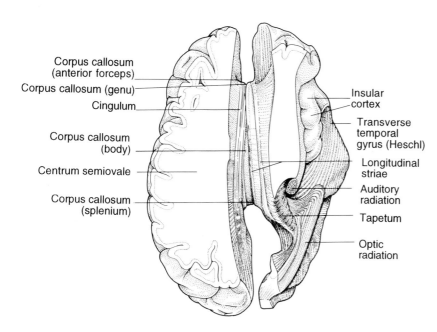

Corpus callosum
(anterior forceps)

Corpus callosum (genu)

Cingulum

Corpus callosum
(body)

Centrum semiovale

Corpus callosum
(splenium)

Insular
cortex

Transverse
temporal
gyrus (Heschl)

Longitudinal
striae

Auditory
radiation

Tapetum

Optic
radiation

Fig. 15.120 Dissection of the superior surface of the hemispheres exposing the corpus callosum, cingulum, longitudinal striae and the optic and auditory radiations. (Redrawn from Carpenter, M. B. (1976) *Human Neuroanatomy*, published by Williams and Wilkins, after Mettler, 1948, with permission.)

hemispheres. It forms the roof of the anterior horn and body of the lateral ventricle and consists of rostrum, genu, body and splenium (Fig. 15.120).

In the cat it provides the sole interhemispheric visual connections (Shounara, 1974), much of whose development is postnatal, lagging behind the visual cortex. Maturation mirrors that of binocular vision (Cragg, 1972, 1975; Ankar and Cragg, 1974; Buisseret and Imbert, 1976).

Whitteridge (1965) showed that the distribution of callosal fibres at the striate–prestriate boundary coincides with regions representing the vertical meridian. He suggested that one of the functions of the corpus callosum was to unite the representation of the two hemifields separated by the chiasmal crossings, at the mid line. This concept must apply to the multiple subzones of the prestriate cortex also. The corpus callosum connects those parts of the striate and prestriate areas in which the mid line of the hemifield is represented. Between each hemisphere V1 is connected to V1, V2 to V2, and so on. The pattern of callosal connection is a guide to the precision of retinal mapping in that area. Thus in V1, which is precisely mapped, a narrow strip of callosal fibres connects to a similar band in V1 of the opposite hemisphere; the strip within V2 and V3 is slightly broader, and the connections to V4 and V5 are diffuse (Zeki and Sandeman, 1976; Zeki, 1993). Elberger (1979) suggested that callosal association fibres are concerned with organization of monocular and binocular regions of the visual fields, and with interocular alignment.

The development of the interhemispheric connec-

tions is influenced by visual experience in the cat. At 2–4 days, callosal axons terminate in the equivalent of areas 17, 18 and 19 (Innocenti, Fiore and Caminiti, 1977), whereas in adult cats they are confined to the striate/prestriate border (Schatz, 1977; Innocenti, 1978).

The broader connections to the striate cortex are retained after monocular deprivation (Innocenti and Frost, 1979), whereas they are expanded asymmetrically with induction of unilateral strabismus (Lund, Mitchell and Henry, 1978; Lund and Mitchell, 1979).

15.12   ORGANIZATION AND FUNCTIONS OF THE VISUAL CORTEX

The simple view of the visual pathway was a series of relays, retinal, geniculate and cortical, consisting of fairly independent conducting pathways whose signals were merely transferred to the cortex for decoding. Newer information has accumulated, based on the electrophysiology of individual neurons ('unit' recording) and demonstration of pathways by a variety of tracer techniques.

The numerical disparity between photoreceptors and retinal ganglion cells is structural evidence of convergence at retinal level, although some macular receptors alone have individual pathways (e.g. a 1:1 relationship between cones, midget bipolar cells and ganglion cells). Collateral synapses between retinal neurons are responsible for the phenomena of lateral inhibition, inhibitory surround and the consequential heightening of contrast between stimulated and

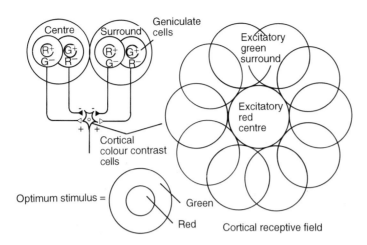

Fig. 15.121 Double-opponent, red-green, colour-contrast cortical cells with concentric receptive fields are highly sensitive to simultaneous colour-contrast. The most common type of geniculate cells can be used synaptically to form a cortical cell. Two or more geniculate cells with overlapping receptive fields form the centre and surround of the concentrically organized colour-contrast cortical cell. Red at the centre of the cortical cells receptive field will excite a 'red on' geniculate cell and the cortical cell itself. Green at the centre will inhibit. Green in the surround of the cortical cells' receptive field will excite a 'green on' geniculate cell and therefore the cortical cell. Red will inhibit. (From Gourass, P. in Kandell and Schwartz.)

unstimulated points. This creates a 'centre-surround' arrangement of receptive fields and provides the fundamental organizational unit whose behaviour is modified at synaptic interfaces along the visual pathway and extending into striate and extrastriate areas. Similar processing of coded information occurs in the lateral geniculate nucleus, where a great complexity of interneuronal connections exists (Fig. 15.121). As mentioned earlier unit recording here also reveals a concentric organization of receptor fields modified slightly from that of the retina, but geniculate neurons are apparently not involved in binocular integration, which almost certainly begins in the columnar arrays of the striate cortex.

In the past two decades the patterns of neuronal structure and function in the striate and prestriate areas of the occipital and neighbouring cortex have been studied intensively by unit recording and axon labelling. Prograde tracing methods include terminal degeneration and autoradiographic labelling; retrograde tracing includes horseradish peroxidase techniques (see Hubel and Wiesel, 1961, 1962, 1965, 1968, 1969, 1972, 1977, 1978; Glees, 1961; Peters and Palay, 1966; Jones and Powell, 1969, 1970; Rossignol and Colonnier, 1971; Gross, Rolha Miranda and Bender, 1972; Le Vay, Wiesel and Hubel, 1980; Gilbert and Wiesel, 1979, 1983). Much of this work has been on cats, but results in monkeys strongly suggest that similar patterns exist in the human cortex.

Briefly, it is clear that there are columnar units or chains of neurons across the thickness of the visual cortex analogous to the 'modules' described by Szentagothai (1975) for other cortical areas. These respond to a precise pattern of stimulation about a point in the retina (the receptive field) and also,

according to the cortical layers activated, to modalities such as luminosity, edges between light and dark, the orientation and speed of movement of such stimuli and their wavelength characteristics. Some neurons within columns show 'ocular dominance' features and respond preferentially to stimulation of the right or left retina. Binocular neurons respond maximally to simultaneous stimulation of corresponding retinal points of the two hemiretinas. Although wavelength-coded units are found in the striate cortex it appears that perception of colour within the visual scene depends on units located in the prestriate cortex.

The anatomical reality of such a columnar cytoarchitecture in the striate cortex has been demonstrated by transport of radioactive tracers such as the amino acid proline, which is transported after intraocular injection to the lateral geniculate nucleus and transsynaptically to the striate cortex (Hubel and Wiesel, 1978) (Fig. 15.122). Studies of terminal degeneration and of synaptic arrangements, partly by electron microscopy, have shown that afferents in the striate cortex (and elsewhere) feed impulses into columnar groups of intermediaries and thence to pyramidal cells to be propagated to subcortical nuclei or to other parts of the cortex.

THE STRIATE CORTEX

The striate cortex exhibits a precise columnar organization centred around its interlamellar connections and forming functional units occupying its thickness (2 mm), from surface to the subjacent white matter (Figs 15.123 and 15.124).

Unit recording from the cells in IVC show them to be driven monocularly, such that there is an

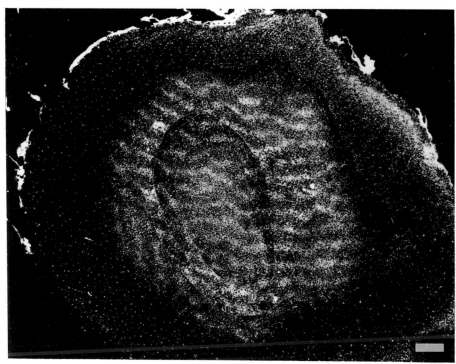

Fig. 15.122 Montage of dark field autoradiography made from sections cut tangential to the operculum of the right hemisphere of a 23-day-old monkey that was monocularly deprived for 21 days. The deprived eye was injected with a mixture of tritiated proline and fucose. The label forms narrow strips which were estimated to occupy, at most, 38% of layer IVC. (From Swindale, N. V., Vital-Durand, F. and Blakemore, C. (1981) *Proc. R. Soc. Lond.*, **213**, 435, with permission.)

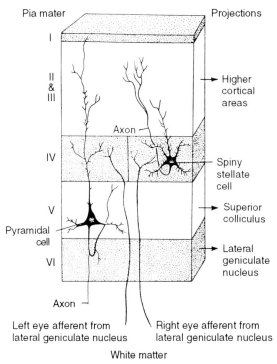

Fig. 15.123 The afferent and efferent connections of the primary visual cortex are made in specific layers of the cortex. (From J. Kelley in Kandell and Schwartz, 1985.)

alternation of inputs from the ipsilateral and contralateral eye along a row of adjacent columns. These monocularly dominated columns are termed **ocular dominance columns** (Fig. 15.125). The cells of IVC show a 'centre-surround' type of opponent organization similar to that of the retinal ganglion cells or lateral geniculate nucleus neurons, and their receptive fields have been termed 'circularly symmetrical'. They respond best for instance to a diffuse patch of light, with a dark surround. They receive from one eye only.

These cells in IVC project to cells in adjacent layers, which show increasingly specialized receptive field behaviour. This is thought to arise from a hierarchical convergence of inputs. Thus the 'circularly symmetrical' cells project to 'simple' cells, and these to complex and hypercomplex cells. The striking difference between their responses is that only the circularly symmetrical cells respond preferentially to pools of diffuse light centred on the receptive field, simple cells and the more complex cells respond preferentially to slits, bars or borders of light, and moreover are sensitive to slit orientation and direction and speed of movement.

Simple cells, which still retain some X- and Y-like features, are found chiefly in IVB whereas **complex**

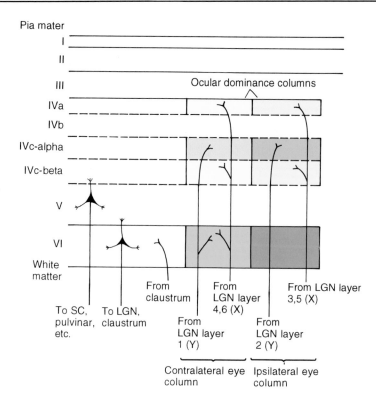

Fig. 15.124 The primary visual cortex receives connections from the various layers of lateral geniculate nucleus and from the claustrum (a thin nucleus that lies just below the insular cortex). Projection from the magnocellular layers of the lateral geniculate nucleus terminate in layer IVc-α (and to a lesser degree in VI), whereas those from the parvocellular layers terminate in layer IVc-β (and to a lesser extent in IVa and VI). Input representing one or other eye is segregated into separate ocular dominance columns. Contralateral and ipsilateral eye columns (vertically oriented columns 500 μm wide and several mm long) lie next to one another in a regular array. The cortex in turn sends an important projection back to the lateral geniculate nucleus (LGN) as well as to the claustrum, superior colliculus (SC), pulvinar and other structures. Projections to the superior colliculus and pulvinar derive from pyramidal cells of layer V. Those to the lateral geniculate nucleus and claustrum derive from the pyramidal cells of layer VI. (Redrawn from Kandell, after Berne and Levy, 1983.)

and **hypercomplex cells** are found outside layer IV, in layers I, III, V and VI. They respond to line stimuli, still exhibiting a centre-surround organization. They are orientation-, movement- and direction-sensitive cells. Complex cells are less orientation specific than simple cells, while hypercomplex cells, which may be further subdivided, respond to a restricted bar length and exhibit inhibitory effects outside the receptive field (Schiller, Finlay and Volman, 1976).

Complex and hypercomplex cells are found above and below layer IV. Some complex cells of layer V project to the tectum (Toyama *et al.*, 1974; Palmer, Rosenquist and Tusa, 1975) while some in layer VI project to the lateral geniculate nucleus (Gilbert and Kelly, 1975; Lund *et al.*, 1975).

Orientation-selective cells are not found in IVC (Hubel and Wiesel, 1968). The proportion of orientation-selective cells increases at increasing eccentricity from the foveal representation (Zeki, 1983). Most studies suggest that orientation-selective cells are not wavelength selective (Dow, 1974; Gouras, 1974; Poggio *et al.*, 1975; Zeki, 1983). Many cells in the striate cortex also code for depth (Poggio, Doby and Talbot, 1977; Poggio and Fischer, 1977).

Complex and hypercomplex cells receive inputs from both eyes and are thus **binocular**. The receptive fields are identical whichever eye is stimulated.

Binocular stimulation within the receptive field of the cell produces a more vigorous response than unilateral stimulation. Fifty per cent of the cells in layers II, III, V and VI are binocular.

In a plane at right-angles to the ocular dominance columns a serial shift in orientation sensitivity of cells in adjacent columns has been demonstrated by studies with penetrating needle electrodes. In the monkey there is a shift in orientation selectivity of about 10° every 20 μm, so that a cycle of 180° is covered by a series of 18 columns.

The organizational unit encompassing a set of right and left dominance columns and a cyle of 180° orientation columns was termed a **hypercolumn** by Hubel and Wiesel, which is conceived to be the functional unit of the retinotopic map, i.e. functionally a comprehensive set of modalities for each corresponding point (Fig. 15.125).

The hypercolumns mentioned above, and containing orientation-selective cells, lie in the cytochrome-oxidase-poor 'interblob' regions of the striate cortex. The cytochrome-oxidase-rich 'blob' regions contain wavelength-selective cells with action spectra showing peak responses in the long (620 nm), middle (500 nm) and short (480 nm) wavelengths (corresponding to the orange-red, green and blue regions of the spectrum). These cells respond when sufficient

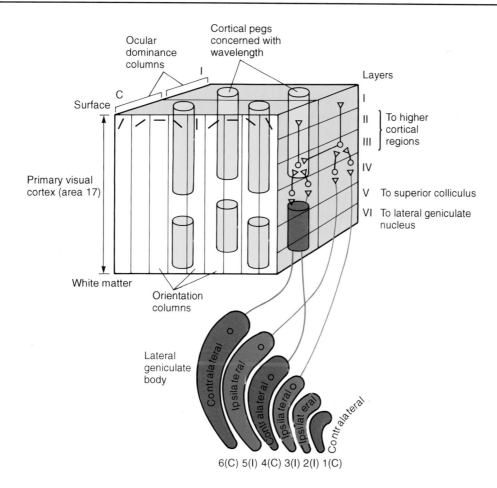

Fig. 15.125 This basic cortical module (*hypercolumn*) in area 17 of the visual cortex contains a complete set of *orientation columns* representing 360° and a set of *ocular dominance columns*. Each hypercolumn also contains several cortical pegs, regions of cortex in which the cells do not have an axis of orientation. Cells in the pegs are concerned with colour. Each layer of the lateral geniculate body receives input from the other *contralateral* (C) or the *ipsilateral eye* and projects in turn to the ipsilateral or contralateral ocular dominance columns. (From Kandell and Schwartz, with permission.)

energy at the selective wavelength falls within its receptive field. In 'void' viewing conditions (i.e. a patch of reflected light with an unilluminated surround), monochromatic light of the appropriate wavelength will stimulate the cell and the perception of colour will be in keeping with the spectral location of the wavelength, i.e. a long wave selective cell will be stimulated by a patch of 620 nm light and this will correlate with the perception of red. In this sense only is the cell 'colour coded', but Zeki (1984) has strongly argued that this appellation is misleading, because in all other circumstances of natural viewing of objects reflecting light of mixed wavelengths it is found that these wavelength-coded cells will respond to targets of any colour, as long as that object reflects sufficient energy at the preferred wavelength. These cells are therefore wavelength-coded but **not** colour coded. Although the existence of truly colour-coded cells in the striate cortex cannot yet be excluded, such

cells are certainly found in V4 of the monkey prestriate cortex.

Other behavioural characteristics of wavelength-coded cells of the striate cortex

In addition to cells with circular receptive fields responsive to a preferred wavelength, cells are found with an opponent organization, responding maximally to, say, long wavelength (red), which are inhibited by middle wavelengths (green), i.e. opponent responses to stimulation by 'colours' (each encountered perceptually as their mutual afterimage in void viewing conditions). These cells have been referred to as 'red on/green off' cells. (From earlier comments, it will be gathered that this terminology is potentially misleading, and their responses would better be referred to the excitatory and inhibitory wavelengths.)

More complex double-opponent cells exist which respond maximally to stimulation of centre and surround by opponent (complementary) colours (i.e. red centre, green surround) which are switched off when the stimulus pattern is reversed (Fig. 15.121). Such responses are thought to result from the convergence of input from lower-order wavelength-sensitive cells.

It has not been excluded that some double-opponent cells could function as colour-coded cells (Michael, 1978).

PRESTRIATE CORTEX

The striate cortex is conceived to be a way station along the visual pathway which segregates different kinds of visual information and projects this to the secondary association areas for further processing (Zeki, 1975). Evidence has accumulated for functional specialization in the various regions of the monkey prestriate cortex as follows: V2, V3, 3a orientation coded; V4 wavelength and colour-coded, some orientation coded; V5 motion and direction sensitive (some colour). This is not to say that cells with other functions are not found in these zones.

Colour-coded cells

Colour-coded cells are found in V4 and V2. These are wavelength-selective cells with properties quite different from those of the striate cortex, although cells with similar 'action spectra' and with a preference for long, middle and short wavelengths are found in both striate and prestriate cortex. However, whereas the striate cells respond to wavelength, independent of target colour in natural viewing conditions, the prestriate colour-coded cells respond specifically to colour and relatively independently of the wavelength composition of the reflected light from an object, as long as it contains the preferred wavelength. Thus, traversing a multicoloured display across the receptive field of a long wavelength (red-coded) cell in V4 results in excitation only when the red targets fall into the receptive field and they do not fire in response to green or blue in natural viewing conditions with the whole field illuminated. This response to the red targets only is still excited when the relative composition of the light reflected from the display is altered, for example decreasing the long wavelength and increasing the middle and short wavelength components. In this way, the colour-coded cells of V4 show 'colour constancy' and therefore mirror everyday perceptual experience. Thus, although the wavelength composition of daylight varies with location and time of day, our perception of the colour of objects varies much less; grass still appears green and cornfields yellow. This colour constancy appears to depend on an input from cells whose receptive fields lie outside the receptive field (as usually defined) of the cell in question. Thus, if a red target, part of a multicoloured display arranged to reflect the standard triplet of energies equivalent to white light, is observed, it will appear white in colour if seen in isolation from the rest of the display; however, it will appear as a vivid red if both the red target and the rest of the display are illuminated and viewed together. This phenomenon was encompassed by Land (1974, 1977) in his Retinex theory of colour vision.

STEREOPSIS

The binocular appreciation of depth (stereopsis) is dependent on the function of both striate and prestriate cortex and the reception of disparity cues arising simultaneously from the two retinas. Points in the visual field further away than a fixated target (beyond the horopter) generate 'divergent disparity' information, while points which are closer (within the horopter) generate convergent disparity information. Binocular cells independently responsive to 'near' or to 'far' disparity have been demonstrated in the cortex.

Objects away from the line of fixation and outside the horopter will be imaged on the right or left hemiretina of each eye and will stimulate disparity cells of the appropriate striate cortex. Objects which lie in the region of the sagittal plane present a different problem because they will be imaged either on both nasal hemiretinas (far disparity), or both temporal hemiretinas (near disparity), and will therefore in each situation stimulate both striate cortices. Disparities of up to 0.5° can be accommodated by the nasotemporal overlap of the retinal projection, but above this degree of disparity integration of information reaching the two hemispheres employs callosal association fibres. Cowey (1985) suggested that the anterior commissure may serve this function for midline stereopsis, but was unable to demonstrate a role for the splenium in the monkey. The nasotemporal overlap in the monkey was confined to a vertical median strip passing through the fovea, 150–250 μm wide and corresponding to 1° of visual angle.

Striate cortex contains cells which are tuned to respond to fine disparities and it is conceived that these project in primates to prestriate area V2, which contains many cells tuned to coarser disparities. Those tuned to changes in disparity caused by moving stimuli are conspicuous in the movement area of the superior temporal sulcus.

Global stereopsis embodies the ability to extract depth information from complex visual scenes, in contrast to the simpler process of **local stereopsis** in which the visual stimulus shows distinct qualitative differences between figure and ground. Clinically, global stereopsis is more affected by lesions of the non-dominant hemisphere (Carmon and Bechtoldt, 1969; Benton and Hecaen, 1970) while lateralization is less certain in relation to local stereopsis. In the monkey large ablations of inferior temporal cortex have only slight effects on global stereopsis (Cowey, 1985).

Some degree of parallel processing by the prestriate cortex is further suggested by the occurrence of other clinical syndromes affecting a narrow aspect of visual processing. Bilateral damage to the ventral aspect of the prestriate cortex produced **cerebral achromatopisa** in the patient of Meadows (1974) who performed poorly on tests of colour vision, while retaining the trichromatic mechanism of the retinocortical projection (Mollon *et al.*, 1980). Bilateral damage to the territory of the posterior cerebral artery may grossly impair detection of movement (Zihl, 1981). The sense of the position of objects in the visual world is impaired by lesions to area 7 of the parietal lobe (Ratcliffe and Davies-Jones, 1972). Higher visual perceptual function involves the attribution of a collective meaning to the multiple sensory responses evoked by a visual stimulus, e.g. face and object recognition. In primates, such tasks may be performed by binocular cells in the inferior temporal cortex with huge receptive fields which straddle the mid line and always include the fovea (see Gross *et al.*, 1981). The cells of the posterior inferior temporal cortex receive projections from V2, V3 and V4 as well as the superior temporal sulcus (Kuypers *et al.*, 1965). Ablation of this region in the monkey impairs visual discriminatory learning tasks for patterns, objects and colours (Gross, Cowey and Manning, 1971; Dean, 1976) without affecting visual fields, grating acuity, critical fusion frequency, the detection of brief flashes or of incremental brightness thresholds (Cowey, 1982). More anterior lesions affect simpler associative functions.

In the rhesus monkey, cortical cells deep in the fundus of the temporal lobe respond electrophysiologically to the presentation of faces in the visual field (Perrett, Rolls and Caan, 1979, 1982). Clinically, bilateral damage to the fusiform, lingual and parahippocampal gyri (i.e. the ventromedial occipitotemporal cortex) results in loss of the ability to identify faces (prosopagnosia).

SUMMARY OF FUNCTION IN THE VISUAL PATHWAY

The processing of visual information about form, colour and spatial relationships is achieved by three independent pathways, which can be traced from the retina to the cortical neurons (Livingstone, 1988). The **magnocellular system** projects to layer IVB of the striate cortex, thence to the thick stripes of V2 and from there to the middle temporal area MT (V5 in the macaque, MT in the owl monkey), an area which analyses information about motion and depth. Neurons in this system have a very fast response time but their responses decay rapidly when the stimulus is maintained, so that the system is particularly sensitive to moving stimuli but not to stationary images. This system is achromatic, and is therefore unable to detect borders on the basis of colour contrast alone.

The **parvocellular system** projects to the 'interblob' region of the striate cortex, which projects in turn to the pale stripes in visual area V2. This system carries high-resolution information about object borders, determined by colour contrast. Neurons in the early stages of this pathway are wavelength-sensitive, but those at higher levels respond to colour-contrast borders but do not carry information about the colours themselves. It is suggested that this system is important for shape perception and the ability to see stationary objects in detail.

Input from both the parvocellular and magnocellular systems projects to the 'blob' areas of the striate cortex and information is passed to the thin stripes of V2 and thence to area V4. This system processes information about colour and luminance but not about movement, shape or depth. It has a several-fold lower acuity than the interblob system and therefore sees objects in colour, but not in detail.

Hubel and Livingstone (1984) have speculated that the segregation of processing for different visual modalities provides an explanation for many visual perceptual phenomena. Thus, it is found that the perception movements or stereopsis (and even of non-stereoscopic depth cues) is lost when equiluminant colour stimuli are used. This is attributed to the properties of the magnocellular system, which is 'colour blind'. It is thought that this system is tuned to detect properties of an object that distinguish it from its background (direction and velocity of motion, depth, lightness and texture, continuity of form) and enable it to be perceived as a whole. The parvocellular system is concerned with the details. In the realm of art, the 'instability' of coloured spots on an equiluminant coloured canvas is interpreted as being due to a failure of the parvocellular system to distinguish borders, so that the magnocellular system cannot signal movement or position of the object. The coloured spot appears to jump around or drift.

DORSAL AND VENTRAL PATHWAYS FOR OBJECT AND SPATIAL VISION

The relationship between the functionally and structurally distinct cortical areas concerned with different components of vision has been summarized by Mishkin, Ungerleider and Macko (1983) on the basis of their own and others' work.

They envisage two separate cortical visual pathways, one specialized for visual object recognition (the 'what' system: Ungerleider, 1986) and the other for spatial location (the 'where' system).

Ventral pathway

The pathway crucial to the visual identification of objects is a multisynaptic occipitotemporal projection which follows the course of the inferior longitudinal fasciculus. This ventral pathway connects the striate, prestriate and inferior temporal areas (Mishkin, 1982). Links between this system and limbic structures in the temporal lobe (Turner, Mishkin and Knapp, 1980) and ventral parts of the frontal lobe (Kuypers et al., 1965) may make cognitive associations between visual objects and other events such as emotions and motor acts possible (Mishkin, Ungerleider and Macko, 1983).

Dorsal pathway

The second pathway is a multisynaptic projection system following the course of the superior longitudinal fasciculus and connecting the striate, prestriate and inferior parietal areas. This dorsal pathway is critical to visual location of objects (Ungerleider and Mishkin, 1982). Links with the dorsal limbic system and dorsal frontal cortex may permit the construction of spatial maps as well as the visual guidance of motor acts triggered by activity in the ventral pathway.

OBJECT VISION

Analysis of the physical properties of an object (such as size, colour, texture and shape) occurs in the subdivisions of the prestriate–posterior temporal complex (Zeki, 1978a–c). Area V1 projects to V2, V2 projects to V3 and thus serially to V4 (contained within OA). Area V4 projects to areas TEO and TE in the inferior temporal cortex (Desimore, Fleming and Gross, 1980). The anterior part of the inferior temporal cortex area TE is the last exclusively visual area in the pathway. This ventral system appears to extract information about stimulus quality from the retinal input to the striate cortex and to assign meaning through connections between area TE and the limbic frontal-lobe systems. Area TE is thought to serve as the highest-order area for the visual perception of objects and also a storehouse of central representations for their later recognition. Bilateral lesions of this area in monkeys lead to the loss of freshly acquired recognition abilities, marked failure to retain learned visual discrimination habits and to acquire new ones postoperatively (Mishkin, 1982). The inferior temporal cortex receives a profuse input from the corpus callosum.

The extremely large visual receptive fields of the inferior temporal neurons (Gross, 1973) appears to provide the neural basis for the ability to recognize an object regardless of orientation or location in the visual field (Gross and Mishkin, 1979). A corollary is, however, that there is a loss of information about visual location.

SPATIAL VISION

The entire posterior parietal cortex (including the dorsal OA) selectively participates in the processing of visuospatial (as distinguished from object-quality) information. The parietal area PG appears to be a polysensory association area handling both visual and tactual modalities relating to the 'macrospace' of vision and the 'microspace' encompassed by the hand. Thus, both visuospatial and tactile discrimination deficits follow lesions to the inferior parietal cortex.

The posterior parietal cortex in the monkey, like the inferior temporal, is totally dependent on striate input for its participation in vision. Area V2 (area OB) projects to visual area MT in the caudal portion of the superior temporal sulcus, mainly within dorsolateral OA. Area MT projects to four additional areas in the upper superior temporal and intraparietal sulci (Ungerleider and Mishkin, 1982). The more anterior one is within parietal area PG. Unlike the inferior temporal cortex, the posterior parietal does not receive a heavy callosal input. Therefore, each posterior parietal area appears organized largely to serve contralateral spatial functions. This may explain the contralateral 'spatial neglect' encountered in humans after unilateral parietal injuries.

A second difference in the organization of visual inputs to these extrastriate association areas was demonstrated in monkeys by selective striate ablation experiments. While inputs from central visual areas are the more important for object recognition functions of the inferior temporal cortex, both central and peripheral visual inputs are important for the visuospatial functions of the parietal cortex.

SYNTHESIS OF OBJECT AND SPATIAL INFORMATION

The separate analysis of visual object and visuospatial information by ventrally and dorsally located systems raises the cognitive question of their ultimate re-integration. It is thought that the connections of both systems to the limbic system and frontal lobe may provide access to sites where this process occurs. Evidence is available that the hippocampal formation is involved with the memorization of object location (Smith and Milner, 1981; Parkinson and Mishkin, 1982).

Some authors have equated the ventral 'what' system and the dorsal 'where' system with the parvocellular and magnocellular pathways. Thus the magnocellular input to layer 4b of the striate cortex (V1) projects directly and indirectly to V5, an area concerned with motion perception, which in turn projects to the parietal cortex which is involved with the spatial aspects of vision. The parvocellular pathway projects to layers 2 and 3 of V1, whose output, both directly and indirectly, is to V4, an area concerned with colour and form. The chief output of V4 is to the inferior temporal cortex. This area is engaged in the highest order of visual perception of objects. Zeki (1993) has questioned the validity of equating the P and M pathways with a 'what' and 'where' system, partly because there is functional overlap between the systems, and because there are interconnections between these pathways at every level which make it difficult to attribute a unique role to one pathway while ignoring the other.

Many cells in layers 2 and 3 of V1 behave in a way suggesting that they receive both magnocellular as well as parvocellular inputs (Hubel and Livingstone, 1990). There are modest connections between layer 4b and layers 2 and 3 of the striate cortex (V1) (Blasdel, Lund and Fitzpatrick, 1985). There are multiple outputs from V1, not only to V4 and V5, but also to V3 and V3a and probably V6; there are reciprocal connections between these extrastriate areas and V1. Fibres in layer 3 of V2 are of sufficient length to connect the thick stripes (M pathway) and the thin stripes and interstripes (P pathway) (Shipp and Zeki, 1989a,b). The outputs from V1 to V3 and V4, with their further projections to the inferior temporal cortex, are sometimes portrayed as an example of the P pathway. But although this is true for V4, V3 receives its inputs from layer 4b of V1 or via the thick stripes of V2 and much of its output is to the parietal cortex, which would be features of the dorsal pathway. Both V3 and V4 are involved with form, but V3 is concerned with dynamic form, and V4 with form in association with colour. In the same way, although V4 has its major projection to the inferior temporal cortex, it also projects, with partial overlap, to an area of parietal cortex contiguous with that receiving a projection from V5. Therefore the parietal cortex receives both P and M pathway projections. Like the projection of V3 to the parietal cortex, that from V4 is from its peripheral parts, which implies a role that does not require the representation of fine detail. However, because of the large receptive fields of neurons in this area, this may not entirely exclude the foveal representation.

15.13 BLOOD SUPPLY OF THE VISUAL CORTEX

The visual cortex is supplied mainly by the posterior cerebral artery, especially its calcarine branch (Figs 15.68–15.79). The middle cerebral artery supplies the anterior end of the calcarine sulcus, and on the lateral surface, near the occipital pole, there is a superior anastomosis between posterior and middle cerebrals, which may account for the sparing of the macula in cases of thrombosis of the posterior cerebral. This view, propounded by Shellshear (1927), is still denied by some, but the consensus of evidence favours it (see Polyak, 1957). Smith and Richardson (1966) have described variations and have related specific branches to retinal topography. These vessels form a rich pial plexus, from which short branches penetrate grey matter, larger ones traversing it to reach the white matter. The latter are end arteries, communicating by capillaries only.

15.14 PRACTICAL CONSIDERATIONS

Division of one optic nerve results in blindness of that eye and a pupil which does not react directly to light, but does consensually, because the motor part of the reflex pathway is intact (Fig. 16.12). The affected pupil will, of course, react to convergence.

Sagittal section of the chiasma results in bitemporal hemianopia (commonly, but not invariably, due to a pituitary tumour). Direct and consensual pupil reactions remain intact. Theoretically the pupil ought to react only when light falls on the temporal retinas, but scatter is difficult to control. Division of uncrossed fibres leads to binasal hemianopia but represents an unusual lesion (e.g. carotid aneurysm in the cavernous sinus).

Central to the chiasma **complete unilateral division of the visual pathway** at any level causes contralateral hemianopia; for example, if the left pathway is divided, loss of the right half visual fields results (temporal of the right side, nasal of the left).

Division of the optic tract produces a contralateral homonymous hemianopia, and it abolishes neither the direct nor the consensual pupil reaction because the chiasmal crossing fibres are intact. It gives rise to Wernicke's hemianopic pupil reaction, i.e. pupils do not react when a narrow beam of light impinges on the blind half retinas, but do so when it falls on the normal halves. (Owing to scattering of light the test is exceedingly difficult to perform.) Lesions of the optic tract and radiation may sometimes be distinguished by ipsilateral ptosis and enlarged pupil when the tract is involved, due to involvement of the ipsilateral oculomotor nerve.

Because pupillary and visual fibres separate in the posterior third of the tract, lesions beyond this usually affect them separately, which explains why Wernicke's hemianopic pupil reaction differentiates a tract lesion from a lesion of the visual pathway behind the point of separation (see above, however).

Destruction of the lateral geniculate nucleus is followed by a contralateral homonymous hemianopia.

Destruction of the visual cortex on one side by, for example, thrombosis of the posterior cerebral artery, causes contralateral homonymous hemianopia. The pupils are unaffected and the macula often spared. If the hemianopia is accompanied by hemiplegia or hemianaesthesia, the lesion is in the posterior part of the internal capsule. Destruction of the geniculocalcarine fibres which curve anteriorly into the temporal lobe results in superior quadrantic hemianopia.

The degree of localization at all levels of the visual pathway entails that even **small lesions in tract, radiation, or striate area** may produce sharply outlined scotomas in corresponding locations in both uniocular visual fields.

A complete hemianopia is much more likely when **lesions involve visual fibres which are tightly packed**, as in the optic tract. In the radiation and occipital cortex, where the fibres are more dispersed, defects such as partial homonymous field defects and quadrantic or smaller scotomas are more usual. Anterior lesions of the optic radiations are less likely to be congruous than posterior lesions.

Because the visual pathway is so extended, and a wide variety of lesions may involve it, visual defects may be of localizing value in diagnosis.

CHAPTER SIXTEEN

Autonomic, aminergic, peptidergic and nitrergic innervation of the eye

16.1 AUTONOMIC NERVOUS SYSTEM

The autonomic nervous system exercises control over the vegetative functions of the body. It consists of two parts, the sympathetic and parasympathetic systems. Generally the viscera are supplied by each system and in such cases the sympathetic and parasympathetic systems exert opposite effects but in differing degree. The autonomic nervous system controls the intrinsic muscles of the eye, vasomotor function, the secretion of tears and the sweat glands of the face.

The autonomic nervous system may be considered as a system of afferent and efferent pathways with a central integrating system. Integration occurs at many levels, which include the cortex, limbic system, hypothalamus, thalamus, brain stem reticular network and spinal cord (Kaada, 1954). The sympathetic and parasympathetic systems share inputs from visceral and somatic sensory afferents.

The outflow system (i.e. the descending nevronal pathway) is stimulated by impulses arising in neurons within the hypothalamus, which may be regarded as the first in a three-neuron pathway. The second-order neurons arise in cell stations in the brain stem and intermediolateral cell column of the spinal cord. Because synapses occur in ganglia outside the central nervous system the second-order and third-order neurons are distinguished as the preganglionic and postganglionic neurons, respectively. The preganglionic neurons are the counterpart of the connector neurons of the somatic system, and the postganglionic neurons, of the somatic lower motor neurons. However, the cell bodies of somatic motor neurons are found within the central nervous system, while those of the autonomic system lie in various ganglia outside it. Sensory fibres affecting somatic and autonomic function travel with autonomic fibres and, like all sensory fibres, have their cell bodies in the posterior root ganglia or the equivalent. They connect by means of the sensory root with neurons situated in the spinal cord or brain stem (Fig. 16.1). The axons of preganglionic neurons emerge as white rami communicantes to reach the motor neurons, which are either in the ganglia of the sympathetic trunks or in ganglia even more peripherally placed, such as the coeliac ganglia. Hence the motor neurons in these ganglia may be equated with the motor nerve cells in the ventral grey column. In the lateral grey column are the somata of the preganglionic or connector neurons of the sympathetic system.

Preganglionic axons are medullated and look whiter than the postganglionic fibres, which are unmedullated. However, the postganglionic parasympathetic fibres of the ciliary ganglion, contained in its short ciliary nerves, are an exception to this, and are in fact medullated. Usually, many postganglionic neurons are activated by a preganglionic neuron, producing mass actions of widely disseminated responses. (For general descriptions of the autonomic nervous system, consult the monographs of White, 1952; Mitchell, 1953; Kuntz, 1953; Pick, 1970; Williams and Warwick, 1980; Miller, 1985.)

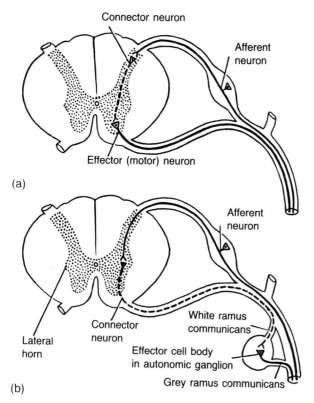

(a)

(b)

Fig. 16.1 (a) A hypothetical somatic reflex pathway; (b) an autonomic reflex pathway. Note general similarity but differences in the sites of the connector and effector cells. In fact, reflex pathways are more complex than this. The somatic 'connector' is rarely, if ever, a single neuron. (From *Last's Anatomy: Regional and Applied*, published by J. & A. Churchill Ltd.)

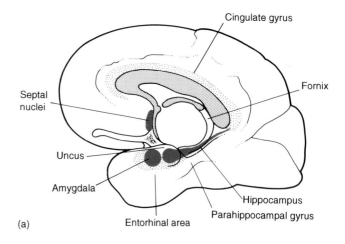

(a)

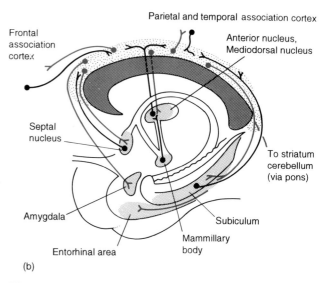

(b)

Fig. 16.2 Main connections of the cingulate gyrus. The cingulate gyrus has connections with cortical association areas and with limbic structures and may act as a mediator between them. (From Brodal, P. (1992) *The Central Nervous System: Structure and Function*, published by Oxford University Press.)

Although the sympathetic and parasympathetic nervous systems have been equated classically with adrenergic and cholinergic neurons, it is now recognized that these efferent pathways and the sensory nerves contain a wide range of neuromodulatory neurons which are intimately involved with the physiopathological responses of the tissues.

LIMBIC SYSTEM

The hypothalamus can be influenced by higher levels of the nervous system such as the orbitofrontal cortex, the cingulate gyrus, hippocampal formation and pyriform area, the preoptic area, septal nuclei and the amygdaloid nucleus (Fig. 16.2). These, together with the mammillary bodies and anterior thalamic nucleus, have been called the 'limbic system' and coincide in part with what was formerly called the rhinencephalon (strictly speaking, those parts of the brain receiving olfactory fibres) (Adey and Tokizane, 1967; Hockman, 1972; DiCara, 1974; Isaacson, 1974; Hall, 1975; Miller, 1985). Although these elements have connections and functions in com-

mon, they do not necessarily perform as a unit, and the term 'system' is misleading.

Some of these structures correspond to the primitive allocortex, which in humans consists of a ring of thin cortical tissue encircling the corpus callosum and brain stem, receiving afferents from specific subcortical nuclei. Whereas the neocortex is concerned with conscious thought and action, the limbic system is concerned with emotions, motivation and affective behaviour (Brodal, 1992).

Stimulation of the limbic cortex has vascular and gastrointestinal effects, and causes excitement and rage; ablation leads to a loss of emotional expression. Hippocampal stimulation gives rise to general excitability, involuntary movement, rage reactions and sexual activity, and stimulation of the amygdala excites a mixture of sympathetic and parasympathetic reactions, including altered respiration, blood pressure and heart rate, pupil constriction or dilatation, defaecation or micturition. Ablation of the amygdala induces placidity. Stimulation of the septal region affects blood pressure, and ablation reduces fear and anxiety (Miller, 1985).

Autonomic activity can be influenced by the cortex, the hippocampus, parts of the thalamus, the basal ganglia, the reticular formation and the cerebellum.

Most of these actions occur through activation of the hypothalamus. Stimulation of the anterior and posterior lobes of the cerebellum causes pupil constriction or dilatation (Dow and Moruzzi, 1985; Snider, 1972).

Hypothalamus

The hypothalamus forms the anterior and lateral walls of the third ventricle, superior and lateral to the optic chiasm. Its superior border is separated from the thalamus by the hypothalamic sulcus. Its other borders are ill-defined. Fulton (1938) recognized the following three nuclear groups (Fig. 16.3):

- anterior;
- middle;
- posterior.

Anterior

The supraoptic nucleus lies lateral to and above the optic chiasm and is connected to the pars inter-

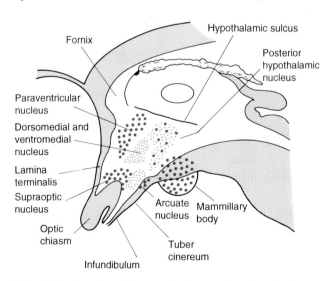

Fig. 16.3 The hypothalamus. Median section through the third ventricle. Some of the major hypothalamic nuclei are shown as red dots whose size indicates the relative size of the neurons of the various nuclei. (From P. Brodal, after Le Gros Clark *et al.* (1936) with permission.)

media and pars posterior of the optic chiasm by the **supraopticohypophyseal tract**. It contains about 750 000 cells and has a parasympathetic function. The paraventricular nucleus lies immediately beneath the ependyma of the anterior wall of the third ventricle: it contains about 55 000 cells. Its cells atrophy after vagotomy or superior cervical sympathectomy (Morton, 1969). The cells of these nuclei are large, pyriform or round in shape.

Middle

The **tuberal nuclei** lie within the tuber cinereum, near its surface, just posterior to the **supraoptic nucleus**. Their multipolar cells are smaller than the other cells of this group. The ventromedial, dorsomedial and lateral hypothalamic nuclei are above the tuberal nuclei.

Posterior

Each mammillary body consists of a medial and a lateral nucleus, of which the medial contains smaller cells and is particularly well developed in humans. They form the termination of the ipsilateral fornix, a thick, arching bundle of fibres originating in the hippocampal region, and are connected directly with the anterior nucleus of the ipsilateral thalamus.

The posterior hypothalamic nucleus lies above and rostral to the mammillary body, and consists of small cells and some scattered large cells.

Other small nuclear groups include the **suprachiasmatic nucleus**, close to the midline above the optic chiasm, and the arcuate nucleus lying ventrally in the third ventricle near the infundibular recess and extending into the medial eminence.

Afferent connections (Fig. 16.4)

The medial forebrain bundle is a diffuse structure, consisting mainly of longitudinal fibres, which carries a large proportion of hypothalamic afferents and efferents from the ventromedial rhinencephalic areas to the preoptic area and possibly to the lateral hypothalamic area and lateral mammillary body. It arises near the anterior commissure and passes to the hypothalamus; also, caudally, to the periaqueductal grey matter of the midbrain (Ransom and Magoun, 1939). Other hypothalamic afferents arise in the cortex, globus pallidus, amygdala, retina, brainstem and spinal cord.

A retinohypothalamic pathway has been demonstrated in various mammals including humans and appears to be concerned with photoneuro-

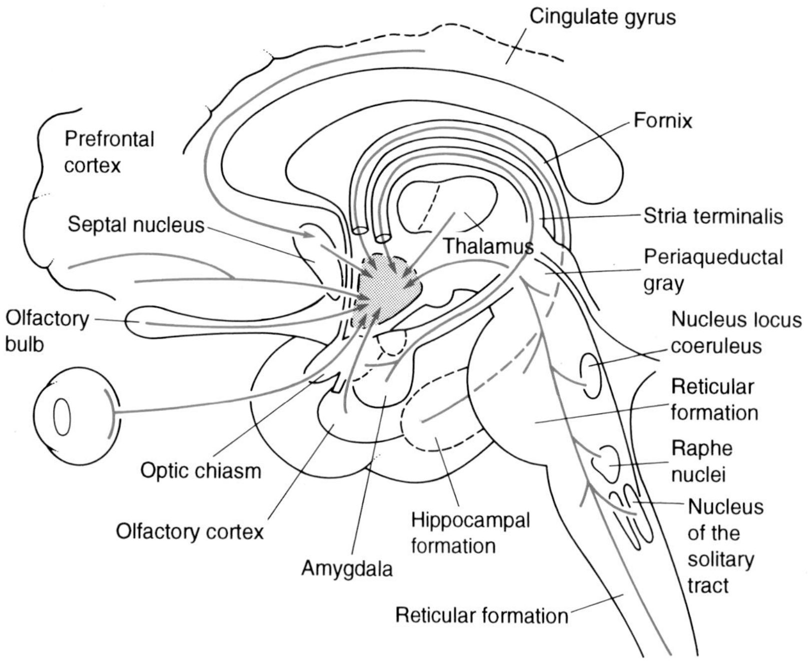

Fig. 16.4 Main afferent connections of the hypothalamus. Arrows indicate the direction of impulse conduction. (From Brodal, P. (1992) *The Central Nervous System: Structure and Function*, published by Oxford University Press.)

endocrine and photoperiodic functions including circadian rhythms (Sadun, 1984).

The hypothalamus receives both direct and indirect olfactory projections, the latter via the amygdala and pyriform cortex. The hippocampal formation sends direct fibres to the hypothalamus, particularly to the mammillary bodies, and secondarily, via the septum. Other hypothalamic connections are from the cingulate gyrus, pyriform cortex and the amygdala (Brodal, 1981). Nauta (1962) identified some fibres from the orbitofrontal cortex to the hypothalamus in the monkey.

Other afferents arising in the midbrain and spinal cord are summarized by Miller (1985).

Efferent connections

Three conspicuous bundles leave the hypothalamus: from the mammillary bodies, from the periventricular nuclei, and from the supraopticohypophyseal tract to the pituitary, by way of its stalk. There are also connections to the spinal cord.

The largest pathway is the **mammillothalamic tract**, which passes from the hypothalamus to the anterior thalamic nucleus. Some fibres also pass to the amygdala, septum, hippocampus and pulvinar (Guillery, 1957; Pasquier and Reinoso-Suarez, 1976; Yoshii, Fujii and Mizokami, 1978).

Fibres can be traced from the ventromedial nucleus of the hypothalamus to the midbrain periaqueductal grey matter and to the pretectal and superior col-

licular regions, the dorsal and ventral tegmental nuclei of Gudden, the raphe nuclei and the nucleus locus coeruleus (Szentagothai *et al.*, 1968; Grofová, Ottersen and Rinvik, 1978). The medial mammillary nucleus also sends a mammillotegmental tract to the midbrain reticular formation.

There are also efferents to the dorsal motor nucleus of the vagus, nucleus of the tractus solitarius and the nucleus ambiguus and to the spinal cord (Conrad and Pfaff, 1976a,b; Saper *et al.*, 1976).

The hypothalamus sends abundant fibres to the posterior lobe of the pituitary gland (the neurohypophysis) via the **supraopticohypophyseal tract**. In humans, there are about 100 000 fibres within the tract, arising chiefly in the supraoptic and paraventricular nuclei (Rasmussen, 1940). The hypophyseal portal system provides a vascular link between the hypophyseal stalk and the anterior lobe, so that the anterior lobe is also under the control of the hypothalamus.

Function of the hypothalamus

The hypothalamus is the coordinating centre for the autonomic system, regulating emotional behaviour, sexual activity and endocrine secretion and adapting the body to environmental change. Its functions include the control of thirst and water balance, body weight, emotions, sleep and arousal, stress and somatic reactions. The hypothalamus controls the endocrine system through the pituitary gland.

In general, the posterior part of the hypothalamus is essential for sympathetic activity; stimulation induces vasoconstriction, heat production, increased metabolism and pupillary dilatation. Its integrity is necessary for the production of 'sham rage'. The anterior part is concerned with parasympathetic activity.

Pituitary gland

Vasopressin (adrenocorticotrophic hormone: ADH) and oxytocin are produced by the neurosecretory cells of the supraoptic and paraventricular hypothalamic nuclei and are transported along the supraopticohypophyseal tract to the fenestrated capillaries of the posterior pituitary, whence they enter the bloodstream. Various releasing factors are synthesized in different regions of the hypothalamus (Fig. 16.5) and are transported in the tuberohypophyseal (tuberoinfundibular) tract, from the tuberal and other regions of the hypothalamus, to the median eminence and infundibular stem of the pituitary. The median eminence lies in the uppermost part of the stalk. Here they are released into the sinusoids of the portal vascular system, the primary blood supply of the anterior lobe (Bernardis, 1974; Reichlin, Baldessarini and Martin, 1978). Most of the arteries supplying the anterior lobe continue upwards in the stalk, without giving rise to capillaries in the gland. Some arteries enter the stalk directly. In the upper part of the stalk they form wide, sinusoidal capillaries whose blood is collected by the hypophyseal portal veins. These pass back into the anterior lobe, where they form a fresh set of sinusoids among the epithelial cells. Thus substances can be transported from the stalk to the anterior lobe (Fig. 16.6).

16.2 PARASYMPATHETIC SYSTEM

The parasympathetic system has two components, cranial and sacral. The preganglionic neurons have their cell bodies in the nuclei of cranial nerves, or in the lateral grey column of the spinal cord (sacral segments 2, 3 and sometimes 4). The postganglionic neurons, however, are in the wall of the viscus innervated. There is an exception to this in the case of part of the cranial outflow, where discrete **ganglia** are established for relay of the preganglionic neuron onto the postganglionic cell body. The ganglia are the ciliary, pterygopalatine, submandibular and optic. Only parasympathetic relay occurs here. All four ganglia also transmit both sensory and sympathetic fibres to share in the peripheral distribution of the branches, but none of these fibres synapses in the ganglia (Fig. 16.7). The postganglionic fibres of the parasympathetic system liberate acetylcholine at their terminals and are called cholinergic. However, both VIPergic and nitrergic fibres are also found in the postganglionic fibres of the pterygopalatine ganglion.

The central pathway arises in cells within the anterior hypothalamus, but their details are poorly known. They terminate in cell clusters in the mid brain, pons and medulla.

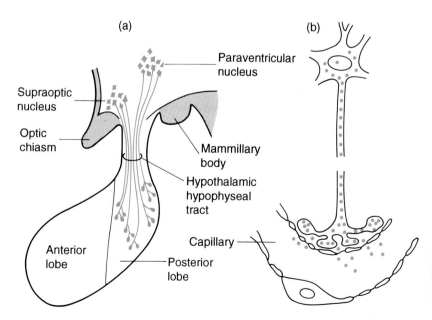

Fig. 16.5 The relationship between the hypothalamus and the pituitary gland. (a) Connections from the hypothalamus to the posterior lobe; (b) axonal transport of peptide hormones (neuropeptides) from the hypothalamus to the pituitary. (From Brodal, P. (1992) *The Central Nervous System: Structure and Function*, published by Oxford University Press.)

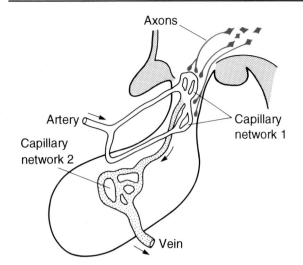

Fig. 16.6 The portal vessels of the pituitary stalk ensure that releasing hormones (factors) are transported from the median eminence in the upper part of the stalk to the epithelial cells of the anterior lobe. (From Brodal, P. (1992) *The Central Nervous System: Structure and Function*, published by Oxford University Press.)

EDINGER–WESTPHAL NUCLEI

The **mid brain outflow** of preganglionic nerve fibres to the ciliary ganglion arises in neurons of the accessory oculomotor nuclei (Figs 16.7 and 16.8). These are located at the level of the anterior quadrigeminal bodies, in the mid line within the periaqueductal grey, just beneath the cerebral aqueduct. The nuclei include the **Edinger–Westphal nuclei**, consisting of medial and lateral visceral cell columns, dorsomedial to the oculomotor complex, the **anterior median nuclei**, near the midline, rostral and ventral to the complex and the **nucleus of Perlia**, lying in the mid line between the somatic oculomotor nuclei, caudal to the anterior median and Edinger–Westphal nuclei. Akert *et al.* (1980) suggested that the ciliary projection arises only in the Edinger–Westphal nuclei, but others have suggested that in humans fibres arise from the ipsilateral Edinger–Westphal nuclei and from the ipsilateral half of the anterior median nucleus (Warwick, 1954; Pierson and

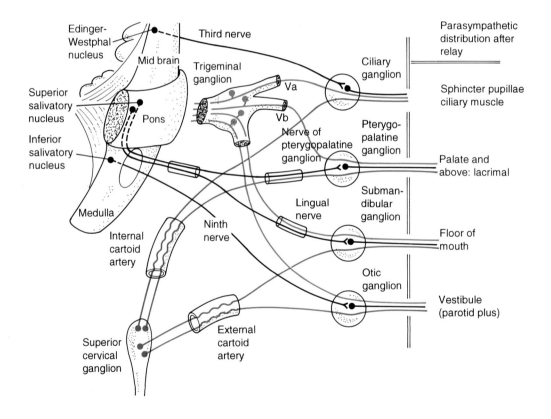

Fig. 16.7 Plan of connections of the cranial parasympathetic ganglia. The otic ganglion lies high up near the skull base but by its connections and branches it is actually the most caudal of the four. Only the parasympathetic roots (in black) relay in the ganglia. They come from three nuclei, one each in the mid brain, pons and medulla. The pontine nucleus (superior salivary nucleus) relays in the middle two ganglia. The sensory roots (shown in blue) come from the trigeminal ganglion, where their cell bodies lie. The third division (Vc) sends branches through the last two ganglia. The sympathetic roots (red) come from cell bodies in the superior cervical ganglion and travel along the internal and external carotid arteries, two on each, to reach their respective ganglia. (From *Last's Anatomy: Regional and Applied*, published by J. & A. Churchill.)

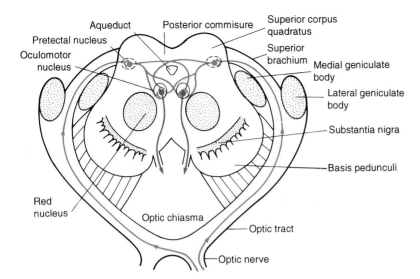

Fig. 16.8 Section through the mid brain and optic chiasm to show the path of pupillary constrictor fibres. Note especially the pretectal nucleus.

Carpenter, 1974; Burde and Loewy, 1980; Burde, 1983). In the monkey, Perlia's nucleus may supply fibres that enter and/or pass through the ciliary ganglion (Burde, 1983).

Jampel and Mindel (1967) found that those cells concerned with pupil constriction are located more ventral and caudal than those involved with ciliary contraction and accommodation. However, later studies (Sillito, 1968; Sillito and Zbrozyna, 1970; Pierson and Carpenter, 1974) suggested that those regions of the visceral nuclei concerned with pupil constriction were the ipsilateral anterior median, and the adjoining rostral part of the Edinger–Westphal nucleus.

THE CILIARY GANGLION

Nerve fibres from the Edinger–Westphal nucleus pass out along the third nerve to the ciliary ganglion and synapse there. From there, postganglionic medullated fibres pass in the short ciliary nerves to sphincter pupillae and ciliary muscles. This medullation of postganglionic axons is exceptional (Fig. 16.9). It may be associated with speed of conduction and in this regard it is interesting to note that in the avian eye the muscles so innervated are necessarily rapid acting, and hence striated. The pathway is also largely concerned with accommodation, which is in some characteristics more somatic than visceral in its activities. This is also in keeping with the unusual nature of ciliary smooth muscle, which differs structurally from vascular and other forms of smooth muscle and has histochemical features resembling extraocular muscle.

According to some authorities, the short ciliary nerves provide a parasympathetic supply addition-

ally to the choroid, but Ruskell considers that this role is served by fibres arising from the pterygopalatine ganglion (personal communication).

There is reciprocal innervation of antagonists. Thus, oculomotor stimulation contracts the sphincter and inhibits the dilator, and likewise the sympathetic is motor to the dilator and inhibitor to the sphincter.

The size and shape of the ciliary ganglion are extremely variable (Grimes and Sallmann, 1960; Elisková, 1973), but its location is constant. The sympathetic root may derive from the plexus on the internal carotid artery which enters the superior orbital fissure. It passes through the ganglion to the short ciliary nerves. Fibres are vasomotor to the iris sphincter and other parts of the eye. In some individuals there may be multiple sympathetic roots,

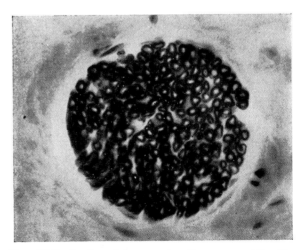

Fig. 16.9 Section of the posterior ciliary nerve of the Rhesus monkey just behind the globe to show medullated fibres (Weigert's stain).

deriving from the internal carotid plexus, or from its continuation along the ophthalmic artery and its branches (Beauvieux and Dupas, 1936; Sinnreich and Nathan, 1981).

The sensory root of the ganglion joins the nasociliary branch of the trigeminal nerve. There may also be direct connections between the short ciliary nerves and the nasociliary nerve, which appear to bypass the ganglion (Sinnreich and Nathan, 1981).

Centrifugal fibres from the occipital cortex to the visceral nuclei are thought to run with the motor pathways to the somatic nuclei. They probably enter the pretectal nuclei more ventrally: Barris (1936) induced miosis in cats on stimulation of occipital areas 18 and 19. Jampel (1959) induced miosis by stimulation of these and other cortical areas. It is of interest that reduced pupil responses are encountered in individuals with suprageniculate lesions (Frydrychowicz and Harms, 1940; Harms, 1951, 1956; Cibis, Campos and Aulhorn, 1975; Hamann *et al.*, 1979; Hamann, Hellner and Jensen, 1981).

The **pontomedullary (bulbar) outflow** of preganglionic fibres (corresponding to the white rami of the thoracic region) are the axons of small neurons in the so-called *salivary nuclei* (see Lewis and Shute, 1959). The neurons in question appear to be situated in or near the cranial extremity of the dorsal vagal nucleus and lie in the column of visceral efferent nuclei for cranial nerves III, VII, IX and X lying immediately ventral to the floor of the ventricular system. It is customary to divide the nucleus into superior and inferior parts but evidence for this is unsatisfactory.

NUCLEI AND CRANIAL NERVES CORRESPONDING TO THE BULBAR OUTFLOW

Superior salivatory (and lacrimal) nuclei

The superior salivatory nucleus lies in the reticular network, dorsolateral to the caudal end of the nucleus of the facial nerve. It is also near to the rostral end of the dorsal nucleus of the vagus, just above the junction of medulla and pons.

Secretomotor fibres leave the brain stem as one of the components of the **nervus intermedius** of the facial nerve, lying between that nerve and the eighth nerve as they emerge at the lower border of the pons. It is a mixed nerve, also carrying sensory fibres for taste and somatic sensation from the anterior two-thirds of the tongue, as well as afferents from the facial muscles, dura and cerebral vessels of the middle cranial fossa (Fig. 16.10a).

Secretomotor fibres leave the nervus intermedius of the facial nerve to join the chorda tympani and run to the submandibular ganglion for relay to sublingual, anterior lingual and submandibular salivary glands.

Vasodilator fibres have been thought to run to the cerebral vessels via the greater petrosal nerve and within the carotid plexus.

Secretomotor distribution

Secretomotor distribution is via the **greater petrosal** nerve, to relay in the pterygopalatine ganglion and supply the lacrimal gland and glands of nose, paranasal sinuses and palate. The fibres pass through the **geniculate ganglion** in the facial canal of the petrous temporal bone, enter the middle cranial fossa, and pass under the trigeminal ganglion to reach the foramen lacerum. Within the fibrocartilage of that foramen these fibres are joined by the sympathetic fibres of the **deep petrosal nerve** from the carotid plexus to form the nerve of the pterygoid canal (**vidian nerve**) which ends in the **pterygopalatine ganglion** in the upper part of the pterygopalatine fossa. This is the relay station for the preganglionic parasympathetic fibres (Fig. 5.30). In the past, it has been stated that the postganglionic fibres enter the nearby **maxillary nerve** and travel by its zygomatic branch to reach the lacrimal gland via the zygomaticotemporal anastomosis with the lacrimal nerve (Fig. 5.29). However, Ruskell (1971) has demonstrated lacrimal rami passing directly to the gland from a retro-orbital plexus composed of direct parasympathetic branches from the **pterygopalatine ganglion** (see below, and also Ruskell, 1968, 1970, 1973).

The pterygopalatine ganglion

The pterygopalatine ganglion is a cone-shaped body 3 mm wide, lying deep in the upper part of the pterygopalatine fossa. It is suspended from the maxillary nerve within a plexus of minute veins, close to the sphenopalatine foramen. Its cells are exclusively those of the parasympathetic postganglionic secretomotor fibres.

Its three roots are:

1. the parasympathetic root from the nerve of the pterygoid canal relaying to give rise to fibres for the lacrimal gland, nasal and sinus mucosae and to the nasopharynx;
2. the sympathetic root from the nerve of the pterygoid canal conveying preganglionic fibres without synapse through the ganglion;

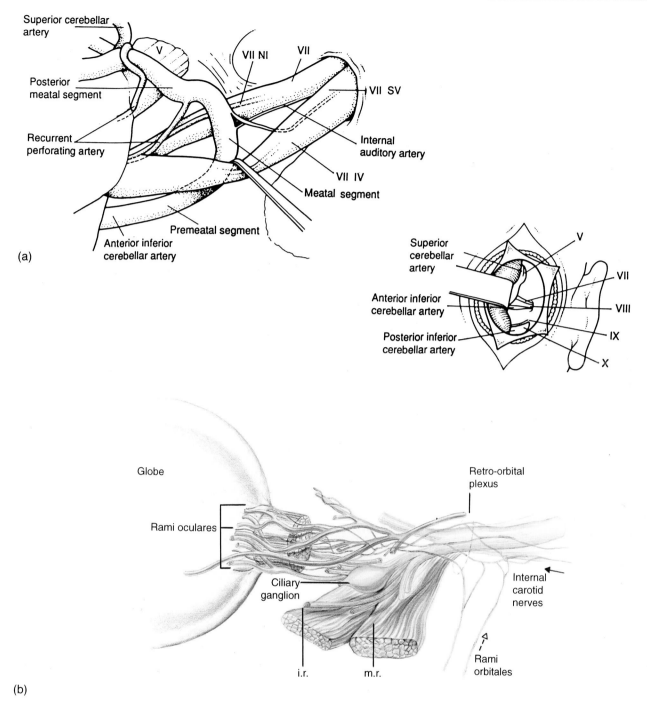

Fig. 16.10 (a) The relationship of the nervus intermedius to the facial nerve. The nervus intermedius (VII N.I.) is seen as it emerges from the brain stem along with the facial (VII) and the vestibulocochlear (VIII SV, VIII IV) nerve trunks. As the nerve courses upwards towards the temporal bone, the nervus intermedius can be seen to join with the facial nerve trunk. Note the relationships of the recurrent and internal auditory branches of the anterior inferior cerebellar artery to this complex. V = trigeminal nerve; IX = glossopharyngeal nerve; X = vagus nerve; VIII SV = cochlear nerve trunks. (From Martin, R. G., Grant, J. L., Peace, D., Theiss, C. and Rhoton, A. L. (1980) *Neurosurgery*, **6**: 483; with permission); (b) the rami oculares in the cynomolgous monkey: a semi-schematic drawing of the orbit from the medial aspect. Autonomic nerves are shown in yellow and their thickness is exaggerated. The ophthalmic artery and its branches are in red. Branches of internal carotid nerves join rami orbitales to form the retro-orbital plexus, its meshes surrounding the orbital nerves intracranially. Orbital branches of the plexus follow the arteries approximately. Three branches proceed towards the globe and they divide to form six rami oculares at the sclera close to the optic nerve. Branches of the oculomotor nerve (oc) are shown passing to the inferior (ir) and medial (mr) rectus muscles. Most of the ciliary nerves are shown severed close to the ciliary ganglion. The retro-orbital plexus is made up of fine autonomic filaments. (This is shown within the dotted circles, which also includes the ocular motor nerve.) (From Ruskell, G. L. (1970a) *Exp. Eye Res.*, **10**, 319, with permission.).

3. the sensory root, which is the largest, and carries twigs from the maxillary nerve and afferents from the nose and nasopharynx, tongue and palate, including taste fibres, destined for the main sensory and spinal nuclei of the fifth nerve.

Its branches are chiefly to nasopharyngeal structures but important fibres enter the orbit to supply:

1. lacrimal gland (parasympathetic);
2. Müller's orbital fibres (sympathetic);
3. periosteum;
4. twigs to the ciliary ganglion, optic nerve sheath, fourth and sixth cranial nerves and posterior ethmoid and sphenoidal sinuses (Hovelacque, 1927; Tanaka, 1932);
5. the ophthalmic artery and its branches;
6. the choroid via the rami oculares.

The parasympathetic supply to the ophthalmic artery and its branches, and to the choroid, derives from the rami orbitales of the pterygopalatine ganglion.

The rami orbitales and retro-orbital plexus

In rabbit, monkey and man, the pterygopalatine ganglion gives rise to the direct lacrimal gland fibres, and to the **rami orbitales**, which pass to the nasal end of the inferior orbital fissure. The latter emerge just within the middle cranial cavity at the anterior end of the cavernous sinus. (This relationship is difficult to visualize and should be confirmed on the skull.) Here they join the internal carotid nerve (sympathetic) to form a plexus of fine autonomic nerves termed the **retro-orbital plexus** (Ruskell, 1965, 1970a). This plexus is present in the fetus (Andres and Kautzky, 1956).

The rami oculares

In the monkey, the retro-orbital gives off four to six efferent fibres, the **rami oculares**, which pass forwards in the dense connective tissue around the oculomotor nerve and enter the orbit through the superior orbital fissure (Fig. 16.10b). These fibres run forwards close to the ophthalmic artery and its branches, and divide and anastomose several times. They advance between the ciliary arteries and nerves and are distributed to the ciliary arteries and to the eyeball itself.

Although the plexus is mixed autonomic, the rami oculares are composed almost entirely of bundles of unmyelinated, postganglionic, parasympathetic fibres derived from the pterygopalatine ganglion. A few rami orbitales from the pterygopalatine ganglion

bypass the retro-orbital plexus and supply the globe directly. Within the rami oculares, a small number of Schwann cells (0.9%) are found among the rami which do not invest nerve axons. Myelinated fibres are present but rare (Ruskell, 1970b).

In the monkey it has been demonstrated, by superior cervical ganglionectomy, that the rami carry no sympathetic fibres. Although this technique does not remove all the sympathetic postganglionic nerve fibres (since there are ectopic ganglia cranial to the superior cervical ganglion (Mitchell, 1953; Bondareff and Gordon, 1966)), it does achieve complete degeneration characteristic of sympathetic vascular terminals without causing neural changes in the rami oculares themselves (Ruskell, 1970b). (In the rabbit, the rami oculares are larger than in the monkey, and they join the long ciliary nerves well before the latter enter the globe. About 13% of their fibres are sympathetic (Ruskell, 1968).)

In the monkey, about 27 rami oculares supply the globe. These are mainly unmyelinated, with an average cross-section of $12 \times 8\ \mu m$, and contain about 24 nerve bundles with 56 axons per bundle. The smallest nerves measure $5 \times 4\ \mu m$, and the largest $30 \times 20\ \mu m$. These rami advance towards the globe between the ciliary nerves and arteries, contributing some unmyelinated fibres to the arteries, and occasional fibres to the ciliary nerves. Numerous unmyelinated nerve axons have been observed amidst the connective tissue of the dural sheath of the optic nerve, but their origins have not been established (Ruskell, personal communication).

Other fibres from the retro-orbital plexus (their rami vasculares) are distributed to each of the major branches of the ophthalmic artery.

Arterial innervation

All the main orbital arteries receive fine branches from the retro-orbital plexus, which may be called the rami vasculares. They run in the adventitia and terminate at the medio-adventitial junction. Some nerves arising from the rami oculares (2–10 nerve bundles in size) run in the adventitia of the ciliary arteries. The arteries receive additional, randomly arranged nerve bundles whose terminals exhibit varicosities rich in vesicles and mitochondria. Most of these bundles contain less than 10 axons; some have up to 40 to 60 axons.

About 9.8% of axon terminals found in the ciliary artery walls are sympathetic in nature. They contain small granular vesicles typical of sympathetic endings and degenerate following cervical ganglionectomy. These fibres are thought to be vasoconstrictor in nature. Other varicose nerve terminals show degenerative changes following pterygopalatine ganglionectomy, and are therefore assumed to be derived from the parasympathetic fibres of the rami oculares. They are regarded as vasodilator in function.

Neural influences on intraocular pressure

Various studies have shown that injection or damage to the pterygopalatine ganglion, pterygopalatine ganglionectomy and greater petrosal neurectomy, all lead to a fall in intraocular pressure (Sluder, 1937; Golding-Wood, 1963; Ruskell, 1970b). This is presumed to be due to section of parasympathetic nerves supplying the choroid. These nerves, which carry coexpressed muscarinic, VIPergic and nitrergic fibres via the rami oculares, are vasodilator to the choroid. Stimulation of the greater petrosal nerve causes a rise in intraocular pressure (Gloster, 1961) although no change in pressure was found by Greaves and Perkins (1956) on stimulation of the facial nerve.

Inferior salivatory nucleus

Secretomotor fibres leave in the IXth cranial nerve and, by local relay in mucous membrane, supply glands of the oropharynx. In the tympanic branch of IX, secretomotor fibres run in the **lesser petrosal nerve** to relay in the otic ganglion and supply the parotid gland.

Dorsal nucleus of vagus

Motor fibres arise in the dorsal nucleus of the vagus, which are destined to relay in the wall of the viscus concerned (heart, lung, intestine).

16.3 SYMPATHETIC SYSTEM

The preganglionic neurons have their cell bodies in the lateral horns of the thoracic and lumbar regions and leave the cord by the white rami communicantes. The cell bodies of the motor postganglionic fibres lie in the lateral chain ganglia or in the peripheral ganglia. Postganglionic fibres are non-medullated and release noradrenaline at their terminals, and are hence termed **adrenergic**. An exception to this rule is the **cholinergic** innervation of the sweat glands.

The sympathetic system supplies pupillodilator fibres, fibres to the orbital smooth muscle (Müller's), vasoconstrictor fibres to vessels and innervates the sweat glands and piloerector muscles of the facial skin.

CENTRAL PATHWAY

The central pathway arises in the posterior hypothalamus and runs an uncertain (and probably polysynaptic) course through the brain stem to reach the ciliospinal centre of Budge in the spinal cord (Harris *et al.*, 1940).

- In the **mid brain** the fibres lie ventrally near the midline.
- In the **pons** the fibres lie ventrally in the periaqueductal grey matter. They may be damaged here in syringobulbia.
- At the level of the **inferior cerebellar peduncle** they shift ventrally and laterally towards the lateral spinothalamic tract.
- In the **medulla** they run through the lateral part of the ventral reticular formation and down the intermediolateral columns of the upper cervical cord where they may be damaged in syringomyelia.
- In the **cord** the sympathetic fibres are found in the first millimetre of the anterolateral column (Kerr and Alexander, 1964; Kerr and Brown, 1964).

There is possibly a partial crossing in the decussation of Forel, the ventral tegmental decussation which is located at the lower border of the mid brain. This decussation also carries rubrospinal fibres across the median raphe. The sympathetic pathway is largely uncrossed below that point. Loewenfeld (1984) has denied the existence of this decussation (Fig. 16.11).

There is probably a distribution of fibres from the sympathetic nuclei of the hypothalamus to the Edinger–Westphal nucleus of the parasympathetic system. Stimulation of this zone results in pupillodilatation by inhibition of pupilloconstrictor tone.

PREGANGLIONIC FIBRES

Preganglionic sympathetic fibres arise in the intermediolateral column of the spinal cord (the so-called dilator centre (Budge and Waller, 1851)) at the junction of its thoracic and cervical regions (and sometimes C8 and T4 in addition). The fibres to the eye are mainly, but not invariably, from the first thoracic segment (TI). Patients have been reported in whom the T1 root has been sectioned without inducing Horner's syndrome and it is assumed that some pupillomotor fibres may leave the cord with the C8 or T2 roots (Miller, 1985). Although most reports state that the white rami travel in the anterior loop of the ansa subclavia to traverse

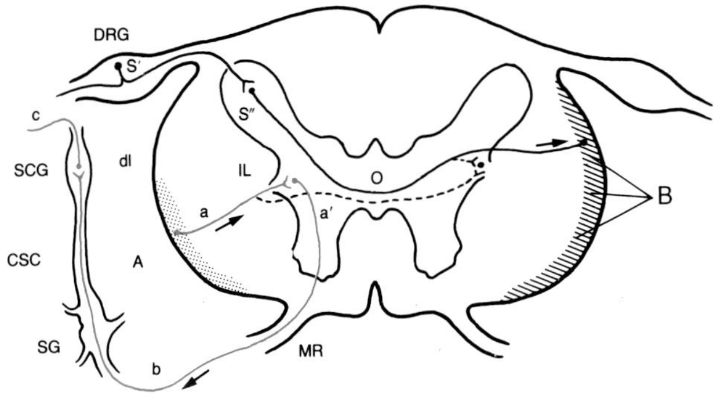

Fig. 16.11 Pupillomotor pathways in the spinal cord (T1 level). Fibres (a) pass from the descending fibres A (stippled) to the ciliospinal centre (of Budge) or intermediolateral cell column (IL), with a minor crosses component (a') to the opposite IL column. Preganglionic fibres (b) from the IL column exit with motor roots (MR) AT C3, T1 and T2 to ascend via the stellate ganglion (SG), cervical sympathetic chain (CSC) to the superior cervical ganglion (SCG) where they synapse with the postganglionic neurons, whose axons continue as the carotid nerve (c). Pupillodilatation produced by pain travels via neurons in the dorsal root ganglion (DRG), which synapse with dorsal horn neuron S''. In the cat and the rabbit the pathway ascends on the opposite side (cross-hatched area B). In humans and other primates direct activation of the ciliospinal centre probably occurs. dl = Dentate ligament.

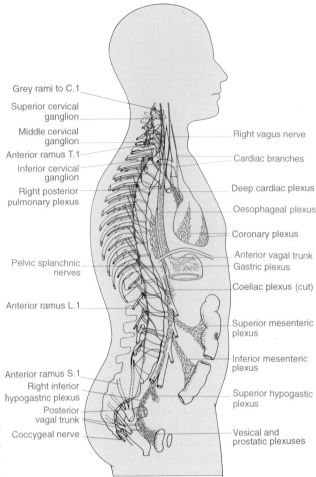

Fig. 16.12 The right sympathetic trunk and its connections with the thoracic, abdominal and pelvic plexuses, *Blue* = parasympathetic fibres, *green* = sympathetic trunk and branches, *red* = white rami communicantes. (Redrawn from Williams, P. L. (ed.) (1995) *Gray's Anatomy*, published by Churchill-Livingstone.)

the inferior/middle ganglion and reach the superior ganglion, Palumbo (1976) has postulated (on the basis of experience with patients undergoing sympathectomy) that pupillomotor sympathetic fibres leave the ventral roots of C8, T1, T2 by a root other than the white rami, and pass by a separate paravertebral route to reach the inferior or stellate ganglion; however, there has been no anatomical confirmation of this. The fibres leave the cord via the white rami communicantes and pass up the cervical sympathetic trunk to the superior cervical ganglion where they synapse with the postganglionic neurons (Fig. 16.12). They travel mainly, but not exclusively, in the anterior loop of the annulus of Vieussens and through the inferior and the middle cervical ganglia without synapse to reach the superior ganglion. The cervical trunk lies in the neck posterior to the carotid sheath and anterior to the transverse processes of the cervical vertebrae.

Stellate ganglion

The stellate ganglion is larger than the middle, and is formed by the fusion of the first thoracic ganglion with the lower two cervical ganglia (the latter may be separate, as an inferior cervical ganglion). Fusion is said to occur in 30–80% of subjects. It lies on or just lateral to the lateral border of the longus colli

between the transverse process of the seventh cervical vertebra and the neck of the first rib, and lies behind the vertebral artery. Below, it is separated from the posterior aspect of the cervical pleura at the apex of the lung by the suprapleural membrane. Here the sympathetic trunk may be vulnerable to damage by an apical tumour of the lung to cause a preganglionic Horner's syndrome, axillary pain and wasting of the muscles of the hand (T1) (Fig. 16.13) (Pancoast's syndrome). Among other branches, the ganglion supplies the plexus on the vertebral artery.

Middle cervical ganglion

The middle cervical ganglion is formed by the fusion of the fifth and sixth cervical ganglia and lies at the

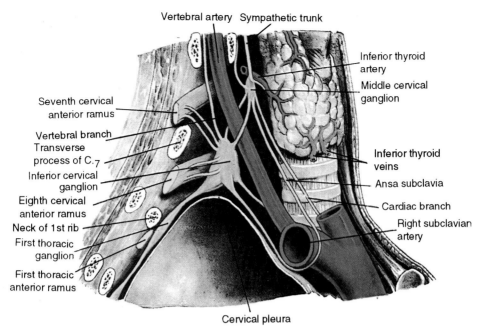

Vertebral artery   Sympathetic trunk

Inferior thyroid
artery

Middle cervical
ganglion

Seventh cervical
anterior ramus

Vertebral branch
Transverse
process of C.7
Inferior cervical
ganglion
Eighth cervical
anterior ramus
Neck of 1st rib
First thoracic
ganglion
First thoracic
anterior ramus

Inferior thyroid
veins

Ansa subclavia

Cardiac branch

Right subclavian
artery

Cervical pleura

Fig. 16.13 The middle and inferior cervical ganglia of the right side, viewed from the right. Note the proximity of the inferior cervical and first thoracic ganglia, usually fused to form a cervicothoracic (stellate) ganglion. (From Williams, P. L. (ed.) (1995) *Gray's Anatomy*, 38th edition, published by Churchill Livingstone.)

level of the sixth cervical vertebra. It is connected to the stellate ganglion by an anterior and posterior cord; the anterior cord is the ansa subclavia which loops around the subclavian artery in intimate relation to the cervical pleura (Williams and Warwick, 1980).

POSTGANGLIONIC FIBRES

Superior cervical ganglion

The superior cervical ganglion, largest of the chain of sympathetic ganglia, is an inch or more in length, and situated near the base of the skull between the internal jugular vein and internal carotid artery. The close relationship of the ganglion to the lower cranial nerves explains their simultaneous involvement in trauma or infections at the base of the skull or in the retroparotid space. The ganglion contains cholinergic preganglionic and adrenergic postganglionic terminals, and catecholamine-containing chromaffin cells (Matus, 1970). Kondo and Fujiwara (1979) have described large, granule-containing cells which may be another kind of aminergic postganglionic fibre. NPY-positive fibres are also found in the sympathetic trunk and NPY may be coexpressed with noradrenaline. It lies at the level of the second and third cervical vertebrae, over their transverse processes. It is a fusion of the ganglia of the first three or four cervical segments, and it sends grey

(postganglionic) rami communicantes to C3 and C4 nerve roots. It contains typical sympathetic cells from which the postganglionic sympathetic fibres arise in far greater number than the synapsing preganglionic neurone (11:1–17:1, Wolff, 1941; 196:1, Ebbesson, 1968). In this way the sympathetic signal is amplified and diffused.

Fibres of distribution of ophthalmic interest

Internal carotid branches

Internal carotid nerve   The internal carotid nerve accompanies the internal carotid artery into the skull through the carotid canal and breaks up into plexuses closely applied to the artery in its course.

Internal carotid plexus   An internal carotid plexus is formed on the lateral side of the artery near the apex of the petrous bone. Fibres from this carotid plexus are distributed in various ways. The largest component of the sympathetic plexus joins the sixth cranial nerve briefly, in the region of the foramen lacerum, before separating to join the ophthalmic nerve and thence the nasociliary nerve. The remaining distribution is:

1. via the **deep petrosal nerve** to join the nerve of the pterygoid canal and thus reach the pterygopalatine ganglion. The fibres traverse the

ganglion without relay and reach the orbit through the inferior orbital fissure, supplying the **orbital Müller's muscle** and possibly the lacrimal gland via the **zygomatic nerve**;

2. to the ophthalmic artery branches, including the lacrimal artery, and also to the sixth nerve;

3. the internal carotid plexus gives off the caroticotympanic nerves in the posterior wall of the carotid canal, which join the tympanic branch of the glossopharyngeal nerve. They form the tympanic plexus on the promontory of the middle ear, lying within the mucous membrane as well as in the bony grooves of the promontory. After traversing the tympanic plexus, the sympathetic fibres rejoin the carotid plexus.

Cavernous plexus   A cavernous plexus on the inferomedial aspect of the artery in the cavernous sinus supplies the eye and almost all the orbit. Fibres are given to all the nerves which enter the orbit (Johnston and Parkinson, 1974; Parkinson, Johnson and Chaudhuri, 1978). Within the cavernous sinus, branches of the sympathetic plexus are distributed with the ophthalmic, anterior cerebral, middle cerebral and anterior choroidal arteries. The posterior communicating artery probably receives fibres from both the internal carotid and the vertebral sympathetic plexuses.

Branches from the cavernous plexus are:

- To the **Gasserian ganglion** and **ophthalmic division** of the fifth nerve, on the underside of which the sympathetic bundle is visible. Fibres distribute with the **nasociliary nerve** via the superior orbital fissure and reach the globe in the **long ciliary nerves**. They are pupillodilator fibres. Occasionally some fibres are carried by the short ciliary nerve (Solnitzky, 1961).

- A small **twig to the ciliary ganglion** which enters the orbit through the superior orbital fissure; it may join the ganglion directly as its sympathetic root; it may unite with the communicating branch from the nasociliary to the ganglion, or it may travel via the ophthalmic nerve and its nasociliary branch. Its fibres pass through the ciliary ganglion without interruption and run in the **short ciliary nerves** to provide **vasoconstrictor fibres** for the blood vessels of the eye (Williams and Warwick, 1980) and also innervate the branched melanocytes of the uveal tract.

- To the **ophthalmic artery** and its branches and to the third and fourth nerves. Branches to the third nerve supply Müller's superior palpebral muscle in the orbit (Raeder, 1924).

Sympathetic ganglion cells have been found in the internal carotid plexus. These should not be forgotten when considering the effects of extirpation of the superior cervical ganglion (Sunderland and Hughes, 1946). The preganglionic neurons in the spinal cord are thus clearly a kind of motor pool (albeit rather scattered) and not an integrative 'centre'. Dilatation of the pupil can be evoked by stimulation of the frontal eye field (Crosby, 1953) and other cortical areas. Although this suggests that the cortex may be involved in reflex pupillodilatation, little is known of the connections of such areas to subcortical or brain stem nuclei, and there is no identifiable 'higher centre' for this function at the cortical level.

A limited supply to the ciliary muscle is now accepted; for a discussion of this controversial subject see Genis-Galvez (1957). Controversy also surrounds a possible sympathetic vasomotor supply in the retina (consult Laties, 1967; Fukuda, 1970). Ruskell (1973) found little evidence of such a supply in primates beyond the optic nerve head, although beta receptors are found on retinal arterioles in some species.

External carotid fibres

Postganglionic sympathetic fibres destined for facial structures leave the upper pole of the superior cervical ganglion almost immediately they are formed and join the external carotid artery.

These **external carotid fibres** course along the external carotid artery and its branches to supply the sweat glands of the face and piloerector muscles, ultimately leaving the blood vessels to be distributed through the terminal branches of the trigeminal nerve.

Vasomotor fibres to the ear and face arise from the third and fourth dorsal thoracic roots, and pilomotor fibres to the secretory glands of the face and scalp arise at the level of fifth and sixth.

16.4   PATH OF THE LIGHT REFLEX

The light reflex consists of a simultaneous and equal constriction of the pupils in response to stimulation of one eye by light. Pupil constriction is elicited with extremely low intensities and is proportional, within limits, to both the intensity and duration of the stimulus. Controversies regarding the pupillary reflex pathway have been admirably reviewed by Loewenfeld (1966) and Lowenstein and Loewenfeld (1962, 1969). These workers favour the view that both rod and cone photoreceptors may serve as the input for the reflex pathway and they regard as improbable

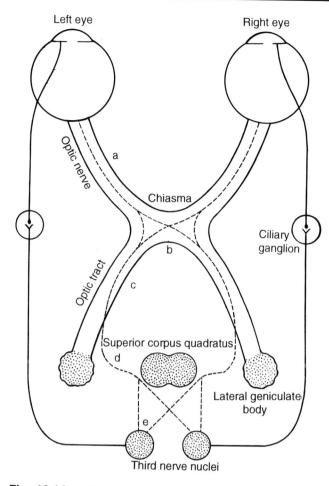

Fig. 16.14 Scheme of the pupillary path (interrupted lines). Section at (a), of the left optic nerve, causes blindness of the left eye, abolition of the direct reaction to light of the left eye with retention of the consensual, and abolition of the consensual reaction of the right eye with retention of the direct. Section at (b), of the chiasma, causes bitemporal hemianopia but abolishes neither the direct nor the consensual pupil reaction. Section at (c), of the left optic tract, causes contralateral (i.e. right) homonymous hemianopia; Wernicke's hemiopic pupil reaction. Section at (d), of the superior brachium on both sides, causes Argyll Robertson pupils. Section at (e), both afferent fibres coming to left nucleus, causes unilateral (left) Argyll Robertson pupil. Section at (e), on both sides, causes bilateral Argyll Robertson pupils. NB: The cell station in the pretectal nucleus is not shown.

the existence of special 'pupillary' receptors or receptors (Fig. 16.14).

AFFERENT TRACT

Two views are expressed as to whether the visual and pupillary fibres are different or identical. Müller's law of specificity of nerve conduction has even been cited to support the view that a dual function is involved and hence separate 'pupillary' and 'visual' fibres must exist. There is no adequate evidence in favour of this view; in particular, the clinical deductions

favouring a duality of receptor, ganglion cell and further pathway ignores the improbability of disease selecting one set of fibres rather than the other. There can be no doubt that the axons subserving the sensation of vision and those concerned with the pupillary reflexes have different pathways and connections. Whether the pupillary pathway is formed by branches of collaterals of retinogeniculate axons is still uncertain (see Ranson and Magoun, 1933; Lowenstein and Loewenfeld, 1984). The assumptions that axons of small diameter are 'pupillary' and the larger ones 'visual' (or vice versa) are both at best poorly supported by evidence.

Pupillary fibres in the optic nerve

The pupillary fibres run in the optic nerve; ablation of the nerve abolishes the direct and also the consensual light reflex i.e. the pupil constriction induced in the fellow eye. The pupillary fibres partially cross in the chiasma, as do the visual, a portion going over to the opposite side while the remainder pass on in the optic tract of the same side. We know that the pupillary fibres cross in the chiasma because section of one optic tract abolishes neither the direct nor the consensual pupil reaction (Miller and Newman, 1981; O'Connor *et al.*, 1982). Experimental division of the chiasma abolishes neither the direct nor the consensual light reflex (Parsons, 1924): hence there **must** be a **posterior** crossing as well (Fig. 16.8).

Pupillary fibres in the optic tract

The pupillary fibres run in the optic tract, incision of which causes Wernicke's hemianopic pupil reaction. They leave the visual fibres at the posterior part of the tract, do not form a cell station at the lateral geniculate body, and run superficially in the superior brachium conjunctivum to the lateral side of the superior colliculus (Bowling and Michael, 1980). Severance of both superior brachia abolishes the reaction of the pupil to light on both sides (Karplus and Kreidl, 1913).

The fibres which enter the superior colliculus are not concerned with the pupillary reflex; destruction of this body down to the aqueduct has no effect on the pupillary reflex.

Pupillary fibres in the mid brain

The pupillary fibres pass into the mid brain at the lateral side of the superior colliculus to reach the pretectal nucleus (an ill-defined collection of small cells anterior to the lateral margin of the superior colliculus), where they have their terminations. The new relay of fibres partially crosses in the posterior commissure and also ventral to the aqueduct, and reaches the sphincter centre of the same and opposite side via the medial longitudinal bundle. In humans the numbers of axons which cross approximately equals those which do not. The 'sphincter centre' is formed by the accessory oculomotor nuclei of Edinger and Westphal.

The pretectal nuclei

Several neuronal subgroups of the pretectal nuclei have been described, although their functional relevance is unclear (Carpenter and Peter, 1970; Scalia, 1972; Carpenter and Pierson, 1973; Kanaseki and Sprague, 1974; Benevento, Rezak and Santos-Anderson, 1977). These are the olivary nucleus, the sublentiform nucleus, the nucleus of the pretectal area, the nucleus of the optic tract, the posterior nucleus and the principal pretectal nucleus (Fig. 16.5).

Retinal fibres end predominantly in the dorso-medial parts of the ipsilateral (and more so the contralateral) **olivary nuclei** and also in the con-tralateral **sublentiform nuclei** (Hendrickson, Wilson and Toyne, 1970; Pierson and Carpenter, 1974; Tigges and O'Steen, 1974; Benevento, Rezak and Santos-Anderson, 1977). There are some projections to the nucleus of the pretectal area.

Efferent neurons have been traced from the ipsilateral and contralateral olivary nuclei and from the sublentiform nuclei to the **visceral nuclei** of the oculomotor complex (Carpenter and Pierson, 1973; Benevento *et al.*, 1977; Burde, 1983).

The literature on the parasympathetic status of the accessory oculomotor nuclei is immense (see War-wick, 1954). Despite some disbelievers, the anatomi-cal and physiological evidence is now undeniable. Many of the cells, if not most, in this small-celled component of the oculomotor complex are con-cerned with accommodation. Attempts to distin-guish pupillomotor and accommodation 'centres' have been few and unconvincing. A study (Sillito and Zbrozyna, 1970) using stimulation techniques in cats suggests that the classical Edinger–Westphal columns are concerned with pupilloconstriction, whereas the majority of the anteriomedian nucleus is not. Some cells are concerned with the vestibulo-ocular reflex.

The visceromotor nuclei of the oculomotor com-plex include not only the Edinger–Westphal nucleus (Edinger, 1885; Westphal, 1887), but also nuclei which are thought to participate in varying degree in pupillomotor control and accommodation.

Probable course of the afferent pupillary fibres (Figs 16.7 and 16.8)

The impulse starts in the rods and cones and relays through the retina to reach the optic nerve; axons partially cross in the chiasma like the visual fibres, accompany the visual fibres in the tract to its posterior third, and there leave the tract as a separate bundle of fibres, probably collaterals of the visual fibres, to enter the superior brachium conjunctivum (Fig. 15.67). They pass into the mid brain lateral to the superior colliculus to synapse in the pretectal nucleus and partially cross to reach the accessory oculomotor nucleus (Edinger–Westphal) of the same and opposite side via the medial longitudinal bundle.

We see, therefore, that there is a double crossing, in the chiasma and in the mid brain.

EFFERENT PATH

The axons of the accessory oculomotor neurons (Edinger–Westphal) extend into the oculomotor nerve and lie on its superficial dorsomedial aspect as it leaves the brain stem (Sunderland and Hughes, 1946). From here they pursue a gently spiralling course medially and downward, so that they lie medially in the nerve as it passes lateral to the petroclinoid ligament and dorsum sellae, and are located in the inferior division of the third nerve as it enters the orbit (Fig. 16.16). The great majority of fibres lie superficially in the oculomotor nerve just under the epimysium, but similar small-diameter myelinated fibres are seen occasionally scattered through the substance of the nerve (Kerr and Hollowell, 1964; Kerr, 1968). From the inferior division of the third nerve, by way of its branch to the inferior oblique, a short and relatively thick nerve trunk reaches the ciliary ganglion. These myelinated, preganglionic, parasympathetic fibres terminate in axosomatic and axodendritic synapses with the ganglionic neurons. The latter project myelinated postganglionic fibres which reach the eyeball through the short ciliary nerves to innervate the sphincter pupillae. It is important to note that the majority (95–97% according to Warwick, 1954) of the fibres in this efferent pathway are concerned with the ciliary muscle, and only 3–5% are pupillomotor.

16.5 THE DARK REFLEX

When illumination to the eye is extinguished rapid reflex pupillary dilatation occurs, in which the initial phase is caused by contraction of the iris dilator muscle and the later phase by sphincter inhibition.

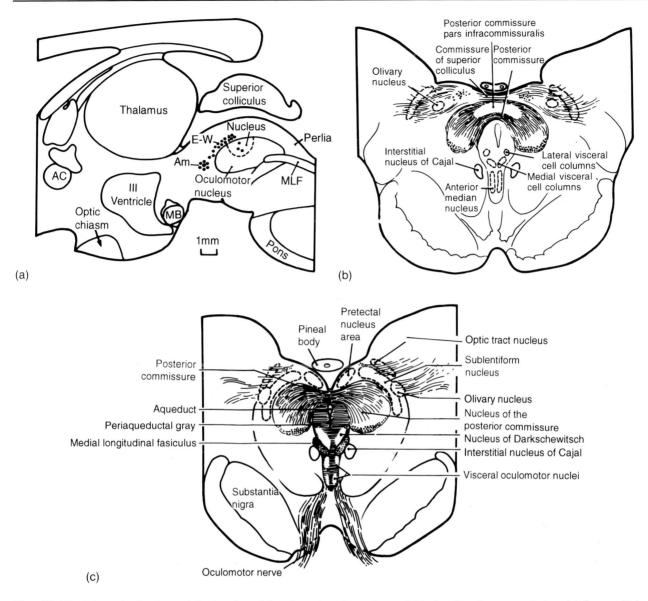

Fig. 16.15 Schematic drawings of the location of the visceral ocular motor nuclei in the dorsal mesencephalon. (a) Parasagittal section showing the rostral–caudal relationships of the anterior median (AM) and Edinger–Westphal (E-W) nuclei and Perlia's nucleus. AC = Anterior commissure; MLF = medial longitudinal fasciculus; MB = mamillary bodies. (Redrawn from Burde, R. M. and Loewy, A. D. (1980) *Brain Res.* **198**, 434–439.) (b) Cross-section of the mesencephalon showing the relationship of the Edinger–Westphal and anterior median nuclei to some of the pretectal nuclei. The Edinger–Westphal nuclei are composed of two cell groups, the lateral and medial visceral cell columns. The anterior median nuclei are located just ventral and rostral to the visceral cell columns of the Edinger–Westphal nuclei and are on either side of the mid line. (Redrawn from Carpenter, M. B. and Pierson, R. J. (1973) *Comp. Neurol.* **149**, 271–300.) (c) Drawing of the major pretectal nuclei and their relationship to the visceral and anterior median oculomotor nuclei. (From Carpenter, M. B. and Pierson, R. J. (1973) *Comp. Neurol.* **149**, 271–300.)

The pupillodilator pathway is clearly inhibited when the eye is illuminated; this inhibition is removed in darkness. The afferent pathway involved must follow the visual fibres to the optic tract, but the subsequent route leading to stimulation of the 'pupillodilator centre' in the cord is uncertain.

Initial response to darkness is sympathetic activation, but there is also a phase which is due to parasympathetic inhibition acting through the Edinger–Westphal and anterior median nuclei. It has been proposed that the 'off' response of the retina relays an inhibitory impulse to the mid brain, which acts on nuclei concerned with pupil constriction (Lowenstein and Loewenfeld, 1962). There is also a slow increase which relates to the progress of dark adaptation.

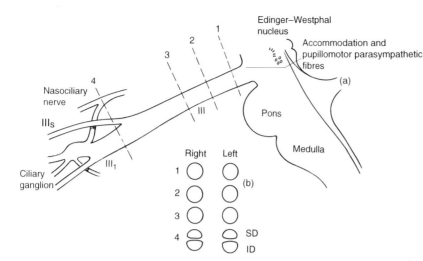

Fig. 16.16 Diagrammatic representation of the pupillomotor and accommodation fibre pathway, in sagittal section. The axons of the Edinger–Westphal neurons leave the mid brain on the dorsal surface of the oculomotor nerve. They follow a spiral course to its inferior division.
III = Oculomotor nerve. (After Kerr.)

Fibres inhibitory to constriction may act on the pretectal or visceral nuclei. It is thought that inhibitory impulses travel via corticothalamo-hypothalamic or corticolimbic pathways to inhibit the mid brain parasympathetic outflow. Electrical stimulation of the diencephalon in sympathectomized cats and monkeys causes pupil dilatation and loss of the light reflex (Lowenstein and Loewenfeld, 1962). Stimulation of the frontal and sensorimotor areas of the brain also causes pupil dilatation. The inhibitory influence originating in the cortex, hypothalamus and reticular-activating system is diminished with fatigue and in sleep, so that the pupil becomes miosed. Stimulation of the hypothalamus may cause mydriasis, lid elevation and a rise in blood pressure (Karplus and Kreidl, 1909; Sano et al., 1970; Balasubramanian et al., 1972; Schvarcz et al., 1972; Kalyanaraman, 1975).

Dilatation in response to arousal or pain is only partly inhibited by sympathectomy (Bechterew, 1883; Kuntz and Richins, 1946) and appears to depend on ascending inhibitory fibres from the cord, that act on the Edinger–Westphal nucleus in the non-human primate. These fibres ascend in the anterolateral funiculus of the cord where they are located superficially, close to the descending sympathetic dilator pathway (Kerr and Brown, 1964). Two ascending pathways have been identified in the brain stem that produce pupillary dilatation when stimulated in sympathectomized cats (Loewy, Araujo and Kerr, 1973), and Kerr (1975) has traced such fibres from the spinal cord to the visceral oculomotor nuclei. It appears established that ascending spinoreticular fibres produce direct inhibition of motoneurons for pupillary constriction.

Stimulation of the hypothalamus induces pupil dilatation even in decerebrate animals (Karplus and Kreidl, 1909; Sano et al., 1970; Kalyanaram, 1975).

Descending sympathetic pathways arise in the posterior and lateral regions of the hypothalamus. More caudally, the pathways come to occupy a lateral position in the brainstem. There are probably some synapses in the pontine and mid brain tegmentums, but some fibres proceed directly without synapse to the ciliospinal centre (Budge and Waller, 1851, 1852; Carmel, 1968).

Kerr and Brown (1964) used microelectrodes to identify descending pupillomotor fibres in non-human primates. They are located superficially in the anterolateral columns of the spinal cord, occupying a ventral position just dorsal to the dentate insertion and extending to a point just lateral to the exit of the ventral roots from the cord. These fibres descend to the cervicothoracic cord, and pass medially to synapse with preganglionic neurons at C8–T2. Stimulation in the monkey routinely causes a mild contralateral mydriasis, so that some crossed connections have been postulated at the level of the ciliospinal centre; these are unlikely to be important in humans. In the cord, the pupillary fibres run together with vasopressor fibres.

Stimulation of wide areas of the limbic system in the cat (cingulate gyrus, subcallosal and postorbital regions, the orbital tubercle and part of the pyriform cortex) produces rapid dilatation of the pupil (Harris, Hodes and Magoun, 1944) and the most active responses have been obtained from the cingulate lobe near the cingulate sulcus.

Dilatation of the pupil has been achieved by stimulation of the frontal lobe (area 8), the occipital lobe and the sensorimotor cortex (Parsons, 1924). This appears to involve activation of the hypothalamus, leading to both dilator muscle stimulation and inhibition of the constrictor muscle.

16.6 CILIOSPINAL REFLEX

Reflex mydriasis to painful stimuli in the neck appears to be mediated by inhibition of the Edinger–Westphal nucleus. The reflex pathway is summarized by Kerr (1968). Afferent impulses are transmitted by small myelinated and unmyelinated fibres to the spinal cord. After synaptic relay in the dorsal horn they pass mainly contralaterally in the most superficial stratum of the lateral aspect of the cord (Fig. 16.12). From this level they ascend to the brain stem to reach the Edinger–Westphal nucleus bilaterally, before or after relay in other structures at the thalamic or hypothalamic level. The effect on the Edinger–Westphal nucleus is one of inhibition. In some subjects the reflex occurs only in response to substantial pain.

16.7 PATH OF THE NEAR REFLEX

When gaze is changed from a distant to a near object three distinct actions are coordinated:

- accommodation;
- pupil constriction;
- convergence.

These synergistic events are termed the 'near reflex'. All three components of the near reflex can be elicited experimentally by stimulation of the occipital association cortex. From the cerebral cortex impulses descend by way of the corticotegmental and corticotectal tracts to relay in the pretectal and possibly tegmental areas. From the relay, fibres run to the Edinger–Westphal nucleus (with those for accommodation located slightly caudal to those for pupilloconstriction), to the motor nuclei of the medial recti and a component passes to the nuclei of the sixth cranial nerve.

There is evidence, mainly from clinical observations, that the fibres mediating pupillary constriction in the near reflex follow a different course to those concerned with the light reflex. It is believed that near reflex fibres approach pretectal nucleus from the ventral aspect and that this explains the loss of the pupil response to light before that to the near reflex (light–near dissociation) as occurs in dorsal compressive or infiltrative lesions of the optic tectum (Parinaud's syndrome). From the Edinger–Westphal nucleus the impulses for pupilloconstriction initiated by light or by the near reflex travel over the same fibres. Those for accommodation follow the same general pathway, with similar relays in the pretectal nucleus and ciliary ganglion, but their final distribution via the short ciliary nerves is to the ciliary muscle.

The near reflex embodies fixation, which consists essentially of an accommodative effort, accompanied by a convergence of the eyeballs. It is, nevertheless, equally possible to alter the focus with one eye, in which case the synergic convergence is absent. The afferent path for the whole reflex must be along the visual pathway to the occipital cortex.

Some believe that the pupillary response may be initiated by convergence itself, with the direct involvement of the occipital cortex. It is believed to begin as proprioceptive impulses in the medial recti, hence via the oculomotor nerve or 1st division of the trigeminal to the mesencephalic nucleus of the trigeminal. From here the impulse passes to the constrictor centre of the oculomotor nerve nucleus, hence via the oculomotor nerve for an unknown distance. Then leaving the oculomotor nerve it misses the ciliary ganglion and makes a cell station in an accessory ganglion, whence it passes to the sphincter pupillae.

16.8 CLINICAL SYNDROMES INVOLVING THE PUPIL

INTERRUPTION OF THE PUPILLARY PATHWAYS

Optic nerve and tract lesions

The effects of optic nerve and tract lesions on the pupillary pathways have been dealt with earlier.

Damage to superior brachium conjunctivum

Bilateral damage to the superior brachium conjunctivum will produce pupils poorly responsive to light and with a retained response to the near reflex (**light–near dissociation**). Compressive lesions of the optic tectum (e.g. pinealoma) may also produce a light–near dissociation by interfering with the function of the pretectal nucleus. It has been suggested that corticotectal fibres to the Edinger–Westphal nucleus subserving the near pupil response lie ventrally and are affected later in the course of the disease. In both situations, the pupil is of normal size or semidilated due to **loss of light-induced pupilloconstrictor tone**.

The Argyll–Robertson pupil

The pupils are small, asymmetric, dilate poorly in the dark and show a light–near dissociation. Loewenfeld (1984) has suggested that the lesion is rostral to the oculomotor nucleus, and thus affects the pupillary-light fibres and spares the accommodation-near fibres. The pupils may be small because of damage to corticotectal fibres inhibitory to the Edinger–Westphal nucleus, resulting in **increased pupilloconstrictor tone**. The iris is also abnormal in appearance and shows stromal atrophy.

Adie's myotonic pupil

In this disorder there is commonly unilateral pupil dilatation which reacts poorly or not at all to light but retains the near-pupil response. The pupil constriction to near may be slowed, and is sustained when the near stimulus is removed. Loewenfeld and Thompson (1967) have suggested that this is due to a ciliary ganglionitis, followed by aberrant regeneration, a reinnervation of the iris sphincter with fibres previously serving the ciliary muscle. As the majority, 95–97%, of parasympathetic postganglionic fibres normally subserve accommodation (Warwick, 1954), there is a predominant reinnervation of the iris sphincter with 'accommodative' fibres and negligible reinnervation with 'pupil-directed' fibres. The typical pupil responses which result are:

1. The pupil response to light is absent or diminished due to deficient reinnervation of the sphincter by pupil fibres subserving the light reflex.
2. A retained response of the pupil to the near reflex is due to aberrant reinnervation of the sphincter by fibres previously destined for the ciliary body (near–accommodation fibres).
3. The pupil contraction to near is asymmetrical due to asymmetry of reinnervation.
4. Pupil response to near is tonic. The pupil constricts slowly because of a numerically deficient innervation and redilates slowly because the partially denervated sphincter muscle is supersensitive to its cholinergic stimulus so that contraction persists. Supersensitivity is readily demonstrated with 0.125% pilocarpine or 2.5% methacholine (Mecholyl).

Damage to the third cranial nerve

The third cranial nerve may be damaged anywhere along its course.

1. Within the brain stem a vascular or intrinsic lesion may produce an oculomotor palsy (1) with contralateral cerebellar signs, due to damage to the red nucleus (Benedekt's syndrome), or (2) with contralateral hemiplegia, due to involvement of the cerebral peduncle (Weber's syndrome) (Fig. 5.8).
2. The nerve may be damaged in the interpeduncular fossa, in its remaining subarachnoid course or in its intracavernous course.
3. It may be damaged at the superior orbital fissure as part of the superior orbital fissure syndrome.
4. Affection of the inferior division of the oculomotor nerve in the orbit, usually traumatic, will cause loss of inferior rectus and oblique action, with an intrinsic (efferent) pupil defect due to involvement of the parasympathetic, preganglionic root of the ciliary ganglion.

If the ciliary ganglion is damaged the pupil will be supersensitive to 0.125% pilocarpine. In the above disorders the pupil is dilated and fails to constrict to direct or consensual light due to loss of efferent parasympathetic sphincter innervation.

Pupil-sparing third nerve palsy

A pupil-sparing third nerve palsy is encountered in diabetes mellitus. The lesion is primarily one of focal demyelination with minimal axonal degeneration. This is caused by intraneural arteriolar closure and it is presumed that the peripheral disposition of the pupil fibres in the oculomotor nerve is the basis for sparing. The nerve is affected in its subarachnoid (Weber, Daroff and Mackey, 1970) or intracavernous portion. In such patients, nerve damage has been found to be located centrally in the nerve, sparing the peripheral visceral fibres (Dreyfus, Hakim and Adams, 1957; Asbury et al., 1970; Weber, Daroff and Mackay, 1970).

SYMPATHETIC LESIONS – HORNER'S SYNDROME

The oculosympathetic pathway may be affected anywhere along its course, causing Horner's syndrome, whose features are:

- Ipsilateral **miosis**, due to dilator paresis.
- Defective dilatation in the dark (Fig. 16.17).
- Partial **ptosis**, due to paresis of the Müller's portion of the levator muscle.
- **Facial anhydrosis** due to loss of sweat gland stimulation. Anhydrosis will occur with central lesions and preganglionic lesions below the base of the skull and the origin of fibres running with the external carotid artery which supply the facial skin. This is a useful localizing sign.
- It is doubtful whether enophthalmos occurs,

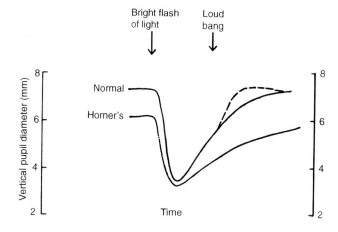

Fig. 16.17 Infrared pupillographic response in Horner's syndrome recorded in darkness. Note that the Horner's pupil is smaller in the dark, but that a bright flash greatly reduces this anisocoria (−normal pupil constrictors). After the flash, the Horner's pupil dilates at a slower rate and lacks the initial fast phase due to contraction of the dilator muscle. A loud, unexpected noise during the recovery phase causes an accelerated dilatation of the normal pupil but does not affect the Horner's pupil. (Courtesy of Dr Shirley Smith.)

because, there is no reason to expect that paresis of the smooth muscle of the orbit, including Müller's portion of the levator muscle, would lead to globe retraction (Koornneef, 1987).

Central lesions

A central lesion may be caused by occlusion of the posterior inferior cerebellar artery (Wallenberg's lateral medullary syndrome), whose features reflect the territory of supply of this artery; thus, (1) ipsilateral Horner's syndrome (central fibres), (2) dysphagia (laryngeal and pharyngeal paralysis – IX and X), (3) ipsilateral facial analgesia (spinal tract and nucleus of trigeminal nerve) and contralateral analgesia of the trunk and extremities (ascending spinothalamic tract), (4) ipsilateral cerebellar ataxia and rotary nystagmus and occasional skew deviation (vestibular nuclei and utricular connections). Central lesions in the cervical cord may be caused by tumour, trauma, demyelination and syringomyelia.

Preganglionic lesions

A root lesion affecting the brachial plexus (and preganglionic fibres) may occur with birth trauma and be associated with Klumpke's paralysis of the ipsilateral arm. Tumours of the chest apex or superior mediastinum may also damage preganglionic fibres in the T1 root (Pancoast's syndrome) or as they enter the sympathetic chain. In the neck, preganglionic fibres may be damaged in relation to the carotid sheath by tumour, inflammation, enlarged lymph nodes and trauma, including surgery and percutaneous carotid angiography.

Postganglionic lesions

Lesions within the cranial cavity affect postganglionic fibres, which are not distributed to facial sweat glands. Such lesions are not usually associated with facial anhydrosis. However, in some subjects sweat glands on the forehead may be innervated by postganglionic fibres running in the internal carotid plexus and in the supraorbital branch of the ophthalmic nerve.

The frequency of lesions at each level has been surveyed by Giles and Henderson (1969). The level of the lesion is often suggested by accompanying signs. Pharmacological differentiation of first, second and third neuron lesions is described by Grimson and Thomson (1975). In brief, complete third neuron section will supersensitize the pupil dilator muscle to topical 1:1000 adrenaline or 1% phenylephrine; hydroxyamphetamine (1%) will fail to release catecholamine from the degenerate nerve endings and the pupil fails to dilate. With a complete second neuron section, the dilator is not supersensitive, but hydroxyamphetamine will cause pupil dilatation by releasing transmitter from intact postganglionic fibres.

16.9 AMINERGIC, PEPTIDERGIC AND NITRERGIC INNERVATION

In recent years it has become apparent that the peripheral nervous system contains not only classical neurotransmitters but also a large number (over 50) of biologically active amines and peptides. In the nervous system generally these transmitters may coexist with each other or with classical neurotransmitters, and may be released simultaneously or selectively. Neuropeptides act as neuromodulators, having an action which is slower in onset, of longer duration and more diffuse in effect than classical neurotransmitters. The means by which they are removed from tissues is not established. Neuropeptides have been identified chemically and immunohistochemically in sensory neurons and among fibres of the sympathetic and parasympathetic nervous systems. Some features of peptidergic, aminergic and nitrergic innervation of the eye are summarized below.

LIDS AND CONJUNCTIVA

The conjunctival vessels in monkeys receives a sympathetic adrenergic supply which is assumed to be vasoconstrictor (Ehinger, 1971; Macintosh, 1974), while a parasympathetic cholinergic supply has been shown in denervation experiments to run with the facial nerve and synapse in the pterygopalatine ganglion. This is regarded as a vasodilator supply (Ruskell, 1985). Although VIP-containing nerves have been identified in rabbit conjunctiva this was not confirmed in human eyes by Miller *et al.* (1983), but there is innervation of the epidermis, hair follicles and lymphoid aggregates in the primate. The meimbomian gland of rhesus and cynonolgous monkeys is also richly innervated, with NPY- and VIPergic fibres closely apposed to the acinar basal laminae, and more sparsely distributed fibres positive for CGRP, TH and SP.

CORNEAL STROMA AND EPITHELIUM

In some species (e.g. rodents) this is richly supplied by sympathetic adrenergic fibres (Tervo and Palkama, 1976). Primary sensory neurons have been shown to contain substance P (Miller *et al.*, 1981; Lehtosalo, Uusitalo and Palakama, 1984), somatostatin, cholecystokinin (Jansco *et al.*, 1981; Stone *et al.*, 1984) and gastrin/bombesin-releasing peptide (Panula *et al.*, 1983). Epithelial serotonergic nerves appear to regulate inward chloride transport which may be modulated by prejunctional dopaminergic receptors (Klyce *et al.*, 1982; Crosson, Beverman and Klyce, 1984). There is no direct evidence of parasympathetic nerve fibres in the cornea.

CHAMBER ANGLE

The chamber angle receives sympathetic, parasympathetic and sensory fibres, most of which are unmyelinated. They are found most frequently in the pericanalicular area as well as in the uveal and corneoscleral meshwork (Ruskell, 1976; Tripathi and Tripathi, 1982). Sympathetic fibres constitute 30% (Nomura and Smelser, 1974) or less (Ruskell, 1976) of the total and their numbers decrease with age and in chronic simple glaucoma (Kurus, 1958; Ehinger, 1971; Wolter, 1959). Some sympathetic nerves immunoreactive to neuropeptide Y and avian pancreatic polypeptide have been demonstrated (Bruun *et al.*, 1984; Stone and Laties, 1983; Stone, Laties and Emson, 1986).

Parasympathetic innervation via the ciliary ganglion was demonstrated by Holland, von Sallman and Collins (1957) while Ruskell (1976, 1985) has emphasized a facial parasympathetic supply in monkeys synapsing in the pterygopalatine ganglion and entering the orbit as the rami orbitales (see also Stone and Laties, 1987). There is also evidence for nerves immunoreactive to vasointestinal polypeptide originating from the pterygopalatine ganglion. Although anterior segment structures receive a sparser supply than the choroid (Uddman *et al.*, 1980) these nerves do innervate the posterior uveal meshwork in the human eye (Stone and Laties, 1987).

Sensory trigeminal fibres containing substance P have been observed in the angle structures of monkeys and humans in both the uveal and corneoscleral parts of the meshwork, the juxtacanalicular tissue, and to either side of Schlemm's canal (Stone and Laties, 1987). A sparse innervation with fibres containing calcitonin gene-related peptide has been noted.

Myelinated trigeminal fibres innervate the mechano-receptor endings of the scleral spur, and there is a nitrergic and VIPergic (parasympathetic), an SP/CGRP-ergic and NPY-ergic innervation of the contractile scleral spur cells (Tamm *et al.*, 1994, 1995).

IRIS

The iris receives sympathetic, parasympathetic and sensory innervation.

Sympathetic innervation

Sympathetic adrenergic fibres densely innervate the iris vasculature, and maintain a constant vasoconstrictor tone (Ehinger, 1966). These are small-diameter fibres with axon varicosities, whose terminals contain small dense-cored vesicles. In the dilator area, these catecholamine-containing fibres form a rich three-dimensional plexus. Fibres innervate the sphincter muscle sparsely and possibly also the iridial melanocytes (Laties, 1974).

In some species sensory fibres immunoreactive for substance P also innervate the iris (especially the sphincter muscle), and their density is increased following sympathetic denervation (Miller *et al.*, 1981; Tervo *et al.*, 1981; Cole *et al.*, 1983; Kessler, Bell and Black, 1983). The possibility of colocalization of amines such as 5-HT and dopamine within sympathetic neurons supplying the iris is discussed by Palkama, Uusitalo and Lehtosalo (1986). Colocalization of substance P with calcitonin gene-related peptidergic fibres occurs; these fibres are numerous in rat iris and ciliary body but less so in the monkey (Terenghi *et al.*, 1985).

Cholinergic innervation

The sphincter muscle, and to a lesser extent the dilator muscle, receive cholinergic innervation (Nishida and Sears, 1969). Although Huhtala *et al.* (1971) found no evidence of parasympathetic innervation of iris blood vessels in the rat, Stjernschantz and Bill (1979) demonstrated a vasoconstriction of iris vessels in the monkey on oculomotor nerve stimulation (and a tendency toward vasodilatation in the ciliary body, which may have reflected increased ciliary muscle activity). Parasympathetic fibres in the iris are small and unmyelinated with small and empty-cored transmitter vesicles.

Serotonergic innervation

Serotonergic fibres have been found in rat and guinea-pig iris (Uusitalo *et al.*, 1982; Palkama, Lehtosalo and Uusitalo, 1984). Palkama has demonstrated dopamine receptors in human iris (Palkama, Uusitalo and Lehtosalo, 1986), while dopaminergic fibres have been demonstrated in the rabbit. Fibres immunoreactive to cholecystokinin, somatomedin and encephalin have been demonstrated in guinea-pig and rat iris (Stone *et al.*, 1984; Bjorklund *et al.*, 1984).

CILIARY BODY

About 1% of the fibres within the ciliary body are sympathetic adrenergic fibres (Ruskell, 1973). They control vasoconstrictor tone of the ciliary vessels. Although sympathetic innervation of the ciliary muscle is small, it is greater in primates, pigs and sheep than in rodents. There are more beta than alpha receptors present, and the effect of beta stimulation is to induce a hypermetropic shift (i.e. to increase tension on the zonule) (Ehinger, 1966; Tornquist, 1966). In the rabbit, the umyelinated, sympathetic adrenergic terminals end in the stroma in contact with the epithelial cells (Uusitalo and Palkama, 1971). Neuropeptide Y, which is associated with sympathetic fibres, has been demonstrated in the stroma of guinea-pig ciliary processes but not intraepithelially (Bruun *et al.*, 1984).

Parasympathetic fibres of oculomotor origin reach the ciliary body by ciliary nerve fibres synapsing in the ciliary ganglion (or less frequently distal to it – Givner, 1939). Other parasympathetic fibres of facial nerve origin synapse in the pterygopalatine ganglion and include small numbers of vasointestinal peptide-reactive fibres in humans which are probably vasodilator. Oculomotor stimulation in the cat and monkey tends to cause vasodilatation, although the effect is not distinguished from a metabolic result of ciliary muscle contraction. In the rabbit there is a cholinergic induced vasoconstriction (Bill and Linder, 1976). Parasympathetic cholinergic axons run in the stromal part of the ciliary processes but their terminals have not been demonstrated to perforate the external limiting membrane and make contact with the epithelium (Uusitalo and Palkama, 1971).

Serotonergic fibres supplying the ciliary processes and substance P-reactive fibres have also been demonstrated in the ciliary body (Klyce *et al.*, 1981; Palkama *et al.*, 1984). Cholecystokinin-positive fibres have been shown in guinea-pig ciliary body (Stone *et al.*, 1984).

Sensory axons are found in the anterior stroma of the monkey ciliary body and pass through the muscle without distributing to it. They are unmyelinated, run in bundles of 3–20 axons each, and measure 0.4–1.6 μm in diameter (Bergmanson, 1977; Lehtosalo *et al.*, 1984). Integrity of sensory neurons is required in some species (e.g. rabbit) to mediate the breakdown of the blood aqueous barrier induced by prostaglandins. Release of substance P or other mediators may be involved.

The ciliary muscle is richly innervated by muscarinic and cholinergic fibres and possesses varicose nerve terminals which are immuno-reactive for CGRP and SP, VIP and NPY. There is also an intrinsic, nitrergic ganglionic plexus located within the reticular and circular parts of the muscle.

CHOROIDAL VESSELS

The choroidal vessels are richly innervated by sympathetic adrenergic fibres which maintain vasoconstrictor tone. There is an equally rich innervation by parasympathetic, vasointestinal peptide-positive and nitrergic vasodilator fibres of facial nerve origin, which reach the eye via the pterygopalatine ganglion in the rami orbitales (Stjernschantz and Bill, 1980; Udmann *et al.*, 1980; Nilsson and Bill, 1984; Uusitalo *et al.*, 1984). Parasympathetic vasodilator fibres also innervate the choroid in primates (Stjernschantz and Bill, 1979). In foveate animals, including humans and some primates, there is an intrinsic ganglionic plexus within the choroid whose fibres are nitrergic and vasointestinal peptidergic, and which is vasodilator in function.

The autonomic supply of the vessels of the optic nerve and proximal retinal arteries is described in Chapter 15.

CHAPTER SEVENTEEN
Development of the human eye

17.1 EMBRYONIC ORIGINS

The heterogeneous tissues that constitute the human eye are derived embryonically from surface ectoderm, neural ectoderm, neural crest, and mesodermal mesenchyme.* During development the final differentiation and arrangement of the different types of cells are controlled by numerous inductive and suppressive interactions, and these complex processes are believed to be mediated by chemical signals that act at the cellular and molecular levels. The specific macromolecules include peptide growth factors which function by modulating the migration, proliferation and differentiation of embryonic cells; for example, transforming growth factor-β has a crucial role in directing the migratory and developmental patterns of cranial neural crest cells (Tripathi

*Mesenchymal cells are a dispersed population of undifferentiated embryonic cells that are stellate shaped and loosely arranged; they are derived from mesoderm or the neural crest.

et al., 1991). Recent experimental data also indicate that the expression of homeobox genes is regulated by different peptide growth factors (Dawid, Sargent and Rosa, 1990; Ruiz i Altaba and Melton, 1990). Homeobox genes (or more correctly homeotic genes) contain a segment of DNA, 180 base-pairs in length, in which the sequence of nucleotides is remarkably similar. This region, known as the homeobox, encodes an almost identical region of some 60 amino acids (the so-called homeobox sequence or homeodomain) in the protein products of these genes. Because the homeodomain recognizes and binds to a specific region of DNA in subordinate genes, thereby activating or repressing their transcription, homeobox genes function as transcription factors. The *MSX-1* or *HOX-7* homeobox gene, for example, codes for a binding protein that induces expression of genes for periocular mesenchyme and, as such, is implicated in normal development of the eye (Monaghan *et al.*, 1991; Beebe, 1994).

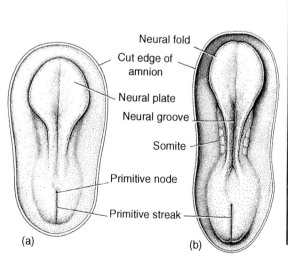

Neural fold
Cut edge of amnion
Neural plate
Neural groove
Somite
Primitive node
Primitive streak

(a)   (b)

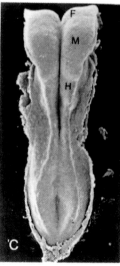

Fig. 17.1 Diagrammatic representation of the dorsal surface of human embryos showing development of the neural plate, neural folds and neural groove. (A) At approximately 19 days of gestation the neural groove is present as a central depression in the neural plate; (B) by day 20 the lateral walls of the neural plate in the mid-region of the embryo have begun to converge and are recognized as the neural folds; (C) SEM of the dorsal surface of a mouse embryo at a developmental stage which corresponds to approximately 20 days' gestation in the human. The neural folds are present in the mid-region of the embryo and the neural groove is present anteriorly and posteriorly. (From: Sadler, T. W. (1990) *Langman's Medical Embryology*, 6th edition, published by Williams and Wilkins, Baltimore.)

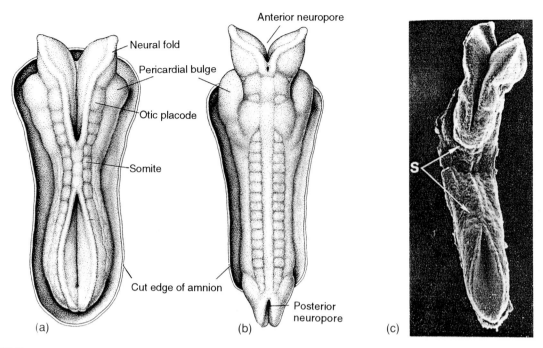

Fig. 17.2 Diagrammatic representation of dorsal view of human embryos at approximately 22 days (a) and 23 days (b) of gestation showing fusion of the neural folds which begins in the mid-region (a) and progresses anteriorly and posteriorly (b); (c) SEM of the dorsal surface of a mouse embryo at a stage corresponding to approximately 22 days' gestation in the human. The neural groove is closing in the cranial (rostral) and caudal directions and is flanked by pairs of somites (S). (From Sadler, T. W. (1990) *Langman's Medical Embryology*, 6th edition, published by Williams and Wilkins, Baltimore.)

DIFFERENTIATION OF THE CENTRAL NERVOUS SYSTEM

Developmentally and functionally the eye is an extension of the central nervous system. In humans the central nervous system differentiates from the ectoderm on the dorsal surface of the developing embryo. The surface ectoderm thickens in the mid-region to form the neural or medullary plate, the cells of which are known as the neural ectoderm. By 18 days of gestation, the neural plate has developed a central depression, the neural groove, and the lateral walls (the so-called neural folds) along the length of the groove grow and converge toward each other (Fig. 17.1). Fusion of the two walls begins in the mid-region of the embryo and progresses both anteriorly and posteriorly, and the developing central nervous system is now recognized as a neural tube

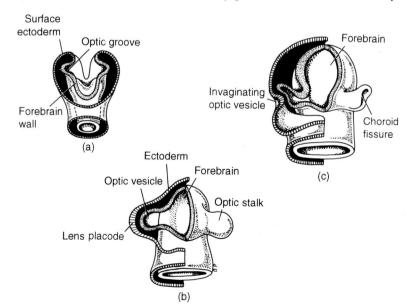

Fig. 17.3 Diagrammatic representation of the cranial region of human embryos at approximately 21 days (a), 27 days (b) and 29 days (c) of gestation. Part of the surface ectoderm has been cut away to reveal the presence of the optic evaginations from the wall of the presumptive forebrain prior to complete closure of the anteriormost region of the neural tube (a), and subsequent development as the optic vesicles (b and c). (From Pansky, B. (1982) *Review of Medical Embryology*, published by McGraw-Hill, Inc., New York.)

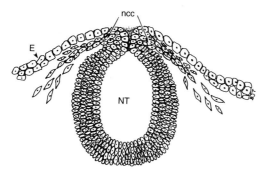

Fig. 17.4 Diagrammatic representation of a cross-section through the dorsal surface of an embryo showing the derivation of neural crest cells (ncc). These cells originate from neuroectoderm located at the crest of the neural folds at about the time the folds fuse to form the neural tube (NT). E = Surface ectoderm. (From Tripathi, B. J., Tripathi, R. C. and Wisdom, J. in Ritch, R., Shields, M. B. and Krupin, T. (eds) (1995) *The Glaucomas*, 2nd edition, published by C. V. Mosby, St Louis.)

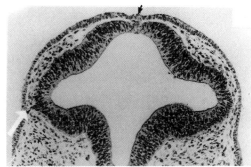

Fig. 17.5 At 3½ weeks of gestation, the optic vesicles appear as hollow hemispherical lateral outgrowths from each side of the forebrain vesicle. Arrow denotes site of the now fused anterior neuropore. (From O'Rahilly, R. and Müller, F. (1992) *Human Embryology and Teratology*, published by Wiley-Liss, New York.)

(Fig. 17.2). However, before closure of the neural tube at the anterior end of the embryo, the neural folds have already developed small lateral grooves which represent the anlage of the future eyes, the optic sulcus (20 days; embryo about 2 mm). The sulcus enlarges to form the optic evaginations (the optic pits internally) which later become the optic vesicles, the convex outer surfaces of which are in contact with the surface ectoderm (Fig. 17.3).

By 24 days (embryo 3 mm) the neural tube remains open only by a small hole, the anterior neuropore. In the human, neuroectodermal cells proliferate from the region of the future crest of the neural folds even before the folds fuse to form the neural tube (Noden, 1982). This produces a population of neural crest cells (Fig. 17.4), which contribute extensively to the development of the eye. The crest cells that remain attached to the neural tube eventually differentiate into the cerebral and spinal ganglia and the roots of the dorsal nerves. However, many of the neural crest cells migrate away from the neural tube and form secondary mesenchyme which differentiates into many body structures including cephalic cartilages, bones and ligaments, leptomeninges, dental papillae, Schwann cells, peripheral sensory and autonomic nerves, ganglia or cranial nerves V, VII, IX and X, spinal ganglia, dermis and melanophores of the skin, as well as many cells of the neuroendocrine system (Tripathi *et al.*, 1995).

THE OPTIC VESICLES

On closure of the neural tube, the optic vesicles enlarge and appear as hollow, symmetrical, hemispherical outgrowths on the lateral side of what is now the forebrain vesicle (Figs 17.3 and 17.5). Dif-

ferential growth is induced because mitoses take place almost entirely in the inner aspect of the neural tube next to the cavity of the primary optic vesicle (ventricular mitoses). The cavity of the hollow optic vesicle communicates with that of the forebrain. Initially, the epithelium of the optic vesicle is high columnar with the nuclei arranged in several layers; later, many layers of cells develop. At first, all of the cells that line the optic vesicle are ciliated on their inner surface; the outer surface of the cells, as well as the inner aspect of the surface ectoderm lying over the vesicle, is covered by a thin basal lamina.

As development proceeds, the breadth of the head increases and so does the distance between the brain and the surface ectoderm. However, the optic vesicle remains in contact with the surface ectoderm and continues to be connected with the forebrain by a constriction, called the optic stalk, most marked dorsally. Meanwhile, the forebrain has developed into the telencephalon (the future cerebral hemispheres) and the diencephalon, and the paired optic stalks arise from the lower region of the side wall of the diencephalon. The cavity of the diencephalon, which will form the third ventricle, is continuous with that of the optic stalk at the region known as the recessus opticus.

Unlike the condition in the adult, the optic vesicles lie laterally and are separated from each other by the broad frontonasal process. In a 19-mm embryo, the direction of growth makes an angle of 65° with the mid-sagittal plane, whereas in the adult the corresponding angle made by the optic nerves is 40°.

At about 27 days of gestation (embryo 4.0–4.5 mm), the surface ectoderm lying over the optic vesicle thickens to form the lens placode (Fig. 17.6), which is surrounded by a thin basal lamina material and is separated from the vesicle by a narrow space that contains fine filamentous material. The

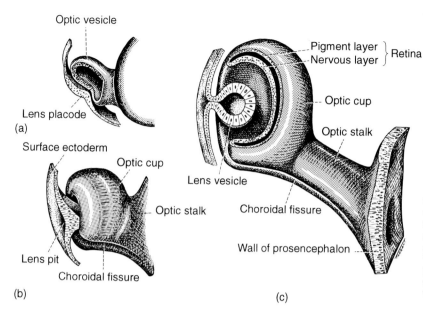

Optic vesicle

Lens placode

(a)

Surface ectoderm

Optic cup

Optic stalk

Lens pit

Choroidal fissure

(b)

Pigment layer ⎫
Nervous layer ⎭ Retina

Optic cup

Optic stalk

Lens vesicle

Choroidal fissure

Wall of prosencephalon

(c)

Fig. 17.6 Diagrammatic representation of development of the human optic cup. The optic vesicle and cup have been partly cut away in (a) and (c) and the lens vesicle is sectioned for clarity. (a) Embryo 4.5 mm; (b) embryo 5.5 mm; (c) embryo 7.5 mm. (From Tripathi, R. C. and Tripathi, B. J. in Davson, H. and Graham, L. T. (eds) (1974) *The Eye*, vol. 5, published by Academic Press, New York.)

interaction of the extracellular elements is thought to induce a gradual invagination of the lens placode and leads to the formation of the lens vesicle. This vesicle initially remains attached to the surface ectoderm by the lens stalk. The formation of the lens vesicle is seen on the surface of the embryo as a small depression, the lens pit or pore. Eventually the lens vesicle separates from the surface ectoderm.

Concurrently, the optic vesicles are developing into optic cups. By 28 days (embryo 7.6–7.8 mm) differential growth and movement of the cells of the optic vesicle cause the temporal and lower walls of the vesicle to move inward against the upper and posterior walls. The two laterally growing edges of the cup eventually meet and fuse. This process of invagination also involves the optic stalk and reduces the lumen of the vesicle to a slit. Where the two laterally growing edges of the cup and the stalk meet ventrally, a fissure results which is known by a variety of names (embryonic, fetal, choroidal or optic fissure).

THE OPTIC FISSURE

The precise events involved in closure of the optic fissure in developing human eyes are not documented, even though this event is crucial to normal development of the eye and optic nerve, and defects in this process result in colobomas, microphthalmia and orbital cysts. However, several studies of experimental animal models have provided more detailed accounts (Geeraets, 1976; Suzuki, Shirai and Majima, 1988; Hero, 1990). The margin of the fissure comprises the inner neural retina that consists of several layers of neuroblastic cells; it is continuous

with the single cell layer of the retinal pigment epithelium at the 'folding point' (Geeraets, 1976). The entire configuration is surrounded by a basal lamina. In the earliest stages of fusion the outer layer of the cup (the future retinal pigment epithelium) becomes inverted into the fissure (Fig. 17.7). These less differentiated cells represent the first site at which the fusion process takes place and, although they are believed to be pigment epithelial cells, they develop melanosomes only after fusion has occurred (Geeraets, 1976; Suzuki, Shirai and Majima, 1988; Hero, 1990). Separation of the fused inner and outer

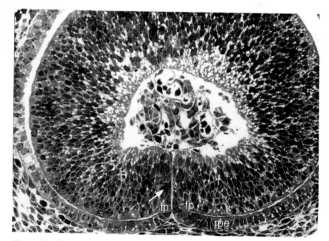

Fig. 17.7 Coronal section of mouse eye late on day 11 of gestation, showing the beginning of closure of the optic fissure. The retinal pigment epithelium (rpe) is inverted at the site of the fissure. R = retina; fp = folding point; arrow denotes cell death. Light micrograph (scale bar = 10 μm). (From Hero, I. (1990), *Invest. Ophthalmol. Vis. Sci.*, **31**, 197; by permission of the Association for Research in Vision and Ophthalmology.)

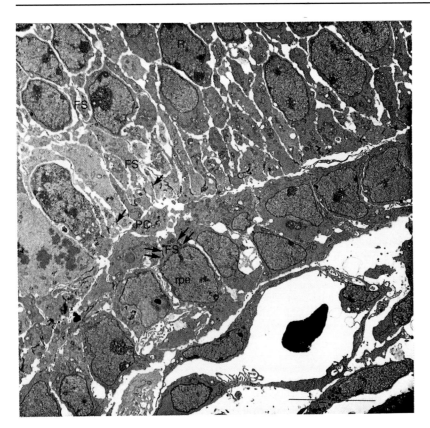

Fig. 17.8 Section through the fusion site (FS) showing the establishment of junctional complexes between adjacent retinal pigment epithelial cells (double arrows) and between adjacent cells of the outer retina (single arrows). A phagocytic cell (PC) is present in the residual ventricular space. Survey transmission electron micrograph (scale bar = 10 μm). (From Hero, I. (1990), *Invest. Ophthalmol. Vis. Sci.*, **31**, 197, by permission of the Association for Research in Vision and Ophthalmology.)

layers that must occur before the opposing margins of the fissure fuse, necessitates the breakdown of the existing intercellular junctions at the folding point (Hero, 1990). As the margins of the optic cup approach each other multifocal appositional contacts develop. Initially the basal lamina is double at these foci but it soon disintegrates and eventually disappears completely. Cytoplasmic processes from the cells lining the fissure form contacts where the basal lamina has disintegrated, and develop junctional complexes. As the neural retina separates from the retinal pigment epithelium at the folding point, a continuous row of intermediate-type junctional complexes develop between adjacent cells of the outermost layer (the presumptive photoreceptors) (Fig. 17.8). Adjacent retinal pigment epithelial cells become joined by zonulae occludentes at their apices, as well as by gap and intermediate junctions along their lateral borders. The fusion process is also characterized by programmed cell death (apoptosis) in both the neural retina and pigment epithelial layers, as well as by the presence of amoeboid-like cells that are actively phagocytic. The amoeboid cells are present in the residual space at the site of fusion and occasionally away from this area as well as within the retina. They are also seen frequently in the primary vitreous. Although the origin of these cells

is not known, it has been suggested that they develop from neuroepithelial cells (Hero, 1990).

Mesenchymal cells of mesodermal origin penetrate the optic cup through the embryonic fissure and presumably contribute to the organization of the primary vitreous. At this stage the optic cup is composed of two layers which are continuous with each other at the margin of the cup and the fissures. The inner layer is much thicker than the outer and will differentiate into all of the cells that constitute the sensory retina. The outer layer will give rise to the retinal pigment epithelium only.

17.2 CORNEA

PRIMARY CORNEAL STROMA

The development of the cornea is triggered by the separation of the lens vesicle from the surface ectoderm at 33 days of gestation (O'Rahilly, 1983). At this stage the ectoderm consists of two layers of epithelial cells that rest on a thin basal lamina. Studies in developing chick embryos have shown that detachment of the lens vesicle induces the basal layer of epithelial cells to secrete collagen fibrils and glycosaminoglycans to fill the space between the lens and the corneal epithelium (Hay and Revel, 1969;

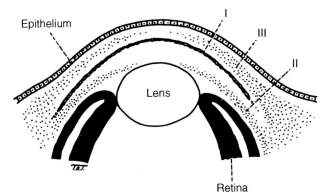

Fig. 17.9 Diagrammatic representation of the three successive waves of ingrowth of neural crest cells associated with differentiation of the anterior chamber. I First wave forms corneal endothelium; II, second wave forms iris and pupillary membrane; III, third wave forms keratocytes. (Modified from Tripathi, R. C. and Tripathi, B. J. in Davson, H. and Graham, L. T. (eds), (1974) *The Eye*, vol. 5, published by Academic Press, New York.)

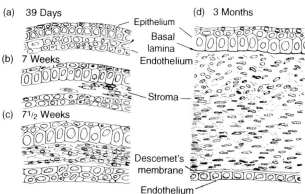

Fig. 17.10 Diagrammatic representation of development of central cornea. (a) At 39 days' gestation a two-layered epithelium rests on its basal lamina and is separated from the endothelium, which consists of two to three layers of cells, by a narrow space; (b) at 7 weeks mesenchymal cells at the periphery migrate between the epithelium and endothelium; (c) by 7½ weeks the mesenchymal cells (future keratocytes) are arranged as four to five incomplete layers and a few collagen fibrils are present; (d) by 3 months of gestation, the epithelium consists of two to three layers of cells, the stroma has 25–30 layers of keatocytes that are arranged more regularly in the posterior half, and a thin, uneven Descemet's membrane is present between the most posterior keratocyte and the now monolayer endothelium. (From Ozanics, V. and Jakobiec, F. A. in Duane, T. D. and Jaeger, E. A. (eds) (1982) *Biomedical Foundations of Ophthalmology*, vol. 1, published by Harper and Row, Philadelphia.)

Dodson and Hay, 1971). The extracellular matrix molecules constitute the primary corneal stroma, which contains only macrophages that engulf the debris remaining after detachment of the lens vesicle. In the human embryo, however, the primary stroma is poorly organized and consists of fine filaments, amorphous material and only a few collagen fibrils. Mesenchymal cells derived from neural crest, which are situated at the margins of the rim of the optic cup, migrate into the developing eye beneath the basal lamina of the corneal epithelium, and form the primordial corneal endothelium. These cells use both the posterior surface of the primary stroma and the fibronectin-containing basal lamina of the anterior lens cells as the substrate for their migration. This event marks the first of three successive waves of ingrowth of neural crest cells into the developing anterior segment of the eye (Fig. 17.9).

CORNEAL EPITHELIUM

In the 17–18-mm embryo (about 40 days gestation), the cornea consists of a superficial squamous cell layer and a basal cuboidal epithelial cell layer, a primary stroma, and a double layer of flattened endothelial cells posteriorly (Fig. 17.10). Scanning electron microscopy shows that by the seventh week of gestation the superficial layer of epithelial cells is pentagonal or hexagonal in shape with a maximal diameter of 10–20 μm (Sellheyer and Spitznas, 1988a–d). Microvilli and fine microplicae are already present on the anterior surface (Fig. 17.11). Ultrastructurally these cells are electron-dense, flat, and contain many glycogen granules. Very rarely,

desmosomes connect the superficial cells with the underlying cuboidal cells (Sellheyer and Spitznas, 1988d). Between the second and third months of gestation most of the superficial cells increase in diameter to 15–20 μm and are covered by microvilli and fine microplicae that are distributed homogeneously over the cell surface. These cells are more electron lucent than previously and do not have as much glycogen. A large number of desmosomes now connect this cell layer with the underlying cells. Beginning at the fourth month, three types of superficial cells can be distinguished: small cells with the largest number of microvilli/microplicae; medium-sized cells with intermediate numbers of surface projections; and large cells with the fewest microvilli and microplicae. These last cells are electron lucent and are believed to be in the process of desquamation (Sellheyer and Spitznas, 1988d). Thus the surface morphology of the human corneal epithelium attains an almost adult appearance by the time the eyelids open at 5–6 months of gestation.

STROMA

Further development of the corneal stroma is preceded by the growth of another wave of

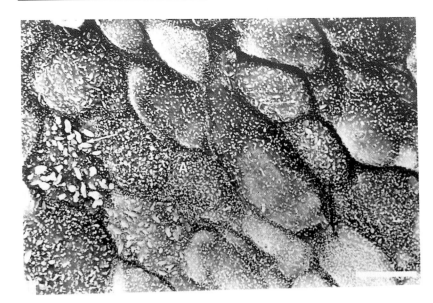

Fig. 17.11 SEM of the anterior surface of the corneal epithelium at the seventh week of gestation. Most cells are covered with fine microvilli and microplicae (A) and a few have coarse microvilli (arrow). Scale bar = 10 μm. (From Sellheyer, K. and Spitznas, M. (1988) *Graefes Arch. Clin. Exp. Ophthalmol.*, **226**, 482, with permission.)

mesenchymal cells from the rim of the optic cup. This proceeds in two directions (Fig. 17.9). At about the 19 mm stage, the cells of the posterior extension grow into the space between the lens epithelium and corneal endothelium, and are destined to form the primary pupillary membrane (see p. 644). At about the same time the extracellular matrix of the primary stroma swells, apparently as a result of hydration of hyaluronic acid, to make space available for the next migratory wave of cells. At approximately 7 weeks gestation (embryo 22–24 mm) the anterior extension of mesenchymal cells migrates between the corneal epithelium and endothelium and will contribute to the further development of the corneal stroma (Fig. 17.10). The central region of the stroma is initially acellular. The ingrowing cells differentiate into stromal fibroblasts or keratocytes that will actively secrete the type I collagen fibrils and the matrix of the mature (secondary) corneal stroma.

Initially, the secondary stroma is rich in fibronectin but this disappears as the mesenchymal cells come to occupy the entire region. The stroma soon attains its maximum width, which is approximately double the normal postembryonic width; this decreases because of dehydration, especially of hyaluronic acid, and compression of the connective tissue. The stellate mesenchymal cells that are dispersed randomly in the stroma gradually change into spindle-shaped cells that are oriented parallel to the corneal surface. This morphogenesis begins posteriorly in the cornea and is followed rapidly by the appearance of collagen fibrils. However, glycosaminoglycans rich in carboxyl and sulphate residues are synthesized before the formation of collagen fibrils. Keratan sulphate is not detected until 6 months of gestation. The collagen fibrils are organized as lamellae, each of which continues to grow by the formation of additional fibrils (interstitial growth); at the same time successive layers of lamellae are formed (appositional growth). Because the lamellae increase in length as well as in width, the diameter and the thickness of the cornea increases.

Centrally, the corneal stroma of an 8-week-old human embryo (30 mm) consists of five to eight rows of cells (Fig. 17.10). The most posterior layers of the stroma are confluent at the periphery with the condensed mesenchymal tissue of the future sclera (see p. 628). The number of stromal cell layers increases rapidly and by the 35 mm stage the cornea consists of two layers of epithelial cells, a stroma with 15 layers of cells and scant collagen fibrils, and an endothelium that is still arranged as a double layer of cells.

DESCEMET'S MEMBRANE AND ENDOTHELIUM

By the third month (embryo 63 mm), the endothelium in the central region of the cornea has become a single layer of flattened cells that rest on their interrupted basal lamina – the future Descemet's membrane (Fig. 17.10). At this stage of development the basal lamina is composed of an electron-lucent zone (lamina lucida, 37.5 nm thick) adjacent to the endothelial cell layer and an electron-dense band (lamina densa, 36.7 nm thick) towards the corneal stroma (Murphy, Alvarado and Juster, 1984). Further differentiation and growth of Descemet's membrane are accomplished by the sequential secretion of a series of individual 'membrane-units' to form a

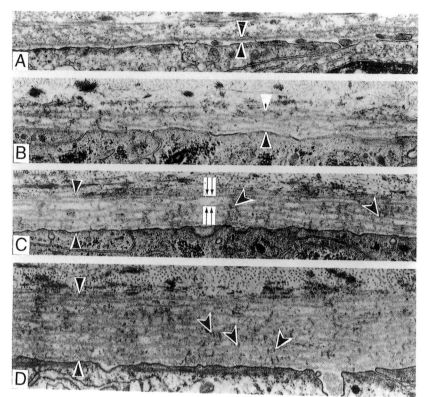

Fig. 17.12 Stages in development of Descemet's membrane as seen by transmission electron microscopy. In each micrograph the stroma is above, the corneal endothelium is below and Descemet's membrane is demarcated by arrowheads. Original magnification ×20 750. (A) In the 12-week-old fetus Descemet's membrane is thin and continuous, and consists of an electron-dense layer adjacent to the stroma and an electron-lucent layer next to the endothelium; (B) approximately three electron-dense layers, each separated by an electron-lucent area, are present in the 16-week-old fetus; (C) by 19 weeks of gestation, the number of lamellae has increased to five. Narrow interlamellar zones are cross-linked by thin linear filaments (arrow) whereas wide zones are devoid of such structures (double arrows); (D) At 26 weeks of gestation Descemet's membrane consists of approximately ten layers with many cross-linking filaments (single arrows). (From Murphy, C., Alvarado, J. and Juster, R. (1984) *Invest. Ophthalmol. Vis. Sci.*, **25**, 1402, by permission of the Association for Research in Vision and Ophthalmology.)

multilayered structure (Fig. 17.12). The process takes place rapidly because, although only one such layer is discernible at 12 weeks of gestation, approximately 10 layers are present by the sixth month and 30–40 layers at birth. At the same time as the deposition of membrane-units is occurring; short thin linear filaments (about 170 nm long and 40 nm in diameter) are laid down perpendicular to and between adjacent layers. It is suggested that these filaments function as cross-linking bridges which bind and pull together the adjacent membrane-unit layers and, during the last trimester of gestation, cause compaction of this region of Descemet's membrane (Murphy *et al.*, 1984). Transmission electron microscopy of flat sections of this region of Descemet's membrane reveals that the fibrils are arranged in a hexagonal fashion and interconnected with nodes and internodes of electron-dense material, thus producing a lamellar pattern of equilateral triangles with sides of about 110 nm. Because of its unique organization, this anterior third of Descemet's membrane is recognized as the 'fetal' banded zone and attains a maximum thickness of about 3 μm at birth. In postnatal life a homogeneous fibrillogranular material, the so-called posterior non-banded zone, constitutes Descemet's membrane, which continues to thicken with age (Tripathi and Tripathi, 1984).

The apices of the endothelial cells are joined by zonulae occludentes in the middle of the fourth month, which corresponds to the onset of production of aqueous humour by the ciliary processes, and the middle layer of wing cells in the epithelium develop. At the sixth month of gestation Descemet's membrane is demarcated clearly, and the stroma consists of an immature extracellular matrix that includes collagen fibrils and numerous active keratocytes (Ozanics and Jakobiec, 1982; Tripathi, Tripathi and Wisdom, 1995).

BOWMAN'S ZONE

Bowman's zone of the anterior stroma is not formed until late in the fourth month of gestation. This region is always acellular; it is presumed that the most superficial keratocytes synthesize and lay down the ground substance and collagen fibrils as they migrate posteriorly in the stroma. What contribution, if any, is made by the primitive epithelium to the development of Bowman's zone is unknown. At this stage of development (17–18 weeks' gestation) the basal lamina of the corneal epithelium consists of a relatively thin lamina lucida (average thickness 41.68 nm) and a fully developed lamina densa (Fig. 17.13). Hemidesmosomes and anchoring filaments are developed only partially. The filaments (average length 474 nm and diameter 17.6 nm) arise at the

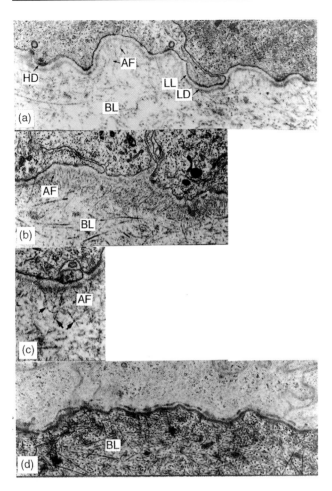

Fig. 17.13 Stages of development of the basal lamina of the corneal epithelium as revealed by transmission electron microscopy (original magnification ×25 000). (a) At 18 weeks of gestation the basal lamina consists of a thin lamina lucida (LL) and a fully developed lamina densa (LD). Anchoring filaments (AF) and hemidesmosomes (HD) are also well developed. BL = Bowman's layer. (b) In the 26-week-old fetus the number of anchoring filaments (AF, shown at higher magnification ×35 000) in (c) has increased and more collagen fibrils are present in Bowman's layer (BL). (d) At one year after birth, the lamina densa is thicker than in the fetal cornea, and densely packed collagen fibrils are present in Bowman's layer (BL). (From Alvarado, J., Murphy, C. and Juster, R. (1983) *Invest. Ophthalmol. Vis. Sci.*, **24**, 1015, by permission of the Association for Research in Vision and Ophthalmology.)

basal surface of the epithelial cells, traverse the lamina densa and lucida and terminate in Bowman's layer (Alvarado, Murphy and Juster, 1983). By 26 weeks of gestation the anchoring filaments with a typical adult appearance are present, especially at the site of hemidesmosomes (Fig. 17.13). At birth the filaments and fibrils are already intermingled with the fully developed collagenous tissue of Bowman's layer (Alvarado, Murphy and Juster, 1983).

The diameter of the unfixed human cornea

increases from 2 mm at 12 weeks' gestation to 3.5 mm at 15 weeks, 4.5 mm at 17 weeks, 5.5 mm at 21 weeks and 9.3 mm at 35 weeks (Ehlers *et al.*, 1968). Once the adult size is attained the turnover and replacement of collagen fibrils is normally extremely slow.

17.3 SCLERA

The sclera is formed by mesenchymal cells that condense around the optic cup. The mesenchymal cells are derived, for the most part, from neural crest cells (Tripathi and Tripathi, 1995). In mammals the caudal region of the sclera is probably derived from paraxial mesoderm because, at the time when neural crest cells are migrating from the neural folds, the caudomedial surface of the optic cup is apposed by mesodermal cells (Noden, 1982). This apposition is maintained throughout the period of crest cell migration and of the development of the cranial and pontine flexures (Figs 17.14 and 17.15).

EARLY DEVELOPMENT

The development of the sclera commences anteriorly before 6.5 weeks of gestation and gradually extends posteriorly (Fig. 17.16). At this stage, eight or nine parallel layers of cells are evident around the rim of the optic cup (Sellheyer and Spitznas, 1988b). Postequatorially, the cells are organized more randomly and the tissue has a more reticular appearance. However, the cells at both sites contain many free ribosomes (often as polyribosomes), a small amount of rough endoplasmic reticulum filled with a flocculent material and a poorly developed Golgi apparatus. In addition, endoplasmic reticulum devoid of ribosomes is associated with the cell plasmalemma and is thought to be of significance for extrusion of procollagen (Sellheyer and Spitznas, 1988b). Glycogen granules and lipid vacuoles, which are the initial energy source, are more numerous in the anteriorly placed cells than in those located around the posterior pole. Occasionally, punctate junctional complexes are present where long cytoplasmic processes of adjacent cells contact each other. Patches of immature collagen fibrils (diameter 27–29 nm) are either associated with the plasma membranes or are distributed randomly in the wide intercellular spaces. No deposits of elastin are present at this early stage in the development of the sclera.

SCLERAL DEMARCATION

By the middle of the seventh week of gestation demarcation of the sclera from the surrounding

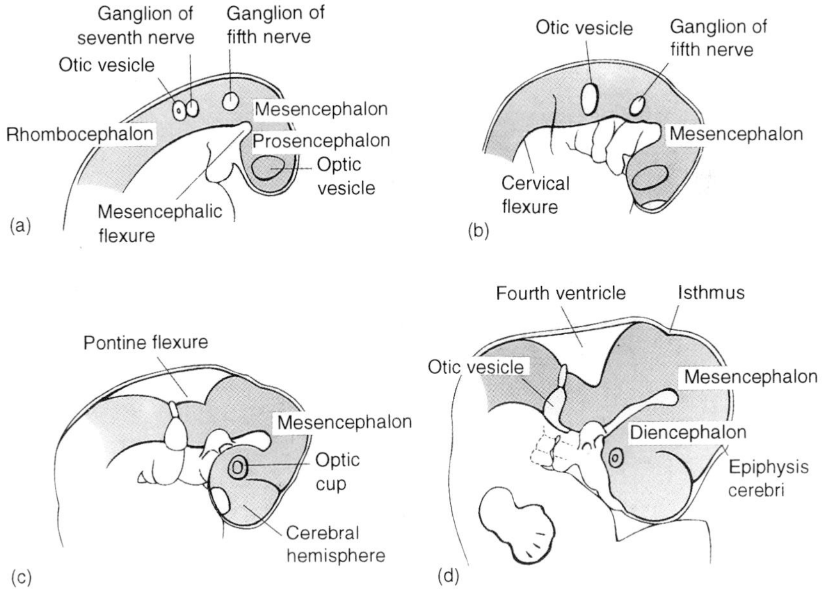

Ganglion of seventh nerve
Ganglion of fifth nerve
Otic vesicle
Rhombocephalon
Mesencephalon
Prosencephalon
Optic vesicle
Mesencephalic flexure
(a)

Otic vesicle
Ganglion of fifth nerve
Mesencephalon
Cervical flexure
(b)

Pontine flexure
Mesencephalon
Optic cup
Cerebral hemisphere
(c)

Fourth ventricle
Isthmus
Otic vesicle
Mesencephalon
Diencephalon
Epiphysis cerebri
(d)

Fig. 17.14 The right lateral side of the embryonic brain at (a) 3½ weeks, (b) 4 weeks, (c) 5 weeks and (d) 6 weeks of gestation, showing the successive development of the mesencephalic, cervical and pontine flexures which bring the caudiomedial surface of the optic cup in apposition with mesodermal tissue of the embryo. (From O'Rahilly, R. and Müller, F. (1992) *Human Embryology and Teratology*, published by Wiley-Liss, New York.)

tissues is apparent (Fig. 17.17). The number of cell layers anteriorly increases to 15 with the increase in cell numbers through mitosis. Towards the choroid the cells are flatter, more elongated, and arranged more compactly than those of the outer aspect of the sclera. The rough endoplasmic reticulum is well developed, especially in the perinuclear cytoplasm where it is associated with the Golgi apparatus. This region of the cytoplasm also contains numerous glycogen granules and lipid vacuoles. The amount of collagen in the intercellular space has increased and the average diameter is now 30–40 nm. Immature elastin deposits, consisting only of microfibrils with a diameter of 10–12 nm, are also present. As the deposition of extracellular matrix components increases, the cytoplasmic processes of neighbouring cells lose contact with each other. The cells in the posterior region of the differentiating sclera resemble those situated anteriorly at the earlier stage of development. Thus the sclera develops not only

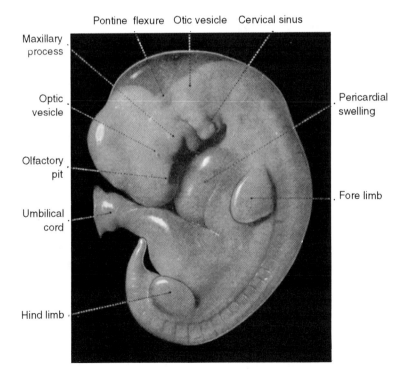

Pontine flexure **Otic vesicle** **Cervical sinus**
Maxillary process
Optic vesicle
Olfactory pit
Umbilical cord
Hind limb
Pericardial swelling
Fore limb

Fig. 17.15 Photograph of a human embryo at approximately 5 weeks of gestation from the left side, showing the flexure of the body.

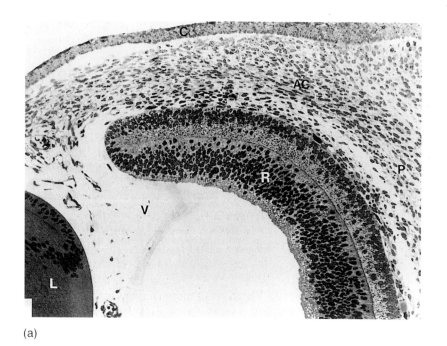

(a)

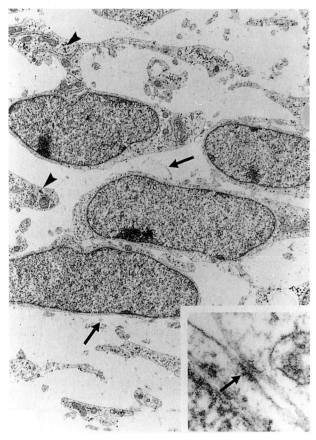

(b)

Fig. 17.16 The peripheral region of the optic cup in a human embryo at 6.4 weeks of gestation. (a) The periocular mesenchyme condenses as parallel layers of cells (AC), marking the beginning of the development of the sclera. Posteriorly (P) the cells are still arranged loosely. C = primitive conjunctiva; R = retina; V = anterior vitreous (detached artifactually); L = lens. Light micrograph, original magnification ×250. (b) The intercellular spaces contain patches of collagen (arrows) and punctate junctional complexes (inset, arrow) are present between juxtaposed cells. Arrowheads indicate glycogen granules. Transmission electron micrographs, original magnification ×6300, inset ×50 000. (From Sellheyer, K. and Spitznas, M. (1988) *Graefes Arch. Clin. Exp. Ophthalmol.*, **226**, 89, with permission.)

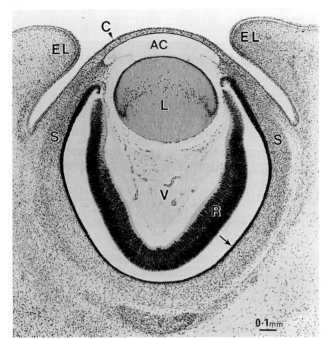

in an anteroposterior direction but also, beginning with this stage, from the inside outward (Sellheyer and Spitznas, 1988b).

During the ninth week of gestation the cells in the posterior region develop long cytoplasmic processes and their long axes become arranged parallel to the choriocapillaris. The amount of collagen in this region increases markedly and the diameter (48 nm) of individual microfibrils is comparable to that seen in the anterior sclera. In addition, deposits of elastin are now recognizable. The scleral fibroblasts also synthesize glycosaminoglycans (dermatan sulphate and chondroitin sulphate). By the eleventh week the differences in the arrangement of the inner and outer portion of the sclera anteriorly are no longer apparent, and the cells have attained an almost adult appearance. At about the same time some undifferentiated mesenchymal cells migrate between the nerve fibres in the optic nerve. These cells become oriented transversely and, through their synthetic activity, form the beginnings of the lamina cribrosa (Fig. 17.18). At the beginning of the fourth month, the sclera in both the pre- and postequatorial regions consists of 30 cell layers; this increases to 50 layers by the sixth month, after which time no further mitoses are seen (Sellheyer and Spitznas, 1988b). The amount of extracellular matrix also increases; the collagen fibrils have a diameter of 100 nm or more

Fig. 17.17 Section through the eye of a 30 mm human embryo (almost 8 weeks of gestation). The number of cell layers in the anterior sclera (S) has increased and its demarcation from the choroid is proceeding posteriorly. C = Cornea; AC = anterior chamber; L = lens; R = neural retina (separated artifactually from the retinal pigment epithelium); EL = eyelids; arrow shows the limbus. Light micrograph, original magnification ×84. (From Tripathi, R. C. and Tripathi, B. J. in Davson, H. and Graham, L. T. (eds) (1974) *The Eye*, vol. 5, published by Academic Press, New York.)

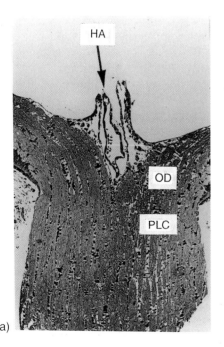

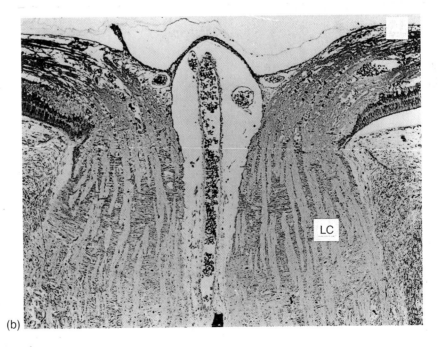

(a)　　　　　　　(b)

Fig. 17.18 Development of the lamina cribrosa. (a) At 12 weeks of gestation, the primitive lamina cribrosa (PLC) consists of mesenchymal cells that have migrated between the nerve fibres in the optic disc (OD) and are oriented transversely. These cells are actively secreting collagen fibrils. HA = Hyaloid artery. Light micrograph, original magnification ×80. (b) By 21 weeks of gestation the lamina cribrosa (LC) is well defined and distinct from the adjacent compact sclera. Light micrograph, original magnification ×80. (From Rhodes, R. H. (1978) *Am. J. Anat.*, **153**, 601, with permission.)

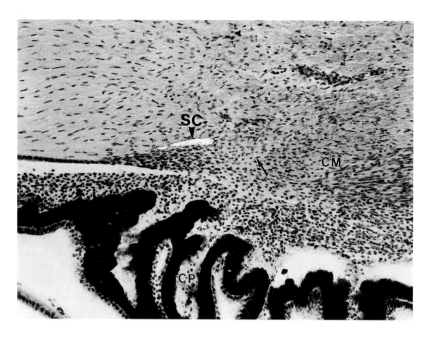

Fig. 17.19 Angular region of a 6-month fetus. The sceral spur (arrow) is present as a wedge-shaped protrusion from the inner aspect of the anterior sclera and provides the site of attachment for the meridional fibres of the developing ciliary muscle (CM). SC = Canal of Schlemm with trabecular meshwork bordering the anterior chamber; CP = ciliary processes. Light micrograph, original magnification ×260. (From Tripathi, R. C. and Tripathi, B. J. in Duane, T. D. and Jaeger, E. A. (eds) (1982) *Biomedical Foundations of Ophthalmology*, vol. 1, published by Harper and Row, Philadelphia.)

and the deposits of elastin have developed their characteristic electron-lucent central cores.

THE SCLERAL SPUR

At approximately 4 months (embryo 70 mm) the inner aspect of the anterior sclera (the inner limbus) develops a fibrous, wedge-shaped protrusion, the scleral spur (Fig. 17.19). The appearance of this structure corresponds to the retraction of the developing ciliary muscle fibres. By the middle of the seventh month the anterior ends of the longitudinal ciliary muscle fibres have established their insertion into the scleral spur. The collagen fibrils and elastic tissue of the spur are oriented circularly (Tripathi *et al.*, 1995).

VASCULAR PLEXUSES

The deep and intrascleral vascular plexuses, the aqueous veins and the collector channels that traverse the sclera at the limbal region are first recognizable at about 12 weeks of gestation. These vessels differentiate from primitive mesoderm, but the factors that govern their arrangement into the fully formed, intricate plexuses are not known (Ozanics and Jakobiec, 1982; Tripathi *et al.*, 1995).

GROWTH FACTORS AND POST-NATAL GROWTH

Because the sclera defines the physical size and shape of the globe, the factors that regulate its development have a major role in defining the ultimate refractive power of the eye. The mRNAs encoding insulin-like growth factor (IGF)-I and -II are both present in the neural crest cells that are destined to form the sclera (Han, D'Ercole and Lund, 1987). However, IGF-II mRNA, which is expressed intensely by the mesenchymal cells as they differentiate into scleral fibroblasts, is not present in the mature sclera or cornea or in the retina (Cuthbertson *et al.*, 1989). Furthermore, the expression of receptors for IGF-II by the mesenchymal cells parallels that of its mRNA which suggests that this growth factor has an autocrine function during development of the sclera.

After birth subsequent growth of the sclera is probably under the control of growth factors that are synthesized and released from the retina (Tripathi *et al.*, 1991). Neonatal deprivation of formed visual input induces myopia although the molecular basis for this regulation is not known. Transduction of a signal, probably a peptide hormone, produced by light falling on the developing neural retina may act as a tissue-specific stimulus for regulation of the growth of the sclera (Stone *et al.*, 1988). The action of light may also prompt the termination of gene expression for IGF-II and its receptor in the sclera. The precise role of other growth modulatory molecules, especially scleral autocrine factor (SAF) and platelet-drived growth factor (PDGF), in the control of scleral fibroblast proliferation in developing human eyes remains to be determined (Tripathi *et al.*, 1991). Experimental studies *in vitro* indicate that SAF has an autocrine function and could be identical, or closely related, to PDGF (Fujioka *et al.*, 1989; Watanabe *et al.*, 1989).

17.4 ANTERIOR CHAMBER AND AQUEOUS OUTFLOW PATHWAY

The slit-like space that results from the ingrowth of the first wave of mesenchymal cells (the future corneal endothelium) and the posterior extension of the second wave of cells (the primary pupillary membrane) from the rim of the optic cup forms the beginnings of the anterior chamber of the eye (Fig. 17.9). Further development of the anterior chamber depends on the differentiation of the structures that border it – namely lateral displacement and deepening of the angular region, differentiation of the angular tissues, differential growth of the cornea that increases its spherical curvature relative to the sclera and the eventual location of the lens behind the developing iris.

ANGLE OF THE ANTERIOR CHAMBER

By approximately 7 weeks of gestation (embryo 22–24 mm), the angle of the anterior chamber is occupied by a nest of loosely organized undifferentiated mesenchymal cells that are destined to develop into the trabecular meshwork (Fig. 17.20). The posterior aspect of the angle is defined by mesodermal cells that are developing into the vascular channels of the pupillary membrane (see p. 659), as well as by loose mesenchymal cells and the pigment epithelium of the forward-growing optic cup which will form the iris (see p. 644). Anteriorly the corneal endothelial cells extend to the angle recess and by, the 15th week

of gestation, these cells meet the anterior surface of the developing iris, thus demarcating the angle of the anterior chamber. At this stage the corneal endothelium lining the chamber angle may be composed of several cell layers, but the cells flatten toward the root of the iris. By the fifth month, the anterior chamber angle is rounded and this configuration persists until about the seventh month. The angle recess shows a progressive deepening that commences at about the third month of gestation (Fig. 17.21) and probably continues for a considerable time after birth (up to the age of 4 years).

As development proceeds the recess of the anterior chamber angle appears to move posteriorly as a result of a differential growth rate of the various tissue elements (Ozanics and Jakobiec, 1982; Tripathi *et al.*, 1995). This process results in the repositioning of the ciliary muscle and processes, which initially overlapped the developing trabecular meshwork, and the entire ciliary body becomes located posteriorly to the meshwork. By 7 months gestation the deepest part of the angle has receded to the level of Schlemm's canal but at the time of birth the apex of the angle is located beyond the canal and is at the level of the scleral spur. The angle at birth differs from that in adulthood because more of the uveal portion of the trabecular meshwork is located anterior to the ciliary muscle and in front of the scleral spur. Additionally, the angle is open to the anterior face of the ciliary body. With the posterior displacement of the angle, the apex (the ciliary band of gonioscopists) is formed primarily by the anterior face of the oblique and circular muscle fibres. The anterior face of the meridional muscle bundle is obscured by the scleral spur (Tripathi *et al.*, 1995).

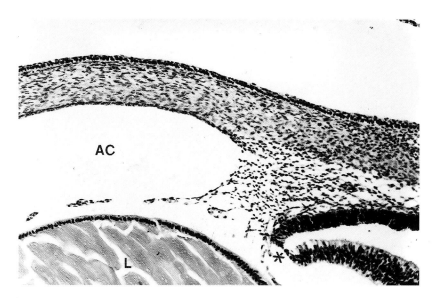

Fig. 17.20 Light micrograph of an eye of an 11-week-old fetus in meridional section. At this stage the angular region is ill defined and occupied by loosely arranged, spindle-shaped cells. The canal of Schlemm is unrecognizable, and the ciliary muscles and processes are not yet formed. The ciliary processes will develop from the neural ectoderm at the rim of the optic cup (asterisk). The corneal endothelium appears continuous with the cellular covering of the primitive iris. AC = Anterior chamber; L = lens. Original magnification ×230. (From Tripathi, R. C. and Tripathi, B. J. in Duane, T. D. and Jaeger, E. A. (eds) (1982) *Biomedical Foundations of Ophthalmology*, vol. 1, published by Harper and Row, Philadelphia.)

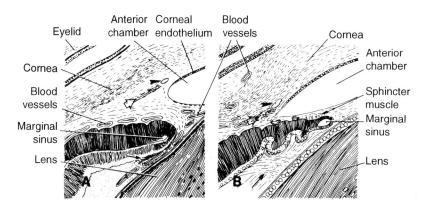

Fig. 17.21 Diagrammatic representation of progressive deepening of the anterior chamber angle in relation to surrounding tissues. (A) At three months' gestation the corneal endothelium extends nearly to the angle recess. An incipient Schlemm's canal (arrowhead) and a more posterior scleral spur condensation (hollow arrow) are present. The pigment epithelium of the forward-growing ectodermal optic cup is indented by blood vessels. (B) At 4 months the angle recess has deepened and the corneal endothelium has receded somewhat. A small aggregate of differentiating sphincter muscle fibre is seen near to the tip of the optic cup. The angle recess is occupied by loose connective tissue separated by many spaces. The iris is further developed and now has a thick root. (From Ozanics, V. and Jakobiec, F. A. in Duane, T. D. and Jaeger, E. A. (eds) (1982) *Biomedical Foundations of Ophthalmology*, vol. 1, published by Harper and Row, Philadelphia.)

TRABECULAR MESHWORK

By the fourth month of gestation the primordium of the trabecular meshwork is recognizable as an approximately triangular or wedge-shaped structure that consists of undifferentiated mesenchymal cells of neural crest origin (Fig. 17.22). The anterior apex of this cell mass lies between the corneal endothelium and the deeper stroma. At this stage the corneal endothelium covers most, if not all, of the anterior face of the trabecular meshwork, thus delineating its

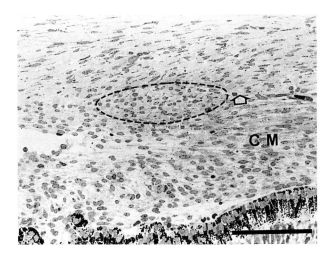

Fig. 17.22 The iridocorneal angle at 16 weeks of gestation in meridional section. The future trabecular meshwork (interrupted line) is distinguishable from the surrounding tissues because the differentiating mesenchymal cells have small rounded nuclei. CM = Ciliary muscle; hollow arrow = future scleral spur. Light micrograph (scale bar = 100 μm). (From Hamanaka, T., Bill, A., Ichinohasma, R. and Ishida, T. (1992) *Exp. Eye Res.*, **55**, 479, with permission.)

border from the anterior chamber. Posteriorly there is no demarcation between those mesenchymal cells destined to form the meshwork proper and those which will differentiate into the ciliary muscle. Based on the shape of the nuclei of the cells in these two regions a demarcation between the corneoscleral region, which has spindle-shaped nuclei, and the ciliary–iris region, which has round nuclei, is thought to be discernible by the 15th week of gestation. There is pronounced mitotic activity in both tissues (Reme and d'Épinay, 1981).

The mesenchymal cells destined to form the trabecular meshwork are attached loosely to each other without junctional specializations and form a reticular network. Electron microscopy reveals that their cytoplasm contains dilated cisternae of endoplasmic reticulum, conspicuous ribosomes and distinct lysosomes (Fig. 17.23). Small patches of collagen fibrils are recognizable between the cells and abundant unmyelinated nerve fibres are also present. Between the fourth and eighth months, the cells elongate and continue to secrete collagen fibrils, elastic tissue and basal lamina material (Reme and d'Épinay, 1981). The cells will also secrete the glycosaminoglycans, proteoglycans, and glycoproteins of the extracellular matrix of the trabecular beams.

The next major change occurs after the development of the scleral spur between the 22nd and 24th fetal weeks (Reme and d'Épinay, 1981). At this time the trabecular meshwork can be divided into the outer corneoscleral portion, which is oriented longitudinally, and the inner uveal meshwork, which has a net-like arrangement. The trabecular beams of the deeper corneoscleral region now have a core of

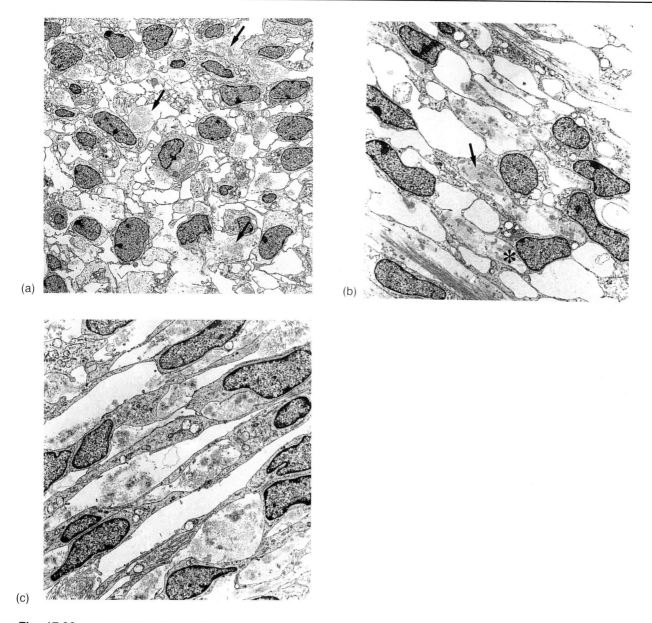

Fig. 17.23 Differentiation of the trabecular meshwork as revealed by transmission electron microscopy. (a) At 15 weeks of gestation patches of collagen fibrils (arrows) are present among the loosely connected mesenchymal cells. (Original magnification × 1666). (b) The corneoscleral trabeculae at 22–24 weeks of gestation. The trabeculae are now oriented longitudinally, and the trabecular cells have numerous cytoplasmic processes. Patches of collagen fibrils (arrow) and elastic tissue (asterisk) are seen in the intercellular spaces. (Original magnification ×2550.) (c) The corneoscleral meshwork at 28–30 weeks of gestation. The trabecular beams consist of a core of collagen fibrils and elastic tissue covered by cells that rest on a tenuous basement membrane. The cortical zone of the beams has not yet formed. (Original magnification ×2500.) (From Reme, C. and d'Épinay, S. L. (1981) *Doc. Ophthalmol.*, **51**, 214, with permission.)

collagen fibrils and elastic tissue surrounded by trabecular cells which rest on a tenuous basal lamina, the future cortical zone. The cells are connected through numerous cytoplasmic processes and align themselves along the framework of extracellular matrix materials that they have secreted. The intercellular spaces enlarge and interconnect to become organized as the intertrabecular and intratrabecular

spaces. However, the uveal meshwork, especially the posterior layer, still consists of mesenchymal cells that are oriented randomly and patches of collagen fibrils scattered in the extracellular compartment. The uveal portion of the meshwork is organized more loosely than is the deeper scleral meshwork. The final development of the shape and orientation of the individual trabecular beams probably depends on

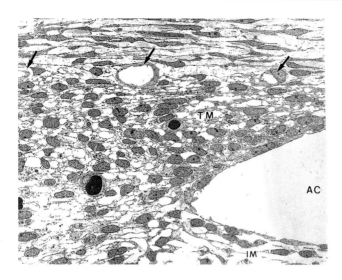

Fig. 17.24 The angular region of a 12-week-old human fetal eye showing a series of venous canaliculi (arrows) at the junction of the anlage of the trabecular meshwork (TM) and the dense corneoscleral tissue (top) which designate the beginning of the development of Schlemm's canal. AC = Anterior chamber; IM = iris stroma mesenchyme. Transmission electron micrograph, original magnification ×1110. (From McMenamin, P. G. (1991) *Exp. Eye Res.*, **53**, 507, with permission.)

mechanical influences such as the direction of the pull exerted on them. Thus the corneoscleral and deep uveal trabeculae are oriented circumferentially as flattened, perforated sheets, whereas the inner uveal trabeculae have a predominantly meridional position of their long axes, with a rounded, cord-like profile arranged in a net-like fashion so as to form a more resilient system (Tripathi, Tripathi and Wisdom, 1995).

Between the 28th and 30th fetal week the corneoscleral beams elongate and the trabecular cells covering each beam are connected by tight junctions and have only slender cytoplasmic processes (Fig. 17.23). The uveal meshwork now has wide intercellular spaces and by the ninth month the uveal trabeculae are well formed. The time at which communication is established between the fetal anterior chamber and the developing intertrabecular spaces is controversial. Classically, this process has been regarded as occurring relatively late in development and as depending on retraction of the corneal endothelium. Recent light and scanning electron microscopic studies of human fetal eyes have shown that, although the profile of the cells extending almost to the apex of the angle resembles corneal endothelium at 12–14 weeks of gestation, the lining is perforated by intercellular gaps of 2–8 μm in diameter (McMenamin, 1989). Furthermore, as development proceeds these lining cells become distinguishable morphologically from corneal endothelial cells. Gradually, as the angle recess deepens and as the trabecular beams differentiate, the open spaces of the meshwork come into direct communication with the anterior chamber. This development can be correlated with the increase in the facility of aqueous outflow (0.09 μl/min/mmHg

before 7 months to 0.3 μl/min/mmHg at 8 months) (Kupfer and Ross, 1971; Pandolfi and Astedt, 1971).

SCHLEMM'S CANAL

Schlemm's canal develops from a small plexus of venous canaliculi by the end of the third month of gestation (Fig. 17.24). These channels are derived from mesodermal mesenchyme and, initially, they function as blood vessels. Whether they arise *in situ* between the developing sclera and trabecular meshwork or are derived initially as blind endings of extensions from the deep scleral plexus of vessels remains open to question. However, the vascular nature of the channels and of the fully developed Schlemm's canal is now confirmed from the demonstration of Weibel–Palade bodies and factor VIII-related antigen in the living endothelial cells (Hamanaka *et al.*, 1992). The presumptive canal of Schlemm has several points of origin around the circumference of the inner limbus and the characteristic single canal is formed by a process of anastomosis (Smelser and Ozanics, 1971; Tripathi and Tripathi, 1989; Hamanaka *et al.*, 1992). The endothelial cells that line the canal of Schlemm are joined by zonulae occludentes junctional complexes. During the fourth month the canal is surrounded by other mesenchymal cells that secrete, and are enmeshed in, basal lamina-like material and foci of collagen fibrils. Eventually this tissue forms the juxtacanalicular region which remains loosely organized toward the trabecular meshwork (Ozanics and Jakobiec, 1982; Tripathi *et al.*, 1995).

At about the beginning of the fifth month, characteristic vacuolar configurations begin to appear in the endothelial cells lining Schlemm's canal (Wulle,

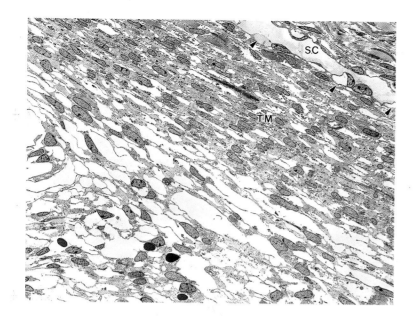

Fig. 17.25 At 22 weeks of gestation Schlemm's canal (SC) is well developed as a single channel. The endothelial lining of its inner wall shows vacuolar configurations (arrowheads), which function in the bulk outflow of aqueous humour across the intact cellular barrier. TM = Corneoscleral trabecular meshwork. Transmission electron micrograph, original magnification ×1110. (From McMenamin, P. G. (1991) *Exp. Eye Res.*, **53**, 507, with permission.)

1972). The vacuolar configurations represent stages in the cyclical formation of transcellular channels that allow for the bulk outflow of aqueous humour across the endothelial barrier (Tripathi, Tripathi and Wisdom, 1995). The development of macrovacuoles corresponds to the time of differentiation of the ciliary processes and the onset of the circulation of aqueous humour. The canal of Schlemm now functions as an aqueous sinus, rather than as a blood vessel (Fig. 17.25).

Up to 6 months of gestation both Schlemm's canal and the scleral spur are located posterior to the deepest part of the angle of the anterior chamber, but by 7 months the angle has receded to the level of the canal. Ultimately, because of growth of the surrounding structures, the canal comes to lie at the apex of the angle and is limited posteriorly by the scleral roll.

17.5 UVEAL TRACT

The uveal tract, which consists of the choroid, ciliary body, and iris, is derived embryonically from vascular channels, neural crest cells and neuroectoderm.

CHOROID

The condensation of neural crest cells that occurs initially around the anterior region of the optic cup and proceeds posteriorly to the optic stalk differentiates into the cells of the ensheathing choroidal stroma. Endothelium-lined blood spaces appear very early in this mesenchymal tissue, and first coalesce anteriorly at the rim of the optic cup to form the

embryonic annular vessel (Ozanics and Jakobiec, 1982). Differentiation of the choriocapillaris begins simultaneously with that of the retinal pigment epithelium during the fourth and fifth weeks of gestation. Only those mesodermal cells that have come into contact with the retinal pigment epithelium form the choriocapillary network (Ozanics and Jakobiec, 1982).

At the beginning of the sixth week of gestation the embryonic human eye is already completely invested

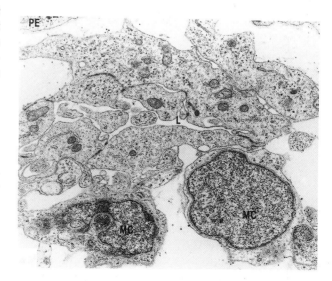

Fig. 17.26 Developing capillary with slit-like lumen (L) in close proximity to the retinal pigment epithelium (PE), which rests on its thin basal lamina (arrow), at 6½ weeks' gestation. MC = Cells of the periocular mesenchyme. Transmission electron micrograph, original magnification ×18 900. (From Sellheyer, K. and Spitznas, M. (1988) *Graefes Arch. Clin. Exp. Ophthalmol.*, **226**, 65, with permission.)

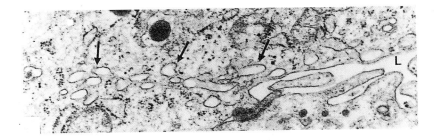

Fig. 17.27 A series of electron-optically empty vesicles (arrows) in an endothelial cell of a primitive capillary of the choriocapillaris in a 6½-week embryo. L = Lumen. Transmission electron micrograph, original magnification ×39 600. (From Sellheyer, K. and Spitznas, M. (1988) *Graefes Arch. Clin. Exp. Ophthalmol.*, **226**, 65, with permission.)

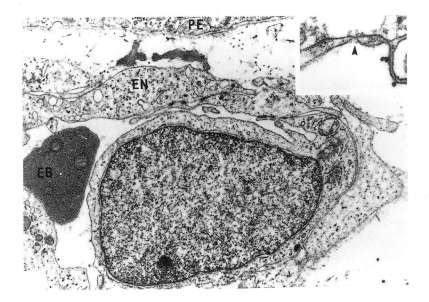

Fig. 17.28 By 7.2 weeks of gestation the capillaries of the choriocapillaris have developed an endothelial lining (EN) with characteristic diaphragmed fenestrations (inset, arrow) towards the retinal pigment epithelium (PE). EB = Erythroblast within lumen. Transmission electron micrographs, original magnification ×18 200 (inset ×75 000). (From Sellheyer, K. and Spitznas, M. (1988) *Graefes Arch. Clin. Exp. Ophthalmol.*, **226**, 65, with permission.)

with a primitive layer of capillaries (Sellheyer, 1990). The lumina of these vessels are narrow or slit-like (Fig. 17.26). The endothelial cells facing Bruch's membrane have abundant cytoplasm that contains numerous electron-optically empty vesicles, most of which are arranged parallel to the luminal and abluminal cell surfaces (Fig. 17.27). These vesicles are presumed to have a secretory function (Sellheyer and Spitznas, 1988a). Adjacent endothelial cells are joined by punctate junctional complexes and zonulae occludentes. Although no typical fenestrations are seen in the endothelial cells on either the retinal or scleral aspect of the capillaries, thin cytoplasmic processes extend from the endothelium into the vessel lumen (the luminal flaps) and exhibit fenestra-like structures (Sellheyer and Spitznas, 1988a).

Choriocapillaris and basal lamina

Diaphragmed fenestrations, characteristic of the choriocapillaris, are first recognized after the seventh week of gestation (Fig. 17.28) and are more numerous during the ninth week. Their development parallels an enlargement of the vessel lumen, thinning of the endothelium, and a decrease in the number of intracytoplasmic vesicles in the cells (Sellheyer and

Spitznas, 1988a). These morphological changes in the endothelial cells are similar to those that occur during angiogenesis of other tissues in the body. Concomitantly, the basal lamina, which until now has been organized only as small patches of extracellular material, becomes well defined, continuous and thicker. Pericytes are detected as early as the sixth week of gestation. Because of the similarity between the ultrastructure of these cells and that of the surrounding periocular mesenchymal cells, it is suggested that pericytes differentiate from the neural crest-derived cells of the adjacent stroma (Sellheyer, 1990).

Development of vasculature

By the end of the second month, arteriolar channels (branches of the future short posterior ciliary arteries) can be distinguished by their narrow lumina and walls of two or more cells (Heimann, 1972). A system of collecting channels also gradually emerges and forms the basis for the rudimentary vortex veins (Fig. 17.29). During the third and fourth months definitive layering of the choroidal vasculature becomes apparent with the development of the outer (sclerad), large vessel layer (of Haller). Small efferent

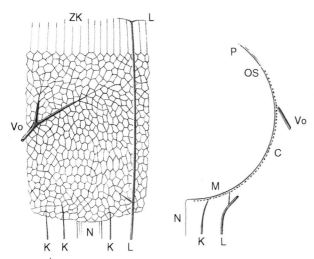

Fig. 17.29 Diagrammatic representation of choroidal vasculature at the end of the second month of gestation. K = Short posterior ciliary arteries; L = long posterior ciliary arteries; N = optic nerve: Vo = vortex vein; ZK = level of future ciliary body; M = site of future macular region; C = choriocapillaris; OS = site of future ora serrata; P = pigment epithelium. (From Heimann, K. (1972) *Ophthalmol. Res.*, **3**, 257, with permission.)

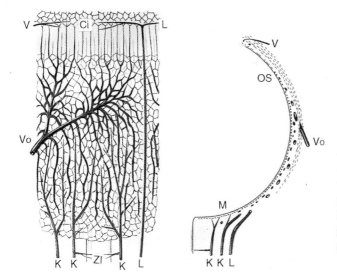

Fig. 17.30 Diagrammatic representation of choroidal vasculature at the end of the fourth month of gestation. K = Short posterior ciliary arteries; L = long posterior ciliary arteries; Zl = formation of the circle of Haller–Zinn; Vo = vortex vein; V = anterior ciliary artery; Ci = beginning of major arterial circle of the iris; M = site of future macular region; OS = site of future ora serrata. (From Heimann, K. (1972) *Ophthalmol. Res.*, **3**, 257, with permission.)

branches of the choriocapillaris join this second, mainly venous, layer which connects with the vortex veins that ultimately pierce through the sclera (Fig. 17.30). Also during the fourth month the long ciliary

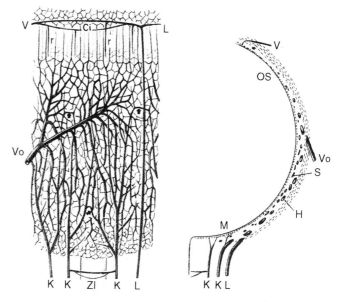

Fig. 17.31 Diagrammatic representation of choroidal vasculature at the end of the sixth month of gestation. K = Short posterior ciliary arteries; L = long posterior ciliary arteries; Zl = circle of Haller–Zinn; Vo = vortex vein; V = anterior ciliary artery; Ci = major arterial circle of the iris; r = recurrent branches: M = site of future macular region; OS = ora serrata; ↓ = interarterial anastomoses; H = Haller's layer; S = Sattler's layer. (From Heimann, K. (1972) *Ophthalmol. Res.*, **3**, 257, with permission.)

arteries form the major arterial circle, and recurrent branches from this vessel extend into the ciliary body by the end of the fifth month. Final anastomosis with the arterial circulation of the choroid is not established, however, until the eighth month of gestation. A third layer (Sattler's) of mostly medium-sized arterioles develops between the choriocapillaris and the outer venous layer during the fifth month of gestation (Fig. 17.31). It is initially confined to the level of the equator and does not reach the developing ciliary body until the sixth month of gestation (Heimann, 1972).

The choroidal stroma

The development of the choroidal stroma begins during the second trimester and by the end of the third month of gestation it is demarcated by the sclera (Ozanics and Jakobiec, 1982). The stroma is organized loosely and contains a few collagen fibrils as well as abundant fibroblasts with prominent endoplasmic reticulum. Elastic tissue is first seen in the fourth month. Melanocytes are derived from cells of neural crest origin and determine the pigmentation of the choroid. Melanosomes are recognized during the seventh month, especially in the region of the outer choroid and suprachoroid.

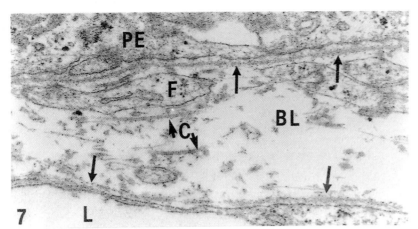

Fig. 17.32 Bruch's membrane (BL) at 9.7 weeks of gestation. Collagen fibrils (C) are present between the basal lamina (arrows) of the retinal pigment epithelium (PE) and of the endothelium of the choriocapillaris. L = lumen; F = process of choroidal firboblast. Transmission electron micrograph, original magnification ×36 500. (From Sellheyer, K. (1990) *Eye*, **4**, 255, with permission.)

BRUCH'S MEMBRANE

At the stage when the optic cup is formed the cells of the retinal pigment epithelium already rest on their thin basal lamina; this is well developed by the sixth week (embryo 12–16 mm) of embryonic life (Fig. 17.26). By this time, the inner layer of collagen fibrils, secreted by numerous fibroblasts, which are present in this region from an early stage, are oriented randomly at the site of the future Bruch's membrane. Four of the five layers of Bruch's membrane are distinguishable by the end of the ninth week of gestation (Fig. 17.32). Fibrils of the central elastic layer are seen by the middle of the third month and become organized as a nearly continuous sheet after mid-term. The outer region of Bruch's membrane is now demarcated by collagen fibrils of the choroidal stroma and the fibroblasts migrate to deeper regions. The outermost component of Bruch's membrane (the basal lamina of the endothelial cells of the choriocapillaris) is the last to be organized (Sellheyer, 1990).

CILIARY BODY

The ciliary epithelium differentiates behind the advancing margin of the optic cup from its two layers of neuroectoderm (Fig. 17.33). Longitudinally oriented indentations juxtaposed to small blood vessels in the choroid are observed in the outer pigmented layer late in the third month. These capillaries are branches from the irregular venous network situated in front of the vessels around the anterior margin of the optic cup (Figs 17.21 and 17.29). At this stage the inner, non-pigmented epithelium is smooth but between the third and fourth months (embryo approximately 65–75 mm) this layer starts to fold in order to follow the contour of, and adhere to, the pigmented layer (Figs 17.21 and

17.34). Approximately 70–75 of these radial folds develop; they are the beginning of the future ciliary processes. During the fourth month capillaries invade the mesenchymal core of the developing

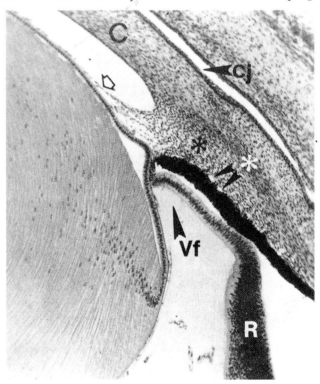

Fig. 17.33 The anterior region of the eye of a fetus at approximately 10½ weeks' gestation. The rim of the optic cup extends anterior to the lens equator. Small vessels (arrowheads) indent the outer (basal) surface of the pigment epithelium but at this stage the inner non-pigmented layer of the optic cup remains smooth. Vitreous fibres (Vf), attached to the inner surface of the cup and to the lens equator, form the faiseau isthmique of marginal bundle of Drault. C = Cornea; cj = conjunctival sac; R = retina; hollow arrow = pupillary membrane; asterisks = anlage of ciliary muscle. Light micrograph. (From Ozanics, V. and Jakobiec, F. A. in Duane, T. D. and Jaeger, E. A. (eds) (1982) *Biomedical Foundations of Ophthalmology*, vol. 1, published by Harper and Row, Philadelphia.)

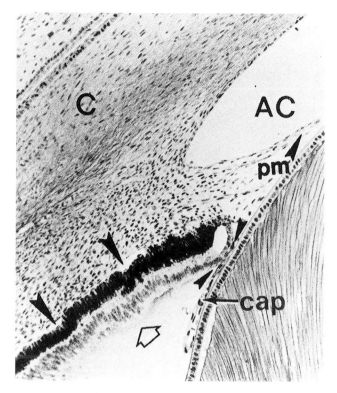

Fig. 17.34 The anterior region of the eye of a fetus at approximately 3 months' gestation. The outer pigmented layer of the optic cup is more undulated with blood vessels (arrowheads) in close proximity. The non-pigmented inner cell layer is also buckling (hollow arrow). C = cornea; AC = anterior chamber; pm = pupillary membrane; cap = capsulopupillary vessel of hyaloid system. Light micrograph. (From Ozanics, V. and Jakobiec, F. A. in Duane, T. D. and Jaeger, E. A. (eds) (1982) *Biomedical Foundations of Ophthalmology*, vol. 1, published by Harper and Row, Philadelphia.)

processes (Fig. 17.35); the growing tips of these vessels consist of a solid bud of endothelial cells. The intracytoplasmic vesicles of the endothelial cells are believed to become confluent with the intercellular spaces, which results in the formation of lumina. The endothelial cells secrete only a patchy basal lamina on their abluminal surface and, as soon as canalization is complete, fenestrations develop in the cytoplasm (Ozanics and Jakobiec, 1982).

The juxtaposed apical surfaces of the double-layered ciliary epithelium initially have cilia that extend into the intercellular space. After the fourth month the two surfaces become joined by gap junctions, desmosomes and fasciae adherens complexes, except in the regions where both epithelial cells possess microvilli (Ozanics and Jakobiec, 1982). Shortly after mid-term, Golgi complexes become prominent in the cytoplasm and their appearance may indicate the synthesis of components of the aqueous humour. Distension of the intercellular spaces between the apposed surfaces of the epithelial layers (noted between the fourth and sixth months) is believed to form a reservoir for the aqueous humour (Wulle, 1967). Interdigitations and membrane infolding of the lateral cell borders occur late in gestation and may indicate the commencement of transport of soluble proteins.

The ciliary muscle

The precursor cells of the ciliary muscle can be identified after the tenth week of gestation as an

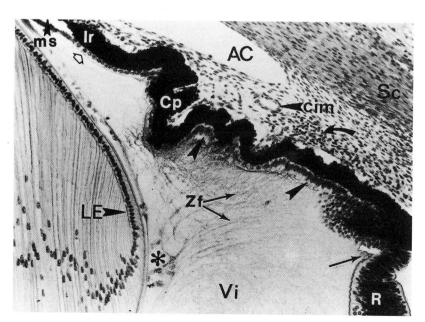

Fig. 17.35 The anterior region of the eye of a fetus at approximately 4 months' gestation. The folding of both the outer pigmented and inner non-pigmented epithelial cell layers has resulted in the formation of immature ciliary processes (Cp), which are at the level of the angle of the anterior chamber (AC). The future iridal portion (Ir) of the cup has a non-pigmented, cuboidal epithelium (hollow arrow), but those cells in the valleys of the primitive processes are columnar (arrowheads). Primitive zonular fibres (Zf) extend between the lens and the ciliary processes. LE = Lens epithelium; ms = marginal sinus; cim = major arterial circle; R = retina; Vi = vitreous with arrow pointing to fetal origin of its base; curved arrow = anlage of ciliary muscle; * = atrophying capsulopupillary membrane. Light micrograph. (From Ozanics, V. and Jakobiec, F. A. in Duane, T. D. and Jaeger, E. A. (eds) (1982) *Biomedical Foundations of Ophthalmology*, vol. 1, published by Harper and Row, Philadelphia.)

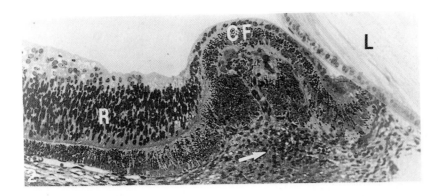

Fig. 17.36 Section through the ciliary body region of an eye from a 12-week-old fetus. Precursors of the ciliary muscle (arrow) are present in the outermost (sclerad) group of cells. CF = Ciliary fold; R = retina; L = lens. Light micrograph, original magnification ×180. (From Sellheyer, K. and Spitznas, M. (1988) *Graefes Arch. Clin. Exp. Ophthalmol.*, **226**, 281, with permission.)

accumulation of loosely arranged mesenchymal cells between the anterior scleral condensation and the primitive ciliary epithelium in the region of the margin of the optic cup (Fig. 17.33). The process of differentiation progresses from the outside inward and commences in the outermost (sclerad) cells during the 12th week (Fig. 17.36). The cytoplasm of the differentiating cells now contains dense bodies, arranged as plaques along the plasmalemma and surrounded by myofilaments (Sellheyer and Spitznas, 1988c) (Fig. 17.37). Individual cells are surrounded by a discontinuous basal lamina. As gestation continues the outer (meridional) portion of the ciliary muscle increases in size; the cells become elongated and arranged parallel to the anterior sclera (Fig. 17.38). The cell outline is now more undulating and the number of filaments within the cytoplasm is increased. At this stage the inner portion of the muscle (that closest to the ciliary epithelium) is less developed, and the cells are relatively immature. However, by four months of gestation the number of dense bodies, filaments and caveolae has increased in these cells, and the undulating outline of neighbouring cells gives rise to an interdigitating pattern (Fig. 17.39). Fibroblasts are present in addition to smooth muscle cells; between the fifth and sixth months these cells become organized and ensheath the ciliary muscle bundles (Sellheyer and Spitznas, 1988c).

During the fifth month the meridional ciliary muscle cells organize into the characteristic triangular shape, and the ends of the fibres are continuous with the developing scleral spur although distinct tendons are not formed until the middle of the seventh month (Ozanics and Jakobiec, 1982). The fibres on the inner aspect of the meridional muscle next become

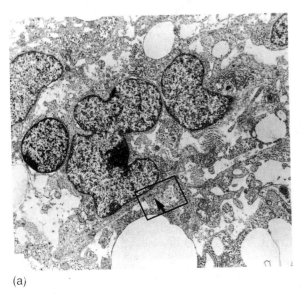

(a)

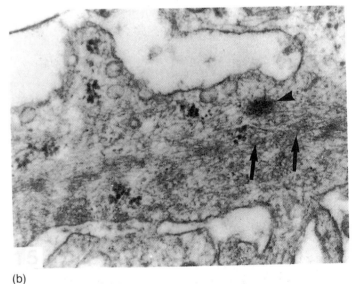

(b)

Fig. 17.37 Differentiation of mesenchymal cells into smooth ciliary muscle at 12 weeks of gestation. (a) Myofilaments (arrows) are recognizable in some cells, and the area enclosed, seen at higher magnification in (b), reveals the presence of dense bodies (arrowhead). Bundles of collagen fibrils are present in the intercellular space. Transmission electron micrographs, original magnifications (a) ×5700 and (b) ×60 000. (From Sellheyer, K. and Spitznas, M. (1988) *Graefes Arch. Clin. Exp. Ophthalmol.*, **226**, 281, with permission.)

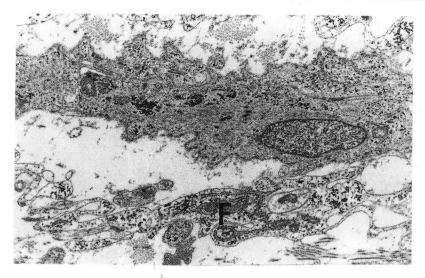

Fig. 17.38 By 14 weeks of gestation the cells of the outer portion of the differentiating ciliary muscle contain many myofilaments and dense bodies. F = fibroblast. Transmission electron micrograph, original magnification ×5700. (From Sellheyer, K. and Spitznas, M. (1988) *Graefes Arch. Clin. Exp. Ophthalmol.*, **226**, 281, with permission.)

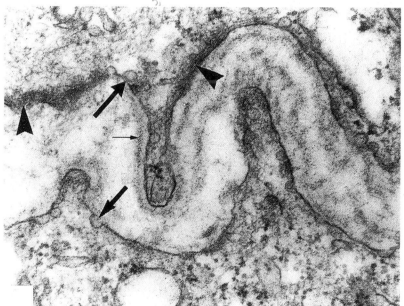

Fig. 17.39 The ciliary smooth muscle cells in an eye of a 4-month-old fetus. Individual cells have surface expansions with which they interdigitate each other. Large arrows = pinocytotic vesicles; small arrow = basal lamina; arrowheads = dense bodies at the cell plasmalemma. Transmission electron micrograph, original magnification ×40 000. (From Sellheyer, K. and Spitznas, M. (1988) *Graefes Arch Clin Exp Ophthalmol*, **226**, 281, with permission.)

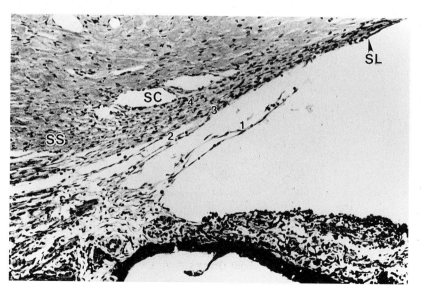

Fig. 17.40 Meridional section of the angle of the anterior chamber in a 9-week-old infant showing the connection of the meridional ciliary muscle cells to the scleral spur (SS) and the relatively poorly developed circular muscle. The angle recess is bridged by the fine iris processes (1) that extend from the iris root and join the uveal meshwork just anterior to its midpoint. The inner uveal trabeculae (2) are well formed and the outer uveal trabeculae pass beneath the scleral spur. SL = Schwalbe's line; 4 = corneoscleral trabeculae; SC = Schlemm's canal. Light micrograph, original magnification ×180. (From Tripathi, B. J., Tripathi, R. C. and Wisdom, J. in Ritch, R., Shields, M. B. and Krupin, T. (eds) (1995) *The Glaucomas*, 2nd edition, published by C. V. Mosby, St Louis.)

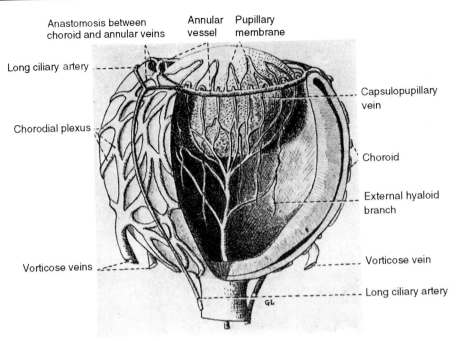

Anastomosis between
choroid and annular veins

Annular
vessel

Pupillary
membrane

Long ciliary artery

Chorodial plexus

Vorticose veins

Capsulopupillary
vein

Choroid

External hyaloid
branch

Vorticose vein

Long ciliary artery

Fig. 17.41 Diagrammatic representation of the vasculature of the embryonic eye at approximately 6 weeks of gestation.

established as the circular portion of the ciliary muscle. However, even at birth, the circular muscle consists only of slender bundles with one or two cell layers (Fig. 17.40), and its development continues for at least 1 year after birth. The third part of the ciliary muscle (the radial portion) lying between the circular and meridional fibres presumably develops soon after the beginning of the differentiation of the circular component. Unlike the fenestrated capillaries of the ciliary processes, adjacent endothelial cells that line the vessels of the ciliary muscle form a continuous lining and are joined by tight junctions.

IRIS

The normal development of the iris depends on complete closure of the embryonic fissure and is associated with the formation of the anterior portion of the tunica vasculosa lentis. The vascular channels of this embryonic structure originally arise at about the sixth week of gestation (embryo 17–18 mm) as blind outgrowths from the annular vessel that encircles the rim of the optic cup (Fig. 17.41), and they extend into the mesenchymal cells covering the anterior surface of the lens. This mesenchymal tissue represents the second wave of neural crest cells that migrated into the developing anterior chamber (Figs 17.9 and 17.33) and ultimately will be incorporated into the iris stroma (Tripathi, Tripathi and Wisdom, 1995).

Vasculature

The long posterior ciliary arteries in the nasal and temporal regions of the ciliary body bifurcate and the resulting branches join the vessels at the periphery of the tunica vasculosa lentis to form the major arterial circle (Fig. 17.41). Later, the major arterial circle also receives branches from the plexus of the anterior ciliary arteries. Vascular loops from both the long posterior ciliary arteries and the major arterial circle supply the pupillary membrane which replaces the most anterior region of the tunica vasculosa lentis.

After the ciliary folds (the prospective ciliary processes) have formed at the end of the third month, both walls of the optic cup at its margin grow forward rapidly (Fig. 17.35). At the 48–50 mm stage the growth of the optic cup separates the thick peripheral region of the tunica vasculosa lentis from the vessels of the pupillary membrane (Ozanics and Jakobiec, 1982; Tripathi et al., 1995). By the end of the fourth month, therefore, the vascular system of the developing iris is arranged into two layers: vessels of the tunica vasculosa lentis posteriorly, and vessels of the iridopupillary membrane anteriorly. Later, during the fifth month, branches from the long ciliary arteries reach the mesenchyme in the mid-region of the iris. The long ciliary arteries also supply several other branches to the developing iris: to the pupillary membrane superficially; to the stroma and, subsequently, the sphincter muscle; and to the ciliary region (the rete of the stroma).

The mesenchymal tissue

The mesenchymal tissue of the iris differentiates earlier than that of the neuroectoderm. At the anterior surface bordering the anterior chamber the cells align with each other to form the anterior border layer. However, no junctional complexes develop; large intercellular gaps remain between adjacent cells which develop long, tenuous cytoplasmic processes. Late in gestation pigmented cells come to lie beneath the anterior border layer. Some mesenchymal cells in the developing stroma become fibroblast-like and secrete collagen fibrils as well as other components of the extracellular matrix (Ozanics and Jakobiec, 1982).

Sphincter and dilator muscles

Further growth and differentiation of the two neuroectodermal layers of the optic cup involves the development of the sphincter and dilator muscles. Basal infoldings in the anterior layer of the epithelium (which is a forward extension of the retinal pigment epithelium) and a reduction in melanogenesis mark the beginning of the formation of the sphincter muscle (Fig. 17.42). By 3 months of gestation fine fibrils are already apparent in the basal (anterior) region of the cells. The cells secrete basal lamina material and, during the fifth month, synthesize myofibrils. The peripheral limit of the muscle is demarcated by an anterior extension of the pigmented epithelial layer into the stroma, the von Michel's spur. Except for the region of the pupillary edge, the muscle bundles become separated from their origin by invading connective tissue septae and

blood vessels during the sixth month of gestation. Although structural changes, such as the development of interdigitations linked by junctions, indicate establishment of cell-to-cell conduction in the seventh month, the muscle does not come to lie free in the posterior stroma until the eighth month (Ozanics and Jakobiec, 1982; Tripathi, Tripathi and Wisdom, 1995).

The first evidence for the development of the dilator muscle is not apparent until the sixth month, when fine fibrils differentiate in the anterior region of the pigmented epithelial cells just peripheral to von Michel's spur. Fibril development gradually proceeds towards the root of the iris. The cytoplasm on the anterior (basal) surface extends into the stroma to accommodate the accumulating myofibrils, and the nuclei and pigment granules are displaced apically (towards the posterior layer of epithelium). The partially differentiated myoepithelial cells continue to develop after birth but the dilator muscle, unlike the sphincter muscle, is not invaded by connective tissue and vessels and does not separate completely from the epithelium.

Pigmented epithelium

The posterior layer of epithelium, covered by its basal lamina, is a continuation of the non-pigmented layer of the ciliary body and consequently of the neuroectoderm that forms the neural retina. Beginning at mid-term the cells gradually become pigmented, a process which commences at the pupillary margin, proceeds toward the periphery and ceases at the root of the iris. Pigmentation is complete by the end of the seventh month. By this time the surfaces of the posterior epithelial cells that border the posterior chamber have also developed infoldings (Ozanics and Jakobiec, 1982).

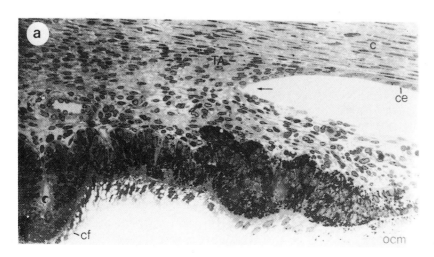

Fig. 17.42 Section through the angular region of a human fetal eye at 15 weeks of gestation. The anterior layer of epithelium at the optic cup margin (ocm) shows a reduction in pigmentation which marks the genesis of the sphincter muscle of the future iris. TA = Anlage of the trabecular meshwork at the apex of the angle recess (arrow); ce = corneal endothelium; cf = ciliary folds. Light micrograph, original magnification ×430. (From McMenamin, P. G. (1989) *Br. J. Ophthalmol.*, **73**, 871, with permission.)

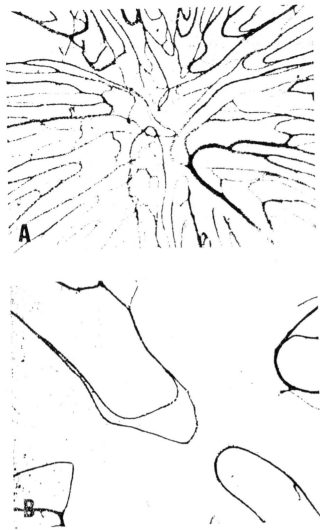

Fig. 17.43 Regression of the pupillary portion of the tunica vasculosa lentis. (A) At 24 weeks of gestation, loss of the connections between the blood vessels in the central region marks the beginning of the reabsorption. (B) By 31 weeks of gestation few vascular channels remain. Light micrographs of flat preparations, original magnification ×40. (From Ko, M.-K., Chi, J. G. and Chang, B.-L. (1985) *J. Ped. Ophthalmol. Strabismus*, **22**, 188, with permission.)

During development the adhesion between the two neuroepithelial layers of the iris is tenuous, especially at the pupillary margin. In this region a dilatation known as the marginal sinus of von Szily can often be recognized (Fig. 17.35). However, this separation is considered to be an artefact (Ozanics and Jakobiec, 1982).

The collarette

The development of the collarette in the iris stroma is related to the arteriovenous loops of the pupillary membrane that are arranged over the sphincter muscle. Starting in the central region, the pupillary portion of the tunica vasculosa lentis regresses during the sixth month (Fig. 17.43). During this process blood flow ceases and the vessel walls of the loops constrict and atrophy (Ko *et al.*, 1985). The regression continues as far as the peripupillary region of the iris. The remains of the vessels and fibroblasts that covered the membrane are phagocytosed by macrophages that invade the tissue. An incomplete arteriovenous anastomosis (the lesser circle) forms at the cillary end of the sphincter muscle; this demarcates the collarette. By the ninth month the superficial vessels central to the collarette have atrophied, and the lesser circle is established as the venous pathway for blood draining from the superficial vessels of the peripheral iris stroma.

The iris is not developed fully at birth: the collarette is closer to the pupil than in the adult, the stroma is thin, and much of the extracellular framework still has to be laid down.

17.6 RETINA

NEURAL RETINA

The differentiation of the neuroectodermal layer of the retina commences early. At 26 days of gestation (embryo 4 mm), the inner layer of the optic vesicle undergoes mitosis to produce three or four compact rows of cells (Rhodes, 1979). Towards the future vitreous cavity the primordial cells of the retina rest on a tenuous basal lamina. At the lateral extent of the optic vesicle, long tapering processes extend from the embryonic retinal cells into the mesenchyme beneath the epidermis. By 32–33 days of gestation (embryo 7 mm) the primordial retina consists of five or six rows of neuroepithelial cells (Fig. 17.44). The nuclei of these cells are segregated at the outer two-thirds of the optic cup (adjacent to the retinal pigment epithelium). Thus, the inner one-third that faces the lens placode is devoid of nuclei and has been termed the inner marginal layer (Rhodes, 1979). This appearance persists until about the seventh week of gestation. The cells of the outermost layer of the nucleated zone (called the ependymal, ventricular, germinative or proliferative layer) have short processes that project into the optic ventricle. Later they develop cilia that invaginate into the surface of the adjacent retinal pigment epithelial cells (Hollenberg and Spira, 1973). These structures disappear at the seventh week and are replaced by precursors of the outer segments of the photoreceptors during the fourth month.

Retinal maturation commences at the posterior pole and proceeds toward the periphery. The

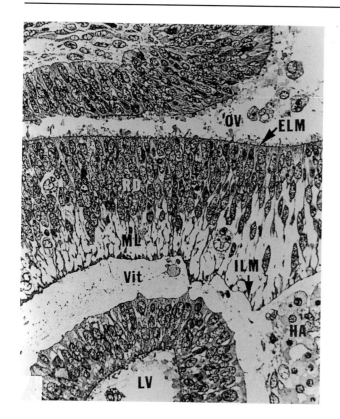

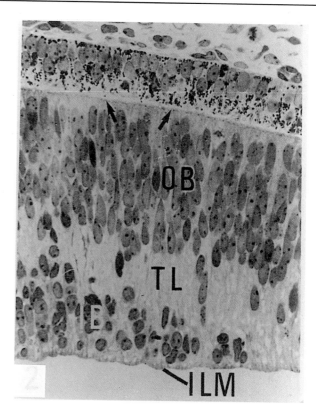

Fig. 17.44 The primordial retina in a human embryo at 32–33 days of gestation. The nuclei of the undifferentiated neuroepithelial cells are segregated towards the outer region of the optic cup. The inner region towards the lens vesicle (LV) is devoid of nuclei and is termed the inner marginal layer (ML). The internal limiting membrane (ILM) separates the retina from the vitreous (Vit) and the external limiting membrane (ELM) constitutes the outer border. Fibrils attached to both the internal limiting membrane and the lens epithelium contribute to the primary vitreous. The hyaloid artery (HA) is present in the embryonic fissure but is not yet incorporated in the vitreous body. OV = Obliterating optic ventricle. Light micrograph, original magnification ×320. (From Rhodes, R. H. (1979) *Am. J. Anat.*, **154**, 195, with permission.)

Fig. 17.45 The retina of a human fetus at 7 weeks of gestation. The outer aggregation of oval nuclei (OB) is separated from the inner spherical nuclei (IB) by the transient layer of Chievitz (TL). The external limiting membrane (arrows) now appears discontinuous. ILM = Internal limiting membrane. Light micrograph, original magnification ×770. (From Spira, A. W. and Hollenberg, M. J. (1973) *Dev. Biol.*, **31**, 1, with permission.)

putative macula is the focal point for the commencement of this centroperipheral sequence of events (Provis *et al.*, 1985). By the end of the embryonic period mitosis is taking place in the germinative layer throughout the entire outer surface of the retina. However, at approximately 14 weeks of gestation, mitosis ceases in the central retina and differentiation of cone photoreceptors commences in a well defined region (the putative fovea) that comprises about 2% of the total retinal area. As gestation progresses the area devoid of mitotic activity increases, so that by 24 weeks dividing cells are present in 62.5% of the retinal surface and are confined to the periphery. By 30 weeks of gestation mitotic activity has ceased completely. However, the surface area of the retina increases at a steady rate of 10–15 mm^2 per week throughout gestation and for the first 3 weeks after birth. This increase in area in the postmitotic phase is attributed to the growth and maturation of individual cells (Provis *et al.*, 1985).

Organization of neuroepithelium

By 4–5 weeks of gestation (embryo 12 mm), the neuroepithelium has become organized into two distinct regions of neuroblastic* cells: inner, towards the vitreous and outer, adjacent to the retinal pigment epithelium. Segregation of nuclei as the inner

*Strictly speaking, the terms 'neuroblasts' and 'glioblasts' should be confined to those postmitotic daughter cells that are committed to differentiate as neurons and glial cells, respectively. Because it remains to be determined at precisely which stage in the development of the retina this occurs, and for the sake of simplicity, neuroblastic cells are defined as undifferentiated neuroepithelial cells in this text.

and outer neuroblastic layers occurs as a result of the inward migration of putative ganglion and Müller cells from the outer layers of the neuroepithelium (Fig. 17.45). This process leaves a region consisting only of tangled cell processes and is known as the transient layer of Chievitz. Based on their morphologic appearance, three types of cell nuclei can be identified (Rhodes, 1979):

1. undifferentiated oval nuclei with compact chromatin and several nucleoli are located predominantly in the outer neuroblastic layer;
2. large, round or oval nuclei with a delicate lacy pattern of chromatin are present mostly in the inner neuroblastic layer (these cells have a relatively large amount of cytoplasm and are the putative ganglion cells);

3. dark, round or oval nuclei that are smallest in size are present in all areas of the developing retina but are most numerous in the inner half of the inner neuroblastic layer; these are putative Müller cells.

The inner marginal layer has become differentiated as the nerve fibre layer and axons from the committed ganglion cells are growing toward the optic nerve head.

The retinal layers

The optic ventricle is still present as a narrow slit in the 20–23 mm stage embryo (7 weeks of gestation) but soon becomes obliterated. During the ninth to twelfth weeks of gestation the layer of Chievitz develops as the definitive inner plexiform layer (Fig. 17.46) and the four major horizontal layers of the retina become distinguishable (Rhodes, 1979). The nuclei of the ganglion cells are now confined to the ganglion cell layer and the axons are aligned as fascicles by processes of Müller cells (Fig.

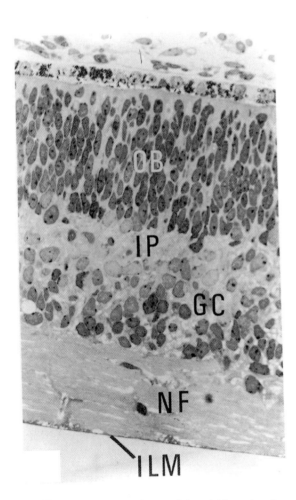

Fig. 17.46 The retina of a human fetus at 10 weeks of gestation. The layer of Chievitz is now recognized as the definitive inner plexiform layer (IP). OB = Outer neuroblastic layer; GC = ganglion cell layer; NF = nerve fibre layer; ILM = internal limiting membrane. Light micrograph, original magnification ×890. (From Spira, A. W. and Hollenberg, M. J. (1973) *Dev. Biol.*, **31**, 1, with permission.)

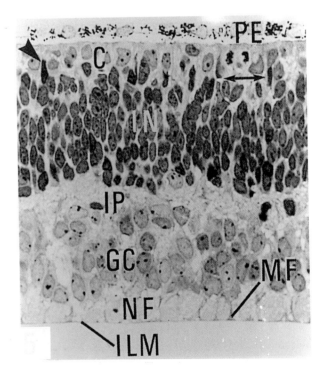

Fig. 17.47 The retina of a human fetus at 12 weeks of gestation showing the nerve fibre layer (NF) penetrated by the radial fibres of the Müller cells (MF). ILM = Internal limiting membrane; GC = ganglion cell layer; IP = inner plexiform layer; IN = inner nuclear layer; C = cones; arrowhead = presumptive cone precursor; double-headed arrow = beginning of outer plexiform layer; PE = retinal pigment epithelium. Light micrograph, original magnification ×980. (From Spira, A. W. and Hollenberg, M. J. (1973) *Dev. Biol.*, **31**, 1, with permission.)

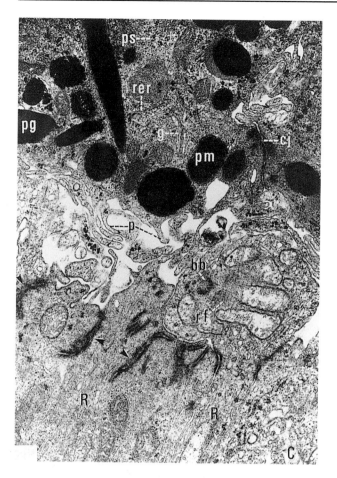

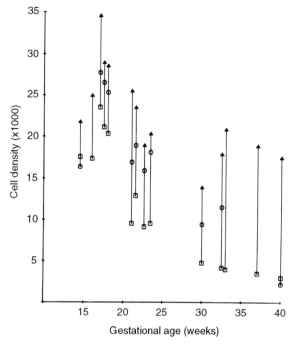

Fig. 17.49 Graph showing the relationship of ganglion cell density with prenatal age in the human fetal retina. (□ = mean; ▲ = maximum; ○ = foveal) The maximum density of cells occurs at approximately 17 weeks of gestation. (From Provis, J. M., van Driel, D., Billson, F. and Russell, P. (1985) *J. Comp. Neurol.*, **233**, 429, with permission.)

Fig. 17.48 The interface between the photoreceptors and the retinal pigment epithelium in a 15-week-old human fetus. The developing rods (R) and cones (C) are joined at their apical–lateral surfaces by junctional complexes of the external limiting membrane (arrowheads). The developing inner segments contain mitochondria, the basal body (bb) of the connecting cilium and associated rootlet fibres (rf). The retinal pigment epithelium (top) has fine processes (p) that extend towards the photoreceptors. Adjacent retinal pigment epithelial cells are joined by junctional complexes (cj) at the apical–lateral borders. Premelanosomes (pm), pigment granules (pg), polysomes (ps), rough endoplasmic reticulum (rer) and a Golgi complex (g) are seen in the cytoplasm. Transmission electron micrograph, original magnification ×27 900. (From Hollenberg, M. J. and Spira, A. W. (1973) *Am. J. Anat.*, **137**, 357, with permission.)

17.47). By the tenth week the outermost cells of the outer neuroblastic layer have begun to differentiate into cones that are characterized by their poorly stained nuclei and abundant cytoplasm (Rhodes, 1979). The adjacent lateral surfaces of these cells are joined by zonulae adherentes junctional complexes, which form the primitive external limiting membrane (Hollenberg and Spira, 1973). The development of the Müller cell processes follows that of the neurons in the inner and outer retina both temporally and spatially; they are prominent be-

tween the cones soon after these photoreceptors enlarge and are morphologically distinct (Rhodes, 1979). Membranous junctional complexes are also present between the outer plasma membrane of the developing photoreceptors and the inner membrane of the retinal pigment epithelial cells (Fig. 17.48); thus the optic ventricle is now occluded completely.

Between about weeks 14–15 and week 17 of gestation, the cell population in the ganglion cell layer increases rapidly (Fig. 17.49). It declines again between weeks 18 and 30, levelling off at 2.2–2.5 million cells (Provis *et al.*, 1985). The decrease in the number of cells towards the end of gestation is accounted for by a period of cell loss (between weeks 14 and 30) due to natural cell death or apoptosis. The ganglion cells in the central retina are initially small (4–10 μm in diameter) and round, whereas those cells at the retinal periphery are mostly fusiform and immature in appearance. With advancing gestational age the soma diameter increases.

Amacrine cells, identifiable by their large pale round nuclei, are first seen scattered at the inner border of the outer neuroblastic layer by week 14 of gestation (embryo approximately 70 mm). Whether these cells differentiate *in situ* or migrate to this

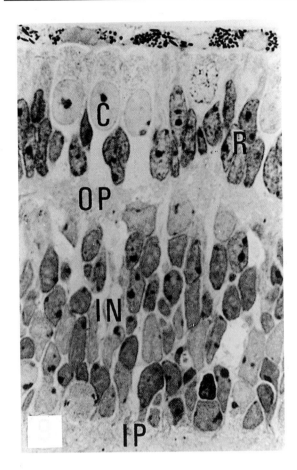

Fig. 17.50 The outer retina in an 18-week-old human fetus. The cones (C) have already elongated and extend foot-processes to the outer plexiform layer (OP). The rods (R) are thinner and less well differentiated. IN = inner nuclear layer; IP = inner plexiform layer. Light micrograph, original magnification ×1850. (From Spira, A. W. and Hollenberg, M. J. (1973) *Dev. Biol.*, **31**, 1, with permission.)

distributed randomly in the cytoplasm. Their orientation as flattened, lamellar discs parallels the development of the horizontal cells.

At 22 weeks of gestation (embryo approximately 120 mm) cells with dark nuclei and condensed peripheral chromatin are dispersed between the cones. These are the cell bodies of the rod photoreceptors. Their developing inner segments initially bulge beyond the external limiting membrane (Hollenberg and Spira, 1973).

Bipolar cells do not differentiate in the inner nuclear layer until week 23, and their elongating dendrites extend to the outer plexiform layer by week 25. Horizontal cells probably develop at about the same time (Rhodes, 1979).

MACULA

Because the putative macula is the focal point for centroperipheral development of the retina, the differentiation of the neurons, glial cells and photoreceptors in the fovea occurs early. However, as judged by its anatomical organization, this area does not reach maturity until 15–45 months after birth (Hendrickson and Yuodelis, 1984). By 15 weeks of gestation the nuclei of the ganglion cells in the putative fovea are well differentiated, as is the inner plexiform layer. Amacrine cell synapses and immature monad bipolar cell synapses, as well as intercellular junctions between all cell types, are already established but dyad bipolar synapses are uncommon (van Driel, Provis and Billson, 1990). Approximately half of the somas in the inner nuclear layer can be identified positively as Müller cells and amacrine cells (accounting for 35% and 11% of the total number of cells, respectively), together with an occasional ganglion cell (1% of the total); most of the remaining cells are probably bipolar cells (van Driel, Provis and Billson, 1990).

At this stage of development the nuclei of the ganglion cells have a round shape (average $6.5 \times 8.5\,\mu m$) and are pale-staining because of a finely dispersed chromatin (van Driel, Provis and Billson, 1990). The abundant cytoplasm is rich in polyribosomes, mitochondria, endoplasmic reticulum (predominantly rough) and microtubules. The Golgi apparatus and centrioles are located in the cytoplasm facing the inner plexiform layer. The broad dendrites of the ganglion cells contain microtubules. Growth cones are present on both the somas and dendrites. The nuclei of the amacrine cells have a characteristic small drumstick-shaped lobe (the nuclear pocket) attached to the remainder of the nucleus by a thin bridge of nuclear material (van

location from the ventricular layer is not clear (Rhodes, 1979). The cones continue to enlarge and by the end of week 17 short synaptic ribbons are present in the basal cytoplasm of these cells; thus, the synaptic structures develop before the outer segments are formed (Hollenberg and Spira, 1973). At week 18 of gestation (96 mm stage) the outer region of the cone cytoplasm takes on a granular appearance because of the accumulation of mitochondria and polysomes (Fig. 17.50). The basal bodies of the cilia are conspicuous at this time. The cell membrane later involutes to envelop the cilium and extends a cylindrical cytoplasmic process toward the apical region of the retinal pigment epithelial cells. Outer segments of the photoreceptors begin to differentiate at 5 months, when multiple infoldings of the plasma membrane develop because of the influence of the ciliary filaments. Initially, as the folds separate from the plasma membrane, they are

Driel, Provis and Billson, 1990). The cytoplasm is mostly vitread to the nucleus and contains many polyribosomes and mitochondria. The round amacrine cell processes arise mostly from the vitreal aspect of the somas and have abundant microtubules. The nuclei of Müller cells are oval in shape and measure, on average, 4.4 × 15.2 μm; often they have indented margins (van Driel, Provis and Billson, 1990). Their somas are located in the mid and vitreal regions of the inner nuclear layer; none are present in the ganglion cell layer at this stage. The Müller cell processes stain darkly because of the abundant filaments and glycogen granules; the processes are already organized in a tree-like arrangement (van Driel, Provis and Billson, 1990).

The fovea

At 22 weeks of gestation, the fovea is a circular to elliptical zone approximately 1.5 mm in diameter and characterized by five to seven layers of cells in the ganglion cell layer, a thin nerve fibre layer, well defined inner plexiform, inner nuclear, and outer plexiform layers and an outer nuclear layer containing exclusively nuclei of cones (Hendrickson and Yuodelis, 1984). The developing horizontal cells can be recognized as a layer of pale, round cells at the outermost edge of the inner nuclear layer. The numerous putative bipolar cells with their round basophilic nuclei lie adjacent to the layer of horizontal cells. The basophilic nuclei of the Müller cells occupy the mid-region of the inner nuclear layer and a heterogeneous population of undifferentiated neurons makes up the remaining inner one-third. In the outer plexiform layer fine neuronal processes make contact with the cones, which now form a single layer of columnar epithelial cells (Fig. 17.51). Neither inner nor outer segments have differentiated

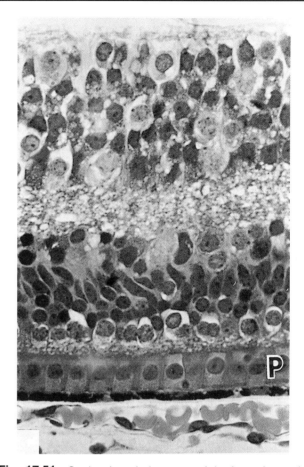

Fig. 17.51 Section through the centre of the future fovea of a 22-week-old fetus. The photoreceptor layer (P) consists exclusively of cones, which lack both inner and outer segments at this stage of development. All of the neuronal and glial cell types are present in the inner nuclear and ganglion cell layers. Light micrograph, original magnification ×130. (From Hendrickson, A. E. and Yuodelis, C. (1984) *Ophthalmology*, **91**, 603, with permission.)

but occasionally the photoreceptors bulge slightly beyond the well defined external limiting membrane. By 24 weeks of gestation the density of cones in the

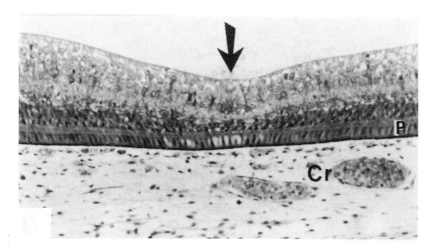

Fig. 17.52 The beginning of the foveal depression in a fetal eye at approximately 24–26 weeks of gestation. Cr = Choroid; P = outer nuclear layer; arrow denotes thinning of inner nuclear and ganglion cell layers. Light micrograph, original magnification ×115. (From Hendrickson, A. E. and Yuodelis, C. (1984) *Ophthalmology*, **91**, 603, with permission.)

future fovea is approximately 38 000/mm²; the maximum rod density (59 200/mm²) occurs in the region surrounding the foveal cone mosaic (Diaz-Araya and Provis, 1992).

The earliest recognizable depression in the central region of the macula is first evident at 24–26 weeks of gestation, apparently caused by thinning of the ganglion cell and inner nuclear layers (Hendrickson and Yuodelis, 1984). At the future foveola the ganglion cell layer is reduced to three or four cells deep, but six layers remain around the depression. Similarly, the inner nuclear layer is reduced to four or five rows of nuclei at the fovea centre and eight to ten rows on the slope (Fig. 17.52). The nerve fibre layer is thicker and Müller cell fibres are prominent. On the nasal slope of the inner nuclear layer an acellular, fibre-containing zone appears and corresponds to the transient layer of Chievitz. Two types of developing bipolar cells are identifiable in the outer third of the inner nuclear layer; one is pale staining and round, the other has a basophilic nucleus and long cytoplasmic processes that extend to the outer plexiform layer. The proximal bases of the cones have begun to taper and turn laterally away from the nucleus; this is the earliest indication of Henle's fibre layer. Pedicles are also now present. The formation of the inner segments of the cones is evident from the accumulation of mitochondria in their cytoplasm bulging beyond the external limiting membrane (Van Driel et al., 1990).

By the seventh month of gestation the inner nuclear layer becomes markedly thinned and the foveal pit is more prominent. The acellular fibrous zone is now present on the temporal as well as the nasal side of the fovea. Major changes have occurred in the cones; both the inner segment and the fibres of Henle's fibre layer have increased in length whereas the width of the inner segments decreases. This allows for an increase in cone density in this region. At 8 months two layers of ganglion cells remain; these reduce to a single layer in the neonate. The inner nuclear layer is thinned to less than three cells thick in the foveola due to lateral displacement (Hendrickson and Yuodelis, 1986).

At birth the transient layer of Chievitz is extremely prominent and consists of axons of bipolar cells passing to the inner plexiform layer. The cones are thinner, and those located beneath the foveal slope appear more mature than the cones at the foveola. Even by 1 week after birth the thick cones still lack outer segments (Fig. 17.53). By 4 months after birth all layers have relocated to the periphery of the foveal slope, leaving the nuclei of the cones almost completely uncovered in the central region or foveola. However, remodelling of the elements at the fovea continues so that the transient layer of Chievitz is not lost completely until nearly 4 years of age (Hendrickson and Yuodelis, 1984). Between birth and 45 months of age the diameter of the cones continues to decrease. The elongation of the foveal cones due to the development of outer segments and basal axon processes (the fibre layer of Henle), and their continued migration toward the foveal pit, results in an increase in cone density from 18/100 μm at 1 week after birth to 42/100 μm in adults (Yuodelis and Hendrickson, 1986).

PERIPHERAL RETINA

The demarcation between the neural epithelium of the ciliary region and the retina at the future ora serrata becomes apparent at about the fourth month

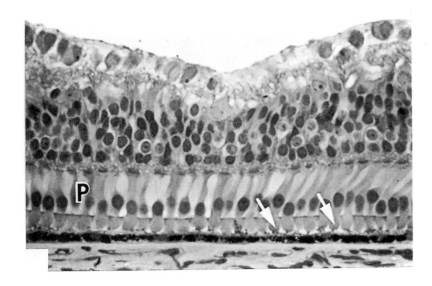

Fig. 17.53 Section through centre of foveal depression in a 5-day-old infant. The photoreceptor layer (P) contains dark-staining cones with prominent nuclei and pale processes of glial cells. The cones have a large round inner segment which bulges above the external limiting membrane (arrows). Small outer segments are barely visible adjacent to the retinal pigment epithelium. Light micrograph, original magnification ×130. (From Hendrickson, A. E. and Yuodelis, C. (1984) *Ophthalmology*, **91**, 603, with permission.)

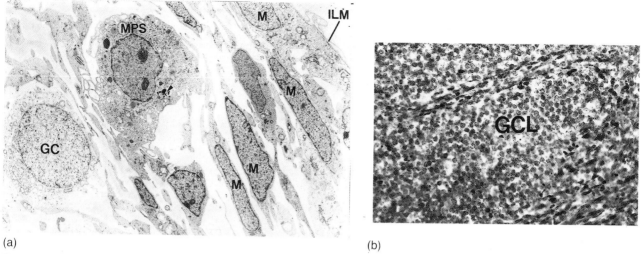

(a)   (b)

Fig. 17.54 Retinal angiogenesis. (a) The inner retina of a fetus at approximately 16–17 weeks' gestation is invaded by spindle-shaped mesodermal cells. (M). MPS = Mononuclear phagocyte; GC = ganglion cell; ILM = internal limiting membrane. Transmission electron micrograph, original magnification ×3900. (b) Whole mount of retina from a fetus of 20 weeks' gestation. Strands of angiogenic mesoderm composed of spindle-shaped cells advance across the surface of the ganglion cell layer (GCL) and represent an early stage of retinal vascularization prior to development of lumina. Light micrograph, original magnification ×730. (From Penfold, P. L., Provis, J. M., Madigan, M. C., van Driel, D. and Billson, F. A. (1990) *Graefes Arch. Clin. Exp. Ophthalmol.*, **228**, 255, with permission.)

of gestation. By the sixth month the peripheral retina has only a thin nerve fibre layer and the ora serrata is established definitively. Between the eighth and ninth months the development of this region is complete in the temporal region, and the indentation or serrated edge of the peripheral retina in other regions of the globe continues to develop after birth. The zone between the ora and the equator enlarges in size until about 2 years of age (Ozanics and Jakobiec, 1982).

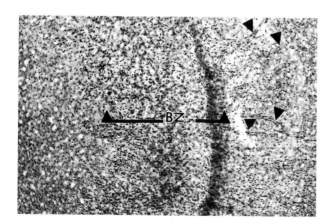

Fig. 17.55 Retinal whole mount from a fetus of 32 weeks' gestation showing the boundary zone (BZ) between the avascular (left) and vascular (right) retina. Arrowheads mark established vessels. Light micrograph, original magnification ×292. (From Penfold, P. L., Provis, J. M., Magidan, M. C., van Driel, D. and Billson, F.A. (1990) *Graefes Arch. Clin. Exp. Ophthalmol.*, **228**, 255, with permission.)

RETINAL ANGIOGENESIS

The terminal portion of the primitive ophthalmic artery invades the embryonic fissure of the human eye at about the 5 mm stage. The fissure closes between the fifth and seventh weeks. The vessel remains in the optic cup and becomes the hyaloid artery. It probably functions, at least initially, to supply the lens and the retina.

At the fourth month of gestation spindle-shaped mesenchymal cells (Fig. 17.54) arise from the hyaloid artery where it enters the optic disc. Initially they permeate the inner layers of the retina as solid cords of undifferentiated cells (Ashton, 1970). The formation of primitive vessels occurs behind the advancing edge of the invading mesenchymal cells (Fig. 17.55); thus a boundary zone, which advances toward the periphery, is established between the avascular and vascularized retina (Penfold *et al.*, 1990). Endothelial cells differentiate first and adjacent cells form junctional complexes, which include both zonulae occludentes and gap junctions. At this stage the lumina are represented only by slit-like openings (Fig. 17.56). As the vessel matures the lumina enlarge and become patent. Pericytes are present from an early stage. The developing vessels are surrounded by basal lamina material continuous with an extracellular matrix rich in collagen fibrils. Processes of astrocytes contact the outer margin of this matrix (Penfold *et al.*, 1990). A prominent feature of the developing vasculature is the association of mononuclear phagocytic cells

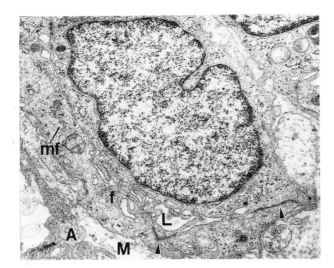

Fig. 17.56 A developing retinal vessel in a human fetus of 16 weeks' gestation. Adjacent endothelial cells are joined by junctional complexes (arrowheads) and enclose a small, slit-like lumen (L). The cytoplasm contains intermediate filaments (mf) and the luminal surface is fimbriated extensively (f). A = Astrocyte; M = collagenous matrix. Transmission electron micrograph, original magnification ×15 200. (From Penfold, P. L., Provis, J. M., Madigan, M. C., van Driel, D. and Billson, F. A. (1990) *Graefes Arch. Clin. Exp. Ophthalmol.*, **228**, 255, with permission.)

(Fig 17.54a), which are thought to have a role in angiogenesis (Penfold *et al.*, 1990).

Retinal vascularization proceeds from the centre to the periphery. By the fifth month patent vessels have extended both superiorly and inferiorly on the temporal aspect of the retina, thus sparing the region of the putative macula. At this stage, vascularization is less extensive on the nasal aspect. Between 24 and 26 weeks of gestation small blood vessels develop in the ganglion cell layer at the foveal slope. By a process of remodelling and retraction of the primitive capillary network, the adult pattern of arterioles, veins and capillaries is established. Primitive capillaries reach the ora serrata by the eighth month but the fully mature pattern of vascularization is not attained until 3 months after birth.

The origin of the intramural pericytes is still obscure; these cells may represent modified endothelial cells that are retained after retraction of the primitive network (Ashton, 1970). However, their presence early in retinal angiogenesis implies that pericytes are present before the process of remodelling is complete and favours the concept that they are derived from neural crest cells.

RETINAL PIGMENT EPITHELIUM

Up to the sixth week of gestation (embryo 20 mm) the outer wall of the optic cup is composed of mitotically

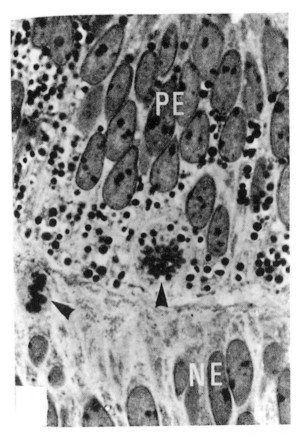

Fig. 17.57 Section through the outer retina of a human fetus at 6½ weeks of gestation showing the pseudostratified pigment epithelium (PE) with numerous melanin granules. Right arrow shows cell division in pigment epithelium, the left arrow cell division in the outer neuroblastic epithelium (NE). Light micrograph, original magnification ×2400. (From Hollenberg, M. J. and Spira, A. W. (1973) Human retinal development: ultrastructure of the outer retina. *Am. J. Anat.*, **137**, 357, with permission.)

active, pseudostratified columnar epithelial cells, the inner surfaces of which are ciliated (Fig. 17.57). The oval nuclei are located in the mid region of the cells. Melanogenesis begins at this time and the cilia disappear. Adjacent cells are already joined by zonulae occludens and zonulae adherens complexes at their apical borders. By 8 weeks (embryo 27–31 mm) the retinal pigment epithelium has become organized as a single layer of hexagonal-shaped columnar cells posteriorly but remains pseudostratified at the periphery. There is no evidence of mitoses and the nuclei are located toward the basal aspect of the cells (Fig. 17.58). Premelanosomes and mature pigment granules are segregated to the inner and outer portions of the cytoplasm, which also contains numerous polysomes, mitochondria and rough endoplasmic reticulum. The apical and basal surfaces that abut the neural retina and choroid, respectively, are smooth. However, the basolateral surfaces have numerous

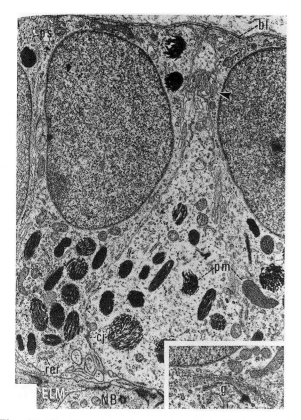

Fig. 17.58 The retinal pigment epithelium of a human fetus at 8 weeks' gestation. The cells contain premelanosomes (pm) in various stages of formation, polysomes (ps), and rough endoplasmic reticulum (rer). The basal cell surface rests on a thin basal lamina (bl) and the apical surface is still smooth. Towards the basal region, processes of adjacent cells interdigitate (arrow), and junctional complexes (cj) are present between adjacent cells at the apical-lateral surface. NB = Outer neuroblastic cells; ELM = external limiting membrane. Inset shows well-developed Golgi (g) complex. Transmission electron micrographs, original magnification ×7700 (inset ×14 900). (From Hollenberg, M. J. and Spira, A. W. (1973) *Am. J. Anat.*, **137**, 357, with permission.)

membrane infoldings that interdigitate (Hollenberg and Spira, 1973).

During the third and fourth months of gestation (77–83 mm stage) the cells become tall cuboidal in shape, and their nuclei spherical. There is an increase in cytoplasmic organelles with more smooth endoplasmic reticulum and a well developed Golgi apparatus present. Most pigment granules are mature or immature, but premelanosomes remain. The terminal web is well established at the lateral apical borders and the inner border shows the beginning of apical processes, which develop before the outer segments of the photoreceptors are formed (Fig. 17.48). By the middle of the fourth month only a few premelanosomes persist and the apical cell processes have become slender microvilli. At this stage the retinal pigment epithelium is believed to be fully functional (Hollenberg and Spira, 1973).

The sequence of differentiation of the retinal pigment is thought to be reflected by the formation of various cytoplasmic structures. Protein synthesis occurs initially, followed by synthesis and melanization of premelanosomes. Infoldings appear on the lateral and basal cell borders later in gestation. Although new cells are added by mitosis during early embryonic life, the increase in the surface area of the retinal pigment epithelium that must take place after birth to accommodate the subsequent growth of the globe is accounted for by enlargement and expansion of individual cells. The functional implications of retinal development are discussed in Chapter 14.

17.7 OPTIC NERVE

The optic stalk forms the initial connection between the optic vesicles and the forebrain. As the

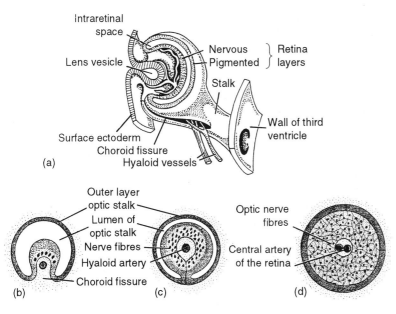

Fig. 17.59 Diagrammatic representations showing closure of the choroidal fissure and transformation of the optic stalk into the optic nerve. (a) Lateral view at approximately 5 weeks of gestation with part of the optic cup, lens vesicle and surface ectoderm cut away for clarity. The hyaloid vessels penetrate the choroidal fissure near the optic stalk, invest the primary vitreous cavity and surround the posterior region of the invaginating lens vesicle. (From Pansky, B. (1982) *Review of Medical Embryology*, published by McGraw Hill, with permission) (b, c, d) Cross-sections of the optic stalk at 6, 7 and 9 weeks of gestation, respectively. After closure of the choroidal fissure, the hyaloid artery (a branch of the primitive ophthalmic artery) is surrounded completely by nerve fibres of retinal ganglion cells growing towards the brain; the basal lamina of the original outer surface of the fissure degenerates (From Sadler, T. W. (1990) *Langman's Medical Embryology*, 6th edition, published by Williams and Wilkins, with permission).

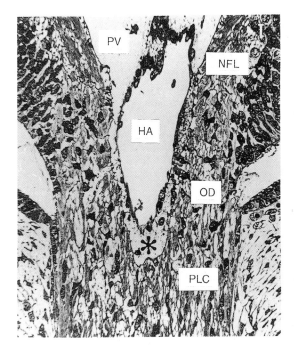

Fig. 17.60 Superoinferior section through a human embryonic eye at 7 weeks of gestation. The optic disc (OD) is formed completely around the hyaloid artery (HA) and the primitive lamina cribrosa (PLC) is traversed by nerve fibres from the nerve fibre layer (NFL) of the retina. * = Canal of the hyaloid artery which is continuous with the cavity filled by primary vitreous (PV). Light micrograph, original magnification ×320. (From Rhodes, R. H. (1978) *Am. J. Anat.*, **153**, 601, with permission.)

vesicles form optic cups (at about the 4–4.5 mm stage; approximately 4 weeks of gestation), the stalk involutes and a shallow groove, the choroidal or embryonic fissure, results (Fig. 17.6). This fissure

accommodates a branch of the primitive ophthalmic artery, the future hyaloid artery (Fig. 17.59). Starting at the forebrain (at the 12–17 mm stage), the lips of the fissure begin to close over the hyaloid artery. This process is complete by 6–7 weeks of gestation (embryo 20 mm). The basal lamina that originally lined the outer surface of the fissure degenerates.

Nerve fibres from the ganglion cells migrate through spaces created by vacuolation and degeneration of some cells in the inner wall of the optic stalk (Figs 17.60 and 17.61). The stalk is filled almost completely with nerve fibres by the 30 mm stage. At this time other cells of the inner layer of the optic stalk transform into glial cells and form an outer mantle; they also give rise to the glial elements of the lamina cribrosa during the eighth week. Enlargement of the temporal side of the eye during the third month shifts the optic nerve nasally; it is now 7–8 mm long and 1.2 mm in diameter. The sheaths of the optic nerve, which are derived from cells of the neural crest, become well defined only between the fourth and fifth months of gestation. Approximately 50% of the growth of the optic disc and nerve has occurred by 20 weeks' gestation, 75% by birth, and 95% before the age of 1 year (Rimmer *et al.*, 1993).

BERGMEISTER'S PAPILLA

Bergmeister's papilla is formed by focal proliferation of glial cells at the optic nerve head by 9 weeks of gestation. This group of cells has a cone-shaped configuration, with its base spread along the internal limiting membrane and the apex extending

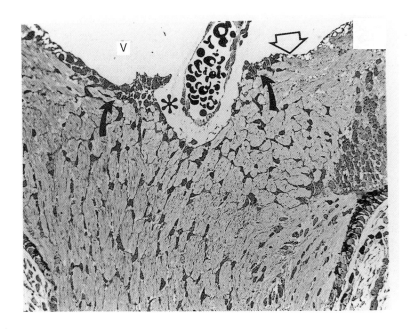

Fig. 17.61 Section through the optic disc of an embryo at 9 weeks' gestation. A group of glial cells located adjacent to the continuity of the hyaloid canal (*) with the vitreous cavity (V) constitute the base of Bergmeister's papilla (arrows). The hollow arrow shows the internal limiting membrane of retina. Light micrograph, original magnification ×320. (From Rhodes, R. H. (1978) *Am. J. Anat.*, **153**, 601, with permission.)

a short distance into the vitreous around the hyaloid canal. The stimulus for the glial cell proliferation is thought to be traction on the vitreal face of the optic disc by the attached vitreous fibrils after growth of the primary vitreous has ceased (Rhodes, 1978). Subsequent focal necrosis and tissue remodelling are responsible for the physiological excavation of the optic cup and also usually involve Bergmeister's papilla, leading to its atrophy. However, Bergmeister's pupilla can remain, together with remnants of the hyaloid artery, on the optic disc with no apparent harmful visual effects.

OPTIC NERVE AXONS

Glioblasts, which differentiate as astrocytes, are present in the optic nerve only up to 10–12 weeks of gestation. At this stage 1.9 million axons, characterized by their round profiles and pale axoplasm containing microtubules, filaments and occasional mitochondria, are present in the optic nerve (Provis *et al.*, 1985). This number of axonal fibres greatly exceeds the number of ganglion cells in the ganglion cell layer and indicates that ganglion cells contribute axons to the optic nerve before their migration in the retina is complete. The number of axons increases rapidly so that at approximately 16 weeks of gestation the fetal optic nerve contains about 3.7 million axons (Fig. 17.62). However, by 33 weeks 70% of the axons have been eliminated and the adult number of fibres (approximately 1.1 million) is established. The rate of loss is not uniform; the maximum number of axons is lost during weeks 16–20, the remainder being eliminated during a more

prolonged period that concludes at about week 30. The decline in axon number is related, at least in part, to the degeneration (pyknosis and apoptosis) of ganglion cells in the fetal retina. The relatively rapid loss of axons may correspond to the segregation of terminals from an initial diffuse projection into discrete laminae in the dorsal lateral geniculate nucleus.

AXONAL CROSSOVER AT THE OPTIC CHIASM

The factors governing the partial crossover of ganglion cell axons at the optic chiasm are poorly defined. Studies *in vitro* of axons from embryonic rat retina reveal that cell membranes prepared from the chiasm midline act as a barrier for presumptive non-crossing axons, but do not influence the growth of fibres that originate from those regions of retina that do not crossover. These findings suggest that repulsive or inhibitory molecules are expressed by certain cells of the chiasm midline (mostly probably radial glial cells) which provide a guidance cue and act specifically on ipsilateral projecting axons (Wizenmann *et al.*, 1993).

MYELINATION

Myelination of the optic nerve fibres starts near the chiasm at about the seventh month and stops at the lamina cribrosa about 1 month after birth.

17.8 VITREOUS

The formation of the vitreous is related to the development and subsequent regression of the hyaloid artery. At 4 weeks of gestation (5–7 mm stage) mesodermal cells invade the cavity of the developing optic cup through the patent optic fissure. These cells differentiate into the hyaloid artery and its branches, the vasa hyaloidae propria, which occupy most of the space between the lens and the neural retina (Figs 17.59a and 17.63). Between the fourth and fifth weeks (embryo 13 mm) the retrolental space becomes filled with the primary vitreous, which consists of fibrillar material, mesenchymal cells and vascular channels (Ozanics and Jakobiec, 1982). The fibrillar content of the extracellular matrix originates from the fibrils that existed between the invaginating lens placode and the inner surface of the optic cup and is therefore ectodermal in origin. It subsequently organizes as a randomly oriented network of collagen fibrils. The mesenchymal cells, which are probably derived from the hyaloid artery

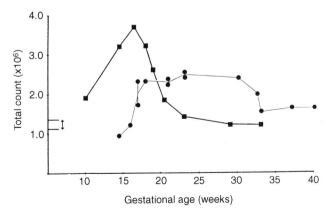

Fig. 17.62 The numbers of cells in the ganglion cell layer (GCL) of the retina (●) and axons in the optic nerve (■), as correlated with gestational age. The double-headed arrow indicates the estimated number of optic nerve fibres in the adult eye (From Provis, J. M., van Driel, D., Billson, F. A. and Russell, P. (1985) *J. Comp. Neurol.*, **236**, 92, with permission).

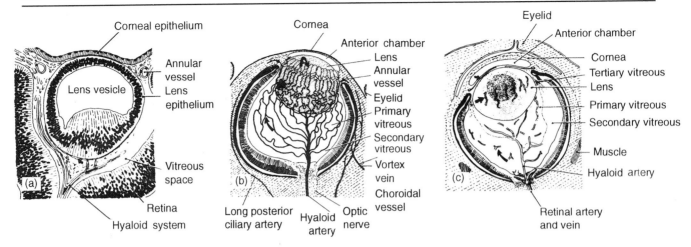

Fig. 17.63 The development of the vitreous. (a) At 5 weeks' gestation, the hyaloid vessels and their branches, the vasa hyaloidae propria, occupy the space between the lens vesicle and the neuroectoderm of the optic cup. A capillary network joins the capsula perilenticula fibrosa, which is composed of ectodermal fibrils associated with vasoformative mesenchyme from the periphery. (b) By the end of the second month the vascular primary vitreous reaches its greatest development. Arborization of the vasa hyaloidae propria (curved arrow) fills the retrolental area and is embedded in collagen fibrils. An avascular secondary vitreous of more finely fibrillar composition forms a narrow zone between the peripheral (outer) branches of the vasa hyaloidae propria and the retina. The hooked arrow points to a vessel of the pupillary membrane. The drawing is a composite of embryos from the 15–30 mm stage. (c) During the fourth month the hyaloid vessels, the vasa hyaloidae propria and the tunica vasculosa lentis atrophy progressively, with the smaller peripheral channels regressing first. The large curved arrow points to remnants of involuted vessels of the superficial portion of the vasa hyaloidae propria in the secondary vitreous. The small curved arrow indicates the location of the pupillary membrane (not drawn). The straight arrow points to remnants of the atrophied capsulopupillary vessels. Zonular fibres (tertiary vitreous) begin to extend from the growing ciliary region towards the lens capsule. Vessels through the centre of the optic nerve connect with the hyaloid artery and vein and send small loops into the retina (open arrow). The drawing is a composite of fetuses from the 75–110 mm stages. (From Ozanics, V. and Jakobiec, F. A. in Duane, T. D. and Jaeger, E. A. (eds) (1982) *Biomedical Foundations of Opthalmology*, vol. 1, published by Harper and Row.)

as well as from the cells that originally invaded the optic cup, differentiate into fibroblasts and mononuclear phagocytes. By the end of the fifth week (16 mm stage) a capillary network develops from the terminal portion of the hyaloid artery and joins the fibrillar capsule on the posterior surface of the lens; this constitutes the posterior vascular capsule. As the developing eye continues to grow the vascular primary vitreous attains its maximum formation by 2 months' gestation (Fig. 17.63).

THE SECONDARY VITREOUS

The secondary vitreous starts to develop at the 13 mm stage and continues until the 70 mm stage. At first it occupies the narrow space between the retina and the posterior (outer) limit of the primary vitreous. The secondary vitreous, which is avascular, consists of a more compact network of type II collagen fibrils with a diameter of 10 nm and primitive hyalocytes. The precise origin of these cells is presumed to be from the phagocytic monocytes of the primary vitreous. The content of hyaluronic acid is very low during the prenatal period, but increases after birth.

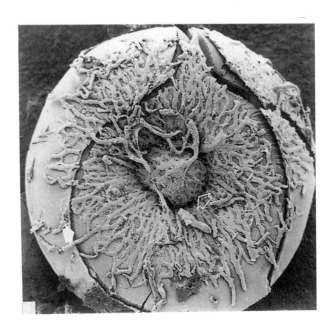

Fig. 17.64 Posterior surface of the lens from a human embryo at 9 weeks of gestation. The network of capillaries constitutes the tunica vasculosa lentis. The cleft (arrow) and sunken centre of the lens (hollow arrow) are due to artefact. Scanning electron micrograph, original magnification ×720. (From Sellheyer, K. and Spitznas, M. (1987) *Graefes Arch. Clin. Exp. Ophthalmol.*, **225**, 377, with permission.)

THE TUNICA VASCULOSA LENTIS

During the ninth week of gestation (embryo 35 mm) vascular elements derived from the annular vessel at the rim of the optic cup extend toward the equator and the anterior surface of the lens (Ozanics and Jakobiec, 1982). They become organized as the capsulopupillary vessels. The entire complex of vascular channels now surrounding the lens constitutes the tunica vasculosa lentis (Fig. 17.64).

The tunica vasculosa lentis reaches its greatest development at about the 40 mm stage. During the third and fourth months (Fig. 17.63) this system atrophies, starting with the capsulopupillary portion at about 10 weeks (45 mm stage). The vasa hyaloidea propria begins to close during the 12th week of gestation (65 mm) and remnants hang like corkscrews from the back of the lens. The process of regression is characterized by a gradual shrinkage of the vessel wall and a reduction in the diameter of the lumina, which eventually leaves thread-like acellular strands of tissue (Ko, Chi and Chang, 1985). By the fourth month atrophy of the hyaloid artery and simultaneous retraction of the primary vitreous have progressed to the extent that they are confined to a narrow central region behind the lens. This area remains throughout life as Cloquet's canal.

THE TERTIARY VITREOUS

At approximately 12 weeks of gestation (embryo 65 mm) a condensation of thicker collagen fibres of the secondary vitreous becomes attached firmly to the internal limiting membrane of the optic cup close to its rim and extends to the equator of the lens. This development of the tertiary vitreous constitutes the embryonic 'zone of origin' or vitreous base, and is known as the marginal bundle of Drualt or the faisceau isthmique. The zonular apparatus of the lens will ultimately develop anterior to these collagen fibrils.

FINAL ORGANIZATION OF VITREOUS

The pupillary membrane and the posterior vascular capsule on the anterior and posterior surfaces of the lens, respectively, finally regress during the fifth month (160 mm). Blood flow in the hyaloid artery ceases at the seventh month of gestation, and the vessel is almost completely atrophied by birth. However, remnants may persist at the posterior lens capsule, near the patellar fossa, as Mittendorf's dots and at the optic disc the remaining attachment is recognized as the area of Martegiani. Finally the

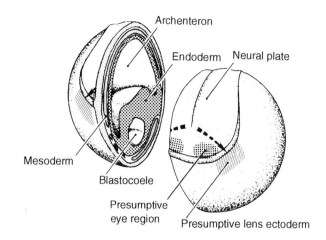

Fig. 17.65 A bisected, developing *Xenopus* egg at the neural plate stage. The boundaries of neural tissue are delineated by the neural folds, with the presumptive eye regions just inside the folds, and the presumptive lens ectoderm just outside of them. Underlying the presumptive lens ectoderm is mesoderm which contributes to the lens-forming response in this species. The inductive influence of the anterior neural plate at this stage is indicated by arrows. (From Grainger, R. M. (1992) *Eye*, **6**, 117, with permission.)

hyalocytes phagocytose debris and then come to occupy a position in the cortex of the vitreous where they begin to synthesize hyaluronic acid.

17.9 LENS AND ZONULES

Determination of lens development is one of the earliest features of embryogenesis. During mid-gastrulation a lens-forming bias is gradually imparted on an extensive region of head ectoderm as a result of the interaction between the surface ectoderm and the underlying chordamesoderm (Albers, 1987; Saha, Clayton and Grainger, 1989). The anlage of the eye subsequently transmits an inductive signal laterally through the neuralized ectoderm to the region of the presumptive lens. At the stage when the neural plate is still open in late gastrulation, the mesoderm located beneath the putative lens ectoderm conveys yet another signal which potentiates the fate of this tissue (Fig. 17.65). Finally, during neurulation, the optic vesicle exerts its effect on the ectoderm (which is now strongly predisposed toward lens formation), invokes the final phase of determination and enhances differentiation. The optic vesicle specifies the precise region of the head ectoderm that will become the lens. However, there is a specific time period during which the surface ectoderm responds to the influence of the optic vesicle. Because growth factors are present at the earliest stage of embryonic development, these are probably the molecules that function

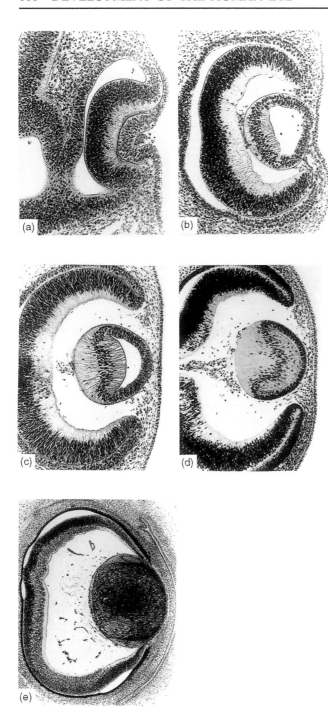

Fig. 17.66 Stages in the formation of the lens. (a) Invagination of the lens placode into the optic cup at 4 weeks' gestation; (b) at 5 weeks' gestation the formation of the lens vesicle is complete; (c) the posterior lens cells increase in length and extend towards the anterior surface of the lens at 6 weeks' gestation; (d) the lumen of the lens vesicle is almost completely obliterated at 7 weeks, and capillaries of the hyaloid system (left of lens) provide vascular supply; (e) the embryonic lens, without a posterior epithelium, is fully formed by 8 weeks of gestation. (From O'Rahilly, R. and Müller, F. (1992) *Human Embryology and Teratology*, published by Wiley-Liss, with permission.)

as the 'signals' between the various germ layers (Tripathi *et al.*, 1991).

LENS PLACODE AND VESICLE

By 27 days of gestation (embryo 4–4.5 mm) elongation of the surface cells has produced a localized area of ectodermal thickening (Fig. 17.6). This region (known as the lens placode) and its underlying basal lamina are separated from the optic vesicle by a narrow space that contains a fine filamentous material (Silver and Wakely, 1974). These extracellular components are thought to have a role in the gradual invagination of the lens placode to form the lens vesicle (at approximately 29 days of gestation) (Fig. 17.66). The formation of the vesicle is marked on the surface of the embryo by a depression known as the lens pit or pore (Fig. 17.6).

Initially the lens vesicle remains attached to the surface ectoderm by the lens stalk (Fig. 17.6) but further differentiation depends on the influence of the optic cup. The vesicle sinks into the orifice of the cup and a zone of extreme attenuation and necrosis develops in the lens stalk. By about 33 days of gestation (8–10 mm stage) the separation is complete and the spherical lens vesicle, approximately 0.2 mm in diameter, comes to lie inside the eye. The apices of the cuboidal cells are now directed toward the central cavity of the lens vesicle, whereas the basal surface is outward and applied to the original basal lamina that envelops the vesicle completely (Fig. 17.67). With continued synthesis and secretion by the lens cells the basal lamina thickens and forms the lens capsule (Tripathi and Tripathi, 1983; 1984).

THE EMBRYONIC NUCLEUS

As the lens vesicle closes, the rate of DNA synthesis of the cells subjacent to the neural retina decreases and their content of cytoplasmic organelles reduces. At the same time they begin to synthesize crystallins (specific lens proteins). Beginning at about 5 weeks (embryo 12 mm) the cells also increase in length (Figs 17.66 and 17.67) and, by extending towards the anterior surface of the lens vesicle, its lumen is obliterated by 45 days of gestation (20 mm stage). These primary lens fibres attach firmly to the apical surface of the anterior lens epithelial cells through fascia adherens tight junctions. The cell nuclei of the fibres, which also migrate anteriorly, eventually disintegrate and disappear. Thus, during the first 2 months of embryogenesis, the posterior cells of the vesicle are responsible for the major growth of the lens (Fig. 17.66). They are preserved as the compact

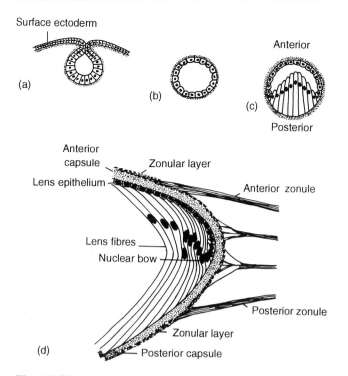

Fig. 17.67 Diagrammatic representations of stages in the development of the lens and its capsule. (a) Formation of lens vesicle from invagination of surface ectoderm together with its basal lamina in an embryo corresponding to 32 days of gestation; (b) separation of the vesicle from the surface ectoderm and its surrounding basal lamina; (c) obliteration of lens vesicle cavity by elongation of posterior cells at about 35 days of gestation; (d) equatorial region of the fully formed lens. With formation of the zonules the lens capsule is augmented by a zonular layer. Attachment of zonules to the anterior, posterior and equatorial regions of the lens periphery becomes apparent at approximately 5½ weeks' gestation. Note the change in polarity of cells from anterior to posterior regions of the lens. (From Tripathi, R. C. and Tripathi, B. J. in Davson, H. (ed.), (1984) *The Eye*, vol. 1A, published by Academic Press, New York.)

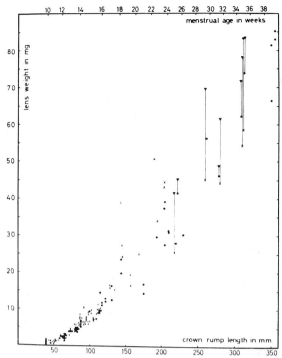

Fig. 17.68 Changes in weight of the lens during development. ▼ = Fresh lenses; ● = formalin fixed lenses; × = ethanol–formalin–acetic acid fixed lenses. The vertical lines indicate the change in weight due to fixation.

core of the lens, known as the embryonic nucleus; the posterior aspect of the lens, therefore, becomes devoid of epithelium (Tripathi and Tripathi, 1983).

THE LENS BOW

The epithelial cells in the pre-equatorial region retain their mitotic and proliferative activity throughout life. The secondary lens fibres formed are displaced inwards toward the embryonic nucleus. They elongate axially towards the two poles, extending directly beneath the epithelium anteriorly and the capsule posteriorly, thereby encircling and covering the primary lens fibres. The nuclei of the newly formed fibres migrate progressively toward the anterior lens surface and, on sectional view, give rise to the distinctive configuration known as the lens bow (Fig. 17.67). During an initial transient stage, the

contralateral fibres that originate from different quadrants of the equatorial region are long enough to reach both the anterior and the posterior poles. This process mandates that the primary fibres lose their original attachments with the lens epithelium anteriorly and their basal lamina posteriorly. However, with successive internalization of fibres and consequent increase in lens volume, new lens fibres can no longer extend from one pole to the other. Instead they meet at radiating lines or sutures that appear as an erect Y anteriorly and an inverted Y posteriorly. The Y sutures, which are first seen at about the 35 mm stage (approximately 8.5 weeks of gestation) persist through the entire thickness of the fetal nucleus, and remain throughout life as a hallmark of lens development. In the infantile and adult nucleus the sutures become more complex. Structurally, the lens develops into three components: the capsule, the epithelium, and the lens cells or fibres.

CHANGES IN LENS SHAPE

The lens undergoes several changes in shape during its embryogenesis. Initially, it is elongated in the anteroposterior direction. However, at the 18–24 mm stage, it is approximately spherical and, with the appearance of secondary lens fibres at the 26 mm stage, the lens becomes wider in its equatorial diameter. The lens then increases rapidly in mass and volume as new fibres are laid down (Fig. 17.68), and expands in both the sagittal and equatorial planes. At birth the lens is almost spheroidal, being slightly wider in the equatorial plane (Bron and Brown, 1994; Brown and Bron, 1996). The factors that govern these changes are unknown but they may be related in part to zonular traction and in part to other factors such as the steady, but small, dehydration of the entire lens that begins *in utero* and continues postnatally (Bours and Fodisch, 1986). The growth of the lens after birth is considered in Chapter 12.

CRYSTALLIN PROTEIN CHANGES

The developing lens possesses other characteristics that distinguish it from the adult structure. For example, the concentration of γ-crystallin in the lens increases steadily throughout fetal life and reaches 23% of the total (crystallin) protein just before birth (Bessems *et al.*, 1990). Its synthesis ceases either just before birth (Thomson and Augusteyn, 1985) or at 5 or 6 years of age (Bours, 1980). The high proportion of γ-crystallin may account, at least in part, for the greater transparency of the most central region of the lens (Bron and Brown, 1996).

The earliest fibres of the zonular apparatus are a continuation of the internal limiting membrane that thickens over the non-pigmented epithelium of the developing ciliary processes. They begin to develop at about the tenth week of gestation (45 mm stage). Later, zonular fibrils are synthesized by the ciliary epithelial cells, and the zonules increase in number, strength and coarseness. By the fifth month the zonules have reached the lens and merge with both the anterior and posterior capsule.

17.10 OCULAR ADNEXAE

By the fourth week of gestation the developing eye is surrounded by neural crest-derived mesenchyme and the invasion of this region of the head by mesodermal mesenchyme is complete. At this time the maxillary and frontonasal processes are beginning to elongate, although differentiation of the periocular skeleton, musculature and connective tissue has not commenced (Noden, 1982).

EYELIDS

The development of the upper lid is evident first as proliferation of the surface ectoderm in the region of

the future outer canthus at 4–5 weeks of gestation (embryo 8–12 mm). During the second month (at approximately 20 mm) both upper and lower eyelids become evident as undifferentiated skin folds that contain mesenchyme of neural crest origin (Fig. 17.17). Later mesodermal mesenchyme invades the lids and differentiates into the palpebral musculature (Noden, 1982). The two lid folds grow towards each other and elongate laterally. The margins contact each other at the beginning of the third month (35–40 mm stage) and fuse at approximately 10 weeks of gestation (embryo 45 mm). At this stage the conjunctival epithelium is already well differentiated. Goblet cells containing sialomucin first appear in the fornix region and extend toward the palpebral region and then the bulbar region (Sellheyer and Spitznas, 1988e; Miyashita, Azuma and Hida, 1992).

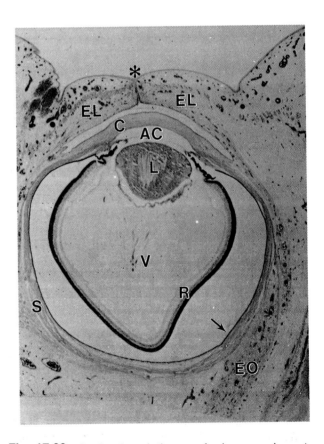

Fig. 17.69 Section through the eye of a human embryo at 16 weeks of gestation. The eyelids (EL) are fused (asterisk) and the extraocular muscles (EO) are developing. C = Cornea; AC = anterior chamber; L = lens; S = sclera; R = neural retina separated artefactually from the retinal pigment epithelium (arrow); V = vitreous cavity. (From Tripathi, B. J., Tripathi, R. C., Livingston, A. M. and Borisuth, N. S. C. (1991) *Am. J. Anat.*, **192**, 442, with permission.)

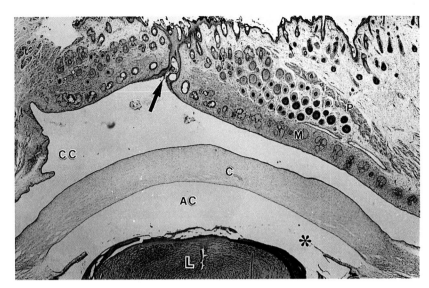

Fig. 17.70 Meridional section of fetal eye at 5 months' gestation. The upper and lower lids now contain meibomian glands (M), palpebral muscles (P) and pilosebaceous units (small arrows), but the lid margins are still fused (large arrow). CC = Conjunctival cul-de-sac; C = cornea; AC = anterior chamber; L = lens; * = pupillary membrane. Light micrograph, original magnification ×24. (From Tripathi, B. J., Tripathi, R. C. and Wisdom, J. in Ritch, R., Shields, M. B. and Krupin, T. (eds), (1995) *The Glaucomas*, 2nd edition, published by C. V. Mosby.)

LACRIMAL GLAND

The lacrimal gland is first seen to arise at about 45 days of gestation (25 mm) as solid cords of epithelial cells proliferating from the basal cells of the conjunctiva located at the temporal region of the upper fornix (Ozanics and Jakobiec, 1982). The surrounding neural crest-derived mesenchymal cells condense around the tips of the cords and differentiate into the acini of the gland. At approximately 3 months (embryo 60–65 mm) the ducts of the gland are formed by vacuolation of the cord cells and the development of lumina. Epidermal growth factor may stimulate tear secretion from the lacrimal gland by promoting the synthesis of prostaglandins, which influence the movement of fluid from the intercellular compartment into the conjunctival sac (Kapalanga and Blecher, 1991).

LID APPENDAGES AND PILOSEBACEOUS GLANDS

The formation of lid appendages and pilosebaceous units takes place between the third and sixth months of gestation (Figs 17.69 and 17.70). The development of the cilia (eyelashes) is apparent initially as a proliferation of the surface epithelial cells into the underlying mesenchyme while maintaining an intact basal lamina; this is followed by differentiation of hair follicles. During the fourth month of gestation the sebaceous glands of Zeis appear as lateral outgrowths from the invaginated epithelial cells. Production of lipid soon commences and it is secreted into the hair shaft; thereafter the canal becomes keratinized. The sebaceous meibomian glands, formed by an ingrowth

of basal epithelial cells at the inner margin, and the sweat glands of Moll that arise from the walls of the hair sacs develop at approximately the 80 mm stage (fourth month) (Ozanics and Jakobiec, 1982).

Between the fifth and sixth months of gestation the eyelids open. This event is normally associated with an increase in the formation of keratohyalin granules in the epidermal cells and with keratinization at the fusion junction. The initiation of keratinization, but not the subsequent differentiation and cornification of the junctional cells, is induced by epidermal growth factor (Nanney *et al.*, 1984). Experimental studies have shown that epidermal growth factor can stimulate precocious eyelid opening by producing keratinization of the epidermis between the upper and lower lids (Carpenter and Cohen, 1979).

EXTRAOCULAR MUSCLES AND ORBITAL CONTENTS

The connective tissue of the orbit, including Tenon's capsule (the fascia bulbi) and the periorbita (modified dura mater), develops from neural crest-derived mesenchyme. Early in embryogenesis the mesodermal condensations of myotomal cells of the preotic somites shift cranially to assume positions near and within the neural crest mesenchyme that is situated medially to the dorsal and caudal aspects of the developing eye (Noden, 1982). These cells give rise to the extraocular muscles (Fig. 17.69); the four muscles innervated by the oculomotor nerve develop from the premandibular condensations, whereas the lateral rectus and the superior oblique muscles differentiate from the maxillomandibular mesoderm.

Classically the development of the extraocular muscles is regarded as beginning at the muscle cone (the annulus of Zinn) around the optic nerve at the apex of the orbit and progressing anteriorly; the tendons start to fuse with the sclera near the end of the third month of gestation (embryo about 60 mm). Recent studies indicate that the muscles differentiate *in situ* from mesenchyme within the orbit (Sevel, 1981). In either event, the undifferentiated cells transform into early myoblasts. Myofibrils with immature Z lines and glycogen granules first appear in the cytoplasm of some myoblasts at approximately 38 days of gestation. Myogenic cells at various stages of development, from myoblasts to muscle fibres, are already present at 40–46 days of gestation. Fusion of the elongated myotubes occurs at the same time as muscle-specific isoenzymes are detectable (Oguni *et al.*, 1992). At about 7 weeks of gestation (22–30 mm stage) the dorsomedial aspect of the superior rectus muscle gives rise to the levator muscle, which grows laterally and over the superior rectus toward the eyelid. By birth the orbital contents are comparable to those in the adult.

BONY ORBIT

Of the seven orbital bones, the first to be laid down is the ethmoid at weeks 6–8 of gestation. The ethmoid and lacrimal bones are derived from the nasal process and the maxillary process contributes to the floor and lateral walls of the orbit. The trochlea begins to consolidate at about 9 weeks of gestation (embryo approximately 40 mm). Except for the lesser wing of the sphenoid, which is initially cartilaginous, all other bones of the orbit are membranous and begin to ossify during the third month. Fusion takes place between the sixth and seventh months.

At first the angle between the orbital axes subtends nearly 180°, but diminishes to approximately 105° at 3 months of gestation. With continued enlargement and repositioning of the head structures and the brain, the eyes become oriented frontally and at birth the angle is 71°. The adult condition of 68° is not achieved until the age of 3 years, by which time the eye has attained its adult size. However, the adult dimensions of the orbit are not reached until adolescence, sometimes as late as 16 years of age.

References and further reading

Abbie, A.A. (1933), The blood supply of lateral geniculate body with note on morphology of choroidal arteries. *J Anat*, **67**, 491.

Abbie, A.A. (1934), The morphology of the fore-brain arteries, with especial reference to the evolution of the basal ganglia. *J Anat*, **68**, 433.

Abbie, A.A. (1938), *Med J Aust*, **2**, 199.

Abdel-Khalek, L.M.R., Williamson, J. and Lee, W.R. (1978), Morphological changes in the human conjunctival epithelium, I: in the normal elderly population. *Br J Ophthalmol*, **62**, 792.

Abd-el-Malek, S. (1938), On the localization of nerve centres of the extrinsic ocular muscles in the oculomotor nucleus. *J Anat*, **72**, 518.

Adams, A.D. (1979), The morphology of human conjunctival mucus. *Arch Ophthalmol*, **97**, 730.

Adey, W.R. and Tokizane, T. (eds.) (1967), Structure and function of the limbic system, in *Progress in Brain Research, vol. 27*, Elsevier, Amsterdam.

Ahnelt, P.K., Kolb, H. and Pflug, R. (1987), Identification of a subtype of cone photoreceptor, likely to be blue sensitive, in the human retina. *J Comp Neurol*, **255**(18), 34.

Aitken, D., Friend, J., Thoft, R.A. *et al.* (1988), An ultrastructural study of rabbit ocular surface transdifferentiation. Invest *Ophthalmol Vis Sci*, **29**, 224.

Aizawa, K. (1958), The depth of the normal anterior chamber. *Acta Soc Ophthalmol*, **62**, 2283.

Akert, K., Glicksman, M.A., Lang, W. *et al.* (1980). The Edinger–Westphal nucleus in the monkey: a retrograde tracer study. *Brain Res*, **184**, 491.

Akiya, S., Uemura, Y. and Fujiwara, T. (1984), Electron microscopic observations on the developing rabbit and human vitreous collagen fibrils by negative staining. *Ophthalmic Res*, **16**, 233.

Albertini, D.F. (1980), Plasma membrane changes during folliculogenesis, in *Biology of the Ovary* (eds P.M. Motta and E.S. Hafex), Martinus Nijoff, Hague, p. 138.

Albrecht, M. and Eisner, G. (1982), The hyalo-capsular zonula. *A von Graefes Arch Klin Exp Ophthalmol*, **218**, 88.

Alcala, J. and Maisel, H. (1985), Biochemistry of lens plasma membranes and cytoskeleton, in *The Ocular Lens: Structure, Function and Pathology* (ed H. Maisel), Marcel Dekker, New York, p. 169.

Aldredge, H., Hershberg, R. and Fisher, C.M. (1970), Oculomotor palsy in diabetes mellitus: a clinicopathological study. *Brain*, **93**, 553.

Alexais, K. and D'Astros, L. (1892), *J Anat Physiol, Paris*, **28**, 519.

Allansmith, M.R., Baird, R.S. and Greiner, J.V. (1979), Vernal conjunctivitis and contact lens-associated giant papillary conjunctivitis compared and contrasted. *Am J Ophthalmol*, **87**, 544.

Allansmith, M.R., Greiner, J.V. and Baird, R.S. (1978), Number of inflammatory cells in the normal conjunctiva. *Am J Ophthalmol*, **86**, 250.

Allansmith, M.R., Kajiyama, G., Abelson, M.B. *et al.* (1976), Plasma cell content of main and accessory lacrimal glands and conjunctiva. *Am J Ophthalmol*, **82**, 819.

Allen, D.P., Low, P.S., Dola, A. *et al.* (1987), Band 3 and ankyrin homologues are present in the eye lens: Evidence for all major erythrocyte membrane components in same non-erythroid cell. *Biochem Biophys Res Commun*, **149**, 266.

Allen, L. (1971a), Stereoscopic fluorescein angiography of the ocular fundus. *J Biol Photogr Assoc*, **39**, 8936.

Allen, L. (1971b), Modified impression fitting. *Int Ophthalmol Clin*, **10**, 747.

Allen, L. (1971c), Cosmetic optics. *Int Ophthalmol Clin*, **10**, 783.

Allen, M., Wright, P. and Reid, L. (1972), The human lacrimal gland. A histochemical and organ culture study of the secretory cells. *Arch Ophthalmol*, **88**, 493.

Allen, M.J. (1956), The influence of age on the speed of accommodation. *Am J Optom*, **33**, 201.

Alley, K. (1977), Anatomical basis for interaction between cerebellar flocculus and brainstem. *Dev Neurosci*, **1**, 109.

Alley, K., Baker, R. and Simpson, J.I. (1975), Afferents to the vestibulo–cerebellum and the origin of the visual climbing fibers in the rabbit. *Brain Res*, **98**, 582.

Allman, J.M., Kaas, J.H., Lane, R.H. *et al.* (1972), A representation of the visual field in the inferior nucleus of the pulvinar in the owl monkey (*Aotus trivirgatus*). *Brain Res*, **40**, 291.

Alm, A. (1977), The effect of sympathetic stimulation on blood flow through the uvea, retina, and optic nerve in monkeys. *Exp Eye Res*, **25**, 19.

Alm, A. and Bill, A. (1970), Blood flow and oxygen extraction in the cat uvea at normal and high intraocular pressures. *Acta Physiol Scand*, **80**, 19.

Alm, A. and Bill, A. (1972), The oxygen supply to the retina. II. Effects of high intraocular pressure on uveal and retinal blood flow in cats. A study with labelled microspheres including flow determinations in brain and some other tissues. *Acta Physiol Scand*, **84**, 306.

Alm, A. and Bill, A. (1973), Ocular and optic nerve blood flow at normal and increased intraocular pressures in monkeys (*Macaca iris*): a study with radioactively labelled microspheres including flow determinations in brain and some other tissues. *Exp Eye Res*, **15**, 15.

Alm, A. and Bill, A. (1987), Ocular circulation, in *Adlers Physiology of the Eye*, 8th edition (eds R.A. Moses and W.M.J. Hart), Mosby, St Louis, p. 183.

Almegard, B. and Andersson, S.E. (1990), Outflow facility in the monkey eye: Effects of calcitonin gene-related peptide, cholecystokinin, galanin, substance P and capsaicin. *Exp Eye Res*, **51**, 685.

Alpern, M. (1969), Movements of the eyes, in *The Eye*, 2nd edition (ed. H. Davson), Academic Press, New York, p. 1.

Alpers, J.B., Berry, R.G. and Paddison, R.M. (1959), *Arch Neurol Psychiatr*, **81**, 409.

Altman, J. and Carpenter, M.B. (1961), Fiber projections of the superior colliculus in the cat. *J Comp Neurol*, **116**, 157.

Alvarado, J., Murphy, C. and Juster, R. (1983), Age-related changes in the basement membrane of the human corneal epithelium. *Invest Ophthalmol Vis Sci*, **24**, 1015.

Alvarado, J., Murphy, C. and Juster, R. (1984), Trabecular meshwork cellularity in primary open angle glaucoma and nonglaucomatous normals. *Ophthalmology*, **91**, 564.

Alvarado, J., Murphy, C., Polansky, J. *et al.* (1981), Age-related changes in trabecular meshwork cellularity. *Invest Ophthalmol Vis Sci*, **21**, 714.

Alvarado, J.A. and Van Horn, C. (1975), Muscle cell types of the cat inferior oblique, in *Basic Mechanisms of Ocular Motility and their Clinical Implications* (eds G. Lennerstrand and P. Bach-y-Rita), Pergamon Press, Oxford, p. 15.

Alvarado-Mallart, R.M. and Pincon-Raymond, M. (1976), Nerve endings on the intramuscular tendons of cat extraocular muscles. *Neurosci Lett*, **2**, 121.

Amalric, P. (1963), Le territoire chorio-rétinien de l'artère ciliaire longue postérieure. Etude clinique. *Bull Soc Ophtalmol Fr*, **63**, 342.

Amalric, P. (1973), Choroidal vessel occlusive syndromes – clinical aspects. *Trans Am Acad Ophthalmol Otolaryngol*, **77**, 291.

Amato, A., Barbour, B., Szatkowski, M. *et al.* (1994), Counter-transport of potassium by the glutamate uptake carrier in glial cells isolated from the tiger salamander retina. *J Physiol*, **479**, 371.

Anderson, D.R. (1969a), Scanning electron microscopy of primate trabecular meshwork. *Am J Ophthalmol*, **71**, 90.

Anderson, D.R. (1969b), Ultrastructure of human and monkey lamina cribrosa and optic nerve head. *Arch Ophthalmol*, **82**, 800.

Anderson, D.R. and Braverman, S. (1976), Re-evaluation of the optic disc vasculature. *Am J Ophthalmol* **82**, 165.

Anderson, D.R. and Hoyt, W.F. (1969), Ultrastructure of intraorbital portion of human and monkey optic nerve. *Arch Ophthalmol*, **82**, 506.

Anderson, D.R., Hoyt, W.F. and Hogan, M.J. (1967), The fine structure of the astroglia in the human optic nerve and optic nerve head. *Trans Am Ophthalmol Soc*, **65**, 275.

Andres, K.H. (1974), Morphological criteria for the differentiation of mechanoreceptors in vertebrates, in *Symposium Mechanorezeption, Abhdlg Rhein Westf Akad Wiss 53*, (ed. J. Schwartzkopff), Westdeutscher Verlag, Opladen, p. 135.

Andres, K.H. and Kautzky, R. (1955), Die Frühentwicklung der vegetativen Hals- und Kopfganglien des Menschen. *Z Anat Entwgesch* **119**, 55.

Andres, K.H. and Kautzky, R. (1956), Kleine vegetative Ganglien in Bereich der Schädelbasis des Menschen. *Dtsch Z Nervenheilk*, **174**, 272.

Andrews, J.S. (1973), The meibomian secretion. *Int Ophthalmol Clin*, **13**, 1.

Ankar, R.L. and Cragg, B.G. (1974), Development of the extrinsic connections of the visual cortex in the cat. *J Comp Neurol*, **154**, 29.

Anseth, A. (1961), Glycosaminoglycans in corneal regeneration. *Exp Eye Res*, **1**, 122.

Aragona, P., Candela, V., Micali, A. *et al.* (1987), Effects of a stable analogue of PGE2 (11-deoxy-13,14 didehydro-16(s)-methylester methyl PGE_2:FCE 20700) on the secretory processes of conjunctival goblet cells of rabbit. *Exp Eye Res*, **45**, 647.

Araki, M. (1977), Observations on the corrosion casts of the choriocapillaris at the posterior pole. *Acta Soc Ophthalmol Jpn*, **80**, 315.

Archambault, L. (1906), Le faisceau longitudinal inférieur et le faisceau optique central. Quelques considerations sur les fibres d'association du cerveau. *Rev Neurol (Paris)*, **4**, 1206.

Archambault, L. (1909), The inferior longitudinal bundle and the geniculocalcarine fasciculus. A contribution to the anatomy of the tract systems of the cerebral hemispheres. *Albany Med Am*, **30**, 118.

Arlt, F. (1863), Veber den Ringmuskel der Augenlider. *A von Graefes Arch Ophthalmol*, **9**, 64.

Armaly, M.F. and Wang, Y. (1975), Demonstration of acid mucopolysaccharides in the trabecular meshwork of the rhesus monkey. *Invest Ophthalmol*, **14**, 507.

Asbury, A.K., Aldredge, H., Hershberg, R. *et al.* (1970), Oculomotor palsy in diabetes mellitus: a clinico-pathological study. *Brain*, **93**, 555.

Ascher, K.W. (1942), The aqueous veins: I. Physiologic importance of the visible elimination of intraocular fluid. *Am J Ophthalmol*, **25**, 1174.

Ascher, K.W. (1949), Aqueous veins and their significance for pathogenesis of glaucoma. *Arch Ophthalmol*, **42**, 66.

Ashton, N. (1951), Anatomical study of Schlemm's canal and aqueous veins by means of Neoprene casts: I. Aqueous veins. *Br J Ophthalmol*, **35**, 291.

Ashton, N. (1952a), Anatomical study of Schlemm's canal and aqueous veins by means of Neoprene casts: II. Aqueous veins (continued). *Br J Ophthalmol*, **36**, 265.

Ashton, N. (1952b), Observation on the choroidal circulation. *Br J Ophthalmol*, **36**, 465.

Ashton, N. (1960), The exit pathway of the aqueous. *Trans Ophthalmol Soc UK*, **80**, 397.

Ashton, N. (1961), Observations on the choroidal circulation. *Br J Ophthalmol*, **54**, 1084.

Ashton, N. (1970), Retinal angiogenesis in the human embryo. *Br Med Bull*, **26**, 103.

Ashton, N., Brini, A. and Smith, R. (1956), Anatomical studies of the trabecular meshwork of the normal human eye. *Br J Ophthalmol*, **40**, 257.

Ashton, N. and Cunha-Vaz, J.G. (1965), Effect of histamine on the permeability of the ocular vessels. *Arch Ophthalmol*, **73**, 211.

Ashton, N. and Smith, R. (1953), Anatomical study of Schlemm's canal and aqueous veins by means of Neoprene casts: III. Arterial relations of Schlemm's canal. *Br J Ophthalmol*, **37**, 577.

Ashton, N. and Tripathi, R.C. (1972), The argyrophilic mosaic of the internal limiting membrane of the retina. *Exp Eye Res*, **14**, 49.

Ashworth, B. (1973), *Clinical Neuro-Ophthalmology*, OUP, Oxford.

Asmussen, G., Kiessling, A. and Wohlrab, F. (1971),

Histochemical characteristics of muscle fibre types in the mammalian extraocular muscles. *Acta Anat*, **79**, 526.

Aster, J.C., Brewer, G. and Maisel, H. (1986), The 4.1-like proteins of the bovine lens: spectrin-binding proteins closely related in structure to red blood cell protein 4.1. *J Cell Biol*, **103**, 115.

Attias, G. (1912), Die Nerven der Hornhaut des Menschen. *A von Graefes Arch Klin Exp Ophthalmol*, **83**, 207.

Auran, J.D., Koester, C.J., Kleiman, N.J. *et al.* (1995), Scanning slit confocal microscopic observation of cell morphology and movement within the normal human anterior cornea. *Ophthalmology*, **102**, 33.

Aurell, G. and Holmgren, H. (1941), Uber das Vorkommen von elastischen Fasem in der Hornhaut des Auges. *Z Zellforsch Mikrosk Anat*, **50**, 446.

Axenfeld, T. (1907), *Ber Versamm Ophthalm Ges Heidelberg*, **34**, 300.

Babizhayev, M.A. and Brodskaya, M.W. (1989), Fibronectin detection in drainage outflow system of human eyes in aging and progression of open-angle glaucoma. *Mech Ageing Dev*, **47**, 145.

Bach-y-Rita, P. and Murata K. (1964), Extra-ocular proprioceptive responses in the VIth nerve of the cat. *Quart J exp Physiol*, **49**, 408.

Bach-y-Rita, P., Collin, C.C. and Hyde, J.E. (1971), *The Control of Eye Movements*, 5th edition, Academic Press, New York.

Bach-y-Rita, P. and Ito, F. (1966), *In vivo* studies on fast and slow muscle fibers in cat extraocular muscles. *J Gen Physiol*, **49**, 1177.

Bahn, C.F., Glassman, R.M., MacCallum, D.K. and Lillie, J.H. (1986), Postnatal development of the corneal endothelium. *Invest Ophthalmol Vis Sci*, **27**, 44.

Bailey, A.J. (1987), Structure, function and aging of the collagens of the eye. *Eye*, **1**, 175.

Bailey, P. and von Bonin, G. (1951), *The Isocortex of Man*, University of Illinois Press, Urbana.

Bairati, A.J. and Orzalesi, N. (1966), The ultrastructure of the epithelium of the ciliary body. *Z Zellforsch*, **69**, 635.

Baker (1900), The Eyeball, in *Norris and Oliver's System of Disease of the Eye*, vol. i, Philadelphia, p. 109. (Cited by Whitnall, 1921.)

Baker, R. *et al.* (1978), Role of the prepositus hypoglossi nucleus in oculomotor function, in *Vestibular Mechanisms in Health and Disease*, Academic Press, London, p. 95.

Baker, R. and Berthoz, A. (1975), Is the prepositus hypoglossi nucleus the source of another vestibulo-ocular pathway? *Brain Res*, **86**, 121.

Baker, R. and Berthoz, A. (1977), Control of gaze by brain stem neurons. *Dev Neurosci*, **1**, 1.

Baker, R., Berthoz, A. and Delgado-Garcia, J. (1977), Monosynaptic excitation of trochlear motoneurons following electrical stimulation of the prepositus hypoglossi nucleus. *Brain Res*, **121**, 157.

Baker, R., Berthoz, A., Delgado-Garcia, J. *et al.* (1978), *Vestibular Mechanisms in Health and Disease*, Academic Press, London.

Baker, R., Gresty, M. and Berthoz, A. (1975), Neuronal activity in the prepositus hypoglossi nucleus correlated with vertical and horizontal eye movement in the cat. *Brain Res*, **101**, 366.

Baker, R. and Highstein, S.M. (1975), Physiological identification of interneurons and motoneurons in the abducens nucleus. *Brain Res*, **91**, 292.

Balasubramaniam, V., Kanaka, T.S., Ramanujam, P.B. *et al.* (1972), Electrophysiological studies during sedative neurosurgery. *Neurology (Madras)*, **20** (Suppl. 2), 175.

Balazs, E.A. (1961), Molecular morphology of the vitreous body, in *The Structure of the Eye* (ed. G.K. Smelser), Academic Press, New York, p. 293.

Balazs, E.A. (1973), The vitreous. *Inst Ophthalmol Clin*, **13**, 169.

Baleydier, C. and Mauguiere, F. (1977), *Exp Brain Res*, **27**, 501.

Bárány, E.H., Berrie, C.P., Birdsall, N.J.M. *et al.* (1982), The binding properties of the muscarinic receptors of the cynomolgus monkey ciliary body and the response to the induction of agonist subsensitivity. *Br J Pharmacol*, **77**, 731.

Bárány, E.H. and Scotchbrook, S. (1954), Influence of testicular hyaluronidase on the resistance to flow through the angle of the anterior chamber. *Acta Physiol Scand*, **30**, 240.

Barmack, N.H., Bell, C.C. and Rence, B.G. (1971), Tension and rate of tension development during isometric responses of extraocular muscle. *J Neurophysiol*, **34**, 1072.

Barris, R.W. (1936), A pupillo-constrictor area in the cerebral cortex of the cat and its relationship to the pretectal area. *J Comp Neurol*, **63**, 353.

Bassnett, S. (1992a), Coincident loss of mitochondria and nuclei during lens fiber differentiation. *Dev Dyn*, **194**, 85.

Bassnett, S. (1992b), Mitochondrial dynamics in differentiating fiber cells of the mammalian lens. *Curr Eye Res*, **11**, 1227.

Batini, C. and Buisseret, P. (1974), Sensory peripheral pathway from extrinic eye muscles. *Arch Ital Biol*, **112**, 18.

Baud, C.A. and Balvoine, C. (1953), The intimate structure of Descemet's membrane and its pathological derivatives. *Br J Ophthalmol*, **126**, 290.

Baurmann, M. (1930), Uber das Ciliafortsatz gefassystem. *Ber Versamm Ophthalm Ges Heidelberg*, **48**, 364.

Beard, C. and Quickert, M.H. (1977), *Anatomy of the Orbit*, 2nd edition, Aesculapius, Birmingham, AL.

Beauvieux, J. and Dupas, J. (1926), Étude anatomo-topographique du ganglion ophthalmique chez l'homme et divers animaux. *Arch Ophtalmol*, **18**, 641.

Beauvieux, J. and Ristitch, K. (1924), Les vaisseaux centraux du nerf optique. *Arch Ophtalmol*, **41**, 352.

Bechterew, A. (1883), Über den verlauf der die pupille verengernden nervenfasern im gehirn und über die localisation eines centrums für die iris und contraction der augenmuskeln. *Pflugers Archiv Ges Physiol Menschen Tiere*, **31**, 60.

Beck, R.W., Savino, P.J., Repka, M.X. *et al.* (1984), Optic disc structure in anterior ischemic optic neuropathy. *Ophthalmology*, **91**, 1334.

Becker, W. and Jurgens, R. (1979), An analysis of the saccadic system by means of double step stimuli. *Vision Res*, **19**, 967.

Beckers, H.J.M., Klooster, J., Vrensen, G.F.J.M. *et al.* (1992), Ultrastructural identification of trigeminal nerve endings in the rat cornea and iris. *Invest Ophthalmol Vis Sci*, **33**, 1979.

Bednarski, A. (1925), De l'excavation physiologique du nerf optique. *Arch Ophthalmol*, **42**, 5.

Bedrossian, E.H. (1958), *D. Phil. Thesis*.

Beebe, D.C. (1994), Homeobox genes and vertebrate eye development. *Invest Ophthalmol Vis Sci*, **35**, 2897.

Beevor, C.E. (1908), *Phil Trans R Soc Lond*, **1**, 1.

Behr, C. (1935), Beitrag zur Anatomie und Klinik des septalen Gewebes und des Arterieneinbaus im Sehnervenstamm. *A von Graefes Arch Ophthalmol*, **134**, 227.

Bell, C. (1822), *Phil Trans R Soc Lond*, **1**, 289.

Belmonte, C., Simon, J. and Gallego, A. (1971), Effects of intraocular pressure changes on the afferent activity of ciliary nerves. *Exp Eye Res*, **12**, 342.

Ben Sira, I. and Riva, C.E. (1975), Fluorescein diffusion in the human optic disc. *Invest Ophthalmol*, **14**, 205.

Bender, D.B. (1981), Retinotopic organization of macaque pulvinar. *J Neurophysiol*, **46**, 672.

Bender, D.B. (1982), Receptive-field properties of neurons in the macaque inferior pulvinar. *J Neurophysiol*, **48**, 1.

Bender, D.B. (1983), Visual activation of neurons in the primate pulvinar depends on cortex but not colliculus. *Brain Res*, **297**, 258.

Bender, M.B. and Bodis-Wollner, I. (1978), Visual dysfunctions in optic tract lesions. *Ann Neurol*, **3**, 187.

Bender, M.B. and Kanzer, M.M. (1939), Dynamics of homonymous hemanopsias and preservative of central vision. *Brain*, **62**, 404.

Bender, M.B. and Strauss, I. (1937), Defects in visual field of one eye only in patients with a lesion of one optic radiation. *Arch Ophthalmol*, **17**, 765.

Bender, M.B. and Weinstein, E.A. (1943), *Arch Neurol Psychiatr*, **49**, 98.

Benedetti, E.L., Dunia, I., Bentzel, C.J. *et al.* (1976), A portrait of plasma membrane specializations in eye lens epithelium and fibers. *Biochim Biophys Acta*, **457**, 353.

Benedetti, E.L., Dunia, I., Ramaekers, F.C.S., *et al.* (1981), Lenticular plasma membranes and cytoskeleton, in *Molecular and Cellular Biology of the Eye Lens*, (ed. H. Bloemendal), John Wiley and Sons, New York, p. 137.

Benevento, L.A. and Fallon, J.H. (1975), The ascending projections of the superior colliculus in the rhesus monkey (*Macaca mulatta*). *J Comp Neurol*, **160**, 339.

Benevento, L.A. and Miller, J. (1981), Visual responses of single neurons in the caudal lateral pulvinar of the macaque monkey. *J Neurosci*, **1**, 1268.

Benevento, L.A. and Rezak, M. (1976), The cortical projections of the inferior pulvinar and adjacent lateral pulvinar in the rhesus monkey (*Macaca mulatta*): an autoradiographic study. *Brain Res*, **108**, 1.

Benevento, L.A., Rezak, M. and Santos-Anderson, R. (1977), An autoradiographic study of the projections of the pretectum in the rhesus monkey (*Macaca mulatta*): evidence for sensorimotor links to the thalamus and oculomotor nuclei. *Brain Res*, **127**, 197.

Bengtsson, B. (1980a), The inheritance and development of cup and disc diameters. *Acta Ophthalmol*, **58**, 733.

Bengtsson, B. (1980b), The alteration and asymmetry of cup and disc diameters. *Acta Ophthalmol*, **58**, 726.

Benton, A.L. and Hecaen, H. (1970), Steroscopic vision in patients with unilateral cerebral disease. *Neurology*, **20**, 1084.

Bergen, M.P. (1981), A literature review of the vascular system in the human orbit. *Acta Morphol Neurol Scand*, **19**, 273.

Bergen, M.P. (1982), Spatial aspects of the orbital vascular system. *Ocular Anat Embryol Teratol*, **1**, 859.

Bergen, M.P. and Los, J.A. (1978), Vascular patterns in the human orbit in relation to the connective tissue septa. *Orb Dis*, **1**, 197.

Berger, E. (1882), Beitrage zur anatomie der zonula zinii. *A von Graefes Arch Klin Exp Ophthalmol*, **28**, 28.

Berger, P.C., Chandler, D.B., Fryczkowski, A.W. and Klintworth, G.K. (1987), Scanning electron microscopy of corrosion casts: application in ophthalmologic research. *Scanning Microsc*, **1**, 223.

Bergland, R.M. and Ray, B.S. (1969), The arterial supply of the human optic chiasm. *Neurosurg*, **31**, 327.

Bergland, R.M., Ray, B.S. and Torack, R.M. (1968), Anatomical variations in the pituitary gland and adjacent structures in 225 human autopsy cases. *J Neurosurg*, **28**, 93.

Bergmanson, J.P.G. (1977), The ophthalmic innervation of the uvea in monkeys. *Exp Eye Res*, **24**, 225.

Bergström, B. (1973), Morphology of the vestibular nerve. 1. Anatomical studies of the vestibular nerve in man. *Acta Otolaryngol*, **76**, 162.

Berman, E.R. (1991), *Biochemistry of the Eye*, Plenum Press, New York.

Bernardis, L.L. (1974), Localization of neuroendocrine functions within the hypothalamus. *Can J Neurol Sci*, **1**, 29.

Bernheimer, S. (1897), Experimentelle Studien zur Kenntniss der Innervation der inneren und ausseren vom Oculomotorius versorgten Muskeln des Auges. *A von Graefes Arch Ophthalmol*, **44**, 481.

Berry, A.C. (1975), Factors affecting the incidence of non-metrical skeletal variants. *J Anat*, **120**, 519.

Bessems, G.J., Bours, J., Hofmann, D. *et al.* (1990), Molecular mass distribution of water-soluble crystallins from the human foetal lens during development. *J Chromatogr*, **529**, 277.

Bill, A. (1962a), Aspects of physiological and pharmalogical regulation of uveal blood flow. *Acta Soc Med Upsalien*, **67**, 122.

Bill, A. (1962b), Autonomic nervous control of uveal blood flow. *Acta Physiol Scand*, **56**, 70.

Bill, A. (1966a), Conventional and uveo-scleral drainage of aqueous humour in the cynomolgus monkey (*Macaca irus*) at normal and high intraocular pressures. *Exp Eye Res*, **5**, 45.

Bill, A. (1966b), The routes for bulk drainage of aqueous humour in the vervet monkey (*Cercopithecus ethiops*). *Exp Eye Res*, **5**, 55.

Bill, A. (1967), Effects of atropine and pilocarpine on aqueous humor dynamics in cynomolgus monkeys (*Macaca irus*). *Exp Eye Res*, **6**, 120.

Bill, A. (1968), A method to determine osmotically effective albumin and gammaglobulin concentrations in tissue fluids, its application to the uvea and a note on the effects of capillary 'leaks' on tissue fluid dynamics. *Acta Physiol Scand*, **73**, 511.

Bill, A. (1975), The drainage of aqueous humor. *Invest Ophthalmol*, **14**, 1.

Bill, A. (1977), Basic physiology of the drainage of aqueous humour. *Exp Eye Res*, **25**, 291.

Bill, A. (1985), Some aspects of the ocular circulation. Friedenwald Lecture. *Invest Ophthalmol Vis Sci*, **26**, 410.

Bill, A. (1991), The 1990 Endre Balazs Lecture: Effects of some neuropeptides on the uvea. *Exp Eye Res*, **53**, 3.

Bill, A. and Bárány, E.H. (1966), Gross facility, facility of conventional routes, and pseudofacility of aqueous humor outflow in the cynomolgus monkey. *Arch Ophthalmol*, **75**, 665.

Bill, A. and Linder, J. (1976), Sympathetic control of cerebral blood flow in acute arterial hypertension. *Acta Physiol Scand*, **96**, 114.

Bill, A. and Svedbergh, B. (1972), Scanning electron microscopic studies of the trabecular meshwork and the canal of Schlemm. An attempt to localise the main resistance to outflow of aqueous humour in man. *Acta Ophthalmol*, **50**, 295.

Bill, A., Tornqvist, P. and Alm, A. (1980), Permeability of the intraocular blood vessels. *Trans Ophthalmol Soc UK*, **100**, 332.

Billings-Gagliardi, S.M., Chan-Palav, V. and Palay, S.L. (1974), *J Neurocytol*, **3**, 619.

Binder, R. (1953), Beitrag zur Kenntnis der Schleimzellen in der Conjunctiva bulbi bei Macacus rhesus. *A von Graefes Arch Ophthalmol*, **153**, 477.

Bito, L.Z., DeRousseau, C.J., Kaufman, P.L. *et al.* (1982), Age-dependent loss of accommodative amplitude in rhesus monkeys: an animal model for presbyopia. *Invest Ophthalmol Vis Sci*, **23**, 23.

Bito, L.Z., Kaufman, P.L., Neider, M. *et al.* (1987), The dynamics of accommodation (ciliary muscle contraction, zonular relaxation, and lenticular deformation) as a function of stimulus strength and age in iridectomized rhesus eyes. *ARVO Suppl: Invest Ophthalmol Vis Sci*, **28**, 318.

Bjorklund, H., Olson, L., Palmer, M. *et al.* (1984), Enkephalin immuno-reactivity in the iris nerves: distribution in normal and grafted irides, persistence and enhanced fluorescence after denervations. *Histochem J*, **80**, 1.

Björkman, A. and Wohlfart, G. (1936), *Z Zellforsch Mikrosk Anat*, **39**, 631.

Blasdel, G.G., Lund, J.S. and Fitzpatrick, D. (1985), Intrinsic connections of macaque striate cortex: axonal projections of cells outside lamina 4C. *J Neurosci*, **5**, 3350.

Blatt, H.L., Rao, G.N. and Aquavella, J.V. (1979), Endothelial cell density in relation to morphology. *Invest Ophthalmol*, **18**, 856.

Blumke, S. and Morganroth, K. Jr (1967), The stereo ultrastructure of the external and internal surface of the cornea. *J Ultrastruct Res*, **18**, 502.

Bock, J. and Schwarz-Karsten, H. (1953), *Ber Dtsch Ophthal Ges*, **58**, 257.

Boeke, J. (1925), Die intrazellulare Lage der Nervenendigungen im Epithelgewebe und ihre Beziehungen zum. *Zellkern Z Zellforsch*, **2**, 391.

Boeke, J. (1927), *Z Zellforsch Mikrosk Anat*, **4**, 448.

Boeke, J. (1933), Innervationsstudien, III. Die Nervenversorgung des M. ciliaris und des sphincter iridis bei Säugern und Vögeln. *Z microsk-anat Forsch*, **33**, 233.

Bondareff, W. and Gordon, B. (1966), Submicroscopic localization of norepinephrine in sympathetic nerves of rat pineal. *J Pharmacol Exp Ther*, **153**, 42.

Boothe, R.G., Dobson, V. and Teller, D.Y. (1985), Postnatal development of vision in human and nonhuman primates. *Annu Rev Neurosci*, **8**, 495.

Borcherding, M.S., Blacik, L.J., Sittig, R.A. *et al.* (1975),

Proteoglycans and collagen fibre organisation in human corneoscleral tissue. *Exp Eye Res*, **21**, 59.

Bormioli, S.P., Sartore, S., Vitadello, M. *et al.* (1980), 'Slow' myosins in vertebrate skeletal muscle. *J Cell Biol*, **85**, 672.

Bors, E. (1926), Uber das zahlenverhaltnis von Nerve und Muskelfasem. *Anat Anz*, **60**, 415.

Bortolami, R., Veggetti, A., Callegari, E. *et al.* (1977), Trigeminal fibres and sensory ganglion cells in the oculomotor nerve of some animals and man. *Boll Soc Ital Biol Sper*, **53**, 214.

Bours, J. (1980), Species specificity of the crystallins and the albuminoid of the ageing lens. *Comp Biochem Physiol*, **65**, 215.

Bours, J. and Fodisch, H.J. (1986), Human fetal lens: wet and dry weight with increasing gestational age. *Ophthalmic Res*, **18**, 363.

Bours, J., Fodisch, H.J. and Hockwin, O. (1987), Age-related changes in water and crystallin content of the fetal and adult human lens, demonstrated by a microsectioning technique. *Ophthalmic Res*, **19**, 235.

Bowling, D.B. and Michael, C.R. (1980), Projection patterns of single physiologically characterized optic tract fibers in the cat. *Nature*, **286**, 899.

Bowman, W. (1848), Observations on the structure of the vitreous humour. *Dublin Quart J Med Sci*, **6**, 102.

Bozler, E. (1948), Conduction, automaticity and tonus of visceral muscle. *Experientia*, **4**, 213.

Brandtzaeg, P. and Baklien, K. (1977), *Ciba Found Symp*, **1**, 77.

Braude, L.S. and Chandler, J.W. (1983), Corneal allograft rejection. The role of the major histocompatability complex. *Surv Ophthalmol*, **27**, 290.

Braun, A., Ehinger, F., Sundler, K. *et al.* (1984), Neuropeptide Y immunoreactive neurons in the guinea pig uvea and retina. *Invest Ophthalmol Vis Sci*, **25**, 1113.

Breitbach, R. and Spitznas, M. (1988), Ultrastructure of the paralimbal and juxtacaruncular human conjunctiva. *A von Graefes Arch Klin Exp Ophthalmol*, **226**, 567.

Briggaman, R.A. (1982), Biochemical composition of the epidermal-dermal junction and other basement membranes. Progress in dermatology. *J Invest Dermatol*, **78**, 1.

Brightman, M.W. (1965), The distribution within the brain of Ferritin injected into cerebrospinal fluid compartments. II Parenchymal distribution. *Am J Anat*, **117**, 193.

Brindley, G.S., Gautier-Smith, P.C. and Lewin, W. (1969), Cortical blindness and the functions of the non-geniculate fibres of the optic tracts. *J Neurol Neurosurg Psychiatry*, **32**, 259.

Brindley, G.S. and Merton, P.A. (1960), The absence of position sense in the human eye. *J Physiol*, **153**, 127.

Brini, A., Porte, A. and Stoeckel, M.E. (1968), Morphologie et structure du vitre adulte, in *Biologie et Chirurgie du Corps Vitre* (eds. A. Brini, A. Bronner, J.P. Gerhard and J. Nordmann), Paul Masson, Paris, p. 1.

Brismar, J. (1974), Orbital phlebography. III. Topography of intra-orbital veins. *Acta Radiol Suppl*, **15**, 577.

Brodal, A. (1969), *Neurological Anatomy*, 2nd edition, OUP, Oxford.

Brodal, A. (1981), *Neurological anatomy in Relation to Clinical Medicine*, 3rd edition, OUP, Oxford.

Brodal, A., Pompeiano, O. and Walberg, F. (1962), The

Vestibular Nuclei and their Connections, in *Anatomy and Functional Correlations*, Charles C. Thomas, Springfield IL.

Brodal, P. (1992), *The Central Nervous System: Structure and Function*, OUP, Oxford.

Brodmann, K. (1909), *J Psychol Neurol, Lpz*, **2**, 137.

Broekhuyse, R.M. (1975), The lipid composition of aging sclera and cornea. *Ophthalmologica*, **171**, 82.

Brolin, S.E., Diderholm, H. and Hammar, H. (1961), An autoradiographic study on cell migration in the eye lens epithelium. *Acta Soc Med Upsalien*, **66**, 43.

Bron, A.J. (1973), Vortex patterns of the corneal epithelium. *Trans Ophthalmol Soc UK*, **93**, 455.

Bron, A.J. (1985), Prospects for the dry eye. *Trans Ophthalmol Soc UK*, **104**, 801.

Bron, A.J. (1986), Lacrimal streams. The demonstration of lacrimal fluid secretion and the lacrimal ductules. *Br J Ophthalmol*, **70**, 241.

Bron, A.J. (1996), Reflections on the tears. A discourse on the classification, diagnosis and management of dry eye. *The Doyne Lecture Eye* (in press).

Bron, A.J. and Brown, N.A.P. (1986), Lens structure and forms of cataract, in *The Lens: Transparency and Cataract* (ed. G. Duncan), Eurage, p.3.

Bron, A.J. and Brown, N.A.P. (1994), Growth of the lens. The lens as a clock, in *Congenital Cataracts* (eds E. Cotlier, S. Lambert and D. Taylor), R.G. Landes Co., Austin, TX.

Bron, A.J. and Goldberg, M.F. (1980), Clinical Features of the Human Limbus. VI European Congress of Ophthalmology, Brighton. *Proc R Soc Med*, **1**, 15.

Bron, A.J. and Seal, D.V. (1986), The defences of the ocular surface. *Trans Ophthalmol Soc UK*, **105**, 18.

Bron, A.J. and Tripathi, R.C. (1969), Anterior corneal mosaic. Further observations. *Br J Ophthalmol*, **53**, 760.

Bron, A.J. and Williams, H.P. (1972), Lipaemia of the limbal vessels. *Br J Ophthalmol*, **56**, 343.

Brooke, M.H. and Kaiser, K.K. (1970), Muscle fibre types: how many and what kind? *Arch Neurol*, **23**, 369.

Brouwer, B. (1918), Klinisch-anatomische Untersuchung uber den oculomotoriuskem. *Zentralbl ges Neurol Psychiat*, **40**, 152.

Brouwer, B. and Zeeman, W.P.C. (1926a), The projection of the retina in the primary optic neuron in monkeys. *Brain*, **49**, 1.

Brouwer, B. and Zeeman, W.P.C. (1926b), *Dtsch Z Nervenheilk*, **89**, 9.

Brown, H.G., Ireland, M. and Kuszak, J.R. (1990), Ultrastructural, biochemical and immunological evidence of receptor-mediated endocytosis in the crystalline lens. *Invest Ophthalmol Vis Sci*, **31**, 2579.

Brown, N.A.P. (1973a), Quantitative slit-image photography of the anterior chamber. *Trans Ophthalmol Soc UK*, **93**, 277.

Brown, N.A.P. (1973b), Lens change with age and cataract; slit-image photography. *Ciba Found Symp*, **19**, 65.

Brown, N.A.P. (1973c), The change in shape and internal form of the lens of the eye on accommodation. *Exp Eye Res*, **15**, 441.

Brown, N.A.P. (1976), Dating the onset of cataract. *Trans Ophthalmol Soc UK*, **96**, 18.

Brown, N.A.P. and Bron, A.J. (1996), *Lens Disorders*. Butterworths, London, Washington.

Brown, N.A.P., Bron, A.J., Ayliffe, W. *et al.* (1987), The objective assessment of cataract. *Eye*, **1**, 234.

Brown, N.A.P., Sparrow, J.M. and Bron, A.J. (1988), Central compaction in the process of lens growth as indicated by lamellar cataract. *Br J Ophthalmol*, **72**, 538.

Browne, J.S. (1976), The contractile properties of slow muscle fibres in sheep extraocular muscles. *J Physiol*, **254**, 535.

Brubaker, R.F., Nagataki, S., Townsend, D.J. *et al.* (1981), The effect of age on aqueous humor formation in man. *Ophthalmology*, **88**, 283.

Brubaker, R.F. and Pederson, J.E. (1982), Ciliochoroidal detachment. *Surv Ophthalmol*, **27**, 281.

Bruckner, R. (1959), Methods of protracted research on the aging of eyes. *Ophthalmologica*, **138**, 59.

Bruesch, S.R. and Arey, L.R. (1942), *J Comp Neurol*, **77**, 631.

Bryson, J.M., Wolter, J.R. and O'Keefe, N.T. (1966), Ganglion cells in the human ciliary body. *Arch Ophthalmol*, **75**, 57.

Budge, J. and Waller, A. (1851), Recherches sur la système nerveaux: action de la partie cervicale du nerf gand sympathique et d'une portion de la moelle épinière sur la dilation de la pupille. *CR Acad Sci (Paris)*, **33**, 370.

Budge, J. and Waller, A. (1852), Prix de physiologie expérimentale de l'année 1852. *CR Acad Sci (Paris)*.

Buisseret, P. and Imbert, M. (1976), Visual cortical cells. Their developmental properties in normal and dark reared kittens. *J Physiol*, **255**, 511.

Bukusoglu, G. and Zieske, J.D. (1988), Characterization of a monoclonal antibody that specifically binds basal cells in the limbal epithelium. *ARVO Suppl: Invest Ophthalmol Vis Sci*, **29**, 192.

Bunt, A.H., Hendrickson, A.E., Lund, J.S. *et al.* (1975), Monkey retinal ganglion cells: morphometric analysis and tracing axonal projections with a consideration of the peroxidase technique. *Neurology*, **164**, 265.

Burde, R.M. (1983), The visceral nuclei of the oculomotor complex. *Trans Am Ophthalmol Soc*, **81**, 532.

Burde, R.M. and Loewy, A.D. (1980), Central origin of oculomotor parasympathetic neurons in the monkey. *Brain Res*, **198**, 434.

Burne, R.A., Mihailoff, G.A. and Woodward, D.J. (1978), Visual cortico-pontine input to the paraflocculus: a combined autoradiographic and horseradish peroxidase study. *Brain Res*, **143**, 139.

Burstein, N.L. and Maurice, D.M. (1978), Cryofixation of tissue surfaces by a propane jet for electron microscopy. *Micron*, **9**, 191.

Busacca, A. (1945), *Elements de Gonioscopie Normale, Pathologique et Experimentale*, Sao Paulo, Brazil: Typografia Rossolillo.

Busacca, A. (1957), *Biomicropscopie Et Histopathologie De L'Oeil*, Druck- und Verlagshaus AG, Zurich.

Busacca, A., Goldmann, H. and Schiff-Wertheimer, P. (1957), *Biomicroscopie Du Corps Vitre Et Du Fond De L'Oeil*, Masson et Cie, Paris.

Buschmann, W., Linnert, D., Hofmann, W. *et al.* (1978), The tensile strength of human zonule and its alteration with age. *A von Graefes Arch Klin Exp Ophthalmol*, **206**, 183.

Bushnell, M.C., Goldbere, M.E. and Robinson, D.L. (1981), Behavioural enhancement of visual responses in monkey cerebral cortex. I. Modulation in posterior parietal cortex related to selective visual attention. *J Neurophysiol*, **46**, 755.

Butler, J.M., Ruskell, G.L., Cole, D.F. *et al.* (1984), Effects of VIIth (facial) nerve degeneration on vasoactive intestinal polypeptide and substance p levels in ocular and orbital tissues of the rabbit. *Exp Eye Res*, **39**, 523.

Butterfield, L.C. and Neufeld, A.H. (1977), Cyclic nucleotides and mitoses in the rabbit cornea following superior cervical ganglionectomy. *Exp Eye Res*, **25**, 427.

Büttner-Ennever, J.A. (1977), Pathways from the pontine reticular formation to structures controlling horizontal and vertical eye movements in the monkey. *Dev Neurosci*, **1**, 89.

Büttner-Ennever, J.A. (1979), Organization of reticular projections onto oculomotor neurones. *Progr Brain Res*, **50**, 619.

Büttner-Ennever, J.A. and Buttner, U. (1978), A cell group associated with vertical eye movements in the rostral mesencephalic reticular formation of the monkey. *Brain Res*, **151**, 31.

Büttner-Ennever, J.A., Buttner, U., Cohen, B. *et al.* (1982), Vertical gaze paralysis and the rostral interstitial nucleus of the medial longitudinal fasciculus. *Brain*, **105**, 125.

Buzzard, F. (1908), A note on the occurrence of muscle spindles in ocular muscles. *Proc R Soc Med*, **1**, 83.

Cajal, S.R. (1909), *Histologie du Systeme Nerveux de l'Homme et des Vertebres*. Norbert Maloine, Paris.

Calasans, O.M. (1953), *Annals of the Faculty of Medicine*, University of Sao Paulo, 27.

Campbell, A.W. (1905), *Histological Studies on the Localisation of Cerebral Function*, CUP, Cambridge.

Campbell, D.G. (1979), Pigmentary dispersion and glaucoma: a new theory. *Arch Ophthalmol*, **97**, 1667.

Campbell, D.G., Simmons, R.J. and Grant, M.W. (1976), Ghost cells as a cause of glaucoma. *Am J Ophthalmol*, **81**, 441.

Campbell, F.W., Robson, J.G. and Westheimer, G. (1959), Fluctuations in accommodation under steady viewing conditions. *J Physiol (Lond)*, **145**, 579.

Campos-Ortega, J.A., Glees, P. and Neuhoff, V. (1968), Ultrastructural analysis of individual layers of the lateral geniculate body of the monkey. *Z Zellforsch Mikrosk Anat*, **87**, 82.

Carew, T.J. and Ghez, C. (1985), Receptors, in *Principles of Neural Science* (eds E.R. Kandel and J.H. Swartz), Elsevier, New York, p. 443.

Carmel, P.W. (1968), Sympathetic deficits following thalamotomy. *Arch Neurol*, **18**, 378.

Carmon, A. and Bechtoldt, H.P. (1969), Dominance of the right cerebral hemisphere. *Neuropsychologia*, **7**, 29.

Carpenter, G. and Cohen, S. (1979), Epidermal growth factor. *Ann Rev Biochem*, **48**, 193.

Carpenter, M.B. (1971), Central oculomotor pathways, in *The Control of Eye Movements* (eds P. Bach-y-Rita, C.C. Collins and J.E. Hyde), Academic Press, New York, p. 67.

Carpenter, M.B. (1976), *Human Neuroanatomy*, Williams & Wilkins, Baltimore.

Carpenter, M.B., Noback, C.R. and Moss, M.L. (1954), *Arch Neurol Psychiatr*, **71**, 714.

Carpenter, M.B. and Peter, P. (1970), Accessory oculomotor nuclei in the monkey. *J Hirnforsch*, **12**, 405.

Carpenter, M.B. and Pierson, R.J. (1973), Pretectal region and the pupillary light reflex: an anatomical analysis in the monkey. *J Comp Neurol*, **149**, 271.

Carpenter, M.B. and Strominger, N.L. (1964), Cerebello-oculomotor fibers in the rhesus monkey. *J Comp Neurol*, **123**, 211.

Carpenter, R.H.S. (1977), *Movements of the Eyes*, Pion Press, London.

Carroll, J.M. and Kuwabara, T. (1968), Ocular pemphigus: an electron microscopic study of the conjunctival and corneal epithelium. *Arch Ophthalmol*, **80**, 683.

Cassebohm, J.F. (1734), *Tractatus Quatuor Anatomici de Aure Humana*, Orphanotrophei, Magdeburg. (Cited by Hayreh and Dass, 1962.)

Castenholz, A. (1970), Untersuchungen zur funktionellen Morphologie der Endstrombahn, in *Technik der vitalmikroskopischen Beobachtung und Ergebnisse experimenteller Studien am Iriskreislauf der Albinoratte*, Franz Steiner Verlag, Wiesbaden.

Castenholz, A. (1971), The vascular system of the albino rat iris and its suitability for vital microscopy and experimental studies on microcirculation. *Ophthalmol Res*, **2**, 358.

Castro-Correira, J. (1967), Studies on the innervation of the uveal tract. *Ophthalmologica*, **154**, 497.

Cereijido, M., Gonzalez-Mariscal, L., Contreras, R.G. *et al.* (1993), The making of a tight junction. *J Cell Sci (Suppl)*, **17**, 127.

Cereijido, M., Robbins, E.S., Dolan, W.J. *et al.* (1978), Polarized monolayers formed by epithelial cells on a permeable and translucent support. *J Cell Biol*, **77**, 853.

Chacko, L.W. (1948), An analysis of fibre-size in the human optic nerve. *Br J Ophthalmol*, **32**, 457.

Chacko, L.W. (1955), *J Anat Soc India*, **4**, 201.

Chaine, G., Sebag, J. and Coscas, G. (1983), The induction of retinal detachment. *Trans Ophthalmol Soc UK*, **103**, 480.

Chalcroft, J.P. and Bullivant, S. (1970), An interpretation of liver cell membrane and junction structure based on observation of freeze-fracture replicas of both sides of the fracture. *J Cell Biol*, **47**, 49.

Chandler, J.W. and Axelrod, A.J. (1980), Conjunctiva-associated lymphoid tissue, in *Immunologic Diseases of the Mucous Membranes* (ed. G.R. O'Connor), Paul Masson, New York, p. 63.

Chandler, J.W. and Gillette, T.E. (1983), Immunologic defence mechanisms of the ocular surface. *Ophthalmology*, **90**, 585.

Chan-Palay, V., Palay, S.L. and Billings-Gagliardi, S.M. (1974), *J Neurocytol*, **3**, 631.

Chapman, G.B. and Spelsberg, W.W. (1963), The occurrence of myelinated and unmyelinated nerves in the iris angle of man and rhesus monkey. *Exp Eye Res*, **2**, 130.

Charcot, J.M. (1879), *Lectures on the Diseases of the Nervous System* (translated by G. Sigerson), Henry C. Lea, Philadelphia, p. 390.

Chase, R. and Kalil, R.E. (1972), Suppression of visual evoked responses to flashes and pattern shift during voluntary saccades. *Vision Res*, **12**, 215.

Chavis, R.M., Welham, R.A.N. and Maisey, M.N. (1978), Quantitative lacrimal scintillography. *Arch Ophthalmol*, **96**, 2066.

Cheng, K. (1963), Cholinesterase activity in human extraocular muscles. *Jpn J Ophthalmol*, **7**, 174.

Cheng, K. and Breinin, G.M. (1966), Fine structure of nerve endings of extraocular muscle. *Arch Ophthalmol*, **74**, 822.

Chi, T., Ritch, R., Stickler, D. *et al.* (1989), Racial differences in optic nerve head parameters. *Arch Ophthalmol*, **107**, 836.

Chouchkov, C. (1978), Cutaneous receptors. *Adv Anat Embryol Cell Biol*, **54**, 1.

Christman, E.H. and Kupfer, C. (1963), Proprioception in extraocular muscle. *Arch Ophthalmol*, **69**, 824.

Chung, C.W., Tigges, M. and Stone, R.A. (1996), Peptidergic innervation of the primate meibomian gland. *Invest Ophthalmol Vis Sci*, **37**, 238.

Cibis, G.W., Campos, E.C. and Aulhorn, E. (1975), Pupillary hemiakinesia in suprageniculate lesions. *Arch Ophthalmol*, **93**, 1322.

Cilimbaris, P.A. (1910), Histologische untersuchungen uber die muskelspindeln der augenmuskeln. *Arch Microsk Anat*, **75**, 692.

Claude, P. (1978), Morphological factors influencing transepithelial permeability: A model for the resistance of the zonula occludens. *J Membr Biol*, **39**, 219.

Claude, P. and Goodenough, D.A. (1973), Fracture faces of zonulae occludentes from 'tight' and 'leaky' epithelia. *J Cell Biol*, **58**, 390.

Cogan, D.G. (1956), *Neurology of the Ocular Muscles*, 2nd edition, Charles C. Thomas, Springfield IL.

Cogan, D.G. (1965), Ophthalmic manifestations of bilateral non-occipital cerebral lesions. *Br J Ophthalmol*, **49**, 281.

Cogan, D.G. (1974), *Ophthalmic Manifestations of Systemic Vascular Disease. Vol III Major Problems in Internal Medicine*, W.B. Saunders, London, p. 132.

Cogan, D.G. and Loeb, D.R. (1949), Optokinetic response and intracranial lesions. *Arch Neurol Psychiatr*, **61**, 183.

Cogan, D.G., Toussaint, D. and Kuwabara, T. (1961), Retinal vascular patterns. IV. Diabetic retinopathy. *Arch Ophthalmol*, **66**, 366.

Cohen, A.I. (1965), The electron microscopy of the normal human lens. *Invest Ophthalmol*, **4**, 433.

Cohen, A.I. (1967), Ultrastructural aspects of the human optic nerve. *Invest Ophthalmol*, **6**, 294.

Cohen, A.I. (1973), Is there a potential defect in the blood brain barrier at the choroidal level of the optic nerve canal? *Invest Ophthalmol*, **12**, 513.

Cohen, B., Büttner-Ennever, J., Waitzman, D. *et al.* (1981), Anatomical connections of a portion of the dorsolateral mesencephalic reticular formation of the monkey associated with horizontal saccadic eye movements. *Soc Neurosci Abstr*, **4**, 776.

Cole, D.F. (1974), Aspects of the intraocular fluids, in *The Eye* (eds H. Davson and L.T. Graham, Jr.), Academic Press, New York, p. 71.

Cole, D.F. (1977), Secretion of the aqueous humour. *Exp Eye Res, Suppl* **1**, 161.

Cole, D.F. (1984), Ocular fluids, in *The Eye*, 3rd edition (ed. H. Davson), Academic Press, New York, p. 269.

Cole, D.F., Bloom, S.R., Burnstock, G. *et al.* (1983), Increase in SP-like immunoreactivity in nerve fibers of rabbit iris and ciliary body one to four months following sympathetic denervation. *Exp Eye Res*, **37**, 191.

Cole, D.F. and Tripathi, R.C. (1971), Theoretical considerations on the mechanism of the aqueous outflow. *Exp Eye Res*, **12**, 25.

Colello, R. (1990), The development of the retinofugal pathway in rodents. D.Phil. Thesis, University of Oxford, Oxford.

Colello, R.J. and Guillery, R.W. (1987), The distribution of axonal profiles within the optic tract of the embryonic mouse. (Supplement.) *Neuroscience*, **22**, S269.

Coleman, D.J. (1970), Unified model for accommodative mechanism. *Am J Ophthalmol*, **69**, 1063.

Coleman, D.J. (1986), On the hydraulic suspension theory of accommodation. *Trans Am Ophthalmol Soc*, **84**, 846.

Coleman, D.J. and Lizzie, F.L. (1979), *In vivo* choroidal thickness measurement. *Am J Ophthalmol*, **88**, 369.

Collewijn, H. (1975), Direction-selective units in the rabbit's nucleus of the optic tract. *Brain Res*, **100**, 489.

Collewijn, H. (1977), Eye and head movements in freely moving rabbits. *J Physiol*, **266**, 471.

Collewijn, H. (1981), *The Oculomotor System of the Rabbit and its Plasticity*, Springer-Verlag, New York.

Collin, J.R.O. (1983), *A Manual of Systematic Eyelid Surgery*, Churchill Livingstone, Edinburgh.

Collonier, M. (1967), *J Anat*, **98**, 327.

Colonnier, M.L. and Guillery, R.W. (1964), Synaptic organisation in the lateral geniculate nucleus of the monkey. *Z Zellforsch Mikrosk Anat*, **62**, 333.

Cone, W. and MacMillan, J.A. (1932), The optic nerve and papilla, in *Cytology and Cellular Pathology of the Nervous System* (ed. W. Penfield), Paul Hoeber, New York, p. 847.

Conel, J.L. (1939), *Post-natal Development of the Human Cerebral Cortex*, Harvard University Press, Boston.

Conrad, L.C.A. and Pfaff, D.W. (1976a), Efferents from medial basal forebrain and hypothalamus in the rat: I. An autoradiographic study of the medial preoptic area. *J Comp Neurol*, **169**, 185.

Conrad, L.C.A. and Pfaff, D.W. (1976b), Efferents from medial basal forebrain and hypothalamus in the rat: II. An autoradiographic study of the anterior hypothalamus. *J Comp Neurol*, **169**, 221.

Cooper, E.R.A., Daniel, P.M. and Whitteridge, D. (1951), Afferent impulses in the oculomotor nerve from the extrinsic eye muscles. *J Physiol*, **113**, 463.

Cooper, H.M. (1986), The accessory optic system in a prosimian primate (*Microcebus murinus*): evidence for a direct retinal projection to the medial terminal nucleus. *J Comp Neurol*, **249**, 28.

Cooper, H.M. and Magnin, M. (1986), A common mammalian plan of accessory optic system organization revealed in all primates. *Nature*, **324**, 457.

Cooper, H.M. and Magnin, M. (1987), Accessory optic system of an anthropoid primate: the gibbon (*Hylobate concolor*): evidence of a direct retinal input to the medial terminal nucleus. *J Comp Neurol*, **259**, 467.

Cooper, S. (1951), *J. Physiol*, **113**, 1.

Cooper, S. and Daniel, P.M. (1949), Muscle spindles in human extrinsic eye muscles. *Brain*, **72**, 1.

Cooper, S., Daniel, P.M. and Whitteridge, D. (1955), Muscle spindles and other sensory endings in the estrinsic eye muscles; the physiology and anatomy of these receptors and of their connexions with the brain stem. *Brain*, **78**, 564.

Cooper, S. and Eccles, J.C. (1930), The isometric responses of mammalian muscles. *J Physiol*, **69**, 377.

Cope, C., Dilley, P.N., Kaura, R. *et al.* (1986), Wettability of the corneal surface: a reappraisal. *Curr Eye Res*, **5**, 777.

Cope, V.Z. (1916), The pituitary fossa and the methods of surgical approach thereto. *Br J Surg*, **4**, 107.

Costello, M.J., McIntosh, T.J. and Robertson, J.D. (1984),

Square array fiber cell membranes in the mammalian lens, in *Proceedings of the 42nd Electron Microscopic Society of America*, San Francisco Press, San Francisco, p. 126.

Costello, M.J., McIntosh, T.J. and Robertson, J.D. (1985), Membrane specializations in mammalian lens fiber cells: distribution of square arrays. *Curr Eye Res*, **4**, 1183.

Cotsarelis, G., Cheng, S.Z., Dong, G. *et al.* (1989), Existence of slow-cycling limbal epithelial basal cells that can be preferentially stimulated to proliferate: Implications on epithelial stem cells. *Cell*, **57**, 201.

Cowan, W.M., Fawcett, J.W., O'Leary, D.D.M. *et al.* (1984), Regressive events in neurogenesis. *Science*, **225**, 1258.

Cowey, A. (1982), Non-sensory visual disorders in man and monkey. *Phil Trans R Soc Lond*, **298**, 3.

Cowey, A. (1985), Disturbances of stereopsis by brain damage. *Brain Mech Spatial Vis*, **1**, 259.

Cragg, B.G. (1972), The development of synapses in cat visual cortex. *Invest Ophthalmol*, **11**, 377.

Cragg, B.G. (1975), The development of synapses in the visual system of the cat. *J Comp Neurol*, **160**, 147.

Cragg, B.G. and Ainsworth, A. (1969), The topography of the afferent projections in circumstriate visual cortex of the monkey studied by the Nauta method. *Vision Res*, **9**, 733.

Crooks, J. and Kolb, H. (1992), Localization of GABA, glycine, glutamate and tyrosine hydroxylase in the human retina. *J Comp Neurol*, **315**, 287.

Crosby, E.C., Humphrey, T. and Lauer, E.W. (1962), *Correlative Anatomy of the Nervous System*, Macmillan, New York.

Crosby, E.C. and Woodburne, R.T. (1943), Nuclear pattern of non-tectal portions of midbrain and isthmus in primates. *J Comp Neurol*, **78**, 441.

Crosson, C.E., Beverman, R.W. and Klyce, D.S. (1984), Microelectrode study of membrane changes associated with sympathetic denervation in the rabbit corneal epithelium. *Invest Ophthalmol Vis Sci*, **25**, 303.

Cruveilhier, J. (1877), *Traite d'Anatomie Descriptive*, Asselin, Paris.

Cserhati, P., Szel, A. and Rohlich, P. (1989), Four cone types characterized by anti-visual pigment antibodies in the pigeon retina. *Invest Ophthalmol Vis Sci*, **30**, 74.

Cunha-Vaz, J.G., Shakib, M. and Ashton, N. (1966), Studies on the permeability of the blood–retinal barrier. I. On the existence, development and site of a blood–retinal barrier. *Br J Ophthalmol*, **50**, 441.

Curcio, C.A. and Allen, K.A. (1990), Topography of ganglion cells in human retina. *J Comp Neurol*, **300**, 5.

Curcio, C.A., Allen, K.A., Sloan, K.R. *et al.* (1991), Distribution and morphology of human cone photoreceptors stained with anti-blue opsin. *J Comp Neurol*, **312**, 610.

Curcio, C.A. and Hendrickson, A.E. (1991), Organization and development of the primate photoreceptor mosaic. *Prog Ret Res*, **10**, 89.

Curcio, C.A., Sloan, K.R., Kalina, R.E. *et al.* (1990), Human photoreceptor topography. *J Comp Neurol*, **292**, 497.

Cushing, H. (1921), The field defects produced by temporal lobe tumors. *Brain*, **341**, 396.

Cuthbertson, R.A., Beck, F., Senior, P.V. *et al.* (1989), Insulin-like growth factor II may play a local role in the regulation of ocular size. *Development*, **107**, 123.

Dacey, D.M. (1993a), Morphology of a small-field bistratified ganglion cell type in the macaque and human retina. *Vis Neurosci*, **10**, 1081.

Dacey, D.M. (1993b), The mosaic of midget ganglion cells in the human retina. *J Neurosci*, **13**, 5334.

Dacey, D.M. (1994), Physiology, morphology and spatial densities of identified ganglion cell types in primate retina. *Ciba Foundation Symposium*, **184**, 12.

Dacey, D.M. and Lee, B.B. (1994), The 'blue-on' opponent pathway in primate retina originates from a distinct bistratified ganglion cell type. *Nature*, **367**, 731.

Dacey, D.M. and Petersen, M.R. (1992), Dendritic field size and morphology of midget and parasol ganglion cells of the human retina. *Proc Natl Acad Sci USA*, **89**, 9666.

Daicker, B. (1972), *Anatomie und Pathologie der Menschlichen Retinociliaren˙ Fundusperipherie. Ein Atlas und Textbuch*, Karger, Basel.

Daicker, B., Guggenheim, R. and Gwyat, L. (1977), Rasterelektronenmikroskopische befunde an Netzhautinnenflachen. II. Hintere Glaskorperabhebung. *A von Graefes Arch Klin Exp Ophthalmol*, **204**, 19.

Daniel, P. (1946), Spiral nerve endings in the extrinsic eye muscles of man. *J Anat*, **80**, 189.

Danis, P.C. (1948), The functional organisation of the third-nerve nucleus in the cat. *Am J Ophthalmol*, **31**, 1122.

Dark, A.J., Durrant, T.E., McGinty, F. *et al.* (1974), Tarsal conjunctiva of the upper eyelid. *Am J Ophthalmol*, **77**, 555.

Dark, A.J., Streeten, B.W. and Jones, D.B. (1969), Accumulation of fibrillar protein in the aging human lens capsule. *Arch Ophthalmol*, **82**, 815.

Darnell, J., Lodish, H. and Baltimore, D. (1990), Molecular cell biology. *Sci Am*, **1**, 1.

Daroff, R.B. and Hoyt, W.F. (1971), Supranuclear disorders of ocular control systems in man: clinical, anatomical and physiological correlations, in *The Control of Eye Movements* (eds P. Bach-y-Rita, C.C. Collins and J.E. Hyde), Academic Press, New York, p. 175.

Daroff, R.B., Troost, B.T. and Leigh, R.J. (1978), Supranuclear disorders of eye movements, in *Neuro-ophthalmology* (ed. J.S. Glaser), J.B. Lippincott Co., Philadelphia, p. 299.

Das, A., Pansky, B. and Budd, G.C. (1987), Demonstration of insulin-specific mRNA in cultured rat retinal glial cells. *Invest Ophthalmol Vis Sci*, **28**, 1800.

Davanger, M. (1975a), The pseudo-exfoliation syndrome. A scanning electron microscopic study. I. The anterior lens surface. *Acta Ophthalmol*, **53**, 809.

Davanger, M. (1975b), The pseudo-exfoliation syndrome. A scanning electron microscopic study. II. The posterior chamber region. *Acta Ophthalmol*, **53**, 821.

Davanger, S., Ottersen, O.P. and Storm-Mathisen, J. (1991), Glutamate, GABA, and glycine in the human retina: an immunocytochemical investigation. *J Comp Neurol*, **311**, 483.

Davanger, S., Storm-Mathisen, J. and Ottersen, O.P. (1994), Colocalization of glutamate and glycine in bipolar cell terminals of the human retina. *Exp Brain Res*, **98**, 342.

Davidowitz, J., Philips, G. and Breinin, G.M. (1977), Organisation of the orbital surface layer in rabbit superior rectus. *Invest Ophthalmol*, **16**, 711.

Davidson, R.M. and Bender, D.B. (1991), Selectivity for

relative motion in the monkey superior colliculus. *J Neurophysiol*, **65**, 1115.

Davson, H. (1980), *Physiology of the Eye*, 4th edition, Churchill Livingstone, London.

Dawid, I.B., Sargent, T.S. and Rosa, F. (1990), The role of growth factors in embryonic induction in amphibians, *Current Topics in Developmental Biology, vol. 24* (ed. M. Nilsen-Hamilton), Academic Press, New York.

Dawson, B.H. (1958), On the blood vessels of the human optic chiasma, hypophysis and hypothalamus. *Brain*, **81**, 207.

De Camilli, P., Vitadello, M., Canevini, M.P. *et al.* (1988), The synaptic vesicle proteins synapsin I and synaptophysin (protein p38) are concentrated both in efferent and afferent nerve endings of the skeletal muscle. *J Neurosci*, **8**, 1625.

de Kater, A.W., Shahsafaei, A. and Epstein, D.L. (1992), Localization of smooth muscle and nonmuscle actin isoforms in the human aqueous outflow pathway. *Invest Ophthalmol Vis Sci*, **33**, 424.

de Kater, A.W., Spurr-Michaud, S.J. and Gipson, I.K. (1990), Localization of smooth muscle myosin-containing cells in the aqueous outflow pathway. *Invest Ophthalmol Vis Sci*, **31**, 347.

De Monasterio, F.M. (1978), *J Neurophysiol*, **41**, 1394.

de Oliveira, F. (1966), Pericytes in diabetic retinopathy. *Br J Ophthalmol*, **50**, 134.

Dean, P. (1976), Effects of inferotemporal lesions on the behaviour of monkeys. *Psychol Bull*, **83**, 41.

Dejong, J.M.B.V., Cohen, B., Matsuo, B. *et al.* (1980), Midsagittal pontomedullary brain stem section: effects on ocular adduction and nystagmus. *Exp Neurol*, **68**, 420.

Delgado-Garcia, J., Baker, R. and Highstein, S.M. (1977), The activity of internuclear neurons identified within the abducens nucleus of the alert cat. *Dev Neurosci*, **1**, 29.

Dell'Osso, L.F., Abel, L.A. and Daroff, R.B. (1977), Inverse latent macro square-wave jerks and macrosaccadic oscillations. *Ann Neurol*, **2**, 57.

Dell'Osso, L.F. and Daroff, R.B. (1974), Functional organization of the ocular motor system. *Aerospace Med*, **45**, 873.

Dell'Osso, L.F. and Daroff, R.B. (1975), Congenital nystagmus waveforms and foveation strategy. *Doc Ophthalmol*, **19**, 155.

Dell'Osso, L.F. and Daroff, R.B. (1990), Eye movement characteristics and recording techniques, in *Neuro-ophthalmology*, 2nd edition (ed. J.S. Glaser), Lippincott, Philadelphia, p. 279.

Dell'Osso, L.F., Daroff, R.B. and Troost, B.T. (1990), Nystagmus and saccadic intrusions and oscillations, in *Neuro-ophthalmology*, 2nd edition (ed. J.S. Glaser), Lippincott, Philadelphia, p. 325.

Demours (1741), Observations anatomiques sur la structure cellulaire du corps vitré. *Memoires de Paris*.

Denonvilliers, C.H. (1837), Propositions et observations d'anatomie, de physiologie et de pathologie. *PhD Thesis*.

Dermietzel, R. (1973), Visualization by freeze-fracturing of regular structures in glial cell membranes. *Naturwissenschaften* 60, 208.

Desimore, R., Fleming, J. and Gross, C.G. (1980), Peristriate afferents to inferior temporal cortex. An HRP study. *Brain Res*, **184**, 41.

Dewulf, A. (1971), *Anatomy of the Normal Human Thalamus*, Elsevier, Amsterdam.

Deyl, J. (1895), *Bull Int Acad Sci Prague*, **12**, 120.

Diaz-Araya, C.M., Madigan, M.C., Provis, J.M. *et al.* (1995), Immunohistochemical and topographic studies of dendritic cells and macrophages in human fetal cornea. *Invest Ophthalmol Vis Sci*, **36**, 644.

Diaz-Araya, C. and Provis, J.M. (1992), Evidence of photoreceptor migration during early foveal development: a quantitative analysis of human fetal retinae. *Vis Neurosci*, **8**, 505.

DiCara, L.V. (ed.) (1974), *Limbic and Autonomic Systems Research*, Plenum Press, New York.

Dichtl, A., Jonas, J.B. and Mardin, C.Y. (1996), Comparison between tomographic scanning evaluation and photographic measurement of the neuroretinal rim. *Am J Ophthalmol*, **121**, 494.

Dickson, D.H. and Crock, G.W. (1972), Interlocking patterns on primate lens fibers. *Invest Ophthalmol*, **11**, 809.

Dickson, D.H. and Crock, G.W. (1975), Fine structure of primate lens fibers in *Cataract and Abnormalities of the Lens*, (ed J.G. Bellows), Grune and Stratton, New York, p. 49.

Dietert, S.E. (1965), The demonstration of different types of muscle fibres in human extraocular muscle by electron microscopy and cholinesterase staining. *Invest Ophthalmol*, **4**, 51.

Dilenge, D., Fischgold, H. and David, M. (1961), L'Artere ophtalmique, aspects angiographiques. *Neurochirurgie*, **7**, 240.

Dilley, P.N. (1985), Contribution of the epithelium to the stability of the tear film. *Trans Ophthalmol Soc UK*, **104**, 381.

Dilley, P.N. and Mackie, I.A. (1981), Surface changes in the anaesthetic conjunctiva in man with special reference to the production of mucus from a non-goblet cell source. *Br J Ophthalmol*, **65**, 833.

Dische, Z. (1970), Biochemistry of connective tissue of the vertebrate eye. *Int Rev Connect Tissue Res*, **5**, 209.

Dische, Z. and Murty, V.L.N. (1974), An insoluble structural glycoprotein, a major constituent of the zonula Zinni. *Invest Ophthalmol Vis Sci*, **13**, 991.

Doane, M.G. (1980), Interactions of eyelids and tears in corneal wetting and dynamics of the normal human eyeblink. *Am J Ophthalmol*, **89**, 507.

Doane, M.G. (1981), Blinking and the mechanics of the lacrimal drainage system. *Ophthalmology*, **88**, 844.

Dodson, J.W. and Hay, E.D. (1971), Secretion of collagenous stroma by isolated epithelium in vitro. *Exp Cell Res*, **65**, 215.

Dollery, C.T., Henkind, P., Kohner, E.M. and Paterson, J.W. (1968), Effect of raised intraocular pressure on the retinal and choroidal circulation. *Invest Ophthalmol*, **7**, 191.

Donaldson, D.D. (1966), A new instrument for the measurement of corneal thickness. *Arch Ophthalmol*, **76**, 25.

Donaldson, G.W.K. (1960), The diameter of the nerve fibres to the extrinsic eye muscles of the goat. *QJ Exp Psychol*, **45**, 25.

Donders, F.C. (1864), On the anomalies of accommodation and refraction of the eye. *New Sydenham Soc*, **1**, 1.

Donovan, A. (1967), The nerve fibre composition of the cat optic nerve. *J Anat*, **101**, 1.

Dow, B.M. (1974), Functional classes of cells and their laminar distribution in monkey visual cortex. *J Neurophysiol*, **36**, 79.

Dow, R., and Morruzzi, G. (1958), *Physiology and Pathology of the Cerebellum*, University of Minnesota Press, Minneapolis.

Dreher, B., Fukada, Y. and Rodiesk, R.W. (1976), Identification, classification and anatomical segregation of cells with X-like and Y-like properties in the lateral geniculate nucleus of old world primates. *J Physiol*, **258**, 433.

Dreher, Z., Robinson, S.R. and Distler, C. (1992), Müller cells in vascular and avascular retinae: a survey of seven mammals. *J Comp. Neurol*, **323**, 59.

Dreyfus, P.M., Hakim, S. and Adams, R.D. (1957), Diabetic ophthalmoplegia: Report of case, with postmortem study and comments on vascular supply of human oculomotor nerve. *Arch Neurol Psychiat*, **77**, 337.

Duane, A. (1912), Normal values of the accommodation at all ages. *Tr MA Section on Ophthalmol*, **1**, 383.

Dubowitz, V. (1985), *Muscle Biopsy: A Practical Approach*, 2nd edition, Baillière, Tindall and Cox, London.

Dubowitz, V. and Pearse, A.G.E. (1960a), A comparative histochemical study of oxidative enzyme and phosphorylase activity in skeletal muscle. *Histochemie*, **2**, 105.

Dubowitz, V. and Pearse, A.G.E. (1960b), Reciprocal relationship of phosphorylase and oxidative enzymes in skeletal muscle. *Nature*, **185**, 701.

Duchenne, G.B.A. (1883), Selections from the clinical works of Dr Duchenne. (Translated and edited by A.V. Poore.) *New Sydenham Soc*, **1**, 1.

Duckworth, W. (1904), *Morphology and Anthropology*. CUP, Cambridge.

Ducournou, D.H. (1982), A new technique for the anatomical study of the choroidal blood vessels. *Ophthalmologica*, **184**, 190.

Duke, J.R. and Siegelman, S. (1961), Acid mucopolysaccharides in the trabecular meshwork of the chamber angle. *Arch Ophthalmol*, **66**, 399.

Duke-Elder, S. (1961), The blood vessels of the orbit, in *System of Ophthalmology: Anatomy of the Visual System* (eds S. Duke-Elder and K. Wybar), Henry Kimpton, London, p. 467.

Duke-Elder, S. and Cook, C. (1963), Normal and abnormal development, in *System of Ophthalmology* (ed. S. Duke-Elder), Henry Kimpton, London.

Duke-Elder, S. and Wybar, K.C. (1961), The anatomy of the visual system, in *System of Ophthalmology*, 2nd edition, (eds S. Duke-Elder and K. Wybar), Henry Kimpton, London.

Dunia, I., Ngoc Lein, D., Manenti, S. and Benedetti, E.L. (1985), Dilemmas of the structural and biochemical organization of lens membranes during differentiation and aging. *Curr Eye Res*, **4**, 1219.

Dursteler, M.R. and Wurtz, R.H. (1988), Pursuit and optokinetic deficits following chemical lesions of cortical areas MT and MST. *J Neurophysiol*, **60**, 940.

Duvernoy, D. (1749), *L'Art de Dissequer Methodiquement les Muscles*, Paris.

Duvernoy, H.M., Delon, S. and Vannson, J.L. (1981), *Brain Res*, **7**, 519.

Duvernoy, H. and Koritke, J.G. (1968), Subependymal vessels of the hyphyseal recess. *J Hirnforsch*, **10**, 227.

Eakins, K.E. and Katz, R. (1971), The pharmacology of extraocular muscle, in *The Control of Eye Movements*, (eds

P. Bach-y-Rita and C.C. Collins), Academic Press, New York, p. 237.

Earley, O. (1991), Morphology and *in vitro* growth dynamics of the human epithelium. An age-related study. *MD Thesis*.

Ebbeson, S.O.E. (1968), Quantitative studies of superior cervical sympathetic ganglia in a variety of primates, including man. II. Neuronal packing density. *J Morphol*, **124**, 181.

Eccles, J.C., Ito, M. and Szentagothai, J. (1967), *The Cerebellum as a Neuronal Machine*, Springer-Verlag, Berlin.

Edinger, L. (1885), Über den verlauf der centralen hirnnervenbahnen mit demonstration von präparaten. *Neurol Zentralbl*, **4**, 309.

Edney, D.P. and Porter, J.D. (1986), Neck muscle afferent projections to the brainstem of the monkey: implications for the neural control of gaze. *J Comp Neurol*, **250**, 389.

Edvinsson, L., Hara, H. and Uddman, R. (1989), Retrograde tracing of nerve fibers to the rat middle cerebral artery with true blue: colocalization with different peptides. *J Cereb Blood Flow Metab*, **9**, 212.

Egeberg, J. and Jensen, O.A. (1969), The ultrastructure of the acini of the human lacrimal gland. *Acta Ophthalmol*, **47**, 400.

Eggers, H.M. (1987), Functional anatomy of the extraocular muscles, in *Biomedical Foundations of Ophthalmology* (eds T.D. Duane and E.A. Jaeger), Harper & Row, Philadelphia.

Eguchi, G. (1964), Electron microscopic studies on lens regeneration: II. Formation and growth of lens vesicle and differentiation of lens fibers. *Embryologia*, **8**, 247.

Ehinger, B. (1964), *Acta Univ Lund*, **20**, 1.

Ehinger, B. (1966a), Adrenergic nerves to the eye and to related structures in man and in the cynmologus monkey (*Macaca irus*). *Invest Ophthalmol*, **5**, 42.

Ehinger, B. (1966b), Ocular and orbital vegetative nerves. *Acta Physiol Scand*, **67**, 1.

Ehinger, B. (1971), A comparative study of the adrenergic nerves to the anterior eye segment of some primates. *Z Zellforsch Mikrosk Anat*, **116**, 157.

Ehlers, N., Mathiessen, M.E. and Anderson, H. (1968), The prenatal growth of the human eye. *Acta Ophthalmol*, **46**, 329.

Eisler, P. (1930), Anatomies des Auges, in *Kurzes Handbuch der Ophthalmologie* (eds F. Schieck and A. Bruckner), Springer-Verlag, Berlin.

Eisner, G. (1971), Autoptische Spaltlampenuntersuchung des Glaskorpers I–III. *A von Graefes Arch Klin Exp Ophthalmol*, **182**, 1.

Eisner, G. (1973a), *Biomicroscopy of the Peripheral Fundus. An Atlas and Textbook*, Springer, Heidelberg.

Eisner, G. (1973b), Autoptische Spaltlampenuntersuchung des Glaskorpers IV–V. *A von Graefes Arch Klin Exp Ophthalmol*, **187**, 1.

Eisner, G. (1975a), Anatomie des Glaskorpers. *A von Graefes Arch Klin Exp Ophthalmol*, **193**, 33.

Eisner, G. (1975b), Clinical examination of the vitreous. *Trans Ophthalmol Soc UK*, **95**, 360.

Eisner, G. (1978), Lichtkoagulation und Glaskorperbildung. Zur Frage der Glaskorperentstehung. *A von Graefes Arch Klin Exp Ophthalmol*, **206**, 33.

Eisner, G. (1989), Clinical anatomy of the vitreous, in *Biomedical Foundations of Ophthalmology* (eds T.D. Duane and E.A. Jaeger), Lippincott, Philadelphia, p. 16:1.

Eisner, G. and Bachmann, E. (1974a), Vergleichend morphologische Spaltlampenuntersuchung des Glaskorpers bei der Katze. *A von Graefes Arch Klin Exp Ophthalmol*, **191**, 343.

Eisner, G. and Bachmann, E. (1974b), Vergleichend morphologische Spaltlampenuntersuchung des Glaskorpers von bei Schaf, Schwein, Hund, Affen und Kaninchen. *A von Graefes Arch Klin Exp Ophthalmol*, **192**, 9.

Eisner, G. and Bachmann, E. (1974c), Vergleichand morphologische Spaltlampenunter suchung des Glaskorpers beim Pferd. *A von Graefes Arch Klin Exp Ophthalmol*, **192**, 1.

Eisner, G. and Bachmann, E. (1974d), Vergleichend morphologische Spaltlampenuntersuchung des Glaskorpers beim Rind. *A von Graefes Arch Klin Exp Ophthalmol*, **191**, 329.

Eisner, G. and van der Zypen, E. (1981), Transivitreal channel related to an intravitreal developmental anomaly. Slit lamp and electron microscopic study. *A von Graefes Arch Klin Exp Ophthalmol*, **217**, 45.

Ekbom, K. and Greits, T. (1970), Carotid angiography in cluster headache. *Acta Radiol Diagn*, **10**, 177.

Elberger, A.J. (1979), The role of the corpus callosum in the development of interocular eye alignment and the organization of the visual field in the cat. *Exp Brain Res*, **36**, 71.

Eliškova, M. (1969), Blood supply of the ciliary ganglion in the rhesus monkey. *Br J Ophthalmol*, **53**, 753.

Eliškova, M. (1973), Blood vessels of the ciliary ganglion in man. *Br J Ophthalmol*, **57**, 766.

Ellingson, B. and Grant, W. (1971), Influence of intraocular pressure and trabeculotomy on aqueous outflow in enucleated monkey eyes. *Invest Ophthalmol*, **10**, 705.

Elliot Smith, G. (1928), The new vision. Bowman lecture. *Trans Ophthalmol Soc UK*, **47**, 64.

Elliot Smith, G. (1930), *J Anat*, **64**, 430.

Elschnig, A. (1901), Der normale Sehnerveneintritt des menschlichen Auges, in *Denkschriften der Mathematish – Naturwissen schaftliche Classe der Kaiserlichen Akademie der Wissenschaften in Wein*, **70**, 219.

Elschnig, A. and Lauber, H. (1907), Uber die sogenannten klumpenzellen der iris. *A von Graefes Arch Ophthalmol*, **65**, 428.

Engelman, T.W. (1867), *Hornhaut des Auges*, Leipzig.

Enoch, I.M. (1976), Retinal stretch and accommodation, in *Current Concepts in Ophthalmology* (eds H.E. Kaufman and T.J. Zimmerman), Mosby, Saint Louis, p. 59.

Enroth-Cugell, C. and Robson, J.G. (1966), The contrast sensitivity of retinal ganglion cells of the cat. *J Physiol*, **187**, 517.

Epling, G.P. (1966), Electron microscopic observations of pericytes in the lungs and hearts of normal cattle and swine. *Anat Rec*, **155**, 513.

Erikson, A. and Svedbergh, B. (1980), Transcellular aqueous humour outflow: a theoretical and experimental study. *A von Graefes Arch Klin Exp Ophthalmol*, **212**, 53.

Erickson-Lamy, K.A., Polansky, J.R., Kaufman, P.L. et al. (1987), Cholinergic drugs alter ciliary muscle response and receptor content. *Invest Ophthalmol Vis Sci*, **28**, 375.

Essner, E. (1971), Localization of endogenous peroxidase in rat exorbital lacrimal gland. *J Histochem Cytochem*, **19**, 216.

Ethier, C.R., Kamm, R.D., Palaszewski, B.A. *et al.* (1986), Calculation of flow resistance in the juxtacanalicular meshwork. *Invest Ophthalmol Vis Sci*, **27**, 1741.

Evinger, C.L., King, W.M., Lisberger, S.G. *et al.* (1975), The role of MLF in eye movements: functional physiology underlying anterior internuclear ophthalmoplegia. *Neurosci Abstr*, **1**, 235.

Falconer, M.A. and Wilson, J.L. (1958), Visual field changes following anterior temporal lobectomy: their significance in relation to 'Meyer's loop' of the optic radiation. *Brain*, **81**, 1.

Famiglietti, E.V.J.R. and Peters, A. (1972), The synaptic glomerulus and the intrinsic neuron in the dorsal lateral geniculate nucleus of the cat. *J Comp Neurol*, **144**, 285.

Farnsworth, P.N. and Burke, P. (1977), Three dimensional architecture of the suspensory apparatus of the lens of the Rhesus monkey. *Exp Eye Res*, **25**, 563.

Farnsworth, P.N., Burke, P.A. and Kestin, W.T. (1978), Suspensory apparatus of the human lens. *ARVO Suppl: Invest Ophthalmol Vis Sci*, **17**, 233.

Farnsworth, P.N., Mauriello, J.A., Burke-Gadomski, P. *et al.* (1976), Surface ultrastructure of the human lens capsule and zonule attachments. *Invest Ophthalmol*, **15**, 36.

Farnsworth, P.N. and Shyne, S.E. (1979), Anterior zonular shifts with age. *Exp Eye Res*, **28**, 291.

Farquahar-Buzzard, E. (1908), The occurrence of muscle spindles in human ocular muscles. *Proc R Soc Med*, **1**, 83.

Faulborn, J. and Bowald, S. (1982), Combined macroscopic, light microscopic, scanning and transmission electron microscopic investigation of the vitreous body. *Ophthalmic Res*, **14**, 117.

Fawcett, D.W. (1966), *The Cell; an Atlas of Fine Structure*, WB Saunders, Philadelphia.

Fawcett, E. (1895), The origin and intracranial course of ophthalmic artery, and the relationship they bear to the optic nerve. *J Anat Physiol Lond*, **30**, 49.

Fawcett, E. and Blachford, J.V. (1906), The circle of Willis: an examination of 700 specimens. *J Anat*, **40**, 63.

Fazakas, S. (1933), *Zentralbl ges Ophthalmol*, **28**, 494.

Feeney, L., Grieshaber, J.A. and Hogan, M.J. (1965), Studies on human ocular pigment, in *The Structure of the Eye* (ed. J.W. Rohen), F.K. Schattauer, Stuttgart, p. 535.

Feeney, L. and Hogan, M. (1961), Electron microscopy of the human choroid. *Am J Ophthalmol*, **51**, 1057.

Feeney, M.L. (1962), Ultrastructure of the nerves in the human trabecular region. *Invest Ophthalmol*, **1**, 462.

Fells, P. (1975), The superior oblique: its actions and anomalies. *Br Orthop J*, **32**, 43.

Fenton, R.H. and Zimmerman, L.W. (1963), Hemolytic glaucoma. An unusual cause of acute open angle secondary glaucoma. *Arch Ophthalmol*, **70**, 236.

Ferrier, D. (1874), The localization of function in the brain. *Proc R Soc Lond*, **22**, 229.

Festal, A.F. (1887), Recherches anatomiques sur les veines de l'orbite. *PhD Thesis*, Paris.

Fincham, E.F. (1925), The changes in the form of the crystalline lens in accommodation. *Trans Optom Soc*, **26**, 16.

Fincham, E.J. (1937), The mechanism of accommodation. *Br J Ophthalmol*, **21**, 8.

Fine, B.S. and Tousimis, A.J. (1961), The structure of the vitreous body and the suspensory ligaments of the lens. *Arch Ophthalmol*, **65**, 95.

Fine, B.S. and Yanoff, M. (1972), *Ocular Histology: A Text and Atlas*, Harper & Row, Philadelphia.

Fine, B.S. and Yanoff, M. (1979), *Ocular Histology: A Text and Atlas*, 2nd edition, Harper & Row, New York and Philadelphia.

Fine, B.S. and Zimmerman, L.E. (1963), Light and electron microscopic observations on the ciliary epithelium in man and rhesus monkey. *Invest Ophthalmol*, **2**, 105.

Fink, A.I., Felix, M.D. and Fletcher, R.C. (1972), The electron microscopy of Schlemm's canal and adjacent structures in patients with glaucoma. *Trans Ophthalmol Soc UK*, **70**, 82.

Fink, A.I., Felix, M.D. and Fletcher, R.C. (1978), The anatomic basis for glaucoma. *Ann Ophthalmol*, **23**, 397.

Fink, W.H. (1956), The development of the orbital fascion. *Am J Ophthalmol*, **42**, 269.

Fischer, A., Mundel, P., Mayer, B. *et al.* (1993), Nitric oxide synthase in guinea pig lower airway innervation. *Neurosci Lett*, **149**, 157.

Fisher, J.H. (1904), *Ophthalmological Anatomy*, Frowde & Hodder, London, 1.

Fisher, R.F. (1969), The elastic constants of the human lens capsule. *J Physiol*, **201**, 1.

Fisher, R.F. (1971), The elastic constant of the human lens. *J Physiol*, **212**, 147.

Fisher, R.F. (1973a), Presbyopia and the changes with age in the human crystalline lens. *J Physiol*, **228**, 765.

Fisher, R.F. (1973b), In *The Human Lens in Relation to Cataract*. (Discussion.) *Ciba Found Symp*, **19**, 114.

Fisher, R.F. (1977), The force of contraction of the human ciliary muscle during accommodation. *J Physiol*, **270**, 51.

Fisher, R.F. (1982), The vitreous and lens in accommodation. *Trans Ophthalmol Soc UK*, **102**, 318.

Fisher, R.F. and Hayes, B.P. (1979), Thickness and volume constants and ultrastructural organization of basement membrane (lens capsule). *J Physiol*, **293**, 229.

Fitzgerald, M.J.J. (1956), The occurrence of a middle superior alveolar nerve in man. *J Anat*, **90**, 520.

Flora, G., Dahl, E. and Nelson, E. (1967), Electron microscopic observations on human intracranial arteries. *Arch Neurol*, **17**, 162.

Floyd, B. B., Cleveland, P. H. and Worthen, D. M. (1985), Fibronectin in human trabecular drainage channels. *Invest Ophthalmol Vis Sci*, **26**, 797.

Flügel, C., Bárány, E.H. and Lütjen-Drecoll, E. (1990), Histochemical differences within the ciliary muscle and its function in accommodation. *Exp Eye Res*, **50**, 219.

Flügel, C., Tamm, E., Lütjen-Drecoll, E. (1992), Age-related loss of Â-smooth muscle actin in normal and glaucomatous human trabecular meshwork of different age groups. *J Glaucoma*, **1**, 165.

Flügel, C., Tamm, E.R., Mayer, B. and Lütjen-Drecoll. (1994), Species differences in choroidal vasodilative innervation: evidence for specific intrinsic nitrergic and VIP-positive neurons in the human eye. *Invest Ophthalmol Vis Sci*, **35**, 592.

Flügel-Koch, C., Kaufman, P. and Lütjen-Drecoll, E. (1994), Association of a choroidal ganglion cell plexus with the fovea centralis. *Invest Ophthalmol Vis Sci*, **35**, 4268.

Foos, R.Y. (1969), Zonular traction tufts of the peripheral retina in cadaver eyes. *Arch Ophthalmol*, **82**, 620.

Foos, R.Y. (1972), Vitreoretinal juncture, topographical variations. *Invest Ophthalmol Vis Sci*, **2**, 801.

Foos, R.Y. (1975), Ultrastructural features of posterior vitreous detachment. *A von Graefes Arch Klin Exp Ophthalmol*, **196**, 103.

Foos, R.Y. and Trese, M.T. (1982), Chorioretinal juncture. Vascularization of Bruch's membrane in peripheral fundus. *Arch Ophthalmol*, **100**, 1492.

Forbes, M.S., Rennels, M.L. and Nelson, E. (1977), Ultrastructure of pericytes in mouse heart. *Am J Anat*, **149**, 47.

Ford, M. and Sarwar, M. (1963), Features of a clinically normal optic disc. *Br J Ophthalmol*, **47**, 50.

Foster, G.E. (1973), PhD Thesis, Liverpool University.

Fox, J.C. and Holmes, G. (1926), Optic nystagmus and its value in the localization of cerebral lesions. *Brain*, **49**, 333.

Francois, J. (1959), Vascularization of the primary optic pathways. *Br J Ophthalmol*, **42**, 65.

Francois, J. (1975), The importance of the mucopolysaccharides in intraocular pressure regulation. *Invest Ophthalmol*, **14**, 173.

Francois, J. and Neetens, A. (1954), Vascularization of the optic pathway: I. Lamina cribrosa and optic nerve. *Br J Ophthalmol*, **38**, 472.

Francois, J., Neetens, A. and Collette, J.M. (1955), Vascular supply of the optic pathway: II. Further studies by micro-arteriography of the optic nerve. *Br J Ophthalmol*, **39**, 220.

Francois, J., Neetens, A. and Collette, J.M. (1956), Vascularization of the optic pathways. IV. Optic tract and external geniculate body. *Br J Ophthalmol*, **40**, 341.

Francois, J., Neetens, A. and Collette, J.M. (1959), Vascularization of the optic radiation and the visual cortex. *Br J Ophthalmol*, **43**, 394.

Francois, J. and Rabaey, M. (1958), Permeability of the capsule for the lens proteins. *Acta Ophthalmol*, **36**, 837.

Franklin, R.M. (1973), Immunohistological studies of human lacrimal gland: localisation of immunoglobulins, secretory component and lactoferrin. *J Immunol*, **110**, 984.

Franklin, R.M. and Bang, B.G. (1980), Mucus-stimulating factor in tears. *Invest Ophthalmol Vis Sci*, **19**, 430.

Franklin, R.M. and Remus, L.E. (1984), Conjunctival-associated lymphoid tissue: evidence for a role in the secretory immune system. *Invest Ophthalmol Vis Sci*, **25**, 181.

Freddo, T.F. (1984), Intercellular junctions of the iris epithelia in *Macaca mulatta*. *Invest Ophthalmol Vis Sci*, **25**, 1094.

Freddo, T.F. (1987), Intercellular junctions of the ciliary epithelium in anterior uveitis. *Invest Ophthalmol Vis Sci*, **28**, 320.

Freddo, T.F. and Raviola, G.R. (1980), The iris stromal cells of adult rhesus monkey: A scanning electron microscope study and a thin section and freeze-fracture analysis of their intercellular junctions. *Proc Int Soc Eye Res*, **1**, 26.

Freddo, T.F. and Raviola, G. (1982a), Freeze-fracture analysis of the interendothelial junctions in the blood vessels of the iris in *Macaca mulatta*. *Invest Ophthalmol Vis Sci*, **23**, 154.

Freddo, T.F. and Raviola, G. (1982b), The homogeneous structure of blood vessels in the vascular tree of *Macaca mulatta* iris. *Invest Ophthalmol Vis Sci*, **22**, 279.

Freddo, T.F. and Sacks-Wilner, R. (1989), Interendothelial junctions of the rabbit iris vasculature in anterior uveitis. *Invest Ophthalmol Vis Sci*, **30**, 1104.

Freddo, T.F., Townes-Anderson, E. and Raviola, G. (1980), Rod-shaped bodies and crystalloid inclusions in ocular vascular endothelia of adult and developing *Macaca mulatta*. *Anat Embryol*, **158**, 121.

Fredericks, C.A., Giolli, R.A., Blanks, R.H.I. et al. (1988), The human accessory optic system. *Brain Res*, **454**, 116.

Freihofer, H.P.M. (1980), Inner canthal and outer orbital distances. *J Maxillofacial Surg*, **8**, 324.

Friberg, L., Olesen, S., Iversen, H.K. et al. (1991), Migraine pain associated with middle cerebral artery dilatation: reversal by sumatriptan. *Lancet*, **338**, 13.

Frieberg, T. (1918), Weitere Untersuchungen uber die Mechanik der Tranehableitung. *Augenheilkunde*, **39**, 266.

Friedenwald, J.F. and Stiehler, R.D. (1935), Structure of the vitreous. *Arch Ophthalmol*, **14**, 789.

Friedenwald, J.S. (1930), Permeability of the lens capsule with special reference to the etiology of senile cataract. *Arch Ophthalmol*, **3**, 182.

Friedenwald, J.S. (1936), Circulation of the aqueous v. mechanism of Schlemm's canal. *Arch Ophthalmol*, **16**, 65.

Friedman, E. and Chandra, S.R. (1972), Choroidal blood flow. III. Effects of oxygen and carbon dioxide. *Arch Ophthalmol*, **87**, 70.

Friedman, E., Kopald, H.H. and Smith, T.R. (1964), Retinal and choroidal blood flow determined with Krypton-85 in anaesthetized animals. *Invest Ophthalmol Vis Sci*, **3**, 539.

Friedman, E. and Oak, S.M. (1965), Choroidal microcirculation *in vivo*. *Bibl Anat*, **7**, 129.

Fries, W. (1981), The projection from the lateral geniculate nucleus to the prestriate cortex of the macaque monkey. *Proc R Soc Lond*, **213**, 73.

Fries, W. and Zeki, S.M. (1983), The laminar origin of the cortical inputs to the fourth visual complex of macaque monkey cortex. *J Physiol*, **340**, 51.

Frund, H. (1911), Die glatte Muskulatur der Orbita und ihre Bedeutung fur die Augensymptome bei Morbus Basedowii. *Beitr Klin Chir*, **73**, 755.

Fry, W.E. (1930), Variations in the intraneural course of the central vein of the retina. *Arch Ophthalmol*, **4**, 180.

Fryczkowski, A.W. (1978), The role of ciliary anterior and posterior arteries in vascularization of the ciliary body and iris. *Klin Oczna*, **48**, 435.

Fryczkowski, A.W. (1988a), Architectonic structure of the blood vessels of the choroid. I. The Peripapillary area. *Klin Oczna*, **90**, 1.

Fryczkowski, A.W. (1988d), Angioarchitecture of the choroid. IV. The equatorial region. *Klin Oczna*, **90**, 46.

Fryczkowski, A.W. (1992), Blood vessels of the eye and their changes in diabetes, in *Scanning Electron Microscopy of Vascular Casts, Methods and Applications* (eds P.M. Motta and H. Fujita), Kluwer Academic Publishers, p. 293.

Fryczkowski, A.W. (1993), Choroidal microvascular anatomy, in *ICG Angiography Book* (ed L.A. Yanuzzi et al.).

Fryczkowski, A.W. and Bruszewska-Fryczkowska, H. (1988c), Angioarchitecture of the choroid. III. The posterior pole. *Klin Oczna*, **90**, 41.

Fryczkowski, A.W., Grimson, B.S. and Peiffer, R.L. (1984), Scanning electron microscopy of vascular casts of the human scleral lamina cribrosa. *Int Ophthalmol*, **7**, 95.

Fryczkowski, A.W., Hodes, B.L. and Walker, J. (1989), Diabetic choroidal and iris vasculature scanning electron microscopy findings. *Int Ophthalmol*, **13**, 269.

Fryczkowski, A.W., Sato, S.E., Mathers, W.D. et al. (1988b), Architectonic structure of the blood vessels of the choroid. II. The submacular area. *Klin Oczna*, **90**, 5.

Fryczkowski, A.W., Sato, S.E., Mathers, W.D. et al. (1988e), Angioarchitecture of the choroid. V. Peripheral choroid. The vortex veins. *Klin Oczna*, **90**, 81.

Fryczkowski, A.W. and Sherman, M.D. (1988), Scanning electron microscopy of human ocular vascular casts: the submacular choriocapillaris. *Acta Anat*, **132**, 265.

Fryczkowski, A.W., Sherman, M.D. and Walker, J. (1991), Observations on the lobular organization of the human choriocapillaris. *Int Ophthalmol*, **15**, 109.

Frydrychowicz, G. and Harms, H. (1940), Ergebnisse pupillomotorischer untersuchungen bei gesunden und kranken. *Verh Dtsch Ophthalmol Ges*, **53**, 71.

Fuchs, A.F. and Kornhuber, H. (1969), Extraocular muscle afferents to the cerebellum of the cat. *J Physiol*, **200**, 713.

Fuchs, A.F. and Lushchei, E.S. (1971), Development of isometric tension in simian extraocular muscle. *J Physiol*, **219**, 153.

Fuchs, E. (1884), Studies on the normal anatomy of the eye. *A von Graefes Arch Ophthalmol*, **30**, 1.

Fuchs, E. (1885), Die periphere Atrophie des Sehnerven. *A von Graefes Arch Ophthalmol*, **31**, 177.

Fuchs, E. (1917), *Textbook of Ophthalmology* (Translated by Duane, A.) 5th English edition, Lippincott, Philadelphia.

Fujino, T. (1961), The blood supply of the lateral geniculate body. *Acta Soc Ophthalmol Jpn*, **65**, 1428.

Fujino, T. (1962), The blood supply of the lateral geniculate body. *Acta Soc Ophthalmol Jpn*, **16**, 24.

Fujioka, M., Shimamoto, N., Kawahara, A. et al. (1989), Purification of an autocrine growth factor in conditioned medium obtained from primary cultures of scleral fibroblasts of the chick embryo. *Exp Cell Res*, **181**, 400.

Fuju, K., Lenkey, C. and Rhoton, A.L. (1980), Microsurgical anatomy of the choroidal arteries. Lateral and third ventricles. *J Neurosurg*, **52**, 165.

Fukuda, M. (1970), Presence of adrenergic innervation to the retinal vessels. A histochemical study. *Jpn J Ophthalmol*, **14**, 91.

Fulton, J.F. (1938), *Physiology of the Nervous System*, OUP, New York, p. 204.

Funk, R. (1991), Ultrastructure of the ciliary process vasculature in cynomolgus monkeys. *Exp Eye Res*, **53**, 461.

Funk, R. and Rohen, J.W. (1987), SEM-studies on the functional morphology of the rabbit ciliary process vasculature. *Exp Eye Res*, **45**, 579.

Funk, R. and Rohen, J.W. (1990), Scanning electron microscopic study on the vasculature of the human anterior eye segment, especially with respect to the ciliary processes. *Exp Eye Res*, **51**, 651.

Furness, J.B., Pompolo, S., Shuttleworth, C.W.R. and Burleigh, D.E. (1992), Light- and electron-microscopic immunochemical analysis of nerve fiber types innervating the taenia of the guinea pig cecum. *Cell Tissue Res*, **270**, 125.

Gabella, G. (1974), The sphincter pupillae of the guinea-pig: structure of muscle cells, intercellular relations and density of innervation. *Proc R Soc Lond, Series B*, **186**, 369.

Gallagher, B. and Maurice, D.M. (1977), Striations of light scattering in the corneal stroma. *J Ultrastruct Res*, **61**, 100.

Gallagher, B.A. (1980), Primary cilia of the corneal endothelium. *Am J Anat*, **159**, 475.

Garey, L.J., Jones, E.G. and Powell, T.P.S. (1968), Interrelationships of striate and extrastriate cortex with the primary relay sites of the visual pathway. *J Neurol Neurosurg Psych*, **31**, 135.

Garner, A. (1986), Ocular angiogenesis, in *International Review of Experimental Pathology* (eds G.W. Richter and M.A. Epstein), Academic Press, New York, p. 249.

Garnier, R.V. (1892), Uber den normalen und pathologischen Zustand der Zonula Zinnii. *Arch Augenheilk*, **24**, 32.

Garron, L. (1963), The ultrastructure of the retinal pigment epithelium with observations on the choriocapillaris and Bruchs membrane. *Trans Am Ophthalmol Soc*, **61**, 545.

Garron, L.K. and Feeney, M.L. (1959), Electron microscopic studies of the human eye. II. Study of the trabeculae by light and electron microscopy. *Arch Ophthalmol*, **62**, 966.

Garron, L.K., Feeney, M.L., Hogan, M.J. *et al.* (1959), Electron microscopic studies of the human eye. I. Preliminary investigations of the trabeculas. *Am J Ophthalmol*, **46**, 27.

Garzino, A. (1953), Le fibre della zonula di Zinn studiate a fresco con il microscopio a contrasto di fase. *Rass Ital Ottalmol*, **22**, 3.

Gattass, R., Oswaldo-Cruz, E. and Sousa, A.P.B. (1979), *Brain Res*, **160**, 413.

Gauthier, G.F. (1969), On the relationship of ultrastructural and cytochemical features to colour in mammalian skeletal muscle. *Z Zellforsch Mikrosk Anat*, **95**, 462.

Gauthier, G.F. (1979), Ultrastructural identification of muscle fiber types by immunocytochemistry. *J Cell Biol*, **82**, 391.

Gauthier, G.F. (1987), The ultrastructure of three fiber types in mammalian skeletal muscle, in *The Physiology and Biochemistry of Muscle as Food* (eds E. Briskey, R.G. Cassens and B.B. Marsh), Madison, Milwaukee.

Geeraets, R. (1976), An electron microscopic study of the closure of the optic fissure in the golden hamster. *Am J Anat*, **145**, 411.

Genis-Galvez, J.M. (1957), Innervation of the ciliary muscle. *Anat Rec*, **127**, 219.

Gerlach, J. (1880) *Anatomie des Auges*, Leipzig.

Gernandt, B.E. (1968), Interactions between extraocular myotatic and ascending vestibular influences. *Exp Neurol*, **20**, 120.

Gernet, H. (1964), Achsenlange und Refraktion lebender Augen von Neugeborenen. *A von Graefes Arch Ophthalmol*, **166**, 530.

Gilbert, C.D. and Kelly, J.P (1975), The projections of cells in cat primary visual cortex. *J Comp Neurol*, **163**, 81.

Gilbert, C.D. and Wiesel, T.N. (1979), Morphology and intracortical projections of functionally characterised neurones in the cat visual cortex. *Nature*, **280**, 120.

Gilbert, C.D. and Wiesel, T.N. (1983), Clustered intrinsic connections in cat visual cortex. *J Neurosci*, **3**, 1116.

Gillette, T.E., Allansmith, M.R., Greiner, J.V. *et al.* (1980), Histologic and immunohistologic comparison of main and accessory lacrimal tissue. *Am J Ophthalmol*, **89**, 724.

Gillette, T.E., Chandler, J.W. and Greiner, J.V. (1982), Langerhans cells of the ocular surface. *Ophthalmology*, **89**, 700.

Gillilan, L.A. (1941), *J Comp Neurol*, **74**, 367.

Gillilan, L.A. (1959), Correlative anatomy of the nervous system. *J Comp Neurol*, **112**, 55.

Gillilan, L.A. (1962), in *Correlative Anatomy of Nervous System* (eds E.C. Crosby *et al.*), Macmillan, New York, p. 1.

Gillilan, L.A (1972), Anatomy and embryology of the arterial system of the brain stem and cerebellum, in *Handbook of Clinical Neurology* (eds I.J. Vinken and G.W. Bruyn), North Holland Publishing Company, Amsterdam, p. 24.

Giolli, R.A. (1963), An experimental study of the accessory optic system in the Cynomolgus monkey. *J Comp Neurol*, **121**, 89.

Giolli, R.A., Blanks, R.H.I. and Torigoe, Y. (1984), Pretectal and brainstem projections of the medial terminal nucleus of the accessory optic system of the rabbit and rat as studied by anterograde and retrograde neuronal tracing methods. *J Comp Neurol*, **227**, 228.

Giolli, R.A., Blanks, R.H.I., Torigoe, Y. *et al.* (1985), Projections of the medial terminal accessory optic nucleus, ventral tegmental nuclei, and substantia nigra of rabbit and rat as studied by retrograde axonal transport of horseradish peroxidase. *J Comp Neurol*, **232**, 99.

Giolli, R.A. and Guthrie, M.D. (1969), The primary optic projections in the rabbit: an experimental degeneration study. *J Comp Neurol*, **136**, 99.

Gipson, I.K. (1989), The epithelial basement membrane zone of the limbus. *Eye*, **3**, 132.

Gipson, I.K. and Anderson, R.A. (1977), Actin filaments in normal and migrating corneal epithelial cells. *Invest Ophthalmol Vis Sci*, **16**, 161.

Gipson, I.K., Spurr-Michaud, S.J. and Tisdale, A.S. (1987), Anchoring fibrils form a complex network in human and rabbit cornea. *Invest Ophthalmol Vis Sci*, **28**, 212.

Gipson, I.K., Westcott, M.J. and Brooksby, N.G. (1982), Effects of cytochalasins B and D and colchicine on migration of the corneal epithelium. *Invest Ophthalmol Vis Sci*, **22**, 633.

Gitlin, G. and Lowental, U. (1969), Is there a commissure of Gudden in man? An examination of the published evidence with a note on the medial root of the human optic tract. *Acta Anat*, **73**, 161.

Givner, I. (1939), Episcleral ganglion cells. *Arch Ophthalmol*, **22**, 82.

Glees, P. (1941), *J Anat*, **75**, 434.

Glees, P. (1961), *The Visual System* (eds R. Jung and H. Kornmuller), Berlin.

Glees, P. and Le Gros Clark, W.E. (1941), The termination of optic fibres in the lateral geniculate body of the monkey. *J Anat*, **75**, 295.

Gloor, B.P., Gloor, M.L., Marshall, J. *et al.* (1980), Healing of mechanical wounds of the corneal endothelium of rhesus monkeys and rabbits, in *The Cornea in Health and Disease. Proceedings of the VIth Congress of the European Society of Ophthalmology*, Academic Press, New York, p. 97.

Gloster, J. (1961), *Br J Ophthalmol*, **45**, 259.

Gnadinger, M.C., Heinmann, R. and Markstein, R. (1973), Choline acetyltransferase in corneal epithelium. *Exp Eye Res*, **15**, 395.

Goldberg, M. and Bushnell, M.C. (1981), Behavioral enhancement of visual responses in monkey cerebral cortex. II. Modulation in frontal eye fields specifically related to saccades. *J Neurophysiol*, **46**, 773.

Goldberg, M.F. (1979), The diagnosis and treatment of sickled erythrocytes in human hyphemas. *Ophthalmic Surg*, **10**, 17.

Goldberg, M.F. and Bron, A.J. (1982), Limbal palisades of Vogt. *Trans Am Ophthalmol Soc*, **80**, 155.

Goldfischer, S., Coltoff-Schiller, B. and Goldfischer, M. (1985), Microfibrils, elastic anchoring components of the extracellular matrix, are associated with fibronectin in the zonule of Zinn and aorta. *Tissue Cell*, **17**, 441.

Golding-Wood, P.H. (1963), *Br Med J*, **i**, 1518.

Goldman, J. and Kuwabara, T. (1968), Histopathology of corneal edema. *Int Ophthalmol Clin*, **8**, 561.

Goldman, J.N. and Benedek, G.B. (1967), The relationship between morphology and transparency in the non-swelling corneal stroma of the shark. *Invest Ophthalmol*, **6**, 574.

Goldman, J.N., Benedek, C.H., Dohlman, C.H. *et al.* (1968), Structural alterations affecting transparency in swollen human corneas. *Invest Ophthalmol*, **7**, 501.

Goldmann, H. (1946), Mitteilung uber den abfluss des kammerwassers beim menschen. *Ophthalmologica*, **112**, 344.

Goldmann, H. (1954), Biomikroskopie des glaskorpers. *Ophthalmologica*, **127**, 334.

Goldnamer, W.W. (1923), *The Anatomy of the Eye and Orbit* (ed. E. Wolff), H.K. Lewis, London.

Gong, H. and Freddo, T.F. (1994), Hyaluronic acid in the normal and glaucomatous human outflow pathway. *ARVO abstract, Invest Ophthalmol Vis Sci*, **35 (suppl.)**, 2083.

Gong, H., Freddo, T.F. and Johnson, M. (1992), Age-related changes of sulfated proteoglycans in the normal human trabecular meshwork. *Exp Eye Res*, **55**, 691.

Gong, H., Trinkaus-Randall, V. and Freddo, T. (1989), Ultrastructural immunocytochemical localization of elastin in normal human trabecular meshwork. *Curr Eye Res*, **8**, 1071.

Gong, H., Tripathi, R.C. and Tripathi, B.J. (1996), Morphology of the aqueous outflow pathway. *Microscopy Research and Technique*, **33**, 336.

Gong, H., Underhill, C.B. and Freddo, T.F. (1994), Hyaluranon in the bovine ocular anterior segment, with emphasis on the outflow pathways. *Invest Ophthalmol Vis Sci*, **35**, 4328.

Gonshor, A. and Melvill Jones, G. (1976), Extreme vestibulo-ocular adaptation induced by prolonged optical reversal of vision. *J Physiol*, **256**, 381.

Gonzalez-Mariscal, L., Chavez-de-Ramirez, B., Lazaro, A. *et al.* (1989), Establishment of tight junctions between cells from different animal species and different sealing capacities. *J Membr Biol*, **107**, 43.

Goodenough, D.A. (1979), Lens gap junctions: a structural hypothesis for nonregulated low-resistance intercellular pathways. *Invest Ophthalmol Vis Sci*, **18**, 1104.

Goodenough, D.A., Dick, J.S.B., II and Lyons, J.E. (1980), Lens metabolic cooperation: a study of mouse lens transport and permeability visualized with freeze substitution autoradiography and electron microscopy. *J Cell Biol*, **86**, 576.

Gordon-Weeks, P.R (1988), The ultrastructure of noradrenergic and cholinergic neurons in the autonomic nervous system, in *Handbook of Chemical Neuroanatomy*, (eds A. Björklund, T. Hökfelt and C. Owman), Elsevier Science BV, Amsterdam, p. 117.

Gordon-Weeks, P.R. and Hobbs, M.J. (1979), A non-adrenergic nerve containing small granular vesicles in the guinea-pig gut. *Neurosci Lett*, **12** 81.

Gouras, P. (1968), *J Physiol*, **199**, 533.

Gouras, P. (1974), Opponent colour cells in different layers of foveal striate cortex. *J Physiol*, **238**, 583.

Graf Spee, F. (1902), Ueber den Bau der Zonulafasem und ihre Anordnung im Menschlichen Auge. *Anat Anz Zbl Ges Wiss Anat*, **21**, 236.

Grant, W.M. (1958), Further studies on facility of flow through trabecular meshwork. *Arch Ophthalmol*, **60**, 323.

Grant, W.M. (1963), Experimental aqueous perfusion in enucleated human eyes. *Arch Ophthalmol*, **69**, 783.

Grantyn, R., Baker, R. and Grantyn, A. (1980), Morphological and physiological identification of excitatory pontine reticular neurons projecting to the cat abducens nucleus and spinal cord. *Brain Res*, **198**, 221.

Graves, B. (1934), Certain clinical features of the normal limbus. *Br J Ophthalmol*, **18**, 305.

Gray, E.G. (1976), Microtubules in the synapses of the retina. *J Neurocytol*, **3**, 361.

Graybiel, A.M. (1977a), Direct and indirect preoculomotor pathways of the brainstem: an autoradiographic study of the pontine reticular formation in the cat. *J Comp Neurol*, **175**, 37.

Graybiel, A.M. (1977b), Organization of oculomotor pathways in the cat. *Dev Neurosci*, **1**, 79.

Grayson, M.C. and Laties, A.M. (1971), Ocular localization of sodium fluorescein: effects of administration in rabbit and monkey. *Arch Ophthalmol*, **85**, 600.

Greeff, R. (1899), Das Wesen der Fuchschen atrophie im sehnerv. *IX Congress International d'Ophthalmologie d'Utrecht*, p. 237.

Greeff, R. (1932), Die Microskopische Anatomie des Sehnerven und der Netzhaut, in *Handbuch der Augenheilkunde 2 und 3 Auflage* (ed. A. Elschnig) Graefe-Saemisch Handbuch der Gesamten Augenheilk 1, 1.

Greider, B. and Egbert, P.R. (1980), Anatomy of the major circle of the iris. ARVO Suppl: *Invest Ophthalmol Vis Sci*, **19**, 256.

Greiner, J.V., Covington, H.I. and Allansmith, M.R. (1977), Surface morphology of the human upper tarsal conjunctiva. *Am J Ophthalmol*, **73**, 892.

Greiner, J.V., Covington, H.I. and Allansmith, M.R. (1979), The human limbus. A scanning electron microscopic study. *Arch Ophthalmol*, **97**, 1159.

Greiner, J.V., Covington, H.I., Fowler, S.A. *et al.* (1982), Cell surface variations of the human upper tarsal conjunctiva. *Ann Ophthalmol*, **14**, 288.

Greiner, J.V., Gladstone, L., Covington, H.I. *et al.* (1980a), Branching of microvilli in the human conjunctival epithelium. *Arch Ophthalmol*, **98**, 1253.

Greiner, J.V., Henriquez, A.S., Covington, H.I. *et al.* (1981), Goblet cells of the human conjunctiva. *Arch Ophthalmol*, **99**, 2190.

Greiner, J.V., Kenyon, K.R., Henriquez, A.S. *et al.* (1980b),

Mucus secretory vesicles in conjunctival epithelial cells of wearers of contact lenses. *Arch Ophthalmol*, **98**, 1843.

Grierson, I. and Howes, R. (1987), Age-related depletion of the cell population in the human trabecular meshwork. *Eye*, **1**, 204.

Grierson, I., Lee, S. and Abraham, S. (1979), A light microscopy study of the effects of testicular hyaluronidase on the outflow system of the baboon (*Papio cynocephalus*). *Invest Ophthalmol Vis Sci*, **18**, 356.

Grierson, I. and Lee, W.R. (1974), Changes in the monkey outflow apparatus at graded levels of intraocular pressure: a qualitative analysis by light microscopy and scanning electron microscopy. *Exp Eye Res*, **19**, 21.

Grierson, I. and Lee, W.R. (1975), Acid mucopolysaccharides in the outflow apparatus. *Exp Eye Res*, **21**, 417.

Grierson, I. and Lee, W.R. (1977), Light microscopic quantitation of the endothelial vacuoles in Schlemm's canal. *Am J Ophthalmol*, **84**, 234.

Grierson, I. and Lee, W.R. (1978), Pressure effects on flow channels in the lining endothelium of Schlemm's canal. *Acta Ophthalmol*, **56**, 935.

Grierson, I., Lee, W.R. and Abraham, S. (1977), Pathways for the drainage of aqueous humour into Schlemm's canal. *Trans Ophthalmol Soc UK*, **97**, 719.

Grierson, I., Lee, W.R. and Abraham, S. (1978a), Further observations on the process of haemophagocytosis in the human outflow system. *A von Graefes Arch Klin Exp Ophthalmol*, **208**, 49.

Grierson, I., Lee, W.R. and Abraham, S. (1978b), The effects of pilocarpine on the morphology of the human outflow apparatus. *Br J Ophthalmol*, **62**, 302.

Grierson, I., Lee, W.R. and McMenamin, P.G. (1981), The morphological basis of drug action on the outflow system of the eye. *Res Clin Forums*, **3**, 1.

Grierson, I. and McMenamin, P.G. (1982), The morphological response of the primate outflow system to changes in pressure and flow, in *Basic Aspects of Glaucoma Research*, F.K. Schattauer Verlag, Stuttgart.

Grignolo, A. (1954a), Researches on the submicroscopic structure of the lens capsule. *G Hal Oftal*, **7**, 300.

Grignolo, A. (1954b), Studies on the submicroscopical structure of the ocular tissues. *Bull Ocul*, **33**, 513.

Grimes, P. and von Sallmann, L. (1960), Comparative anatomy of ciliary nerves. *Arch Ophthalmol*, **64**, 81.

Grofová, I., Ottersen, O.P. and Rinvik, E. (1978), Mesencephalic and diencephalic afferents to the superior colliculus and periaqueductal gray substance demonstrated by retrograde axonal transport of horseradish peroxidase in the cat. *Brain Res*, **146**, 205.

Gross, C.G. (1973), *Handbook of Sensory Physiology VII/3* (ed. R. Jung), Springer-Verlag, Berlin, p. 451.

Gross, C.G., Bruce, C.J., Desimone, R. *et al.* (1981), Cortical visual areas of the temporal lobe, in *Cortical Sensory Organization* (ed. C.N. Woolsey), Humana Press, New York, p. 187.

Gross, C.G., Cowey, A. and Manning, F.J. (1971), Further analysis of visual discrimination deficits following foveal prestriate and inferotemporal lesions in rhesus monkeys. *J Comp Physiol Psychol*, **76**, 1.

Gross, C.G. and Mishkin, M. (1979), *Lateralization in the Nervous System* (eds S. Harped, R.W. Daty, L. Goldstein *et al.*), Academic Press, New York, p. 109.

Gross, G.G., Rolha Miranda, C.E. and Bender, M.B. (1972),

Visual properties of neurons in inferotemporal cortex of the macacque. *J Neurophysiol*, **35**, 96.

Grozdanovic, Z., Baumgarten, H.G. and Bruning, G. (1992), Histochemistry of NADPH-diaphorase, a marker for neuronal nitric oxide synthase, in the peripheral autonomic nervous system in the mouse. *Neuroscience*, **48**, 225.

Gudden, B. (1874), Uber die Kreuzung der Fasem im Chiasma nervorum opticorum. *A von Graefes Arch Ophthalmol*, **20**, 249.

Guggenmoos-Holzmann, I., Engel, B., Henke, V. *et al.* (1989), Cell density of human lens epithelium in women higher than in men. *Invest Ophthalmol Vis Sci*, **30**, 330.

Guillery, R.W. (1957), Degeneration in the hypothalamic connexions of the albino rat. *J Anat (Lond.)*, **91**, 91.

Guillery, R.W. (1971a), *Exp Brain Res*, **12**, 184.

Guillery, R.W. (1971b), Patterns of synaptic interconnections in the dorsal lateral geniculate nucleus of cat and monkey. A brief review. *Vision Res*, **3**, 211.

Guillery, R.W (1991), Rules that govern the development of the pathways from the eye to the optic tract in mammals, in *Development of the Visual System* (eds D.M. Lam and C.J. Shatz), MIT Press, Cambridge, MA, p. 153.

Guillery, R.W. and Colonnier, M. (1970), Synaptic patterns in the dorsal lateral geniculate nucleus of the monkey. *Z Zellforsch Mikrosk Anat*, **103**, 90.

Guillery, R.W., Hickey, T.L., Kaas, J.H. *et al.* (1984), Abnormal central visual pathways in the brain of an albino green monkey (*Cercopithecus aethiops*). *J Comp Neurol*, **226**, 165.

Guillery, R.W., Polley, E.H. and Torrealba, F. (1982), The arrangement of axons according to fiber diameter in the optic tract of the cat. *J Neurosci*, **2**, 714.

Guillery, R.W. and Walsh, C. (1987), Changing glial organisation relates to changing fibre order in the developing optic nerve of ferrets. *J Comp Neurol*, **265**, 203.

Gullstrand, A. (1912), Die nemspaltlampe in der ophtalmologischen praxis. *Klin Monatsbl Augenheilk*, **50**, 483.

Gurwitsch, M. (1883), Ueber die Anastomosen zwischen den Gesichts- und Orbitalvenen. *A von Graefes Arch Ophthalmol*, **29**, 31.

Guzek, J.P., Holm, M. and Cotter, J. (1987), Risk factors for intraoperative complications in 1000 extracapsular cataract cases. *Ophthalmology*, **94**, 461.

Halata, Z. (1975), The mechanoreceptors of the mammalian skin: Ultrastructure and morphological classification. *Adv Anat Embryol Cell Biol*, **50**, 1.

Halata, Z., Rettig, T. and Schulze, W. (1985), The ultrastructure of sensory nerve endings in the human knee joint capsule. *Anat Embryol*, **172**, 265.

Hall, E. (1975), The anatomy of the limbic system, in *Neural Integration of Physiological Mechanisms and Behavior* (eds G.J. Mogenson and F.R. Calaresu), University of Toronto Press, Toronto, p. 68.

Haller, A. (1754), Arteriarum oculi historia et tabulae arteriarum oculi. Gottingen. Cited by François *et al.* (1954), *Br J Ophthalmol*, **38**, 472.

Hamada, R. (1974), Aspect ultrastructural des cellules et du tissu conjonctif corneen normal. *Arch Ophthalmol (Paris)*, **35**, 23.

Hamanaka, T., Bill, A., Ichinihasama, R. *et al.* (1992), Aspects of the development of Schlemm's canal. *Exp Eye Res*, **55**, 479.

Hamann, K.-U., Hellner, K., Müller-Jensen, A. *et al.* (1979), Videopupillographic and VER investigations in patients with congenital and acquired lesions of the optic radiation. *Ophthalmologica*, **178**, 348.

Hamann, K.-U., Hellner, K.A. and Jensen, W. (1981), The dynamics and latency of the pupillary response in cases of homonymous hemianopia. *Neuro-ophthalmology*, **2**, 23.

Hamasaki, D., Ong, J. and Marg, E. (1956), The amplitude of accommodation in presbyopia. *Am J Optom Arch Am Acad Optom*, **33**, 2.

Hammar, H. (1965), An autoradiographic study on cell migration in the eye lens epithelium from normal and alloxan diabetic rats. *Acta Ophthalmol*, **43**, 442.

Han, V.K., d'Ercole, A.J. and Lund, P.K. (1987), Cellular localization of somatomedin (insulin-like growth factor) messenger RNA in the human fetus. *Science*, **236**, 193.

Handelman, G.H. and Koretz, J.F. (1982), Appendix: Mathematical derivation of a human accommodation model. *Vision Res*, **22**, 924.

Hanna, C., Bicknell, D.S. and O'Brien, J.E. (1961), Cell turnover in the adult human eye. *Arch Ophthalmol*, **65**, 695.

Hannover, A. (1845) Entdeckung des Baues des Glaskörpers. *Arch Anat Physiol und Wiss Med*.

Hara, K., Lütjen-Drecoll, E., Prestele, H. *et al.* (1977), Structural differences between regions of the ciliary body in primates. *Invest Ophthalmol Vis Sci*, **16**, 912.

Hardebo, J.E., Suzuki, N., Ekblad, E. *et al.* (1992), Vasoactive intestinal polypeptide and acetylcholine coexist with neuropeptide Y, dopamine-β-hydroxylase, substance P or calcitonin gene-related peptide in neuronal subpopulations in cranial parasympathetic ganglia of rat. *Cell Tissue Res*, **267**, 291.

Harding, C.V., Donn, A. and Srinivasan, B.D. (1959), Incorporation of thymidine by injured lens epithelium. *Exp Cell Res*, **18**, 582.

Harding, C.V., Reddan, J.R., Unakar, N.J. *et al.* (1971), The control of cell division in the ocular lens. *Int Rev Cytol*, **31**, 215.

Harding, J. (1991), *Cataract: Biochemistry, Epidemiology and Pharmacology*, Chapman & Hall, London.

Harding, J.J. (1993), Pathophysiology of cataract. *Curr Opin Ophthalmol*, **4**, 14.

Harding, J.J. and Crabbe, M.J.C. (1984), The lens: development, proteins, metabolism and cataract, in *The Eye*, 3rd edition (ed. H. Davson), Academic Press, London, p. 207.

Harding, J.J. and Dilley, K.J. (1976), Structural proteins of the mammalian lens: a review with emphasis on changes in development, aging and cataract. *Exp Eye Res*, **22**, 1.

Harker, D.U. (1972), The structure and innervation of sheep superior rectus and levator palpebrae extraocular muscles. *Invest Ophthalmol*, **11**, 956.

Harman, I.J. and Teuber, H.L. (1959), The geniculo-calcarine system of MR. A case of cortical blindness. Paper read at Spring Meeting of American Anatomists, Seattle, 1959. (Cited by Teuber *et al.* 1960.)

Harms, H. (1951), Hemianopische pupillenstarre. *Klin Monatsbl Augenheilkd*, **118**, 133.

Harms, H. (1956), Möglichkeiten und grenzen der pupil-lometrischen perimetrie. *Klin Monatsbl Augenheilkd*, **129**, 518.

Harris, A.J., Hodes, R. and Magoun, H.W. (1944), The afferent path of the pupillo-dilator reflex in the cat. *J Neurophysiol*, **7**, 231.

Harris, H.A. (1933), *Bone Growth in Health and Disease*, OUP, Oxford, 1.

Hart, R.W. (1972), Theory of neural mediation of intra-ocular dynamics. *Bull Math Biol*, **34**, 113.

Harting, J.K., Hall, W.C., Diamond, I.T. *et al.* (1973), Anterograde degeneration study of the superior colliculus in *Tupaia glis*: evidence for a subdivision between superficial and deep layers. *J Comp Neurol*, **148**, 361.

Harting, J.K., Huerta, M.F., Frankfurter, A.J. *et al.* (1980), Ascending pathways from the monkey superior colliculus. An autoradiographic analysis. *J Comp Neurol*, **192**, 853.

Hassler, R. (1955), *Sixth Latin-American Congress on Neurosurgery*, Montevideo, p. 254.

Hatton, J.D. and Ellisman, M.H. (1981), The distribution of orthogonal arrays and their relationship to intercellular junctions in neuroglia of the freeze-fractured hypothalamo-neurohypophysical system. *Cell Tissue Res*, **215**, 309.

Hay, E.D. and Revel, J.P. (1969), Fine structure of the developing avian cornea, in *Monographs in Developmental Biology, vol. 1* (eds A. Wolsky and P.S. Chen), Karger, Basel.

Haye, C., Clay, C. and Bignaud, J. (1970), L'exploration radiologique de l'orbite. *Arch Ophthalmol*, **30**, 179.

Hayreh, S.S. (1962), The ophthalmic artery. III. Branches. *Br J Ophthalmol*, **46**, 212.

Hayreh, S.S. (1963), Blood supply and vascular disorders of the optic nerve. *Ann Inst Barraquer*, **4**, 7.

Hayreh, S.S. (1964), The orbital vessels of rhesus monkey. *Exp Eye Res*, **3**, 16.

Hayreh, S.S. (1972), Blood supply and vascular disorders of the optic nerve, in *The Optic Nerve* (ed. J.S. Cant), Henry Kimpton, London, p. 59.

Hayreh, S.S. (1974a), The choriocapillaris. *A von Graefes Arch Klin Exp Ophthalmol*, **192**, 165.

Hayreh, S.S. (1974b), The long posterior ciliary arteries. An experimental study. *A von Graefes Arch Klin Exp Ophthalmol*, **192**, 197.

Hayreh, S.S. (1974c), Sub-macular choroidal vascular pattern. Experimental fluorescein fundus angiographic studies. *A von Graefes Arch Klin Exp Ophthalmol*, **192**, 181.

Hayreh, S.S. (1974d), Anatomy and physiology of the optic nerve head. *Trans Am Acad Ophthalmol Otolaryngol*, **78**, 240.

Hayreh, S.S. (1974e), Recent advances in fluorescein fundus angiography. *Br J Ophthalmol*, **58**, 39.

Hayreh, S.S. (1975a), Segmental nature of the choroidal vasculature. *Br J Ophthalmol*, **59**, 631.

Hayreh, S.S. (1975b), *Anterior Ischemic Optic Neuropathy*, Springer, New York.

Hayreh, S.S. (1976), Choroidal circulation in health and in acute vascular occlusion, in *Vision and Circulation* (ed. S. Cant), Henry Kimpton, London, p. 157.

Hayreh, S.S. (1990), *In vivo* choroidal circulation and its watershed zones. *Eye*, **4**, 273.

Hayreh, S.S. and Baines, J.A.B. (1972a), Occlusion of the posterior ciliary artery. I. Effects on choroidal circulation. *Br J Ophthalmol*, **56**, 719.

Hayreh, S.S. and Baines, J.A.B. (1972b), Occlusion of the posterior ciliary artery. II. Chorioretinal lesions. *Br J Ophthalmol*, **56**, 736.

Hayreh, S.S. and Baines, J.A.B. (1973), Occlusion of the vortex veins. An experimental study. *Br J Ophthalmol*, **57**, 217.

Hayreh, S.S. and Dass, R. (1962a), The ophthalmic artery. I. Origin and intra-cranial and intra-canicular course. *Br J Ophthalmol*, **46**, 65.

Hayreh, S.S. and Dass, R. (1962b), The ophthalmic artery II. Intra-orbital course. *Br J Ophthalmol*, **46**, 165.

Hayreh, S.S. and Scott, W.E. (1978), Fluorescein iris angiography. II. Disturbances in iris circulation following strabismus operation on the various recti. *Arch Ophthalmol*, **96**, 1390.

Hayreh, S.S. and Vrabec, F. (1966), The structure of the head of the optic nerve in the rhesus monkey. *Am J Ophthalmol*, **61**, 136.

Hedges, T.R., Jr., Baron, E.M., Hedges, T.R., III and Sinclair, S. H. (1994), The retinal venous pulse. Its relation to optic disc characteristics and choroidal pulse. *Ophthalmology*, **101**, 542.

Heegaard, S. (1994), Structure of the human vitreoretinal border region. *Ophthalmologica*, **208**, 82.

Heide, W., Fahle, M., Koenig, E. *et al.* (1990), Impairment of vertical motion detection and downgaze palsy due to rostral midbrain infarction. *J Neurol*, **23**, 432.

Heide, W., Koenig, E. and Dichgans, J. (1990), Optokinetic nystagmus, self-motion senation and their after-effects in patients with occipito-parietal lesions. *Clin Vision Sci*, **5**, 145.

Heimann, K. (1972), The development of the choroid in man. *Ophthalmic Res*, **3**, 257.

Heine, L. (1898), Beitrage zur Physiologie und Pathologie der Linse Graefes. *Arch Ophthalmol*, **46**, 525.

Helveston, E.M., Merriam, W.W., Ellis, F.D. *et al.* (1982), The trochlea: a study of the anatomy and physiology. *Ophthalmology*, **89**, 124.

Henderson, T. (1908), The anatomy of the so-called ligamentum pectinatum iridis and its bearing on the physiology and pathology of the eye. *Trans Ophthalmol Soc UK*, **28**, 47.

Hendrickson, A.E. (1982), *Cytochemical Methods in Neuroanatomy* (eds V. Chan-Palay and S. Palay), Liss, New York, p. 1.

Hendrickson, A.E. (1985), Dots, stripes and columns in monkey visual cortex. *Trends Neurosci*, **9**, 229.

Hendrickson, A.E. (1994), Primate foveal development: a microcosm of current questions in neurobiology. *Invest Ophthalmol Vis Sci*, **35**, 3129.

Hendrickson, A.E., Wilson, J.R. and Ogren, M.P. (1978), The neuroanatomical organization of pathways between the dorsal internal geniculate nucleus and visual cortex in old world and new world primates. *J Comp Neurol*, **182**, 123.

Hendrickson, A.E., Wilson, M.E. and Toyne, M.J. (1970), The distribution of optic nerve fibers in *Macaca mulatta*. *Brain Res*, **23**, 425.

Hendrickson, A.E. and Yuodelis, C. (1984), The morphological development of the human fovea. *Ophthalmology*, **91**, 603.

Henkind, P. (1964), Angle vessels in normal eyes: A gonioscopic evaluation and anatomic correlation. *Br J Ophthalmol*, **48**, 551.

Henkind, P. (1967), Radial peripupillary capillaries of the retina. I. Anatomy: human and comparative. *Br J Ophthalmol*, **51**, 115.

Henkind, P. and Levitzky, M. (1969), Angioarchitecture of the optic nerve: I. The papilla. *Am J Ophthalmol*, **68**, 979.

Henle, J. (1853), Handbuch der topographischen Anatomie. *Immunol Rev*, **1**, 1.

Henle, J. (1876) *Handbuch der Gefasslehre des Menschen. 2. Aufl.* Vieweg Sohn, Braunschweig.

Henn, V. and Buttner, U. (1982), Disorders of horizontal gaze, in *Functional Basis of Ocular Motility Disorders* (eds G. Lennerstrand, D.S. Gee and E.L. Keller), Pergamon Press, Oxford.

Henn, V., Büttner-Ennever, J.A. and Hepp, K. (1982), The primate oculomotor system. I. Motoneurons. *Hum Neurobiol*, **1**, 77.

Henn, V., Hepp, K. and Büttner-Ennever, J.A. (1982), The primate oculomotor system. II Premotor system. *Hum Neurobiol*, **1**, 87.

Henn, V., Young, L.R. and Finley, C. (1974), Vestibular nucleus units in alert monkeys are also influenced by moving visual fields. *Brain Res*, **71**, 144.

Henry, J.G.M. (1959), Contribution a l'etude de l'anatomie des vaisseaux de l'orbite et de la loge caverneuse – par injection de matieres plastiques – du tendon de Zinn et de la capsule de Tenson. *PhD Thesis*, Paris.

Henschen, S.E. (1893), *Brain*, **16**, 170.

Hepp, K. and Henn, V. (1979), Neuronal activity preceding rapid eye movements in the brainstem of the alert monkey. *Progr Brain Res*, **50**, 645.

Hepp, K., Henn, V. and Jaeger, J. (1982), Eye movement related neurons in the cerebellar nuclei of the alert monkey. *Exp Brain Res*, **45**, 253.

Herbert, J., Cavallaro, T. and Martone, R. (1991), The distribution of retinol-binding protein and its mRNA in the rat eye. *Invest Ophthalmol Vis Sci*, **32**, 302.

Herman, L.H. (1966), *Anat Rec*, **154**, 1.

Hermann, H. and Lebeau, P.L. (1962), ATP level, cell injury and apparent epithelium-stroma interaction in the cornea. *J Cell Biol*, **13**, 465.

Hernandez, M.R. (1992), Ultrastructural immuno-cytochemical analysis of elastin in the human lamina cribrosa. Changes in elastic fibers in primary open-angle glaucoma. *Invest Ophthalmol Vis Sci*, **33**, 2891.

Hernandez, M.R., Luo, X.X., Andrzejewska, W. *et al.* (1989), Age-related changes in the extracellular matrix of the human optic nerve head. *Am J Ophthalmol*, **107**, 476.

Hernandez, M.R., Luo, X.X., Igoe, F. *et al.* (1987), Extracellular matrix of human lamina cribrosa. *Am J Ophthalmol*, **104**, 567.

Hernandez, M.R., Wang, N., Hanley, N.M. *et al.* (1991), Localization of collagen types I and IV mRNAs in human optic nerve head by in situ hybridization. *Invest Ophthalmol Vis Sci*, **32**, 169.

Hero, I. (1990), Optic fissure closure in the normal cinnamon mouse. *Invest Ophthalmol Vis Sci*, **31**, 197.

Hess, A. (1961), A structure of slow and fast extrafusal muscle fibers in the extraocular muscles and their nerve endings in guinea pigs. *J Cell Comp Physiol*, **58**, 63.

Hess, A. (1967), The structure of vertebrate slow and twitch muscle fibers. *Invest Ophthalmol*, **6**, 217.

Hess, A. and Pilar, G. (1963), Slow fibers in the extraocular muscles of cat. *J Physiol*, **169**, 780.

Hess, C. (1911), Pathologie und Therapie des Linsensystems, in *Graefe-Saemisch Handbuch*, 3rd edition *Graefe-Saemisch Handbuch der Gesamten Augenheilk* **1**, 35.

Hewitt, A. and Adler, R. (1989), The retinal pigment epithelium and interphotoreceptor matrix: structure and specialized functions, in *Retina* (eds S.J. Ryan and T. Ogden), C.V. Mosby, St Louis, p. 57.

Hickam, J.R., Frayser, R. and Ross, J.C. (1963), A study of retinal venous blood oxygen saturation in human subjects by photographic means. *Circulation*, **27**, 375.

Hickey, T.L. and Guillery, R.W. (1979), Variability of laminar patterns in the human lateral geniculate nucleus. *J Comp Neurol*, **183**, 221.

Hikosaka, O., Igusa, Y. and Imai, H. (1978), Firing pattern of prepesitus hypoglossi and adjacent reticular neurones related to vestibular nystagmus in the cat. *Brain Res*, **144**, 395.

Hikosaka, O. and Wurtz, R.H. (1980), Discharge of substantia nigra neurons decreases before visually guided saccades. *Soc Neurosci Abstr*, **6**, 15.

Hiles, D.A., Biglan, A.W. and Fetheroff, E.C. (1979), Central corneal endothelial cell counts in children. *WHO*, **5**, 292.

Hill, J.C., Bethell, W. and Smirinaul, H.J. (1974a), Lacrimal drainage – a dynamic evaluation. I. Mechanics of tear transport. *Can J Ophthalmol*, **9**, 411.

Hill, J.C., Bethell, W. and Smirinaul, H.J. (1974b), Lacrimal drainage – a dynamic evaluation. II. Clinical aspects. *Can J Ophthalmol*, **9**, 417

Hines, M. (1931), *Am J Anat*, **47**, 1.

Hines, M. (1942), Recent contributions to localization of vision in the central nervous system. *Arch Ophthalmol*, **28**, 913.

Hirano, N. (1941), Nervöse Innervation des Corpus ciliare des Menschen. *A von Graefes Arch Ophthalmol*, **142**, 549.

Hirsch, M., Montcourrier, P., Pouliquen, Y. *et al.* (1982), Quick-freezing technique using a 'slamming' device for the study of corneal stromal morphology. *Exp Eye Res*, **34**, 841.

Hirsch, M., Renard, G., Faure, J.P. *et al.* (1977), Study of the ultrastructure of the rabbit corneal endothelium by the freeze-fracture technique: Apical and lateral junctions. *Exp Eye Res*, **25**, 277.

Hockman, C.C. (ed.) (1972), *Limbic System Mechanics and Autonomic Function*, Charles C. Thomas, Springfield, IL.

Hockwin, O., Poonawalla, N., Noll, E. *et al.* (1973), Durchlässigkeit der isolierten Rinderlinsenkapsel für Aminosäuren und wasserlösliche Eiweisse *Graefes. Arch Ophthalmol*, **188**, 175.

Hoddevik, G.H., Brodal, A., Kawamura, K. *et al.* (1977), The pontine projection to the cerebellar vermal visual area studied by means of the retrograde azonal transport of horseradish peroxidase. *Brain Res*, **123**, 209.

Hodson, S. and Mayes, K.R. (1979), Intercellular spaces in chemically fixed corneal endothelia are related to solute pump activity not to solvent coupling. *J Physiol (Lond)*, **294**, 627.

Hodson, S.A. and Miller, F. (1976), The bicarbonate ion pump in the endothelium which regulates the hydration of rabbit cornea. *J Physiol*, **263**, 563.

Hoffman, F. (1972), The surface of epithelial cells of the cornea under the scanning electron microscope. *Ophthal Res*, **3**, 207.

Hoffmann, K.P. and Distler, C. (1989), Quantitative analysis of visual receptive fields of neurons in nucleus of the optic tract and dorsal terminal nucleus of the accessory optic tract in macaque monkey. *J Neurophysiol*, **62**, 416.

Hoffmann, K.P., Distler, C., Erickson, R.G. *et al.* (1988), Physiological and anatomical identification of the nucleus of the optic tract and dorsal terminal nucleus of the accessory optic tract in monkeys. *Exp Brain Res*, **69**, 635.

Hofmann, H. and Lambeck, F. (1969), The response of neuromuscular blocking agents on extraocular muscle and intraocular pressure. *Proc R Soc Med*, **62**, 1217.

Hogan, M. and Feeney, L. (1963a), The ultrastructure of the retinal vessels. II. The small vessels. *J Ultrastruct Res*, **9**, 29.

Hogan, M.F. (1961), Ultrastructure of the choroid. Its role in the pathogenesis of chorioretinal diseases. *Trans Pacific Coast Oto-ophthalmol Soc*, **42**, 61.

Hogan, M.J. (1963), The vitreous, its structure and relation to the ciliary body and retina. *Invest Ophthalmol*, **2**, 418.

Hogan, M.J., Alvarado, J.A. and Weddell, J.E. (1971a), The cornea, in *Histology of the Human Eye*, WB Saunders, Philadelphia, p. 55.

Hogan, M.J., Alvarado, J.A. and Weddell, J.E. (1971b), *Histology of the Human Eye*, WB Saunders, Philadelphia.

Hogan, M.J. and Feeney, L. (1963b), Ultrastructure of the retinal blood vessels: I The large vessels. *J Ultrastruct Res*, **9**, 10.

Holland, M.G., Von Sallmann, L. and Collins, E.M. (1956), A study of the innervations of the chamber angle. *Am J Ophthalmol*, **42**, 148.

Holland, M.G., Von Sallman, L. and Collins, E.M. (1957), A study of the innervation of the chamber angle: II. The origin of trabecular axons revealed by degeneration experiments. *Am J Ophthalmol*, **44**, 206.

Hollander, H. and Martinex-Milan, L. (1975), Autoradiographic evidence for a topographically organized projection from the striate cortex to the lateral geniculate nucleus in the rhesus monkey (*Macacca mulatta*). *Brain Res*, **100**, 407.

Hollenberg, M. and Burt, W. (1969), The fine structure of Bruch's membrane in the human eye. *Can J Ophthalmol*, **4**, 296.

Hollenberg, M.J. and Spira, A.W. (1973), Human retinal development: ultrastructure of the outer retina. *Am J Anat*, **137**, 357.

Hollins, M. (1974), Does the central human retina stretch during accommodation? *Nature*, **251**, 729.

Holly, F.J. and Lemp, M.A. (1971), Wettability and wetting of corneal epithelium. *Exp Eye Res*, **11**, 239.

Holly, F.J. and Lemp, M.A. (1977), Tear physiology and dry eyes. *Surv Ophthalmol*, **22**, 69.

Holmberg, A. (1955), Studies of the ultrastructure of the non-pigmented epithelium in the ciliary body. *Acta Ophthalmol*, **33**, 377.

Holmberg, A. (1959a), Differences in the ultrastructure of normal human and rabbit ciliary epithelium. *Arch Ophthalmol*, **62**, 952.

Holmberg, A. (1959b), The fine structure of the inner wall of Schlemm's canal. *Arch Ophthalmol*, **62**, 956.

Holmberg, A. (1965), Schlemm's canal and the trabecular meshwork: an electron microscopic study of the normal structure in man and monkey (*Cerocipthecus ethiops*). *Doc Ophthalmol*, **19**, 339.

Holmes, G. and Lister, W.T. (1915), *Brain*, **39**, 34.

Hoogenraad, T.U., Jennekens, F.G.I. and Tan, K.E.W.P. (1979), Histochemical fibre types in human extraocular muscles, an investigation of inferior oblique muscle. *Acta Neuropathol*, **45**, 73.

Horton, J.C. (1984), Cytochrome oxidase patches: a new cytoarchitecture feature of monkey visual cortex. *Phil Trans R Soc Lond, Series B*, **304**, 199.

Horton, J.C., Greenwood, M.M. and Hubel, D.H. (1979), Non-retinotopic arrangement of fibres in the cat optic nerve. *Nature*, **282**, 720.

Horton, J.C. and Hubel, D.H. (1981), Regular patchy distribution of cytochrome oxidase staining in primary visual cortex of macaque monkey. *Nature*, **292**, 762.

Hovelacque, A. (1927), *L'anatomie des Nerfs Craniens et Rachidiens*, Paris.

Hovelacque, A. and Reinhold, P. (1917), *Rev Anthropol*, **27**, 277.

Howe, L. (1907), *The Muscles of the Eye*, New York.

Hoyt, W.F. (1969), Correlative functional anatomy of the optic chiasm. *Clin Neurosurg*, **17**, 189.

Hoyt, W.F. and Luis, O. (1963), The primate chiasm: details of visual fibre organization studied by silver impregnation techniques. *Arch Ophthalmol*, **70**, 69.

Hubel, D.H. and Livingstone, M.S. (1984), Anatomy and physiology of a colour system in the primate visual cortex. *J Neurosci*, **4**, 309.

Hubel, D.H. and Livingstone, M.S. (1990), Color and contrast sensitivity in the lateral geniculate body and primary visual cortex of the macaque monkey. *J Neurosci*, **10**, 2223.

Hubel, D.H. and Wiesel, T.N. (1961), Integrative action in the cat's lateral geniculate body. *J Physiol*, **155**, 385.

Hubel, D.H. and Wiesel, T.N. (1962), Receptive fields, binocular, interaction and functional architecture in the cat's visual cortex. *J Physiol*, **160**, 106.

Hubel, D.H. and Wiesel, T.N. (1965), Receptive fields and functional architecture in two non-striate visual areas of the cat. *J Neurophysiol*, **28**, 229.

Hubel, D.H. and Wiesel, T.N. (1968), Receptive fields and functional architecture of monkey striate cortex. *J Physiol*, **195**, 215.

Hubel, D.H. and Wiesel, T.N. (1969), Anatomical demonstration of columns in the monkey striate cortex. *Nature*, **221**, 747.

Hubel, D.H. and Wiesel, T.N. (1972), Laminar and columnar distribution of geniculo-cortical fibres in the macaque monkey. *J Comp Neurol*, **146**, 421.

Hubel, D.H. and Wiesel, T.N. (1977), Functional architecture of macaque monkey visual cortex. *Br Orth J*, **198**, 1.

Hubel, D.H. and Wiesel, T.N. (1978), Distribution of inputs from the two eyes in the striate cortex of the squirrel monkeys. *Soc Neurosci Abstr*, **4**, 632.

Huber, A. (1975), Angiography in diagnosis of orbital disease. *Mod Probl Ophthalmol*, **14**, 120.

Hudspeth A.J and Yee, A.G. (1973), The intercellular junctional complexes of retinal pigment epithelia. *Invest Ophthalmol*, **12**, 354.

Hughes, B. (1954), *The Visual Fields: A Study of the Applications of Quantitative Perimetry to the Anatomy and Pathology of the Visual Pathways*, Blackwell Scientific, Oxford, p. 67.

Huhtala, A., Tervo, T., Huikuri, K.T. *et al.* (1971), Effects of denervations on the acetylcholinesterase-containing and fluorescent nerves of the rat iris. *Acta Ophthalmol*, **54**, 85.

Hutchinson, A.K., Rodrigues, M.M. and Grossniklaus, H.E (1995), Iris, in *Biomedical Foundations of Ophthalmology*, (eds T.D. Duane and E.A. Jaeger), J.B. Lippincott Co., Philadelphia.

Huxley, H.E. (1971), The structural basis of muscle contraction. *Proc R Soc Lond*, **178**, 131.

Hykin, P.G. and Bron, A.J. (1992), Age-related morphological changes in lid margin and meibomian gland anatomy. *Cornea*, **11**, 334.

Hyrtl, J. (1875), *Lehrbuch der Anatomie des Menschen*, **13**, Auf Braumuller, Vienna, p. 972.

Igusa, Y., Sasaki, S. and Shimazu, H. (1980), Excitatory premotor burst neurons in the cat pontine reticular formation related to the quick phase of vestibular nystagmus. *Brain Res*, **182**, 451.

Ikui, H., Minatsu, T., Maeda, J. *et al.* (1960), Fine structure of the blood vessels of the iris; light and electron microscopic studies. *Kyushu J Med Sci*, **11**, 113.

Ikui, H., Tominaga, Y. and Mimura, K. (1964), The fine structure of the central retinal artery and vein in the optic nerve of the human eye and the pathological changes found occurring therein in hypertension and arteriosclerosis. *Acta Soc Ophthalmol Jpn*, **68**, 899.

Ingvar, S. (1923), On thalamic evolution. Preliminary note. *Acta Med Scand*, **59**, 696.

Innocenti, G.M. (1978), Postnatal development of interhemispheric connections of the cat visual cortex. *Arch Ital Biol*, **116**, 463.

Innocenti, G.M., Fiore, L. and Caminiti, R. (1977), Exuberant projection into the corpus callosum from the visual cortex of newborn cats. *Neurosciences*, **4**, 237.

Innocenti, G.M. and Frost, D.O. (1979), Effects of visual experience on the maturation of the efferent system to the corpus callosum. *Nature*, **280**, 231.

Inomata, H., Bill, A. and Smelser, G. (1972), Aqueous humor pathways and sites of outflow resistance through the trabecular meshwork and into Schlemm's canal of the cynomolgus monkey (*Macaca irus*). *Am J Ophthalmol*, **73**, 760.

Inoue, S., Leblond, C.P., Rico, P. *et al.* (1989), Association of fibronectin with the microfibrils of connective tissue. *Am J Anat*, **186**, 43.

Isaacson, R.L. (1974), *The Limbic System*, Plenum Press, New York.

Ishikawa, T. (1962), Fine structure of the human ciliary muscle. *Invest Ophthalmol*, **1**, 587.

Ishikawa, T. (1963), Fine structure of retinal vessels in man and macaque monkey. *Invest Ophthalmol*, **2**, 1.

Isomura, G. (1977), Nerve supply for anomalous ocular muscle in man. *Anat Anz*, **142**, 225.

Ito, T. and Shibasaki, S. (1964), Lichtmikroskopische untersuchungen uber die glandula lacrimalis des menschen. *Arch Histol Jap*, **25**, 117.

Iwamoto, T. (1961), Electron microscopic studies on the cells in the normal human iris stroma. *Acta Soc Ophthalmol Jpn*, **65**, 1296.

Iwamoto, T. (1964), Light and electron microscopy of the

presumed elastic components of the trabeculae and scleral spur of the human eye. *Invest Ophthalmol Vis Sci*, **3**, 144.

Iwamoto, T. and Smelser, G.K. (1965a) Electron microscope studies on the mast cells and blood and lymphatic capillaries of the human corneal limbus. *Invest Ophthalmol*, **4**, 815.

Iwamoto, T. and Smelser, G.K. (1965b) Electron microscopy of the human corneal endothelium with reference to transport mechanisms. *Invest Ophthalmol*, **4**, 270.

Iwanoff, A. and Arnold, J. (1874), Mikroscopische Anatomie des Uveal traktus und der Linse, in *Handbuch der gesamten Augenheilkunde* (eds A. Graefe and T. Saemisch), Wilhelm Engelmann, Leipzig, p. 265.

Iwasaki, M., Myers, K.M., Rayborn, M.E. *et al.* (1992), Interphotoreceptor matrix in the human retina: cone-like domains surround a small population of rod photoreceptors. *J Comp Neurol*, **319**, 277.

Jacobs, D.S. and Blakemore, C. (1988), Factors limiting the postnatal development of visual acuity in the monkey. *Vision Res*, **28**, 947.

Jakobiec, F.A. and Ozanics, V. (1982), General topographic anatomy of the eye. *Arch Ophthalmol*, **1**, 1.

Jakus, M.A. (1956), Studies on the cornea. II The fine structure of Descemet's membrane. *J Biophys Biochem*, **2**, 241.

Jakus, M.A. (1961), The fine structure of the human cornea, in *The Structure of the Eye* (ed. G.K. Smelser), Academic Press, London, p. 343.

Jakus, M.A. (1964), *Ocular Fine Structure*, Churchill Livingstone, Edinburgh, p. 1.

Jampel, R.S. (1959), Representation of the near-response on the cerebral cortex of the macaque. *Am J Ophthalmol*, **48**, 573.

Jampel, R.S. and Mindel, J. (1967), The nucleus for accommodation in the midbrain of the macaque. *Invest Ophthalmol*, **6**, 40.

Jänig, W. and Morrison, J.F.B. (1986), Functional properties of spinal visceral afferents supplying abdominal and pelvic organs, with special emphasis on visceral nociception, in *Progress in Brain Research* (eds F. Cervero and J.F.B. Morrison), Elsevier, Amsterdam, p. 87.

Jansco, G., Hokfelt, T., Lundberg, J.M. *et al.* (1981), Immunohistochemical studies on the effect of capsaicin on spinal and medullary peptide and monoamine neurons using antisera to substance P, gastin/CCK, somatostatin, VIP, enkephalin, neurotensin and 5-hydroxytryptamine. *J Neurocytol*, **10**, 963.

Jayaraman, A., Batton, R.R. and Carpenter, M.B. (1977), Nigrotectal projection in the monkey: an autoradiographic study. *Brain Res*, **135**, 147.

Jennekens, F.G.I., Tan, K.E.W.P. and Hoogenraad, T.U. (1976), Enzyme-histochemistry of normal external ocular muscles. *Ophthalmologica*, **173**, 326.

Jester, J., Rodrigues, M.M. and Sun, T.-T. (1984), Change in epithelial keratin expression during healing of rabbit corneal wounds. *Invest Ophthalmol Vis Sci*, **26**, 828.

Jo, A. and Trauzettel, H. (1974), Topographische Beziehungen der vehen in des Orbita. *Verh Anat Ges*, **68**, 539.

Johnson, S.B., Coakes, R.L. and Brubaker, R.F. (1978), A simple photogrammatic method of measuring anterior chamber volume. *Am J Ophthalmol*, **85**, 469.

Johnson, S.B., Passmore, J.A. and Brubaker, R.F. (1977), The fluorescein distribution volume of the anterior chamber. *Invest Ophthalmol*, **16**, 633.

Johnston, J.A. and Parkinson, D. (1974), Intracranial sympathetic pathways associated with the sixth cranial nerve. *J Neurosurg*, **39**, 236.

Johnston, J.B. (1909), The morphology of the forebrain vesicle in vertebrates. *J Comp Neurol*, **19**, 593.

Johnston, M.C., Noden, D.M., Hazelton, R.D. *et al.* (1979), Origins of ocular and periocular tissues. *Exp Eye Res*, **29**, 27.

Johnstone, M.A. and Grant, W.M. (1973), Pressure-dependent changes in structures of the aqueous outflow system of human and monkey eyes. *Am J Ophthalmol*, **75**, 365.

Johnstone, M.C., Bhakdinaronk, A. and Reid, Y.C. (1973), In *Fourth Symposium on Oral Sensation and Perception Development in the Fetus and Infant* (ed. J.F. Bosma), WHO, Geneva, p. 37.

Jokl, A. (1927), *Vergleichende Untersuchungen Uber Den Bau Und Die Entwicklung Des Glaskorpers Und Seiner Inhaltsgebilde Bei Wirbeltieren Und Beim Menschen*, Almquist und Wiksells, Uppsala-Stockholm.

Jonas, J.B. and Fernández, M.C. (1994), Shape of the neuroretinal rim and position of the central retinal vessels in glaucoma. *Br J Ophthalmol*, **78**, 99.

Jonas, J.B., Fernández, M.C. and Naumann, G.O.H. (1991), Correlation of the optic disc size to glaucoma susceptibility. *Ophthalmology*, **98**, 675.

Jonas, J.B., Fernández, M.C. and Naumann, G.O.H. (1992b), Glaucomatous parapapillary atrophy. Occurrence and correlations. *Arch Ophthalmol*, **110**, 214.

Jonas J.B., Gusek, G.C., Guggenmoos-Hölzmann, I. *et al.* (1987), Optic nerve head drusen associated with abnormally small optic discs. *Int Ophthalmol*, **11**, 79.

Jonas, J.B., Gusek, G.C. and Naumann, G.O.H. (1988), Optic disc, cup and neuroretinal rim size, configuration and correlations in normal eyes. *Invest Ophthalmol Vis Sci*, **29**, 1151.

Jonas, J.B. and Naumann, G.O.H. (1991), The anatomical structure of the normal and glaucomatous optic nerve, in *Glaucoma Update IV* (ed. G.K. Krieglstein), Springer-Verlag, Berlin–Heidelberg–New York, p. 66.

Jonas, J.B. and Schiro D. (1993), Normal retinal nerve fiber layer visibility correlated to rim width and vessel caliber. *A von Graefes Arch Klin Exp Ophthalmol*, **231**, 207.

Jonas, J.B., Schmidt, A.M., Müller-Bergh, J.A., Schlötzer-Schrehardt, U.M. and Naumann, G.O.H. (1992a), Human optic nerve fiber count and optic disc size. *Invest Ophthalmol Vis Sci*, **33**, 2012.

Jones, E.G. (1985), *The Thalamus, Lateral Geniculate Nucleus*, Plenum Press, New York, p. 453.

Jones, E.G. and Powell, T.P.S. (1969), Connexions of the somatic sensory cortex of the rhesus monkey. I. Ipsilateral cortical connexions. *Brain*, **92**, 477.

Jones, E.G. and Powell, T.P.S. (1970), An anatomical study of converging sensory pathways within the cerebral cortex of the monkey. *Brain*, **93**, 793.

Jones, L.T. (1961), An anatomical approach to problems of the eyelids and lacrimal apparatus. *Arch Ophthalmol*, **66**, 111.

Jones, R. (1971), The effect of pH on AB staining of sialomucin and sulphomucin at selected epithelial tissue sites. *PhD Thesis*, Institute of Medical Laboratory Technology, University of London.

Jones, R.F. and Maurice, D.M. (1966), New methods of measuring the rate of aqueous flow in man with fluorescein. *Exp Eye Res*, **5**, 208.

Judge, S.J. and Miles, F.A. (1981), Gain changes in accommodative vergence induced by alteration of the effective interocular separation, in *Progress in Oculomotor Research* (eds A.F. Fuchs and W. Becker), Elsevier, Amsterdam, p. 587.

Jumblatt, M.M. and Neufeld, A.H. (1981), Characterisation of cyclic AMP-mediated wound closure of the rabbit corneal epithelium. *Curr Eye Res*, **1**, 189.

Jurand, A. and Yamada, T. (1967), Elimination of mitochondria during Wolffian lens degeneration. *Exp Cell Res*, **46**, 636.

Kaada, B.R. (1951), Somato-motor, autonomic and electrocorticographic responses to electrical stimulation of 'rhinencephalic' and other structures in primates, cat and dog: Study of responses from limbic, subcallosal, orbito-insular, piriform and temporal cortex, hippocampus-fornix and amygdala. *Acta Physiol Scand*, **24** (Suppl. 83), 1.

Kaas, J.H., Huerta, M.F., Weber, J.T. *et al.* (1978), Patterns of retinal terminations and laminar organization of the lateral geniculate nucleus of primates. *J Comp Neurol*, **182**, 517.

Kaczurowski, M.I. (1964), I. Zonular fibers of the human eye. *Am J Ophthalmol*, **58**, 1030.

Kaczurowski, M.I. (1967), II. The surface of the vitreous. *Am J Ophthalmol*, **63**, 419.

Kahn, N.M. (1969), Blood supply of the midbrain. PhD thesis, London University.

Kalyanaraman, S. (1975), Some observations during stimulation of the human hypothalamus. *Confin Neurol*, **37**, 189.

Kanai, A. and Kaufman, H.E. (1973), Aging changes of collagen fibres. *Ann Ophthalmol*, **5**, 285.

Kanaseki, T. and Sprague, J.M. (1974), Anatomical organization of pretectal nuclei and tectal laminae in the cat. *J Comp Neurol*, **158**, 319.

Kapalanga, J. and Blecher, S.R. (1991), Histological studies on eyelid opening in normal male mice and hemizygotes for the mutant gene Tabby (Ta) with and without epidermal growth factor treatment. *Exp Eye Res*, **52**, 155.

Kaplan, E. and Shapley, R.M. (1982), X and Y cells in the lateral geniculate nucleus of macaque monkeys. *J Physiol*, **330**, 125.

Kapoor, R. , Bornstein, P. and Sage, E. H. (1986), Type VIII collagen from bovine Descemet's membrane: structural characterization of a triple-helical domain. *Biochemistry*, **25**(13), 3930.

Karasaki, S. (1964), An electron microscopic study of wolffian lens regeneration in the adult newt. *J Ultrastruct Res*, **11**, 246.

Karplus, J.P. and Kreidl, A. (1909), Gehirn und sympathicus: I. Mitteilung zwischenhirnbasis und halssympathicus. *Arch Anat Physiol*, **129**, 138.

Karplus, J.P. and Kreidl, A. (1913), *Pflugers Arch*, **145**, 115.

Kase, M., Miller, D.C. and Noda, H. (1980), Discharges of Purkinje cells and mossy fibers in the cerebellar vermis of the monkey during saccadic eye movements and fixation. *J Physiol*, **300**, 539.

Kato, T. (1938), Uber histologische untersuchungen der augenmuskeln von menschen und saugetieren. *Okajimas Folia Anat Jpn*, **16**, 131.

Kaufman, H.E., Capella, J.A. and Robbins, J.E. (1966), The human corneal endothelium. *Am J Ophthalmol*, **61**, 835.

Kawamura, K.A., Brodal, A. and Hoddevik, G. (1974), The projection of the superior colliculus onto the reticular formation of the brainstem. An experimental anatomical study in the cat. *Exp Brain Res*, **19**, 1.

Kaye, G.I. and Pappas, G.D. (1962), Studies on the cornea I. The fine structure of the rabbit cornea and the uptake and transport of colloidal particles by the cornea *in vivo*. *J cell Biol*, **12**, 457.

Kaye, G.I., Pappas, G.D. and Donn, A. (1961), An electron microscope study of the rabbit corneal endothelium in relation to its uptake and transport of colloidal particles. *Anat Rec*, **139**, 244.

Kayes, J. (1967), Pore structure of the inner wall of Schlemm's canal. *Invest Ophthalmol*, **6**, 381.

Kayes, J. (1975), Pressure gradient changes in the trabecular meshwork of monkeys. *Am J Ophthalmol*, **79**, 549.

Kayes, J. and Holmberg, A. (1960), The fine structure of Bowman's layer and the basement membrane of the corneal epithelium. *Am J Ophthalmol*, **50**, 1013.

KazSoong, H. and Fairley, J.A. (1985), Actin in human corneal epithelium. *Arch Ophthalmol*, **103**, 565.

Keene, D.R., Maddox, B.K., Kuo, H.J. *et al.* (1991), Extraction of extendable beaded structures and their identification as fibrillin-containing extracellular matrix microfibrils. *J Histochem Cytochem*, **39**, 441.

Kefalides, N.A. (1978), *Biology and Chemistry of Basement Membranes*, Academic Press, New York, p. 215.

Keller, E.L. (1974), Participation of medial pontine reticular formation in eye movement generation in monkey. *J Neurophysiol*, **37**, 316.

Keller, E.L. (1977), Control of saccadic eye movements by midline brain stem neurons. *Dev Neurosci*, **1**, 327.

Keller, E.L. (1982), Neuronal discharge in the vermis of the cerebellum and its relation to saccadic eye movement generation, in *Functional Basis of Ocular Motility Disorders* (eds G. Lennerstrand, D.S. Zee and E.L. Keller), Pergamon Press, Oxford.

Keller, E.L. and Crandall, W.F. (1981a), Neural activity in the nucleus reticularis tegmenti pontis in the monkey related to eye movements and visual stimulation. *Ann NY Acad Sci*, **374**, 249.

Keller, E.L. and Crandall, W.F. (1981b) Optokinetic and vestibular responses in medial pontine nucleus neurons in alert monkey. *Soc Neurosci Abstr*, **7**, 623.

Keller, E.L. and Crandall, W.F. (1983), Neuronal responses to optokinetic stimuli in pontine nuclei of behaving monkey. *J Neurophysiol*, **49**, 169.

Kenyon, K.R. (1969), The synthesis of basement membrane by the corneal epithelium in bulbous keratopathy. *Invest Ophthalmol*, **8**, 156.

Kerr, F.W. (1968), The pupil-functional anatomy and clinical correlation. *Neuro-ophthalmol*, **4**, 49.

Kerr, F.W. and Alexander, S. (1964), Descending autonomic pathways in the spinal cord. *Arch Neurol*, **10**, 249.

Kerr, F.W. and Brown, J.E. (1964), Pupillomotor pathways in the spinal cord. *Arch Neurol*, **10**, 262.

Kerr, F.W. and Hollowell, O.W. (1964), Location of pupillomotor and accommodation fibres in the oculomotor nerve; experimental studies on paralytic mydriasis. *J Neurol Neurosurg Psych*, **27**, 473.

Kerr, F.W. and Lysak, W.R. (1964), Somatotopic organisation of trigeminal–ganglion neurones. *Arch Neurol*, **11**, 593.

Kerr, F.W.L. (1975), The ventral spinothalamic tract and other descending systems of the ventral funiculus of the spinal cord. *J Comp Neurol*, **159**, 335.

Kessing, S.V. (1966), Investigations of the conjunctival mucin. Quantitative studies of the goblet cells of conjunctiva. *Acta Ophthalmol*, **44**, 439.

Kessing, S.V. (1968), Mucous gland system of the conjunctiva. A quantitative normal anatomical study. *Acta Ophthalmol Suppl*, **95**, 1.

Kessler, J.A., Bell, W.O. and Black, I.B. (1983), Interactions between the sympathetic and sensory innervation of the iris. *J Neurosci*, **3**, 1301.

Kestenbaum, A. (1963), *Applied Anatomy of the Eye*, Grune & Stratton, New York.

Khodadhoust, A.A., Silverstein, A.M., Kenyon, K.R. *et al.* (1968), Adhesions of regenerating corneal epthelium. The role of basement membrane. *Am J Ophthalmol*, **65**, 339.

Kier, E.L. (1966), Embryology of the normal optic canal and its anomalies. *Invest Radiol*, **1**, 346.

King, W.M. and Fuchs, A.F. (1977), Neuronal activity in the mesencephalon related to vertical eye movements. *Dev Neurosci*, **1**, 319.

King, W.M., Lisberger, S.G. and Fuchs, A.F. (1976), Response of fibers in medial longitudinal fasciculus (MLF) of alert monkeys during horizontal and vertical conjugate eye movements evoked by vestibular or visual stimuli. *J Neurophysiol*, **39**, 1135.

Kinoshita, J.H., Kern, H.L. and Merola, L.O. (1961), Factors affecting the action transport of calf lens. *Biochim Biophys Acta*, **47**, 458.

Kinsey, V.E. and Reddy, D.V.N. (1965), Studies on the crystalline lens. XI. The relative role of the epithelium and capsule in transport. *Invest Ophthalmol*, **4**, 104.

Kistler, J. and Bullivant, S. (1980), Lens gap junctions and orthogonal arrays are unrelated. *FEBS Lett*, **111**, 73.

Kistler, J. and Bullivant, S. (1987), Protein processing in lens intercellular junctions: Cleavage of MP70 to MP38. *Invest Ophthalmol Vis Sci*, **28**, 1687.

Kjallman, L. and Frisen, L. (1986), The cerebral ocular pursuit pathways. A clinicoradiological study of small-field optokinetic nystagmus. *J Clin Neur Ophthalmol*, **6**, 209.

Klein, B. (1966), Regional and aging characteristics of the normal choriocapillaris in flat preparations. *Am J Ophthalmol*, **61**, 1191.

Klyce, S.D., Neufeld, A.H. and Zadunaisky, J.A. (1973), The activation of chloride transport by epinephrine and Db cyclic-AMP in the cornea of the rabbit. *Invest Ophthalmol*, **12**, 127.

Klyce, S.D., Palkama, A., Harkonen, M. *et al.* (1981), Neuronal serotonin stimulates chloride transport in the rabbit corneal epithelium. *Invest Ophthalmol Vis Sci*, **20**, 194.

Klyce, S.D., Palkama, K.A., Harkonen, M. *et al.* (1982), Serotonin stimulates chloride transport in the rabbit corneal epithelium. *Invest Ophthalmol Vis Sci*, **23**, 181.

Knepper, P.A., Hvizd, M.G., Goossens, W. *et al.* (1989), GAG profile of human TM in primary open-angle glaucoma. *ARVO abstract, Invest Ophthalmol Vis Sci*, **30(suppl.)**, 224.

Knoche, H. and Addicks, K. (1976), Electron microscopic studies of the pressoreceptor fields of the carotid sinus of the dog. *Cell Tissue Res*, **173**, 77.

Knoche, H., Walther-Wenke, G. and Addicks, K. (1977), Die Feinstruktur der barorezeptorischen Nervenendigungen in der Wand des Sinus caroticus der Katze. *Acta Anat*, **97**, 403.

Knoche, H., Wiesner-Menzel, L. and Addicks, K. (1980), Ultrastructure of baroreceptors in the carotid sinus of the rabbit. *Acta Anat*, **106**, 63.

Ko, M.-K., Chi, J.G. and Chang, B.-L. (1985), Hyaloid vascular pattern in the human fetus. *J Pediatr Ophthalmol Strabismus*, **22**, 188.

Kobayashi, M. (1958), Electron microscopic studies on the lacrimal gland. Report 2. The lacrimal gland of the human eye. *Acta Soc Ophthalmol Jpn*, **62**, 2208.

Koeppe, L. (1918), Clinical observations with the slit-lamp and corneal microscope. *Arch Ophth*, **96**, 242.

Kohler, A. and Tobgy, A.F. (1929), Mikroskopische Untersuchungen einiger Augenmedien mit ultra-violettem und mit polarisertem Licht. *A von Graefes Arch Klin Exp Ophthalmol*, **99**, 263.

Kokott, W. (1934), Das Spaltlinienbild der Sklera, *Klin Monatsbl Augenheilk*, **92**, 117.

Kokott, W. (1938), Uber mechanisch-funktionelle Strukturen des Auges. *A von Graefes Arch Ophthalmol*, **138**, 424.

Kolb, H. (1991), Anatomical pathways for color vision in the human retina. *Vis Neurosci*, **7**, 61.

Kolb, H. and DeKorver, L. (1991), Midget ganglion cells of the parafovea of the human retina: a study by electron microscopy and serial section reconstructions. *J Comp Neurol*, **303**, 617.

Kolb, H., Fernandez, E., Schouten, J. *et al.* (1994), Are there three types of horizontal cell in the human retina? *J Comp Neurol*, **343**, 370.

Kolb, H., Linberg, K.A. and Fisher, S.K. (1992), Neurons of the human retina: a Golgi study. *J Comp Neurol*, **318**, 147.

Kolega, J., Manabe, M. and Sun, T.T. (1989), Basement membrane heterogeneity and variation in corneal epithelial differentiation. *Differentiation*, **42**, 54.

Kondo, H. and Fujiwara, S. (1979), Granule-containing cells in the human superior cervical ganglion. *Acta Anat*, **103**, 192.

Konigsmark, B.W., Kalyanaraman, U.P., Cory, P. *et al.* (1969), An evaluation of techniques in neuronal population estimates: the sixth nerve nucleus. *Johns Hopkins Hosp Bull*, **125**, 146.

Koontz, M.A. and Hendrickson, A. (1987), Stratified distribution of synapses in the inner plexiform layers of primate retina. *J Comp Neurol*, **263**, 581.

Koornneef, L. (1974), The first results of a new anatomical method of approach of the human orbit following a clinical enquiry. *Acta Morphol Neurol Scand*, **12**, 259.

Koornneef, L. (1976), Spatial aspects of orbital musculofibrous tissue in man. *PhD Thesis*, Amsterdam.

Koornneef, L. (1977), *Spatial Aspects of Orbital Musculofibrous Tissue in Man*, Swets & Zeitlinger, Amsterdam.

Koornneef, L. (1987), Orbital connective tissue. In *Biomedi-*

cal Foundations of Ophthalmology (eds T.D. Duane and E.A. Jaeger), Harper & Row, New York, p. 1.

Koretz, J.F. (1994), Accommodation and presbyopia, in *Principles and Practice of Ophthalmology. Basic Sciences* (eds D.M. Albert and F.A. Jakobiec), W.B. Saunders Co., Philadelphia, p. 270.

Koretz, J.F., Bertasso, A.M., Neider, M.W. *et al.* (1988), Preliminary characterization of human crystalline lens geometry as a function of accommodation and age. Non-invasive assessment of the visual system. *OSA Technical Digest Series*, **3**, 130.

Koretz, J.F. and Handelman, G.H. (1982), Model of the accommodative mechanism in the human eye. *Vision Res*, **22** 917.

Koretz, J.F. and Handelman, G.H. (1983), A model for accommodation in the young human eye. The effects of elastic anisotropy on the mechanism. *Vision Res*, **23**, 1679.

Koretz, J.F. and Handelman, G.H. (1986), Modeling age-related accommodative loss in the human eye. *Int J Math Modeling*, **7**, 1003.

Koretz, J.F. and Handelman, G.H. (1988), How the human eye focuses. *Sci Am*, **259**, 92.

Koretz, J.F., Handelman, G.H. and Brown, N.A.P. (1984), Analysis of human crystalline lens curvature as a function of accommodative state and age. *Vision Res*, **24**, 1141.

Koretz, J.F., Kaufman, P.L., Neider, M.W. *et al.* (1989), Accommodation and presbyopia in the human eye – aging of the anterior segment. *Vision Res*, **29**, 1685.

Koshland, M.E. (1975), Structure and function of the J chain. *Adv Immunol*, **20**, 41.

Krauhs, J.M. (1979), Structure of rat aortic baroreceptors and their relationship to connective tissue. *J Neurocytol*, **8**, 401.

Krause, W. (1861), Ganglienzellen im Orbiculus ciliaris in *Anatomische Untersuchungen* (ed W. Krause), Hannover, p. 1.

Krause, W. (1867), Termination of the nerves in the conjunctiva. *J Anat Physiol Lond*, **1**, 346.

Krekeler, F. (1923), Die Struktur der Sklera in den verschiedenen Lebensaltern. *WHO*, **93**, 144.

Kreutziger, G.O. (1968), Freeze etching of intercellular junctions of mouse liver, in *Proceedings of the 26th Annual Meeting of the Electron Microscopy Society of America* (ed C.J. Arcenaux), Clator's Publishing Division, Baton Rouge, New Orleans, p. 234.

Kreutziger, G.O. (1976), Lateral membrane morphology and gap junction structure in rabbit corneal endothelium. *Exp Eye Res*, **23**, 285.

Krey, H.F. (1975), Segmental vascular patterns of the choriocapillaris. *Am J Ophthalmol*, **80**, 198.

Krstic, R. and Postic, G. (1978), Ultrastructure of specific endothelial organelles (SEO) of the iris capillaries in glaucoma simplex. *Microvasc Res*, **5**, 141.

Krümmel, H. (1938), Die Nerven des menschlichen Ziliarkörpers. *A von Graefes Arch Ophthalmol*, **138**, 845.

Kuffler, S.W. and Gerard, R.W. (1974), The small-nerve motor system to skeletal muscle. *J Neurophysiol*, **10**, 383.

Kuhn, R.A. (1961), *Am J Roentgenol*, **86**, 1040.

Kuhnel, W. (1968a), Comparative histological, histochemical and electron-microscopical investigations on lacrimal glands. VI. Human lacrimal gland. *Z Zellforsch Mikrosk Anat*, **89**, 550.

Kuhnel, W. (1968b), Comparative histological, histochemical and electron-microscopic studies on the lacrimal glands. II. Goat. *Z Zellforsch Mikrosk Anat*, **86**, 430.

Kuhnel, W. (1968c), Comparative histological histochemical and electron-microscopical investigations of the lacrimal glands. V. Cattle. *Z Zellforsch Mikrosk Anat*, **87**, 504.

Kuhnel, W. (1968d), Comparative histological, histochemical, and electron-microscopical investigations of the lacrimal glands. IV. Dog. *Z Zellforsch Mikrosk Anat*, **88**, 23.

Kuhnel, W. (1968e), Comparative histological, histochemical and electron-microscopical investigations of the lacrimal glands. III. Sheep. *Z Zellforsch Mikrosk Anat*, **87**, 31.

Kuhnt, H. (1879), Zur Kenntniss des Sehnerven und der Netzhaut. *A von Graefes Arch Ophthalmol*, **25**, 179.

Kuhnt, H. (1890), *Jena Z Med Naturn*, **24**, 177.

Kummer, W., Fischer, A., Mundel, P. *et al.* (1992), Nitric-oxide synthase in VIP-containing vasodilator nerve fibers in the guinea pig. *Neuroreport*, **3**, 653.

Kuntz, A. (1953), *The Autonomic Nervous System*, 4th edition, Baillière, Tindall & Cox, London.

Kuntz, A. and Richins, C.A. (1946), Reflex pupillodilator mechanisms: an experimental analysis. *J Neurophysiol*, **9**, 1.

Kunzle, H. and Akert, K. (1977), Efferent connections of cortical area 8 (frontal eye field) in *Macaca fascicularis*. A reinvestigation using the autoradiographic technique. *J Comp Neurol*, **173**, 147.

Kupfer, C. (1960), Motor innervation of extraocular muscle. *J Physiol*, **153**, 522.

Kupfer, C. (1962a), The projection of the macula in the lateral geniculate nucleus of man. *Am J Ophthalmol*, **54**, 597.

Kupfer, C. (1962b), Relationship of ciliary body meridional muscle and corneoscleral trabecular meshwork. *Arch Ophthalmol*, **68**, 818.

Kupfer, C., Chumbley, L. and De Downer, J.C. (1967), Quantitative histology of optic nerve, optic tract and lateral geniculate nucleus of man. *J Anat*, **101**, 393.

Kupfer, C. and Ross, K. (1971), The development of the outflow facility in the human eye. *Invest Ophthalmol*, **10**, 513.

Kuru, Y. (1967), Meningeal branches of the ophthalmic artery. *Acta Radiol*, **6**, 241.

Kurus, E. (1955), Über ein Ganglienzellsystem der menschlichen Aderhaut. *Klin Monatsbl Augenheilk*, **127**, 198.

Kurus, E. (1958), Versuch einer morphologischen analyse der function und dysfunction der intraocularen druck-regulierung. *Klin Monatsbl Augenheilk*, **132**, 201.

Kuszak, J.R. (1995), The development of lens sutures, in *Progress in Retinal and Eye Research* (eds N.N. Osborne and G.J. Chader), Elsevier Science Ltd/Pergamon Press, Oxford, p. 567.

Kuszak, J.R., Bertram, B.A., Mascai, M.S. *et al.* (1984), Sutures of the crystalline lens: A review. *Scanning Electron Microsc*, **III**, 1369.

Kuszak, J.R., Bertram, B.A. and Rae, J.L. (1986), The ordered structure of the crystalline lens, in *Cell and Developmental Biology of the Eye. Development of Order in the Visual System* (eds S.R. Hilfer and J.B. Sheffield), Springer-Verlag, New York, p. 35.

Kuszak, J.R., Brown, H.G. and Deutsch, T.A. (1993b),

Anatomy of aged and cataractous crystalline lenses, in *Principles and Practice of Ophthalmology*, (eds D.A. Albert and F.A. Jacobiec), W.B. Saunders Co., Philadelphia, p. 564.

Kuszak, J.R., Deutsch, T.A. and Brown, H.G. (1993), Anatomy of aged and senile cataractous lenses, in *Principles and Practice of Ophthalmology*, 1st ed. (eds F.A. Jakobiec and D. Albert), W.B. Saunders, Philadelphia p.564.

Kuszak, J.R., Ennesser, C.A., Bertram, B.A. *et al.* (1989), The contribution of cell-to-cell fusion to the ordered structure of the crystalline lens. *Lens Eye Toxic Res*, **6**, 639.

Kuszak, J.R., Khan, A.R. and Cenedella, R.J. (1988), An ultrastructural analysis of plasma membrane in the U18666A cataract. *Invest Ophthalmol Vis Sci*, **29**, 261.

Kuszak, J.R., Maisel, H. and Harding, C.V. (1978), Gap junctions of chick lens fibre cells. *Exp Eye Res*, **27**, 495.

Kuszak, J.R., Mascai, M.S., Bloom, K.J. *et al.* (1985), Cell-to-cell fusion of lens fibre cells *in situ*: correlative light, scanning electron microscopic and freeze-fracture studies. *J Ultrastruct Res*, **93**, 144.

Kuszak, J.R., Novak, L.A. and Brown, H.G. (1995), An ultrastructural analysis of the epithelial-fiber interface (EFI) in primate lenses. *Exp Eye Res*, **61**, 579.

Kuszak, J.R., Peterson, K.L. and Brown, H.G. (1996), Electron microscopic observations of the crystalline lens. *Microsc Res Tech*, **33**, 441.

Kuszak, J.R., Peterson, K.L., Sivak, J.G. *et al.* (1994), The interrelationship of lens anatomy and optical quality. II. Primate lenses. *Exp Eye Res*, **59**, 521.

Kuszak, J.R. and Rae, J.L. (1982), Scanning electron microscopy of the frog lens. *Exp Eye Res*, **35**, 449.

Kuszak, J.R., Sivak, J.G. and Weerheim, J.A. (1991a), Lens optical quality is a direct function of lens sutural architecture. *Invest Ophthalmol Vis Sci*, **32**(7), 2119. [published erratum appears in *Invest Ophthalmol. Vis Sci* (1992), **33**, 2076.

Kuwabara, T. (1968), Microtubules in the lens. *Arch Ophthalmol*, **79**, 189.

Kuwabara, T. (1975), The maturation of the lens cell: a morphologic study. *Exp Eye Res*, **20**, 427.

Kuwabara, T. (1978), Current concepts in anatomy and histology of the cornea. *Contact Lens Intraoc Lens Med J*, **4**, 101.

Kuwabara, T. and Cogan, D. (1963), Retinal vascular patterns. VI. Mural cells of the retinal capillaries. *Arch Ophthalmol*, **69**, 492.

Kuwabara, T. and Cogan, D.G. (1960), Studies of retinal vascular patterns. I. Normal architecture. *Arch Ophthalmol*, **64**, 904.

Kuwabara, T. and Imaizumi, M. (1974), Denucleation process of the lens. *Invest Ophthalmol Vis Sci*, **13**, 973.

Kuwabara, T., Perkins, D.G. and Cogan, D.G. (1976), Sliding of the epithelium in experimental wounds. *WHO*, **15**, 4.

Kuypers, H.G.J.M. and Lawrence, D.G. (1967), Cortical projections to the red nucleus and the brain stem in the rhesus monkey. *Brain Res*, **4**, 151.

Kuypers, H.G.J.M., Szwarcbart, M.K., Mishkin, M. *et al.* (1965), Occipito-temporal corticocortical connections in the rhesus monkey. *Exp Neurol*, **11**, 245.

Kuzetsova, L.V. (1963), *Trudy Sestaj Naunnej Konterencii po Vozrastroj Morfologu Fysiologu i Biochimu*, Moskva.

Lai, Y.L. (1967), The biopsy of human iris. *Folia Ophthalmol Jpn*, **18**, 1060.

Laing, R.A., Neubauer, L., Oak, S.S. *et al.* (1984), Evidence for mitosis in the adult corneal endothelium. *Ophthalmology*, **91**, 1129.

Laing, R.A., Sandstrom, M.M., Berrospi, A.R. *et al.* (1976), Changes in the corneal endothelium as a function of age. *Exp Eye Res*, **22**, 587.

Lamers, W.P.M.A. (1962), *De Innervatie Van Het Trabeculum Corneosclerale*, Nijmegen, Centrale Drukkerij.

Land, E.H. (1974), The retinex theory of colour vision. *Proc R Inst Gt Brit*, **47**, 23.

Land, E.H. (1977), *Sci Am*, **237**, 108.

Landis, D.M. and Reese, T.S. (1974), Arrays of particles in freeze-fractured astrocytic membranes. *J Cell Biol*, **60**, 316.

Landon, D.N. (1981) In *Skeletal Muscle Pathology* (eds F.L. Mastaglia and J. Walton), Churchill Livingstone, Edinburgh.

Langham, M.E. and Palewicz, K. (1977), The pupillary, the intra-ocular pressure and the unsomotor responses to noradrenaline in rabbits. *J Physiol*, **267**, 339.

Langham, M.E. and Taylor, I.S. (1956), Factors affecting the hydration of the cornea in the excised eye and the living animal. *Br J Ophthalmol*, **40**, 321.

Lasjaunias, P., Brismar, J., Morret, J. *et al.* (1978), Recurrent cavernous branches of the ophthalmic artery. *Acta Radiol Suppl*, **19**, 553.

Laties, A.M. (1967), Central retinal artery innervation. Absence of adrenergic innervation to the intraocular branches. *Arch Ophthalmol*, **77**, 405.

Laties, A.M. (1974), Ocular melanin and adrenergic innervation of the eye. *Appl Ergonomics*, **72**, 560.

Laties, A.M. and Jacobowitz, D. (1966), *Anat Rec*, **156**, 383.

Latkovic, S. and Nilsson, S.G. (1979), The ultrastructure of the normal conjunctival epithelium of the guinea pig. II. The superficial layer of the perilimbal zone. *Acta Ophthalmol*, **57**, 123.

Lauber, H. (1908), Beitrage Entwicklungsgeschichte und anatomie der iris. *A von Graefes Arch Ophthalmol*, **63**, 1.

Lauber, H. (1936a), Die Aderhaut (Choroidea), in *Handbuch der Mikroskopischen Anatomie*, (ed. W. von Möllendorf), Springer, Berlin, p. 91.

Lauber, H. (1936b), Der Strahlenkörper (*Corpus ciliare*). D. Die Nerven des Strahlenkörpers, in *Handbuch der mikroskopischen Anatomie* (ed. W. von Möllendorf), Springer, Berlin, p. 134.

Laule, A., Cable, M.K., Hoffman, C.E. *et al.* (1978), Endothelial cell population changes of human cornea during life. *Arch Ophthalmol*, **96**, 2031.

Lauweryns, B., van den Oord, J.J., De Vos, R. *et al.* (1993a), A new epithelial cell type in the human cornea. *Invest Ophthalmol Vis Sci*, **34**, 1983.

Lauweryns, B., van den Oord, J.J. and Missotten, L. (1993b), The transitional zone between limbus and peripheral cornea. An immunohistochemical study. *Invest Ophthalmol Vis Sci*, **34**, 1991.

Lauweryns, B., van den Oord, J.J., Volpes, R. *et al.* (1991), Distribution of very late activation integrins in the human cornea. *Invest Ophthalmol Vis Sci*, **32**, 2079.

Lazorthes, G. (1978), Vascularisation et Circulation Cerebrales, *Maroc-Med.* **1**, 11.

Lazorthes, G., Pouches, J., Bastides, G. *et al.* (1958), *Rev Neurol (Paris)*, **99**, 617.

Le Double, F. (1897), *Traites des Varietes du Systeme Musculaire de l'Homme*, Paris.

Le Gros Clark, W.E. (1926), The mammalian oculomotor nucleus. *J Anat*, **60**, 426.

Le Gros Clark, W.E. (1932), The structure and connections of the thalamus. *Brain*, **55**, 406.

Le Gros Clark, W.E. and Penman, G.G. (1934), The projections of the retina in the lateral geniculate body. *Proc R Soc Lond*, **114**, 291.

Le Vay, S., Wiesel, T.N. and Hubel, D.H. (1980), The development of ocular dominance columns in normal and visually deprived monkeys. *J Comp Neurol*, **191**, 1.

Leber, T. (1865), Untersuchungen uber den Verlauf und Zusammenhang der Gefasse im Menschlichen Auge. *A von Graefes Arch Ophthalmol*, **11**, 1.

Leber, T. (1872), *Graefe-Saemisch Handbuch Gesamten Augenheilk*, **18**, 25.

Leber, T. (1903), Der Abfluss der Augenflussigkeit. *A von Graefes Arch Klin Exp Ophthalmol*, **2**, 271.

Lee, B., Godfrey, M., Vitale, E. *et al.* (1991), Linkage of Marfan syndrome and a phenotypically related disorder to two different fibrillin genes. *Nature*, **52**, 330.

Lee, J.P. and Olver, J.M. (1990), Anterior segment ischaemia, *Eye*, **4**, 1.

Lee, R.E. and Davison, P.F. (1981), Collagen composition in ocular tissues of the rabbit. *Exp Eye Res*, **32**, 737.

Lee, W.R. and Grierson, I. (1982), In *The Pathology of Ocular Disease*, Marcel Dekker, New York, p. 525.

Lee, W.R., Murray, S.B., Williamson, J. *et al.* (1981), Human conjunctival surface mucins. A quantitative study of normal and diseased (KCS) tissue. *Graefes Arch Ophthalmol*, **215**, 209.

Lehtosalo, J., Uusitalo, H. and Palakama, A. (1984), Sensory supply of the anterior uvea: a light and electron microscope study. *Exp Brain Res*, **55**, 562.

Lehtosalo, J., Uusitalo, H., Stjernschantz, J. *et al.* (1984), Substance P-like immunoreactivity in the trigeminal ganglion. A fluorescence, light and electron microscope study. *Histochem J*, **80**, 421.

Leichnetz, G.R. (1981), The prefrontal cortico-oculomotor trajectories in the monkey: a possible explanation for the effects of stimulation/lesion experiments on eye movement. *J Neurol Sci*, **49**, 387.

Leigh, R.J. (1989), The cortical control of ocular pursuit movements. *Rev Neurol (Paris)*, **145**, 605.

Leigh, R.J. and Zee, D.S. (1991), *The Neurology of Eye Movements*, 2nd edition, F.A. Davis Co, Philadelphia.

Lele, P.P. and Grimes, P. (1960), The role of neural mechanisms in the regulation of intraocular pressure in the cat. *Exp Neurol*, **2**, 199.

Lemp, M.A. and Weiler, H.H. (1983), How do tears exit? *Invest Ophthalmol Vis Sci*, **24**, 619.

Lende, R.A. and Poulos, D.A. (1970), Functional localization in the trigeminal ganglion in the monkey. *J Neurosurg*, **32**, 336.

Lennerstrand, G. (1974), Electrical activity and isometric tension in motor units of the cat's inferior oblique muscle. *Acta Physiol Scand*, **91**, 458.

Lennerstrand, G. (1975), Motor units in eye muscles, in *Basic Mechanisms of Ocular Motility and their Clinical Implications* (eds G. Lennerstrand and P. Bach-y-Rita), Pergamon Press, Oxford, p. 119.

Lennerstrand, G. (1986), Contractile properties and histochemistry of extraocular muscle in the pigmented and albino guinea pig. *Acta Ophthalmol*, **63**, 723.

Lennerstrand, G. and Bach-y-Rita, P. (1975) In *Basic Mechanisms of Ocular Motility and Their Clinical Implications* (eds G. Lennerstrand and P. Bach-y-Rita), Pergamon Press, Oxford, p. 119.

Lesueur, L., Arne, J.L., Mignon-Conte, M. *et al.* (1994), Structural and ultrastructural changes in the development process of premature infants' and children's corneas. *Cornea*, **13**, 331.

Leuenberger, P.M. (1973), Lanthanum hydroxide tracer studies on rat corneal endothelium. *Exp Eye Res*, **15**, 85.

Leventhal, A.G., Rodieck, R.W. and Dreher, B. (1981), Retinal ganglion cell classes in the Old World monkey: morphology and central projections. *Science*, **213**, 1139.

Leventhal, A.G., Schall, J.D., Ault, S.J. *et al.* (1988), Class-specific cell death shapes the distribution and pattern of central projection of cat retinal ganglion cells. *J Neurosci*, **8**, 2011.

Levitzky, M. and Hendkind, P. (1969), Angioarchitecture of the optic nerve: II. Lamina cribrosa. *Am J Ophthalmol*, **68**, 986.

Lewis, G.P., Erickson, P.A., Kaska, D.D. and Fisher, S.K. (1988), An immunocytochemical comparison of Müller cells and astrocytes in the cat retina. *Exp Eye Res*, **47**, 839.

Lewis, P.R. and Shate, C.C.D. (1959), Selective staining of visceral efferents in the rat brain stem by a modified koelle technique. *Nature*, **183**, 1743.

Ley, A.P., Holmberg, A.S. and Yamashita, T. (1960), Histology of zonulysis with alpha-trypsinogen employing light and electron microscopy. *Am J Ophthalmol*, **49**, 67.

Li, Z.Y., Streeten, B.W. and Wallace, R.N. (1991), Vitronectin localizes to pseudoexfoliative fibers in ocular conjunctival sites by immunoelectron microscopy. *ARVO Suppl: Invest Ophthalmol Vis Sci*, **32**, 777.

Lichter, P.R. (1969), Iris processes in 340 eyes. *Am J Ophthalmol*, **68**, 872.

Lieberman, A.R. (1974), Neurons with presynaptic perikarya and presynaptic dendrikes in the rats geniculate nucleus. *Brain Res*, **59**, 35.

Lieberman, M.F., Maumenee, A.E. and Green, W.R. (1976), Histologic studies of the vasculature of the anterior optic nerve. *Am J Ophthalmol*, **82**, 405.

Lim, C.H. and Ruskell, G.L. (1978), Corneal nerve access in monkeys. *A von Graefes Arch Klin Exp Ophthalmol*, **208**, 15.

Lim, W.C. and Webber, W.A. (1975), A light and transmission electron-microscopic study of the rat iris in pupillary dilation and constriction. *Exp Eye Res*, **21**, 433.

Linberg, K.A. and Fisher, S.K. (1986), An ultrastructural study of interplexiform cell synapses in the human retina. *J Comp Neurol*, **243**, 561.

Linberg, K.A. and Fisher, S.K. (1988), Ultrastructural evidence that horizontal cell axon terminals are presynaptic in the human retina. *J Comp Neurol*, **268**, 281.

Lindgren, E. (1957), Radiologic examination of the brain and spinal cord. *Acta Radiol Suppl*, **151**, 1.

Linsenmayer, T.F., Fitch, J.M., Gross, J. *et al.* (1985), Are the collagen fibrils in the avian cornea of two different collagen types. *Ann NY Acad Sci*, **460**, 232.

Linsenmeier, R.A., Grishnan, L.J., Jakiela, M.G. *et al.* (1982), *Vision Res*, **22**, 1173.

Liotet, S., Van Bijsterveld, O.P., Kogbe, O. *et al.* (1987), A new hypothesis on tear film stability. *Ophthalmologica*, **195**, 119.

Lisberger, S.G. and Fuchs, A.F. (1974), Response of flocculus Purkinje cells to adequate vestibular stimulation in the alert monkey: fixation vs. compensatory eye movements. *Brain Res*, **69**, 347.

Lisberger, S.G. and Fuchs, A.F. (1978a), Role of primate flocculus during rapid behavioral modification of vestibuloocular reflex. I. Purkinje cell activity during visually guided horizontal smooth-pursuit eye movements and passive head rotation. *J Neurophysiol*, **41**, 733.

Lisberger, S.G. and Fuchs, A.F. (1978b), Role of primate flocculus during rapid behavioral modification of vestibuloocular reflex. II. Mossy fiber firing patterns during horizontal head rotation and head movement. *J Neurophysiol*, **41**, 764.

Livingstone, M.S. (1988), Art illusion and the visual system. *Sci Am*, **1**, 68.

Livingstone, M.S. and Hubel, D.H. (1981), Regions of poor orientation tuning coincide with patches of cytochrome oxidase staining in monkey striate cortex. *Neurosci Abstr*, **7**, 357.

Livingstone, M.S. and Hubel, D.H. (1982), Thalamic inputs to cytochrome oxidase-rich regions in monkey visual cortex. *Proc Natl Acad Sci USA*, **79**, 6098.

Livingstone, M.S. and Hubel, D.H. (1984), Anatomy and physiology of a color system in the primate visual cortex. *J Neurosci*, **4**, 309.

Llinas, R. and Wolfe, J.W. (1977), Functional linkage between the electrical activity in the vermal cerebellar cortex and saccadic eye movements. *Exp Brain Res*, **29**, 1.

Lo, W.K. (1987), *In vivo* and *in vitro* observations on permeability and diffusion pathways of tracers in rat and frog lenses. *Exp Eye Res*, **45**, 393.

Lo, W.K. and Harding, C.V. (1983), Tight junctions in the lens epithelia of human and frog: freeze-fracture and protein tracer studies. *Invest Ophthalmol Vis Sci*, **24**, 396.

Lo, W.K. and Harding, C.V. (1984), Square arrays and their role in ridge formation in human lens fibers. *J Ultrastruct Res*, **86**, 228.

Lo, W.K. and Harding, C.V. (1986), Structure and distribution of gap junctions in lens epithelium and fibre cells. *Cell Tissue Res*, **244**, 253.

Locket, N.A. (1968), The dual nature of human extraocular muscle. *Br Orthoptic J*, **26**, 2.

Lockhart, R.D. and Brandt, W. (1938), Length of striated muscle fibers. *J Anat*, **72**, 470.

Loewy, A.D., Araujo, J.C. and Kerr, F.W.L. (1973), Pupillodilator pathways in the brain stem of the cat: anatomical and electrophysiological identification of a central autonomic pathway. *Brain Res*, **60**, 65.

Logan-Turner, A.L. (1901), *The Accessory Sinuses of the Nose*, Green, London, 1.

Logan-Turner, A.L. (1908a), The relation of disease of the nasal accessory sinuses to diseases of the eye, *Lancet*, **ii**, 396.

Logan-Turner, A.L. (1908b), *BMJ*, **ii**, 730.

Lombardi, G. and Passerini, A. (1967), The orbital veins. *Am J Ophthalmol*, **64**, 440.

Lombardi, G. and Passerini, A. (1968), Venography of the orbit: technique and anatomy. *Br J Radiol*, **41**, 282.

Lopping, B. and Weale, R.A. (1965), Changes in corneal curvature following ocular convergence. *Vision Res*, **5**, 207.

Lorente de no, R. (1933), Vestibulo-ocular reflex arc. *Arch Neurol*, **30**, 245.

Los, J.A. (1970), A new method of three dimensional reconstruction of microscopical structures based on photographic technic. *Acta Morphol Neurol Scand*, **8**, 273.

Los, J.A. (1971a), A method for ultra-thin sectioning of microscopical structures in a predetermined direction. *Acta Morphol Neerl Scand*, **9**, 13.

Los, J.A. (1971b), A new method of three-dimensional reconstruction of microscopical structures based on photographic techniques. *Acta Morphol Neerl Scand*, **8**, 273.

Lowenfeld, I.E. (1966), Pupillary movements associated with light and near vision: an experimental review of the literature, in *Recent Developments in Vision Research* (ed. M. Whitcomb), National Academy of Sciences, National Research Council, Washington, DC, p. 17.

Lowenfeld, I.E. (1984), *The Pupil: Anatomy, Physiology and Clinical Applications*, Wayne State University Press, Detroit.

Lowenstein, O. and Lowenfeld, I.E. (1959), Scotopic and photopic thresholds of the pupillary light reflex in normal man. *Am J Ophthalmol*, **48**, 87.

Lowenstein, O. and Lowenfeld, I.E. (1969), The pupil, in *The Eye*, 2nd edition (ed. H. Davson), Academic Press, New York, p. 231.

Lund, J.S., Lund, R.D., Hendrickson, A.E. *et al.* (1975), The origin of efferent pathways from the primary visual cortex, area 17, of the macaque monkey as shown by retrograde transport of horseradish peroxidase. *J Comp Neurol*, **164**, 287.

Lund, R.D. (1975), Variations in the laterality of the central projections of retinal ganglion cells. *Exp Eye Res*, **21**, 193.

Lund, R.D. (1978), *Development and Plasticity of the Brain*, OUP, Oxford.

Lund, R.D. and Hankin, M.H. (1995), Pathfinding by retinal ganglion cell axons: transplantation studies in genetically and surgically blind mice. *J Comp Neurol*, **356**, 481.

Lund, R.D. and Mitchell, D.E. (1979), Asymmetry in the visual callosal connections of strabismic cats. *Brain Res*, **167**, 176.

Lund, R.D., Mitchell, D.E. and Henry, G.H. (1978), Squint-induced modification of callosal connections in cats. *Brain Res*, **144**, 169.

Lütjen-Drecoll, E., Futa, R. and Rohen, J.W. (1981), Ultrahistochemical studies on tangential sections of the trabecular meshwork in normal and glaucomatous eyes. *Invest Ophthalmol Vis Sci*, **21**, 563.

Lütjen-Drecoll, E. and Kaufman, P.L. (1979), Echothiopate-induced structural alterations in the anterior chamber angle of the cynomolgus monkey. *Invest Ophthalmol Vis Sci*, **18**, 918.

Lütjen-Drecoll, E., Rittig, M., Rauterberg, J. *et al.* (1989), Immunomicroscopical study of type VI collagen in the trabecular meshwork of normal and glaucomatous eyes. *Exp Eye Res*, **48**, 139.

Lütjen-Drecoll, E., Shimizu, T., Rohrbach, M. *et al.* (1986), Quantitative analysis of 'plaque material' in the inner and outer wall of Schlemm's canal in normal and glaucomatous eyes. *Exp Eye Res*, **42**, 443.

Lütjen-Drecoll, E., Tamm, E. and Kaufman, P.L. (1988a),

Age changes in rhesus monkey ciliary muscle: light and electron microscopy. *Exp Eye Res*, **47**, 885.

Lütjen-Drecoll, E., Tamm, E. and Kaufman, P.L. (1988b), Age related loss of morphologic response to pilocarpine in rhesus monkey ciliary muscle. *Arch Ophthalmol*, **106**, 1591.

Luyckx, J. (1966), Mesure des composantes optiques de l'oeil du nouveau-né par échographie ultrasonique. *Arch Ophthalmol, Paris*, **26**, 159.

Lynch, J.C., Mountcastle, V.B., Tablot, W.H. *et al.* (1977), Parietal lobe mechanisms for directed visual attention. *J Neurophysiol*, **40**, 362.

Lyness, R.W. (1986), An investigation into some aspects of the histopathology of extraocular muscles. *MD Thesis*, University of Belfast.

Maciewicz, R., Phipps, B.S., Foote, W.E. *et al.* (1983), The distribution of substance P-containing neurons in the cat Edinger-Westphal nucleus: relationship to efferent projection systems. *Brain Res*, **270**, 217.

Maciewicz, R.J. and Spencer, R.F. (1977), Oculomotor and abducens internuclear pathways in the cat. *Dev Neurosci*, **1**, 99.

Macintosh, S.R. (1974), The innervation of the conjunctiva in monkeys. An electron microscopic and nerve degeneration study. *A von Graefes Arch Klin Exp Ophthalmol*, **192**, 105.

Maddox, E.C. (1886), Investigations on the relationship between convergence and accommodation of the eyes. *J Anat*, **20**, 475.

Magenis, R.E., Maslen, C.L., Smith, L. *et al.* (1991), Localization of the fibrillin (FBN) gene to chromosome 15 and band 21.1. *Genomics*, **11**, 346.

Maggiore, L. (1917), *Ann Ottalm*, **40**, 317.

Maggiore, L. (1924), *Ann Ottalm*, **52**, 625.

Magoun, H.W. and Ransom, M. (1942), The supra optic decussations in the cat and monkey. *J Comp Neurol*, **76**, 435.

Mai, J.K. (1978), The accessory optic system and the retino-hypothalamic system. A review. *J Hirnforsch*, **19**, 213.

Maioli, M.G., Squatrito, S. and Domeniconi, R. (1989), Projections from visual cortical areas of the superior temporal sulcus to the lateral terminal nucleus of the accessory optic system in macaque monkeys. *Brain Res*, **498**, 389.

Maisel, H. (1977), Filaments of the vertebrate lens. *Experientia*, **33**, 525.

Maisel, H., Alcala, J., Kuszak, J. *et al.* (1981), Maturation of the lens fiber cell: some morphological and biochemical correlates.

Maisel, H., Lieska, N. and Bradley, R. (1978), Isolation of filaments of the chick lens. *Experientia*, **34**, 352.

Malmfors, T. (1965), *Acta Physiol Scand*, **65**, 259.

Malpeli, J.G. and Baker, F.H. (1975), The representation of the visual field in the lateral geniculate nucleus of *Macaca mulatta*. *J Comp Neurol*, **161**, 569.

Mandell (1967), Corneal contour of the human infant. *Arch Ophthalmol*, **77**, 345.

Mann, I. (1957), *Developmental Abnormalities of the Eye*, 2nd edition, Lippincott, Philadelphia.

Mann, I.C. (1927a) *The development of the human eye*, 3rd edition. Br. Med. Assoc., London.

Mann, I.C. (1927b), *Trans Ophthalmol Soc UK*, **47**, 142.

Mann, R.M., Riva, C.E., Cranstoun, S.D. *et al.* (1993), Nitric oxide and choroidal blood flow (chBF) regulation. *ARVO Suppl: Invest Ophthalmol Vis Sci*, **34**, 1394.

Mannhardt, F. (1871), *A von Graefes Arch Ophthalmol*, **17**, 11.

Manni, E., Bortolami, R. and De Sole, C. (1966), Eye muscle proprioception and the semilunar ganglion. *Exp Neurol*, **16**, 226.

Manni, E., Bortolami, R. and De Sole, C. (1967), *Boll Soc Ital Biol Sper*, **43**, 66.

Manni, E., Bortolami, R. and Derck, P.L. (1970a), Presence of cell bodies of the afferents from the eye muscles in the semilunar ganglion. *Arch Ital Biol*, **108**, 106.

Manni, E., Bortolami, R. and Deriu, P.L. (1970b), Superior oblique muscle proprioception and the trochlear nerve. *Exp Neurol*, **26**, 543.

Manni, E., Bortolami, R., Pettorossi, V.E. *et al.* (1978), Afferent fibres and sensory ganglion cells within the oculomotor nerve in some mammals and man. II. Electrophysiological investigations. *Arch Ital Biol*, **116**, 16.

Manni, E., Palmieri, G. and Marini, R. (1971a), Peripheral pathway of the proprioceptive afferents from the lateral rectus muscles of the eye. *Exp Neurol*, **30**, 46.

Manni, E., Palmieri, G. and Marini, R. (1971b), Extraocular muscle proprioception and the descending trigeminal nucleus. *Exp Neurol*, **33**, 195.

Manni, E., Palmieri, G. and Marini, R. (1974), Central pathway of extraocular muscle proprioception. *Exp Neurol*, **42**, 181.

Manni, E. and Pettorossi, V.E. (1976), Somatotopic localization of the eye muscle afferents in the semilunar ganglion. *Arch Ital Bio*, **114**, 178.

Marchi, V. (1882), Über die Terminalorgane der Nerven (Golgi's nervenkorperchen) in den Sehnen der Augenmuskeln. *A von Graefes Arch Ophthalmol*, **28**, 203.

Marino, R. and Rasmussen, T. (1968), Visual field changes after temporal lobectomy in man. *Neurology*, **18**, 825.

Marrocco, R.T. and Brown, J.B. (1975), Correlation of receptive field properties of monkey LGN cells with the conduction velocity of retinal afferent input. *Brain Res*, **92**, 137.

Marshall, J., Beaconsfield, M. and Rothery, S. (1982), The anatomy and development of the human lens and zonules. *Trans Ophthalmol Soc UK*, **102**, 423.

Marshall, J. and Grindle, C.F.J. (1978), Fine structure of the cornea and its developments. *Trans Ophthalmol Soc UK*, **98**, 320.

Marshall, G.E., Konstas, A.G. and Lee, W.R. (1990), Immunogold localization of type IV collagen and laminin in the aging human outflow system. *Exp Eye Res*, **51**, 691.

Marshall, G.E., Konstas, A.G. and Lee, W.R. (1991), Immunogold ultrastructural localization of collagens in the aged human outflow system. *Ophthalmology*, **98**, 692.

Martinez, A.J., Hay, S. and McNeer, K.W. (1976), Extraocular muscles: light microscopy and ultrastructural features. *Acta Neuropathol*, **34**, 237.

Martola, E.L. and Baum, J.L. (1968), Central and peripheral corneal thickness. A clinical study. *Arch Ophthalmol*, **79**, 28.

Mason, C.A. and Lincoln, D.W. (1976), Visualisation of retino-hypothalmic projection in the rat by cobalt precipitation. *Cell Tissue Res*, **168**, 117.

Mathers, L.H. (1971), Tectal projection to the posterior thalamus of the squirrel monkey. *Brain Res*, **35**, 295.

Mathers, L.H. and Rapisardi, S.C. (1973), Visual and somatosensory receptive fields of neurons in the squirrel monkey pulvinar. *Brain Res*, **64**, 65.

Matsuda, H. (1968), Electron microscopic study on the corneal nerve with special reference to its endings. *Jpn J Ophthalmol*, **12**, 163.

Matsuda, H. and Sugiura, S. (1971), Ultrastructure of 'tubular body' in the endothelial cells of the ocular blood vessels. *Invest Ophthalmol Vis Sci*, **9**, 919.

Matsusaka, T. (1975), Tridimensional views of the relationship of pericytes to endothelial cells of capillaries in the human choroid and retina. *J Electron Microsc*, **24**, 13.

Matthews, M.R., Cowan, W.M. and Powell, T.P. (1960), Transneuronal cell degeneration in the lateral geniculate nucleus of the macaque monkey. *J Anat*, **94**, 145.

Matus, A.I. (1970), Ultrastructure of the superior cervical ganglion fixed with zinc iodide and osmium tetroxide. *Brain Res*, **17**, 195.

Maunsell, J.H.R. and Van Essen, D.C. (1983), The connection of the middle temporal visual area (MT) and their relationship to a cortical hierarchy in the macaque monkey. *J Neurosci*, **3**, 2563.

Maurice, D.M. (1953), Preliminary notes Intracellular spacing of the corneal endothelium. *Biochim Biophys Acta*, **11**, 311.

Maurice, D.M. (1957), The structure and transparency of the cornea. *J Physiol*, **136**, 263.

Maurice, D.M. (1962), The cornea and sclera, In *The Eye* (ed. H. Davson), Academic Press, New York, p. 289.

Maurice, D.M. (1969), The cornea and sclera, in *The Eye*, 2nd edition (ed. H. Davson), Academic Press, London, p. 489.

Maurice, D.M. (1973), The dynamics and drainage of tears. *Int Ophthalmol Clin*, **13**, 103.

Maurice, D.M. (1984), The cornea and sclera, in *The Eye*, 3rd edition (ed. H. Davson), Academic Press, London, p. 1.

Maurice, D.M. and Giardini, A.A. (1951), A simple optical apparatus for measuring the corneal thickness, and the average thickness of the human cornea. *Br J Ophthalmol*, **35**, 169.

Maurice, D.M. and Riley, M.V. (1968), The biochemistry of the cornea, in *The Biochemistry of the Eye* (ed. C.N. Graymore), Academic Press, New York, p. 1.

Mayer, J.C.A. (1777), *Anatomische Beschneibung der Blutgefasse des menschlichen korpers*, Springer-Verlag, Berlin, p. 1.

Mayr, R., Gottschall, J., Gruber, H. *et al.* (1975), Internal structure of cat extraocular muscle. *Anat Embryol (Berl)*, **148**, 25.

Mayr, R., Stockinger, L. and Zenker, W. (1966), Elektronenmikroskopische untersuchungen an unterschiedlich innervierten muskelfasem der ausseren augenmuskulatur des rhesesaffen. *Z Zellforsch Mikrosk Anat*, **75**, 434.

Mays, L.E. and Porter J.D. (1984), Neural control of vergence eye movements: activity of abducens and oculomotor neurones. *J Neurophysiol*, **52**, 743.

Mays, L.E. and Sparks, D.L. (1980a), Saccades are spatially, not retinocentrically, coded. *J Neurophysiol*, **44**, 1163.

Mays, L.E. and Sparks, D.L. (1980b), Dissociation of visual and saccade-related responses in superior colliculus neurons. *J Neurophysiol*, **43**, 207.

McConnell, E.M. (1953), The arterial blood supply of the human hypophysis cerebri. *Anat Rec*, **115**, 175.

McCulloch, C. (1954), The zonule of Zinn: its origin course and insertion, and its relation to neighboring structures. *Trans Am Ophthalmol Soc*, **52**, 525.

McCullough, C.M. (1986), The zonule of Zinn: its origin, course and insertion and its relation to neighbouring structures. *Trans Am Ophthalmol Soc*, **52**, 525.

McDonald, J.E. and Brubacker, S. (1971), Meniscus-induced thinning of tear films. *Am J Ophthalmol*, **72**, 139.

McEwen, W.K. (1958), Application of Poiseville's law to aqueous outflow. *Arch Ophthalmol*, **60**, 290.

McLoon, L.K. and Wirtschafter, J.D. (1991), Regional differences in the orbicularis oculi muscle: conservation between species. *J Neurol Sci*, **104**, 197.

McMahon, R.T., Tso, M.O.M. and McLean, I.W. (1975), Histologic localization of sodium fluorescein in human ocular tissue. *Am J Ophthalmol*, **80**, 1058.

McMasters, R.E., Weiss, A.H. and Carpenter, M.B. (1966), Vestibular projections to the nuclei of the extraocular muscles. Degeneration resulting from discrete partial lesions of the vestibular nuclei in the monkey. *Am J Anat*, **118**, 163.

McMenamin, P.G. (1989), Human fetal iridocorneal angle: a light and scanning electron microscopic study. *Br J Ophthalmol*, **73**, 871.

McMenamin, P.G. (1991), A quantitative study of the prenatal development of the aqueous outflow system in the human eye. *Exp Eye Res*, **53**, 507.

McMenamin, P.G., Lee, W.R. and Aitken, D.A.N. (1986), Age-related changes in the human outflow apparatus. *Ophthalmology*, **93**, 194.

McNutt, N.S. and Weinstein, R.S. (1970), The ultrastructure of the nexus. A correlated thin-section and freeze-cleave study. *J Cell Biol*, **47**, 666.

Meadows, J.C. (1974), Disturbed perception of colours associated with localized cerebral lesions. *Brain*, **97**, 615.

Meek, K.M., Elliott, G.F. and Nave, C. (1986), A synchrotron X-ray diffraction study of bovine cornea stained with cupromeronic blue. *Collagen Rel Res*, **6**, 203.

Meek, K.M. and Leonard, D.W. (1993), Ultrastructure of the corneal stroma: a comparative study. *Biophys J*, **64**, 273.

Meikle, T.H. and Sprague, J.M. (1964), *Int Rev Neurobiol*, **6**, 150.

Melanowski, W.H. and Stachow, A. (1958), Recherches sur la structure chimique de la sclerotique de l'oeil humain selon l'age, in XVIII International Congress of Ophthalmology Bruxelles. *Acta Ophthalmol Suppl*, **1**, 397.

Merkel, F. (1885), *Handbuch der topographischen Anatomie*; 2nd edition.

Merkel, F. (1887), Der musculus superciliaris. *Anat Anz*, **2**, 17.

Merkel, F. and Orr, A.W. (1892), Das Auge des Neugeborenen an einem schematischen Durchschnitt erlautert. (Anatomische Hefte.) *Arb Anat Inst Wiesbaden*, **1**, 271.

Merrillees, N.C.R., Sunderland, S. and Hayhow, W. (1950), Neuromuscular spindles in the extraocular muscles in man. *Anat Rec*, **108**, 23.

Mettler, F.A. (1935), Cortigofugal fiber connections of the

cortex of *Macaca mulatta* occipital region. *J Comp Neurol*, **61**, 221.

Meyer, A. (1907), The connections of the occipital lobes and the present status of the cerebral visual affections. *Trans Assoc Am Phys*, **22**, 7.

Meyer, F. (1887), Zur Anatomie der Orbitalarterien. *Morph Jahrbuch*, **12**, 414.

Meyer, P.A.R. (1989), The circulation of the human limbus. *Eye*, **3**, 121.

Meyer, P.A.R. and Watson, P.G. (1987), Low dose fluorescein angiography of the conjunctiva and episclera. *Br J Ophthalmol*, **71**, 2.

Michael, C.R. (1978), Colour vision mechanisms in monkey striate cortex: dual opponent cells with concentric receptive fields. *J Neurophysiol*, **41**, 572.

Michaelson, I.C. and Campbell, A.C.P. (1940), The anatomy of the finer retinal vessels and some observations on their significance in certain retinal diseases. *Trans Ophthalmol Soc UK*, **60**, 71.

Mikulicich, A. and Young, R. (1963), Cell proliferation and displacement in the lens epithelium of young rats injected with tritiated thymidine. *Invest Ophthalmol*, **2**, 344.

Milam, A.H., De Leeuw, A.M., Gaur, V.P. *et al.* (1990), Immunolocalization of cellular retinoic acid binding protein to Müller cells and/or a subpopulation of GABA-positive amacrine cells in retinas of different species. *J Comp Neurol*, **296**, 123.

Miledi, R. and Slater, C.R. (1969), Electron-microscopic structure of denervated skeletal muscle. *Proc R Soc Lond, Series B*, **174**, 253.

Miles, F.A., Braitman, D.J. and Dow, B.M. (1980), Long-term adaptive changes in primate vestibulo-ocular reflex. IV. Electrophysiological observations in flocculus of adapted monkeys. *J Neurophysiol*, **43**, 1477.

Miles, F.A. and Fuller, J.H. (1975), Visual tracking and the primate flocculus. *Science*, **189**, 1000.

Millard, C.B., Tripathi, B.J. and Tripathi, R.C. (1987), Age-related changes in protein profiles of the normal human trabecular meshwork. *Exp Eye Res*, **45**, 623.

Miller, A., Costa, M., Furness, J.B. *et al.* (1981), Substance P immunoreactive sensory nerves supply the rat iris and cornea. *Neurosciences*, **23**, 243.

Miller, A.S., Coster, D.J., Costa, M. *et al.* (1983), Vasoactive intestinal peptide immunoreactive nerve fibres in the human eye. *Aust J Ophthalmol*, **11**, 185.

Miller, D. and Benedek, G. (1973), *Intraocular Light Scattering*, Charles C. Thomas, Springfield, IL, p. 1.

Miller, J.E. (1967), Cellular organization of rhesus extraocular muscle. *Invest Ophthalmol*, **6**, 18.

Miller, J.E. (1971), Recent histologic and electron microscopic findings in extraocular muscle. *Trans Am Acad Ophthalmol Otolaryngol*, **75**, 1175.

Miller, J.E. (1975), Aging changes in extraocular muscle, in *Basic Mechanisms of Ocular Motility and their Clinical Implications* (eds G. Lennerstrand and P. Bach-y-Rita), Pergamon Press, Oxford, p. 47.

Miller, N.R. (1982), *Walsh and Hoyts Clinical Neuro-ophthalmology*, 4th edition, Williams & Wilkins, Baltimore.

Minckler, D.S. (1980), The organization of nerve fibre bundles in the primate optic nerve head. *Arch Ophthalmol*, **98**, 1630.

Minckler, D.S., McLean, I.W. and Tso, M.O.M. (1976), Distribution of axonal and glial elements in the rhesus optic nerve head studied by electron microscopy. *Am J Ophthalmol*, **82**, 179.

Minkowski, M. (1913), Experimentelle Untersuchungen uber die Beziehungen der Grosshirn rinde und der Netzhaut zu den primaren optischen Zentren, besunders zum Corpus geniculatum externum. *Arb Hirnanat Inst Zurich*, **7**, 255.

Mishima, S. (1965), Some physiological aspects of the precorneal tear film. *Arch Ophthalmol*, **73**, 233.

Mishima, S. (1982), Clinical investigations on the corneal endothelium. *Am J Ophthalmol*, **93**, 1.

Mishima, S., Gasset, A., Klyce, S. *et al.* (1966), Determination of tear flow. *Invest Ophthalmol*, **5**, 264.

Mishima, S. and Maurice, D.M. (1961), The oily layer of tear film and evaporation from the corneal surface. *Exp Eye Res*, **1**, 39.

Mishkin, M. (1982), A memory system in the monkey. *Phil Trans R Soc Lond, Series B*, **298**, 85.

Mishkin, M., Ungerleider, L.G. and Macko, K.A. (1983), Object vision and spatial vision: two cortical pathways. *Trends Neurosci*, **6**, 414.

Misotten, L. (1964), L'Ultrastructure des tissues oculaires. *Bull Soc Belge Ophthalmol*, **136**, 199.

Mitchell, G.A.G. (1953), *The Anatomy of the Autonomic Nervous System*, Churchill Livingstone, London.

Miyashita, K., Azuma, N. and Hida, T. (1992), Morphological and histochemical studies of goblet cells in developing human conjunctiva. *Jpn J Ophthalmol*, **36**, 169.

Modak, S.H (1972), A model for transcriptional control in terminally differentiating lens fibre cells, in *Cell Differentiation* (eds R. Harris, P. Allin and D. Viza), Munksgaard, Copenhagen, p. 339.

Modak, S.P. and Bollum, F.J. (1972), Detection and measurement of single-strand breaks in nuclear DNA in fixed lens sections. *Exp Cell Res*, **75**, 544.

Modak, S.P., Morris, G. and Yamada, T. (1968), DNA synthesis and mitotic activity during early development of chick lens. *Dev Biol*, **17**, 544.

Mohler, C.W. and Wurtz, R.H. (1976), Organisation of monkey superor colliculus intermediate layer cells discharging before eye movements. *J Neurophysiol*, **39**, 722.

Mohler, C.W. and Wurtz, R.H. (1977), Role of striate cortex and superior colliculus in the visual guidance of saccadic eye movements in monkeys. *J Neurophysiol*, **40**, 74.

Mollier, G. (1938), A quadruple stain for the demonstration of smooth and striated muscles and their relationship to the connective tissue. *A Wissensch Mikr*, **55**, 472.

Mollon, J.D., Newcombe, F., Polden, P.G. *et al.* (1980), On the presence of three cone mechanisms in a case of total achromatopsia, in *Colour Vision Deficiencies*, vol. 5 (ed. G. Verriest), Hilger, Bristol, p. 130.

Molnar, L. (1970), Refraktions anderung des Auges im Laufe des Lebens. *Augenheilkunde*, **156**, 326.

Monaghan, A.P., Davidson, D.R., Sime, C. *et al.* (1991), The Msh-like homeobox genes define domains in the developing vertebrate eye. *Development*, **112**, 1053.

Montagna, W. (1967), *Advances in the Biology of the Skin*, New York.

Morgan, M.W. and Harrigan, R.F. (1951), *Am J Optom*, **28**, 242.

Morris, J.L. (1993), Cotransmission from autonomic vasodilator neurons supplying the guinea-pig uterine artery. *J Auton Nerv Syst*, **42**, 11.

Morrison, J.C. and Van Buskirk, E.M. (1983), Anterior collateral circulation in the primate eye. *Ophthalmology*, **90**, 707.

Morrison, J.C. and Van Buskirk, E.M. (1984), Ciliary process microvasculature of the primate eye. *Am J Ophthalmol*, **97**, 372.

Morrison, J.C. and Van Buskirk, E.M. (1986), Microanatomy and modulation of the ciliary vasculature. *Trans Ophthalmol Soc UK*, **105**, 13.

Morton, A. (1969), A quantitative analysis of the normal neuron population of the hypothalamic magnocellular nuclei in man and of their projections to the neurohypophysis. *J Comp Neurol*, **136**, 143.

Moseley, H., Grierson, I. and Lee, W.R. (1983), Mathematical modelling of aqueous humour outflow from the eye through the pores in the lining endothelium of Schlemm's canal. *Clin Phys Physiol Meas*, **4**, 47.

Moses, R.A. (1977), The effects of intraocular pressure on resistance to outflow. *Surv Ophthalmol*, **22**, 88.

Moses, R.A. and Arnzen, R.J. (1980), The trabecular mesh: a mathematical analysis. *Invest Ophthalmol Vis Sci*, **19**, 1490.

Moskowitz, M.A. (1984), The neurobiology of vascular head pain. *Ann Neurol*, **16**, 157.

Motais, E. (1887), *L'Appareil Moteur de L'Oeila*, Delahaye & Lecrosnier, Paris.

Motter, B.C. and Mountcastle, V.B. (1981), The functional properties of the light-sensitive neurons of the posterior parietal cortex studied in waking monkeys: foveal sparing and opponent vector organization. *J Neurosci*, **1**, 3.

Mountcastle, V.B. and Henneman, (1952), *J Comp Neurol*, **97**, 409.

Mountcastle, V.B., Lynch, J.C., Georgopoulos, A. *et al.* (1975), Posterior parietal association cortex of the monkey: command functions for operations within extrapersonal space. *J Neurophysiol*, **38**, 871.

Mousa, G.Y. and Trevithick, J.R. (1977), Differentiation of rat lens epithelial cells in tissue culture: II. Effects of cytochalasins B and D on actin organization and differentiation. *Dev Biol*, **60**, 14.

Mukuno, K. (1968), Fine structure of the human extraocular muscles. 3. Neuromuscular junction in the normal human extraocular muscles. *Acta Soc Ophthalmol Jpn*, **72**, 104.

Müller, F. (1977), The development of the anterior fulcate and lacrimal arteries in the human. *Anat Embryol*, **150**, 207.

Müller, H. (1859a), Über Ganglienzellen im Ziliarmuskel des Menschen. *Verh Physik-med Ges Würzburg*, **10**, 107.

Müller, H. (1859b) Über glatte Muskelfasern und Nervengeflechte der Choroidea im menschlichen Auge, *Verh Physik-med Ges Würzburg*, **10**, 107.

Murphy, C., Alvarado, J. and Juster, R. (1984), Prenatal and postnatal growth of the human Descemet's membrane. *Invest Ophthalmol Vis Sci*, **25**, 1420.

Murphy, C.G., Andersen, J.Y., Newsome, D.A. and Alvarado, J.A. (1987), Localization of extracellular proteins of the human trabecular meshwork by indirect immunofluorescence. *Am J Ophthalmol*, **104**, 33.

Mustafa, G.Y. and Gamble, H.J. (1979), Changes in axonal numbers in developing human trochlear nerve. *J Anat*, **128**, 323.

Muther, T.F. and Friedland, B.R. (1980), Autoradiographic localization of carbonic anhydrase in the rabbit ciliary body. *J Histochem Cytochem*, **28**, 1119.

Mwasi, L.M. and Raviola, G. (1985), Morphology and permeability properties of blood capillaries in extraocular muscles of macaque monkey. *A von Graefes Arch Klin Exp Ophthalmol*, **223**, 9.

Namba, T., Nakamura, T. and Grob, D. (1986), Motor nerve endings in human extraocular muscle. *Neurology*, **18**, 403.

Nanney, L.B., Magid, M., Stoscheck, G.M. *et al.* (1985), Comparison of epidermal growth factor binding and receptor distribution in normal human epidermis and epidermal appendages. *J Invest Dermatol*, **83**, 385.

Nathan, H. and Goldhammer, Y. (1973), The rootlets of the trochlear nerve. Anatomical observations in human brains. *Acta Anat*, **84**, 590.

Nathan, H., Ovaknine, M.D. and Kosary, I.Z. (1974), The abducens nerve. Anatomical variations in its course. *J Neurosurg*, **41**, 561.

Nathan, H. and Turner, J.W.A. (1942), *Brain*, **65**, 343.

Nauta, W.J.H. (1962), Neural associations of the amygdaloid complex in the monkey. *Brain*, **85**, 505.

Neider, M., Crawford, K., Kaufman, P.L. *et al.* (1990), In vivo videography of the rhesus monkey accommodative apparatus. Age-related loss of ciliary muscle response to central stimulation. *Arch Ophthalmol*, **108**, 69.

Neiger, M. (1960), Connective structures of the orbit and the fat body of the orbit. *Acta Anat*, **39**, 107.

Nesterov, A.P. (1970), Role of the blockade of Schlemm's canal in pathogenesis of primary open angle glaucoma. *Am J Ophthalmol*, **70**, 691.

Neuhuber, W.L. and Clerc, N. (1990), Afferent innervation of the esophagus in cat and rat, in *The Primary Afferent Neuron* (eds W. Zenker and W.L. Neuhuber), Plenum, New York, p. 93.

Newman, E.A. (1987), Distribution of potassium conductance in mammalian Müller (glial) cells: a comparative study. *J Neurosci*, **7**, 2423.

Newman, E.A. (1994), A physiological measure of carbonic anhydrase in Müller cells. *Glia*, **11**, 291.

Newman, E.A. and Odette, L.L. (1984), Model of electroretinogram b-wave generation: a test of the K^+ hypothesis. *J Neurophysiol*, **51**, 164.

Newman, S.A. and Miller, N.R. (1983), The optic tract syndrome: neuro-ophthalmologic considerations. *Arch Ophthalmol*, **101**, 1241.

Nichols, B., Chiappino, M.L. and Dawson, C.R. (1985), Demonstration of the mucous layer of the tear film by electron microscopy. *Invest Ophthalmol Vis Sci*, **26**, 464.

Nichols, B., Dawson, C.R. and Togni, B. (1983), Surface features of the conjunctiva and cornea. *Invest Ophthalmol Vis Sci*, **24**, 570.

Nichols, F.T., Mawad, M., Mohr, M. *et al.* (1990), Focal headache during balloon inflation in the internal carotid and middle cerebral arteries. *Stroke*, **21**, 555.

Niesel, P. (1982), Visible changes of the lens with age. *Trans Ophthalmol Soc UK*, **102**, 327.

Nilssen, S., Linder, J. and Bill, A. (1980), Ocular effects of vasoactive intestinal polypeptide (VIP) and facial nerve stimulation, in *Proceedings of the International Seminar on Selected Topics of Eye Research* (ed. M. de Vincentiis), Baccini & Chiappi, Florence, p. 53.

Nilsson, S.F.E. and Bill, A. (1984), Vasoactive intestinal

polypeptide (VIP): effects in the eye and on regional blood flows. *Acta Physiol Scand*, **121**, 385.

Nilsson, S.F.E., Linder, J. and Bill, A. (1985), Characteristics of uveal vasodilation produced by facial nerve stimulation in monkeys, cats and rabbits. *Exp Eye Res*, **40**, 841.

Nilsson, S.F.E., Sperber, G.Ö. and Bill, A. (1986), Effects of vasoactive intestinal polypeptide (VIP) on intraocular pressure, facility of outflow and formation of aqueous humor in the monkey. *Exp Eye Res*, **43**, 849.

Nishida, S. (1982), Scanning electron microscopy of the zonular fibers in human and monkey eyes. *ARVO Suppl: Invest Ophthalmol Vis Sci*, **1**, 357.

Nishida, S. and Sears, M.L. (1969), Dual innervation of the iris sphincter muscle of the albino guinea pig. *Exp Eye Res*, **8**, 467.

Noback, C.R. and Laemle, L.K. (1970), Structural and functional aspects of the visual pathways of primates, in *The Primate Brain, Advances in Primatology* (eds C.R. Noback and W. Montana), Appleton-Century-Crofts, New York, p. 55.

Noden, D.M. (1978), The control of avian cephalic neural crest cytodifferentiation. I Skeletal and connective tissue. *Dev Biol*, **67**, 296.

Noden, D.M. (1982), Periocular mesenchyme: neural crest and mesodermal interactions, in *Ocular Anatomy, Embryology, and Teratology* (ed. F.A. Jakobiec), Harper and Row, Philadelphia.

Nomura, T. and Smelser, G.K. (1974), The identification of adrenergic and cholinergic nerve ending in the trabecular meshwork. *Invest Ophthalmol Vis Sci*, **13**, 525.

Nordmann, J. and Roth, A. (1967), Aspect biomicroscopique du corps vitre selon la position. *Bull Soc Ophthalmol, Fr*, **67**, 939.

Norn, M.S. (1966), Mucous thread in inferior conjunctival fornix. Quantitative analyses of the normal mucous thread. *Montpellier Med*, **44**, 33.

Norn, M.S. (1974), External eye: methods of examination. *Scriptor*, **1**, 1.

Noske, W., Stamm, C.C. and Hirsch, M. (1994), Tight junctions of the human ciliary epithelium: regional morphology and implications on transepithelial resistance. *Exp Eye Res*, **59**, 141.

Nutt, A.B. (1955), The significance and surgical treatment of congenital ocular palsies. *Ann R Coll Surg Engl*, **16**, 30.

Nyberg-Hansen, R. (1966), Functional organization of descending supraspinal fibre systems to the spinal cord. Anatomical observations and physiological correlations. *Ergeb Anat Entwickl Gesch*, **39**, 1.

Obata, H., Horiuchi, H., Miyata, K. *et al.* (1994), Histopathological study of the meibomian glands. *Nippon Ganka Gakkai Zasshi*, **98**, 765.

Ober, M. and Rohen, J.W. (1979), Regional differences in the fine structure of the ciliary epithelium related to accommodation. *Invest Ophthalmol Vis Sci*, **18**, 655.

O'Connor, P.S., Kasdon, D., Tredici, T.J. *et al.* (1982), The Marcus Gunn pupil in experimental optic tract lesions. *Ophthalmology*, **89**, 160.

Oda, K. (1986), Motor innervation and acetylcholine receptor distribution of human extraocular muscle fibers. *J Neurol Sci*, **74**, 125.

Ogden, T. (1989a), The glia of the retina, in *Retina* (eds S.J Ryan and T. Ogden), C.V. Mosby, St Louis, p. 53.

Ogden, T. (1989b), Topography of the retina, in *Retina* (eds S.J. Ryan and T. Ogden), C.V. Mosby, St Louis, p. 32.

Ogren, M. and Hendrickson, A. (1976), Pathways between striate cortex and subcortical regions in *Macaca mulatta* and *Saimiri sciureus*: evidence for a reciprocal pulvinar connection. *Exp Neurol*, **53**, 780.

Oguni, M., Setogawa, T., Matsu, H. *et al.* (1992), Timing and sequence of the events in the development of extraocular muscles in staged human embryos: ultrastructural and histochemical study. *Acta Anat*, **143**, 195.

Ohnishi, Y. and Kuwabara, T. (1979), Breakdown site of blood–aqueous barrier in the ciliary epithelium. *RVO Suppl: Invest Ophthalmol Vis Sci*, **18**, 241.

Olsen, E.G. and Davanger, M. (1984), The healing of human corneal endothelium. *Acta Ophthalmol*, **62**, 885.

Olver, J.M. (1990), Functional anatomy of the choroidal circulation, methyl methacrylate casting of human choroid. *Eye*, **4**, 262.

Olver, J.M. and Lee, J.P. (1989), The effects of strabismus surgery on anterior segment circulation. *Eye*, **3**, 318.

Olver, J.M. and McCartney, A.C.E. (1989), Orbital and ocular micro-vascular casting in man. *Eye*, **3**, 588.

Olver, J.M., Spalton, D.J. and McCartney, A.C.E. (1990), Microvascular study of the retrolaminar optic nerve in man: the possible significance in anterior ischaemic optic neuropathy. *Eye*, **4**, 7.

Oppel, O. (1963), Microskopische Untersuchungen uber die Anzahl und Kaliber der markhaltigen nervenfasem im Fasciculus opticus des Menschen. *A von Graefes Arch Ophthalmol*, **166**, 19.

Optican, L.M. (1982), Saccadic dysmetria, in *Functional Basis of Ocular Motility Disorders* (eds G. Lennerstrand, D.S. Zee and E.L. Keller), Pergamon Press, Oxford.

Optican, L.M. and Robinson, D.A. (1980), Cerebellar-dependent adaptive control of primate saccadic system. *J Neurophysiol*, **44**, 1058.

Optican, L.M., Zee, D.S. Miles, F.A. *et al.* (1980), Oculomotor deficits in monkeys with floccular lesions. *Soc Neurosci Abstr*, **6**, 474.

O'Rahilly, R. (1983), The timing and sequence of events in the development of the human eye and ear during the embryonic period proper. *Anat Embryol*, **168**, 87.

Orzalesi, N., Riva, A. and Testa, F. (1971), *J Submicrosc Cytol*, **3**, 283.

Osborne, N.N. (1983), The occurrence of serotonergic nerves in the bovine cornea. *Neurosciences*, **35**, 15.

Osterberg, G. (1935), Topography of the layer of rods and cones in the human retina. *Acta Ophthalmol Suppl*, **6**, 1.

Packer, O., Hendrickson, A.E. and Curcio, C.A. (1990), Developmental redistribution of photoreceptors across the *Macaca nemestrina* (pigtail macaque) retina. *J Comp Neurol*, **298**, 472.

Paget, D.M. (1945) The circle of Willis, in *Intra-Cranial Arterial Aneurysms* (ed. W.E. Dandy), New York.

Palkama, A., Lehtosalo, J. and Uusitalo, H. (1984), 5-hydroxytryptamine receptors in the cornea and ciliary processes of the rat and human eyes. *Ophthal Res*, **16**, 207.

Palkama, A., Uusitalo, H. and Lehtosalo, J. (1986), Innervation of the anterior segment of the eye: with special reference to functional aspects. *Neurohistochemistry*, **1986**, 587.

Palkama, A., Uusitalo, H., Lehtosalo, J. *et al.* (1984), 5-HT nerves in the anterior segment of the eye & the effect of ketanserin in intraocular pressure (IOP) in normal and sympathectomized animals, in *Proceedings of the International Seminar on Selected Topics of Eye Research* (ed. M. di Vincentiis), Baccini & Chiappi, Firenze, p. 70.

Palmer, L.A., Rosenquist, A.C. and Tusa, R. (1975), Visual receptive fields in the lam LGNd, MIN and PN of the cat. *Neurosci Abstr*, **1**, 54.

Palumbo, L.T. (1976), A new concept of the sympathetic pathways to the eye. *Ann Ophthalmol*, **8**, 947.

Panda-Jonas, S., Jonas, J.B., Jakobczyk, M. and Schneider, U. (1994), Retinal photoreceptor count, retinal surface area, and optic disc size in normal human eyes. *Ophthalmology*, **101**, 519.

Pandolfi, M. and Astedt, B. (1971), Outflow resistance in the fetal eye. *Acta Ophthalmol (Kbh)*, **49**, 344.

Panula, P., Hadjiconstantinou, M., Yang, H.Y.T. *et al.* (1983), Immunohistochemical localization of tombesin/gastrin-releasing peptide and substance P in primary sensory neurons. *J Neurosci*, **3**, 2021.

Papaconstantinou, J. (1967), Molecular aspects of lens cell differentiation. *Science*, **156**, 338.

Paranko, J., Kallsjoki, M., Pelliniemi, L. *et al.* (1986), Transient co-expression of cytokeratin and vimentin in differentiating rat sertoli-cells. *Dev Biol*, **117**, 35.

Parkinson, D. (1972), Anatomy of the cavernous sinus. *Neuro-ophthalmol*, **6**, 73.

Parkinson, D., Johnston, J. and Chaudhuri, A. (1978), Sympathetic connections to the fifth and sixth cranial nerves. *Anat Rec*, **191**, 221.

Parkinson, J.K. and Mishkin, M. (1982), *Soc Neurosci Abstr*, **8**, 23.

Parmigiani, C.M. and McAvoy, J.W. (1989), A morphometric analysis of the development of the rat lens capsule. *Curr Eye Res*. **8**, 1271.

Parsons, J.H. (1924), The physiology of pupil reactions. *Trans Ophthalmol Soc UK*, **44**, 1.

Partlow, G.D., Colonnier, M. and Szabo, J. (1977), Thalamic projections of the superior colliculus in the rhesus monkey, *Macaca mulatta*. A light and electron microscopic study. *J Comp Neurol*, **73**, 285.

Pasquier, D.A. and Reinoso-Suarez, F. (1976), Direct projections from hypothalamus to hippocampus in the rat demonstrated by retrograde transport of horseradish peroxidase. *Brain Res*, **108**, 165.

Patel, S., Marshall, J. and Fitzke, F.W. (1993), Shape and radius of posterior corneal surface. *Refract Corneal Surg*, **9**, 173.

Payrau, P., Pouliquen, Y., Faure, J.P. *et al.* (1967), *La Transparence de la Cornee. Les Mechanismes de ses Alterations*. Paul Masson, Paris, p. 1.

Peachey, L.D. (1971), The structure of the extraocular muscle fibers of mammals; in *The Control of Eye Movements* (eds P. Bach-y-Rita, C.C. Collins and J.E. Hyde), Academic Press, New York, p. 47.

Pederson, R.A., Abel, L.A. and Troost, B.T. (1982), Eye movements. *Ocular Anat Embryol Teratol*, **31**, 927.

Penfold, P.L., Provis, J.M., Madigan, M.C. *et al.* (1990), Angiogenesis in normal human retinal development: the involvement of astrocytes and macrophages. *Graefe's Arch Clin Exp Ophthalmol*, **228**, 255.

Perez, G.M. and Keyser, R.B. (1986), Cell body counts in human ciliary ganglia. *Invest Ophthalmol Vis Sci*, **27**, 1428.

Perkins, E.S. (1961), Sensory mechanisms and intraocular pressure. *Exp Eye Res*, **1**, 160.

Perlmutter, D. and Rhoton, A.L. (1976), Microsurgical anatomy of the anterior cerebral-anterior communicating recurrent artery complex. *J Neurosurg*, **45**, 259.

Perrett, D.I., Rolls, E.T. and Caan, W. (1979), Temporal lobe cells of the monkey with visual responses selective for faces. *Neurosciences*, **53**, 53.

Perrett, D.I., Rolls, E.T. and Caan, W. (1982), Visual neurones responses to faces in the monkey temporal cortex. *Exp Brain Res*, **1**, 1.

Peschell, M. (1905), Die strukturlosen Augenmembranen im Ultramikroskop. *A von Graefes Arch Ophthalmol*, **60**, 557.

Peter, J.B., Bernard, R.J., Edgerton, V.R. *et al.* (1972), Metabolic profiles of three fiber types of skeletal muscle in guinea pigs and rabbits. *Biochemistry*, **11**, 2627.

Peters, A. and Palay, S.L. (1966), The morphology of laminae A and A1 of the dorsal nucleus of the lateral geniculate body of the cat. *J Anat*, **100**, 451.

Petersen, R.A., Lee, K.J. and Donn, A. (1965), Acetylcholinesterase in the rabbit cornea. *Arch Ophthalmol*, **73**, 370.

Petersen, S.E., Robinson, D.L. and Currie, J.N. (1989), Influences of lesions of parietal cortex on visual spatial attention in humans. *Exp Brain Res*, **76**, 267.

Peterson, W.S. and Jocson, V.L. (1974), Hyaluronidase effects on aqueous outflow resistance. Quantitative and localising studies in the rhesus monkey eye. *Am J Ophthalmol*, **77**, 573.

Peterson, W.S., Jocson, V.L. and Sears, M.L. (1971), Resistance to aqueous outflow in the rhesus monkey eye. *Am J Ophthalmol*, **72**, 445.

Petras, J.M. (1971), Connections of the parietal lobe. *J Psychiatr Res*, **8**, 189.

Pfeifer, R.A. (1925), *Trans Pacif Coast Oto-ophthalmol Soc*, **43**, 1.

Pfeifer, R.A. (1925), Myelogenetisch-anatomische Untersuchungen uber den zentralen, in *Abschnitt der Schleitung Monograph a.d. G.d. Neurol. u. Psychiat*, Springer-Verlag, Berlin.

Pfister, R.R. (1973), The normal surface of corneal epithelium: a scanning electron microscopic study. *Invest Ophthalmol*, **12**, 654.

Pfister, R.R. (1975a), The normal surface of conjunctiva epithelium. A scanning electron microscopic study. *Invest Ophthalmol*, **14**, 267.

Pfister, R.R. (1975b), The healing of corneal epithelial abrasions in the rabbit: a scanning electron microscope study. *Invest Ophthalmol*, **14**, 648.

Pfister, R.R. and Burstein, N.L. (1976), The normal and abnormal human corneal epithelial surface: a scanning electron microscopic study. *WHO*, **1**, 1.

Phillips, A.J. (1972), *Br J Physiol Opt*, **27**, 141.

Phillipson, B.T. (1969), Distribution of protein within the normal rat lens. *QJ Exp Psychol*, **8**, 258.

Phillipson, B.T., Hanninen, L. and Balazs, E.A. (1975), Cell contacts in human bovine lenses. *Exp Eye Res*, **21**, 205.

Piatigorsky, J., Webster, H. and Wolberg, H. (1972),

Cell elongation in the cultured embryonic chick lens epithelium with and without protein synthesis. *J Cell Biol*, **55**, 82.

Pick, J. (1970), *The Autonomic Nervous System*, Lippincott, Philadelphia.

Pierobon Bormioli, S., Torresan, S., Sartore, S. *et al.* (1979), Immunohistochemical identification of slow-tonic fibers in human extrinsic eye muscles. *Invest Ophthalmol Vis Sci*, **18**, 303.

Pierson, R. and Carpenter, M.B. (1974), Anatomical analysis of pupillary reflex pathways in the rhesus monkey. *J Comp Neurol*, **158**, 121.

Pilar, G. and Hess, A. (1966), Differences in internal structure and nerve terminals of the slow and twitch muscle fibers in the cat superior oblique. *Anat Rec*, **154**, 243.

Pleyer, U., Hartmann, C. and Sterry, W. (1997) Aeolus Press, Buren, The Netherlands, p. 1 (in press).

Podhoranyi, G. (1966), Uber die Becherzellen der Bindehaut. *A von Graefes Arch Ophthalmol*, *169*, 285.

Poggio, G.F., Baker, F.H., Mansfield, R.J.W. *et al.* (1975), Spatial and chromatic properties of neurons subserving foveal and parafoveal vision in rhesus monkeys. *Brain Res*, **100**, 25.

Poggio, G.F., Doty, J.R. and Talbot, W.H. (1977), Foveal striate cortex of behaving monkey: single-neuron responses to square-wave gratings during fixation of gaze. *J Neurophysiol*, **40**, 1369.

Poggio, G.F. and Fischer, B. (1977), Binocular interaction and depth sensitivity in striate and prestriate cortex of behaving rhesus monkey. *J Neurophysiol*, **40**, 1392.

Poirier, P. (1911), *Traite d'Anatomie Humaine*, 3rd edition, no. 5: *Les Organes du Sens*.

Pola, J. and Wyatt, H.J. (1980), Target position and velocity: the stimuli for smooth pursuit eye movements. *Vision Res*, **20**, 523.

Polgar, J., Johnson, M.A., Weightman, D. *et al.* (1973), Data on fibre size in thirty-six human muscles – an autopsy study. *J Neurol Sci*, **19**, 307.

Polyak, S.L. (1934), Projection of the retina upon the cerebral cortex, based upon experiments with monkeys. *Proceedings of the Association for Research in Nervous and Mental Diseases*, Williams & Wilkins, Baltimore, p. 535.

Polyak, S.L. (1941), *The Retina*, University of Chicago Press, Chicago.

Polyak, S.L. (1957), In *The Vertebrate Visual System* (ed. H. Kluver), University of Chicago Press, Chicago, p. 1390.

Polyak, S.L. (1957), *The Vertebrate Visual System*. University of Chicago Press, Chicago.

Porte, A., Brini, A. and Stoeckel, M.E. (1975), Fine structure of the lens epithelium. *Ann Ophthalmol*, **7**, 623.

Porter, A. (1984), Localization of neurons providing afferent and efferent innervation of monkey extraocular muscles. *Soc Neurosci Abstr*, **1**, 1.

Porter, J.D. (1986), Brainstem terminations of extraocular muscle primary afferent neurons in the monkey. *J Comp Neurol*, **247**, 133.

Porter, J.D., Burns, L.A. and May, P.J. (1989), Morphological substrate for eyelid movements: innervation and structure of primate levator palpebrae superioris and orbicularis oculi muscle. *J Comp Neurol*, **287**, 64.

Porter, J.D., Guthrie, B.L. and Sparks, D.L. (1983), Innervation of monkey extraocular muscles: localization of sensory and motor neurons by retrograde transport of horseradish peroxidase. *J Comp Neurol*, **218**, 208.

Porter, J.D. and Spencer, R.F. (1982), Localization and morphology of cat extraocular muscle afferent neurones identified by retrograde transport of horseradish peroxidaase. *J Comp Neurol*, **204**, 56.

Posner, M.I., Walker, J.A., Friedrich, F.J. *et al.* (1984), *J Neurosci*, **4**, 1863.

Pow, D.V., Crook, D.K. and Wong, R.O. (1994), Early appearance and transient expression of putative amino acid neurotransmitters and related molecules in the developing rabbit retina: an immunocytochemical study. *Vis Neurosci*, **11**, 1115.

Precht, W. (1978), *Neuronal Operations in the Vestibular System*, Springer-Verlag, New York.

Precht, W. (1979), Vestibular mechanisms. *Ann Rev Neurosci*, **2**, 265.

Precht, W. (1982), Anatomical and functional organization of optokinetic pathways, in *Functional Basis of Ocular Motility Disorders* (eds G. Lennerstrand, D.S. Zee and E.L. Keller), Pergamon Press, Oxford, p. 18.

Priestley-Smith, J.B. (1890), On the size of the cornea in relation to age, sex, refraction and primary glaucoma. *Trans Ophthalmol Soc UK*, **10**, 68.

Probst, M. (1906), Uber die zentralen sinnesbahnen und die sinneszentren des menschlichen gehirnes. *Sber Akad Wiss Wien*, **115**, 103.

Provis, J.M. (1987), Patterns of cell death in the ganglion cell layer of the human fetal retina. *J Comp Neurol*, **259**, 237.

Provis, J.M., van Driel, D., Billson, F.A. *et al.* (1985a), Development of the human retina: patterns of cell distribution and redistribution in the ganglion cell layer. *J Comp Neurol*, **233**, 429.

Provis, J.M., van Driel, D., Billson, F.A. *et al.* (1985b), Human fetal optic nerve: overproduction and elimination of retinal axons during development. *J Comp Neurol*, **238**, 92.

Prydal, J.I. (1990), *Invest Ophthalmol Vis Sci*, **30**, 470.

Prydal, J.I. and Campbell, F.W. (1992), Study of precorneal tear film thickness and structure by interferometry and confocal microscopy. *Invest Ophthalmol Vis Sci*, **33**, 1996.

Purpura, D.P. and Yahr, M.D. (1966), *The Thalamus*, Columbia University Press, New York.

Quain, R. (1900), *Elements of Anatomy*, Vol. III (eds E.A. Schaffer and G.D. Thane), London.

Quain, R. (1908), *Quain's Elements of Anatomy*, 11th edition (eds E.A. Schafer and G.D. Thane), Longmans, Green & Co, London.

Quigley, H.A. (1986), Pathophysiology of the optic nerve in glaucoma, in *Glaucoma* (eds J.A. McAllister and R.P. Wilson), Butterworth, London, p. 30.

Quigley, H.A. and Addicks, E.M. (1981), Regional differences in the structure of the lamina cribrosa and their relation to glaucomatous optic nerve damage. *Arch Ophthalmol*, **99**, 137.

Quigley, H.A., Addicks, E.M., Green, W.R. *et al.* (1981), Optic nerve damage in human glaucoma II. The site of injury and susceptibility to damage. *Arch Ophthalmol*, **99**, 635.

Quigley, H.A., Coleman, A.L. and Dorman-Pease, M.E.

(1991), Larger optic nerve heads have more nerve fibers in normal monkey eyes. *Arch Ophthalmol*, **109**, 1443.

Quigley, H.A., Hohman, R.M., Addicks, E.M. *et al.* (1983), Morphologic changes in the lamina cribrosa correlated with neural loss in open angle glaucoma. *Am J Ophthalmol*, **95**, 673.

Rabl, C. (1903), *Uber den Bau und Entwicklung der Linse*, Leipzig.

Raczkowsky, D. and Diamond, I.T. (1978), Cells of origin of several efferent pathways from the superior colliculus in Galago senegalensis. *Brain Res*, **146**, 351.

Radius, R.L. (1981), Regional specificity in anatomy at the lamina cribrosa. *Arch Ophthalmol*, **99**, 478.

Radius, R.L. and Anderson, D.R. (1979a), The course of axons through the retina and optic nerve head. *Arch Ophthalmol*, **97**, 1154.

Radius, R.L. and Anderson, D.R. (1979b), The histology of retinal nerve fiber layer bundles and bundle defects. *Arch Ophthalmol*, **97**, 948.

Radius, R.L. and Gonzales, M. (1981), Anatomy of the lamina cribrosa in human eyes. *Arch Ophthalmol*, **99**, 2159.

Rae, A.S.L. (1961), Bilateral infarction of calcarine cortex with lateral geniculate degeneration. *Confin Neurol*, **21**, 225.

Rae, J.L. and Kuszak, J.R. (1983), The electrical coupling of epithelium and fibers in the frog lens. *Exp Eye Res*, **36**, 317.

Rae, J.L. and Stacey, T.R. (1979), Lanthanum and procion yellow as extracellular markers in the crystalline lens of the rat. *Exp Eye Res*, **28**, 1.

Raeder, J.G. (1924), Paratrigeminal paralysis of oculo-pupillary sympathetic. *Brain*, **47**, 149.

Rafal, R.D. and Grimm, R.J. (1981), Progressive supranuclear palsy: functional analysis of the response to methysergide and antiparkinsonian agents. *Neurology*, **31**, 1507.

Rafal, R.D. and Posner, M.I. (1987), Deficits in human visual spatial attention following thalamic lesions. *Proc Natl Acad Sci USA*, **84**, 7349.

Rafferty, N.S. (1963), Studies of an injury induced growth in the frog lens. *Anat Rec*, **146**, 299.

Rafferty, N.S. (1967), Proliferative response in experimentally injured frog lens epithelium: autoradiographic evidence for movement of DNA synthesis toward injury. *J Morphol*, **121**, 295.

Rafferty, N.S. (1972a), The cytoarchitecture of normal mouse lens epithelium. *Anat Rec*, **173**, 225.

Rafferty, N.S. (1972b), Mechanism of repair of lenticular wounds in Rana pipiens: I. Role of cell migration. *J Morphol*, **133**, 409.

Rafferty, N.S. and Goossens, W. (1977), Ultrastructure of traumatic cataractogenesis in the frog: a comparison with mouse and human lens. *Am J Anat*, **148**, 385.

Rafferty, N.S. and Goossens, W. (1978), Cytoplasmic filaments in the crystalline lens of various species: functional correlations. *Exp Eye Res*, **26**, 177.

Rafferty, N.S. and Scholz, D.L. (1984), Polygonal arrays of microfilaments in epithelial cells of the intact lens. *Curr Eye Res*, **3**, 1141.

Rafferty, N.S. and Scholz, D.L. (1989), Comparative study of actin filament patterns in lens epithelial cells. Are these determined by the mechanism of lens accommodation? *Curr Eye Res*, **8**, 569.

Ramaekers, F.C.S. and Bloemendal, H. (1981), Cytoskeletal and contractile structures in lens cell differentiation, in *Molecular and Cellular Biology of the Eye Lens* (ed. H. Bloemendal), John Wiley and Sons, New York, p. 85.

Ramrattan, R.S., van der Schaft, T.L., Mooy, C.M *et al.* (1994), Morphometric analysis of Bruch's membrane, the choriocapillaris, and the choroid in aging. *Invest Ophthalmol Vis Sci*, **35**(6), 2857.

Ranson, S.W. (1943), *The Anatomy of the Nervous System*, W.B. Saunders, Philadelphia.

Ranson, S.W. and Magoun, H.W. (1933), *Arch Neurol Psychiat*, **30**, 1193.

Ranson, S.W. and Magoun, H.W. (1939), The hypothalamus. *Ergeb Physiol*, **41**, 56.

Rao, V., Friend, J., Thoft, R.A. *et al.* (1987), Conjunctival goblet cells and mitotic rate in children with retinol deficiency and measles. *Arch Ophthalmol*, **105**, 378.

Raphan, T. and Cohen, B. (1978), Brainstem mechanisms for rapid and slow eye movements. *Ann Rev Physiol*, **40**, 527.

Rapuano, C.J., Fishbaugh, J.A. and Strike, D.J. (1993), Nine point corneal thickness measurements and keratometry readings in normal corneas using ultrasound pachymetry. *Insight*, **18**, 16.

Rasmussen, A.T. (1940), Effects of hypophysectomy and hypophysial stalk resection on the hypothalamic nuclei of animals and man. *Res Publ Ass Nerv Ment Dis*, **20**, 245.

Rasmussen, L. and Windle, W.F. (1960), *Neural Mechanisms of the Auditory and Vestibular Systems*, Charles C. Thomas, Springfield, IL.

Ratcliffe, G. and Davies-Jones, G.A.B. (1972), Defective localization in focal brain wounds. *Brain*, **95**, 49.

Raviola, G. (1971), The fine structure of the ciliary zonule and ciliary epithelium with special regard to the organization and insertion of the zonular fibrils. *Invest Ophthalmol*, **10**, 851.

Raviola, G. (1974), Effects of paracentesis on the blood–aqueous barrier: an electron microscope study on *Macaca mulatta* using horseradish peroxidase as a tracer. *Invest Ophthalmol*, **13**, 828.

Raviola, G. (1977), The structural basis of the blood ocular barriers. *Exp Eye Res Suppl*, **27**, 27.

Raviola, G. and Raviola, E. (1975), Intercellular junctions in the ciliary epithelium of the rhesus monkey. *Anat Rec*, **181**, 539.

Raviola, G. and Raviola, E. (1981), Paracellular route of aqueous outflow in the trabecular meshwork and canal of Schlemm. *Invest Ophthalmol Vis Sci*, **21**, 52.

Raviola, G., Sagaties, M.-J. and Miller, C. (1987), Intercellular junctions between fibroblasts in connective tissues of the eye in Macaque monkeys. *Invest Ophthalmol Vis Sci*, **28**, 834.

Reddan, J., Weinsieder, A. and Wilson, D. (1979), Aqueous humor from traumatized eyes triggers cell division in the epithelia of cultured lenses. *Exp Eye Res*, **28**, 267.

Rees, P.M. (1967), Observations on the fine structure and distribution of presumptive baroreceptor nerves at the carotid sinus. *J Comp Neurol*, **131**, 517.

Reese, A.B. (1934), Ciliary processes; their relationship to intra-ocular surgery. *Am J Ophthalmol*, **17**, 422.

Reese, T.S. and Karnovsky, M.J. (1967), Fine structural localization of a blood–brain barrier to exogenous peroxidase. *J Cell Biol*, **34**, 207.

Reichlin, S., Baldessarini, R.J. and Martin, J.B. (eds) (1978), *The Hypothalamus*, Raven Press, New York.

Reinstein, D.Z., Silverman, R.H., Rondeau, M.J. *et al.* (1994), Epithelial and corneal thickness measurements by high-frequency ultrasound digital signal processing. *Ophthalmology*, **101**, 140.

Reme, C. and d'Épinay, S.L. (1981), Periods of development of the normal human chamber angle. *Doc Ophthalmol*, **51**, 241.

Ren, Z.X., Brewton, R.G. and Mayne, R. (1991), An analysis by rotary shadowing of the mammalian vitreous humor and zonular apparatus. *J Ultrastruct Biol*, **106**, 56.

Renard, G., Hirsch, M., Galle, P. *et al.* (1976), Ciliated cells of corneal endothelium. Functional and morphological aspects compared to cilia of other organs. *Arch Ophtalmol, Paris*, **36**, 59.

Renard, G., Lemasson, C. and Saraux, H. (1965), *Anatomie de l'Oeil et de ses Annexes*, Paul Masson, Paris.

Rentsch, F.J. and Van der Zypen, E. (1971), Altersbedingte veranderungen der sog. Membrana limitons interna des ziliakorpers im menschlichen auge. *Aging Dev*, **1**, 70.

Retziu, S. (1871), Om membrana limitans retinae interna. *Nord Med Ark*, **111**, 1.

Revel, J.P. and Karnovsky, M.J. (1967), Hexagonal array of subunits in intercellular junctions of the mouse heart and liver. *J Cell Biol*, **33**, 450.

Rhodes, R.H. (1978), Development of the human optic disc: light microscopy. *Am J Anat*, **153**, 601.

Rhodes, R.H. (1979), A light microscopic study of the developing human neural retina. *Am J Anat*, **154**, 195.

Rhodin, J.A.G. (1968), Ultrastructure of mammalian venous capillaries, venules and small collecting veins. *J Ultrastruct Res*, **25**, 452.

Rhoton, A.L., Harris, F.S. and Renn, W.H. (1977), Microsurgical anatomy of the sellar region and cavernous sinus. *Neuro-ophthalmol*, **9**, 1.

Rhoton, A.L., Obayashi, S. and Hollinshead, W.A.H. (1968), *J Neurosurg*, **29**, 609.

Richmond, F.J.R., Johnston, W.S.W., Baker, R.S. *et al.* (1984), Palisade endings in human extraocular muscles. *Invest Ophthalmol Vis Sci*, **25**, 471.

Ridgeway, E.B. and Gordon, A.M. (1975), Muscle activation: effects of small length changes on calcium release in single fibers. *Science*, **189**, 881.

Rimmer, S., Keating, C., Chou, T. *et al.* (1993), Growth of the human optic disk and nerve during gestation, childhood, and early adulthood. *Am J Ophthalmol*, **116**, 748.

Ring, H. and Fujino, T. (1967), Observations on the anatomy and pathology of the choroidal vasculature. *Arch Ophthalmol*, **78**, 431.

Ringel, S.P., Engel, W.K., Bender, A.N. *et al.* (1978a), Histochemistry and acetylcholine receptor distribution in normal and denervated monkey extraocular muscles. *Neurology*, **28**, 55.

Ringel, S.P., Wilson, W.B., Barden, M.T. *et al.* (1978b), Histochemistry of human extraocular muscle. *Arch Ophthalmol*, **96**, 1067.

Risco, J.M., Grimson, B.S. and Johnson, P.T. (1981), Angioarchitecture of the ciliary artery circulation of the posterior pole. *Arch Ophthalmol*, **99**, 864.

Rittig, M., Lutjen-Drecoll, E., Rauterberg, J. *et al.* (1990), Type-VI collagen in the human iris and ciliary body. *Cell Tissue Res*, **259**, 305.

Robinson, D.A. (1965), The mechanics of human smooth pursuit eye movement. *J Physiol*, **180**, 569.

Robinson, D.A. (1972), Eye movements evoked by collicular stimulation in the alert monkey. *Vision Res*, **12**, 1795.

Robinson, D.A. (1973), Models of the saccadic eye movement control system. *Kybernetik*, **14**, 71.

Robinson, D.A. (1975), Oculomotor control signals, in *Basic Mechanisms of Ocular Motility and their Clinical Implications* (eds G. Lennerstrand and P. Bach-y-Rita), Pergamon Press, Oxford, p. 337.

Robinson, D.A. (1982a), Plasticity in the oculomotor system. *Fed Proc*, **41**, 2153.

Robinson, D.A. (1982b), A model of cancellation of the vestibulo-ocular reflex, in *Functional Basis of Ocular Motility Disorders* (eds G. Lennerstrand, D.S. Zee and E.L. Keller), Pergamon Press, Oxford.

Robinson, D.A. and Fuchs, A.F. (1969), Eye movements evoked by stimulation of frontal eye fields. *J Neurophysiol*, **32**, 637.

Robinson, D.L. and McClurkin, J.W. (1989), in *The Neurobiology of Saccadic Eye Movements* (eds R.H. Wurtz and M.E. Goldberg), Elsevier, New York, p. 337.

Robinson, D.L., McClurkin, J.W. and Kertzman, C. (1990), Orbital position and eye movement influences on visual responses in the pulvinar nuclei of the behaving macaque. *Exp Brain Res*, **82**, 235.

Robinson, D.L. and Petersen, S.E. (1992), The pulvinar and visual salience. *TINS* **15**, 127.

Robinson, D.L. and Wurtz, R.H. (1976), Use of an extra retinal signal by monkey superior colliculus neurons to distinguish real from self-induced stimulus movement. *J Neurophysiol*, **39**, 852.

Rodrigues, M.M., Hackett, J. and Donohoo, P. (1987), Iris, in *Biomedical Foundations of Ophthalmology*, vol. 1 (eds T.D. Duane and E.A. Jaeger), Harper & Row, Philadelphia.

Rodrigues, M.M., Rowden, G., Hackett, J. *et al.* (1981), Langerhans cells in the normal conjunctiva and peripheral cornea of selected species. *Invest Ophthalmol Vis Sci*, **21**, 759.

Rodrigues, M.M., Sivalingham, E. and Weinreb, S. (1976), Histopathology of 150 trabeculectomy specimens in glaucoma. *Trans Ophthalmol Soc UK*, **96**, 245.

Rodriguez-Boulan, E. and Nelson, W.J. (1989), Morphogenesis of the polarized epithelial cell phenotype. *Science*, **245**, 718.

Rogers, J.H. and Hunt, S.P. (1987), Carbonic anhydrase-II messenger RNA IN neurons and glia of chick brain: mapping by *in situ* hybridization. *Neurosci*, **23**, 343.

Rohen, H. (1964), *Das Auge und seine Hilfsorgene*.

Rohen, J.W. (1952), Der ziliarkorper als functionelles system. *Morph Jahrbuch*, **92**, 415.

Rohen, J.W. (1956), Über den Ansatz der Ciliarmuskulatur im Bereich des Kammerwinkels. *Ophthalmologica*, **131**, 51.

Rohen, J.W. (1961), Comparative and experimental studies on the iris of primates. *Am J Ophthalmol*, **52**, 384.

Rohen, J.W. (1964), Ciliarkorper (Corpus ciliare) in *Handbuch der mikroskopischen Anatomie des Menschen*. pt. 4, *Haut und Sinnesorgane. Das Auge und seine Hilfsorgane*, 3rd edition (eds W.V. Mollendorf and W. Bargmann), Springer-Verlag, New York, p. 189.

Rohen, J.W. (1979), Scanning electron microscopic studies of the zonular appartus in human and monkey eyes. *Invest Ophthalmol Vis Sci*, **18**, 133.

Rohen, J.W. (1989), Altersveranderungen im Bereich des vorderen Augensegments, in *Handbuch der Gerontologie*, 3rd edition (eds D. Platt, O. Hochwin and H.-J. Merte), p. 68.

Rohen, J.W., Futa, R. and Lütjen-Drecoll, E. (1981), The fine structure of the cribriform meshwork in normal and glaucomatous eyes as seen in tangential sections. *Invest Ophthalmol Vis Sci*, **21**, 574.

Rohen, J.W., Kaufman, P.L., Eichhorn, M. *et al.* (1989), Functional morphology of accommodation in the racoon. *Exp Eye Res*, **48**, 523.

Rohen, J.W. and Lütjen-Drecoll, E. (1971), Age changes of the trabecular meshwork in human and monkey eyes, in *Ageing and Development, vol. 1*, (eds H. Bredt and J.W. Rohen), Schattauer Verlag, Stuttgart, p.1.

Rohen, J.W. and Lütjen-Drecoll, E. (1981), Ageing- and non-ageing processes within the connective tissues of the anterior segment of the eye, in *Biochemical and Morphological Aspects of Ageing* (ed. W.E.G. Müller and J.W. Rohen), Franz Steiner Verlag GmbH, Wiesbaden, p. 157.

Rohen, J.W., Lütjen-Drecoll, E. and Bárány, E.H. (1967), The relation between the ciliary muscle and the trabecular meshwork and its importance for the effect of miotics on aqueous outflow resistance. A study in two contrasting monkey species, *Macaca irus* and *Cercopithecus aethiops*. *A von Graefes Arch Klin Exp Ophthalmol*, **172**, 23.

Rohen, J.W. and Rentsch, F.J. (1969), Der Konstruktive Bau des Zonula apparates beim Menschen und dessen-funktionelle Bedeutung Grundlagen fur eine neue Akkommodation. *Graefes Arch Klin Exp Ophthalmol*, **178**, 1.

Rohen, J.W. and Unger, H.H. (1959), Zur morphologie und pathologie der kammerbucht des auges. *Abhandlg Mainz Akad D Wiss U Lit, Mathem-Naturwiss Klasse*, **3**, 1.

Rohen, J.W. and Witmer, R. (1972), Electron microscopic studies on the trabecular meshwork in glaucoma simplex. *A von Graefes Arch Klin Exp Ophthalmol*, **183**, 251.

Rohrschneider, K., Burk, R.O.W., Kruse, F.E. and Völcker, H.E. (1994), Reproducibility of the optic nerve head topography with a new laser tomographic scanning device. *Ophthalmology*, **101**, 1044.

Roll, P., Reich, M. and Hofmann, H. (1975), Der Verlauf der Zonulafasern. *A von Graefes Arch Klin Exp Ophthalmol*, **195**, 41.

Ron, S. and Robinson, D.A. (1973), Eye movements evoked by cerebellar stimulation in the alert monkey. *J Neurophysiol*, **36**, 1004.

Rones, B. (1958), A mechanistic element in trabecular function. *Am J Ophthalmol*, **45**, 189.

Ronne, H. (1914), Die anatomische projektion der maula im corpus geniculatum externa. *Zentralbl ges Neurol Psychiat*, **22**, 469.

Rosengren, B. (1928), Zur Frage der mechanik der mechanik der tranenbleiking. *Acta Ophthalmol*, **6**, 367.

Ross, R. and Bornstein, P. (1969), The elastic fiber: I. The separation and partial characterization of its macromolecular components. *J Cell Biol*, **40**, 366.

Rossignol, S. and Collonier, M. (1971), A light microscope study of degeneration patterns in cat cortex after lesions of the lateral geniculate nucleus. *Vision Res*, **3**, 329.

Rothstein, H. (1968), Experimental techniques for the investigation of the amphibian lens epithelium, in *Methods in Cell Physiology* (ed D.M. Prescott), Academic Press, New York, p. 45.

Rothstein, H., Reddan, J.R. and Weinsieder, A. (1965), Response to injury in the lens epithelium of the bullfrog: II. Spatio-temporal patterns of DNA synthesis and mitosis. *Exp Cell Res*, **37**, 440.

Rothstein, H., Weinsieder, A. and Blaiklock, R. (1964), Response to injury in the lens epithelium of the bullfrog, *Rana catesbeina*. *Exp Cell Res*, **35**, 548.

Rouviere, H. (1967), *Anatomie Humaine Descriptive et Topographique. Dixieme ed. Rev. augm. par A. Delmas, T.I. Tete et cou*. Paul Masson, Paris.

Rowlerson, A.M. (1987), Fibre types in extraocular muscles. *ESA Symposium Text*, **1**, 19.

Rucker, C.W. (1958), The concept of a semidecussation of the optic nerves. *Arch Ophthalmol*, **59**, 159.

Ruiz i Altaba, A. and Melton, D.A. (1990), Axial patterning and the establishment of polarity in the frog embryo. *Trends Genet*, **6**, 57.

Ruskell, G.L. (1965), *The Structure of the Eye*. Schattauer, Stuttgart.

Ruskell, G.L. (1968), The fine structure of nerve terminations in the lacrimal glands of monkeys. *J Anat*, **103**, 65.

Ruskell, G.L. (1970a), An ocular parasympathetic nerve pathway of facial nerve origin and its influence on intraocular pressure. *Exp Eye Res*, **10**, 319.

Ruskell, G.L. (1970b), The orbital branches of the pterygo-palatine ganglion and their relationship with internal carotid nerve branches in primates. *J Anat*, **106**, 323.

Ruskell, G.L. (1971a), The distribution of autonomic post-ganglionic nerve fibres to the lacrimal gland in monkeys. *J Anat*, **109**, 229.

Ruskell, G. (1971b), Facial parasympathetic innervation of the choroidal blood vessels in monkeys. *Exp Eye Res*, **12**, 166.

Ruskell, G.L. (1972), Dual innervation of the central artery of the retina in monkeys, in *The Optic Nerve* (ed. J.S. Cant), Henry Kimpton, London, p. 48.

Ruskell, G.L. (1973), Sympathetic innervation of the ciliary muscle in monkey. *Exp Eye Res*, **16**, 183.

Ruskell, G.L. (1975), Nerve terminals and epithelial cell variety in the human lacrimal gland. *Cell Tissue Res*, **158**, 121.

Ruskell, G.L. (1976), The source of nerve fibres of the trabeculae and adjacent structures in monkey eyes. *Exp Eye Res*, **23**, 449.

Ruskell, G.L. (1978), The fine structure of innervated myotendinous cylinders in extraocular muscles of Rhesus monkeys. *J Neurocytol*, **7**, 693.

Ruskell, G.L. (1979), The incidence and variety of Golgi tendon organs in extraocular muscles of the Rhesus monkey. *J Neurocytol*, **8**, 639.

Ruskell, G.L. (1982), Innervation of the anterior segment of the eye, in *Basic Aspects of Glaucoma Research* (ed E. Lütjen-Drecoll), Schattauer Verlag, Stuttgart, p. 49.

Ruskell, G.L. (1983), Fibre analysis of the nerve to the inferior oblique muscle in monkeys. *J Anat*, **137**, 445.

Ruskell, G.L. (1984a), Sheathing of muscle fibres at neuromuscular junctions and at extra-junctional loci in human extra-ocular muscles. *J Anat*, **138**, 33.

Ruskell, G.L. (1984b), Quelques observations sur les fuseaux des muscles oculo-moteurs humains. *J Fr Ophthalmol*, **7**, 665.

Ruskell, G.L. (1985a), Innervation of the conjunctiva. *Trans Ophthalmol Soc UK*, **104**, 390.

Ruskell, G.L. (1985b), Facial nerve distribution to the eye. *Am J Optom Physiol Optics*, **62**, 793.

Ruskell, G.L. and Griffiths, T. (1979), Peripheral nerve pathway to the ciliary muscle. *Exp Eye Res*, **28**, 277.

Ruskell, G.L. and Simons, T. (1992), The internal carotid artery has a sleeve of increased innervation density within the cavernous sinus in monkeys. *Brain Res*, **595**, 116.

Ruskell, G.L. and Wilson, J. (1983), Spiral nerve endings and dapple motor end plates in monkey extraocular muscles. *J Anat*, **136**, 85.

Rutnin, U. (1967), Fundus appearance in normal eyes. I. The choroid. *Am J Ophthalmol*, **64**, 821.

Saari, M. (1972a), Fine structure of the microcirculatory bed of the pig iris. *Ann Med Exp Biol Fenn*, **50**, 12.

Saari, M. (1975), Ultrastructure of the microvessels of the iris in mammals with special reference to their permeability. *Albrecht von Graefes Arch Klin Exp Ophthalmol*, **194**, 87.

Sacks, J.G. (1985), The levator-trochlear muscle. A supernumerary orbital structure. *Arch Ophthalmol*, **103**, 540.

Sadun, A. (1984), An undescribed human visual pathway mediating circadian rhythms. Presented at the 5th International Neuro-ophthalmology Society Meeting, Antwerp, Belgium, May 14–18.

Saha, M.S., Clayton, L. and Grainger, R.M. (1989), Embryonic lens induction: more than meets the optic vesicle. *Diff Dev*, **28**, 153.

Sakai, L.Y., Keene, D.R. and Engvall, E. (1986), Fibrillin, a new 350-kd glycoprotein, is a component of extracellular microfibrils. *J Cell Biol*, **103**, 2499.

Sakai, L.Y. *et al.* (1991), Purification and partial characterisation of fibrillin, a cysteine-rich structural component of connective tissue microfibrils. *J Biol Chem*, **266**, 14763.

Salamon, G., Guerinel, G., Louis, R. *et al.* (1965), Etude radio-anatomique de l'artere ophthalmique. *Ann Radiol*, **8**, 557.

Salamon, G., Raybund, C. and Griscoli, F. (1971), Anatomical study of the blood vessels of the orbit, in *Proceedings of the Second Congress of the European Association of Radiology*, Amsterdam, p. 284.

Salatapek, M. and Banks, M.S. (1978), Infant sensory assessment: vision. *Acta Ophthalmol Suppl*, **1**, 1.

Salzmann, M. (1912), *The Anatomy and Histology of the Human Eyeball in the Normal State. Its Development and Senescence* (translated by E.V.L. Brown), University of Chicago Press, Chicago.

Sanders, K.M. and Ward, S.M. (1992), Nitric-oxide as a mediator of nonadrenergic noncholinergic neurotransmission. *Am J Physiol*, **262**, G379.

Sanderson, K.J. (1971), The projection of the visual field to the lateral geniculate and medial interlaminar nuclei in the cat. *J Comp Neurol*, **143**, 101.

Sano, K., Mayanagi, Y., Sekino, H. *et al.* (1970), Results of stimulation and destruction of the posterior hypothalamus in man. *J Neurosurg*, **33**, 689.

Saper, C.B., Loewy, A.D., Swanson, L.W. *et al.* (1976), Direct hypothalamo-autonomic connections. *Brain Res*, **117**, 305.

Sappey, P.C. (1867), *Anatomie Descriptive*, 4th edition, Paris.

Sappey, P.C. (1888), *Traite d'Anatomie Descriptive*, 4th edition. *Part 2: Myologie–angiologie*, Delahaye & Lecrosnier, Paris.

Sarks, S.H. (1976), Ageing and degeneration in the macular region: a clinico-pathological study. *Br J Ophthalmol*, **60**, 324.

Sartore, S., Mascarello, F., Rowlerson, A. *et al.* (1987), Fibre types in extraocular muscles: a new myosin isoform in the fast fibres. *J Muscle Res Cell Motil*, **8**, 161.

Sasaki, K. (1963), Electrophysiological studies on oculomotor neurons in the cat. *Jpn J Physiol*, **13**, 287.

Sato, K. (1965), Studies on the swelling and the uptake of radio-active sulphate in the rabbit corneal stroma after removal of the epithelium and endothelium. *Jpn J Ophthalmol*, **9**, 92.

Savino, P.J., Paris, M., Schatz, N.J. *et al.* (1978), Optic tract syndrome. A review of 21 patients. *Arch Ophthalmol*, **96**, 656.

Sawaki, Y. (1977), Retino-hypothalamic projection: electrophysiological evidence for the existence in female rats. *Brain Res*, **120**, 336.

Scalia, F. (1972), The termination of retinal axons in the pretectal region of mammals. *J Comp Neurol*, **145**, 223.

Schaeffer, J.P. (1924), Some points in the regional anatomy of the optic pathway with special reference to tumors of the hypophysis cerebri; and resulting ocular changes. *Anat Rec*, **28**, 243.

Schall, B.F., Burns, M.S. and Bellhorn, R.S. (1980), Potential ultrastructural sites of unusual permeability in the feline iris. *ARVO Suppl: Invest Ophthalmol Vis Sci*, **19**, 35.

Schatz, C.J. (1977), Anatomy of interhemispheric connections in the visual system of Boston Siamese and ordinary cats. *J Comp Neurol*, **173**, 497.

Schenker, H.W. and Yablonski, M.E. (1981), Fluorophotometric study of epinephrine and timolol in human subjects. *Arch Ophthalmol*, **99**, 1212.

Schiefferdecker, P. (1904), Eine Eigentümlichkeit im Baue der Augenmuskeln. *Dtsch med Wschr*, **30**, 725.

Schiller, P.H., Finlay, B.L. and Volman, S.F. (1976), Quantitative studies of single cell properties in monkey striate cortex I. Spatiotemporal organization of receptive fields. *J Neurophysiol*, **39**, 1288.

Schiller, P.H. and Malpeli, J.G. (1978), Functional specificity of lateral geniculate nucleus laminae of the rhesus monkey. *J Neurophysiol*, **41**, 788.

Schiller, P.H. and Stryker, M. (1972), Single unit recording and stimulation in superior colliculus of the alert rhesus monkey. *J Neurophysiol*, **35**, 915.

Schimmelpfennig, B.H. (1982), Nerve structures in human central corneal epithelium. *A von Graefes Arch Klin Exp Ophthalmol*, **218**, 14.

Schlemm, F.S. (1830), Bulbus oculi. *Theoret-Prakt Handb Chirurgie*, **3**, 332.

Schmidt, I. (1971), The Wolfflin spots on the iris. *Am J Optom*, **48**, 573.

Schnyder, H. (1984), The innervation of the monkey accessory lateral rectus muscle. *Brain Res*, **296**, 139.

Schurr, P.H. (1951), Angiography of the normal ophthalmic artery and choroidal plexus of the eye. *Br J Ophthalmol*, **35**, 473.

Schwalbe, G. (1870), Untersuchungen uber die Lymphbahnen des Auges und Ihre Begrenzungen. *Arch Microsk Anat*, **6**, 261.

Schwarcz, J.R., Driollet, R., Rios, E. *et al.* (1972), Stereotactic hypthalamotomy for behaviour disorders. *J Neurol Neurosurg Psychiatr*, **35**, 356.

Schwarz, W. (1953a), Elektronenmikroskopische Untersuchungen uber die Differenzierung der Cornea- und Sklera-fibrillen des Menschen. *Z Zellforsch Mikrosk Anat*, **38**, 78.

Schwarz, W. (1953b), Elektronenmikroskopische Untersuchungen uber den Aufbau der Sklera und der Cornea des Menschen. *Z Zellforsch Mikrosk Anat*, **38**, 26.

Schwarz, W. (1956), Electron microscopic studies of the vitreous body. *Anat Anz*, **1**, 102.

Schwarz, W. (1971), In *Anatomie der Kornea*, Bergmann, Munich, p. 1.

Schweinitz, G.D.E. (1923), The Bowman lecture. Concerning certain ocular aspects of pituitary body disorders, mainly exclusive of the usual central and peripheral hemianopic. *Trans Ophthalmol Soc UK*, **43**, 12.

Scott, B.L. and Pease, D.C. (1959), *Am J Anat*, **104**, 1.

Scott, J.E. (1980), Localization of proteoglycans in tendon by electron microscopy. *Biochem J*, **187**, 887.

Scott, J.E. and Haigh, M. (1985), Proteoglycan-Type I collagen fibril interactions in bone and non-calcifying tissues. *Biosci Rep*, **5**, 71.

Sears, M.L. and Teasdall Stone, H.H. (1959), Stretch effects in human ocular muscle: An electromyographic study. *Bull Johns Hopkins Hosp*, **104**, 174.

Sebag, J. and Balasz, E.A. (1984), Pathogenesis of CME–anatomic considerations of vitreo-retinal adhesions. *Surv Ophthalmol*, **28**, 493.

Sebag, J. and Balasz, E.A. (1985), Human vitreous fibres and vitreoretinal disease. *Trans Ophthalmol Soc UK*, **104**, 123.

Sebag, J., Balasz, E.A. and Flood, M.T. (1984), The fibrous structure of the human vitreous. *Ophthalmologia*, **88**, 62.

Segawa, K. (1964), Electron microscopy of dendritic cells in the human corneal epithelium. *Arch Ophthalmol*, **72**, 650.

Segawa, K. (1975), Ultrastructural changes of the trabecular tissues in primary open angle glaucoma. *Jpn J Ophthalmol*, **19**, 317.

Segawa, K. (1979), Electron microscopic changes of the trabecular tissue in primary open angle glaucoma. *Ann Ophthalmol*, **11**, 49.

Seland, J.S. (1974), Ultrastructural changes in the normal human lens capsule from birth to old age. *Acta Ophthalmol*, **52**, 688.

Sellheyer, K. (1990), Development of the choroid and related structures. *Eye*, **4**, 255.

Sellheyer, K. and Spitznas, M. (1987), Ultrastructure of the human posterior tunica vasculosa lentis during gestation. *Graefe's Arch Clin Exp Ophthalmol*, **225**, 377.

Sellheyer, K. and Spitznas, M. (1988a), The fine structure of the developing human choriocapillaris during the first trimester. *Graefe's Arch Clin Exp Ophthalmol*, **226**, 65.

Sellheyer, K. and Spitznas, M. (1988b), Development of the human sclera. *Graefe's Arch Clin Exp Ophthalmol*, **226**, 89.

Sellheyer, K. and Spitznas, M. (1988c), Differentiation of the ciliary muscle in the human embryo and fetus. *Graefe's Arch Clin Exp Ophthalmol*, **226**, 281.

Sellheyer, K. and Spitznas, M. (1988d), Surface differentiation of the human corneal epithelium during prenatal development. *Graefe's Arch Clin Exp Ophthalmol*, **226**, 482.

Sellheyer, K. and Spitznas, M. (1988e), Ultrastructural observations on the development of the human conjunctival epithelium. *Graefe's Arch Clin Exp Ophthalmol*, **226**, 489.

Sesemann, E. (1869), Die Orbitalvenen des Menschen und ihr Zusammenhang mit den oberflachlichen venen des Kopfes. *Arch Anat Physiol Wiss Med*, **2**, 154.

Sevel, D. (1981), Reappraisal of the origin of human extraocular muscles. *Ophthalmology*, **88**, 1330.

Shakib, M. and Cunha-Vaz, J.G. (1966), Studies on the permeability of the blood–retinal barrier: IV. Junctional complexes of the retinal vessels and their role in the permeability of the blood–retinal barrier. *Exp Eye Res*, **5**, 229.

Shapley, R.M. and Perry, V.H. (1986), Cat and monkey retinal ganglion cells and their visual functional roles. *Trends Neurosci*, **9**, 229.

Sharpe, J.A. and Deck, J.H.N. (1978), Destruction of the internal sagittal stratum and normal smooth pursuit. *Ann Neurol*, **4**, 473.

Shaw, E.L., Rao, G.N., Arthur, E.J. *et al.* (1978), The functional reserve of corneal endothelium. *Trans Am Acad Ophthalmol Otolaryngol*, **85**, 640.

Shellshear, J.E. (1927), *Brain*, **50**, 236.

Sherrard, E.S., Novakovic, P. and Speedwell, Z. (1987), Age-related changes of the corneal endothelium and stroma as seen *in vivo* by specular microscopy. *Eye*, **1**, 197.

Sherrington, C.S. (1897), Further note on the sensory nerves of muscles. *Proc R Soc Lond*, **61**, 247.

Sherrington, C.S. (1905), *Proc R Soc Lond, Series B*, **76**, 160.

Sherwood, M.B., Grierson, I., Millar, L. *et al.* (1989), Long-term morphologic effects of anti-glaucoma drugs on the conjunctiva and Tenon's capsule in glaucomatous patients. *Ophthalmology*, **96**, 327.

Shimizu, K. (1978), Segmental nature of the angioarchitecture of the choroid, *Excerpta Medica*, Amsterdam, New York, Oxford; 215.

Shimizu, K. and Kazuyoshi, U. (1978), *Structure of the Ocular Vessels* Igaku-Shoin, Tokyo, New York.

Shiose, Y. (1970), Electron microscopic studies on blood–retinal and blood–aqueous barriers. *Jpn J Ophthalmol*, **14**, 73.

Shipp, S.D. and Zeki, S.M. (1989a), The organization of connections between areas V5 and V1 in macaque monkey visual cortex. *Eur J Neurosci*, **1**, 309.

Shipp, S.D. and Zeki, S.M. (1989b), The organization of connections between areas V5 and V2 in macaque monkey visual cortex. *Eur J Neurosci*, **1**, 333.

Shipp, S.D. and Zeki, S.M. (1984), Specificity of connexions is related to cytochrome oxidase architecture in area V2 of macaque monkey visual cortex. *J Physiol*, **352**, 23.

Shounara, K. (1974), An attempt to relate the origin and distribution of commissural fibers to the presence of large and medium pyramids in layer III in the cat's visualcortex. *Brain Res*, **67**, 13.

Siah, P.B. (1983), Influence of aging and the sympathetic nervous system on aqueous humor dynamics in man; a fluorophotometric and tonographic study. *D Phil Thesis*.

Siebinga, I., Vrensen, G.F.J.M., De Mul, F.F.M. *et al.* (1991), Age-related changes in local water and protein content of human eye lenses measured by Raman microspectroscopy. *Exp Eye Res*, **53**, 233.

Siemmerling, E. (1888), Ein fall von gummoser erkrankung der hirnbasis mit betheiligung des chiasma nervorum opticorum. *Arch Psychiatr Nervkrankh*, **19**, 423.

Sigelman J. and Ozanics, V. (1982), Retina, in *Ocular Anatomy, Embryology, and Teratology* (ed. F. Jakobiec), Harper and Row, Philadelphia, p. 441.

Sillito, A.M. (1968), The location and activity of pupil-loconstrictor neurones in the mid-brain of the cat. *J Physiol (Lond)*, **194**, 39P.

Sillito, A.M. and Zbrozyna, A.W. (1970), The localization of pupilloconstrictor function within the mid-brain of the cat. *J Physiol (Lond)*, **211**, 461.

Silver, P.H.S. and Wakely, J. (1974), The initial stage in the development of the lens capsule in chick and mouse embryo. *Exp Eye Res*, **19**, 73.

Simionescu, M., Simionescu, N. and Palade, G.E. (1975), Segmental differentiations of cell functions in the vascular endothelium. *J Cell Biol*, **67**, 863.

Simionescu, N., Simionescu, M. and Palade, G.E. (1978), Open junctions in the endothelium of the post-capillary venules of the diaphragm. *J Cell Biol*, **79**, 27.

Simons, K. and Fuller, S.D. (1985), Cell surface polarity in epithelia. *Ann Rev Cell Biol*, **1**, 243.

Simpson, J.I. (1984), The accessory optic system. *Ann Rev Neurosci*, **7**, 13.

Simpson, J.I. and Alley, K.E. (1974), Visual climbing fiber input to rabbit vestibulo-cerebellum: A source of direction specific information. *Brain Res*, **82**, 302.

Sinclair, D. (1967), *Cutaneous Sensation*, OUP, Oxford, p. 1.

Singh, S. and Dass, R. (1960), The central artery of the retina: II A study of its distribution and anastomoses. *Br J Ophthalmol*, **44**, 280.

Sinnreich, Z. and Nathan, H. (1981), The ciliary ganglion in man. *Anat Anz*, **150**, 287.

Sivanandasingham, P. (1973), *PhD Thesis*, London University.

Sjostrom, M., Angquist, K.A., Bylund, A.C. *et al.* (1982), Morphometric analyses of human muscle fiber types. *Muscle Nerve*, **5**, 538.

Skuta, G.L. (1987), Zonular dialysis during extracapsular cataract extraction in pseudoexfoliation syndrome. *Arch Ophthalmol*, **105**, 632.

Sliney, D. and Wolbarsht, M. (1980), *Safety with Lasers and Optical Sources*, Plenum Press, New York, p. 336.

Sluder, G. (1937), *Nasal Neurology, Headaches and Eye Disorders*. Mosby, St. Louis.

Smelser, G.K. (1960), Morphological and functional development of the cornea, in *The Transparency of the Cornea* (eds W.S. Duke-Elder and E.S. Perkins), Blackwell Scientific, Oxford, p. 23.

Smelser, G.K. and Ozanics, V. (1965), New concepts in anatomy and histology of the cornea, in *The Cornea World Congress* (eds J.H. King and J.W. McTigue), Butterworth, Washington, p. 1.

Smelser, G.K. and Ozanics, V. (1971), The development of the trabecular meshwork in primate eyes. *Am J Ophthalmol*, **71**, 366.

Smith, C.G. and Richardson, W.F.G. (1966), The course and distribution of the arteries supplying the visual (striate) cortex. *Am J Ophthalmol*, **67**, 139.

Smith, M.L. and Milner, B. (1981), *Neuropsychologia*, **19**, 781.

Smith, R.S. (1971), Ultrastructural studies of the blood–aqueous barrier. I. Transport of an electron dense tracer in the iris and ciliary body of the mouse. *Am J Ophthalmol*, **71**, 1066.

Smith, R.S. and Rudt, L.A. (1973), Ultrastructural studies of the blood–aqueous barrier. II. The barrier to horse-radish peroxidase in primates. *Am J Ophthalmol*, **76**, 937.

Smith, R.S. and Rudt, L.A. (1975), Ocular vascular and epithelial barriers to microperoxidase. *Invest Ophthalmol*, **14**, 556.

Snider, R.S. (1972), Some cerebellar influences on autonomic function; in *Limbic System Mechanism and Autonomic Function* (ed. C.H. Hockman), Charles C. Thomas, Springfield, IL, p. 87.

Snip, R.C., Thoft, R.A. and Tolentino, F.I. (1979), Epithelial healing rates of the normal and diabetic human cornea. *ARVO Suppl: Invest Ophthalmol Vis Sci*, **18**, 73.

Snyder, S.H. (1992), Nitric oxide and neurons. *Curr Opin Neurobiol*, **2**, 323.

Soemmering, S.T. (1801), *Abbildungen des Menschlichen Auges. Frankfurt a. main 50.* (Cited by Gurwitsch, 1883.)

Solnitzky, O. (1961), Horner's syndrome: its diagnostic significance. *Georgetown Univ Med Cent Bull*, **14**, 204.

Sondermann, R. (1933), Uber Entstehung Morphologie und Funcktion Des Schlemmchen-Kanals. *Acta Ophthalmol*, **11**, 280.

Sorsby, A. and Sheridan (1960), The eye at birth: measurements of the principle diameters in forty-eight cadavers. *J Anat*, **94**, 192.

Spalding, J.M.K. (1952), Wounds of the visual pathway. I The visual radiation. *J Neurol Neurosci Psych*, **15**, 99.

Speakman, J.S. (1960), Drainage channels in the trabecular wall of Schlemm's canal. *Br J Ophthalmol*, **44**, 513.

Spencer, L.M., Foos, R.Y. and Straatsma, B.R. (1969), Meridronal folds and meridional complexes of the peripheral retina. *Trans Am Acad Ophthalmol Otolaryngol*, **73**, 204.

Spencer, R.F., Evinger, C. and Baker, R. (1982), Electron microscopic observations of axon collateral synaptic endings of cat oculomotor motoneurons stained by intracellular injection of horseradish peroxidase (HRP). *Brain Res*, **234**, 423.

Spencer, R.F. and Porter, J.D. (1981), Innervation and structure of extraocular muscles in the monkey in comparison to those of the cat. *J Comp Neurol*, **198**, 649.

Spencer, R.F. and Porter, J.D. (1988), Structural organization of the extraocular muscles, in *Neuroanatomy of the Oculomotor System* (ed. J.A. Buttner-Ennever), Elsevier, Amsterdam, p. 33.

Spencer, W.H. *Ophthalmic Pathology*, 3rd edition, *vol. 1*, WB Saunders, Philadelphia.

Spencer, W.H. (1978), Drusen of the optic disk and aberrant axoplasmic transport. The XXXIV Edward Jackson Memorial Lecture. *Am J Ophthalmol*, **85**, 1.

Spencer, W.H., Alvarado, J. and Hayes, T.L. (1968), Scanning electron microscopy of human ocular tissues: the trabecular meshwork. *Invest Ophthalmol*, **7**, 651.

Sperling, S. and Jacobson, S.R. (1980), The surface coat on human corneal endothelium. *Acta Ophthalmol*, **58**, 96.

Spira, A.W. and Hollenberg, M.J. (1973), Human retinal

development: ultrastructure of the inner retinal layers. *Dev Biol*, **31**, 1.

Spiro, A.J. and Beilin, R.L. (1969), Human muscle spindle histochemistry. *Arch Neurol*, **20**, 271.

Spitznas, M. and Hogan, M.J. (1970), Outer segments of photoreceptors and the retinal pigment epithelium. Interrelationships in the human eye. *Arch Ophthalmol*, **84**, 810.

Spitznas, M., Luciano, L. and Reale, E. (1970), Fine structure of rabbit scleral collagen. *Am J Ophthalmol*, **69**, 414.

Spitznas, M. and Reale, E. (1975), Fracture faces of fenestrations and junctions of endothelial cells in human choroidal vessels. *Invest Ophthalmol Vis Sci*, **14**, 98.

Srinivasan, B.D. and Iwamoto, T. (1973), Electron microscopy of rabbit lens nucleoli. *Exp Eye Res*, **16**, 9.

Srinivasan, B.D., Worgul, B.V., Iwamoto, T. *et al.* (1977), The conjunctival epithelium. II. Histochemical and ultrastructural studies on human and rat conjunctiva. *Ophthal Res*, **9**, 65.

St Helen, R. and McEwan, W.K. (1961), Rheology of the human sclera. I An elastic behaviour. *Am J Ophthalmol*, **52**, 539.

Stahelin, L.A. (1972), Three types of gap junctions interconnecting intestinal epithelial cells visualized by freeze-etching. *Proc Natl Acad Sci USA*, **69**, 1318.

Stallard, H.B. (1950), *Eye Surgery*, Williams & Wilkins, Baltimore, p. 499.

Stanfield, J.P. (1960), *Exp Neurol*, **2**, 25.

Stark, W.J. and Streeten, B.W. (1984), The anterior capsulotomy of extracapsular cataract extraction. *Ophthalmic Surg*, **15**, 911.

Steele, E.J. and Blunt, M.J. (1956), The blood supply of the optic nerve and chiasma in man. *J Anat*, **90**, 486.

Steiger, H.J. and Büttner-Ennever, J. (1978), Relationship between motoneurons and internuclear neurons in the abducens nucleus: a double retrograde tracer study in the cat. *Brain Res*, **148**, 181.

Stein, B.M. and Carpenter, M.B. (1967), Central projections of portions of the vestibular ganglia innervating specific parts of the labyrinth in the rhesus monkey. *Am J Anat*, **120**, 281.

Steinberg, R.H., Wood, I. and Hogan, M.J. (1977), Pigment epithelial ensheathment and phagocytosis of extrafoveal cones in human retina. *Phil Trans Roy Soc Lond (Biol)*, **277**, 459.

Stenström, S. (1946), Untersuchungen uber die Variation und Kovariation der optischen Elemente des menschlichen Auges. *Acta Ophthalmol*, **26**, 1.

Stern, W.H. and Ernest, J.T. (1974), Microsphere occlusion of the choriocapillaris in rhesus monkey. *Am J Ophthalmol*, **78**, 438.

Steuhl, K.P. (1989), Ultrastructure of conjunctival epithelium. *Dev Ophthalmol*, **19**, 1.

Steuhl, K.P., Sitz, U., Knorr, M. *et al.* (1995), Age-dependent distribution of Langerhans cells within human conjunctival epithelium. *Ophthalmologe*, **92**, 21.

Stevenson, T.C. (1963), Intrascleral nerve loops: a clinical study of frequency and treatment. *Am J Ophthalmol*, **55**, 935.

Stibbe, E.P. (1928), A comparative study of the nictitating membrane of birds and mammals. *J Anat*, **62**, 159.

Stieve, E. (1949), The structure of the human ciliary muscle, its changes during life and its influence on accommodation. *Anat Anz*, **97**, 69.

Stieve, R. (1930), Uber die caruncula lacrymalis des Menschen. *Arch Microsk Anat*, **1**, 29.

Stingl, G., Tamaki, K. and Katz, S.I. (1980), Origin and function of epidermal Langerhans cells. *Immunol Rev*, **53**, 149.

Stjernschantz, J. and Bill, A. (1979), Effect of intracranial stimulation of the oculomotor nerve on ocular blood flow in the monkey, cat and rabbit. *Invest Ophthalmol Vis Sci*, **18**, 99.

Stjernschantz, J. and Bill, A. (1980), Vasomotor effects in facial nerve stimulation: non-cholinergic vasodilation in the eye. *Acta Physiol Scand*, **109**, 45.

Stone, J. and Hansen, S.M. (1966), The projection of the cats retina on the lateral geniculate nucleus. *J Comp Neurol*, **126**, 601.

Stone, R.A. and Kuwayama, Y. (1989), The nervous system and intraocular pressure, in *The Glaucomas* (eds R. Ritch, M.B. Shields and T. Krupin), CV Mosby, St. Louis, p. 257.

Stone, R.A., Kuwayama, Y. and Laties, A.M. (1987), Regulatory peptides in the eye. *Experientia*, **43**, 791.

Stone, R.A., Kuwayama, Y., Laties, A.M. *et al.* (1984), Guinea pig ocular nerves contain peptide of the cholecystokinin/gastrin family. *Exp Eye Res*, **39**, 387.

Stone, R.A. and Laties, A.M. (1983), Pancreatic polypeptide-like immunoreactive nerves in the guinea pig eye. *Invest Ophthalmol Vis Sci*, **24**, 1620.

Stone, R.A. and Laties, A.M. (1987), Neuroanatomy and neuroendocrinology of the chamber angle; in *Glaucoma Update III* (ed. G.K. Kriegelstein), Springer, Berlin, p. 1.

Stone, R.A., Laties, A.M. and Emson, P.C. (1986), Neuropeptide Y and the ocular innervation of rat, guinea pig, cat and monkey. *Neuroscience*, **17**, 1207.

Stone, R.A., McGlinn, A.M., Kuwayama, Y. *et al.* (1988), Peptide immunoreactivity of the ciliary ganglion and its accessory cells in the rat. *Brain Res*, **475**, 389.

Stone, R.A., Tervo, T., Tervo, K. and Tarkkanen, A. (1986), Vasoactive intestinal polypeptide-like immunoreactive nerves to the human eye. *Acta Ophthalmol*, **64**, 12.

Stopford, J.S.B. (1916), The arteries of the pons and medulla oblongata. Part I. *J Anat Physiol Lond*, **50**, 131.

Stopford, J.S.B. (1917), The arteries of the pons and medulla oblongata. Part II. *J Anat Physiol Lond*, **51**, 250.

Stotler, W.A. (1937), *Proc Soc Exp Biol Med*, 36, 576.

Straatsma, B.R., Foos, R.Y. and Spencer, L.M. (1969), The retina – topography and clinical correlations. Symposium on the retina and retinal surgery. *New Orleans Acad J Ophthalmol*, **1**, 1.

Straatsma, B.R., Landers, M.B. and Kreiger, A.E. (1968), The ora serrata in the adult human eye. *Arch Ophthalmol*, **80**, 3.

Streeten, B.W. (1992), Anatomy of the zonular apparatus, in *The Biomedical Foundations of Ophthalmology* (eds T.D. Duane and E.A. Jaeger), Harper and Row, Philadelphia, p. 1.

Streeten, B.W. (1995), The ciliary body, in *Biomedical Foundations of Ophthalmology* (eds T.D. Duane and E.A. Jaeger), J.B. Lippincott, Philadelphia.

Streeten, B.W. and Eshaghian, J. (1978), Human posterior subcapsular cataract. *Arch Ophthalmol*, **96**, 1653.

Streeten, B.W. and Gibson, S.A. (1988), Identification of extractable proteins from the bovine ocular zonule: major zonular antigens of 32 kd and 250 kd. *Curr Eye Res*, **7**, 139.

Streeten, B.W., Licari, P.A., Marucci, A.A. *et al.* (1981), Immunohistochemical comparison of ocular zonules and the microfibrils of elastic tissue. *Invest Ophthalmol Vis Sci,* **21,** 130.

Streeten, B.W. and Pulaski, J.P. (1978), Posterior zonules and lens extraction. *Arch Ophthalmol,* **96,** 132.

Streeten, B.W., Swann, D.A., Licari, P.A. *et al.* (1983), The protein composition of the ocular zonules. *Invest Ophthalmol Vis Sci,* **24,** 119.

Sudakevitch, T. (1947), The variations in the trunks of the posterior ciliary arteries. *Br J Ophthalmol,* **31,** 738.

Sugiura, S., Waku, I. and Kondo, E. (1962), Comparative anatomical and embryological studies on polygonal cell system in basal epithelial layer of cornea. *Acta Soc Ophthalmol Jpn,* **66,** 1010.

Sullivan, D.A., Wickham, L.A., Krenzer, K.L., Rocha, E.M. and Toda, I. (1996), Aqueous tear deficiency in Sjögren's syndrome: possible causes and potential treatment, in *Oculodermal Diseases – Immunology of Bullous Oculo-Muco-Cutaneous Disorders,*

Sun, T.-T. and Vidrich, A. (1981), Keratin filaments of corneal epithelial cells. *Vision Res,* **21,** 55.

Sunderland, S. and Hughes, E.S.R. (1946), The pupilloconstructor pathway and the nerves to the ocular motor muscles in man. *Brain,* **69,** 301.

Sur, M. and Sherman, S.M. (1982a), Linear and nonlinear W-cells in C-laminae of the cat's lateral geniculate nucleus. *J Neurophysiol,* **47,** 869.

Suzuki, H. and Kato, E. (1966), Binocular interaction of cat's lateral geniculate body. *J Neurophysiol,* **29,** 909.

Suzuki, N., Hardebo, J.E., Kåhrström, J. *et al.* (1990), Neuropeptide Y co-exists with vasoactive intestinal polypeptide and acetylcholine in parasympathetic cerebrovascular nerves originating in the sphenopalatine otic, and internal carotid ganglia in the rat. *Neuroscience,* **36,** 507.

Suzuki, T., Shirai, S. and Majima, A. (1988), Morphological study on the mechanism of closure of the embryonic fissure. *Acta Soc Ophthalmol Jpn,* **92,** 238.

Svedbergh, B. (1974), Effects of artificial intraocular pressure elevation on the outflow facility and ultrastructure of the chamber angle in the vervet monkey (*Cercopithecus ethiops*). *Acta Ophthalmol,* **52,** 829.

Svedbergh, B. (1976), Aspects of the aqueous humor drainage. Functional ultrastructure of Schlemm's canal, the trabecular meshwork and the corneal endothelium at different intraocular pressures. *Acta Univ Upsalien,* **256,** 71.

Svedbergh, B., Lütjen-Drecoll, E., Ober, M. *et al.* (1978), Cytochalasin B-induced structural changes in the anterior ocular segment of the cynomolgus monkey. *Invest Ophthalmol Vis Sci,* **17,** 718.

Svedburgh, A. (1975), Effects of intraocular pressure elevation on the corneal endothelium in the vervet monkey. *Montpellier Med,* **53,** 839.

Swann, D.A. (1980), Chemistry and biology of vitreous body. *Int Rev Exp Pathol,* **22,** 1.

Sweeney, D.S., Vannas, A., Holden, B.A. *et al.* (1985), Evidence for sympathetic neural influence on human corneal epithelial function. *WHO,* **63,** 215.

Swegmark, G. (1969), Studies with impedance cyclography on human ocular accommodation at different ages. *Montpellier Med,* **47,** 1186.

Szalay, J., Nunziata, B. and Henkind, P. (1975), Permeability of iridial blood vessels. *Exp Eye Res,* **21,** 35.

Szel, A., Diamantstein, T. and Rohlich, P. (1988), Identification of the blue-sensitive cones in the mammalian retina by anti-visual pigment antibody. *J Comp Neurol,* **273,** 593.

Szent-Gyorgyi, A. (1917), Untersuchungen uber den bau des glaskorpers. *Arch Microsk Anat,* **89,** 324.

Szentágothai, J. (1942), Die innere Gliederung des Oculomotorius Kernes. *Arch Psychiat Nervkrankh,* **115,** 127.

Szentágothai, J. (1943), *Arch Psychiatr Nervkrankh,* **116,** 721.

Szentágothai, J. (1950), The elementary vestibulo-ocular reflex arc. *J Neurophysiol,* **1,** 395.

Szentágothai, J. (1963), The structure of the synapses in the lateral geniculate body. *Acta Anat,* **55,** 166.

Szentágothai, J. (1970), Glomerular synapses, complex synaptic arrangements and their operational significance, in *The Neurosciences (Second Study Program)* (ed. F.O. Schmitt), Rockefeller University Press, p. 427.

Szentágothai, J. (1975), The 'module-concept' in cerebral cortex architecture. *Brain Res,* **95,** 475.

Szentágothai, J., Flerkó, Mess, B. and Halász, B. (1968), *Hypothalamic Control of the Anterior Pituitary,* 2nd edition, Akadémiai Kiakó, Budapest.

Takakusaki, I. (1969), Fine structure of the human palpebral conjunctiva with special reference to the pathological changes in vernal catarrh. *Arch Histol Jpn,* **30,** 247.

Talmadge, E.K. and Mawe, G.M. (1993), NADPH-diaphorase and VIP are colocalized in neurons of gallbladder anglia. *J Auton Nerv Syst,* **43,** 83.

Tamm, E.R., Croft, M.A., Jungkunz, W. *et al.* (1992a), Age-related loss of ciliary muscle mobility in the rhesus monkey. Role of the choroid. *Arch Ophthalmol,* **110,** 871.

Tamm, E.R., Flügel, C., Baur, A. *et al.* (1991), Cell cultures of human ciliary muscle: Growth, ultrastructural and immunocytochemical characteristics. *Exp Eye Res,* **53,** 375.

Tamm, E.R., Flügel, C., Stefani, F.H. *et al.* (1992b), Contractile cells in the human scleral spur. *Exp Eye Res,* **54,** 531.

Tamm, E.R., Flügel, C., Stefani, F.H. *et al.* (1994), Nerve endings with structural characteristics of mechanoreceptors in the human scleral spur. *Invest Ophthalmol Vis Sci,* **35,** 1157.

Tamm, E.R., Flügel-Koch, C., Mayer, B. *et al.* (1995a), Nerve cells in the human ciliary muscle: Ultrastructural and immunocytochemical characterization. *Invest Ophthalmol Vis Sci,* **36,** 414.

Tamm, E.R., Koch, T.A., Mayer, B. *et al.* (1995b), Innervation of myofibroblast-like scleral spur cells in human and monkey eyes. *Invest Ophthalmol Vis Sci,* **36,** 1633.

Tamm, E.R., Lütjen-Drecoll, E. and Rohen, J.W. (1990), Age-related changes of the ciliary muscle in comparison with changes induced by treatment with prostaglandin $F_{2\hat{A}}$: An ultrastructural study in rhesus and cynomolgus monkeys. *Mech Ageing Dev,* **51,** 101.

Tamm, S., Tamm, E. and Rohen, J.W. (1992), Age-related changes of the human ciliary muscle. A quantitative morphometric study. *Mech Ageing Dev,* **62,** 209.

Tanguchi, Y. (1962), Fine structure of blood vessels in the ciliary body. *Jpn J Ophthalmol,* **6,** 93.

Tarkhan, A.A. (1934), Innervation of the extrinsic ocular muscles. *J Anat*, **68**, 293.

Tarlov, E. and Tarlov, S.R. (1971), The representation of extraocular muscles in the oculomotor nuclei: experimental studies in the cat. *Brain Res*, **34**, 37.

Tarlov, E. and Tarlov, S.R. (1972), Anatomy of the two vestibulo-oculomotor projection systems. *Prog Brain Res*, **37**, 489.

Tarlov, E. and Tarlov, S.R. (1975), Synopsis of current knowledge about association projections from the vestibular nuclei, in *The Vestibular System*, Academic Press, New York, p. 55.

Tawara, A., Varner, H.H. and Hollyfield, J.G. (1989), Distribution and characterization of sulfated proteoglycans in the human trabecular tissue. *Invest Ophthalmol Vis Sci*, **30**, 2215.

Teal, P.K., Morin, J.D. and McCulloch, C. (1972), Assessment of the normal disc. *Trans Am Ophthalmol Soc*, **70**, 164.

Ten Tuscher, M.P.M., Klooster, J., Van der Want, J.J.L *et al.* (1989), The allocation of nerve fibers to the anterior segment and peripheral ganglia of rats: I. The sensory innervation. *Brain Res*, **494**, 95.

Teravainen, H. (1968), Electron microscopic and histochemical observations on different types of nerve endings in the extraocular muscles of the rat. *Z Zellforsch Mikrosk Anat*, **90**, 372.

Teravainen, H. (1969), Localization of acetylcholinesterase activity in myotendinous and myomyous junctions of the striated skeletal muscles of the rat. *Experientia*, **25**, 524.

Terenghi, G., Polak, J.M., Ghatei, P.K. *et al.* (1985), Distribution and origin of calcitonin gene-related peptide (CGRP) immunoreactivity in the sensory innervation of the mammalian eye. *J Comp Neurol*, **233**, 506.

Tervo, K., Tervo, T., Eranko, L. *et al.* (1981), Immunoreactivity for substance P in the Gasserian ganglion, ophthalmic nerve and anterior segment of the rabbit eye. *Histochem J*, **13**, 435.

Tervo, T. and Palkama, A. (1976), Adrenergic innervation of the rat corneal epithelium. *Invest Ophthalmol Vis Sci*, **15**, 147.

Testut, (1905), *Traité d'anatomie humaine, 5th edition*, Paris.

Thanos, S., Moore, S. and Hong, Y. (1996), Retinal microglia, in *Progress in Retinal and Eye Research*, (eds N.N. Osborne, and G.J. Chader), Elsevier Science Ltd, Oxford, p. 331.

Theodossiadis, G.P. (1971), Uber die vaskularisation in der regio praelaminaris der papilla optica. *Klin Monatsbl Augenheilk*, **158**, 646.

Thoft, R.A. and Friend, J. (1977), Biochemical transformation of regenerating surface epithelium. *Invest Ophthalmol Vis Sci*, **16**, 14.

Thoft, R.A. and Friend, J. (1983), The X,Y,Z hypothesis of corneal epithelial maintenance. *Invest Ophthalmol Vis Sci*, **24**, 1442.

Thomson, J.A. and Augusteyn, R.C. (1985), Ontogeny of human lens crystallins. *Exp Eye Res*, **40**, 393.

Thurston, S.E., Leigh, R.J., Crawford, T. *et al.* (1988), Two distinct deficits of visual tracking caused by unilateral lesions of cerebral cortex in humans. *Ann Neurol*, **23**, 266.

Tiedemann, (1824), *Z Physiol*, **1**, 237.

Tien, L., Rayborn, M.E. and Hollyfield, J.G. (1992), Characterization of the interphotoreceptor matrix surrounding rod photoreceptors in the human retina. *Exp Eye Res*, **55**, 297.

Tiffany, J.M. (1990a), Measurement of wettability of the corneal epithelium. 2. Contact angle method. *Acta Ophthalmol*, **68**, 182.

Tiffany, J.M. (1990b), Measurement of wettability of the corneal epithelium. 1. Particle attachment method. *Acta Ophthalmol*, **68**, 175.

Tigges, J. and O'Steen, W.K. (1974), Termination of retinofugal fibers in squirrel monkey: a reinvestigation using autoradiographic methods. *Brain Res*, **79**, 489.

Tilton, R.G., Kilo, C. and Williamson, J.R. (1979), Pericyte-endothelial cell relationships in cardiac and skeletal muscle capillaries. *Microvasc Res*, **18**, 325.

Toda, N. (1993), Mediation by nitric-oxide of neurally-induced human cerebral-artery relaxation. *Experientia*, **49**, 51.

Tomasi, T.B. (1976), *The Immune System of Secretions*, Prentice Hall, New Jersey, p. 1.

Tomii, S. and Kinoshita, S. (1994), Observations of human corneal epithelium by tandem scanning confocal microscope. *Scanning*, **16**, 305.

Tonjum, A.M. (1974), Permeability of horseradish peroxidase in rabbit corneal epithelium. *Acta Ophthalmol*, **52**, 650.

Torczynski, E. (1981), Preparation of ocular specimens for histopathologic examination. *Ophthalmology*, **88**, 1367.

Torczynski, E. (1987), Choroid and suprachoroid, in *Biomedical Foundations of Ophthalmology* (eds T.D. Duane and E.A. Jaeger), Lippincott, Philadelphia, p. 1.

Torczynski, E. and Tso, M.O.M. (1976), The architecture of the choriocapillaris at the posterior pole. *Am J Ophthalmol*, **81**, 428.

Toris, C.B. and Pederson, J.E. (1987), Aqueous humor dynamics in experimental iridocyclitis. *Invest Ophthalmol Vis Sci*, **28**, 477.

Tornquist, G. (1966), Effect of cervical stimulation on accommodation in monkeys, an example of a beta-adrenergic, inhibitory effect. *Acta Physiol Scand*, **67**, 363.

Tornqvist, P. and Alm, A. (1979), Retinal and choroidal contribution to retinal metabolism *in vivo*. A study in pigs. *Acta Physiol Scand*, **106**, 351.

Torre, M. (1953), Nombre et dimension des unites motrices dans les muscles extrinseques de l'oeil et, en general, dans les muscles squelettiques relies a des organes de sens. *Schweiz Arch Neurol*, **72**, 362.

Torrealba, F., Guillery, R.W., Eysel, U. *et al.* (1982), Studies of retinal representations within the cat's optic tract. *J Comp Neurol*, **211**, 377.

Tousmis, A.J. and Fine, B.S. (1959), Ultrastructure of the iris: an electron microscopic study. *Am J Ophthalmol*, **48**, 397.

Toussaint, D., Kuwabara, T. and Cogan, D.G. (1961), Retinal vascular patterns: II. Human retinal vessels studied in three dimensions. *Arch Ophthalmol*, **65**, 575.

Townes-Anderson, E. and Raviola, G. (1978), Degeneration and regeneration of autonomic nerve endings in the anterior part of rhesus monkey ciliary muscle. *J Neurocytol*, **7**, 583.

Townes-Anderson, E. and Raviola, G. (1981a), Development of the blood–ocular barriers in the rhesus monkey. *ARVO Suppl: Invest Ophthalmol Vis Sci*, **20**, 78.

Townes-Anderson, E. and Raviola, G. (1981b), The formation and distribution of intercellular junctions in the rhesus monkey optic cup: the early development of the cilio-iridic and sensory retinas. *Dev Biol*, **85**, 209.

Toyama, K., Matsunami, K., Ohno, T. *et al.* (1974), An intracellular study of neuronal organization in the visual cortex. *Exp Brain Res*, **21**, 45.

Tozer, F.M. and Sherrington, C.S. (1910), Receptors and afferents of the third, fourth and sixth cranial nerves. *Proc R Soc Lond*, **82**, 450.

Tranum-Jensen, J. (1975), The ultrastructure of the sensory end-organs (baroreceptors) in the atrial endocardium of young mini-pigs. *J Anat*, **119**, 255.

Traquair, H.M. (1916), The anatomical relations of the hypophysis and the chiasma. *Ophthalmoscope*, **14**, 562.

Traquair, H.M. (1957), *Br Orthopt J*, **7**, 1.

Trayhurn, P. and Van Heyningen, R. (1972), The role of respiration in the energy metabolism of the bovine lens. *Biochem J*, **129**, 507.

Trayhurn, P. and Van Heyningen, R. (1973a), The metabolism of amino acids in the bovine lens: their oxidation as a source of energy. *Biochem J*, **136**, 67.

Trayhurn, P. and Van Heyningen, R. (1973b), The metabolism of glutamine in the bovine lens: glutamine as a source of glutamate. *Exp Eye Res*, **17**, 149.

Treffers, W.F. (1982), Human endothelial wound repair; *in vitro* and *in vivo*. *Ophthalmologica*, **89**, 605.

Trinkaus-Randall, V., Tong, M., Thomas, P. *et al.* (1993), Confocal imaging of the alpha 6 and beta 4 integrin subunits in the human cornea with aging. *Invest Ophthalmol Vis Sci*, **34**, 3103.

Tripathi, B.J., Li, T., Li, J., *et al.* (1997) Age-related changes in trabecular cells *in vitro*. *Exp Eye Res*, in press.

Tripathi, B.J., Millard, C.B. and Tripathi, R.C. (1990), Qualitative and quantitative analyses of sialic acid in the human trabecular meshwork. *Exp Eye Res*, **51**, 601.

Tripathi, B.J., Tripathi, R.C., Livingston, A.M. *et al.* (1991), The role of growth factors in the embryogenesis and differentiation of the eye. *Am J Anat*, **192**, 442.

Tripathi, B.J., Tripathi, R.C. and Wisdom, J. (1995), Embryology of the anterior segment of the human eye, in *The Glaucomas* 2nd edition (eds R. Ritch, M.B. Shields and T. Krupin), Mosby, St Louis.

Tripathi, B.J., Tripathi, R.C., Yang, C. *et al.* (1991), Synthesis of a thrombospondin-like cytoadhesion molecule by cells of the trabecular meshwork. *Invest Ophthalmol Vis Sci*, **32**, 177.

Tripathi, R.C. (1968), Ultrastructure of Schlemm's canal in relation to aqueous outflow. *Exp Eye Res*, **8**, 335.

Tripathi, R.C. (1969), Ultrastructure of the exit pathway of the aqueous. *PhD Thesis*, University of London.

Tripathi, R.C. (1971), Mechanism of the aqueous outflow across the trabecular wall of Schlemm's canal. *Exp Eye Res*, **11**, 116.

Tripathi, R.C. (1972a), Aqueous outflow pathway in normal and glaucomatous eyes. *Br J Ophthalmol*, **56**, 157.

Tripathi, R.C., (1972b), Ultrastructure of the normal cornea, in *Corneal Grafting* (ed. T.A. Casey), Butterworth, London and Washington, p. 38.

Tripathi, R.C. (1974), Comparative physiology and anatomy of the aqueous outflow pathway; in *The Eye* (ed. H. Davson), Academic Press, London, p.163.

Tripathi, R.C. (1977a), The functional morphology of the outflow systems of ocular and cerebrospinal fluids. *Exp Eye Res Suppl*, **25**, 65.

Tripathi, R.C. (1977b), Pathologic anatomy of the outflow

pathway of aqueous humour in chronic simple glaucoma. *Exp Eye Res*, **25(suppl.)**, 403.

Tripathi, R.C. (1977c), Uveoscleral drainage of aqueous humour. *Exp Eye Res Suppl*, **25**, 305.

Tripathi, R.C. and Cole, D.F. (1976), Uveoscleral drainage in the rabbit. *AVRO Suppl: Invest Ophthalmol Vis Sci*, **1**, 1.

Tripathi, R.C. and Tripathi, B.J. (1982), Functional anatomy of the anterior chamber angle, in *Biomedical Foundations of Ophthalmology* (eds T.D. Duane and E.A. Jaeger), Lippincott, Philadelphia, p. 10:1.

Tripathi, R.C. and Tripathi, B.J. (1984a), Anatomy of the human eye, orbit and adnexa, in *The Eye*, 3rd edition (ed. H. Davson), Academic Press, London, pp. 40, 157.

Tripathi, R.C. and Tripathi, B.J. (1984b), Morphology of the normal, aging and cataractous human lens. I. Development and morphology of the adult and aging lens. *Lens Res*, **1**, 1.

Trojanowski, J.Q. and Jacobson, S. (1976), A real and laminar distribution of some pulvinar cortical efferents in rhesus monkey. *J Comp Neurol*, **169**, 371.

True-Gabelt, B., Polansky, J.R. and Kaufman, P.L. (1987), Ciliary muscle muscarinic receptors, ChAt and AChE in young and old rhesus monkeys. *ARVO Suppl: Invest Ophthalmol Vis Sci*, **28**, 65.

Tseng, S.C.G., Jarvinen, J.J., Nelson, W.G. *et al.* (1982), Correlation of specific keratins with different types of epithelial differentiation: monoclonal antibody studies. *Cell*, **30**, 361.

Tso, M.O.M., Shih, C.-Y. and McLean, I.W. (1975), Is there a blood brain barrier at the optic nerve head? *Arch Ophthalmol*, **93**, 815.

Tsuchida, U. (1906), Über die Ursprungskerne der Augenbewegungsnerven und über die mit diesen in Beziehung stehenden bahnen im Mittel- und Zwishenhirn; normalanatomische, embryologische, pathologisch-anatomische und vergleichend-anatomische Untersuchungen. *Arb Hirnanat Inst Zürich*, **2**, 1.

Tsuchida, U. (1932), On the oculomotor nucleus. *Arb Hirnanat Inst Zurich*, **1**, 1.

Turner, B.H., Mishkin, M. and Knapp, M. (1980), Organization of the amygalopetal projections from modality specific cortical association areas in the monkey. *J Comp Neurol*, **191**, 515.

Tusa, R.J. and Ungerleider, L.G. (1988), Fiber pathways of cortical areas mediating smooth pursuit eye movements in monkeys. *Ann Neurol*, **23**, 174.

Tusa, R.J. and Zee, D.S. (1989), Cerebral control of smooth pursuit and optokinetic nystagmus; in *Current Neuro Ophthalmology* (eds S. Lessell and J.T.W. van Dalen), Year Book Medical Publishers, Chicago, p. 115.

Uddman, R., Alumets, J., Ehinger, B. *et al.* (1980a), Vasoactive intestinal peptide nerves in ocular and orbital structures of the cat. *Invest Ophthalmol Vis Sci*, **19**, 855.

Uddman, R., Alumets, J., Ehinger, B. *et al.* (1980b), Vasoactive intestinal peptide nerves in ocular and orbital structure of the cat. *Invest Ophthalmol Vis Sci*, **19**, 878.

Uemura, T. and Cohen, B. (1973), Effects of vestibular lesions on vestibulo-ocular reflexes and posture in monkeys. *Acta Ophthalmol Suppl*, **315**, 1.

Ueno, K. (1961), Some controversial points on the fine structure of the human iris. Negation of the existence of the continuous anterior endothelium and the fine structure of the dilator pupillae muscle and of the pigment epithelium, *Kyushu J Med Sci*, **12**, 43.

Uga, S. (1968), Electron microscopy of the ciliary muscle. *Acta Soc Ophthalmol Jap*, **72**, 1019.

Unger, H.Y. and Rohen, J.W. (1958), Kammerbucht und Akkamodation. *Anat Anz*, **105**, 93.

Unger, H.Y. and Rohen, J.W. (1959), Studies on the histology of the inner wall of Schlemm's canal. *Am J Ophthalmol*, **48**, 204.

Unger, W.G (1989), Mediation of the ocular response to injury and irritation: Peptides versus prostaglandins, in *The Ocular Effects of Prostaglandins and other Eicosanoids. Proceedings in Clinical and Biological Research* (eds L.Z. Bito and J. Stjernschantz), Alan R Liss, New York, p. 293.

Ungerleider, L.G. and Christensen, C.A. (1977), Pulvinar lesions in monkeys produce abnormal eye movements during visual discrimination training. *Brain Res*, **136**, 189.

Ungerleider, L.G. and Christensen, C.A. (1979), Pulvinar lesions in monkeys produce abnormal scanning of a complex visual array. *Neuropsychologia*, **17**, 493.

Ungerleider, L.G., Desimone, R., Galkin, T.W. *et al.* (1984), Subcortical projections of area MT in the macaque. *J Comp Neurol*, **223**, 368.

Ungerleider, L.G. and Mishkin, M. (1982), In *Analysis of Visual Behavior* (eds D.J. Ingle and R.S.W. Goodale), MIT Press, Cambridge, p. 549.

Uusitalo, H., Lehtosalo, J., Laakso, J. *et al.* (1982), Immunohistochemical and biochemical evidence for 5-hydroxytryptamine containing nerves in the anterior part of the eye. *Exp Eye Res*, **35**, 671.

Uusitalo, H., Lehtosalo, J., Palkama, A. *et al.* (1984), Vasoactive intestinal polypeptide (VIP)-like immunoreactivity in the human and guinea pig choroid. *Exp Eye Res*, **38**, 435.

Uusitalo, R. and Palkama, A. (1971), Evidence for the nervous control of secretion in the ciliary processes. *Prog Brain Res*, **34**, 513.

Uyama, M., Ohkuma, H. Itotagawa, S. *et al.* (1980), Pathology of choroidal circulatory disturbances. Part I. Angioarchitecture of the choroid, observations on plastic cast preparations. *Acta Soc Ophthalmol Jpn*, **84**, 1893.

Valu, L. (1962), Über die Innervation des Uvea-Trabekel-Systems. *Graefes Arch Klin Exp Ophthalmol*, **164**, 496.

Valu, L. (1963), Innervation of the uveal–trabecular system. *Szemeszet Ophthalmol Hung*, **100**, 8.

Van Buren, J.M. and Baldwin, M. (1958), The architecture of the optic radiation in the temporal lobe of man. *Brain*, **81**, 15.

van Crevel, H. and Verhaart, W.J.C. (1963), The rate of secondary degeneration in the central nervous system. II. The optic nerve of the cat. *J Anat*, **97**, 451.

van der Hoeve, J. (1920), Die Bedeutung des Gesichtsfeldes fur die Kenntnis des Verlaufs und der Endigung der Sehnervenfasern in der Netzhaut. *Graefes Arch Ophthalmol*, **102**, 184.

van der Werf, F (1993), Innervation of the lacrimal gland in the cynomolgus monkey. A retrograde tracing and immunohistochemical study. (Thesis), in *Autonomic and Sensory Innervation of Some Orbital Structures in the Primate*, van der Werf, F. Universiteit van Amsterdam, Amsterdam, p. 51.

Van der Zypen, E. (1967), Licht- und elektronenmikroskopische Untersuchungen über den Bau und die Innervation des Ziliarmuskels bei Mensch und Affe (*Cercopithecus aethiops*). *Graefes Arch Klin Exp Ophthalmol*, **174**, 143.

Van der Zypen, E. and Rentsch, F.J. (1971), Alters bedingte Veranderungen am ciliarepithel des menschlichen. *Auges Altern Entwicklung*, **1**, 37.

van Driel, D., Provis, J.M. and Billson, F.A. (1990), Early differentiation of ganglion, amacrine, bipolar, and Müller cells in the developing fovea of human retina. *J Comp Neurol*, **291**, 203.

Van Heyningen, R. (1969), The lens: metabolism and cataract. In *The Eye*, 2nd edition (ed. H. Davson), Academic Press, New York, p. 381.

Vannas, S. and Teir, H. (1960), Observations on structure and age changes in the human sclera. *Acta Ophthalmol*, **38**, 268.

Vantrappen, L., Geboes, K., Missotten, L. *et al.* (1985), Lymphocytes and Langerhans cells in the normal human cornea. *Invest Ophthalmol*, **26**, 285.

Vardi, N. and Sterling, P. (1994), Subcellular localization of GABAA receptor on bipolar cells in macaque and human retina. *Vision Res*, **34**, 1235.

Varner, H.H., Rayborn, M.E., Osterfeld, A.M. and Hollyfield, J.G. (1987), Localization of proteoglycan within the extracellular matrix sheath of cone photoreceptors. *Exp Eye Res*, **44**, 633.

Vegge, T. (1963), Ultrastructure of normal human trabecular endothelium. *Acta Ophthalmol*, **41**, 193.

Vegge, T. (1967), The fine structure of the trabeculum cribiforme and the inner wall of Schlemm's canal in the normal human eye. *Z Zellforsch Mikrosk Anat*, **77**, 267.

Vegge, T. (1971), An electron microscopic study of the permeability of iris capillaries to horseradish peroxidase in the vervet monkey (*Cercopithecus aethiops*). *Z Zellforsch Mikrosk Anat*, **121**, 74.

Vegge, T. (1972), A study of the ultrastructure of the small iris vessels in the vervet monkey (*Cerocopithecus aethiops*). *Z Zellforsch*, **123**, 195.

Vegge, T. and Ringvold, A. (1969), Ultrastructure of the wall of human iris vessels. *Z Zellforsch Mikrosk Anat*, **94**, 19.

Vidic, B. (1968), The origin and the course of the communicating branch of the facial nerve to the lesser petrosal nerve in man. *Anat Rec*, **162**, 511.

Vignaud, J., Clay, C. and Aubin, M.L. (1972), Orbital arteriography. *Radiol Clin North Am*, **10**, 39.

Vignaud, J., Clay, C. and Bilaniuk, L.T. (1974), Venography of the orbit. *Radiology*, **110**, 373.

Vignaud, J., Hasso, A.N., Lasjaunias, P. *et al.* (1974), Orbital vascular anatomy and embryology. *Radiology*, **111**, 617.

Vignaud, J., Salamon, G., Lasjaunias, P. *et al.* (1975), Vascular studies of the orbit. Magnification using 0.1 mm focal spot. *Mod Probl Ophthalmol*, **14**, 87.

Villard, H. (1896), Recherches sur l'histologie de la conjonctive normal. *Montpellier Med*, **5**, 651.

Virchow, H. (1910), Mikroskopische Anatomie der auberen Augenhaut und des Lidapparates, in *Handbuch der gesamten Augenheilkunde*, (eds A. Graefe and T. Saemisch), p. 1.

Vogt, A. (1921), *Atlas of Slit-Lamp Microscopy of the Living Eye*; 1st edition Julius Springer, Berlin.

Vogt, A. (1924), *Klin Monatsbl Augenheilk*, **66**, 321.

Vogt, A. (1941), *Spaltlampenmikroskopie des Lebenden Anges*. Schwetz Fruck- und Veriabshaus, Zurich.

von Düring, M. and Andres, K.H. (1988), Structure and functional anatomy of visceroreceptors in the mammalian respiratory system, in *Progress in Brain Research* (eds W. Hamann and A. Iggo), Elsevier, Amsterdam, p. 139.

Von Economo, C. and Koskinas, G.N. (1925), *Die Cytoarchitecktonik der Himrinde*, Springer, Berlin.

Von Haller, A. (1781), *Iconum Anatomicarum Corporis Humani Fasc* (cited by Meyer, 1887); 7th edition, Van den Hoeck, Gottingen.

Von Noorden, G.K. and Middleditch, P.R. (1975), Histological observations in the normal monkey lateral geniculate nucleus. *Invest Ophthalmol Vis Sci*, **14**, 55.

Von Pflugk, A. (1909), Die Fixierung der Wirbeltierlingen insbesondere der Linse des neugeborenen. *Menschen Klin Monatsbl Augenheilk*, **47**, 1.

von Sallmann, L., Fuortes, M.G.F., Macri, F.J. *et al.* (1958), Study of afferent electric impulses induced by intraocular pressure changes. *Am J Ophthalmol*, **45**, 211.

Voss, H. (1957), Beitrage zur mikroskopischen Anatomie der Augenmuskeln des Menschen (Faserdicke, muskel Spindeln, Ringbinden). *Anat Anz*, **104**, 345.

Vossius, A. (1883), Beitrage zur Anatomie des N. Opticus. *A von Graefes Arch Ophthalmol*, **29**, 119.

Vrabec, F. (1952), Sur une question de l'endothelium de la surface antérieure de l'iris humain. *Ophthalmologica*, **123**, 210.

Vrabec, F. (1954), L'innervation du systeme trabeculaire de l'angle irien. *Ophthalmologica*, **128**, 359.

Vrabec, F. (1961), The topography of encapsulated terminal sensory corpuscles of the anterior chamber angle of the goose eye, in *The Structure of the Eye* (ed. G.K. Smelser), Academic Press, New York, p. 325.

Vrabec, F. (1965), On the development and senile changes of the innervation of the trabecular meshwork in humans, in *The Structure of the Eye* (ed J.W. Rohen), Schattauer Verlag, Stuttgart, p. 215.

Vrabec, F. (1976), Glaucomatous cupping of the human optic disc. A neuro-histological study. *A von Graefes Arch Klin Exp Ophthalmol*, **198**, 223.

Waardenburg, P.J. (1951), A new syndrome combining developmental anomalies of eyelids, eyebrows, and nose root, with pigmentary defects of iris and head hair with congenital deafness. *Am J Hum Genet*, **3**, 195.

Waespe, W. and Henn, V. (1977a), Neuronal activity in the vestibular nuclei of the alert monkey during vestibular and optokinetic stimulation. *Exp Brain Res*, **27**, 523.

Waespe, W. and Henn, V. (1977b), Vestibular nuclei activity during optokinetic after-nystagmus (OKAN) in the alert monkey. *Exp Brain Res*, **30**, 323.

Waggener, J.D. (1964), Electron microscope studies of brain barrier mechanisms. *J Neuropathol Exp Neurol*, **23**, 174.

Waitzman, D.M. and Cohen, B. (1979), Unit activity in the mesencephalic formation (MRF) associated with saccades and positions of fixation during a visual attention task. *Soc Neurosci Abstr*, **5**, 389.

Walberg, F. (1958a), On the termination of rubrobulbar fibers. Experimental observations in the cat. *J Comp Neurol*, **110**, 65.

Walberg, F. (1958b), Descending connections to the lateral reticular nucleus. An experimental study in the cat. *J Comp Neurol*, **109**, 363.

Walberg, F. (1961), Fastigiofugal fibers to the perihypoglossal nuclei in the cat. *Exp Neurol*, **3**, 525.

Walker, A.E. (1938), *The Primate Thalamus*, University of Chicago Press, Chicago.

Wallace, R.N., Streeten, B.W. and Hanna, R.B. (1991), Rotary shadowing of elastic system microfibrils in the ocular zonule, vitreous, and ligamentum nuchae. *Curr Eye Res*, **10**, 99.

Walls, G.L. (1962), The evolutionary history of eye movements. *Vision Res*, **2**, 69.

Walls, G.L. (1963), *The Vertebrate Eye*, Haffner, New York.

Walsh, C. and Guillery, R.W. (1985), Age-related fiber order in the optic tract of the ferret. *J Neurosci*, **5**, 3061.

Walsh, C. and Polley, E.H. (1985), The topography of ganglion cell production in the cat's retina. *J Neurosci*, **5**, 741.

Walsh, F.B., Hoyt, W.F. and Miller, N.R. (1969), *Walsh and Hoyt's Clinical Neuro-ophthalmology*, Williams & Wilkins, Baltimore.

Walter, J.G. (1778), *Epistola anatomica: De venis occuli summatim. Berolins Lateinisches Original mit deutscher Uebersetzung.* (Cited by Gurwitsch, 1883.)

Wanko, T., Lloyd, B.J. and Matthews, J. (1964), The fine structure of human conjunctiva in the perilimbal zone. *Invest Ophthalmol*, **3**, 285.

Ward, F.O. (1858), *Outlines of Human Osteology*, 2nd edition, Renshaw, London, 1.

Waring, G.O., Bourne, W.M., Edelhauser, H.F. *et al.* (1982), The normal corneal endothelium. Normal and pathologic structure and function. *Ophthalmologica*, **89**, 531.

Warwick, R. (1951), A juvenile skull exhibiting duplication of the optic canals. *J Anat*, **85**, 289.

Warwick, R. (1953), Representation of the extra-ocular muscles in the oculomotor nuclei of the monkey. *J Comp Neurol*, **98**, 449.

Warwick, R. (1954), The ocular parasympathetic nerve supply and its mesencephalic sources. *J Anat*, **88**, 71.

Warwick, R. (1955), The so-called nucleus of convergence. *Brain*, **78**, 92.

Warwick, R. (1956), Oculomotor organisation. *Ann R Coll Surg Engl*, **19**, 36.

Warwick, R. (1964), Oculomotor organization, in *The Oculomotor System* (ed. M.B. Bender), Harper & Row, Philadelphia, p. 173.

Watanabe, K., Fujioka, M., Takeshita, T. *et al.* (1989), Scleral fibroblasts of the chick embryo proliferate by an autocrine mechanism in protein-free primary cultures: differential secretion of growth factors depending on the growth state. *Exp Cell Res*, **182**, 321.

Watts, J.W. (1934), *J Anat*, **68**, 534.

Watzke, R.C., Soldevilla, J.D. and Trune, D.R. (1993), Morphometric analysis of human retinal pigment epithelium: correlation with age and location. *Curr Eye Res*, **12**, 133.

Weale, R.A. (1982), *A Biography of the Eye: Development, Growth, Age*, H.K. Lewis, London.

Weber, J.T. and Giolli, R.A. (1986), The medial terminal nucleus of the monkey: evidence for a 'complete' accessory optic system. *Brain Res*, **365**, 164.

Weber, R.B., Daroff, R.B. and Mackey, E.A. (1970), Pathology of oculomotor nerve palsy in diabetics. *Neurology*, **20**, 835.

Weddell, G. (1941), The pattern of cutaneous innervation in relation to cutaneous sensibility. *J Anat*, **75**, 346.

Weddell, G., Palmer, E. and Pallie, W. (1955), Nerve endings in mammalian skin. *Biol Rev*, **30**, 159.

Weekers, R. and Grieten, J. (1961), The measurement of the depth of the anterior chamber in clinical practice. *Bull Soc Belge Ophthalmol*, **129**, 361.

Weekers, R., Grieten, J. and Lavergne, G. (1961), Study of the dimensions of the human antérior chamber. *Ophthalmologica*, **142**, 650.

Weekers, R., Grieten, J. and Lekiux, M. (1963), Etude des dimensions de la chambre antérieure de l'oeil humain: IV. L'intumescence cristallinienne et ses consequences chirurgicales. *Ophthalmologica*, **146**, 57.

Wegawa, K. (1975), Ultrastructural changes of the trabecular tissues in primary open angle glaucoma. *Jpn J Ophthalmol*, **19**, 317.

Wei, Z.G., Sun, T.T. and Lavker, R.M. (1990), Conjunctival goblet cells have proliferative capabilities. *ARVO Suppl: Invest Ophthalmol Vis Sci*, **32**, 734.

Weibel, E.R. (1974), On pericytes, particularly their existence on lung capillaries. *Microvasc Res*, **8**, 218.

Weimar, V. (1960), Healing processes in the cornea; in *The Transparency of the Cornea* (eds W.S. Duke-Elder and E.S. Perkins), Blackwell Scientific, Oxford, p. 111.

Weinsieder, A., Briggs, R., Reddan, J. *et al.* (1975), Induction of mitosis in ocular tissue by chemotoxic agents. *Exp Eye Res*, **20**, 33.

Weinsieder, A., Rothstein, H. and Drebert, D. (1973), Lenticular wound healing: evidence for genomic activation. *Cytobiologie*, **7**, 406.

Weiss, L. (1895), Uber das Wachstum des Auges. *Klin Monatsbl Augenheilk*, **33**, 218.

Weiss, L. (1897), Uber das Wachstum des menschlichen Auges und uber die Veranderung der Muskelinsertionen am wachsenden Auge (Anatomische Hefte). *Arb Anat Inst Wiesbaden*, **8**, 191.

Weiss, R.A., Eichner, R. and Sun, T.T. (1984), Monoclonal antibody analysis of keratin expression in epidermal diseases: A 48 kD and a 56 kD keratin as molecular markers for keratinocyte hyperproliferation. *J Cell Biol*, **98**, 1397.

Weiter, J.J. and Ernest, J.T. (1974), Anatomy of the choroidal vasculature. *Am J Ophthalmol*, **78**, 583.

Welt, K. and Zacharias, K. (1970), Development of the periorbital structures in man. *Anat Anz*, **127**, 511.

Wen, R. and Oakley, B. (1990), K(+)-evoked Müller cell depolarization generates b-wave of electroretinogram in toad retina. *Proc Natl Acad Sci USA*, **87**, 2117.

Wendland, J.P. and Nerenberg, S. (1960), The geniculocalcarine pathway in the temporal lobe. *Univ Minn Med Bull*, **31**, 482.

Werb, A. (1984), Senile ptosis. *Trans Ophthalmol Soc UK*, **104**, 22.

Westall, C.A. and Schor, C.M. (1985), Asymmetries of optokinetic nystagmus in amblyopia: the effect of selected retinal stimulation. *Vision Res*, **25**, 1431.

Westheimer, G. and Blair, S.M. (1973), Oculomotor defects in cerebellectomized monkeys. *Int Ophthalmol*, **12**, 618.

Westheimer, G. and Blair, S.M. (1974), Unit activity in accessory optic system in alert monkeys. *Int Ophthalmol*, **13**, 533.

Westphal, C. (1887), Über einen fall von chronischer progressive lähmung des augenmusklen (ophthalmoplegia externa) nebst beschreibung von ganglienzellengruppen im bereich des oculomotoriuskerns. *Arch Psychiatr Nervenkr*, **98**, 846.

White, J.C. (1952), *Automonic Nervous System*, 3rd edition, Henry Kimpton, London.

Whitfield, L.C. (1967), *The Auditory Pathway*, Edward Arnold, London.

Whitnall, S.E. (1911), *J Anat Physiol, Lond*, **36**, 1.

Whitnall, S.E. (1932), *The Anatomy of the Human Orbit and Accessory Organs of Vision*, 2nd edition, OUP, Oxford, p. 303.

Whitteridge, D. (1965), Area 18 and the vertical meridïan of vision, in *Functions of the Corpus Callosum* (ed. E.G. Ettlinger), Churchill Livingstone, Edinburgh.

Wieczorek, D.F., Periasamy, M., Butler-Browne, G.S. *et al.* (1985), Co-expression of multiple myosin heavy chain genes, in addition to a tissue-specific one, in extraocular musculature. *J Cell Biol*, **101**, 618.

Wiedenmann, B. and Huttner, W.B. (1989), Synaptophysin and chromogranins/secretogranins: Widespread constituents of distinct types of neuroendocrine vesicles and new tools in tumor diagnostics. *Virchows Arch B Cell Pathol*, **58**, 95.

Wiederholt, M., Sturm, A. and Lepple-Wienhues, A. (1994), Relaxation of trabecular meshwork and ciliary muscle by release of nitric oxide. *Invest Ophthalmol Vis Sci*, **35**, 2515.

Wieger, (1883) *Ueber den canalis Petiti und ein Ligamentum hyaloideocapsulare.* Inaug. Diss, Strassburg.

Wigham, C.G. and Hodson, S.A. (1987), Physiological changes in the cornea of the aging eye. *Eye*, **1**, 190.

Wilbrand, H.L. and Saenger, A. (1906), Die Neurologie des Auges, in *Handbuch for Nerven und Augenarzte*, Weisbaden-Munschen.

Wilcox, L.M. Jr., Keough, E.M., Connolly, R.J. *et al.* (1981), Comparative extraocular muscle blood flow. *J Exp Zool*, **215**, 87.

Wiley, L., SunderRay, N., Sun, T.T. *et al.* (1991), Regional heterogeneity in human corneal and limbal epithelia: An immunohistochemical evaluation. *Invest Ophthalmol Vis Sci*, **32**, 594.

Willekens, B. and Vrensen, G. (1982), The three dimensional organization of the lens fibers in the rhesus monkey. *Graefes Arch Klin Exp Ophthalmol*, **219**, 112.

Williams, D.R. (1988), Topography of the foveal cone mosaic in the living human eye. *Vision Res*, **28**, 433.

Williams, P.L. and Warwick, R. (1975), *Functional Neuroanatomy of Man*, Churchill Livingstone, Edinburgh.

Williams, P.L. and Warwick, R. (1980), *Gray's Anatomy*, 36th edition, Churchill Livingstone, Edinburgh.

Williams, R.W. (1991), The human retina has a cone-rich rim. *Vis Neurosci*, **6**, 403.

Wilson, D.J., Jaeger, M.J. and Green, W.R. (1987), Effects of extracapsular cataract extraction on the lens zonules. *Ophthalmology*, **94**, 467.

Wilson, E.M. and Melvill Jones, G. (1979), *Mammalian Vestibular Physiology*, Plenum Press, New York.

Wilson, H.R., Mets, M.B., Nagy, S.E. and Kressel, A.B. (1988a), Albino spatial vision as an instance of arrested visual development. *Vision Res*, **29**, 979.

Wilson, H.R., Mets, M.B., Nagy, S.E. and Ferrera, V.P. (1988b), Spatial frequency and orientation tuning of spatial visual mechanisms in human albinos. *Vision Res*, **28**, 991.

Wilson, M.E. and Toyne, M.J. (1970), Retino-tectal and cortico-tectal projections in *Macaca mulatta*. *Brain Res*, **24**, 395.

Wilson, T.M., Strang, R. and Mackenzie, E.T. (1977), The response of the choroidal and cerebral circulations to changing arterial P_{CO_2} and acetazolamide in the baboon. *Invest Ophthalmol Vis Sci*, **16**, 576.

Wilson, V.J. and Yoshida, M. (1969), Monosynaptic inhibition of neck motoneurones by the medial vestibular nucleus. *Exp Brain Res*, **9**, 240.

Winckler, G. (1937), *Arch Anat Histol Embryol*, **23**, 219.

Wistow, G.J. and Piatigorsky, J. (1988), Lens crystallins: the evolution and expression of proteins for a highly specialized tissue. *Immunol Rev*, **57**, 479.

Witusek, W. (1966), Types of physiological excavation of the optic nerve head. *Ophthalmologica*, **152**, 57.

Wizenmann, A., Thanos, S., Boxberg, Y.V. *et al.* (1993), Differential reaction of crossing and non-crossing rat retinal axons on cell membrane preparations from the chiasm midline: an *in vitro* study. *Development*, **117**, 725.

Wobman, P.R. and Fine, B.S. (1972), The clump cells of Koganei. A light and electron microscopic study. *Am J Ophthalmol*, **73**, 90.

Wohlfart, G. (1935) Untersuchungen über die Gruppierring von Muskelfasern verschiedener Grösse und Struktur innerhalb der primaren Muskelfaserbundel in der Skelemuskulatur, sowie Beobachtungen über die Innervation diesen Bundel. *Z Mikrosk Anat Forsch*, **37**, 621.

Woinow, M. (1874), Ueber die Brechungscoefficient der ver schiedenen Linsenschichten. *Klin Monatsbl Augenheilk*, **12**, 407.

Wolf, J. (1968a), Inner surface of regions in the anterior chamber taking part in the regulation of intraocular tension, including the demonstration of the covering viscous substance. *Doc Ophthalmol*, **25**, 113.

Wolf, J. (1968b), The secretory activity and the cuticle of the corneal endothelium. *Doc Ophthalmol*, **25**, 150.

Wolff, E. (1939), Some aspects of the blood supply of the optic nerve. *Trans Ophthalmol Soc UK*, **59**, 157.

Wolff, E. (1951), Unicellular sebaceous glands in the basal layer of the normal human epidermis. *Lancet*, **888**.

Wolff, E. (1953), The so-called medial root of the optic tract is essentially a visual commissure. *Brain*, **76**, 455.

Wolff, E. (1954), *The Anatomy of the Eye and Orbit*, 4th edition, H.K. Lewis, London, p. 12.

Wolff, E. (1976), *The Anatomy of the Eye and Orbit*, 7th edn (ed. R. Warwick), H.K. Lewis, London.

Wolff, G.A. Jr (1941), The ratio of preganglionic neurons to postganglionic neurons in the visceral nervous system. *J Comp Neurol*, **75**, 235.

Wolfrum, M. (1908), Beitrage zur Anatomie und Histologie der Aderhaut beim Menschen und bei hoheren Wirbeltieren. *A von Graefes Arch Ophthalmol*, **67**, 307.

Wollschlaeger, P., Wollschlaeger, G., Ide, C. *et al.* (1971), Arterial blood supply of the human optic chiasm and surrounding structures. *Ann Ophthalmol*, **3**, 862.

Wolter, J. (1960), Nerves of the human choroid. *Arch Ophthalmol*, **64**, 120.

Wolter, J.R. (1953), The innervation of the ciliary muscle of man. *Ber Versamm Ophthalm Ges Heidelberg*, **58**, 327.

Wolter, J.R. (1957a), Innervation of the corneal endothelium of the eye of the rabbit. *Arch Ophthalmol*, **58**, 246.

Wolter, J.R. (1957b), The human optic papilla: a demonstration of new anatomic and pathologic findings. *Am J Ophthalmol*, **44**, 48.

Wolter, J.R. (1959), Neuropathology of the trabeculum in open angle glaucoma. *Arch Ophthalmol*, **62**, 99.

Wong-Riley, M.T.T. (1979), Changes in the visual system of monocularly sutured or enucleated cats demonstrable with cytochrome oxidase histochemistry. *Brain Res*, **171**, 11.

Wood Jones, F. (1949), *Buchanant Manual of Anatomy*, 8th edition, Ballière, Tindall, & Cox, London.

Woodhead-Galloway, J. (1981), The body as engineer. *New Scientist*, **90**, 772.

Woodlief, N.F. (1980), Initial observations on the ocular microcirculation in man. I. The anterior segment and extraocular muscles. *Arch Ophthalmol*, **98**, 1268.

Woodlief, N.F. and Eifrig, D.E. (1982), Initial observations on the ocular microcirculation in man. The choriocapillaris. *Ann Ophthalmol*, **14**, 176.

Woollard, H.H. (1931), *J Anat*, **65**, 225.

Woollard, H.M. (1926), Notes on the retina and lateral geniculate body in Tupaia, Tarsius, Nycticebus and Hapale. *Brain*, **49**, 77.

Woolsey, C.N. (1964), In *Cerebral Localisation and Organisation* (eds G. Shatterbrand and C.N. Woolsey), Madison, USA.

Wooten, G.F. and Reis, D.S. (1972), Blood flow in extraocular muscle of cat. *Arch Neurol*, **26**, 153.

Worgul, B.V. (1992), Lens, in *The Biomedical Foundations of Ophthalmology* (eds T.D. Duane and E.A. Jaeger), Harper and Row, Philadelphia, p. 1.

Worgul, B.V. and Merriam, G.R. Jr (1979), The effect of endotoxin induced intraocular inflammation on the rat lens epithelium. *Invest Ophthalmol Vis Sci*, **18**, 401.

Worgul, B.V., Merriam, G.R. Jr, Szechter, A. *et al.* (1976), Lens epithelium and radiation cataract. I. Preliminary studies. *Arch Ophthalmol*, **94**, 996.

Worgul, B.V. and Rothstein, H. (1977), On the mechanism of radiocataractogenesis. *Medikon*, **6**, 5.

Wright, P. and Mackie, I.A. (1977), Mucus in the healthy and diseased eye. *Trans Ophthalmol Soc UK*, **97**, 1.

Wulle, K.G. (1967), Zelldifferenzierungen im Ciliarepithel während der menschichen Fetalentwicklung und ihre Beziehungen zur Kammerwasser bildung. *Graefe's Arch Clin Exp Ophthalmol*, **172**, 170.

Wulle, K.G. (1972), Electron microscopy of the fetal development of the corneal endothelium and Descemet's membrane of the human eye. *Invest Ophthalmol*, **11**, 897.

Wulle, K.G. and Lerche, W. (1969), Zur Feinstrukur der embryonalen menschlichen Linsenblase. *A von Graefes Arch Klin Exp Ophthalmol*, **173**, 141.

Wurtz, R.H. and Albano, J.E. (1980), Visual motor function of the primate superior colliculus. *Ann Rev Neurosci*, **3**, 189.

Wurtz, R.H., Goldberg, M.E. and Robinson, D.L. (1980), *Prog Psychobiol Physiol Psychol*, **9**, 43.

Wybar, K. (1954), A study of choroidal circulation of the eye in man. *J Anat*, **88**, 94.

Xuerer, G.P., Prichard, M.M. and Daniel, P.M. (1954), *QJ Exp Psychol*, **39**, 119.

Yamamoto, M., Shimoyama, I. and Highstein, S.M. (1978), Vestibular nucleus neurons relaying excitation from the anterior canal to the oculomotor nucleus. *Brain Res*, **148**, 31.

Yamamoto, R., Bredt, D., Snyder, S.H. *et al.* (1993), The localization of nitric oxide synthase in the rat eye and related cranial ganglia. *Neuroscience*, **54**, 189.

Yamamoto, T. (1966), Electron microscopic observation of human optic nerves. *Jpn J Ophthalmol*, **10**, 40.

Yanoff, M. and Fine, B.S. (1972), *Ocular Histology*, Harper & Row, New York, p. 391.

Yanoff, M. and Fine, B.S. (1989), *Ocular Pathology: A Text and Atlas*, 3rd edition, Lippincott, Philadelphia.

Ye, H., Yang, J. and Hernandez, M.R. (1994), Localization of collagen type III mRNA in normal human optic nerve heads. *Exp Eye Res*, **58**, 53.

Yee, A.G. and Revel, J.P. (1975), Endothelial cell junctions. *J Cell Biol*, **66**, 200.

Yee, R.W. (1985), Changes in the normal corneal endothelial cellular pattern as a function of age. *Curr Eye Res*, **4**, 671.

Yeh, S., Scholz, D.L., Liou, W. *et al.* (1986), Polygonal arrays of actin filaments in human lens epithelial cells. *Invest Ophthalmol Vis Sci*, **27**, 1535.

Yoneya, S. and Tso, M.O.M. (1984), Patterns of the choriocapillaris. *Int Ophthalmol*, **6**, 95.

Yoneya, S. and Tso, M.O.M. (1987), Angioarchitecture of the human choroid. *Arch Ophthalmol*, **105**, 681.

Yoshii, N., Fujii, M. and Mizokami, T. (1978), Hypothalamic projection to the pulvinar-LP complex in the cat: a study by the HRP-method. *Brain Res*, **155**, 343.

Young, H.M., Furness, J.B., Shuttleworth, C.W.R. *et al.* (1992), Colocalization of nitric oxide synthase immunoreactivity and NADPH diaphorase staining in neurons of the guinea-pig intestine. *Histochemistry*, **97**, 375.

Young, R.W. (1991), *Age-Related Cataract*. Oxford University Press, Oxford.

Yukie, M. and Iwai, E. (1981), Direct projection from the dorsal lateral geniculate nucleus to the prestriate cortex in macaque monkeys. *J Comp Neurol*, **201**, 81.

Yuodelis, C. and Hendrickson, A. (1986), A qualitative and quantitative analysis of the human fovea during development. *Vis Res*, **26**, 847.

Zagorski, Z. (1980), Replication capacity of the regenerating human corneal endothelium in organ culture, in *Wundheilung des Auges und ihre Komplikationer* (eds G.O.H. Naumann and B.P. Gloor), Bergmann, Munchen, p. 223.

Zaki, W. (1960), The trochlear nerve in man. Study relative to its origin, its intracerebral traject and its structure. *Arch Anat Histol Embryol*, **45**, 105.

Zampighi, G.A., Hall, J.E., Ehring, G.R. *et al.* (1989), The structural organization and protein composition of lens fiber junctions. *J Cell Biol*, **108**, 2255.

Zander, E. and Weddell, G. (1951), Observations on the innervation of the cornea. *J Anat*, **85**, 68.

Zee, D.S., Yamazaki, A., Butler, P.H. *et al.* (1981), Effect of ablation of flocculus and paraflocculus on eye movements in primate. *J Neurophysiol*, **46**, 878.

Zeki, S.M. (1969), Representation of central visual fields in prestriate cortex of monkeys, *Brain Res*, **14**, 271.

Zeki, S.M. (1970), Interhemispheric connections of prestriate cortex of monkeys. *Brain Res*, **19**, 63.

Zeki, S.M. (1971), Cortical projections from two prestriate areas in the monkey. *Brain Res*, **34**, 19.

Zeki, S.M. (1975), The functional organisation of projections from striate to prestriate visual cortex in the rhesus monkey. *Cold Spring Harbor Symp Quant Biol*, **40**, 591.

Zeki, S.M. (1977), Simultaneous anatomical demonstration of the representation of the vertical and horizontal meridians in areas V2 and V3 of rhesus monkey visual cortex. *Phil Trans R Soc Lond, Series B*, **195**, 517.

Zeki, S.M. (1978a), The cortical projections of foveal striate cortex in the rhesus monkey. *J Physiol (Lond)*, **277**, 227.

Zeki, S.M. (1978b), Functional specialisation in the visual cortex of the rhesus monkey. *Nature*, **274**, 423.

Zeki, S.M. (1978c), The third visual complex of rhesus monkey prestriate cortex. *J Physiol (Lond)*, **277**, 245.

Zeki, S.M. (1978d), Uniformity and diversity of structure and function in rhesus monkey prestriate visual cortex. *J Physiol (Lond)*, **277**, 273.

Zeki, S.M. (1983), The distribution of wavelength and orientation selective cells in different areas of monkey visual cortex. *Proc R Soc Lond*, **217**, 449.

Zeki, S.M. (1984a), The construction of colours by the cerebral cortex. *Proc R Inst Gt Brit*, **56**, 231.

Zeki, S.M. (1984b), The specialization of function and the function of specialization in the visual cortex, in *Recent Advances in Physiology* (ed. P.F. Baker), Churchill Livingstone, Edinburgh.

Zeki, S.M. (1993), *A Vision of the Brain*. Blackwell Scientific Publications, Oxford.

Zeki, S.M. and Sandeman, N. (1976), Combined anatomical and electrophysiological studies on the boundary between the second and third visual areas of rhesus monkey visual cortex. *Proc R Soc Lond*, **194**, 555.

Zenker, W. and Anzenbacher, H. (1964), On the different forms of myo-neural junction in two types of muscle fiber from the external ocular muscles of the rhesus monkey. *J Cell Comp Physiol*, **63**, 273.

Zhang, Y.L., Tan, C.K. and Wong, W.C. (1994), Localisation of substance P-like immunoreactivity in the ciliary ganglia of monkey (*Macaca fascicularis*) and cat: A light- and electron-microscopic study. *Cell Tissue Res*, **276**, 163.

Zieske, J.D. and Wasson, M. (1992), Colocalization of alpha-enolase and epidermal growth factor receptor in adult and developing rat cornea. *RVO Suppl: Invest Ophthalmol Vis Sci*, **33**, 819.

Zihl, J. (1981), Untersuchungen von Sehfunktionen bei Patienten mit einer Schadigung des zentralen visuellen systems unter besonderer Berucksichtigung der Restitution dieser Funktionen. Post-doctoral thesis, Ludwig-Maximilians Universitat, Munchen.

Zimmerman, D.R., Trueb, B., Winterhalter, K.H. *et al.* (1986), Type VI collagen is a major component of the human cornea. *FEBS Lett*, **197**, 55.

Zimmerman, L.E. (1957), Demonstration of the hyaluronidase-sensitive acid mucopolysaccharide. In trabecula and iris in routine paraffin sections of adult eyes; a preliminary report. *Am J Ophthalmol*, **44**, 1.

Zimmerman, L.E. (1958), Further histochemical studies of acid mucopolysaccharides in the intraocular tissues. *Am J Ophthalmol*, **43**, 299.

Zinn, J.G. (1755), *Descriptio Anatomica Oculi Humani*, van den Hoeck, Gottingen.

Zinn, J.G. (1780), *Descriptio Anatomica Oculi Humani*, 2nd edition (ed. H.A. Wrisberg), van den Hoeck, Gottingen, p. 194.

Zinn, K.M. and Benjamin-Henkind, J. (1982), Retinal pigment epithelium, in *Ocular Anatomy, Embryology, and Teratology* (ed. F. Jakobiec), Harper and Row, Philadelphia, p. 533.

Zypen, E. van der (1970), Licht- und elektronenmikroscokopische Untersuchungen uber die Alterveranderungen am M. ciliaris im menschlichen Auge. *A von Graefes Arch Klin Exp Ophthalmol*, **179**, 332.

Index

Page numbers in **bold** type refer to figures; those in *italic* refer to tables.